T0138996

SECOND EDITION

ASBESTOS

RISK ASSESSMENT,
EPIDEMIOLOGY,
AND HEALTH EFFECTS

SECOND EDITION

ASBESTOS

RISK ASSESSMENT, EPIDEMIOLOGY, AND HEALTH EFFECTS

RONALD F. DODSON
SAMUEL P. HAMMAR

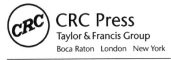

CRC Press
Taylor & Francis Group
Boca Raton London New York

CRC Press is an imprint of the
Taylor & Francis Group, an **informa** business

CRC Press
Taylor & Francis Group
6000 Broken Sound Parkway NW, Suite 300
Boca Raton, FL 33487-2742

© 2011 by Taylor & Francis Group, LLC
CRC Press is an imprint of Taylor & Francis Group, an Informa business

First issued in paperback 2017

No claim to original U.S. Government works
Version Date: 20110428

ISBN 13: 978-1-138-07670-9 (pbk)
ISBN 13: 978-1-4398-0968-6 (hbk)

Library of Congress Cataloging-in-Publication Data

Asbestos : risk assessment, epidemiology, and health effects / edited by Ronald F. Dodson, Samuel P.
  Hammar. -- 2nd ed.
     p. cm.
  Includes bibliographical references and index.
  ISBN 978-1-4398-0968-6
  1. Asbestos--Toxicology. 2. Asbestosis. I. Dodson, Ronald F. II. Hammar, Samuel P.

RA1231.A8A74 2011
615.9'2539224--dc22   2010048219

Visit the Taylor & Francis Web site at
http://www.taylorandfrancis.com

and the CRC Press Web site at
http://www.crcpress.com

Dr. Dodson dedicates the book to the memory of his parents, Benjamin F. Dodson and Vera I. Dodson. Their inspiration and encouragement were motivation for both the personal and professional facets of his life. He also dedicates the book to his wife, Sandy, who has always provided a loving, stabilizing, and encouraging presence.

Dr. Hammar dedicates the book to his beloved Mother, Ella Hammar, who was the hardest working person he has ever known. He also dedicates the book to his special friend, Lee Hewitt, who greatly encouraged him during the process of developing the Second Edition.

Contents

Preface

Asbestos is a generic term for the fibrous form of a group of silicate minerals. The term *asbestos* is often limited to the six regulated forms defined in regulatory guidelines. These terms provide a common basis for communication regarding the applicably defined fibrous forms of minerals that are commonly found in commercial products. Asbestos is used in products because of its physical attributes, which, in the past, have given it the designation as "a magic mineral." Asbestos is lightweight and offers excellent insulation properties, fireproofing, and increased tensile strength as a component of other products. Other important features of asbestos that have made it a material of choice in many commercial applications is its relative inexpensiveness and ease of application. From a health effect standpoint, inhalation of asbestos fibers can result in a variety of cancers and other pathological responses, including fibrotic diseases. A unique feature of asbestos fibers as compared with most other inhaled dusts is their carcinogenicity.

The physical properties of asbestos resulted in its widespread use in many products. Contrary to popular opinion, the United States has not yet joined over 50 countries in the world where asbestos-containing products have been banned. Thus, imported products with asbestos components are still being sold commercially. The remaining asbestos in place from previous applications is an issue that society will be dealing with for decades. The other important issue when dealing with potential asbestos exposure consists often of even knowing that a given material contains asbestos.

Asbestos is a potential threat to health when it becomes friable or disturbed, thus creating aerosolized and respirable fibrous dust. Asbestos and asbestos-like particulates are components of various minerals mined for a wide array of products. These are not often considered to contain asbestos because asbestos is not added for any commercial application and is often simply a component of the mined vein. Thus, unsuspected exposures may occur from disturbance of these products.

The complexities resulting from asbestos exposure and the resultant understanding of health-related effects require a working understanding of a multidisciplinary nature. The first edition of this book offered one of the first volumes that specifically brought specialists from different disciplines together to provide the reader with a single resource for answering complex questions regarding asbestos-related issues. The second edition expands the successful approach used in the first edition by adding additional chapters and expanding the content of the previous chapters to make this an all-inclusive thesis on the subject of asbestos and asbestos-related public health issues. Internationally recognized authors were invited to contribute sections where their expertise was brought together with that of other outstanding specialists into one cohesive document.

The historical overview of asbestos and the awareness that it constitutes a risk to human health set the basis for understanding what we know and what we are still learning about asbestos and human health. The evolving laboratory techniques that offer reproducible observations as to the presence/quantitation of asbestos in various physical and aerosol samples provide the reader with quick references as to the state-of-the-art use of instrumentation and procedures applicable to answering specific questions.

The main point of entry for asbestos dust is via the respiratory system. It is critical the reader has a basic understanding as to how and what dust reaches what levels of the respiratory system and how our lungs are designed to protect against inhaled particulates when they are capable of doing so without being overwhelmed.

Considerable information exists regarding tissue burden of asbestos, but to appreciate the appropriate interpretation of the data, one must appreciate the limitations of the techniques or count schemes as applied. This fundamental understanding is critical if one is to fully appreciate what is reported in a tissue sample by first being able to determine what was included in a count scheme and what was "overlooked." The concept that fiber length alone is a predictor of the potential for pathogenic responses attempts to foolishly oversimplify the various mechanisms by which an inhaled fiber may induce a disease. Ignoring the fact that short fibers are the primary form of asbestos reaching extrapulmonary sites creates a false aura that one can pick one's favorite length of fiber and then make the disease somehow fit that particulate dimension.

The fact that the physical features of asbestos alone do not explain all components of asbestos-induced diseases is clearly appreciated by the reader once he or she has evaluated the chapter on molecular mechanisms. The pathological complexities of asbestos-related disease have resulted in the second edition containing specific chapters on asbestosis, pleural disease, lung cancer, cancers outside of the lung (excluding mesothelioma), and mesothelioma. The state-of-the-art overview regarding interpretation of diagnostic information in the clinical chapters provides a complete reference for the healthcare specialist. The findings from studies of various groups of individuals exposed to asbestos form the basis of the extensive detail provided to the reader in the chapter discussing asbestos-related epidemiology. The results of known exposures are discussed as applicable to the development of specific diseases. As with all of the chapters, a basis is provided to the reader from which various views are considered, based on the variations of the questions asked.

The significance of asbestos as a pathologically active dust necessitates that special emphasis be given to clinical monitoring and resultant interpretations. These issues are addressed in practical terms for the practicing clinical professional as they pertain to diagnostic interpretations. Furthermore, an additional chapter offers an overview as to what the clinical educator or postgraduate clinical specialist should consider as part of the adaptation to good clinical practice regarding asbestos-related issues.

All specialists involved with asbestos-related issues need to be aware of the regulatory guidelines and their intended applicability. Specialists from the two major regulatory agencies have provided the readers with a quick reference of the governing documents applicable to asbestos as well as insight into the regulatory process governing asbestos-related issues.

Readers of the first edition of our book have commended the usefulness of the interdisciplinary approach of the book. This second edition has taken those positive comments and provides the reader with an updated and expanded state-of-the-art discussion concerning important interdisciplinary factors associated with asbestos-related issues in an easy to use reference document.

Acknowledgments

Drs. Hammar and Dodson would like to make special recognition of Ms. Michaele Stoll for her contribution in the development of the Second Edition of *Asbestos: Risk Assessment, Epidemiology, and Health Effects*. Michaele provided editorial assistance both via continuing interactions with each of the authors as well as intensive review of the drafts of each chapter. Her knowledge of terminology regarding asbestos-related diseases enabled the editors to rely heavily on her attention to detail in the critique of the submitted documents. Dr. Hammar also would like to acknowledge the assistance of Ms. Nancy Bennett in his office for providing additional support needed during the process of developing the Second Edition.

Editors

Ronald F. Dodson, PhD, received his BA in biology and general sciences (double major) from East Texas State College and an MA in biology and chemistry from East Texas State University. His doctorate was from the Life Sciences Division of Texas A&M University with an emphasis in biological electron microscopy. After a postdoctoral appointment in anatomy at the University of Texas Health Science in San Antonio, he joined the faculty of Baylor College of Medicine in Houston where he conducted ultrastructural research. Dr. Dodson was recruited to join the faculty of the University of Texas Health Center where he was charged with beginning a research effort. His academic career at the Health Center included serving in administrative positions, including chief of Department of Cell Biology/Environmental Sciences, chairman of the same department, associate director for research, vice president for research, and codirector of the Texas Institute for Occupational Safety and Health. He was awarded the status of professor of biology with tenure at the University of Texas at Tyler in the early 1980s. Dr. Dodson has also directed an EPA/Texas Department of Health (Model Accreditation governed) training division and holds licenses through the Texas Department of Human Health Services as an inspector/manager planner and supervisor/contractor (restricted) as applicable in the areas of asbestos-related activities.

Dr. Dodson was invited to serve on the EPA, NIOSH, and IOM groups where he offered his perspective on asbestos-related issues. He has served on the advisory board for the Texas Department of Health, which was charged with developing the first state regulation in Texas for governing asbestos-related work activities in public buildings. His laboratory was one of only a few academic laboratories in the country that also participated in the AHERA/NIST accreditation program in analytical transmission electron microscopy. Dr. Dodson presently serves as a member of the advisory board of the School of Rural Public Health of Texas A&M University School of Medicine.

Dr. Dodson has served as a peer reviewer for numerous scientific journals and granting agencies. He has published over 100 scientific contributions on dust-related health issues with most of those focusing on asbestos. He has presented numerous papers at scientific meetings and agency-sponsored meetings as well as other professional societies where asbestos-related issues are of interest. His laboratory has developed some of the preparative techniques that have permitted them to evaluate tissue burden of asbestos in a number of types of samples. He has published much of the world's literature on asbestos content in extrapulmonary sites and has authored numerous articles where total fiber burden in a sample (including short fibers) were quantified. He has authored some of the limited number of research publications where lavage and sputum materials were evaluated for ferruginous body content and uncoated asbestos fibers. Dr. Dodson holds the status of fellow in the American Heart Association and fellow in the College of Chest Physicians. Dr. Dodson was selected as the Eminent Scientist and Outstanding Scholar of the Year in 2001 and as the Millennium Golden International Award Winner by the International Research Promotion Council (Asia-Pacific Chapter) for his works as applicable to asbestos-related health issues in developing countries.

Dr. Dodson retired in 2005 from his two academic appointments and created his own consulting company: Dodson Environmental Consulting, Inc. In this position, he continues to provide consultative evaluation of tissue samples, write scientific documents, and conduct scientific research into asbestos-related issues.

Samuel P. Hammar, MD, is a board-certified anatomic and clinical pathologist who specializes in lung disease, cancer, and diagnostic techniques used to investigate cancer. He obtained a BA degree in chemistry in 1965 and attended the University of Washington Medical School from 1965 to 1969 where he obtained his MD degree. He did his training in pathology at the University of Washington School of Medicine, including time in experimental pathology and electron microscopy.

For the past 25 years, Dr. Hammar has been primarily interested in asbestos-related lung disease, especially mesothelioma. He is a member of the U.S.–Canadian Mesothelioma Panel, a member of the International Mesothelioma Pathology Group, and a member of the International Mesothelioma Interest Group. In conjunction with Dr. Dodson, Dr. Hammar has done extensive research into asbestos-related disease and sees asbestos-induced lung disease on a regular basis as a practicing pathologist in Bremerton, Washington, the home of the Puget Sound Naval Shipyard.

Dr. Hammar is particularly interested in all aspects of mesothelioma. In association with his friend and colleague, Dr. Ronald Dodson, they have conducted extensive studies concerning the concentration and type of asbestos in extrapulmonary sites. Dr. Hammar and Dr. Dodson are currently evaluating the concentration/type of asbestos in the "normal" visceral and parietal pleura and in mesothelioma tumor tissue, hyaline plaque, and lung tissue.

Dr. Hammar and Dr. Dodson consider themselves extremely fortunate to study asbestos-induced diseases and hope to contribute to the knowledge of such diseases. Dr. Hammar considers himself fortunate to be able to provide information to patients and their families who are suffering from asbestos-related diseases.

Dr. Hammar may be reached via e-mail at hammar.dsl@hotmail.com or by telephone at 360-479-7707 (work) or 360-434-7546 (cellular phone).

Contributors

Daniel T. Crane
Occupational Safety and Health Administration
U.S. Department of Labor
Sandy, Utah

Ronald F. Dodson
Dodson Environmental Consulting, Inc.
ERI Consulting, Inc.
Tyler, Texas

Gary K. Friedman
Pulmonary Division, Texas Lung Institute
The University of Texas Health
  Science Center
Houston, Texas

Samuel P. Hammar
Diagnostic Specialties Laboratory
PAKC/DSL, Inc., P.S.
Bremerton, Washington

Douglas W. Henderson
Department of Surgical Pathology
Flinders Medical Centre
Adelaide, South Australia

Sonja Klebe
Department of Anatomical Pathology
Flinders Medical Centre
Adelaide, South Australia

James Leigh
Sydney School of Public Health
University of Sydney
Sydney, Australia

Richard A. Lemen
United States Public Health Service (Ret.)
Canton, Georgia

Jeffrey L. Levin
Department of Occupational Health Sciences
The University of Texas Health
  Science Center
Tyler, Texas

Adele Cardenas Malott
U.S. Environmental Protection Agency
Dallas, Texas

James R. Millette
MVA Scientific Consultants
Duluth, Georgia

Paul P. Rountree
Department of Occupational Health Sciences
The University of Texas Health
  Science Center
Tyler, Texas

CHAPTER **1**

The History of Asbestos Utilization and Recognition of Asbestos-Induced Diseases

Douglas W. Henderson and James Leigh

CONTENTS

1.1 WHAT IS ASBESTOS?

"Asbestos"—derived from the Greek for *inextinguishable* or *unquenchable*—is a commercial term applied to a variety of hydrated fibrous silicates that have (i) the capacity to add tensile strength when added to other materials (such as cement to produce asbestos cement); (ii) resistance to fire; (iii) poor thermal conductivity (insulating properties); and (iv) resistance to corrosion by acids and alkalis (especially the amphibole varieties of asbestos). Because of these properties, it was once regarded as a "magic mineral"[1]—used in approximately 3000–4000 different products—but it is now regarded as a deadly threat to health ("killer dust"[1]) and has been banned in more than 50 nations, although its use continues, most notably in the "developing world" and especially in Asia.

Asbestos is conventionally divided into two broad groups (Table 1.1)[2]: (i) the serpentine group that contains only a single member, namely, chrysotile, the name of which is derived from the Greek for gold (*chrysos*) and fiber (*tilos*); and (ii) the amphiboles, which include crocidolite, amosite, and the (usually) noncommercial amphiboles, namely, tremolite, actinolite, and anthophyllite (the last of these being mined at the Paakkila mine in Finland until it was closed and at a few other sites). The serpentine chrysotile is characterized by curly fibers that tend to matt together, whereas the amphiboles are characterized by straight needle-like fibers with a capacity for longitudinal splitting.[2–4]

1

Table 1.1 Chemical Composition of Asbestos Fiber Types

Asbestos Type	Chemical Formula
Serpentine	
Chrysotile	$Mg_3Si_2O_5(OH)_4$
Amphiboles: commercial	
Crocidolite	$Na_2(Fe_3{}^{2+})(Fe_2{}^{3+})Si_8O_{22}(OH)_2$
Amosite	$(Fe, Mg)_7Si_8O_{22}(OH)_2 \; Fe > 5$
Amphiboles: noncommercial	
Tremolite	$Ca_2Mg_5Si_8O_{22}(OH)_2$
Anthophyllite	$(Mg, Fe)_7Si_8O_{22}(OH)_2 \; Mg > 6$
Actinolite	$Ca_2(Mg, Fe)_5Si_8O_{22}(OH)_2$

1.2 PREINDUSTRIAL HISTORY OF ASBESTOS

Accounts of past and continuing use of asbestos can be found in many standard texts and journal articles.[3–7] One of the best-documented and referenced accounts of its preindustrial usage can be found in Rachel Maines' book *Asbestos and Fire: Technological Trade-offs and the Body at Risk*,[7] although her argument in later sections of the book is open to dispute (see later discussion).

The occasional and sometimes colorful use of asbestos has extended from Neolithic times until the twenty-first century. In this setting, asbestos (anthophyllite) has been found in Neolithic pottery in Finland from about 2500 BCE[3]—apparently added to confer tensile strength when added to clay—and its use has also been recorded in other Neolithic sites, including Central Russia, Norway, and Lappland.[8] However, in the Western literature, the earliest known documented reference to what might have been asbestos has been attributed by some to Theophrastus (ca. 372–287 BCE)— a student of Aristotle and his successor at the Lyceum in Athens[8]—in his book *De Lapidibus* [On Stones],[9] compiled in about 300 BCE. In Chapter II.17, he wrote:

> In the mines at Scapte Hyle a stone was once found which was like rotten wood in appearance. Whenever oil was poured on it, it burnt, but when the oil had been used up, the stone stopped burning, as if it were itself unaffected.

(Scapte Hyle was a mining district in Thrace opposite the island of Thasos in the Northern Aegean.[9]) In commentary on this description, Theophrastus' twentieth-century translators/editors Caley and Richards[9] set forth the following commentary:

> Moore [in *Ancient Mineralogy*, p. 153] thought that Theophrastus was really referring to asbestos. The color of the stone makes this unlikely, though its structure makes it less improbable, since some forms of decayed wood do have a fibrous structure like asbestos. We know from statements of various early authors that asbestos was known in antiquity, and that it was mainly used for the manufacture of incombustible cloth, though evidently wicks for oil lamps were also made of it. Moreover, direct evidence of the use of asbestos by the ancients has been obtained in modern times by the discovery of ancient garments woven from this mineral. It is, however, unlikely that Theophrastus is alluding to asbestos, since the mineral does not occur in the locality mentioned. There were only two known sources of asbestos in Greece and its vicinity in ancient times: Karystos at the southern extremity of the island of Euboea, and a place to the southeast of Mt. Troodos on Cyprus, where the abandoned workings are still to be seen today.
>
> It is much more probable that Theophrastus [was] referring to the well-known brown fibrous lignite, which in appearance and in other respects very often closely resembles rotten wood. Lignite of various kinds is known to occur in the region named by Theophrastus....Lignite of the kind to which he apparently refers often contains in its natural state as much as 20 per cent of water; thus it cannot readily be ignited...

Maines[8] refers to Chinese, Singhalese, and Indian sources concerning the use of asbestos in antiquity. She[8] mentions Lih-tsze who wrote near the end of the fifth century BCE concerning a fireproof cloth that was cleaned by fire. It is also claimed that Herodotus recorded the use of asbestos in a cremation shroud.[5,10,11]

Gaius Plinius Secundus (23–79 CE), better known as Pliny the Elder, certainly refers to asbestos in book XXXVI.xxi of his *Natural History* where he commented:[12]

> Asbestos looks like alum and is completely fire-proof; it also resists all magic potions, especially those concocted by the Magi.

Maines[8] refers to book XIX.iv:

> Chapter IV. Also a linen has now been invented that is incombustible. It is called "live" linen, and I have seen napkins made of it glowing on the hearth at banquets and burnt more brilliantly clean by the fire than they could be by being washed in water. This linen is used for making shrouds for Royalty, which keep the ashes of the corpse separate from the rest of the pyre.

Having stated this, it appears that Pliny thought that asbestos was a plant that grew

> …in the deserts and sun-scorched regions of India where no rain falls, the haunts of deadly snakes, and it is habituated to living in burning heat; it is rarely found, and is difficult to weave into cloths because of its shortness.…The Greek name for it is asbestinon, derived from its peculiar properties.

It is sometimes claimed that Pliny had warned of the dangers of asbestos and that slaves who worked with the material wore masks to protect against the dust.[6] However, Maines[8] asserts that no reference can be found to the wearing of masks by "slaves" who worked with this material—so that the often-repeated claim on this issue appears to be in error. It seems more likely that the masks were worn by artisans who worked with cinnabar, not asbestos, and Pliny apparently did not state that the artisans were slaves (Book XXXIII.xli).[8]

It is said that Pausanias (ca. 175 CE) recorded a gold lamp made by Callimachus of Athens for the goddess Minerva, which had a wick made of Carpasian linen—"the only linen which is not consumed by fire."[10] Over a thousand years later, in *The Travels*, Marco Polo[13] described cloths used by Tartars in the Khanate Province of Ghinghintalas during the Yüan dynasty:

> When the stuff found in this vein…has been dug out of the mountain and crumbled into bits, the particles cohere and form fibres like wool.…Then this wool-like fibre is carefully spun and made into cloths. When the cloths are first made, they are far from white. But they are thrown into the fire and left there for a while; and there they turn as white as snow. And whenever one of these cloths is soiled or discoloured, it is thrown into the fire and left there for a while, and it comes out as white as snow.…One of these cloths is now at Rome; it was sent to the Pope by the Great Khan as a valuable gift.… (pp. 89–90).

Marco Polo's account clearly indicated that asbestos is a mineral in character as opposed to the hair of a mythical fire-resistant salamander as widely supposed in Medieval superstition.

It has been claimed that the Emperor Charlemagne (ca. 742–814 CE) had a tablecloth made of asbestos thrown into the fire after dinner to the amazement of his guests, but this story seems apocryphal.[8] However, Maines[8] refers to an account by Ibn al-Fatiq, who recorded that tenth-century Christian pilgrims to Jerusalem were sold small pieces of what appears to have been asbestos, claimed to have been fragments of the True Cross, the divine and magical properties of which were proven by their incombustibility.

Much later, the chevalier Jean Albini (1762–1834)—nephew of Galvani and a professor of physics at the University of Bologna—used asbestos cloth to make a fire-resistant suit that he exhibited in several European cities and at the Royal Institution in London in 1829.[14]

1.3 ASBESTOS FROM THE BEGINNING OF THE INDUSTRIAL ERA

A useful account of the modern history of asbestos has been set forth by Frank[15] and by Hammar and Dodson.[3] By about 1850, chrysotile deposits had been found around Thetford in Canada and at about that time the fire-resistant properties of asbestos were demonstrated by a forest fire in the mid-1870s, where the rocky outcrops of asbestos deposits did not burn, unlike the trees.[15] According to Frank,[15] approximately 50 tons of asbestos were mined in Quebec by 1876, and by the 1950s more than 900,000 tons were mined each year.[15] In the early nineteenth century, asbestos was noted in South Africa, particularly in the North West area of Cape Province, and the name crocidolite was assigned to the blue-gray stone ("wooly stone").[15] According to Frank's[15] account, serious production of asbestos in South Africa did not get underway until the early twentieth century, with production far less than in Canada, and less than approximately 10,000 tons each year until 1940. In the Transvaal area, amosite (reportedly an acronym for *Asbestos Mines of South Africa*)[3,15] was mined, and approximately 80,000 tons of amosite were produced each year by 1970.

Other nations with significant production of asbestos include Russia, where chrysotile was discovered in 1720 in the region of the Ural Mountains near the Tagyl River.[16] The deposit was soon mined, and an asbestos cloth produced therefrom was presented to Peter the Great in 1722.[16] However, by 1735, production was discontinued "...due to lack of practical importance of the deposit...."[16] In 1765, an anthophyllite deposit was discovered south of Ekaterinburg, in a hill subsequently called Asbestoyaya.[16] Still later, the Bazhenovskoye chrysotile deposit was found in late 1884, and mining began in 1886[17] (the Vosnessenskiy mine)[16,17]—where production of chrysotile still continues around the *monogorod* town of Asbest.[*] Other chrysotile deposits were later found in the middle and southern Urals.[16]

Major chrysotile asbestos production continues in Kazakhstan (chrysotile), Zimbabwe (initially the Shabata deposits and then the Shabani mine from about 1950[3]), Brazil, and, more recently, China.[15]

Asbestos was also mined in Italy (e.g., chrysotile at the Balangero mine). In the United States, small deposits of asbestos were mined in Vermont, Arizona, and California as well as even smaller deposits of anthophyllite in North Carolina and Georgia.[15] The use of asbestos in the United States[18] is shown in Table 1.2 for the years 1920–2003.

In Australia, approximately 47 tonnes of amphiboles were mined at Jones' Creek, near Gundagai, New South Wales between 1880 and 1889, and approximately 35 tonnes of chrysotile were mined at Anderson's Creek, Tasmania between 1890 and 1899. South Australia was the first state to mine crocidolite in a very small mine at Robertstown in 1916. During the twentieth century, there was a gradual increase in asbestos production, with more chrysotile than amphiboles mined until 1939. After commencement of mining at Wittenoom in Western Australia (WA)[19] in 1937, crocidolite dominated production until final closure in 1966. New South Wales, the first state to mine asbestos, also produced the largest tonnages of chrysotile (until 1983) as well as smaller quantities of amphiboles (until 1949). With the closure of the crocidolite mine at Wittenoom in 1966, Australian asbestos production declined to a pre-1952 level. Exports declined from 1967. Imports of chrysotile also began to decline. The earliest records of asbestos imports date from 1929: the main sources of raw asbestos imports were Canada (chrysotile) and South Africa (crocidolite and amosite). About twice as much chrysotile was imported as was mined, and half as much crocidolite was imported than was mined. After Wittenoom was closed, a small amount (122 tonnes) of crocidolite was mined in South Australia. In New South Wales, the chrysotile mine at Baryulgil continued production. In 1971, the chrysotile deposits at Woodsreef near Barraba, New South Wales, began to be exploited, and exports of asbestos fiber expanded as production increased; this operation was opencast with dry milling.

Australian production of asbestos decreased in 1981 because of the drop in world demand for asbestos and the increased operating costs at the Woodsreef mine. This mine ceased production in

---

[*] A monogorod town is one based on and exists because of a single industry, such as Togliatti in the former Soviet Union, which came into existence for the specific purpose of automobile production.

Table 1.2   Asbestos Production, Imports, and Consumption for the United States, 1920–2003, by 10- and 5-Year Intervals, with Data for 2003

Year	Production	Imports	Exports	Consumption
1920	1500	151,000	600	152,000
1930	4000	189,000	700	192,000
1940	17,000	224,000	4000	237,000
1950	38,000	640,000	17,000	660,000
1960	41,000	607,000	5000	643,000
1970	114,000	589,000	35,000	668,000
1975	89,000	489,000	33,000	545,000
1980	80,000	327,000	49,000	359,000
1985	57,000	142,000	46,000	154,000
1990	20,000	41,000	29,000	32,000
1995	9000	22,000	17,000	15,000
2000	5000	15,000	19,000	1000
2003	–	4500	3500	4600

Note: All data are in metric tons. Apparent consumption calculated as production + imports – exports, with no adjustment to account for changes in government and industry stocks: negative values indicate shipments from stocks. The values in the U.S. Geological Survey are stated to be reasonably accurate to the first three digits so that the numbers listed above have been rounded off to the nearest 50 tonnes for values <1000 to 500 for values in the range of 1000–10,000 and to the nearest 1000 tones for numbers >10,000: this being so, some of the values do not add up exactly.

Source: Data are from U.S. Geological Survey (USGS). See, Virta, R.L. Worldwide asbestos supply and consumption trends from 1900 through 2003: U.S. Geological Survey Circular 1298, 80 pages, 2006, available only online, accessible at http://www.usgs.gov/pubprod and Larson, T., Melnikova, N., Davis, S.I., Jamison, P. *Int. J. Occup. Environ. Health*, 13, 398–403, 2007.

1983 when the dry milling plant could not meet dust control regulations. Tables 1.3 and 1.4 set forth data for the production, importation, and consumption of asbestos in Australia.[20]

In this context, it has been asserted by some authors such as Price and Ware[21] and Kelsh et al.[22] (with no cited supporting evidence) that "… the Australian high rates of [malignant mesothelioma] are not unexpected due to widespread environmental exposures to high levels of amphibole asbestos including crocidolite."[21] In reality, in Australia most mesotheliomas are attributable to specifically identifiable asbestos exposure, especially amphibole-containing exposures, whether occupational (direct and bystander) or nonoccupational, and including low-dose exposures from identified point sources of exposure.[23] Studies on airborne asbestos fiber concentrations in the general urban environment have not demonstrated environmental exposures significantly in excess of those recorded for other nations. For example, a 1990 report from the Western Australian Advisory Committee on Hazardous Substances[24] found that among schools in WA—mainly schools in Perth, the capital city of the Australian State where the Wittenoom Blue Asbestos Industry was located—the airborne concentrations of asbestos fibers were less than 0.002 fiber per milliliter, perhaps even less than that figure by one order of magnitude (i.e., below the working detection limit).* These fiber levels in the

---

* All but 1 of the 13 schools inspected had asbestos cement roofs; a visual inspection was carried out, and samples were taken from each of the roofs and samples were also taken from gutters, downpipes, and soil. The condition of the roofs was assessed and ranked on a scale of 1–5, the score of 1 indicating that the condition was virtually as good as new, whereas 5 corresponded to extensive deterioration. The roofs ranged in size from small to very large, and they had been in place for 10–34 years. Only one achieved a ranking of 1 (time of construction unknown); all others had scores of 2–5, and the highest scores correlated with the longest times since construction. The percentage of asbestos content for the

Table 1.3   Production and Imports of Asbestos in Australia, 1930–1983

Years	Chrysotile Production	Chrysotile Imports	Crocidolite Production	Crocidolite Imports	Amosite Production	Amosite Imports
1930–1939	1200	–	400	–	50	–
1940–1949	3000	–	5600	–	750	–
1950–1959	11,500	314,100	63,250	2800	1	107,500
1960–1969	8850	329,000	86,550	–	–	81,450
1970–1979	394,350	388,000	–	–	–	87,900
1980–1983	160,400	64,650	–	–	–	8500

Note: Data have been rounded off to the nearest 50 tonnes.
Source: Based on data from the Bureau of Mineral Resources and modified from Leigh, J., Driscoll, T. *Int. J. Occup. Environ. Health*, 9, 206–17, 2003.

Table 1.4   Production, Imports, Exports, and Apparent Consumption in Tonnes of Asbestos (All Types) for Australia, 1930–1985

Years	Production	Imports	Exports	Apparent Consumption
1930–1939	1600	51,550	1200	52,000
1940–1949	9350	140,000	2400	146,900
1950–1959	74,750	314,100	51,400	337,400
1960–1969	95,400	434,700	44,700	485,400
1970–1979	394,350	555,600	45,500	704,450
1980–1985	160,400	104,300	109,800	154,950
Total	740,300	1,602,800	450,000	1,888,000

Note: Values have been rounded off to the nearest 50 tonnes and therefore may not add up exactly.
Source: Based on data from the Bureau of Mineral Resources and modified from Leigh, J., Driscoll, T. *Int. J. Occup. Environ. Health*, 9, 206–17, 2003.

"general environment" are comparable with those recorded in other nations (e.g., see Health Effects Institute–Asbestos Research[25] and World Health Organization[26]).

Major producers of asbestos now include Canada (which exports most of its chrysotile asbestos production), Russia, and China (most of which is used for domestic consumption in those two nations).[21] Russian production in 2000 was approximately 700,000 tonnes followed by 450,000 tonnes in China and 335,000 tonnes in Canada (see Table 1.5 for data for 1975). In 2000, the worldwide production of asbestos was 2,130,000 tonnes, mostly chrysotile from Canada, Russia, and China, with a sharp decline in production thereafter (see Table 1.6 for data for 2003). As mentioned in the first paragraph of this chapter, more than 50 nations (including the United Kingdom,

roof samples ranged from 0% to 40% in one sample, and most samples contained 10% to 20%. Crocidolite was detected in 6 of 18 roof samples (only in roofs 30 years old or older), and amosite was identified in 14 of 18; all samples contained chrysotile. High-volume air sampling (approximately 10 m^3) was carried over 24 h out at three sites whenever possible at each of seven schools—a classroom, a veranda, and a remote open site such as a sports field—using a vertical elutriar/37 mm cassette/vacuum pump and was studied by both phase-contrast light microscopy and scanning electron microscopy. Despite more than 100 h of scanning, not a single fiber was found in 20 samples; a single amosite fiber attached to a 3.25-μm nonfibrous particle and assessed as nonrespirable was found at one school. Not one fiber was found on air sampling either in central Perth or in a rural town some 100 km east of Perth (York). Air sampling carried out in 1989 in a railways workshop in Perth—where there were more than "8 acres" of asbestos cement roofing more than 60 years old—revealed a concentration of more than 0.01 fibers/mL in one sample from the "asbestos shed" used for asbestos removal (as assessed by phase-contrast light microscopy: PCLM); two other samples with fiber concentrations of 0.05 and 0.02 fibers/mL (PCLM) from the same "shed" were then assessed by scanning electron microscopy: in one of these samples, only 1 of 16 fibers was asbestos, and there were no asbestos fibers in the other.

Table 1.5   Ten Major Producers and/or Importers of Asbestos in 1975, Plus Data for the United States

Country	Production	Imports	Exports	Consumption
Soviet Union (Russia + Kazakhstan)	**1,900,000**	–	613,000	1,287,000
Canada	**1,056,000**	5000	1,086,000	–25,000
West Germany	–	**386,000**	74,000	312,000
South Africa	**355,000**	29,000	368,000	15,000
Southern Rhodesia	**262,000**	–	260,000	2000
Japan	5000	**253,000**	2000	256,000
China	**150,000**	–	–	150,000
Italy	**147,000**	66,000	81,000	132,000
France	–	**139,000**	2000	137,000
United Kingdom	–	**139,000**	2000	137,000
United States	90,000	**489,000**	33,000	545,000
World total	4,213,000	2,746,000	2,628,000	4,331,000

Note: Apparent consumption calculated as production + imports – exports, with no adjustment to account for changes in government and industry stocks: negative values indicate shipments from stocks. The values listed above have been rounded off to the nearest 1000 tonnes: this being so, some of the values do not add up exactly. The values in bold indicate whether the country was a major producer or importer of asbestos.
Source: Data are from U.S. Geological Survey (USGS). See citation in the source to Table 1.2.

Europe,[27] Scandinavia, Australia, and apparently Japan) have now banned the use of all forms of asbestos, apart from a few special applications for which no substitute is available.

It appears that on a per capita basis, the greatest production or importation of asbestos is in Russia and the former Soviet Republics including Kazakhstan and in Thailand[15] (Table 1.6). Apart from those nations with asbestos bans in place, the countries with the lowest per capita consumption include Canada and the United States[15] (Table 1.6).

Japan has been an importer of asbestos as opposed to a significant producer. Little asbestos was used in Japan during the Second World War because of the Allies' blockade, but the use of asbestos in Japan accelerated after 1945. One consequence is that the rise of asbestos-related diseases in Japan appears to have taken place later than similar rises in western industrialized nations. In 1960, 77,000 tons of asbestos were imported into Japan, reaching a peak of 352,316 tons in 1974.[28]

The major uses of asbestos are as follows:[15]

- The use of asbestos (both chrysotile and the commercial amphiboles)—as an insulating and fire-resistant material in a variety of circumstances that include commercial buildings, ships (naval vessels including submarines,* merchant ships, and passenger liners), power stations, and locomotives and as insulation around steam pipes and in boilers of all types and furnaces and ovens, and the list goes on.
- The use of both chrysotile or crocidolite or amosite in differing proportions in asbestos cement building materials, including asbestos cement walls; the use of thick asbestos blocks in wet areas of houses and in the roofs of houses, for example, in the eaves; and as corrugated asbestos cement roofing material itself. Such high-density asbestos products were based on the capacity of asbestos fibers to add tensile strength to such materials, their lightness in terms of weight, and their fire resistance and insulating properties.
- The use of chrysotile in particular for brake blocks/linings and gaskets.
- Asbestos textiles (chrysotile) for the production of asbestos blankets and fire-resistant and insulating suits, for example, for firemen and workers in foundries as well as asbestos rope.

* The present authors' files include cases of mesothelioma among workers involved in the dismantling of German U-boats after the Second World War, in Barrow-in-Furness.[29]

Table 1.6   Producers and/or Importers of Asbestos in 2003, Showing Data for
            the Nations Listed in Table 1.5,[a] with the Addition of Further
            Producers/Consumers

Country	Production	Imports	Exports	Consumption
Russia	**878,000**	1000	450,000	429,000
Kazakhstan	**355,000**	3000	184,000	174,000
Canada	**194,000**	205	175,000	20,000
Germany	–	100	–	100
South Africa	6000	1000	4000	3000
Zimbabwe[b]	**147,000**	1	99,000	5000
Japan	–	23,000	20	23,000
China	**350,000**	145,000	3000	492,000
France	–	5	–	–5
United Kingdom	–	25	–	25
United States	–	5000	4000[c]	5000[c]
Brazil	**194,00**0	29,000	144,000	78,000
India	19,000	**176,000**	3000	192,000
Ukraine	–	**156,000**	–	156,000
Thailand	–	**133,000**	125	133,000
World total	2,146,000	1,067,000	1,067,000	2,109,000

Note:
[a] Data for Italy are not listed in the USGS values for 2003 (see footnote for Table 1.5).
In this table, data for metric tonnage >1000 have been rounded off to the nearest
1000; data for metric tonnage <300 have been rounded to nearest 5, except for
Zimbabwe (importation of 1 metric ton).
[b] Zimbabwe has only a small manufacturing capacity for asbestos products so that the
calculated apparent consumption probably includes approximately 43,000 tonnes
going into stocks and 5000 tonnes of estimated consumption.
[c] Includes exports and reexports of asbestos; for the United States, the apparent consumption is assumed by the USGS to equal the imports.
Source: Data are from U.S. Geological Survey (USGS). See citation in the source to
Table 1.2.

- The use of asbestos filters, for example, in gas masks and as a filter for wine.
- Other occasional or idiosyncratic uses such as blue asbestos mattresses, the use of asbestos in fire-
resistant paints, and the production of asbestos paper (asbestos was also used in the production of
"ordinary" paper).

The use of asbestos in ships is particularly noteworthy. Ships of all types are particularly vulnerable
to fire at sea with problems in the evacuation of passengers and crew from vessels on fire.[7] One of
the most notorious examples concerned the *Morro Castle* in 1934, when it appears the captain was
murdered by a member of the crew who then set fire to the forecastle of the ship.[7] The first mate,
who had assumed command, appears to have been very inexperienced and steered the ship toward
the nearest port, but in doing so headed the ship into the wind, which then blew the fire back along
the vessel, resulting in the deaths of some 137 people.[7]

1.4 EVOLUTION OF KNOWLEDGE CONCERNING
ASBESTOS-RELATED DISEASES

1.4.1 Asbestosis

By definition, asbestosis refers to diffuse interstitial fibrosis affecting lung parenchyma, induced
by the inhalation and deposition of asbestos fibers.[30–33]

Castleman[6] refers to mention by the Viennese physician Netolitzky of the "...emaciation and pulmonary problems in asbestos weavers..." in his *Handbuch der Hygiene* (1897), and in Great Britain, the first reference to the injurious effects of asbestos seems to have been made by the lady inspectors of factories in 1898. Castleman[6] sets forth the following quotation concerning their observations:

In the case of one particular asbestos works...far from any precaution having been taken, the work (sifting, mixing, and carding) appeared to be carried on with the least possible attempt to subdue the dust....

Reportedly, an inspection in 1906 revealed a "...thick, foglike atmosphere of dust...the atmosphere is of a thick whitey-yellow consistency...."[6]

The first patient with asbestosis for whom a record seems to exist was a 33-year-old man seen in 1899 by Dr. H. Montague Murray at the Charing Cross Hospital in London.[5] Before his death in 1900, the patient was the sole survivor of 10 men who had worked together in the carding room of an asbestos factory (all the others had died at around 30 years of age). Murray's case was never published in detail in the mainstream medical literature, but in evidence to the Departmental Committee on Industrial Diseases in 1906, Murray referred to the presence of spicules of asbestos in sections of the lung.[5]

Germany never produced raw asbestos on a significant scale, perhaps explaining why fatalities from asbestosis were not reported there until 1914, but products manufacture did take place.[34] According to Proctor,[34] asbestos at about that time was often called *Bergflachs* in Germany ("mountain flax"), and asbestosis was known as *Bergflachslunge*. In 1914, Fahr recorded the presence of crystals in the lung tissue of German patients with asbestosis.

In 1918, a statistician with the Prudential Insurance Company referred to premature mortality among asbestos workers, after which those workers were refused life insurance.[6]

In 1924, Cooke[35] published the first account of asbestosis in the English language literature. Detailed descriptions followed in 1927,[10,36] complete with high-quality photomicrographs of asbestos bodies (then referred to as "curious bodies"[36]). Cooke's[35] case appears to have been that of Nellie Kershaw who worked for Turner Brothers Asbestos Company from the age of 13 years and intermittently after she was aged 26 years, until her total disablement at 31 years and her death when she was 33 years old.[6] It seems that a doctor's certificate referred to her having sustained "asbestos poisoning," but Turner and Newall (T&N) Industries repudiated that diagnosis and noted that no such condition was listed among the compensable diseases in the Workmen's Compensation Act[6] (one of the first in a long litany of denial and suppression of information and then derisory *ex gratia* payments to the partners of those who had died—vividly described in Tweedale's[1] book *Magic Mineral to Killer Dust: Turner & Newall and the Asbestos Hazard*—subject to an undertaking that there would be no further claim against the company for a particular case.) Castleman's[6] book *Asbestos: Medical and Legal Aspects*[6] discusses further reports on asbestosis in the medical literature in Great Britain.

In 1930, Merewether and Price completed an investigation into the asbestos textile industry in the United Kingdom.[6] They found that approximately 26% of workers examined had asbestosis and a further 21 of 363 cases had "precursive signs" of the disease. They also found that the severity of the asbestosis and its speed of development appeared to correlate with the intensity of the exposure.

A memorable publication was that by Wood and Gloyne[37] in 1934. These authors reviewed 100 cases of asbestosis and outlined the circumstances in which asbestosis was encountered:

The picture of pulmonary asbestosis is that of a pneumoconiosis occurring in a factory in which few precautions have been taken to protect the workers from a danger, the gravity of which was not realised. Happily these conditions are now a thing of the past....There is thus good reason to believe that the disease is now under control [*sic*].

It is also worth pointing out that one of the asbestosis cases reported by Wood and Gloyne[37] concerned an 18-year-old van boy who mixed asbestos in an open yard for a period of approximately 2.5 years.

In 1938, Dreessen et al.[38] published an extensive study of asbestosis in the asbestos textile industry in Charleston, South Carolina, where Canadian commercial chrysotile was used almost exclusively (in this regard, chrysotile appears to be less potent for the induction of almost any asbestos disease than the amphiboles, with the exception of the asbestos textile industry). Dreessen et al.[38] suggested that an airborne asbestos dust concentration less than 5 million particles per cubic foot (mppcf) would probably prevent the development of asbestosis. However, as acknowledged by Dreessen et al.[38] themselves, their study was flawed because approximately 150 workers in the factory had been replaced by other workers "with little or no previous asbestos exposure" approximately 15 months before the study began (apparently, many of the 150 workers who left did so because they had asbestosis, and although efforts were made to trace them, less than half could be examined). Accordingly, there was an "abnormally large percentage of workers with less than five years of employment" in that industry at the time of the study. Nonetheless, Dreessen et al.[38] suggested their standard of 5.0 mppcf or less was appropriate until better data could be derived, and it became a widely used standard (it was introduced into Victoria in Australia in about 1945). In this regard, to convert million particles per cubic foot into asbestos fibers per milliliter of air, a conversion factor of approximately 3 is generally used, so that 5.0 mppcf corresponds to approximately 15 fibers per milliliter,[39] but a number of studies have used a variety of different conversion factors, so there are problems in extrapolating from counts expressed as million particles per cubic foot to airborne asbestos fiber concentrations in terms of fibers per milliliter.[27,39] In fact, the *Dreessen Standard* did not prevent the development of asbestosis in many workers exposed to airborne asbestos fibers at a level of 5.0 mppcf or even substantially less.

On pages 43–44 of their report, Dreessen et al.[38] also recommended the following:

- Control of dust at the point of origin with dust-removal devices.
- Replacement of dust-laden air by clean air by the use of exhaust systems attached to the equipment.
- The use of "approved types of respirators."
- "Periodic studies of the condition of the working environment…to determine whether the control methods adopted are constantly adequate. This requires the dust concentrations to be determined for each operation."

It is notable that in many work situations—in both industry and especially at various points of end use of asbestos-containing materials such as work in the building construction industry—no systematic measurements of airborne dust/fiber concentrations were carried out.

In 1968, the British Occupational Hygiene Society (BOHS) proposed a limit of 2 fibers per milliliter of air for amosite and chrysotile (immediately introduced by government) to reduce the incidence of asbestosis in a workforce to 1%.[1,40] In 1970, a British government-issued note advised workplace inspectors that no action was required when fiber levels were less than 2 fibers per milliliter; that for fiber concentrations in the range 2–12 fibers per milliliter, further readings should be taken; and only when the levels were more than 12 fibers per milliliter over a 10-min average should the use of exhaust ventilator and respirators be advised.[1] The BOHS did not attempt to set a standard for control of mesothelioma or lung cancer. Flaws in the proposed standard were apparent in the published report (e.g., failure to include ex-workers causing bias and taking clinical findings on trust).[40] The whole BOHS process in 1966–1968 has since been critically evaluated and the standard shown to have been too high by a factor of approximately 10.[40]

1.4.2 Asbestos-Related Lung Cancer

In 1938, three German papers and a review from Austria reported evidence of a link between asbestosis and lung cancer,[34] and Nordmann[41] referred to this occurrence as *der Berufskrebs der*

Asbestarbeiter (the occupational cancer of asbestos workers). In his book, *The Nazi War on Cancer*, Proctor[34] comments in the chapter on *Occupational Carcinogenesis* that the German reports were the most convincing at that time, although anecdotal autopsy reports of lung cancer in patients with asbestosis had been reported earlier, beginning in the mid-1930s.[42–45] Proctor[34] mentions that Franz Koelsch noted in 1938 that the 12 cases of asbestosis-related lung cancer reported by that time "…while suggestive, did not prove the link," whereas Ludwig Teleki in Vienna expressed greater confidence ("…extremely likely…"). Nordmann[41] thought that approximately 12% of asbestosis patients would develop lung cancer. In 1939, Wedler stated that "…there was not the slightest doubt ('…kaum ein Zweifel daran…') that asbestos in the lungs could cause cancer,"[34] and a 1942 review remarked on the reluctance ("…grosse Zurückhaltung…") of English and American scientists to acknowledge the link. In 1941, Nordmann and Sorge[46] induced lung tumors in mice subjected to inhalation of chrysotile asbestos (*Chrysotilasbest*): a photograph of the apparatus used for this experiment is reproduced on page 112 of Proctor's[34] book. In 1943, the German government designated lung cancer in association with any degree of asbestosis as a compensable disease.[34,47] In a world preoccupied with other issues, no attention seems to have been given to this matter, and the analysis of the association between asbestos/asbestosis and lung cancer languished until 1955 when it was further revived by Doll.[48]

In 1991, Enterline[47] commented on the gap of approximately 12 years between the recognition of the link between asbestos in Germany, and the publication of Doll's[48] paper in 1955:

> A lack of experimental and epidemiological evidence played a major role in delaying a consensus [on asbestos and lung cancer]. Other important factors included a rejection of science conducted outside of the U.S. during this period, particularly a rejection of German scientific thought during and after WWII, and a rejection of clinical evidence in favor of epidemiological investigations. Individual writers rarely changed their minds on the subject of asbestos as a cause of cancer.

During the 1930s and 1940s, assessment of causation of cancer was approached largely from a clinical (e.g., case series) and experimental approach, whereas epidemiologic investigations were in their infancy (including studies on the role of tobacco smoke in the causation of lung cancer).

In opening his 1955 paper, Doll[48] stated that some 61 cases of lung cancer had been recorded in association with asbestosis: the "…large number…" of cases was considered suggestive but did not prove that "…lung cancer is an occupational hazard among asbestos workers." He placed stronger emphasis on (i) Merewether's 1949 observation that lung cancer was found at autopsy in 31 of 235 cases of asbestosis (13.2%) but only 91 of 6884 cases of silicosis (1.3%); and (ii) Gloyne's finding at autopsy of lung cancer in 17 of 121 cases of asbestosis (14.1%) in comparison with 55 of 796 cases of silicosis (6.9%). In Doll's[48] study, lung cancer was found at autopsy in 18 cases among 105 deceased workers at one asbestos factory, 15 of the cases being associated with asbestosis. In addition,[48]

> One hundred and thirteen men who had worked for at least 20 years in places where they were liable to be exposed to asbestos were followed up and the mortality among them compared with that which would have been expected on the basis of the mortality experience of the whole male population. Thirty-nine deaths occurred in the group whereas 15.4 were expected. The excess was entirely due to excess deaths from lung cancer (11 against 0.8 expected)….* All the cases of lung cancer were confirmed histologically and all were associated with presence of asbestos.

---

* Some notable aspects of Doll's paper include the following: (i) for the 18 lung cancers in "… a large asbestos works…," there were eight deaths in the first half of the period 1935–1952, all associated with asbestosis, whereas there were 10 deaths during the second half, seven associated with asbestosis and three without; (ii) the consistent association with asbestosis in the follow-up study is unsurprising, given that all the workers were involved in "scheduled areas" (dusty trades) for at least 20 years; and (iii) there was no adjustment for smoking. In addition, at that time there was no way to estimate how much the risk of lung cancer would decline with reducing exposures (i.e., it is obvious that the follow-up for the second half of the period studied was substantially shorter than for the first half). Tweedale[1] has given a graphic account of the industry's attempts to prevent publication of Doll's paper.

...the average risk among men employed for 20 or more years has been of the order of 10 times that experienced by the general population. The risk has become progressively less as the duration of employment under the old dusty conditions has decreased.

Causation of lung cancer by asbestos is specifically discussed in Chapter 6.

1.5 ASBESTOS EXPOSURE AND MESOTHELIOMA: HISTORICAL KNOWLEDGE

The causal relationship between asbestos and mesothelioma had been well established by the late 1960s, and at that time it was recognized that mesothelioma could follow exposures to asbestos that were nonoccupational in character—brief, transient, and low dose—including, for example, the development of mesothelioma from asbestos exposures related to "handyman"-type work on asbestos cement building materials; and the development of mesothelioma from bystander, environmental, and neighborhood-type exposures was described in 1965.[49,50]

Two cases of mesothelioma were described by Wedler in 1943,[51,52] two by Cartier in Canada in 1952,[53] and three by van der Schoot in Holland in 1958.[54] However, the relationship between asbestos exposure (most notably crocidolite [blue asbestos] exposure) and pleural mesothelioma was more firmly established in 1960 in the seminal paper by Wagner et al.[55*]

Of the 33 cases comprising that series of mesotheliomas,[55] several did not involve *direct* occupational exposures to asbestos but rather *indirect/environmental* exposures. For example, Case 3 involved a 53-year-old woman who "lived her whole life in a location near an asbestos mill." Cases 5, 6, 8, and 9 also involved patients who lived in the vicinity of mines. Case 15 was a 42-year-old woman whose mother also had mesothelioma and who "lived at mine until age of 20; went to school near cobbing sheds." Case 20 concerned a 53-year-old woman who "spent [her] whole life in village on wagon route to Kimberley." Case 21 was a 44-year-old man "who lived in the vicinity of mines until the age of 16; often on dumps as a child." Case 23 was a 63-year-old woman who "lived in the vicinity of the mines until the age of 30." Case 24 was a 35-year-old man who "lived in the vicinity of a mill from the age of 1–7; played on the dumps as a child." Case 25 was a 50-year-old woman who "lived in a mining area from the age of 10 to 18 years; after 1918 spent whole life in same town as case 24" (the 35-year-old man referred to earlier).

Smither et al.[66] and McCaughey et al.[67] recorded further cases of asbestos-related mesothelioma in 1962 in the *British Medical Journal*, and the comment was made that the asbestos exposures for some cases of mesothelioma had been "minimal."[35] The first case of asbestos-related mesothelioma in Australia was published in 1962 in the *Medical Journal of Australia*.[68] In the same year, Wagner et al.[69] published studies on the mucin histochemistry of mesothelioma[70] and on the induction of mesothelioma in experimental animals by asbestos (in the journal *Nature*[69]). In 1962, the third edition of Hunter's *The Diseases of Occupations* referred to the remarkable association of mesothelioma with asbestos, citing the 1960 Wagner study. At that time, there were no clear distinctions between the potency of different asbestos fiber types for the induction of mesothelioma.[†]

---

* In 1991/1992, Wagner set out the story of how he came to discover the relationship between asbestos and mesothelioma.[56,57] He commented on the fiber types implicated in the causation of mesothelioma:[57]

"1990: There is overwhelming evidence that crocidolite is the main fiber associated with mesotheliomas. Amosite has been associated with a few mesotheliomas in South Africa and a few more in the United States, but these cases are minimal when compared with those caused by crocidolite."

In fact, by 1990, amosite had been implicated in the causation of mesothelioma in the United States,[58] Europe (Denmark),[59] Australia,[60] and Japan[61] and is now recognized as the most common fiber type implicated in mesothelioma causation in the United States, especially in insulation workers.[62–65]

† The amphibole hypothesis was developed later during the 1980s and published most clearly in the paper by Mossman et al.[71] in the journal *Science* in 1990. It has been the subject of debate in the literature during the 1990s,[72–80] but most authorities (including the authors of this chapter) now recognize the differential potency of the amphiboles (crocidolite, amosite, noncommercial amphiboles, notably tremolite) versus chrysotile for the causation of mesothelioma in particular.[4,27,81]

In the United States, Selikoff and his coworkers documented the risks of cancer, and specifically mesothelioma, from asbestos exposure in 1964 and 1965 in the *Journal of the American Medical Association*[82] and in the *New England Journal of Medicine*[83] as well as the induction of mesothelioma in hamsters by asbestos, including amosite.[84]

In their 1964 paper in the *Journal of the American Medical Association* dealing with neoplasia and asbestos exposure among insulation workers, Selikoff et al.[82] also commented:

A particular variety of environmental exposure may be of even greater concern. Asbestos exposure in industry will not be limited to the particular craft that uses the material. The floating fibers do not respect job classifications. Thus, for example, insulation workers undoubtedly share their exposure with their workmates in other trades: intimate contact with asbestos is possible for electricians, plumbers, sheet-metal workers, steamfitters, laborers, carpenters, boiler makers, and foremen; perhaps even the supervisory architect should be included.

In 1965, Newhouse and Thompson[49,50] described the occurrence of mesotheliomas as a consequence of (i) domestic (household contact) asbestos exposure among the wives who shook out and laundered the asbestos-contaminated work clothes of their partners and (ii) neighborhood exposures to asbestos. For example, these authors[50] referred to the following in relation to neighborhood exposures:

The factory where more than a fifth of the series were employed opened in 1913, having been situated nearer the City of London for the previous seven years. There were three affected female patients living within half a mile of the factory during the seven years it was in production at its first site. At the time it opened, they were children between five and seven years old. At the present site, there were eight patients living with a half mile radius of the factory. One, a male, was born within a quarter of a mile of the factory in 1922 and remained at the same address for 16 years. The other seven were females and aged between six and 13 when the factory opened. They remained in the area for only between three and seven years, except for one who remained at the same address until she died 48 years later....

Thus, among those with no occupational or domestic exposures to asbestos there are 11 (30.6%) of the patients in the mesothelioma series and five (7.6%) in the control series who lived within half a mile of the factory at its present and previous sites.... The difference in the proportion of patients in the two series who lived in the vicinity of the factory and had no other exposure to asbestos is statistically significant ($\chi^2 = 7.85$, $P < 0.01$).

Including the 11 patients who lived near the asbestos factory there are 51 who had been exposed to asbestos. In 39, exposure first occurred before 1930, in the remaining 12 before 1943. The interval between first exposure and onset of symptoms varied between 16 and 55 years (mean 37.5). The duration of exposure also varied widely, ranging from five weeks to over 50 years.

In the same paper, Newhouse and Thompson[50] commented:

There seems little doubt of the risk of both occupational and domestic exposure of asbestos. Wagner et al. (1950) [*sic*: it should have been 1960] described patients with no other exposure except living as a child in the vicinity of the asbestos mines.

They[44] also referred to mesotheliomas as a consequence of household contact exposure:

...among the women [with mesothelioma] only 10 worked in the asbestos factories and a further 17 had nonindustrial exposures, seven in the home and 10 living near asbestos factories [p. 586].... The group of nine, seven women and two men, whose relatives worked with asbestos, are of particular interest. The most usual history was that of the wife who washed her husband's dungarees or work clothes. In one instance we were told that the husband, a docker, came home 'white with asbestos' every evening for three or four years and she brushed him down. The two men in the group, when boys of eight or nine years old, had sisters who were working at the asbestos factory where others of this series were employed. One of these girls worked as a spinner from 1925 to 1936. In 1947 she died of asbestosis. The press report of the inquest states, 'she used to return home from work with dust on her clothes.' Her brother had no other exposure to asbestos... (p. 584).

In a 1968 review on the *Geographic Pathology of Pleural Mesothelioma* published in the monograph *The Lung* by the International Academy of Pathology, Churg and Selikoff[85] commented as follows:

> The tumor [mesothelioma] is more often seen in workers who have only moderate or small amount of asbestos in their lungs, and who show little, if any, clinical or radiologic evidence of pulmonary fibrosis. This amount of asbestos may be inhaled not only by professional asbestos workers, but also by those who handle products containing only a small proportion of asbestos, those who do not handle asbestos at all but merely work alongside asbestos workers such as craftsmen employed in the building industry—carpenters, electricians, etc.—those who have relatives who carry asbestos home in their work clothes and those who live close to asbestos plants. Taken together, this is a large group which can contribute significantly to the incidence of mesothelioma. Beyond that is the general population, particularly the urban population, which, as has been recently been demonstrated, inhales small amounts of asbestos. Reports from Cape Town, South Africa, Miami and Pittsburgh, United States, London, England, and areas of Finland indicate that at least a few asbestos bodies are present in the lungs of 20 to 57% of adults dying in these locations. Because the minimal carcinogenic dose of asbestos has not been established, the significance of this slight exposure is not known. However, the use of asbestos is increasing very rapidly both in quantity (from 500,000 tons per year in 1930 to nearly four million in 1965) and in diversity of applications (over 3000 applications now known). The current cases of mesothelioma due to asbestos must be ascribed to the dust inhaled some 30 years ago. The 8-fold increase in asbestos production over these 30 years suggests that there may be an appreciable prevalence of mesothelioma in the years to come, not only among those occupationally exposed but perhaps also among the general population.

1.6 TRADE-OFFS (COST–BENEFIT ARGUMENTS): A DEFENSE OF ASBESTOS?

One of the defenses of the asbestos industry and its apologists is that human life in all its complexity involves the balancing of myriad benefits versus risks; for example, treatment of diseases with almost any pharmaceutical drug involves probabilistic assessment of the benefit expected for the treatment in question versus nonresponsiveness and, more importantly, the risk and severity of side effects (a drug that causes bone marrow aplasia only rarely would clearly require more critical assessment than another drug that caused most of those who take it to sneeze once or twice only).[27] In the case of asbestos, the argument is advanced that the benefits from its past (and in some nations continuing) use far outweighed the disadvantage of the diseases that it caused among a minority of those exposed to it (at older ages than other competitive risks such as fire[7])—even taking into account the fact that lung cancer has a poor prognosis overall and the mortality rate for malignant mesothelioma approaches 100%.

The trade-off argument is sometimes buttressed by specific examples, some apocryphal. A few eclectic quasi-anecdotal examples follow:

- Maines[7] quotes Morgan and Gee[86] to the effect that "…the Challenger [space shuttle] disaster was a consequence of substituting a non-asbestos-containing putty…to seal the O-rings of the craft." However, this seems to be an urban myth adduced to emphasize the allegedly baleful consequences of non-use of asbestos. It seems that the O-rings never contained asbestos and weren't 'putty'." The late quantum physicist Richard Feynman was a member of the commission appointed by President Ronald Reagan to investigate the Challenger disaster, and he pointed out that the cause appeared to be loss of resilience of the rubber O-rings at low temperatures. Accordingly, in his biography of Feynman, *Genius: Richard Feynman and Modern Physics*,[87] James Gleick wrote:

  > Feynman noted that there were well-known problems with the rubber O-rings that sealed the joints between sections of the tall solid-fuel rockets…they were *ordinary rubber rings,* thinner than a pencil yet thirty-seven feet long, the circumference of the rocket. They were meant to take the pressure of hot gas and form a seal by squeezing tight into the metal joint.…Feynman pressed Molloy on why resiliency

was crucial: a soft metal like lead, squeezed into the gap, would not be able to hold a seal amid the vibration and changing pressure. "If this material weren't resilient for say a second or two," Feynman said, "that would be enough to be a very dangerous situation?" ... [emphasis in italics added]...

DR FEYNMAN:...I took this stuff that I got out of your seal and I put it in ice water, and I discovered that when you put some pressure on it for a while and then undo it doesn't stretch back. It stays the same dimension. In other words, for a few seconds at least and more seconds than that, there is no resilience in this particular material when it is at a temperature of 32 degrees [Fahrenheit]....I believe that has some significance for our problem....

When...tests were finally performed on behalf of the commission...they showed that failure of the cold seals had been virtually inevitable—not a freakish event, but a consequence of the plain physics of materials....

- The terrorist attack on the World Trade Center in New York on September 11, 2001, is cited as another example: one of the World Trade Towers had asbestos insulation up to the fortieth floor (about half later replaced), whereas the other did not. The fire generated by 90,000 L of aviation fuel would have burned at approximately 1000°C, and the lightweight structural steel used for construction of the towers (a "perimeter tube" design) would have softened at approximately 450°C, losing half its tensile strength at approximately 650°C. Eagar and Musso[88] commented that:

  ...the building was not able to withstand the intense heat of the jet fuel fire. While it was impossible for the fuel-rich diffuse-flame fire to burn at a temperature high enough to melt the steel, its quick ignition and intense heat caused the steel to lose at least half its strength and to deform, causing buckling or crippling. This weakening and deformation caused a few floors to fall, while the weight of the stories above them crushed the floors below, initiating a domino collapse.

- Taking into account these circumstances and the structural damage inflicted by the initial impact of the aircraft, it seems that nothing would have prevented or significantly delayed the collapse of the towers. Conversely, there has been concern about the possible potential health hazards from the asbestos in the dust created when the buildings collapsed, although any risk from the asbestos appears to be extremely low.

At a less anecdotal level, Maines' book *Asbestos & Fire: Technological Trade-offs and the Body at Risk*[7] seems to argue that the health consequences were worthwhile as a trade-off against deaths from fire. For example, she states:

In 1948, of the approximately 10,000 Americans who died from fire every year,* almost 40% were children—approximately 10 deaths per day of children of elementary school age or younger. In 1999, the latest year for which the Centers for Disease Control (CDC) have published statistics, 2355 persons died of mesothelioma and 449 of asbestosis, none of whom were under the age of 15. More *children* died every year from fire, before we built the fire safety system that includes asbestos, than *adults* are now dying from asbestos-related disease.

She also comments that asbestos building materials and fire safety systems for which asbestos materials were an important component "...successfully reduced the annual rate of fire deaths in the US from 9.1 per 100,000 in 1913 to 1.0 in 1998." Yet in Table 1.2 where she lists the fire deaths—including the rate per 100,000 people versus asbestos use—it is evident that the fire death rate fell from 6.2 down to 3.3 during the years 1947–1970, and for each of those years, the use of asbestos was at its peak, at more than one billion pounds weight for each of those years, with peak use of almost 1.59 billion pounds in 1965 and 1.47 billion for 1970 (the 2 years when the use was maximal). Subsequently, between 1975 and 1990, asbestos use declined from 197,308,000 pounds down to 91,156,736 pounds, but during those years of declining use, the fire death rate per 100,000 declined further from 2.9 to 2.0—so that the reduction in fire deaths appears to have been explicable at least in part by factors other than asbestos use (e.g., general improvements in building construction and less use of inflammable materials such as wood as well as fire detectors, sprinkler systems, more efficient fire brigade systems, etc.).

---

* In her Table 1.2, she gives a value of 7688.

The "trade-offs" defense is beset with a number of problems from the perspective of history and ethics (discussed in some detail by Smith[89] in the 1992 book *Malignant Mesothelioma*):

- As discussed by Smith,[89] there are significant ethical problems in justifying trade-offs in human life—which can essentially involve a pricing of life—although such trade-offs obviously do occur (as examples he cites skyscraper construction, rescue of humans from life-threatening situations where the rescuers' lives are put at risk, and decision making on resource allocation in medicine). He states:[89]

  We can deduce…that to argue that the benefits of asbestos to society outweigh any harm caused to a "small" number of workers is fallacious, because it attempts to equate *incommensurable* values on some imaginary scale of utility.* That even a small number of workers die for the benefit of the production of certain consumer products [even if those products save lives] does not make this situation morally right. At best, it is a socially necessary evil that should [be] eliminated as soon as possible by technical advances.

- As shown clearly in Castleman's[6] and Tweedale's[1] books, the asbestos industry was aware of the capacity of asbestos to cause serious disease in the form of asbestosis since the 1930s. Yet the record was one of denial or suppression of the information then available, which was usually not communicated to the workers—raising the issue of consent of the workers to be put at risk by their employment. As Smith[89] states:

  Where there is uncertainty about the risks to health of workers, or a possible threat to the environment, workers and society have an *unqualified, unconditional* right to be informed of those risks in an impartial and understandable way.…

Maines[7] comments on what she calls *The Conspiracy of Silence Hypothesis* (p. 160):

  It is an article of faith in the anti-asbestos literature that the dangers of asbestos disease were deliberately kept from all but a privileged few, thus preventing workers from understanding the risks they took in the workplace.…A conspiracy of silence that results in seven hundred publications surely cannot be considered a success, as a spokesman from Johns-Manville pointed out in 1978.…Anyone with an interest in the subject, which apparently did not often include the staff or elected representatives of the insulators or building trades unions, could have learned about these risks as workers in other occupations learned about lead, mercury, gasoline, and other known hazards. An hour in a public library at any time after 1926 would have revealed all of the "secrets" the asbestos products manufacturers were allegedly trying to conceal.

Of course, there was (and continues to be) a serious imbalance between the resources and information available to individual workers and their union representatives versus the employing corporations. If such corporations were in possession of such information, there was (and still is) an overriding and unbreakable obligation for them to communicate that information to those potentially affected by their products.

Smith[89] comments:

  Governments, whose role is the protection of their citizenry, have a moral obligation to ensure safe working conditions, and even in the worst-case scenario, where there are unavoidable dangers, they are obliged to monitor industrial activities closely and to eliminate dangers whenever possible. One can argue that *all* participants in industrial activity (corporations, governments at all levels, and union organizations) have a responsibility to address these issues. Even so, failure to fulfill the most fundamental role of government—the protection of human life—has no bearing on the moral responsibility of asbestos (or other) mine operators. X's failure to fulfill one obligation cannot excuse Y from fulfillment of another obligation. Thus, one of the strongest arguments advanced by the asbestos industry in its own defence is logically unsound and morally fallacious."

- An exposure standard designed to prevent asbestosis had been developed by 1938,[38] although it was flawed and did not prevent the development of this disease (but adherence to the standard would have reduced the frequency and severity of asbestosis). Dreessen et al.[38] had set forth various steps to be taken to reduce exposure to comply with the standard (which included monitoring of airborne dust levels). But in many industries, including the building construction industry and some shipyards, no such measurements were ever carried out. Here, one can comment that enforcement of occupational standards is as strong an obligation of government as compliance is for industry.

---

* It also begs the question: Who decides?

- Of course, another defense that has been raised in relation to the causation of mesothelioma is that industry could not have been aware of this risk before 1960 and even for some time thereafter. In response to this claim, one can comment: (i) by 1962, it had been recognized that mesotheliomas had been recorded in those whose exposures seemed to have been "minimal"; and (ii) as stated in footnote on page 367 of *Malignant Mesothelioma*,[89]

  …an industry cannot reasonably claim immunity [from] blame or moral accountability for its failure or inability to anticipate a hitherto unforeseen form of occupational disease X, if its control measures have been inadequate to prevent known occupational diseases Y or Z resulting from its activities or products. This is because the industry is already culpable on the basis of prevailing knowledge and it cannot realistically expect absolution simply because its actions (or inactions) have some unpredictable consequences.

1.7 THE GLOBAL BURDEN OF ASBESTOS-RELATED DISEASES

The greatest concern over asbestos-related diseases in industrialized nations now focuses on cancer, especially malignant mesothelioma—including concern over likely future cases of asbestos-induced cancer for developing nations where asbestos use continues and where there are few controls on occupational dust exposures (or a failure to enforce existing standards) and also where there are few restrictions on tobacco smoking (relevant to lung cancer; see Chapter 6). It has been estimated that annual deaths from asbestos-related diseases are in the order of 90,000–100,000 worldwide and the final total is likely to be somewhere in the order of 5,000,000 or more.* Because of the long latency interval between first exposure to asbestos and the subsequent diagnosis of the disorder, mcsothelioma cases and deaths are expected to continue until 2030–2050, even in those countries that have implemented bans on all forms of asbestos. For France only, Banaei et al.[90] estimated that "…between 1997 and 2050, the most optimistic and pessimistic trends of future exposure will lead to the deaths from mesothelioma of between 44,480 and 57,020 men…," leading to a corresponding loss of some 877,200 to 1,171,500 person-years of life.

As other examples, it has been estimated that there are approximately 6000 deaths annually from mesothelioma in the United States,[91] and some 2156 deaths from mesothelioma were recorded in the United Kingdom for 2007.*

For the year 2003, the Australian Mesothelioma Register recorded 535 cases of mesothelioma among men and 110 cases in women, with a total of 645 cases, corresponding values for 2005 are 485 (men) and 112 (women).[92] Particularly notable is the increase in the number of cases in women, from 22 in 1982 to 112 in 2005.[92] A similar trend for a rising incidence of mesothelioma in women has been recorded in the United Kingdom[93] (see also Strickler et al.[94] for the United States). This trend indicates that the claim advanced by some authors[95]—that the mesothelioma rate in women has remained unchanged over decades, despite increased use of asbestos, and that this unchanging rate is the "background" (environmental) rate and is evidence of a "threshold" level of asbestos exposure for mesothelioma induction—is wrong. There is general agreement that mesothelioma induction by asbestos is governed by a cumulative dose–response relationship *with no identified threshold* (e.g., see the World Health Organization Monograph *Environmental Health Criteria 203: Chrysotile Asbestos*[26] and Hodgson and Darnton[81]).

On the basis of the data for Britain, France, Germany, Italy, The Netherlands, and Switzerland, Peto et al.[96] predicted in 1999 that the number of men who would die from mesothelioma in Western Europe each year would almost double over the ensuing 20 years, from approximately 5000 in 1998 to approximately 9000 around 2018. The numbers would then decline, but they predicted a total of

---

* See Takala J. ILO's role in the global fight against asbestos. European Asbestos Conference, 2003. http://www.hvbg.de/e/asbest/konfrep/konfrepe/repbeitr/takala_en.pdf; http://www.hse.gov.uk/statistics/causdis/mesothelioma/. See also the 2010 Collegium Ramazzini statement (Collegium Ramazzini Web site: http://www.collegiumramazzini.org/news.asp).

Table 1.7   Estimates of Mesothelioma Incidence in 30 Nations

Country	Incidence Rate[a]	Country	Incidence Rate[a]	Country	Incidence Rate[a]
Australia	32[b]	France	10–13	Austria	5.6
Great Britain	30	Finland	>10	Poland	4
Belgium	29	Canada	9	Slovakia	4
Netherlands	23	Cyprus	9	Slovenia	4
Italy	17	United States	9	Spain	4
Norway	16	Hungary	8	Estonia	3
New Zealand	15	Turkey	7.8	Israel	3
Denmark	13	Croatia	7.4	Latvia	3
Germany	13	Japan	7	Lithuania	3
Sweden	12	Romania	6	Macedonia	3

Note:
[a] Incidence rate = estimated crude incidence rate per million of the population per year.
[b] For 2003.
Source: Modified from estimates in Bianchi C, Bianchi T. Malignant mesothelioma: global incidence and relationship with asbestos. *Ind Health 2007*; 45: 379–87.

approximately 250,000 deaths in men for the period 1995–2029. Subsequently, Pelucchi et al.[97] suggested the total number of deaths is likely to be less than the estimate of 250,000. When asbestos-related lung cancers are added to the mesothelioma burden at an estimated ratio of one or two lung cancers for every mesothelioma (see Chapter 6), the total number of asbestos-related cancer deaths is still likely to be in the vicinity of 500,000 or more.

Crude incidence rates for mesothelioma for some 30 nations are shown in Table 1.7.[98]

1.8 SUMMARY

Asbestos-related diseases have imposed significant morbidity and mortality across industrialized nations for about the last 80 years and will continue to do so for decades to come as a consequence of past exposures to asbestos during the 1950s to the 1980s and beyond—in part because of the latency interval between exposure and subsequent disease such as asbestosis, lung cancer, and malignant mesothelioma. In addition, the use of chrysotile asbestos continues, especially in developing and now Asian nations (chrysotile is still mined in and exported from Russia, Brazil, Canada, and Zimbabwe, and mining for domestic usage continues in Russia, Kazakhstan, China, and Brazil). The nations that continue to import asbestos include India, Sri Lanka, Indonesia, Thailand (one of the highest per capita users), Nigeria, Angola, Uruguay, and Ecuador. Many of the nations to which asbestos is exported have poor surveillance and controls on occupational exposures, and the situation in many such countries is compounded by high frequency of cigarette smoking in the population (see Chapter 6).

Conflict-of-Interest Statement: The authors have prepared reports on causation and/or diagnosis of benign asbestos-related disorders, such as asbestosis as well as lung cancer and mesothelioma, for Courts in Australia, for example, the Dust Diseases Tribunal in New South Wales and in other Australian Courts, and in the United Kingdom and, for JL, the United States, and have given courtroom testimony on these disorders. Neither author has any affiliation with the asbestos industry or any nonprofessional group that lobbies for or against the industry.

REFERENCES

1. Tweedale G. *Magic Mineral to Killer Dust: Turner & Newall and the Asbestos Hazard*. Oxford: Oxford University Press; 2000.
2. Craighead JE, Gibbs A, Pooley F. Mineralogy of asbestos. In: Craighead JE, Gibbs AR, editors. *Asbestos and Its Diseases*. Oxford: Oxford University Press; 2008, pp. 23–38.
3. Hammar SP, Dodson RF. Asbestos. In: Tomashefski JF Jr, editor. *Dail and Hammar's Pulmonary Pathology*. 3rd ed. Vol. 1. New York: Springer; 2008, pp. 950–1031.
4. Hammar SP, Henderson DW, Klebe S, Dodson RF. Neoplasms of the pleura. In: Tomashefski JF Jr, editor. *Dail and Hammar's Pulmonary Pathology*. 3rd ed. Vol. 2. New York: Springer; 2008, pp. 558–734.
5. Henderson DW, Shilkin KB, Whitaker D. Introduction and historical aspects: With comments on mesothelioma registries. In: Henderson DW, Shilkin KB, Langlois SL, Whitaker D, editors. *Malignant Mesothelioma*. New York: Hemisphere; 1992, pp. 1–22.
6. Castleman BI. *Asbestos: Medical and Legal Aspects*. 4th ed. New York: Aspen; 1996.
7. Maines R. *Asbestos & Fire: Technological Trade-Offs and the Body at Risk*. New Brunswick: Rutgers University Press; 2005.
8. Maines R. Asbestos before 1880: From natural wonders to industrial material. In: *Asbestos & Fire: Technological Trade-Offs and the Body at Risk*. New Brunswick: Rutgers University Press; 2005, pp. 24–44.
9. Theophrastus. On stones. Columbus (OH): Ohio State University; ca. 300 BCE.
10. Cooke WE. Pulmonary asbestosis. *Br Med J* 1927;2:1024–5.
11. Cooke WE. Asbestos dust and the curious bodies found in pulmonary asbestosis. *Br Med J* 1929;2:578–80.
12. Pliny the Elder. *Natural History. A Selection* [Healy JF, Trans.]. Harmondsworth: Penguin Classics; 1991.
13. Marco Polo (ca. 1299). *The Travels* [Latham R, Trans.]. Harmondsworth: Penguin; 1979.
14. Murray R. Asbestos: A chronology of its origins and health effects. *Br J Ind Med* 1990;47:361–5.
15. Frank AL. The history of the extraction and uses of asbestos. In: Dodson RF, Hammar SP, editors. *Asbestos: Risk Assessment, Epidemiology, and Health Effects*. Boca Raton: CRC Press; 2006, pp. 1–8.
16. Kashansky SV. A 300-year history of the discovery of asbestos in the Urals. In: Peters GA, Peters BJ, editors. *Sourcebook on Asbestos Diseases*. Vol. 20. Charlottesville: Lexis; 1999, pp. 129–44.
17. Zorina LI, Kashansky SV. The Bazhenovskoye chrysotile asbestos deposits. In: Peters GA, Peters BJ, editors. *Sourcebook on Asbestos Diseases*. Vol. 19. Charlottesville: Lexis; 1999, pp. 193–204.
18. Larson T, Melnikova N, Davis SI, Jamison P. Incidence and descriptive epidemiology of mesothelioma in the United States, 1999–2002. *Int J Occup Environ Health* 2007;13:398–403.
19. Layman L. The blue asbestos industry at Wittenoom in Western Australia: A short history. In: Henderson DW, Shilkin KB, Langlois SL, Whitaker D, editors. *Malignant Mesothelioma*. New York: Hemisphere; 1992, pp. 305–27.
20. Leigh J, Driscoll T. Malignant mesothelioma in Australia 1945–2002. *Int J Occup Environ Health* 2003;9:206–17.
21. Price B, Ware A. Asbestos exposure and disease trends in the 20th and 21st centuries. In: Craighead JE, Gibbs AR, editors. *Asbestos and Its Diseases*. Oxford: Oxford University Press; 2008, pp. 375–96.
22. Kelsh MA, Craven VA, Teta MJ, et al. Mesothelioma in vehicle mechanics: is the risk different for Australians? *Occup Med (Lond)* 2007;57:581–9.
23. NOHSC. The incidence of mesothelioma in Australia 1997 to 1999: Australian Mesothelioma Register Report 2002. Canberra: National Occupational Health and Safety Commission; 2002.
24. Western Australian Advisory Committee on Hazardous Substances. Asbestos cement products. Report by the Western Australian Advisory Committee on Hazardous Substances: Perth: Western Australian Advisory Committee on Hazardous Substances; 1990.
25. Health Effects Institute–Asbestos Research. *Asbestos in Public and Commercial Buildings: A Literature Review and Synthesis of Current Knowledge*. Cambridge (MA): Health Effects Institute–Asbestos Research; 1991.
26. World Health Organization. *Environmental Health Criteria 203: Chrysotile Asbestos*. Geneva: World Health Organization; 1998.

27. World Trade Organization Dispute Settlement Report WT/DS135. European communities—Measures concerning asbestos and asbestos-containing products. Geneva: World Trade Organization; 2000. See also World Trade Organization Dispute Settlement Reports 2001. Vol. VIII (DSR 2001: VIII). Cambridge: Cambridge University Press; 2004, pp. 3303–4047.

28. Morinaga K, Kishimoto T, Sakatani M, Akira M, Yokoyama K, Sera Y. Asbestos-related lung cancer and mesothelioma in Japan. *Ind Health* 2001;39:65–74.

29. Edge JR, Choudhury SL. Malignant mesothelioma of the pleura in Barrow-in-Furness. *Thorax* 1978;33:26–30.

30. Churg A. Nonneoplastic disease caused by asbestos. In: Churg A, Green FHY, editors. *Pathology of Occupational Lung Disease*. 2nd ed. Baltimore: Williams & Wilkins; 1998, pp. 277–338.

31. Mossman BT, Churg A. Mechanisms in the pathogenesis of asbestosis and silicosis. *Am J Respir Crit Care Med* 1998;157:1666–80.

32. De Vuyst P, Gevenois PA. Asbestosis. In: Hendrick DJ, Burge PS, Beckett WS, Churg A, editors. *Occupational Disorders of the Lung: Recognition, Management, and Prevention*. London: Saunders; 2002, pp. 143–62.

33. Sporn TA, Roggli VL. Asbestosis. In: Roggli VL, Oury TD, Sporn TA, editors. *Pathology of Asbestos-Associated Diseases*. 2nd ed. New York: Springer; 2004, pp. 71–103.

34. Proctor RN. *The Nazi War on Cancer*. Princeton (NJ): Princeton University Press; 1999.

35. Cooke WE. Fibrosis of the lungs due to the inhalation of asbestos dust. *Br Med J* 1924;2:147.

36. McDonald S. Histology of pulmonary asbestosis. *Br Med J* 1927;2:1025–6.

37. Wood WB, Gloyne SR. Pulmonary asbestosis: A review of 100 cases. *Lancet* 1934;2:1383–5.

38. Dreessen WC, Dallavalle JM, Edwards TI, Miller JW, Sayers RR. A study of asbestosis in the asbestos textile industry. U.S. Treasury Department, Public Health Service: Public Health Bulletin no. 241. Washington (DC): U. S. Government Printing Office; 1938.

39. Henderson DW, Rödelsperger K, Woitowitz H-J, Leigh J. After Helsinki: A multidisciplinary review of the relationship between asbestos exposure and lung cancer, with emphasis on studies published during 1997–2004. *Pathology* 2004;36:517–50.

40. Greenberg M. The 1968 British Occupational Hygiene Society chrysotile asbestos hygiene standard. In: Peters GA, Peters BJ, editors. *Sourcebook on Asbestos Diseases: Medical, Technical, and Historical Aspects*. Vol. 14. Charlottesville: Michie; 1997, pp. 219–57.

41. Nordmann M. Der Berufskrebs der Asbestarbeiter. *Z Krebsforsch* 1938;47:288–302.

42. Lynch KM, Smith WA. Pulmonary asbestosis: III. Carcinoma of lung in asbesto-silicosis. *Am J Cancer* 1935;24:56–64.

43. Gloyne SR. Two cases of squamous carcinoma of the lung occurring in asbestosis. *Tubercle* 1935–1936;17:5–10.

44. Egbert DS, Geiger AJ. Pulmonary asbestosis and carcinoma: Report of a case with necropsy findings. *Am Rev Tuberc* 1936;34:143–50.

45. Gloyne SR. A case of oat cell carcinoma of the lung occurring in asbestosis. *Tubercle* 1936–1937;18:100–1.

46. Nordmann M, Sorge A. Lungenkrebs durch Asbestsatub im Tierversuch. *Z Krebsforsch* 1941;51:170.

47. Enterline PE. Changing attitudes and opinions regarding asbestos and cancer 1934–1965. *Am J Ind Med* 1991;20:685–700.

48. Doll R. Mortality from lung cancer in asbestos workers. *Br J Ind Med* 1955;12:81–6.

49. Newhouse ML, Thompson H. Mesothelioma of pleura and peritoneum following exposure to asbestos in the London area. *Br J Ind Med* 1965;22:261–9.

50. Newhouse ML, Thompson H. Epidemiology of mesothelial tumors in the London area. *Ann N Y Acad Sci* 1965;132:579–88.

51. Wedler HW. Uber den Lungenkrebs bei Asbestose. *Dtsch Arch Klin Med* 1943;191:189–209.

52. Wedler HW. Asbestose und Lungenkrebs. *Dtsch Med Wochenschr* 1943;69:575.

53. Cartier P. In Smith WE. Survey of some current British and European studies of occupational tumor problems. *Arch Ind Hyg Occup Med* 1952;5:242–63 [a contribution to the discussion, p. 62].

54. Van der Schoot HC. Asbestosis en pleuragezwellen. *Ned Tijdschr Geneeskd* 1958;102:1125–6.

55. Wagner JC, Sleggs CA, Marchand P. Diffuse pleural mesothelioma and asbestos exposure in the North Western Cape Province. *Br J Ind Med* 1960;17:260–71.

56. Wagner JC. The discovery of the association between blue asbestos and mesotheliomas and the after-math. *Br J Ind Med* 1991;48:399–403 [in Danish].

57. Wagner JC. Foreword. In: Henderson DW, Shilkin KB, Langlois SLP, Whitaker D, editors. *Malignant Mesothelioma*. New York: Hemisphere; 1992, pp. xvii–xxv.

58. Omenn GS, Merchant J, Boatman E, Dement JM, Kuschner M, Nicholson W, et al. Contribution of environmental fibers to respiratory cancer. *Environ Health Perspect* 1986;70:51–6.

59. Otte KE, Sigsgaard TI, Kjaerulff J. Massive exposure to asbestos and malignant mesothelioma, familial accumulation. *Ugeskr Laeger* 1990;152:3013–4.

60. Barnes R, Rogers AJ. Unexpected occupational exposure to asbestos. *Med J Aust* 1984;140:488–90.

61. Morinaga K, Kohyama N, Yokoyama K, Yasui Y, Hara I, Sasaki M, et al. Asbestos fiber content of lungs with mesotheliomas in Osaka, Japan: A preliminary report. *IARC Sci Publ* 1989:438–43.

62. Dodson RF, O'Sullivan M, Corn CJ, McLarty JW, Hammar SP. Analysis of asbestos fiber burden in lung tissue from mesothelioma patients. *Ultrastruct Pathol* 1997;21:321–36.

63. Langer AM, Nolan RP. Asbestos in the lungs of persons exposed in the USA. *Monaldi Arch Chest Dis* 1998;53:168–80.

64. Levin JL, McLarty JW, Hurst GA, Smith AN, Frank AL. Tyler asbestos workers: Mortality experience in a cohort exposed to amosite. *Occup Environ Med* 1998;55:155–60.

65. Roggli VL, Vollmer RT. Twenty-five years of fiber analysis: What have we learned? *Hum Pathol* 2008;39:307–15.

66. Smither WJ, Gilson JC, Wagner JC. Mesotheliomas and asbestos dust. *Br Med J* 1962;2:1194–5.

67. McCaughey WTE, Wade OL, Elmes PC. Exposure to asbestos dust and diffuse pleural mesothelioma. *Br Med J* 1962;2:1397.

68. McNulty JC. Malignant pleural mesothelioma in an asbestos worker. *Med J Aust* 1962;2:953–4.

69. Wagner JC. Experimental production of mesothelial tumours of the pleura by implantation of dusts in laboratory animals. *Nature* 1962;196:180–1.

70. Wagner JC, Munday DE, Harington JS. Histochemical demonstration of hyaluronic acid in pleural mesotheliomas. *J Pathol Bacteriol* 1962;84:73–8.

71. Mossman BT, Bignon J, Corn M, Seaton A, Gee JB. Asbestos: Scientific developments and implications for public policy. *Science* 1990;247:294–301.

72. Mossman BT. Mechanisms of asbestos carcinogenesis and toxicity: The amphibole hypothesis revisited. *Br J Ind Med* 1993;50:673–6.

73. Cullen MR. The amphibole hypothesis of asbestos-related cancer: Gone but not forgotten. *Am J Public Health* 1996;86:158–9 [editorial].

74. Stayner LT, Dankovic DA, Lemen RA. Occupational exposure to chrysotile asbestos and cancer risk: A review of the amphibole hypothesis. *Am J Public Health* 1996;86:179–86.

75. Wagner JC. Asbestos-related cancer and the amphibole hypothesis: I. The first documentation of the association. *Am J Public Health* 1997;87:687–8.

76. Stayner LT, Dankovic DA, Lemen RA. Asbestos-related cancer and the amphibole hypothesis: II. Stayner and colleagues respond. *Am J Public Health* 1997;87:688.

77. Langer AMP, Nolan RPP. Asbestos-related cancer and the amphibole hypothesis: III. The amphibole hypothesis: neither gone nor forgotten. *Am J Public Health* 1997;87:688–9.

78. Mossman BT, Gee JBL. Asbestos-related cancer and the amphibole hypothesis: IV. The hypothesis is still supported by scientists and scientific data. *Am J Public Health* 1997;87:689–90.

79. Cullen MR. Asbestos-related cancer and the amphibole hypothesis: V. Cullen responds. *Am J Public Health* 1997;87:690–1.

80. Stayner LT, Dankovic DA, Lemen RA. Asbestos-related cancer and the amphibole hypothesis: VI. Stayner and colleagues respond. *Am J Public Health* 1997;87:691.

81. Hodgson JT, Darnton A. The quantitative risks of mesothelioma and lung cancer in relation to asbestos exposure. *Ann Occup Hyg* 2000;44:565–601.

82. Selikoff IJ, Churg J, Hammond EC. Asbestos exposure and neoplasia. *JAMA* 1964;188:22–6.

83. Selikoff IJ, Churg J, Hammond EC. Relation between exposure to asbestos and mesothelioma. *N Engl J Med* 1965;272:560–5.

84. Smith WE, Miller L, Churg J, Selikoff IJ. Mesotheliomas in hamsters following intrapleural injection of asbestos. *J Mt Sinai Hosp N Y* 1965;32:1–8.

85. Churg J, Selikoff IJ. Geographic pathology of pleural mesothelioma. In: Liebow AA, Smith DE, editors. *The Lung*. Baltimore: Williams & Wilkins; 1968, pp. 284–97.

86. Morgan WKC, Gee JBL. Asbestos-related diseases. In: Morgan WKC, Seaton A, editors. *Occupational Lung Diseases*. Philadelphia: Saunders; 1994, pp. 308–73.

87. Gleick J. *Genius: Richard Feynman and Modern Physics*. London: Abacus; 1992.

88. Eagar TW, Musso C. Why did the World Trade Center collapse?: Science, engineering and speculation. *JOM* 2001;53:8–11. http://www.tms.org/pubs/journals/JOM/0112/Eagar/eagar-.html

89. Smith JW. The asbestos industry: A perspective on the bioethics of industrial activity and disasters. In: Henderson DW, Shilkin KB, Langlois SL, Whitaker D, editors. *Malignant Mesothelioma*. New York: Hemisphere; 1992, pp. 351–61.

90. Banaei A, Auvert B, Goldberg M, Gueguen A, Luce D, Goldberg S. Future trends in mortality of French men from mesothelioma. *Occup Environ Med* 2000;57:488–94.

91. Lemen RA. Epidemiology of asbestos-related diseases and the knowledge that led to what is known today. In: Dodson RF, Hammar SP, editors. *Asbestos: Risk Assessment, Epidemiology, and Health Effects*. Boca Raton (FL): CRC Press; 2006, pp. 201–308.

92. Safe Work Australia. Mesothelioma in Australia: Incidence 1982 to 2005; deaths 1997 to 2006. Canberra: Commonwealth of Australia; June 2009.

93. Peto J, Rake C, Gilham C, Hatch J. *Occupational, Domestic and Environmental Mesothelioma Risks in Britain: A Case–Control Study*. London: HSE Books; 2009.

94. Strickler HD, Goedert JJ, Devesa SS, Lahey J, Fraumeni JFJ, Rosenberg PS. Trends in US pleural mesothelioma incidence rates following Simian Virus 40 contamination of early Poliovirus vaccines. *J Natl Cancer Inst* 2003;95:38–45.

95. Price B, Ware A. Mesothelioma trends in the United States: An update based on Surveillance, Epidemiology, and End Results Program data for 1973 through 2003. *Am J Epidemiol* 2004;159:107–12.

96. Peto J, Decarli A, La Vecchia C, Levi F, Negri E. The European mesothelioma epidemic. *Br J Cancer* 1999;79:666–72.

97. Pelucchi C, Malvezzi M, La Vecchia C, Levi F, Decarli A, Negri E. The mesothelioma epidemic in Western Europe: An update. *Br J Cancer* 2004;90:1022–4.

98. Bianchi C, Bianchi T. Malignant mesothelioma: global incidence and relationship with asbestos. *Ind Health* 2007;45:379–87.

CHAPTER **2**

Asbestos Analysis Methods

James R. Millette

CONTENTS

2.1 INTRODUCTION

The value of a standard method is that it defines procedures in such a way that different laboratories working independently will achieve similar results when using the same method. There are more than 30 different "standard" methods available for the analysis of asbestos in a variety of media. The methods include those for determining the amount of asbestos in air, water, bulk building materials, surface dust, carpet, soil, and specific product materials such as vermiculite and talc. Some methods, although in draft or interim forms, have become generally recognized and used as standard methods by the analytical community. Governmental agencies, such as the Occupational Safety and Health Administration (OSHA), the National Institute of Occupational Safety and Health

(NIOSH), the U.S. Environmental Protection Agency (EPA), the California Air Resources Board (CARB), and the New York State Department of Health, have promulgated some of the methods. Consensus standards groups such as the American Society for Testing and Materials (ASTM), the International Standards Organization (ISO), and the American Water Works Association (AWWA) have published other methods. A number of methods have gained acceptance after being published in the scientific literature. Which method to use in a particular situation depends on the media to be tested and level of information required.

Because the concern with asbestos is related to its fibrous nature, microscopy is the chief analytical tool used for its analysis. Different microscopes have advantages and disadvantages with regard to cost and the ability to provide information about asbestos fibers. Polarized light microscopy (PLM) is the standard way to analyze for asbestos in bulk materials. Phase-contrast microscopy (PCM) is the instrumental technique used for many occupational air sample analyses. Transmission electron microscopy (TEM) and, in some cases, scanning electron microscopy (SEM) are used for all types of samples when small fibers are involved or specific identification of individual asbestos fibers is desired.

2.2 SAMPLE COLLECTION

The collection of samples for analysis depends on the media to be tested and the specific procedures for sample collection are usually provided in the particular analysis method. In general, air samples are collected on membrane filters, water samples in glass or plastic bottles, surface dust by microvacuum or wipe samplers, and solid materials such as building materials, soil and specific products in plastic bags or rigid plastic containers. Air samples are collected on either mixed cellulose ester (MCE) or polycarbonate (PC) filters using either 37- or 25-mm air cassettes. To be quantitative, air samples must be collected with a measured amount of air volume, and surface dust samples must be collected from measured areas of a surface.

2.3 POLARIZED LIGHT MICROSCOPY

A PLM (Figure 2.1) is a compound light microscope that contains a piece of polarizing material in the light path below the sample and another in the light path above the sample. The "PLM method" uses a stereo light microscope (Figure 2.2) to help in taking apart a bulk sample and a polarizing light microscope to identify the fibers among the binders and fillers. Work in the 1980s by McCrone[1,2] established the procedures for asbestos fiber identification by PLM. The PLM identification of asbestos fibers depends on several optical crystallographic properties: refractive indices, dispersion staining, birefringence, sign of elongation, and extinction angle.

The *refractive index* of a substance is numerically equal to the ratio of the velocity of light in a vacuum to its velocity in a substance.[1] The velocity (of light) in any given substance depends on composition; in general, the higher the atomic number of the atoms involved, the lower the velocity and the higher the index.[1] *Dispersion staining* produces its color, not by any chemical interaction but by virtue of the difference between the dispersion of refractive index for a particle and the liquid medium in which the particle is immersed.[1] *Birefringence* refers to the difference between the two refractive indices at right angles to the axis of the microscope.[2] Elongated particles are said to have a positive *sign of elongation* when they have a greater refractive index in the parallel direction than in the perpendicular direction.[1] *Extinction* refers to the behavior on rotation of the microscope stage when a crystalline substance is observed between crossed polarizing sheets. Each particle will show alternate brightness (polarization colors) and darkness (extinction). The particle shows parallel extinction when a prominent direction, for example, length of a fiber, is oriented parallel to the polarizer or analyzer vibration direction in its darkness position.[2]

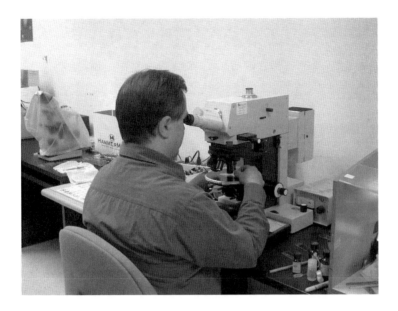

Figure 2.1 Analyst using a PLM for asbestos analysis.

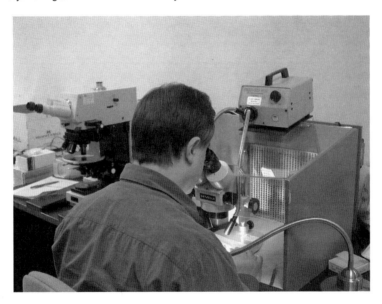

Figure 2.2 Analyst using a stereo-binocular microscope in a HEPA-filtered hood to examine a bulk sample for asbestos.

Because of the size of the wavelength of light, PLM methods of identification are limited to fibers approximately 1 μm in diameter (Figure 2.3).

2.4 BULK ASBESTOS METHODS

The U.S. EPA has defined asbestos-containing material as any material or product that contains more than 1% asbestos.[3,4] The bulk analysis procedure most often specified is the "Method

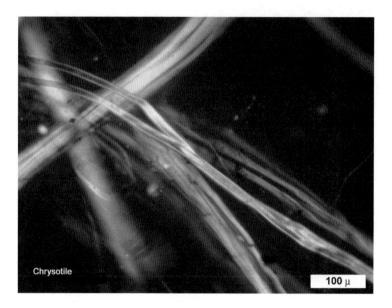

Figure 2.3 Image of asbestos as seen with a PLM.

for the Determination of Asbestos in Bulk Building Materials (EPA-600/R-93/116)" published in 1993.[5] Although it is generally accepted as an improvement over the U.S. EPA "Interim Method for the Determination of Asbestos in Bulk Insulation Samples (EPA-600/M4-82-020)" published in December 1982,[6] the 1993 method has never been formally adopted by the EPA. The NIOSH 9002 and the OSHA ID-191 methods involve similar procedures as the 1993 EPA bulk method.[7,8]

Bulk asbestos analysis performed by PLM methods involves identifying the type of asbestos present on the basis of optical properties and then estimating the relative amount of asbestos in relation to the rest of the bulk sample. The estimates are given in terms of volume percents or, in some cases, area percents. PLM analysts practice with samples of known asbestos percentages until they can visually estimate the values on a consistent basis. The PLM visually estimated asbestos percent values do not necessarily correspond to the weight percent of asbestos in a product. When all components of a bulk material have similar densities, the volume percent value is expected to be similar to the weight percent value. However, if the sample contains 12% chrysotile asbestos by weight in a binder of a denser material such as calcium carbonate (limestone), then the PLM analytical result may show 30% to 40% asbestos by volume. Similarly, if a sample contains 45% to 50% chrysotile asbestos by weight in a material that contains the same weight of a lighter component such as cellulose (paper fibers), then the PLM analytical result may show 5% to 10% asbestos by volume. In most asbestos-containing materials, the precise determination of the percent of asbestos by weight is not of great importance because once a material is shown to contain more than 1% asbestos, it is considered a regulated asbestos-containing building material. In most building products such as insulation, fireproofing, acoustical plasters, and pipe covering where asbestos was intentionally added, the amount of asbestos present is significantly more than 1%.

In some materials such as some ceiling tiles, floor tiles, caulks, paints, and joint compounds, the amount of asbestos may have been added in the low range (approximately 1%). For these materials, special procedures should be used. One special procedure is called "point counting."[9] In this procedure, the particles of the sample material are dispersed on a microscope slide and 400 nonempty points on the slide randomly selected for examination. If, on one of the points, an asbestos fiber happens to line up with the center of the microscope eyepiece crosshairs, the fiber is counted. Percentage of asbestos is calculated on the basis of the number of positive "hits" during the count. Counting three asbestos fibers out of 400 nonempty points, for instance, corresponds to an asbestos percent of 0.75%. A stratified point-counting method is available as a method in the Certification Manual of the New York State Department of Health Environmental Laboratory Approval Program (ELAP).[10,11] The item states: "For samples containing high amounts of asbestos, the stratified point-count technique invokes labor-saving semi-quantitative counting rules. The stratified method is based on the premise that accurate quantitation is unnecessary for materials that contain substantial amounts of asbestos. In contrast, extensive analytical effort is still required for samples that contain positive but small amounts of asbestos."[10] Although more quantitative, the point-count technique has been criticized as not being statistically valid at the 1% level.[12] For a sample in which a value of exactly 1% was determined by the 400 point-count procedure, repeated point-count analyses would be expected to fall variously within the range of 0.27% to 2.6% asbestos on the basis of Poisson statistics. To provide a more statistically valid analysis when low levels of asbestos may be present, matrix reduction is used to concentrate the asbestos fibers. When possible, combustible material is ashed away, acid-soluble material is dissolved away, and density separation is used to prepare the sample of bulk material so that low levels of asbestos fibers can be readily found. Electron microscopy can also be used to help provide quantitative values for low levels of asbestos. The EPA 1993 bulk method, the NIOSH 9002, the OSHA ID-191, and the ELAP Item 198.4 all contain some discussion of matrix reduction and use of electron microscopy.[13] A bulk microscopy method that incorporates various forms of matrix reduction for particular sample product types and use of electron microscopy is being drafted concurrently by task groups in both ASTM and ISO. A comparison of several of the bulk methods is shown in Table 2.1.

Table 2.1 Comparison of Common Methods for Measuring Asbestos in Bulk Building Materials

	EPA-600/ M4-82-020 1982	EPA-600/ R-93/116 1993	NIOSH 9002	OSHA ID-191	ASTM and ISO Bulk in Progress
Instrument	Stereo + PLM XRD	Stereo + PLM and TEM	Stereo + PLM	Stereo + PLM with mention of SEM and TEM	PLM and TEM
Sample preparation	As is and some matrix reduction	As is and some matrix reduction, gravimetric	As is and some matrix reduction	As is and organic and carbonate matrix reduction	As is and detailed matrix reduction, gravimetric
Magnification	×1–1000	×1–20,000	×10–400	–	×1–20,000
Minimum fiber diameter	Approximately >1 µm	Approximately >1 µm	Approximately >1 µm	Approximately >1 µm	Approximately >1 µm
AR	NA	Generally >10:1	NA	3:1 with mention of 100:1	Not known at this time
Measurement	Volume or areal estimation	Visual estimation	Areal estimation	Areal estimation	Volume estimation + weight measure
Identification	Refractive indices, dispersion staining, birefringence, sign of elongation, and extinction angle	Refractive indices, dispersion staining, birefringence, sign of elongation, and extinction angle	Refractive indices, dispersion staining, birefringence, sign of elongation, and extinction angle	Refractive indices, dispersion staining, birefringence, sign of elongation, and extinction angle; mention of SEM and TEM	Refractive indices, dispersion staining, birefringence, sign of elongation, and extinction angle + TEMID
Reporting	% asbestos	% asbestos and possible weight percent	% asbestos	% asbestos	Volume or areal and percent asbestos or weight percent

AR, aspect ratio.

2.5 PCM: AIR ANALYSIS

The PCM (Figure 2.4) is a compound light microscope that illuminates a specimen with a hollow cone of light. The cone of light is narrow and enters the field of view of the objective lens. Within the objective lens is a ring-shaped device that introduces a phase shift of a quarter of a wavelength of light. This illumination causes minute variations of refractive index in a transparent specimen to become visible. The phase-contrast mode pushes the ability of the light microscope to see fibers as thin as 0.25 μm in diameter, but it does so at the expense of identification. PCM is not used to identify asbestos fibers.

The most commonly used PCM method, NIOSH 7400, requires a positive PCM (dark) with green or blue filter, an adjustable field iris, ×8 to 10 eyepieces, and a ×40 to 45 phase objective (total magnification is approximately ×400).[14] Most PCM analysts use binocular PCMs. Within one of the eyepieces there is a Walton–Beckett-type graticule, which forms an analysis area of approximately 0.00785 mm^2 at the specimen plane. The other U.S. Government–promulgated PCM method, OSHA ID-160, has similar requirements.[15] Under the PCM methods, fibers are counted when they are greater than 5 μm in length and have an aspect ratio (AR) (length to width) of at least 3:1. The NIOSH 7400 method "A" counting rules used for counting asbestos fibers have no upper limit on the diameter of the fiber counted. A fiber that appears to be partially obscured by a particle is counted as one fiber. If the fiber ends emanating from a particle do not seem to be from the same fiber and each end meets the length and AR criteria, they are counted as separate fibers. Results of the PCM methods are given in terms of fibers per cubic centimeter of air. According to the current regulations (as of June 2009) promulgated by OSHA, an employer shall ensure that no employee is exposed to an airborne concentration of asbestos in excess of 0.1 fiber per cubic centimeter of air as an 8-h time-weighted average as determined by the OSHA ID-160 method or by an equivalent method (e.g., NIOSH 7400).[16] OSHA has also established a short-term excursion limit. Under this rule, an employer shall ensure that no employee is exposed to an airborne concentration of asbestos in excess of 1.0 fiber per cubic centimeter of air (1 f/cc) as averaged over a sampling period of 30 min as determined by the OSHA ID-160 method or by an equivalent method.[17] The only method considered to be an equivalent method by OSHA at this time is the NIOSH 7400 method

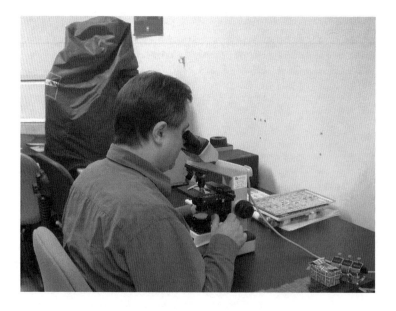

Figure 2.4   Analyst using a PCM for asbestos analysis.

(with NIOSH 7402 in some cases). To be considered by OSHA to be equivalent, a method must pass the equivalency test found in 29CFR1910 (General Industry Asbestos Standard).

2.6 TRANSMISSION ELECTRON MICROSCOPY

The TEM (Figure 2.5) uses electromagnetic coils as lenses to form magnified images with an electron beam in the same way that a light microscope uses glass lenses and a light beam to form images. Electrons can be accelerated with high potential energies, which produce a beam with a very small wavelength and thus allow much higher magnifications than can be achieved with the wavelengths of light. The commonly used TEM methods call for a TEM that can operate at an accelerating potential of 80,000 (80 kV) to 120,000 V. If operating properly at 80 to 120 kV, a TEM is easily capable of obtaining a direct screen magnification of approximately ×100,000 with a resolution better than 10 nm. This allows the smallest asbestos fibers, which are approximately 20 nm (0.02 μm) in diameter, to be examined. In addition to the analysis of fiber morphology by TEM (Figure 2.6), selected area electron diffraction (SAED) and x-ray energy dispersive spectroscopy (EDS) can be used to gain information about a particle's crystal structure and elemental composition. TEM with SAED and EDS is referred to as analytical electron microscopy. Examples of a chrysotile SAED pattern and EDS spectra from reference asbestos minerals are shown in Figures 2.7 and 2.8.

The NIOSH 7402 method is the complementary TEM method for the PCM 7400 method.[18] With 7402, fibers greater than 5 μm in length and having an AR (length to width) of at least 3:1 and a width of at least 0.25 μm are characterized by SAED and EDS. These fibers are then classified as nonasbestos or asbestos. The type of asbestos is also determined. A value of percent asbestos is determined and this percentage applied to PCM results of the same sample. No concentration of fibers per cubic centimeter is reported under Method 7402. The ASTM method for the PCM analysis of workplace exposures, D4240, has been removed from official ASTM practice, and a new method with the inclusion of some TEM procedures for the identification of the fibers found in mines and quarries has been published.[19] The ASTM Method, D7200-06: Standard Practice for Sampling and Counting Airborne Fibers, Including Asbestos Fibers, in Mines and Quarries, by PCM and TEM,

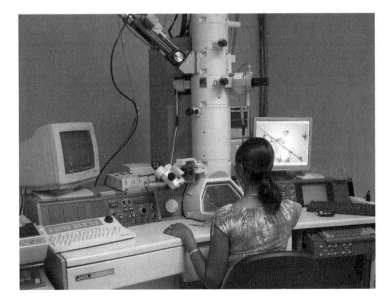

Figure 2.5 Analyst using a TEM for asbestos analysis.

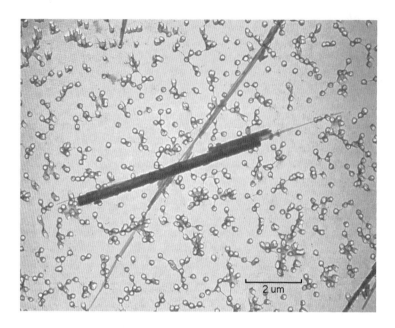

Figure 2.6 Image of crocidolite and chrysotile asbestos fibers as seen with a TEM. Crocidolite is the thicker fiber; chrysotile is longer and thin. The circles are carbon replicas of the PC filter.

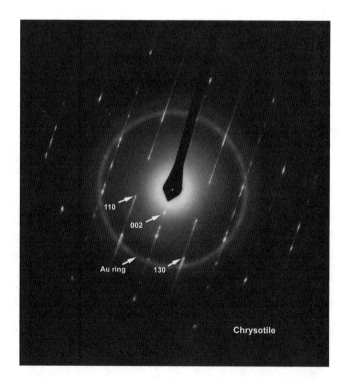

Figure 2.7 Chrysotile SAED pattern. The gold ring results from coating the fiber with a thin layer of gold and is used for calibration.

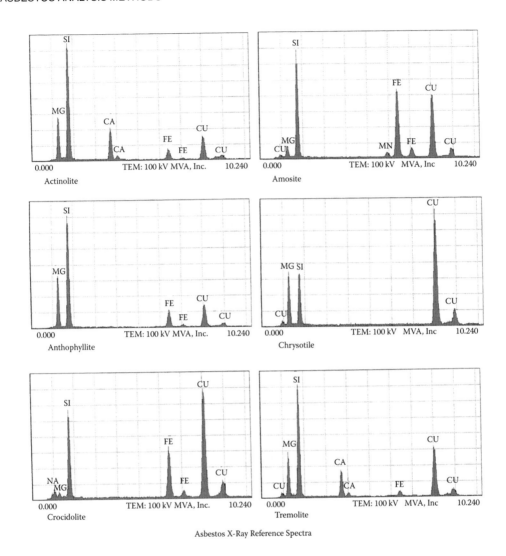

Asbestos X-Ray Reference Spectra

Figure 2.8   EDS x-ray spectra for NIST reference asbestos fibers.

is currently being studied by NIOSH for consideration by OSHA.[20] Under the D7200 method, three classes of elongated particles are established. During PCM analysis, fibers longer than 5 μm with an AR of 3:1 are classified in Class 1 if they show curvature, split ends, or a bundle appearance. Fibers that are greater than 10 μm or less than 1 μm in width are classified as Class 2. All other particles that meet the basic NIOSH definition of a fiber are classified as Class 3. According to the method, if the sum of Classes 1 and 2 are greater than 50% of the total, the data indicate the possibility of an asbestos fiber population. The analyst is to proceed with TEM analysis. Changing the classification criterion of Class 2 to fibers that are greater than 10 μm and less than 1 μm in width is being considered by ASTM.

Early TEM measurements of airborne asbestos such as those used by Nicholson involved the collection of fibers on a membrane filter followed by an indirect-transfer method.[21,22] In the TEM specimen procedure known as the "rubout" method, air samples collected using mixed cellulose ester filters were ashed in a low-temperature plasma asher and the residual ash dispersed in a solution of nitrocellulose. The dispersion was "rubbed out" or spread as uniformly as possible on an optical microscope slide. After the solvent had evaporated, a portion of the film containing the particles from the filter residue was mounted on a TEM grid for examination. The value of asbestos was reported in terms of nanograms per cubic meter of air. The values were determined by summing the masses of the fibers that were calculated from the TEM dimensions of each fiber and an appropriate density for the type of asbestos found.

In 1978, Samudra et al.[23] published the first methodology for determination of the numerical concentration of asbestos fibers in ambient atmospheres using a direct preparation method. The provisional methodology developed under contract for the U.S. EPA recommended air sampling using a 0.4-μm pore size PC filter and preparation of TEM specimen grids by carbon coating followed closely by chloroform extraction to remove the filter polymer. The Samudra methodology was never taken beyond the provisional status.

In the early 1980s, Yamate et al.[24] at the Illinois Institute of Technology Research Institute were asked under contract by EPA to take the methods that were being used by various laboratories and put together a TEM method for airborne asbestos. Their document, which circulated in draft form in 1984, was never officially adopted by EPA. Although it remained in draft form, it became the generally accepted method for TEM analysis of airborne asbestos. As a fiber definition, it used the minimum AR of 3:1 from the NIOSH and OSHA methods but had no minimum fiber length. However, fibers less than 1 mm at the fluorescent screen magnification level were characterized as being 1 μm. At the analysis magnification of ×20,000, the 1-mm size corresponded to 0.5 μm. In addition to asbestos fibers, the method classified asbestos-containing objects as bundles, clusters, and matrices (see Table 2.2 for a comparison of fiber definitions used by several airborne asbestos analysis methods). Yamate et al.[24] also included the concept of levels of analysis because he realized that analytical tools available with the analytical electron microscope provided progressively more specific identification of asbestos fibers depending on the amount of time devoted to the task. The method's levels are known among the TEM asbestos analytical community as Yamate Level 1, Level 2, and Level 3. Level 1, requiring the least amount of identification, was designed for those situations where the airborne particulate was well characterized. If a particular process was known to emit only chrysotile, Level 1 permitted identification on the basis of morphology alone. For Level 2, asbestos identification was determined by morphology and visual diffraction characteristics for chrysotile. For amphiboles, Level 2 included some x-ray elemental information. Asbestos identification in Yamate Level 3 began with the identification steps in Level 2 and added diffraction pattern indexing to more specifically identify the amphibole.

The Yamate method also contained a section for the situation where an air filter was overloaded. The preparation was an indirect procedure where a portion of the filter was ashed and the ash suspended in water. A second filter was prepared with a portion of the suspension and then processed using the same direct procedures described in the main method.

On October 22, 1986, President Reagan signed into law the Asbestos Hazard Emergency Response Act (AHERA).[25] The Act required that EPA describe the methods used to determine completion of response actions such as the abatement of school buildings. Following the deliberations of a panel of asbestos analysis experts, the "Interim TEM Analytical Methods" were published in the Federal Register on October 30, 1987, as Appendix A to Subpart E of the EPA's "Asbestos-containing Materials in Schools; Final Rule and Notice." Following an asbestos abatement and before the protective plastic barriers are removed, leaf blowers and fans are used to aggressively stir the air and resuspend any settled dust while five area air samples are collected. For abatement clearance, the five area air samples collected inside the containment were to be compared with five or more area air samples collected outside the containment. No aggressive disturbance of the air outside the containment was to be done. If there was no statistical difference between the two sets of samples, the abated area was cleared and prepared for reoccupancy. A simplified version of the Yamate draft method was needed to create a rapid method for the clearance of school buildings. The AHERA method maintained many of the method particulars of the Yamate method but

Table 2.2 Comparison of Fiber Definitions Used in Measuring Asbestos in Air

Fiber—NIOSH 7400 (PCM)	Longer than 5 μm with a length to width ratio equal to or greater than 3:1.
Fiber—NIOSH 7402 (TEM)	All particles with a diameter greater than 0.25 μm that meet the definition of a fiber (AR greater than or equal to 3:1, longer than 5 μm).
Fiber—OSHA ID-160 (PCM)	A particle that is 5 μm or longer, with a length to width ratio of 3:1 or longer.
Fiber—Yamate (TEM)	Particle with an AR of 3:1 or greater and with substantially parallel sides.
Fiber—AHERA (TEM)	A structure greater than or equal to 0.5 μm in length with an AR (length to width) of 5:1 or greater and having substantially parallel sides.
Fiber (fiber)—ISO 10312 (TEM)	An elongated particle that has parallel or stepped sides. For the purposes of this international standard, a fiber is defined to have an AR equal to or greater than 5:1 and a minimum length of 0.5 μm.
Bundle—NIOSH 7400 (PCM)	Not defined in method.
Bundle—NIOSH 7402 (TEM)	Not defined in method.
Bundle—OSHA ID-160 (PCM)	Not defined in method.
Bundle—Yamate (TEM)	Paniculate composed of fibers in a parallel arrangement, with each fiber closer than the diameter of one fiber.
Bundle—AHERA (TEM)	A structure composed of three or more fibers in a parallel arrangement with each fiber closer than one fiber diameter.
Bundle—ISO 10312 (TEM)	A structure composed of parallel, smaller diameter fibers attached along their lengths. A fiber bundle may exhibit diverging fibers at one or both ends.
Cluster—NIOSH 7400 (PCM)	Not defined in method.
Cluster—NIOSH 7402 (TEM)	Not defined in method.
Cluster—OSHA ID-160 (PCM)	Not defined in method.
Cluster—Yamate (TEM)	Particulate with fibers in a random arrangement such that all fibers are intermixed and no single fiber is isolated from the group.
Cluster—AHERA (TEM)	A structure with fibers in a random arrangement such that all fibers are intermixed and no single fiber is isolated from the group. Groupings must have more than two intersections.
Cluster—IS010312 (TEM)	A structure in which two or more fibers, or fiber bundles, are randomly oriented in a connected grouping.
Matrix—NIOSH 7400 (PCM)	Not defined in method.
Matrix—NIOSH 7402 (TEM)	Not defined in method.
Matrix—OSHA ID-160 (PCM)	Not defined in method.
Matrix—Yamate (TEM)	Fiber or fibers with one end free and the other end embedded or hidden by a particulate.
Matrix—AHERA (TEM)	Fiber or fibers with one end free and the other end embedded in or hidden by a particulate. The exposed fiber must meet the (AHERA) fiber definition.
Matrix—ISO10312 (TEM)	A structure in which one or more fibers, or fiber bundles, touch, are attached to or partially concealed by a single particle or connected group of nonfibrous particles.

simplified the counting and recording for a rapid clearance procedure. As in the Yamate method, structures were counted. A structure was defined as a microscopic bundle, cluster, fibers, or matrix that may contain asbestos. A matrix was defined as a fiber or fibers with one end free and the other end embedded in or hidden by a particulate. The exposed fiber must meet the fiber definition. Under the AHERA method, an asbestos fiber was defined as a structure greater than or equal to 0.5 μm in length with an AR (length to width) of 5:1 or greater and having substantially parallel sides. Individual dimensions of structures or fibers are not recorded under the AHERA method, but information about the overall structure size is classified as either between 0.5 and 5.0 μm or greater than 5.0 μm. The size data are not used to determine compliance with the AHERA regulations but is included so that if an area does not pass, the project manager might infer something about the source of the contamination. Many large structures found in the air would suggest improper cleaning, whereas small structures could have come from a source external to the cleaning effort. During the deliberations of the expert panel, the question was raised about whether all 10 samples needed to be analyzed if no asbestos structures were found on the five inside-the-containment samples. On the basis of experience of some of the panel in finding occasional asbestos fibers on blank (unused) PC filters, it was decided that a sample was clearly above the blank filter level if it had a filter loading greater than 70 structures per millimeter square (str/mm^2). In the real-world abatement industry, the 70 str/mm^2 became the generally recognized clearance level, and contractors were and still are normally instructed to reclean if the average of the five inside samples exceeded that value. Only rarely today is the comparison made of the five inside and five outside samples. Those few cases are usually where a contractor believes that asbestos contamination outside the containment area is contributing to the air within the abatement area.

2.7 SCANNING ELECTRON MICROSCOPY

In 1987 when the AHERA method mandated the use of TEM, the scanning electron microscope was determined to be inadequate for building clearance (Figure 2.9). The reasons given in the AHERA document were as follows: (1) currently available methodologies were not validated for the analysis of asbestos fibers, (2) SEM was limited in its ability to identify the crystalline structure of a particular fiber, (3) the National Bureau of Standards found that the image contrast of the microscopes was difficult to standardize between individual scanning electron microscopes, and (4) no current laboratory accreditation program existed for accrediting SEM laboratories.[25] NBS had determined that the only SEM method recognized at that time, the Asbestos International Association protocol,[26] had inherent difficulty when examining certain types of asbestos. As of 2009, there are still no laboratory accreditation programs for SEM laboratories. In the United States, no standard SEM method is in use for asbestos, although it is mentioned in the OSHA ID-160 method. However, there is interest internationally, and the ISO 14966 method for SEM analysis of inorganic fibrous particles that includes asbestos (Figure 2.10), ceramic fibers, and glass fibers in air was approved in 2002.[27]

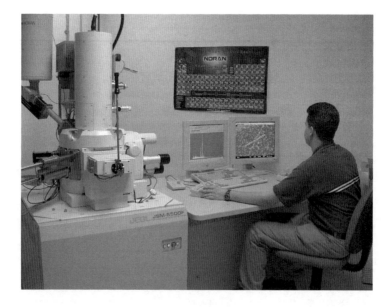

Figure 2.9 Analyst using an SEM for asbestos analysis.

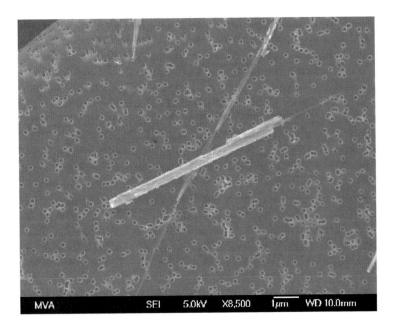

Figure 2.10 Image of crocidolite and chrysotile asbestos fibers as seen with an SEM. Same fibers as shown in Figure 2.6.

2.8 TEM BEYOND AHERA

In 1987 when the AHERA method was published in the Federal Register as an interim method, it contained a provision that the method would be updated by the National Institute of Standards and Technology (NIST). As of 2009, no updated version of the method has been published by NIST or any other federal agency. The AHERA method became the generally accepted TEM method for the analysis of asbestos in air. However, its lack of specific size data for individual asbestos structures was considered a deficiency for some situations. A Yamate Level 2 analysis was requested on occasions when information about fiber size was needed. In March 1988, the CARB issued Method 427 for the determination of paniculate asbestos emissions from stationary sources using stack sampling, light microscopy, and electron microscopy.[28] Although the NIOSH 7400 PCM method may be used with the CARB 427 method, it is evident that the TEM portion is the focus of the method. Recording of fiber size data is done on the basis of the Yamate method.

A more complete TEM airborne asbestos analysis procedure developed largely by Dr. Chatfield of Chatfield Technical Consulting was released in 1995 by the ISO.[29] The International Standard 10312 contains counting rules which expand on the Yamate and AHERA concept of asbestos structures. Clusters and matrices are subdivided into dispersed and compact structures. A dispersed cluster contains asbestos fibers that can be measured and reported separately, whereas a compact cluster has fibers too intertwined to be reported individually. In this method, cluster and matrix components are identified, measured, and recorded separately up to a maximum of nine substructures. The ISO 10312 was followed in 1998 by the ASTM Standard Test Method D6281-98, which was a translation of the ISO 10312 method into ASTM format with a few improvements and changes.[30] The ASTM Method D6281 was reapproved in 2002 as D6281-02. For samples that contain any appreciable amount of asbestos, analysis by either ISO 10312 or ASTM D6281 is considerably more time consuming than an AHERA analysis and therefore more expensive. The data produced by ISO 10312/ASTM D6281 were designed to allow another analyst to review the data of the original analyst and understand how the asbestos structures were present on the filter grid. The method of data recording was designed to allow reevaluation of the counting data as new medical evidence or regulatory requirements become available. From the results of an ISO 10312 (or ASTM D6281) analysis, it should be possible to determine several different airborne asbestos structure concentration values on the basis of a number of fiber size classifications. For instance, it should be possible to extract what a structure per cubic centimeter concentration would have been if the sample had been analyzed by AHERA counting rules. Some precision data have been determined for the ASTM D6281 method (also applicable to ISO 10312). The ASTM interlaboratory studies found relative standard deviations of 0.1 for amphibole fibers (amosite) and 0.5 for chrysotile fibers.

Both ISO 10312 and ASTM D6281 have an annex, which describes procedures for the determination of concentrations of asbestos fibers and bundles longer than 5 μm and of PCM-equivalent (PCME) asbestos fibers. For improved analytical sensitivity and statistical precision, the larger fiber counts are done at lower magnifications so more area of the filter may be examined. The U.S. EPA has set a risk-based cleanup benchmark for asbestos in air for their World Trade Center (WTC) Test and Clean Program. The EPA risk-based benchmark for PCME asbestos fibers analyzed by TEM (ISO 10312 or ASTM D6281) is 0.0009 s/cc.[31] A comparison of four common asbestos methods for the analysis of air samples is shown in Table 2.3.

In 1999, ISO 13794 (indirect air) was published.[32] The asbestos structure and the fiber counting procedures in this method are the same as those presented in ISO 10312 and ASTM D6281. ISO 13794 provides an indirect-transfer procedure so overloaded filters can be analyzed. The filter preparation methods described in both ISO 10312 and ASTM D6281 are direct-transfer procedures. In steps similar to the Yamate indirect preparation procedure, a portion of the original filter is ashed and the ash suspended in water. A second filter is prepared with a known portion of the suspension and then processed using the same direct procedures described in ISO 10312 and ASTM D6281. Although the method states "This International Standard is applicable to measurement of airborne asbestos in a wide range of ambient air situations, including the interior atmospheres of buildings, and for detailed evaluation of any atmosphere in which asbestos fibers are likely to be present," the user is cautioned that comparison of results using this indirect-transfer procedure with those from a direct-transfer procedure may not be done *a priori*.[32] The best study of the differences between direct and indirect air sample preparation remains the study by Chesson and Hatfield.[33] Their findings supported the generally accepted opinion that TEM analysis of air samples using indirect-transfer methods provides estimates of the total airborne asbestos structure concentration that are higher than those using direct-transfer methods. They concluded that no single factor can be used to convert measurements made by one method to a value that is comparable with measurements made by the other. They also concluded that the breakdown of larger structures into smaller ones

Table 2.3 Comparison of Common Methods for Measuring Asbestos in Air

	NIOSH 7400	NIOSH 7402	AHERA	ISO
Instrument	PCM	TEM	TEM	TEM
Filter preparation	Direct	Direct	Direct	Direct: 10312; Indirect: 13794
Magnification	×450	×10,000	~×20,000	~×20,000
Fiber length	$L > 5$ μm	$L > 5$ μm	$L > 0.5$ μm	$L > 0.5$ μm
Fiber diameter	$W > 0.25$ μm	$W > 0.25$ μm	$W > 0.002$ μm	$W > 0.002$ μm; PCME: $L > 5$ μm, $W > 0.25$ μm
AR	>3:1	>3:1	>5:1	>5:1 or 3:1
Counting	Fibers	Fibers	Structures	Structures and fibers
Identification	None	Morphology, crystal structure, elements	Morphology, crystal structure, elements	Morphology, crystal structure, elements
Reporting	Fibers/cm³	% asbestos	All asbestos str/cm³ and >5 μm structures	All asbestos str/cm³ and >5 μm fibers and PCME fibers/cm³

during indirect preparation does not appear to be sufficient to explain the difference in measured concentrations. Interference by debris and association of unattached structures may also be important. They recommended additional research was needed to determine which transfer method more accurately reflects biologically meaningful airborne asbestos concentrations.

2.9 WATER ANALYSIS

There are three standard methods available for the analysis of drinking water for asbestos: the EPA 100.1, the EPA 100.2, and the AWWA 2570.[34–36] These methods are all TEM methods and are compared in Table 2.4.[37] The EPA has set a maximum contaminant level of seven million fibers longer than 10 μm/L of drinking water and has listed both the 100.1 and 100.2 methods as acceptable for the analysis of water-borne asbestos. The EPA 100.1 method is a research report produced in 1984 before the EPA drinking water regulations and describes counting procedures that include asbestos fibers longer than 0.5 μm. The EPA 100.2 describes counting only those fibers longer than 10 μm. Guidance as to the modifications of EPA 100.1 necessary to comply with the EPA drinking water regulations was published by Feige et al.[38] Some precision data for the water method were described in EPA 100.1. An interlaboratory comparison study with six laboratories found relative standard deviations for amphibole fibers (crocidolite) of 25% and for chrysotile fibers of 29%.[34] The ELAP Certification Manual Item 198.2 describes a modification to Method 100.2 required for New York State Department of Health compliance.[39] In the modification, the ozone generator is considered optional *only* if all samples are filtered within 48 h.

2.10 SURFACE DUST ANALYSIS

In 1989, the ASTM subcommittee D22.07 began work on methods for the analysis of asbestos in settled dust.[40] Three ASTM methods are currently available for the analysis of surface dust for asbestos. These methods include two microvacuum methods: ASTM D5755-02 (structure count) and D5756-02 (mass) and one wipe method, ASTM D6480-99.[41–43] An EPA carpet method, EPA/600/J-93/167, was developed during a research study that was published as an article in 1993.[44] The EPA number was assigned in 2001. The three ASTM methods are nondestructive, whereas the carpet method requires that a piece be cut from the carpet and sent to the laboratory. Some precision data have been determined for the ASTM D5755 method. The ASTM interlaboratory study found a relative standard deviation of 0.5 for samples of WTC dust containing chrysotile fibers. A comparison of the four surface (settled) dust methods is shown in Table 2.5.

Table 2.4   Comparison of Common Methods of Measuring Asbestos in Water

	EPA 100.1	EPA 100.2	AWWA 2570
Instrument	TEM	TEM	TEM
Filter preparation	Indirect PC	Indirect (PC and MCE)	Indirect (PC and MCE)
Magnification	~×20,000	~×20,000	~×20,000
Fiber length	$L > 0.5$ μm	$L > 10$ μm	$L > 0.5$ μm
Fiber diameter	$W > 0.002$ μm	$W > 0.002$ μm	$W > 0.002$ μm
AR	>5:1	>5:1	>5:1
Counting	Fibers	Fibers	Fibers
Identification	Morphology, crystal structure, elements	Morphology, crystal structure, elements	Morphology, crystal structure, elements
Reporting	Millions of asbestos fibers per liter (MFL)	MFL > 10 μm	MFL

Table 2.5   Comparison of Common Methods for Measuring Asbestos in Surface Dust

	ASTM D5755-02	ASTM D5756-02	ASTM D6480-99	EPA/600/J-93/167
Instrument	TEM	TEM	TEM	TEM
Sample preparation	Microvacuum (indirect)	Microvacuum (indirect)	Wipe (indirect)	Piece of carpet (indirect)
Magnification	~×20,000	~×20,000	~×20,000	~×20,000
Fiber length	$L > 0.5\ \mu m$	$L > 0.5\ \mu m$	$L > 0.5\ \mu m$	$L > 0.5\ \mu m$
Fiber diameter	$W > 0.002\ \mu m$	$W > 0.002\ \mu m$	$W > 0.002\ \mu m$	$W > 0.002\ \mu m$
AR	>5:1	>5:1	>5:1	>5:1
Counting	Asbestos structures	Asbestos structures	Asbestos structures	Asbestos structures
Identification	Morphology, crystal structure, elements	Morphology, crystal structure, elements	Morphology, crystal structure, elements	Morphology, crystal structure, elements
Reporting	Asbestos s/cm²	Asbestos μg/cm²	Asbestos s/cm²	Asbestos s/cm² of carpet

Because dust particles can be arranged in layers more than one particle thick, direct preparation techniques are of limited value for TEM because the electron beam must be able to penetrate the sample. Indirect preparation procedures are used for all four methods. The results of the analysis are expressed in numbers or mass of asbestos structures per square centimeter of surface sampled. The number count methods were originally designed with an analytical sensitivity of approximately 1000 str/cm² but can achieve much better sensitivities on clean surfaces. A nominal analytical sensitivity for the mass determination is 0.24 pg of asbestos/cm². There is some disagreement on how to interpret the surface dust asbestos data.[45–53] The U.S. EPA has set risk-based cleanup benchmarks for asbestos in settled dust for their WTC Test and Clean Program. The EPA risk-based benchmarks for asbestos analyzed according to the ASTM D5755 method (microvacuum count) are 5000 s/cm² for accessible areas (e.g., floors) and 50,000 s/cm² for infrequently accessed areas (e.g., behind a bookshelf). At EPA's Libby, Montana site, an action level of 5000 s/cm² in generally accessible areas has been established for triggering cleanup in a residential dwelling.

Because the amount and the type of surface dust collected by each method differ, it is clear that results of one settled dust method cannot be necessarily compared directly with data from another. For instance, the bulk carpet method, EPA/600/J-93/167, is an analysis of the total amount of dust in a carpet. Because carpets are known to be excellent traps for dust and dirt, the amount of asbestos in the carpet may be considerably higher than that collected from the surface of the same carpet using the D5755 microvacuum method. It is not appropriate to compare bulk carpet values with results of the D5755 method or with the EPA risk-based cleanup benchmarks, although both are given in terms of structures per square centimeter. In one set of tests, the EPA/600/J-93/167 results were found to be approximately 100 times higher than that of the D5755 type analysis because the bulk carpet method involves all dirt trapped in the carpet and the microvacuum method only analyzed the top, readily releasable dust.[44] Asbestos in dust deep in the carpet may not be releasable under normal activities and may only be of concern when the carpet is being removed. Asbestos fibers that are in a sticky film on a surface and therefore not readily releasable are collected by the D6480 wipe method. The wipe method gives an index of all asbestos fibers on a surface regardless of how stuck they are, whereas the microvacuum method gives an index of the readily releasable fibers.

2.11 SOIL ANALYSIS

Soil is a difficult medium for the analysis of asbestos because soil minerals are not easily separated from the asbestos fibers. In a method used by the U.S. EPA Region 1, sieving is used to enhance the ability to find asbestos fibers that are then identified using essentially the standard PLM bulk analysis procedure.[54] The Australian Standard Bulk Method for the qualitative identification of asbestos in bulk samples has a section specifically for soil samples.[55] The entire sample is screened through a 10-mm (1 cm) sieve. The less than 10-mm fraction is then sieved through a 2-mm sieve. The less than 2-mm fraction is spread to a thickness of no more than 1 to 3 mm. Using a combination of low- and high-power stereomicroscopy, all fractions are examined for fibers that are then identified by PLM with dispersion staining. The fibrous particles that are found are weighed, or the length and widths of each fiber bundle are estimated. The method describes a reporting limit of 0.1 g/kg or 0.01%.

The chrysotile flotation method described by Falini et al.[56] in 2003 appeared to be a method that could separate asbestos from soil without drastically changing the fiber size distribution. However, studies of the Falini et al.[56] method concluded that the chrysotile flotation method does not provide an effective and efficient way to completely and cleanly separate asbestos with a range of fiber sizes from soils. Although the method may be gentle enough to maintain the integrity of the asbestos fibers (i.e., without fiber length reduction), the processing lost the longer and thicker fibers, thus not maintaining the integrity of the fiber size distribution. In the CARB 435 method, "Determination of Asbestos Content of Serpentine Aggregate," the sample aggregates are crushed to produce a material with a nominal size of less than three-eighths of an inch.[57] The samples are further crushed using a Braun mill or equivalent to produce a material of which the majority shall be less than 200 Tyler mesh (76-μm diameter). Asbestos identification is done by PLM and the determination of the amount of asbestos is done using a 400-point count. Crushing of the samples is necessary because all particles must fit under the coverslip on the microscope slide and be of a uniform size for point counting. The lower detection limit is described as 0.25% (1 asbestos fiber/400 nonempty points). However, there is considerable statistical uncertainty in this value.[12]

Currently, soil methods designed around both grinding and sieving are under consideration. It is thought that crushing or grinding the soil sample will produce a more homogeneous mixture, which should improve the precision of the analysis. However, interlaboratory comparison studies done among West Coast laboratories have shown that the type of crusher and other factors need more investigation to achieve the level of precision needed. Although the sieving approach is thought to be more difficult in terms of achieving good quantitative results than the grinding approach, it should provide information about the fiber sizes, which is lost during a repertory grinding step. A soil method that uses sieving, PLM, and TEM is currently under development by the ASTM Subcommittee D22.07.

A more complicated procedure, which looks at airborne asbestos fibers that might be released from soil, is called the Superfund method.[58,59] The soil sample is placed in a rotating drum, and air samples are collected in a vertical elutriator. The samples are analyzed by TEM according to procedures on the basis of the ISO 10312 method. The counting procedure may be modified to count "protocol" fibers. Protocol fibers are asbestos fibers with certain length and width characteristics as determined by studies in biological systems. At one point in time, fibers longer than 40 μm were thought to be of greatest interest, and the method was modified to count more grid openings at a lower magnification for better counting statistics. A comparison of the two soil methods is shown in Table 2.6.

Table 2.6   Comparison of Common Methods for Measuring Asbestos in Soil

	EPA Superfund	EPA Region 1 CARB 435
Instrument	TEM	PLM
Sample preparation	Elutriator	Sieving crushing
Magnification	~×20,000	×10–1000
Fiber length; diameter	$L > 0.5$ μm; $W > 0.002$ μm	$W > {\sim}1$ μm
AR	>5:1	>3:1
Counting	Structures	Areal % point count
Identification	~ISO 10312	Optical
Reporting	Various	% asbestos

2.12 VERMICULITE ANALYSIS

Vermiculite is also a special case for bulk asbestos analysis. Sometimes referred to as "The Cincinnati Method," the EPA research method for the sampling and analysis of fibrous amphibole in vermiculite attic insulation uses a flotation step to separate the vermiculite from the more dense amphiboles.[60] The fibrous amphiboles found in Libby, Montana, vermiculite can be hand picked from the "sinks" using a stereomicroscope and weighed to get a direct weight percent estimate. The method includes a TEM portion for the analysis of amphibole fibers that might be present in the "suspended particle" fraction of the water used in the flotation step. Criteria for examination of the TEM specimens are specified in ISO 10312 or ISO 13794. Early in 2004, EPA held a day and a half workshop for a panel of experts to meet and propose a method to determine whether Libby amphibole is present in a sample of vermiculite attic insulation. The objective of the method is to be accurate with respect to identifying Libby amphibole, to be affordable to the average homeowner, and to be adaptable to most current commercial fiber analysis laboratories. This more routine vermiculite method, on the basis of the Cincinnati research method, was expected to be released in late 2004. The routine method is still currently under development.

2.13 METHODS FOR ASBESTOS ANALYSIS IN OTHER MEDIA

In addition to media such as air, water, soil, and dust, methods for analyzing asbestos in clothing, talc, and biological specimens have appeared in the scientific literature.[61–64] Only a few of the many scientific papers that contain descriptions of asbestos analysis methods are referenced here. Sample preparation procedures are generally different for each type of sample matrix, but the type of microscopy to be used and the counting rules are usually borrowed from one of the standard methods described earlier.

2.14 ASBESTOS DEFINITIONS AND TERMINOLOGY

The definition of a "Federal Asbestos Fiber" depends on the federal agency involved. The OSHA uses a definition of a fiber that is at least 5 μm long with an AR (length to width) of 3:1. The EPA uses a definition of a fiber that is at least 0.5 μm long with a 5:1 AR. The ISO and the ASTM TEM methods use a definition of a fiber that is 0.5 μm long with a 5:1 AR definition in their main procedure and provide an annex, which describes counting fibers greater than 5 μm long with an AR of 3:1. Other ARs such as 10:1 and 20:1 have been suggested for defining an asbestos fiber but have not been adopted.

From the microscopic analyst's point of view, an asbestos fiber is defined by the counting method being used. Under the AHERA counting rules, a fiber is a structure having a minimum length greater than 0.5 μm and an AR (length to width) of 5:1 or greater and substantially parallel sides. The appearance of the end of the fiber, that is, whether it is flat, rounded, or dovetailed, is to be noted. However, AHERA does not use information about fiber ends, nor does it say whether to record this information. Under Section 3.22 of the ISO 10312 counting rules (and a similar section in ASTM D6281), a fiber is defined as an elongated particle that has parallel or stepped sides.

Individual chrysotile fibers, called fibrils, are too thin to be seen by the light microscope during the PCM analysis by NIOSH 7400. The fibers of chrysotile that are seen in the light microscope are actually bundles of fibrils. During the analysis by TEM using the NIOSH 7402 method that considers only elongated particles longer than 5 μm in length and greater than 0.25 μm in width with a 3:1 AR, the chrysotile "fibers" are more correctly listed as bundles. As stated in the ISO 10312 method: "For chrysotile, PCME fibers will always be bundles."[29] During the analysis by TEM using the AHERA method, chrysotile fibrils are listed as fibers. These AHERA chrysotile "fibers" (actually fibrils less than 0.05 μm in diameter) are not visible with the light microscope. Similar terminology is used in the water and dust methods. With the exception of the NIOSH 7402 method, all TEM chrysotile fibers are actually fibrils and not visible with the light microscope.

2.15 PCM EQUIVALENCY

The U.S. NIOSH 7400 standard method uses PCM and involves counting only those fibers that can be seen with the light microscope (thicker than 0.25 μm) and longer than 5 μm. The TEM companion method NIOSH 7402 considers the same fiber characteristics as the 7400 method, but because the TEM can resolve thin asbestos fibers, 7402 analysis is restricted to fibers greater than 0.25 μm. The TEM fibers analyzed under NIOSH 7402 are then PCME fibers. However, the NIOSH 7402 method is not established to provide concentrations of asbestos fibers. The determination and reportable value from 7402 is a percentage of asbestos fibers of all fibers in the PCME range in the sample. This percentage can thereby be applied to 7400 values to determine asbestos fiber concentrations in fibers per cubic centimeter. Other TEM methods (primarily ISO 10312 and occasionally AHERA) have been used to determine PCME concentrations. It is important when interpreting the data to understand the differences in counting rules between methods. Appendix B of Method NIOSH 7400 contains a description of the asbestos fiber counting rules (referred to as "A" rules) as they apply to labeled objects in Figure 2.2 of the 7400 method. For Object 2 in Figure 2.2, the method states: "Although the object has a relatively large diameter (>3 μm), it is counted as a fiber under the rules. There is no upper limit on the fiber diameter in the counting rules." The ISO 10312 method defines a PCME fiber as "any particle with parallel or stepped sides, with an AR of 3:1 or greater, longer than 5 μm and which has a diameter between 0.2 and 3.0 μm." Using the ISO 10312 method for PCME counting will, therefore, not provide a count of PCM fibers equivalent to the NIOSH 7400 method, unless it is modified so that fibers of all diameters are included.

More serious cautions are appropriate for the attempt to use AHERA counts to estimate PCME concentrations. It is important to realize that the NIOSH 7400 method includes fibers associated with other particles. For Object 6 in Figure 2.2, the NIOSH 7400 method states: "A fiber partially obscured by a particle is counted as one fiber. If the fiber ends emanating from a particle do not seem to be from the same fiber and each end meets the length and AR criteria, they are counted as separate fibers." The AHERA method counts all asbestos objects as structures. Objects that contain one or more fibers partially obscured by a particle are counted as matrices. Under the NIOSH PCM method, several fibers meeting the length and AR criteria, which are overlapping but do not seem to be part of the same bundle, would be counted as separate fibers. Under the AHERA TEM method, these would all be counted as one cluster. If an analyst tries to use the AHERA data to estimate a PCME fiber count and chooses only those structures identified as bundles greater than 5 μm, they will miss PCME fibers that are parts of matrices or clusters. Because AHERA uses a 5:1 AR while the PCM method uses a 3:1 ratio, an AHERA count would not have included fibers more than 5 μm with only a 3:1 AR. Considering the differences in the two methods, it is not appropriate to attempt to estimate PCME fiber concentrations from AHERA data. However, an AHERA analysis in which no asbestos structures are found is considered to be consistent with no PCME fibers detected. It would be a most unusual sample to have no AHERA countable asbestos structures but still have some large fibers with ARs between 3:1 and 5:1.

2.16 CLEAVAGE FRAGMENTS

Most asbestos methods dictate the counting of the asbestos forms of six minerals: one serpentine type (chrysotile) and five amphiboles (amosite, anthophyllite, actinolite, crocidolite, and tremolite).

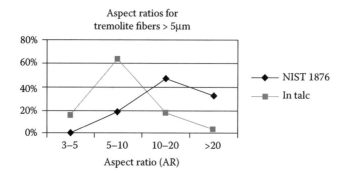

Figure 2.11   Comparison of ARs for tremolite fibers from the Standard Reference Material 1876, tremolite asbestos, and tremolite from a talc sample.

Elongated particles with ARs greater than 3:1 or 5:1 that did not come from a population of asbestos fibers are sometimes called cleavage fragments. The distinction of how to tell an asbestos fiber from a cleavage fragment is currently being debated within the scientific community. A population of fibers as observed in a bulk sample having the asbestiform habit is generally recognized by several characteristics.[5] These include mean ARs in the range from 20:1 to 100:1 or higher for fibers longer than 5 μm. Asbestos is characterized by very thin fibrils, usually less than 0.5 μm in width, and two or more of the following:

- Parallel fibers occurring in bundles
- Fiber bundles displaying splayed ends
- Matted masses of individual fibers
- Fibers showing curvature

It is more difficult to classify individual fibers as to asbestiform or cleavage fragments because individual fibers do not exhibit all the characteristics of a population. With the exception of the requirements given in the TEM standard methods that the asbestos fibers have substantially parallel or stepped sides, there is little specific information for the analyst in the way of asbestos or cleavage fragment differentiation. Research has shown that a population of cleavage fragment particles has a smaller mean AR than a population of commercial asbestos fibers. However, the AR distributions of the two populations can overlap and, on an individual basis, some fibers could be classified either way. In Figure 2.11, the ARs of tremolite fibers found in a talc sample are compared with the ARs determined from the NIST standard reference tremolite asbestos sample SMR 1876. The population of tremolite fibers in talc is considered to be nonasbestiform because the mean AR is less than 20:1. However, some individual tremolite fibers in talc like the one shown in Figure 2.12 would be counted as an asbestos fiber under standard methods if found by itself. There is particular difficulty in using bulk characteristics of amphibole asbestos fibers found in air samples. Air sample filters produced from standard reference amosite asbestos fibers contain many fibers but very few parallel fibers occurring in bundles, fiber bundles displaying splayed ends, matted masses of individual fibers, or fibers showing curvature.

2.17 AMPHIBOLES

For most standard asbestos methods, "asbestos" means chrysotile and the asbestiform varieties of the five amphiboles: crocidolite (riebeckite), amosite (cummingtonite–grunerite), anthophyllite, tremolite, and actinolite. The ISO 10312 method is more open-ended in its definition of asbestos

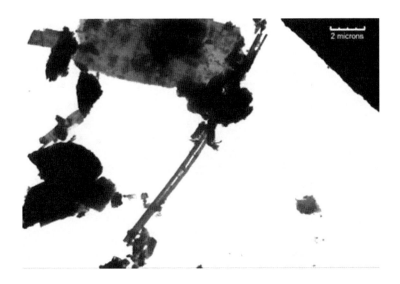

Figure 2.12   TEM image of a tremolite fiber found in a talc sample.

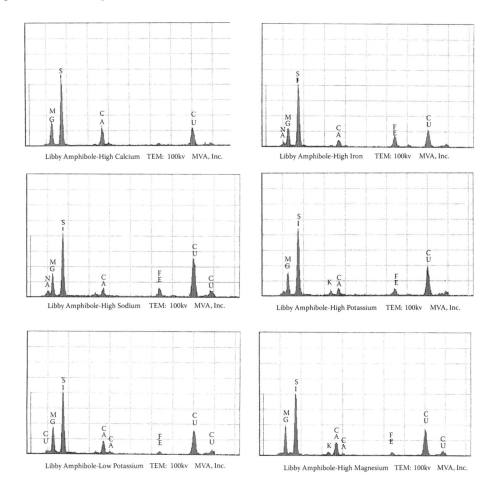

Figure 2.13   EDS x-ray spectra for Libby amphiboles.

with the statement "the most common asbestos varieties are:" (the varieties listed on page 42). Other amphiboles can also exhibit asbestiform habits. The difference between nonregulated asbestiform amphiboles and those that are regulated is the amount of elemental substitution that occurred when the mineral was formed in the earth. The different amphibole names as defined by different elemental compositions are described in Leake et al.[65] Among the amphiboles present in vermiculite from Libby, Montana are tremolite, richterite, and winchite.[66–69] The specific mineralogical determinations were made after extensive mineralogical studies. Distinguishing between tremolite, richterite, and winchite by PLM is difficult because the minerals have very similar optical properties. Figure 2.8 shows the elemental spectra produced by NIST reference asbestos materials using TEM–EDS methodology. As seen in Figure 2.13, the elemental spectra from several Libby amphibole fibers are similar to tremolite or actinolite reference materials but differ in small amounts of sodium and potassium.

The association of amphibole fibers with some chrysotile ores was reported by Addison and Davies.[70] Ilgren and Chatfield[71] reported finding tremolite in the ore from the Jeffrey Mine in Quebec, Canada. Williams-Jones et al.[72] reported that the bulk of the amphibole in the Jeffery Mine in Quebec, Canada was in the form of tremolite and actinolite.

The quantitative analysis for low levels of amphibole fibers in chrysotile or chrysotile-containing products requires that the sample be prepared in a way that eliminates the chrysotile and concentrates the amphibole fibers so they may be detected. This is done first with an ashing at 600°C to aid digestion by opening the chrysotile fibers and to eliminate any organic material such as cellulose fibers. The ashing is followed by an acid digestion step, which is followed by a base digestion step. The residue can then be analyzed by x-ray diffraction or TEM. Using this analysis, low levels (less than 1%) of tremolite and/or actinolite have been found in a number of chrysotile-containing products including, sheet gaskets, packing, brakes, and dryer felt.

ACKNOWLEDGMENTS

The author thanks Bryan Bandli, Randy Boltin, Pronda Few, Al Harmon, Whitney Hill, Bill Turner, Beth Wortman, and Catherine Debban for their help in providing figures and editing assistance for this chapter.

REFERENCES

1. McCrone WC. *The Asbestos Particle Atlas.* Ann Arbor (MI): Ann Arbor Science Publishers Inc; 1980. p. 21.
2. McCrone WC. *Asbestos Identification.* Chicago (IL): McCrone Research Institute; 1987.
3. Asbestos Hazard Emergency Response Act. *Fed Regist* 1987;52(210):41845.
4. National Emission Standards for Hazardous Air Pollutants. Asbestos NESHAP revision, final rule. *Fed Regist* 1990;55(224):48405.
5. U.S. Environmental Protection Agency. Method for the determination of asbestos in bulk building materials. EPA-600/R-93/116. Washington (DC): U.S. Environmental Protection Agency; July 1993.
6. U.S. Environmental Protection Agency. Test method: interim method for the determination of asbestos in bulk insulation samples. EPA-600/M4-82-020. Washington (DC): U.S. Environmental Protection Agency; December 1982.
7. National Institute of Occupational Safety and Health, NIOSH 9002. Asbestos (bulk) by polarized light microscopy (PLM)—Method 9002, Issue 2. *NIOSH Manual of Analytical Methods.* 4th ed. Washington (DC): U.S. Department of Health & Human Services; 1994. p. 94.
8. National Institute of Occupational Safety and Health, OSHA ID-191. Polarized light microscopy of asbestos—non-mandatory 1915.1001 App K, Occupational Safety and Health Standards for Shipyard Employment, Subpart Z: toxic and hazardous substances. *Fed Regist* 1994;59(113):40964.

9. Perkins RL. Point-counting technique for friable asbestos-containing materials. *Microscope* 1990;38:29–39.

10. New York State Department of Health, ELAP Item 198.1. Polarized-light microscope methods for identifying and quantitating asbestos in bulk samples. New York State Department of Health Environmental Laboratory Approval Program Certification Manual. Albany (NY): New York State Department of Health; 2003.

11. Webber JS, Janulis RJ, Carhart LJ, Gillespie MD. Quantitating asbestos content in friable bulk samples: Development of a stratified point-count method. *Am Ind Hyg Assoc J* 1990;51(8):447–52.

12. Chatfield EJ. A validated method for gravimetric determination of low concentrations of asbestos in bulk materials. In: Beard ME, Rook HL, editors. *Advances in Environmental Measurement Methods for Asbestos*. ASTM STP 1342. West Conshohocken (PA): American Society for Testing and Materials; 2000. p. 90–110.

13. New York State Department of Health, ELAP Item 198.4. Transmission electron microscope method for identifying and quantitating asbestos in non-friable organically bound samples. New York State Department of Health Environmental Laboratory Approval Program Certification Manual. Albany (NY): New York State Department of Health; 1997.

14. National Institute of Occupational Safety and Health, NIOSH 7400. Asbestos and other fibers by phase contrast microscopy (PCM)—Method 7400. *NIOSH Manual of Analytical Methods*. 4th ed. Washington (DC): U.S. Department of Health & Human Services; 1994 [NIOSH Publication no. 94-113].

15. Crane D. Occupational Safety and Health Administration, OSHA ID-160. Asbestos in air; United States Department of Labor, US Government Printing Office, Washington, DC; July 1997.

16. U.S. Department of Labor. Occupational Safety and Health Standards, Asbestos Standard. 29 CFR, 1910.1001(c)(1). *Congressional Federal Register*, US Government Printing Office, Washington, DC.

17. U.S. Department of Labor. Occupational Safety and Health Standards, Asbestos Standard. 29 CFR, 1910.1001(c)(2). *Congressional Federal Register*, US Government Printing Office, Washington, DC.

18. National Institute of Occupational Safety and Health, NIOSH 7402. Asbestos fibers by transmission electron microscopy (TEM)—Method 7402, *NIOSH Manual of Analytical Methods*. 4th ed. Washington (DC): U.S. Department of Health & Human Services; 1994 [NIOSH Publication 94-126].

19. American Society for Testing and Materials. Standard practice for sampling and counting airborne fibers, including asbestos fibers, in mines and quarries, by phase contrast microscopy and transmission electron microscopy. ASTM D7200. West Conshohocken (PA): American Society for Testing and Materials; 2006.

20. Harper M, Lee EG, Doorn SS, Hammond O. Differentiating non-asbestos amphibole and amphibole asbestos by size characteristics. *J Occup Environ Hyg* 2008;5:761–70.

21. Nicholson WJ, Rohl AN, Ferrand EF. Asbestos air pollution in New York City. In: *Proceedings of the Second International Clean Air Congress, Washington, DC, December 1970*. New York: Academic Press; 1971. p. 136–139.

22. U.S. Environmental Protection Agency. Asbestos contamination of the air in public buildings. EPA-450/3-76-004. Research Triangle Park (NC): U.S. Environmental Protection Agency; 1975.

23. Samudra A, Harwood CF, Stockham JD. Electron microscope measurement of airborne asbestos concentration: A provisional methodology manual. EPA 600/2-77-178. Washington (DC): Office of Research and Development; 1978.

24. Yamate G, Agarwall SC, Gibbons RD. Methodology for the measurement of airborne asbestos by electron microscopy. EPA Draft Report Contract no. 68-02-3266. Washington (DC): Office of Research and Development; 1984.

25. Asbestos Hazard Emergency Response Act. Appendix A to Subpart E—Interim transmission electron microscopy analytical methods. U.S. EPA, 40 CFR Part 763. Asbestos-containing materials in schools, final rule and notice. *Fed Regist* 1987;52(210):41857–94.

26. Asbestos International Association. Method for the determination of airborne asbestos fiber and other inorganic fibers by scanning electron microscopy. AIA Health and Safety Publication, Recommended Technical Method 2 (RTM2). London, UK: Asbestos International Association; 1982.

27. International Standards Organization, ISO 14966. Ambient air: determination of numerical concentration of inorganic fibrous particles—Scanning electron microscopy method. Geneva, Switzerland: International Standards Organization; 2002.

28. California Air Resources Board, CARB 427. Determination of asbestos emissions from stationary sources, Method 427. Sacramento, CA: California Air Resources Board; March, 23, 1988.

29. International Standards Organization, ISO 10312. Ambient air: determination of asbestos fibers—Direct-transfer transmission electron microscopy procedure. Geneva, Switzerland: International Standards Organization; 1995.

30. American Society for Testing and Materials. Standard test method for airborne asbestos concentration in ambient and indoor atmospheres as determined by transmission electron microscopy direct transfer. ASTM D6281-04. West Conshohocken (PA): American Society for Testing and Materials; 2004.

31. U.S. Environmental Protection Agency. World Trade Center Indoor Dust Test and Clean Program Plan, final version. New York, NY: U.S. Environmental Protection Agency Region 2; November 2005.

32. International Standards Organization, ISO 13794. Ambient air: determination of asbestos fibers—Indirect transmission electron microscopy method. Geneva, Switzerland: International Standards Organization; 1999.

33. Chesson J, Hatfield J. Comparison of airborne asbestos levels determined by transmission electron microscopy using direct and indirect transfer techniques. EPA 560/5-89-004. Washington, DC: U.S. Environmental Protection Agency; 1990.

34. Chatfield EJ, Dillon MJ. U.S. Environmental Protection Agency, EPA Method 100.1. Analytical method for the determination of asbestos fibers in water. EPA 600/4-84-043. Washington, DC: U.S. Environmental Protection Agency; 1984.

35. Brackett KA, Clark PJ, Millette JR. U.S. Environmental Protection Agency, Method 100.2. Determination of asbestos structures over 10 µm in length in drinking water. EPA/600/R-94/134. Washington, DC: U.S. Environmental Protection Agency; 1994.

36. American Water Works Association. Asbestos. In: *Standard Methods for the Examination of Water and Wastewater*. American Public Health Association. Washington, DC. 18th ed., Section 2570; 1994, p. 10–15.

37. Millette JR, Few P, Krewer JA. Asbestos in water methods: EPA's 100.1 and 100.2 and AWWA's Standard Method 2570. In: Beard ME, Rook HL, editors. *Advances in Environmental Measurement Methods for Asbestos*. ASTM STP 1342. West Conshohocken (PA): American Society for Testing and Materials; 2000, p. 227–241.

38. Feige MA, Clark PJ, Brackett KA. Guidance and clarification for the current U.S. EPA test method for asbestos in drinking water. *Environ Choices Tech Suppl* 1993:13–4.

39. New York State Department of Health. Revision to waterborne asbestos analysis. ELAP Item 198.2. New York State Department of Health Environmental Laboratory Approval Program Certification Manual. Albany, NY: New York State Department of Health; 1997.

40. Beard ME, Millette JR, Webber JS. Developing ASTM standards, monitoring asbestos. Standardization news. *Am Soc Testing Mater* 2004;32(4);26–29.

41. American Society for Testing and Materials. Standard test method for microvacuum sampling and indirect analysis of dust by transmission electron microscopy for asbestos structure number surface loading. ASTM D5755-02. West Conshohocken (PA): American Society for Testing and Materials; 2002.

42. American Society for Testing and Materials. Standard test method for microvacuum sampling and indirect analysis of dust by transmission electron microscopy for asbestos mass surface loading. ASTM D5756-02. West Conshohocken (PA): American Society for Testing and Materials; 2002.

43. American Society for Testing and Materials. Standard test method for wipe sampling of surfaces, indirect preparation, and analysis for asbestos structure number concentration by transmission electron microscopy. ASTM D6480-99. West Conshohocken (PA): American Society for Testing and Materials; 1999.

44. Millette JR, Clark PJ, Brackett KA, Wheeles RK. Methods for the analysis of carpet samples for asbestos. U.S. Environmental Protection Agency, EPA/600/J-93/167. *Environ Choices Tech Suppl* 1993(March/April): 21–24.

45. Millette JR, Hays SM. *Settled Asbestos Dust: Sampling and Analysis*. Boca Raton: Lewis Publishers; 1994.

46. Hatfield RL, Krewer JA, Longo WE. A study of the reproducibility of the micro-vac technique as a tool for the assessment of surface contamination in buildings with asbestos-containing materials. In: Beard ME, Rook HL, editors. *Advances in Environmental Measurement Methods for Asbestos*. ASTM STP 1342. West Conshohocken (PA): American Society for Testing and Materials; 2000, p. 301–312.

47. Lee RJ, VanOrden DR, Stewart IM. Dust and airborne concentrations—Is there a correlation? In: Beard ME, Rook HL, editors. *Advances in Environmental Measurement Methods for Asbestos*. ASTM STP 1342. West Conshohocken (PA): American Society for Testing and Materials; 2000, p. 313–322.

48. Ewing WM. Further observations of settled asbestos dust in buildings. In: Beard ME, Rook HL, editors. *Advances in Environmental Measurement Methods for Asbestos.* ASTM STP 1342. West Conshohocken (PA): American Society for Testing and Materials; 2000, p. 323–332.

49. Fowler DP, Price BP. Some statistical principles in asbestos measurement and their application to dust sampling and analysis. In: Beard ME, Rook HL, editors. *Advances in Environmental Measurement Methods for Asbestos.* ASTM STP 1342. West Conshohocken (PA): American Society for Testing and Materials; 2000, p. 333–349.

50. Crankshaw OS, Perkins RL, Beard ME. An overview of settled dust analytical methods and their relative effectiveness. In: Beard ME, Rook HL, editors. *Advances in Environmental Measurement Methods for Asbestos.* ASTM STP 1342. West Conshohocken (PA): American Society for Testing and Materials; 2000, p. 350–365.

51. Millette JR, Mount MD. Applications of the ASTM asbestos in dust method D5755. In: Beard ME, Rook HL, editors. *Advances in Environmental Measurement Methods for Asbestos.* ASTM STP 1342. West Conshohocken (PA): American Society for Testing and Materials; 2000, p. 366–377.

52. Chatfield EJ. Correlated measurements of airborne asbestos-containing particles and surface dust. In: Beard ME, Rook HL, editors. *Advances in Environmental Measurement Methods for Asbestos.* ASTM STP 1342. West Conshohocken (PA): American Society for Testing and Materials; 2000, p. 378–402.

53. Hays SM. Incorporating dust sampling into the asbestos management program. In: Beard ME, Rook HL, editors. *Advances in Environmental Measurement Methods for Asbestos.* ASTM STP 1342. West Conshohocken (PA): American Society for Testing and Materials; 2000, p. 403–410.

54. U.S. Environmental Protection Agency. The protocol for screening soil and sediment samples for asbestos content used by the U.S. Environmental Protection Agency, Region 1 Laboratory, Boston, MA; 1997.

55. Australian Standard Method for the Qualitative Identification of Asbestos in Bulk Samples. AS 4964-2004. Australia: Council of Standards; March 24, 2004.

56. Falini G, Foresti E, Gazzano M, Gualtieri IG, Pecchini G, Renna E, Roveri N. A new method for the detection of low levels of free fibres of chrysotile in contaminated soils by x-ray powder diffraction. *J Environ Monit* 2003;5:654–60.

57. California Resources Board (CARB) Method 435. Determination of asbestos content of serpentine aggregate. Sacramento, CA: California Air Resources Board; 1991.

58. Berman DW, Chatfield EJ. Interim superfund method for the determination of asbestos in ambient air. EPA 540/2-90/005a. Washington, DC: U.S. Environmental Protection Agency; May 1990.

59. Berman DW, Kolk AJ. Superfund method for the determination of releasable asbestos in soils and bulk materials [interim version]. Prepared for the U.S. EPA, Office of Solid Waste and Emergency Response, Contract 68-W9-0059. Washington, DC: U.S. Environmental Protection Agency; July 1995.

60. U.S. Environmental Protection Agency. Research method for sampling and analysis of fibrous amphibole in vermiculite attic insulation. Cincinnati Method, EPA/600/R-04/004. Washington, DC: U.S. Environmental Protection Agency; January, 2004.

61. Chatfield E. Analytical protocol for determination of asbestos contamination of clothing and other fabrics. *Microscope* 1990;38:221–2.

62. Kramer T, Millette JR. A standard TEM procedure for identification and quantitation of asbestiform minerals in talc. *Microscope* 1990;38:457–68.

63. Krewer JA, Millette JR. Comparison of sodium hypochlorite digestion and low-temperature ashing preparation techniques for lung tissue analysis by TEM. *Proceedings of the Microbeam Analysis 1986, 21st Conference on Microbeam Analysis Society*, Albuquerque, NM, San Francisco Press, Inc.; August 1986.

64. Dodson RF, Williams MG, Corn CJ, Idell S, McLarty, JW. Usefulness of combined light and electron microscopy: Evaluation of sputum samples for asbestos to determine past occupational exposure. *Mod Pathol* 1989;2(4):320–2.

65. Leake BE, Woolley AR, Arps CES, Birch WD, Gilbert MC, Grice JD, et al. Nomenclature of the amphiboles: Report of the sub-committee on amphiboles of the International Mineralogical Association, Commission on New Minerals and Mineral Names. *Can Mineral* 1997;35:219–46.

66. Wylie AG, Verkouteren JR. Amphibole asbestos from Libby, Montana: Aspects of nomenclature. *Am Mineral* 2000;85:1540–2.

67. Bandli BR, Gunter ME. Identification and characterization of mineral and asbestos particles using the spindle stage and the scanning electron microscope: The Libby, Montana, U.S.A. amphibole-asbestos as an example. *Microscope* 2000;49:191–9.

68. Meeker GP, Bern AM, Brownfield IK, Lowers HA, Sutley SJ, Hoefen TM, et al. The composition and morphology of amphibole from the Rainy Creek Complex, near Libby, Montana. *Am Mineral* 2003;88:1955–69.

69. Bandli BR, Gunter ME, Twamley B, Foit FF, Cornelius SB. Optical, compositional, morphological, and x-ray data on eleven particles of amphibole from Libby, Montana, U.S.A. *Can Mineral* 2003;41:1241–53.

70. Addison J, Davies LST. Analysis of amphibole asbestos in chrysotile and other minerals. *Ann Occup Hyg* 1990;34(2):159–75.

71. Ilgren E, Chatfield E. Coalinga fibre—A short, amphibole-free chrysotile. *Indoor Built Environ* 1998;7:18–31.

72. Williams-Jones AE, Normand C, Clark JR, Vali H, Martin RF, Dufresne A, Nayebzadeh A. Controls of amphibole formation in chrysotile deposits: evidence from the Jeffery Mine, Asbestos, Quebec. In: *The Health Effects of Chrysotile Asbestos: Contribution of Science to Risk-Management Decisions.* Canadian Mineralogist Special Publication 5. Québec, Canada: Mineralogical Association of Canada; 2001. p. 89–104.

CHAPTER 3

Analysis and Relevance of Asbestos Burden in Tissue

Ronald F. Dodson

CONTENTS

The objective of this chapter is to provide the reader with the tools for best understanding the content from past and future publications regarding asbestos burden.

3.1 RESPIRATORY SYSTEM AND WHY IT IS VULNERABLE TO INHALED DUST

To appreciate the significance of asbestos in body tissues, it is first relevant to understand how it got there and the normal functioning of the major portal of entry for dust into the body—the respiratory system. The design of the respiratory system has evolved into highly functional anatomical regions. The upper airways are designed to warm, moisten, and filter the incoming air. These can be thought of primarily as conducting tubes or conduits for two-directional airflow. In the ideal situation, the first contact with the external air is as it passes through the nasal cavity. As with the other conducting passageways, the nasal chambers create directional changes in airflow (via the angular changes in the passages) and are provided at initial levels with hairs to further initiate turbulence. During exercise or talking, humans shift to "mouth breathing," thus bypassing the nasal passages, and the inhaled air and its dust component go directly through the mouth to the trachea. There are some 32 branches of the conducting airways in the normal adult lung before reaching the distal acinus.[1]

These anatomical branching impacts the direction of airflow, which further serves to increase the potential for dust entrapment. This is because any deviation in the direction of airflow, particularly when it creates "whirlpools" or changes in velocity of flow, increases the chances of sedimentation to occur among the suspended dust particles. These currents can induce perpendicular flow to the walls of the airways, which results in the dust being brought into physical contact with the surfaces. The result of this anatomical design combined with the fact that most surfaces of the conducting airways are lined with "sticky" substances results in highly efficient entrapment of many inhaled particles in the upper airways. The entrapment of larger particles on the mucosa (lining) of the major bronchi is especially prominent where both the direction of flow and the air velocity change abruptly.[1] Lippmann et al.[2] reviewed this process and noted the result of decreasing airway sizes distally, combined with the increasing number of tubes in total cross section, results in decreases in air velocity. The impact of these physical events is that the larger particles get deposited by impaction. At the level of the smallest airways where there are the lowest velocities, the particle entrapment is via sedimentation and diffusion.[2]

The importance of entrapment of inhaled dusts in the conducting airways is critical in preventing it from reaching the lower respiratory tract and potentially compromising the functional respiratory units of the lung. The lung is particularly vulnerable to the toxic gases and dusts in the environment as it represents the largest surface within the body exposed to the external environment.[3] The lungs are responsible for providing oxygen to all cells in the body and for elimination of carbon dioxide produced by these cells. The critical impact of the lungs on the well-being of all parts of the body is emphasized by Witschi[3] in that it is the "only organ in the body in man to receive within 1 minute from one to five times the circulating blood volume." To achieve this objective, the normal lung "filters about 12,000 liters of air per day to 'extract' the fuel needed for survival"[4] and is perfused with more than 6000 L of blood per day to permit normal gas exchange critical for the function of the cells that make up the body.

The functional unit that makes up the majority of the lung parenchyma is the terminal and respiratory bronchioles and the alveoli or air sacs that give the lung its sponge-like appearance (Figures 3.1 and 3.2) when viewed by the eye. Ochs et al.[5] reported that the average number of alveoli in six adult lungs was 480 million. Weibel[6] equated this very large internal surface as being nearly that of a tennis court. The morphological composition of air sacs and associated lung parenchyma is illustrated in Figure 3.1. The three-dimensional morphology includes the alveoli, the smaller airways, and the associated circulatory components resulting in the lung appearing to be composed of small sack-like structures. The thin lining surrounding the lung tissue is the visceral pleura, which is made up of flattened mesothelium, whereas the predominate cell types of the alveoli are type I and type II pneumocytes (Figure 3.2). Type II pneumocytes are secretory cells that contribute the surfactant lining material necessary to maintain inflation of the air sacks. Type I pneumocytes are cells that form a thin lining over the surface of the air sack and are designed to permit gases (oxygen and carbon dioxide) to be exchanged across the air–blood barrier with the circulating blood that perfuses throughout the numerous small blood capillaries that traverse the regions between the alveoli and the small airways. The surface of the alveoli are designed to be relatively sterile, and inhaled materials are prevented from reaching this level only if the previously described entrapments at the upper airways remove the inhaled particulates from the incoming air. When the alveoli and the surface of small airways are compromised by the presence of inhaled particulates, defense cells from the interstitium are mobilized as a defensive response. Turino[7] appropriately described

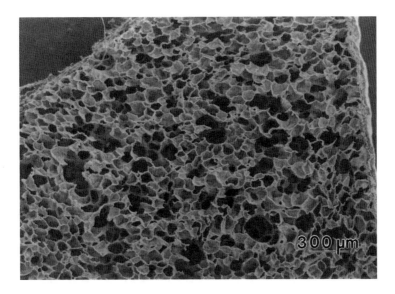

Figure 3.1 The lung parenchyma as seen in this lower magnification scanning electron micrograph shows the three-dimensional morphology of the alveoli, smaller airways, and associated circulatory components that result in the lung appearing to be comprised of small sack-like structures.

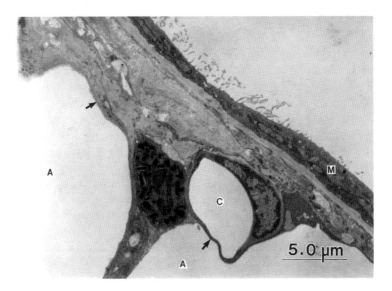

Figure 3.2 This low-magnification transmission electron micrograph shows the thin visceral pleural surface consisting of a layer of mesothelial cells (M). The alveoli (A) are lined by type I (arrow) and type II pneumocytes. A cross section through an interstitial capillary (C) shows the close association between the vascular space and the alveolar spaces.

the lung parenchyma as a "dynamic matrix" that is comprised predominately of collagen, elastin, glycosaminoglycans, and fibronectin. The appropriate balance of these components combined with the proper functional capabilities of the cells that make up the lung parenchyma are critical for a healthy lung. Response to inhaled dusts can acutely or chronically alter the balance and result in reduced lung function and, if sufficiently vigorous and widespread, result in permanent loss of normal respiratory functions in the reactive areas of the lung.

3.2 DUST ELIMINATION FROM THE LUNG

The potential for dust entrapment in the larger airways has been discussed. The effectiveness of the upper airway defense/filtration mechanisms is that the majority of dust particles larger than 3 µm in diameter never reach the lower respiratory system or alveolar surfaces.[8] Gross and Detreville[8] projected the defense mechanisms of the lung function at a level of 98%–99% efficiency for trapping or removing inhaled particulates. The inefficiency for the removal of 1%–2% of inhaled dusts under such assumptions would account for the resultant development of pneumoconiosis (dust diseases). The defense mechanisms of the lung are divided between levels of anatomical divisions. The conducting airways are lined with a sticky blanket of mucus. Columnar lining cells making up a part of the surface lining of the larger conducting airways have specialized hairlike extensions from their surfaces called *cilia*. There are several hundreds of these per cell, and their role is to expedite the movement of the mucous layer and entrapped particulates from the level of deposit to the next higher levels toward the pharynx for elimination as a component of sputa. The cilia beat approximately 1000 times per minute in a coordinated scheme to assure rapid upward movement of the surface layer and any entrapped materials.[9] The combined function of entrapment of particulates in the mucus and the effective transport of the entrapped dusts and mucus with the assistance of the "beating" underlying cilia form a critical clearance mechanism from the lung often referred to as the mucociliary escalator.

The lowest level of the respiratory tract consists of the alveoli that comprise the majority of the lung parenchyma. These fragile-appearing air sacs consist of thin-walled structures formed by the close apposition of a cytoplasmic extension of an epithelial cell on the airway side, an area of basement membrane, and the thin wall of the smallest circulatory blood vessel in the body—the capillary. The extremely thin wall of this region gives it a "spiderweb" appearance in sections when viewed by light microscopy. It is specifically designed anatomically to permit the effective exchange of gases from the air–blood–air compartments. The morphological appearance of the delicate nature of the wall of this structural unit at the light microscopy level led some to consider it initially to be acellular. In reality, the components of the two cell types which populate the air–blood barrier (Figures 3.3 and 3.4) form a total thickness ranging from 0.2 to 0.5 µm, which is up to 20–50 times thinner than a sheet of airmail paper.[4,6] For proper gas exchange to occur, these sacs must remain open, with minimal congestion and with maintenance of normal wall integrity to assure flexibility for contraction and expansion of the lower lung parenchyma. The surfaces of normal alveoli are protected from foreign material by the previously described defense filtrations that occur in the conducting airways. The alveolar surfaces are ideally maintained in a sterile state. In normal tissue, secreted glycolipoprotein (surfactant) from type II alveolar cells assists in assuring a low surface tension on the surface of the alveoli and helps prevent them from collapsing at low lung volumes (Figures 3.3 and 3.5).[10] In contrast with the micrograph shown in Figure 3.3, the air–blood barrier in the section from an experimental animal model (Figure 3.4) shows the leakage of horseradish peroxidase (arrow) through the barrier onto the surface of the alveolar sac. If congestion occurs in the air sacs as a result of an inflammatory response of defense cells to inhaled particulates or if the walls of the sacks become thickened so that gas exchange is difficult, their functional state as the major respiratory units responsible for proper lung function in the lung is compromised. Particulates that reach this lowest level of the respiratory system represent a population of the smallest structures in the inhaled dusts. These have successfully bypassed the upper level defense mechanisms and reached a respiratory level where clearance is less effective.

The primary response to dust particles that reach the alveoli is a "call up" of macrophages. These defense cells migrate from the interstitium onto the surface of alveoli. The cells convert to a cellular form capable of functioning in an aerobic environment and display chemotaxis features that permit them to move along the alveolar surface to deposited particulates (Figure 3.6). Macrophages are the major defense mechanisms of the lower respiratory tract and function by attempting to clear

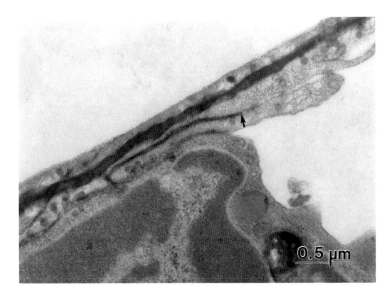

Figure 3.3 This transmission electron micrograph shows the boundaries of the alveolar–air–blood barrier. The dark material illustrates the penetration of the tracer horseradish peroxidase to the level of the junctions between the alveolar cells (arrow) that prevents its leakage into the airway.

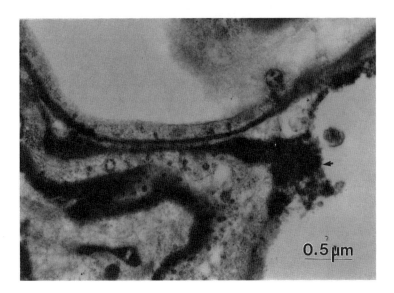

Figure 3.4 In contrast with the micrograph shown in Figure 3.3, the air–blood barrier in this section from an experimental animal model shows the leakage of horseradish peroxidase (arrow) through the barrier onto the surface of the alveolar sac. The change was induced as an early response to asbestos exposure.

the alveoli of infectious, toxic, and allergic particulates that have evaded the mechanical defenses of the nasal passages, glottis, and mucociliary transport system.[11] Pulmonary macrophages attempt to ingest and isolate foreign particulates (Figure 3.7) and contain internal chemical packages that work to denature or "digest" some ingested microorganisms. Werb[12] states "like a chameleon, the macrophage senses alterations in its environment-changes in oxygen tension, the presence of different cells such as lymphocytes, foreign materials, microorganisms or changes in plasma proteins and hormones. Not only is it adaptive to its own environment, but the changes in the structure and

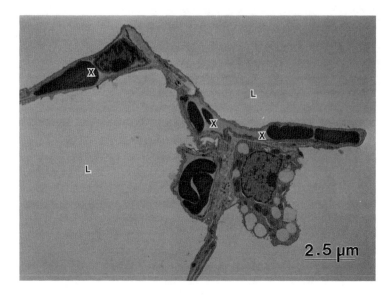

Figure 3.5 The delicate architecture of the alveolar level is shown in this transmission electron micrograph. The thin cellular separation between the blood compartment and the capillary.

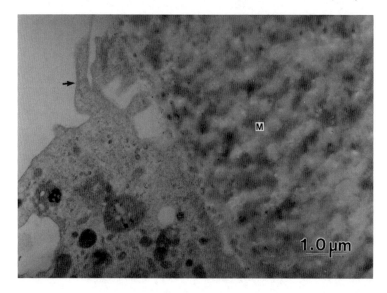

Figure 3.6 This micrograph illustrates the cross section of an activated macrophage that has been cultured on medium (M). The stimulated macrophage shows surface projections (arrow) that extend from the cell surface and provide the mechanism by which the cells move toward a stimulus either on culture medium or in tissue.

functional properties of the macrophage, in general, are reversible. Considering that the macrophage is long lived, with its half-life estimated to be on the order of weeks or months, this cycle of phenotypic response may repeat many times. Macrophages respond to a call for chemotaxis when the fortifications that defend us against an onslaught of microorganisms and other foreign materials have been breached."

A population of macrophages is capable by some yet to be understood mechanisms of relocating to the surface of the more proximal levels of the airways where the more rapid clearance of

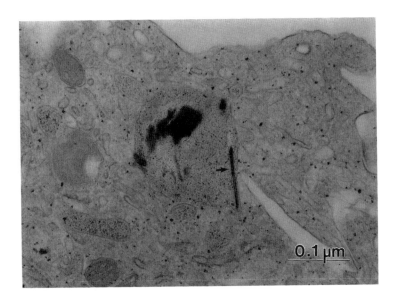

Figure 3.7   This small amosite fiber (arrow) in this transmission electron micrograph is being isolated within a siderosome of a macrophage.

macrophages and their phagocytized dust particles occur via the mucociliary escalator. Camner et al.[13] studied the efficiency of clearance for various sized particles and found that the deeper the particulates were inhaled, the longer the time was required to clear them from the lung. The average retention after 24 h was around 100% for particles deposited in generations 13–16 (ciliated bronchioles) and around 20% in generations 0–12 (both large and small ciliated airways). It should be recognized that clearance is an ongoing event; thus, periods of elevated dust accumulation may not be totally represented by tissue burden at the time of sampling, particularly if the period from last exposure has covered an appreciable period of months or years.

The impact of smoking and asbestos as combined causal agents of disease in man is discussed in appreciable detail in the section on clinical issues. However, it is appropriate to note that exposure to tobacco smoke alters the cellular composition of the upper airways (resulting in squamous cell metaplasia and goblet cell hyperplasia) and negatively impacts on the effectiveness of the mucociliary escalator to properly function. Lippmann et al.[2] noted "cigarette smoking and bronchitis produce a proximal shift in the deposition pattern" and "if the particles penetrate the epithelium, either bare or within macrophages, they may be sequestered within cells or enter the lymphatic circulation and be carried to pleural, hilar, and more distant lymph nodes." Animal studies conducted to assess the effect of smoking and clearance were conducted by the research group led by Dr. Andrew Churg. In a study using a guinea pig model,[14] it was determined that "cigarette smoking impedes asbestos clearance, largely by increasing retention of short fibers." They further concluded "increased pulmonary fiber burden may be important in the increased disease rate seen in asbestos workers who smoke." In a companion work,[15] the observations "implied that failure of macrophages clearance and subsequent rerelease of fibers into the medium may at least partially explain the changes in fiber sizes and eventually increases in tissue fiber concentrations in smoke-exposed animals." Thus, clearance in a smoker of all types of dust including asbestos[16,17] is less efficient than in a nonsmoker.[2] Churg and Stevens[18] found that in the case of asbestos-exposed individuals, asbestos recovered from the airway mucosa or parenchyma of smokers was shorter than that in nonsmokers. They concluded that smoking led to enhanced retention of short fibers. The other observation was that many more short fibers were cleared over time in individuals who did not have compromised clearance.

3.3 DUST OVERLOADING AND THE IMPACT ON THE RESPIRATORY TRACT

The process as described for clearance from the lung represents the ideal response to dust inhalation and its rapid elimination from the lung. In many instances, exposure to dust can result in periods of "dust overloading" of the defense mechanisms.[19–22] This phenomenon is due to alterations in the capabilities of macrophages to respond to dust burden partly because of overwhelming the phagocytic component and the number of macrophages stimulated to meet the elevated burden of inhaled dust. This results in "macrophage congestion," including congestion at the level of the alveoli and small airways. This results in some macrophages not being able to leave the congested area. These phagocytic cells eventually die and release the ingested particulates, which in turn trigger an influx of more phagocytic cells in response to the freed dust. Oberdorster[19] suggested impaired alveolar macrophage-mediated lung clearance and the accumulation of high levels of pulmonary dust can result in adverse chronic effects, including inflammation, fibrosis, and tumors. For example, it has been shown that poorly soluble, nonfibrous particles (carbon black, coal dust, diesel soot, nonasbestiform talc, and titanium dioxide) elicit tumors in rats when deposition overwhelms the clearance mechanisms of the lung creating the condition of overloading.[23] The impact of elevated dust burden and the risk of developing permanent pathological changes in the respiratory system lie in part with the level of inherent toxicity associated with the accumulated dust. There is increasing appreciation that the same macrophages that provide front line defense in the lower respiratory system carry a liability for inducing injury to lung tissue. The impact of compound exposures of asbestos have been shown in an animal model where Coin et al.[24] found that after three consecutive inhalation exposures to chrysotile, there were asbestos fibers retained at the 6-month evaluation of the tissue. The "three exposures to chrysotile caused a large increase in DNA synthesis in the epithelium of the terminal bronchioles and more proximal airways. When compared with a single exposure, the triple exposure caused an enhanced inflammatory response and a prolonged period of increased DNA synthesis in the proximal alveolar region. Hyperplastic, fibrotic lesions subsequently developed in the same region and persisted for at least 6 months after exposure." Compound exposures to amosite in an animal model likewise resulted in a newer area of responsiveness involving appreciable neutrophil component, while reactive areas to the earlier exposure were typified as being represented by a majority of cells being macrophages.[25]

Pinkerton et al.[26] evaluated the tissue response after chronic exposures using Fisher 344 rats. They concluded "that during exposure to asbestos fibers, macrophages and alveolar epithelial cells contain statistically significant amounts of asbestos and are associated with histological changes indicating marked epithelial injury. Increased amounts of fibers are also localized in the lung interstitium with continued exposure to asbestos and are associated with progressive interstitial fibrotic reaction. After cessation of exposure, macrophages and epithelial cells are cleared of fibers and resolve toward normal proportions. However, significant clearance of fibers from the lung interstitium does not occur after cessation of exposure, and there is a continuing process of fibrogenesis."

Data from such studies emphasize the need to separate assumptions on the basis of findings from one exposure in animal models from the responses after actual compound exposures that occur in occupationally exposed humans. It is through animal models that many concepts of asbestos-induced pathogenicity have been described. Differences in chrysotile and amphibole risks for induction of disease are described in the chapter involving molecular biological interactions. There are several unique features that suggest that amphiboles may carry more of a risk for inducing malignancy, not the least of which is the potential for inhalation of longer fibers when compared with chrysotile (see section on asbestos characteristics). Indeed, some animal models have been interpreted as indicating chrysotile is less pathogenically active, whereas other studies have shown it to be an appreciably active form of asbestos. For example, Reeves et al.[27] found variations in tumorigenicity between fiber types after exposure, stating that "Two pulmonary cancers were produced in rats exposed to inhalation of crocidolite. Local injection into the pleural or peritoneal cavities caused 5 mesotheliomas in rats after chrysotile treatment and 6 mesotheliomas in rats and rabbits after crocidolite treatment. Guinea pigs and hamsters developed no tumors in this experiment, and with the dose used, there were no tumors in any species in the amosite group." Kimizuka et al.[28] found that "chrysotile induced more prominent cell (leukocyte or macrophages) necrosis and alveolar wall thickening. These findings indicate chrysotile asbestos induces stronger cell reactions in the alveolar wall and is more noxious than amosite."

Hesterberg et al.[29] tested the effects of chronic inhalation in rats of X607 (a rapidly dissolving synthetic vitreous fiber) with those previously reported for RCF1 (a refractory ceramic synthetic vitreous fiber) and chrysotile fiber. As will be discussed in detail within the section on fiber length and pathogenicity, a reference point for the potential pathogenicity of a fiber is its durability/biopersistence in tissue. The study reported that RCF1 and chrysotile asbestos "induced pulmonary fibrosis and thoracic neoplasms (chrysotile induced 32% more pulmonary neoplasms than RCF1). Lung deposition and fiber lengths did not explain the toxicological differences between the three fibers." The authors stated that from their data, "chrysotile dissolution was negligible." Rodelsperger[30] pointed out a reasonable concern when attempting to extrapolate data from rat models (and potential all rodent models) to human experiences regarding the carcinogenic potency of fibers in that "the life span of rats is too low to measure the elimination rate of bio-persistent fibers sufficiently." It is also true that animals have a more rapid clearance rate than humans and obviously smaller airways for more efficient filtration of dusts than occurs in the larger passageways of humans.

The macrophage is a cell type characterized by Brody[31] as being on the "one hand a potential defender of the alveolar environment and on the other hand as a central mediator of lung disease." Simplistically, the surfaces of alveolar sacs in the ideal state are devoid of cells and debris, and when inhaled dust such as asbestos stimulates the call up of macrophages and neutrophils,[32,33] the balance of the alveolar environment changes, potentially resulting in long-term or permanent pathological alterations. The anatomical area that normally consists of open spaces for gas exchange becomes filled with defense cells and fluid. As the macrophages interact with the inhaled dust, the potential exists for there to be a release of oxidants,[34,35] chemoattractants for other inflammatory cells,[36,37] proteases,[38,39] and growth factors that stimulate fibroblasts to replicate from these cells[40–42] and to secrete collagen.[43] The latter two events are pivotal in the induction of fibroproliferative disorders in the lung such as intra-alveolar/interstitial fibrosis[40] or in the case of asbestos-induced fibrosis (asbestosis). Bowden[44] reported that these combinations of deleterious events associated with macrophages in the lung are direct contributors to the development of emphysema and interstitial fibrosis.

Secretions from macrophages occur in the normal process of phagocytosis of bacteria, virus, or dust particles. However, if the dust particulates are particularly toxic, the macrophage may be killed, and the release of internal chemicals occurs immediately. If dust overloading occurs, the macrophages may not be able to escape from the airway because of lack of clearance. When the macrophages reach the end of their life expectancy, they release the dust, which triggers the call up of more macrophages, enzymes, and other chemicals that negatively interact with the cell wall and adjacent cells. Such a scenario would be expected to occur with generation after generation of newly attracted macrophages and thus result in a constant reinforcement of the negative events as described earlier. In part, this concept should be considered as a factor in the continuing development of fibrosis in an asbestotic lung, which can progress long after the individual's contact with asbestos had ceased. Thus, as summarized by Brain,[45] "though the macrophages serve as the first line of defense for the alveolar surface, they may also be capable of injuring the host while exercising their defensive role."

3.4 RELOCATION OF PARTICULATES FROM THE LUNG VIA THE LYMPHATICS

The most efficient mechanism for dust clearance from the lung follows a pathway that back up the same route as it entered the airways by the mechanisms described. However, there is another route for clearance or relocation of particulates from the lung, and that is by lymphatic drainage into lymph nodes via lymphatic channels.[2,46–51] The drainage of lymphatics from the lung have long been appreciated as indicated by the evidence of silicotic nodules forming in lymph nodes of silica-exposed individuals[52,53] as well as observations from numerous animal models as described in detail in a recent publication from our laboratory.[54] In one interesting animal study, Oberdorster et al.[55] studied the transfer of amosite fibers from the lower respiratory system in a dog model. The project incorporated both neutron activated amosite fibers as well as detection of the fibers by scanning electron microscopy at a period of 24 h after exposure. The assessment included both thoracic lymph nodes and postnodal lung lymph. The authors concluded that there was "a fast translocation of fibers from the airspaces of the lung to the lymph nodes and even into postnodal lymph." The findings indicated that the "structures of the peripheral lung and lymph node itself act like size selective filters, permitting only the fine fibre-fraction to penetrate." This conclusion is consistent with our findings of the actual fiber burden in the lung and lymph nodes from exposed humans.[54] Oberdorster et al.[55] further concluded that "fibres below about 9 μm in length and below about 0.5 μm in diameter can be cleared into the postnodal lymph and thus can reach any organ of the body."

The awareness of the communication routes between the lung and the lymphatics is well appreciated as typified by the use of the Naruke lymph node map used by the American Joint Commission for staging the spread of primary carcinomas of the lung.[56]

Furthermore, the characterization as to which level of the lung is drained by the various anatomically located nodes in the chest cavity is described by Netter[57] in his illustrated anatomical text. It is ironic that, previously, only theoretical concepts have been offered regarding asbestos relocation from the lung to the lymph nodes and thus as potential routes to extrapulmonary sites. However, a recent study[54] from our laboratory provides quantitative data regarding fiber burden and characterization of the fibers found in the lymph nodes as compared with that in lung tissue. The observations are described in applicable sections under topics regarding asbestos in extrapulmonary sites and the relevance of short fibers in assessing accurate tissue burdens.

Dust overload of the usual clearance mechanisms previously described results in the translocation of a portion of the dust to extrapulmonary sites via the lymphatics and lymph nodes as discussed by Cullen et al.[58] The logic of this explanation is that usual clearance route via the mucociliary escalator of dust from the deeper lung is impaired/overwhelmed. Relocation of dust from the lung to the lymph node and the lymphatic drainage has resulted in these sites becoming "reservoirs of retained material" or, in the case of the nodes, as "repositories for dust."[8,59] With sufficient dust accumulation the lymph nodes become "densely mineralized and stony hard."[8] If dust accumulated in the nodes has appreciable cytotoxicity, pathological changes can occur, including the formation of nodules.[53] This same route through the lymphatic system has been suggested as the mechanism by which asbestos fibers relocate to extrapulmonary sites,[60,61] a concept for which we have now offered quantitative validation.[54]

Another interesting issue regarding relocation of fibrous dust from the lung to lymph nodes and other extrapulmonary sites involves the influence of mixed dust on the process. Davis et al.[62] evaluated the influence of nonfibrous dusts on translocation of respirable size asbestos. The scientists studied translocation and clearance in a rat model after 1 year of exposure and 2 years of follow-up. They acknowledged that rat pleural lining differs from humans in thickness and morphological complexity. Thus, mechanisms of translocation through the visceral pleura may be appreciably different between rats and humans. However, when combining the exposure of chrysotile or amosite with titanium dioxide or quartz, they observed differing levels of reactions and end points (tumor formation). Quartz "greatly increased fibrosis above that produced by the asbestos types alone." The occurrence of pulmonary tumors and mesothelioma in animals receiving asbestos and other dusts was increased. The authors observed the "presence of particulate dusts made little difference in the amounts of amosite fibre retained in the lung tissue, but, with chrysotile, titanium dioxide appeared to increase retention while quartz reduced it."

A recent evaluation by Pintos et al.[63] from two case–control studies assessed the risk of mesothelioma and occupational exposure to asbestos and man-made vitreous fibers. Not surprisingly, the findings revealed "in workers with exposure levels lower than historical cohort studies and across a wide range of industries, a strong association was found between asbestos, especially when it was amphibole, and mesothelioma." The investigators determined that "subjects exposed to both asbestos and MMVF had particularly high risks, an unexpected result."

The subject of reactions in mixed exposures to nonfibrous and/or mixed fibrous dusts is beyond the focus of this chapter; however, it is useful to remember that most exposures in humans are to mixed dusts. It is also useful to recognize that although the molecular mechanisms discussed in the various sections may emphasize characteristics of fibrous dusts, many of the same mechanisms may have applicability to respired dusts that are of the same elemental composition but not in a fibrous form. A potential synergistic effect between various fibrous and nonfibrous dusts cannot be ruled out as a mechanism resulting in increased risk for development of disease.

3.5 MORPHOLOGICAL FEATURES OF ASBESTOS THAT DETERMINE ITS POTENTIAL FOR INHALATION

Asbestos minerals have been used by intent in more than 3000 commercial applications.[64] Asbestos is sometimes a component of minerals mined for many different products that are considered as not containing asbestos or having less than a "regulated percent of content 1%," which trigger the regulatory definition of asbestos-containing material. Thus, millions of individuals are exposed to asbestos-containing products in the workplace or through secondary or bystander exposures from occupational settings. The widespread use of asbestos results from their unique properties including high tensile strength, flexibility, insulating properties, fire resistance, and resistance to strong chemicals—both alkaline and acidic.[65] These attributes in the past made asbestos an important commercial contributor to the economic development of industrialized societies.[66] The problem arises that when asbestos is disturbed, it results in fibers breaking down into respirable-sized dust particles. This fibrous dust is easily inhaled and can cause pathological damage to the lung (e.g., asbestosis, lung cancer, mesothelioma) and extrapulmonary sites.[67]

The term *asbestos* refers to a group of six different fibrous forms of minerals and is generally used in society as a generic nomenclature. The mineral name and the name given to the asbestos and nonasbestos form of anthophyllite, actinolite, and tremolite are the same. The most widely used form of asbestos in commercial applications (90%–95%) is chrysotile, which is a serpentine form of mineral.[68–70] The other five forms of asbestos (amosite, crocidolite, actinolite, tremolite, and anthophyllite) are the asbestiform habits of the amphibole family of mineral groups. The nonfibrous form of these minerals can break along cleavage planes and create elongated cleavage fragments[71] that are sometimes confused with the fibrous form in that they are morphologically similar in appearance, particularly by light microscopy. Although an in-depth discussion of the differentiation between the cleavage fragment and the asbestiform habit is outside the scope of this chapter, suffice it to say that the former is not considered "asbestos" under the definition of regulated fibers. This is not to imply that cleavage fragments of these minerals may not carry their own risk to health if sufficient numbers are inhaled, as will be emphasized later in this chapter.

Amosite and crocidolite were used in commercial applications in the United States while use of anthophyllite was limited. In the past, actinolite, tremolite, and anthophyllite have been considered "noncommercial asbestos types." However, their presence in products containing minerals such as vermiculite and talc provides a vehicle for their widespread use, even if the exposures are often less intense than those occurring in occupational exposures to commercial forms of asbestos. Compounding the issue of exposure to noncommercial amphiboles is that often the individual has had no idea the product contained asbestiform structures. Tremolite asbestos is considered as a mineral component (often referred to as a contaminant) of Canadian chrysotile. Tremolite asbestos within chrysotile asbestos mined from Canada[64] is suggested by some investigators to be an important factor in diseases associated with exposures to Canadian chrysotile.[72] All types of asbestos have a silicon tetroxide (SiO_4) tetrahedral as backbone of the crystal lattice. Chrysotile is a magnesium silicate (Figure 3.8) that is assembled in nature with the layers of linked silica tetrahedral alternating with the layers of magnesium oxide–hydroxide octahedral (brucite). The double layering in this type of structure rolls up onto itself to form hollow tubes or scrolls that are morphologically characteristic of chrysotile. The impact of this internal organization as reflected in the physical features of the fiber is that the longer the fiber becomes, the more likely it is to coil or curl (Figure 3.9). Thus, the fiber when seen in cross section displays a true diameter at any one point, which is thinner than the functional diameter of the fiber in an air stream. This greater functional diameter because of morphological curvature of a fiber within an airstream results in less potential for the inhalation of longer, more curved fibers than comparable length straight fibers. The amphiboles, on the other hand, contain aggregates of cations (calcium, sodium, iron, and magnesium) between the strips of linked silica tetrahedral in the form of parallel chains (Figures 3.10–3.12). The variations of the percentage and types of cations determine the type of amphibole asbestos. All amphiboles, because of the repeating crystalline units, tend to be straight even as the fiber (crystal) increases in length (Figure 3.13). Thus, the functional diameter tends to be similar to the actual diameter in an air stream. It is therefore easier to inhale longer fibers of amphiboles than equivalent length longer fibers of chrysotile. This difference alone favors the retention of amphiboles in the lung as short or small entities having a greater potential to be more rapidly cleared.[73] The other side of this issue is that greater numbers of smaller entities may be inhaled over a shorter period of time and lead to dust overloading as previously described. The smaller entities are (as will be extensively described in later sections) the dust particles that are more likely to reach extrapulmonary sites. A final point regarding the smaller entities is that their combined surface area/reactive surface may well exceed that contributed by the larger (in the case of asbestos, longer) structures. A chronic inhalation study

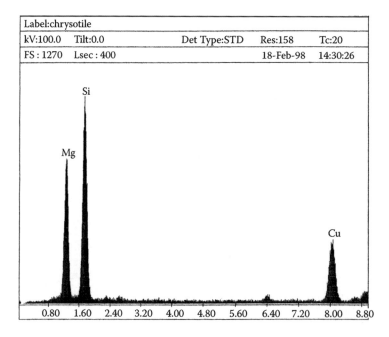

Figure 3.8 This x-ray energy dispersive spectrum (XEDS) illustrates the major elemental components of chrysotile—silicon and magnesium. The copper spike is from the grid that supports the sample preparation.

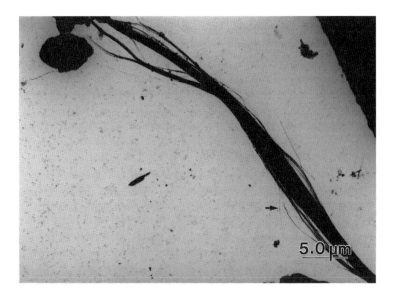

Figure 3.9 The large bundle of chrysotile fibers was obtained from digested lung tissue of a chrysotile miner. The curved morphology of the chrysotile is evident even in this large bundle. There are a number of areas on the bundle that show the fraying characteristic that can result in separation into smaller units including separation to the fibrillar level (arrow). (Tissue provided courtesy of Dr. Andrew Churg.)

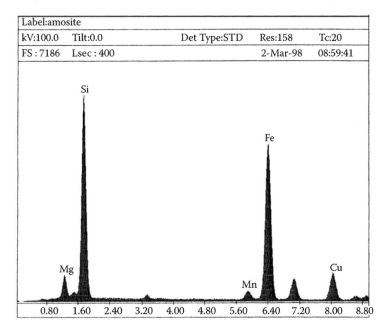

Figure 3.10 This x-ray energy dispersive spectrum (XEDS) shows the elemental composition of a major commercial amphibole (amosite asbestos) that is a ferromagnesium silicate.

by Hesterberg et al.[29] compared the biologic effects in rats of a rapidly dissolving synthetic vitreous fiber with a refractory ceramic synthetic vitreous fiber and chrysotile (Jeffrey Mine, Canada). At the selected end point, the rapidly dissolving synthetic vitreous fiber group did not show fibrosis or tumors, whereas the refractory ceramic synthetic vitreous fiber group and the chrysotile-exposed group showed pulmonary fibrosis and tumors with chrysotile inducing "32% more pulmonary

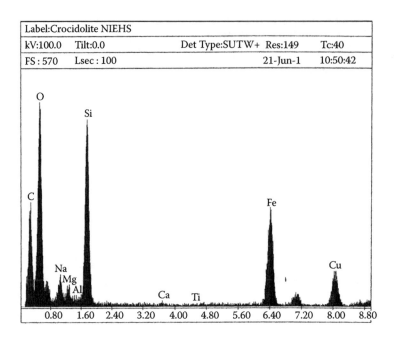

Figure 3.11   This sample of crocidolite (commercially used blue asbestos) was obtained from the National Institute of Environmental Health Sciences and illustrates the usual elemental composition of this type of asbestos as a ferromagnesium silicate with a sodium (Na) component.

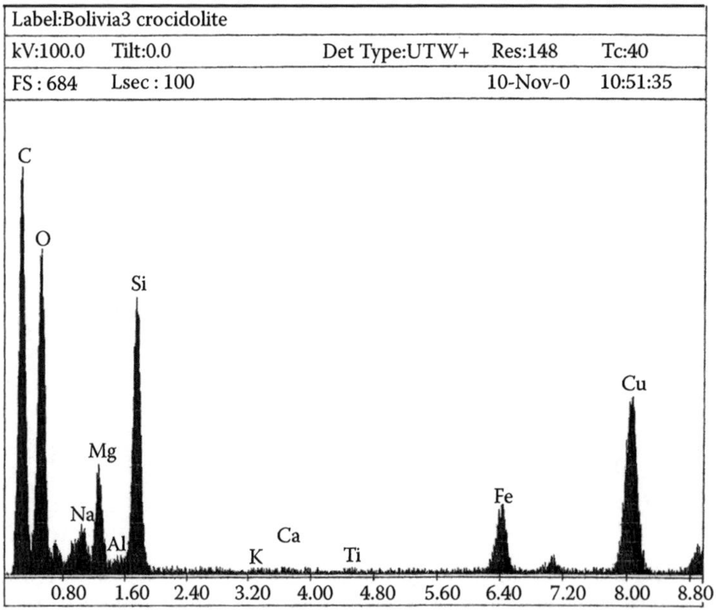

Figure 3.12   The x-ray energy dispersive spectrum (XEDS) illustrates the variability of the elemental composition of amphiboles, which can occur in different mineralogical formations. The crocidolite analyzed in this spectrum is referred to as "Bolivian Blue" and illustrates different magnesium to silica ratio when compared with the standard South African crocidolite illustrated in Figure 3.11.

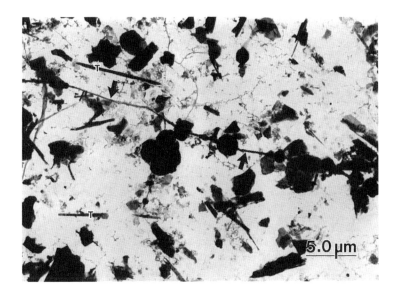

Figure 3.13 The long chrysotile cored asbestos body shown in the center of the photograph (arrow) illustrates tendencies in several areas for a curvature to occur in the fiber. This contrasts with the straight fibers seen as uncoated tremolite asbestos (T) within the field. This tissue sample was from an individual who had been a chrysotile asbestos miner exposed to both chrysotile and tremolite in their work environment. (Material courtesy of Dr. Andrew Churg.)

neoplasms than RCF1"—the refractory ceramic fibers. The issue of interpreting chrysotile biopersistence in animal models should be reviewed with the concerns offered by Pezerat that "aggressive pretreatment of fibers, inducing many faults and fragility in the fibers' structure, may lead to rapid hydration and breaking of long fibers in the lungs."[74] A review of alterations that some procedures may induce in the process of isolating ferruginous bodies/fibers from lung and other samples will be discussed in the section of this chapter on tissue preparation.

There are important differences in surface charges associated with differences in composition of various types of asbestos as has been discussed by Hamilton,[75] Valerio et al.,[76] and Xu et al.[77] Likewise, there are differences in surface cations among the amphibole forms, which result in potential for chemical reactions to occur. Some reactions can produce harmful by-products, including the formation of reactive radicals. A recent study by MacCorkle et al.[78] evaluated the response of cultured human fibroblasts after exposure to amphiboles and several types of chrysotile. They observed that the individual fibers were engulfed into the cytoplasm where they "induced significant mitotic aberrations leading to chromosomal instability and aneuploidy." The observation indicated that the "intracellular asbestos fibers induced aneuploidy and chromosome instability by binding to a subset of proteins that include regulators of the cell cycle, cytoskeleton, and mitotic process." The precoating of fibers with protein complexes blocked the measurable asbestos-induced changes associated with surface reactions without affecting the uptake by the cells. The mechanisms that resulted in the damaging interactions in this study involved surface reactions that did not appear to be dependent on the type of asbestos, which is in contrast with the Fenton–iron-driven reactions that have been emphasized as important in amphibole generation of damaging free radicals because of iron content, particularly with crocidolite and amosite.

These features are discussed in greater detail in the chapter on molecular mechanisms of asbestos interactions with cells and the lung milieu. The significance of asbestos to become a respirable dust is inherent in that the fibers and bundles can dissociate into shorter or thinner units during traumatic disturbance, which can occur in airflow or exerted physical pressure. The upper limits of respirability in humans has been given for a rounded structure as 10 μm in diameter[79,80] and for a

fibrous particulate as 3.5 μm in diameter.[79] The potential for inhaling fibrils (the thinnest unit structure) is evident when recognizing that from our experience the measurements for such structures
by analytical transmission electron microscopy (ATEM) for the most commonly used commercial
types of asbestos are 0.02–0.08 μm for chrysotile, 0.06–0.35 μm for amosite, and 0.04–0.15 μm
for crocidolite. It is evident that bundles or fibers composed of multiple fibrils are well within the
respirable range for fibrous dust (Figure 3.14). It should be recognized that the filtration and entrapment processes as described earlier result in many fibrous particulates being trapped higher up the
respiratory system and rapidly eliminated. However, the potential for inhalation is a relative issue on
the basis of the overall numbers common in many exposures to fibrous dust as the distributions in
sizes (diameters) that can comprise the aerosolized dust in the individual's breathing zone are often
mixed. Smaller diameter and shorter fibrous particulates are more readily inhaled to a greater depth
in the respiratory system and may be inhaled in far greater numbers than the larger counterparts.[81]

The issue of fiber size and the potential for inducing irreversible changes in human and/or animal models have been discussed regarding respirability and the inherent physical potential for being
more readily cleared/translocated in portions of this section and in subsequent sections of this chapter. However, the impact of surface area as a factor in determination of the potential for inducing
molecular/biochemical reactions has received limited attention. One study evaluating the impact
of fiber type and surface area was conducted by Timbrell et al.[82] The study involved tissue specimens obtained from postmortem lungs of individuals who had amphibole exposure at mining sites,
including Paakkila (Finland—anthophyllite), Wittenoom (Australia—crocidolite), North Western
Cape Province (NW Cape, South Africa—crocidolite), and Transvaal (South Africa—amosite and
crocidolite). The authors observed that when "mass was used as a parameter of fiber quantity, the fiber
concentrations in specimens showing a given degree of fibrosis increased progressively: Wittenoom <
NWCape < Transvaal < Paakkila. Significantly, however, when surface area was used as the parameter, the fiber concentrations in specimens showing a given degree of fibrosis were approximately
equal: Wittenoom = NW Cape = Transvaal = Paakkila. But when the number was used as the
parameter, the fiber concentrations in specimens showing a given degree of fibrosis decreased progressively: Wittenoom » NW Cape » Transvaal » Paakkila. These trends in the concentrations of

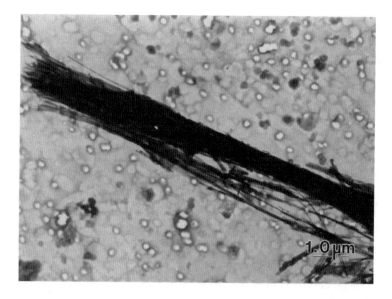

Figure 3.14   This bundle of chrysotile asbestos was isolated by digestion techniques from an occupationally
exposed individual. The disassociation of the bundle into smaller units including fibrils is evident
in the micrograph.

retained fiber required to produce the same degree of fibrosis are the consequence of large differences in fiber size between the four locations, rather than the differences in type of amphibole. Long-resident chrysotile fibres exhibited roughly the same fibrogenicity per unit of surface area as amphibole fibres, and this was also true for quartz grains."

As discussed in the sections involving macrophagic/clearance response, the repetitious exposures to such dusts may trigger an ongoing inflammatory response resulting in pathological changes in the tissue.

3.6 FERRUGINOUS BODIES IN TISSUE

The term ferruginous body means "iron-rich" body. These structures when found in lung tissue are indicators that the defense cells of the lung—the alveolar macrophages—have interacted with a particulate and deposited an iron-rich coating on its surface. If these structures are created on asbestos fibers, they are appropriately called "asbestos bodies." The first reports of these golden brown structures in lung tissue were by Marchand[83] in 1906. These structures were first recognized by Cooke[84] in 1929, who used the name "curious bodies." In 1931, Gloyne[85] proved that the cores of these structures were asbestos fibers by exposing guinea pigs to asbestos dust. After 6 months, Gloyne[85] found varying degrees of maturing ferruginous bodies in their lung tissue. He also reported a ferruginous body in the lung tissue of a gray rat caught on an asbestos factory premises. Gloyne[86] warned of the complexity of identifying a ferruginous body formed in tissue sections by noting "there is difficulty previously mentioned that an elongated structure such as an asbestosis body rarely lies entirely in one plane." This is a point well remembered today before tending to call anything that stains positively with an iron stain a ferruginous body (implying it is consistent with an asbestos body as seen by light microscopy).

There is universal agreement that the coating that forms on asbestos fibers is deposited through interactions with macrophages (Figure 3.15) and appears to preferentially involve deposition on the longer fibers that do not become internalized within the phagocyte. The shorter fibers that can be phagocytized within the macrophages are often found in "iron-rich" organelles as indicated by the

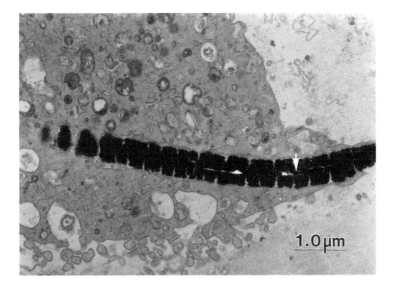

1.0 µm

Figure 3.15 The section of the asbestos body seen in this field is surrounded by a macrophage. The asbestos fiber in the center of the body (arrow) is surrounded by the iron–protein coat deposited through surface interactions with macrophages.

Perls-positive nature of the regions. However, the shorter fibers do not morphologically exhibit coatings when isolated from the tissue. In 1970, Davis[87] reported in animal models that the "first coating material of the asbestos bodies seems to be some form of acid mucopolysaccharide, but this coating soon becomes impregnated with ferritin or hemosiderin to form the well-known Perls-positive bodies." In 1972, Governa and Rosanda[88] suggested that mucopolysaccharides might act as a matrix for iron deposition on the coating (Figure 3.16). Not all animal species readily form asbestos bodies, if at all,[89] and the formation of such bodies in man also varies between individuals.[90–92]

The common link in stimulating the formation of asbestos bodies in tissue is the presence of asbestos fibers longer than 8 μm (with most being over 20 μm in length), with the majority of asbestos fibers in lung being much shorter and uncoated.[90–92] It is evident that diameters and surface irregularities may play a role in the selection process as suggested by the appearance of fibrous cores where the ferruginous coating had been removed[92] and because asbestos bodies represent only a portion of the longer fiber burden within the tissue at a given time.[91] It should be noted that other fibrous and nonfibrous inhaled structures stimulate formation of ferruginous bodies. Gross et al.[93] introduced the term "pseudo-asbestos bodies" or "unusual ferruginous bodies" to designate these structures. Fibrous aluminum silicate, silicon carbide whiskers, cosmetic talc, and glass fibers can stimulate ferruginous body formation in animals.[94] Holmes et al.[95] used sized fiberglass to stimulate "pseudo-asbestos body" formation in hamster lung. In human tissue, Churg and Warnock[96] reported ferruginous bodies on cores of sheet silicates (talc, mica, or kaolinite) and carbon. Dodson et al.[97–99] demonstrated ferruginous bodies from human material could form on iron-rich fibers, carbon filaments, fibrous talc, and various sheet silicates (Figures 3.17–3.20). Initially, it may seem that the previously mentioned types of ferruginous bodies would make it difficult to differentiate an asbestos body by light microscopy. Churg[91] correctly observed that when a ferruginous body seen by light microscopy as a beaded structure formed on a clear, elongated, transparent, usually straight core, that structure is with a high degree of certainty an asbestos body. In fact, a trained reader can easily distinguish the vast majority of nonasbestos ferruginous bodies by use of the light microscope. Asbestos bodies have been found in tissue outside of the lung.[100,101] The most common location for such observations has been the lymph nodes.[102–104] The question was raised if asbestos bodies could

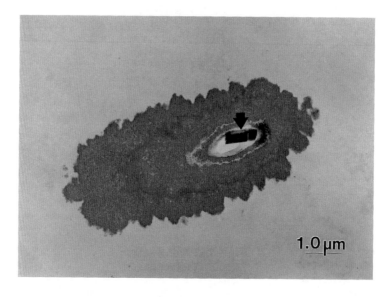

Figure 3.16 This cross-sectional view of an asbestos body reveals the central asbestos core (arrow) as surrounded by layers of iron-rich coating.

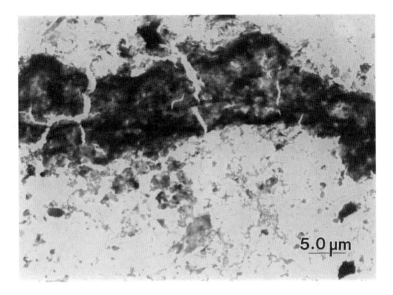

Figure 3.17   The ferruginous body seen in this field is formed on an iron-rich fiber.

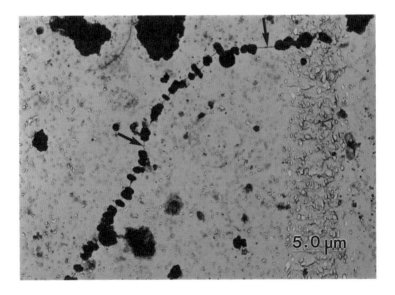

Figure 3.18   The core of this ferruginous body is formed on a graphite (organic) filament (arrow).

form in extrapulmonary sites on uncoated asbestos fibers relocated from the lung, or was it necessary that they be relocated as mature bodies? In a study from our laboratory, a guinea pig model was used to compare the coating efficiency of fibers introduced into the lung tissue as compared with reactions to fibers from the same preparation injected into the spleen and liver in other groups of animals.[105] The liver and the spleen were found to independently exhibit the inherent capability to form ferruginous bodies, but at a much less efficient rate than within the lung tissue.

The presence of asbestos bodies in sections from lung tissue offers an important indicator of past asbestos exposure. The Pneumoconiosis Council of the College of American Pathologists and the National Institute for Occupational Safety and Health stated that the "minimal criteria that permitted the diagnosis of asbestosis in tissue were demonstration of discrete foci of fibrosis in the

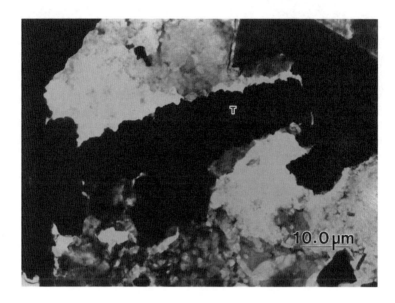

Figure 3.19   A talc fiber (T) forms the core material of this ferruginous body.

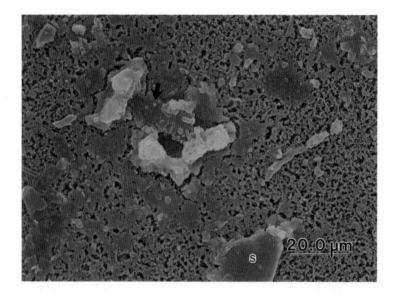

Figure 3.20   The ferruginous bodies seen in this scanning electron micrograph indicate that ferruginous coatings can occur on nonfibrous dusts. One of the bodies was formed on a central core of a thick rectangular dust particle (arrow), whereas the second ferruginous body was formed on a "plate-like" silicate (S) particle.

walls of respiratory bronchioles associated with the accumulations of asbestos bodies."[106] Crouch and Churg,[107] in recognizing the relative insensitivity of tissue sections for detection of ferruginous bodies, stated that "the demonstration of a single asbestos body on casual inspection of several lung sections implies asbestos exposure many times above background." Compounding the issue of using tissue sections for the identification of asbestos bodies is that the plane of section may only strike one level of the body and not permit visualization of the core material or if the structure is formed on an elongated core.

3.7 DESTRUCTIVE TESTING METHODS USED IN SAMPLING TISSUE AND FLUIDS FOR ASBESTOS BODIES AND UNCOATED ASBESTOS FIBERS

Although light microscopic evaluation of tissue sections in determination of the pathological processes is important, histologic evaluation of tissue sections offers a relatively insensitive method for determining asbestos body and fiber concentrations. Thus, a method that provides an expansion of the amount of tissue sampled involves destruction of relatively large amounts of tissue and collection of the particulates from that tissue on a flat surface for analysis. Some techniques used for tissue sampling include sample filtration,[108] low-temperature ashing,[109] and high-temperature ashing.[110] Additional options for tissue destruction include digestion with ozone,[111,112] strong bases,[113,114] sodium hypochlorite, and/or hydrogen peroxide.[115–117] It is important that any tissue preparation where the tissue is destroyed avoids inducing sufficient trauma to cause ferruginous bodies to fragment or asbestos bundles to dissociate into smaller units resulting in a falsely elevated asbestos tissue burden.[118–120]

Ashcroft and Heppleston[113] compared the effects on longer and uncoated fibers induced by drying the tissue before maceration. Their conclusions were: "this effect (of fractures) is evident microscopically on comparing suspension prepared from dried and wet portions of the same lung and it may exaggerate the fibre count. The numbers of fibres from wet and dried asbestotic lung tissue were compared in five cases, a sample of tissue from each being divided into two approximately equal-sized portions showing uniform pathological features." "All five specimens show higher coated fibre counts after drying, and in three specimens the uncoated fibre count is also increased."[113] The concern for breakage of the ferruginous bodies and uncoated asbestos fibers was further expressed by the European Respiratory Society Task Force.[121] The ERS Task Force Report[121] cautions that the potential not only exists for creation of artifacts in fiber/ferruginous body content of tissue due to drying of the tissue before low temperature ashing, but the "uncontrolled use of ultrasound to disperse the residue may break the fibres, resulting in higher counts and smaller sizes. Fibres may be lost during repeated centrifugation."

Dement et al.[122] concluded the following regarding fiber analysis: "The use of indirect sample transfer for transmission electron microscopy (TEM) of asbestos has been shown to break up the airborne fibers into smaller units. Depending upon the treatment, the observed concentration of fibers and their size distribution change drastically. There is no biological justification for such a violent treatment, and the measured entity is not a biologically justifiable measured quantity. Therefore the use of indirect sample transfer method for asbestos sampling should be discouraged, and the more gentle direct transfer method should be used."

To safeguard against this occurrence, it has been recommended that two separate samples are taken from each site (when adequate tissue permits). One sample is completely dried and the other samples pooled and used for the digestion procedure.[119] This approach permits determination of wet to dry ratio as used in determining ferruginous bodies or uncoated asbestos fiber per gram of wet or dry tissue. If there is not enough adequate tissue for two comparative samples (dry/wet), then it is advisable the individual sample is maintained/processed in a wet state, and data are given as fibers per gram of wet tissue or deparaffinized wet tissue (if tissue is extracted from paraffin blocks), unless there will be concern for induced changes in the characteristics of the tissue burden as per the previous discussions. Clarification of the sampling scheme and tissue status is critical if comparisons are to be made with the findings of others. When adequate tissue exists, multiple sites should be sampled. The wet samples are weighed and pooled for digestion. It is preferable to use multiple tissue samples to compensate for variations of ferruginous body/fiber burden within various areas of the tissue. The larger number of samples compensates for random sampling issues, although often single or several small tissue samples may be all that are available. Under such conditions, the use of digestion techniques and the screening of digested material for ferruginous bodies by light microscopy and for uncoated asbestos fibers by electron microscopy offer the best evidence concerning past exposure.[122] If a small sample contains asbestos bodies or fibers, it is reasonable that similar "hot" areas are present in the lung. If a small sample is negative, then the concern is that random sampling error has resulted in the tissue not being representative of the general lung/tissue burden.

The method for digesting tissue[123] in our laboratory incorporates a modification of the Smith and Naylor[124] bleach digestion technique. The procedure permits the maximum disruption of tissue but with minimal trauma to particulates obtained from the tissue through the application of the most "direct" mode of sample preparation. This is in contrast with "indirect methods" of preparations that often involve additional manipulations of the sample. These may include the filter being ashed to remove more organic debris and the redispersion of the material collected from the ashed preparation as a suspension into an additional liquid for redispersion. In the direct method, the tissue is digested with the material collected on the filter remaining in place throughout the additional treatment, thus avoiding additional manipulations and possible loss or disruption of asbestos bodies or fibers. This is critical because data on the basis of laboratory suspensions of pure chrysotile asbestos indicate fiber size distribution may be greatly affected by indirect preparation procedures with the greatest impact being an increased number of short fibers below 2.5 μm.[65] These would not be included in a count of fibers longer than 5 μm, although they may have been this length or longer in the tissue before the traumatic influence of the preparative procedures. Thus, the indirect method is suspect of splitting and fragmenting chrysotile fibers or bundles and, potentially, ferruginous bodies.

The original bleach digestion procedure[124] works well for some tissues, but the development of the modified version was deemed necessary to digest tissue with considerable mucus content, thus reducing the amount of residual tissue material trapped on the surface of the filter. This procedure also allows digestion of sputum and lavage material to the degree that ferruginous bodies and uncoated asbestos fibers can be quantified.[125,126] The use of a digested aliquot permits sampling of tissue with the least inherent variation in procedures that could contribute to sampling errors. The procedure used in our facility is to sample a portion of the aliquot for ferruginous body content of the tissue by collecting a measured amount of the solution on a mixed cellulose ester (MCE) filter. This membrane filter is easily cleared by acetone vapor resulting in a transparent film being left on the surface of a glass slide. This preparation can then be screened by light microscopy for identification of ferruginous bodies. It is critical that the core material of the ferruginous bodies be easily seen to distinguish asbestos bodies from nonasbestos ferruginous bodies. The data from this preparation provide the information used for determining ferruginous body numbers per gram of digested tissue. Such information can be compared with data from a given laboratory for tissue burden per gram wet or dry for tissue from the general population with findings from lung samples from individuals with defined asbestos exposures.

In the technique used in our laboratory, a second sample of the aliquot is passed through a smooth surfaced polycarbonate filter (0.2 μm pored). The material is prepared for evaluation by analytical transmission electron microscopy (ATEM). The pore size chosen for the collection of material is critical if one desires to include the thinner and shorter fibers in a count because considerable numbers of short and long, thin fibers in an aqueous solution can pass through a pore size as small as 0.4 μm in diameter.[127] The counterpoint is that if the digestion procedure selected has not dissolved the majority of the tissue components, the membrane will rapidly occlude even with a 0.4-μm pored filter. This is of concern when the objective of the preparation is to determine uncoated asbestos fiber burden in the tissue as the residue can easily obscure smaller, thinner fibers. This issue is of much less concern when the collection of material to be assessed is for asbestos body content because asbestos bodies are large and easily seen when compared with uncoated asbestos fibers. Selected filters from each polycarbonate lot should be screened for inherent contamination by TEM. These data are used as part of the basis for establishment of laboratory background levels for asbestos in a laboratory. Each solution used in the preparation of the tissue should be prefiltered before use to further protect against introduction of asbestos from nontissue sources. The use of a polycarbonate filter which has a smooth surface with defined pores as opposed to an irregular sur-faced MCE filter for collecting digestate material has recently been further supported by findings in the study of Webber et al.[128] Their study evaluated the performance of membrane filters used for TEM analysis of asbestos. They concluded that "unless substantial care is used in the collapsing of MCE filters with an acetone hot block, grid preparations can suffer and fiber recoveries can be compromised." They further observed that in some phases of etching, the surface of the MCE as part of the preparation for TEM sampling can lead to the loss of short fibers. The comparison of the MCE and the polycarbonate filters for TEM preparations resulted in their conclusion that the latter were favored because of advantages of "straightforward preparation, improved solvents, and reduced contamination" of the PC filters.

3.8 INSTRUMENTATION USE IN TISSUE ANALYSIS FOR ASBESTOS

A discussion regarding the use of the light microscope in determining asbestos burden in tissue requires description of several applications. First, sections cut from paraffin blocks can be mounted on glass slides and screened for ferruginous bodies in H&E or iron stained preparations. This is an insensitive method, and the evaluation of digested material by light microscopy for asbestos bodies on a filter is more sensitive because the content of much more tissue is evaluated. The use of light microscopy for determination of uncoated asbestos fibers collected from tissue is of limited to no value. Most inhaled fibers are below the level of resolution of the light microscope, and those seen can only be categorized as fibers because distinction between fiber types (asbestos and nonasbestos) cannot be made.[81] The more definitive instruments for asbestos fiber identification are the analytical scanning electron microscope (SEM) and the ATEM.

As pointed out in the Health Effects Institute report on Asbestos in Public and Commercial Buildings,[65] "the scanning electron microscope appears at first review to be a suitable instrument for analysis of fibers collected on a filter (in this case from air samples). SEMs are less costly than analytical transmission electron microscopes, specimen preparations are relatively simple, and they can be equipped with an x-ray energy dispersive analyzer for determination of elemental composi-tions of particles. They have an acceptable level of resolution to permit identification of the asbestos particles." It is not possible to provide a better description as to the limits of the SEM than provided in the Health Effects Institute report as quoted in the following: "Detection of a small asbestos fiber on the surface of an air filter, using any type of microscope, requires that both resolution and con-trast be sufficient. When the SEM is operated at high magnification, a compromise must be made between image resolution and the signal presented to the image-forming system. This compromise leads to a routine detectability for small diameter fibers on the viewing screen that is often only slightly better than that achieved in the PCOM (i.e., approximately 0.2 µm).[129–133] The full resolution of the instrument can be achieved; permitting the detection of the smallest asbestos fibers, but only if each field of view is photographed using a time exposure of about 1 min or more. To produce real-time images at the magnification required, the beam current must be increased, and at the required high-beam currents, the resolution is degraded.[134] Real-time operation is required because each fiber must be identified. The image quality can be improved by using heavy metals, such as gold, to coat the surface of the filter, but this coating compromises the interpretation of the x-ray spectra on which fiber identification is based and may even obscure objects on the filter. Energy dispersive x-ray analysis (EDXA) is the only technique available in the SEM by which fibers can be identi-fied. Identification of fibers by this technique alone has some serious limitations. The approximate chemical composition, derived from an EDXA spectrum, is frequently not sufficient to discrimi-nate between asbestos varieties and some other relatively common minerals.[135] In addition, when attempts are made to identify a fiber by the use of EDXA, contributions to the EDXA spectrum may be made by other particulates close to the fiber under examination. The composite EDXA spectrum thus obtained can lead to ambiguities in identification. Definitive identification of asbestos fibers can often be achieved only by a combination of chemical and electron diffraction data, and this combination of identification techniques is available only in the analytical TEM."[65]

The most accurate instrument for detecting and analyzing asbestos fiber types in a sample and appropriately providing their dimensions is the ATEM. The data derived from fibers collected on a membrane filter from an air sample or from a tissue preparation require the same levels of resolution and analytical interpretation provided only by the ATEM. The Asbestos Hazard Emergency Response Act (Title II of the Toxic Substance Control Act 15, U.S.C. Sections 2641–2654) defines ATEM as the "state-of-the-art" instrument and required the use of ATEM for final clearance in many abatement projects in schools. As of August 1, 1990, laboratories performing analysis for abatement clearance in U.S. schools were required to be accredited by the National Voluntary Laboratory Accreditation Program. This accreditation includes assurance that analysis by ATEM is done consistently and that other laboratories likewise use the same magnification for analysis, including the same dimension fibers in any count scheme, analyzing the fibers in the same way, and reporting the data in the same way. Another important part of the National Voluntary Laboratory Accreditation Program is that of quality assurance. Steps were described earlier as to how our laboratory carries out quality assurance to ensure analysis of the tissue is not altered because of contamination within the laboratory or from other sources. Once particulates to be analyzed, including asbestos fibers, are collected on a filter, it is irrelevant as to whether they are from air, water, or tissue. The only major difference is that considerable numbers of fibers can be lost (as per the concern of the indirect method of tissue preparation) or obscured on the filter surface by debris, thus preventing the analyst from detecting smaller particulates. The count scheme under the Asbestos Hazard Emergency Response Act includes structures (fibers) that are greater than or equal to 0.5 µm in length, have an aspect ratio of at least 5:1, and have parallel sides (in the case of fibers) for most of their length. The analysis includes defining the morphology, the elemental composition (EDXA), and the crystalline characteristics (selected area diffraction). This contrasts with the light microscope counting scheme where fibers counted are 5 µm or longer, have parallel sides for most of their length, and where there is no differentiation as to the type of fiber counted. The power of the ATEM to provide the most accurate information as to uncoated asbestos fiber burden in tissue is only as useful as the quality of the preparation permits and the utilization of the instrument at a sufficient magnification to permit detection of short and long, thin asbestos fibers. The analytical scheme of counting should include fibers below 5 µm, the population of fibers that make up the majority of fibers in human lung and extrapulmonary sites,[54,81,136] if the overall representation of fiber burden is to be achieved. To ignore fibers less than 5 µm in a count scheme provides a biased base of information that starts with a decision to exclude most chrysotile in air or tissue samples.

3.9 USEFULNESS OF SPUTUM AND LAVAGE AS INDICATORS OF PAST ASBESTOS EXPOSURE

Sputum is collected as phlegm produced as a normal process of clearance from the respiratory system. A marker of sputum as being from the deeper regions of the lung is the presence of pulmonary macrophages. As described in the section on clearance mechanisms, macrophages are capable of reaching the mucociliary escalator and bring associated (in the case of asbestos bodies) or ingested dust particles (smaller fibers) to the back of the throat for elimination via swallowing or expectoration. Sputum can be collected via spontaneous or induced methods. In the latter, a mist of salt water triggers a cough reflex to clear more sputum. Smokers produce more sputum, whereas nonsmokers are poor sputum producers. Asbestos bodies formed in the lung can be found in the mucus or macrophage-laden material in the sputum of occupationally exposed individuals. Greenberg et al.[137] evaluated asbestos body production in a group of former amosite workers for approximately a year. Sputa was screened cytologically. One-third of sputa samples from workers contained asbestos bodies that were most numerous in induced sputum samples. Bignon et al.[138] reported an absence of asbestos bodies in sputum when the asbestos body concentration in lung parenchyma was under 1000/cm^3. McLarty et al.,[139] in a further review of the amosite-exposed cohort, concluded that the presence of asbestos bodies in sputa was related to radiographic findings of interstitial fibrosis (asbestosis) and pleural fibrosis and to spirometric findings of restrictive lung disease. Age and cigarette smoking were also related to the number of asbestos bodies found in sputum samples. Modin et al.[140] reviewed the findings of asbestos bodies in sputa and bronchial washings obtained as screening in a general hospital/clinic setting and concluded that finding ferruginous bodies in either sample was a highly specific marker for past asbestos exposure and reflected the presence of a significant asbestos load within the lung. Paris et al.[141] reviewed three consecutive sputum samples collected from 270 retired workers in a textile and friction materials factory. In this study, 53% of samples were positive for ferruginous bodies. The authors concluded that the prevalence of asbestos bodies in sputa was not related to sex, smoking status, or latency.

Sebastien et al.[142] evaluated sputa samples from a cohort of vermiculite miners and millers who were exposed to ore that contained the amphibole tremolite as well as other fibrous amphiboles. Two sputa samples were collected from all but three of the 173 workers. Chest radiographs were scored according to the 1980 ILO classification. They reported that 75% of the workers had from "one to nearly 4000 asbestos bodies in their sputum, and their concentration in sputum and cumulative exposure (intensity × duration) were significantly related." The authors stated "the finding that the radiographic changes were better explained by the sputum index than by cumulative exposure."

Dodson et al.[143] determined asbestos body and uncoated asbestos fiber content in 12 randomly selected sputa samples from former amosite asbestos workers and 12 individuals from the general population with no history of asbestos exposure. The sputa was digested by the procedure previously described by Williams et al.,[123] after which samples were screened by light microscopy and TEM for asbestos bodies/fibers. The inconsistency of finding asbestos bodies in sputa, even from occupationally exposed individuals, was reflected in that none of the 12 sputa samples from former amosite workers contained asbestos bodies, nor were any asbestos bodies found in samples from the general population. However, 10 of 12 samples from the amosite group contained uncoated amosite fibers as detected by electron microscopic evaluation. One short chrysotile fiber was found in our sputum samples from the general population group. The finding of uncoated fibers and no asbestos bodies in sputa from exposed individuals was not surprising because asbestos bodies are larger and less easily brought upward by macrophages than uncoated fibers that are more easily carried upward in mucus or are moved upward within macrophages that have ingested the fibers. Screening for uncoated fibers by electron microscopy increased the sensitivity of sputa analysis for identifying past occupational exposure to asbestos.

The techniques for assessing the various content (including dust particles) in bronchoalveolar lavage (BAL) fluid were developed after the creation of the fiber-optic bronchoscope in the late 1960s. The technique by definition is "a procedure that recovers cellular and noncellular components from the epithelial surface of the lower respiratory tract and differs from bronchial washings that typically refer to aspiration of secretions or small amounts of instilled saline from the large airways."[144] The BAL technique provides clinicians a new mechanism by which they can sample the lung milieu and the free cells that populate the lower respiratory tract. Begin[145] reviewed the array of diseases about which additional information could be learned via application of the BAL technique, including those categorized as inflammatory and interstitial in nature. One particular application is the sampling of lower airway contents for dust particles.

De Vuyst et al.[146–149,156] provided much of our data concerning the usefulness of lavage assessment in asbestos-exposed individuals. A comparison of the asbestos body content of lavage material was made with content of lung samples from the same individuals, most of whom were undergoing thoracotomy procedures for lung cancer.[148] Their findings were the absence of or low asbestos body (AB) counts (<1 AB /mL BAL fluid) corresponded in about 70% of cases to concentrations of less than 1000 AB/g of dry lung tissue and in 100% of the cases to tissue concentrations of less than 10,000 AB/g. In subjects with BAL containing greater than 1 AB/mL of BAL, it was found that 85% of cases contained more than 1000 AB/g of dry lung tissue. Those individuals with greater than 10 AB/mL of BAL fluid were all found to contain lung burdens of greater than 10,000 AB/g of dry lung tissue. In an earlier companion study, the sensitivity of BAL fluid analysis for indicating past exposure to asbestos was supported; in the study, 28 of 28 individuals with obvious exposures were found to have ABs in lavage material.[147] Among 40 controls, only five were found to have ABs in BAL fluid, and the burden was reported to be 1 AB/mL of BAL fluid. De Vuyst et al.,[146] in another study that included assessment of BAL fluid from white-collar workers, blue-collar workers, and subjects with definite exposure to asbestos, found that ABs were a marker of exposure to asbestos and not an asbestos-induced disease. Asbestos bodies were more likely to be found in BAL fluid from "patients presenting with asbestos-related diseases but in whom exposure is not confirmed by the occupational history (65 of 78 cases)." Sebastien et al.[150] studied BAL fluid from 69 patients with suspected asbestos-related diseases who subsequently underwent lung biopsy or autopsy. They concluded that when the BAL fluid "exceeds 1 AB/mL, it can be quite confidently predicted, however, that the parenchymal concentration is in excess of 1000 AB/g (dry weight) and that the patient has experienced a nontrivial asbestos exposure."

Schwartz et al.[151] concluded that asbestos bodies found in lavage fluid are a reproducible assay for exposure but have little utility in most clinical settings to predict disease presence. Similarly, Oriowski et al.[152] found that the extent of pleural plaques correlated neither with frequency or duration of exposure nor to the number of asbestos bodies in BAL fluid in subjects free of lung parenchymal abnormalities determined by high-resolution computerized tomography. One must remember when reviewing the correlation of asbestos bodies in BAL fluid that they represent only a population of longer fibers (>8 µm) in the lung and tell nothing about the overall burden of longer, uncoated, or shorter asbestos fibers. Furthermore, asbestos-related diseases often occur long after first exposure and not infrequently a considerable time from last exposure. Thus, asbestos bodies in BAL fluid may confirm a level of past exposure to longer fibers but not offer insight to the quantity of the overall fiber burden in the past. Because asbestos bodies form months to years after exposure, their presence can be detected in BAL fluid long before the latency period required for the development of asbestos-induced diseases, for example, often 15–50 years. Asbestos bodies in BAL fluid through representation of a higher percentage of longer fibers in the lung indicates an increased likelihood of occupational exposure to asbestos because asbestos fibers found in general populations are usually short and uncoated.[153,154]

The information discussed to this point regarding past levels of asbestos exposure as determined from BAL fluid is based on asbestos body content determined by light microscopy. Additional information regarding past exposure can be obtained from BAL samples analyzed by electron microscopy just as the sensitivity of sputum samples is expanded when uncoated fiber composition is included in an analysis. Gellert et al.[155] compared findings by light and electron microscopy of BAL fluid from 15 subjects with exposure to asbestos, 3 of whom had clinical and radiological evidence of asbestosis compared with asbestos BAL fluid concentrations findings in 13 urban-dwelling control subjects. Asbestos fibers were confirmed in BAL fluid from 11 of 15 exposed persons ranging between 133 and 3700 fibers per milliliter of lavage fluid, with the range of asbestos bodies per milliliter of lavage fluid being 0–333. Five exposed subjects with no asbestos bodies detected by light microscopy were found to have uncoated asbestos fibers by electron microscopy (range = 133–2711 fibers/mL of lavage fluid). Only one sample from the control group was found to have a "few" asbestos fibers in the BAL fluid.

The use of BAL fluid has been shown to be of value for assessment of exposures to particular fiber types, including exposures in secondary settings.[156] These include lavage material analyzed from a woman (household contact) with bilateral pleural and diaphragmatic plaques whose only source of exposure was while washing the clothing of her husband who had been an asbestos sprayer. The second individual had been a coal miner for much of his adult life. The presence of crocidolite fibers in the lavage material was attributed to the individual's daily use of personal protection masks during work in the coal mine. These masks were reported to have been used from 1920 to 1970 and contained crocidolite. The third case was of a mason who for 44 years lived in a region of Turkey where exposure to tremolite, as found in his lavage material, was known to occur as a result of environmental exposures. The final case consisted of an individual who had "all of the possible asbestos-related diseases except lung cancer." These were attributed to a short but intense exposure that had occurred 47–51 years before the diagnosis of the specific diseases. Dodson et al.[98] found ferruginous bodies formed on a variety of particulates inhaled by foundry workers. These included fibrous and nonfibrous structures. The most common nonasbestos cores of elongated ferruginous bodies consisted of sheet silicates, graphite (carbon), and iron-rich fibers. Dodson et al.[157] reported that the greatest specificity is obtained for correlating past exposures to asbestos by using a combination of light microscopic quantitation of asbestos bodies correlated with the uncoated asbestos fiber burden as determined by ATEM evaluation of BAL fluid samples.

The high incidence of malignant mesothelioma in villages in Turkey (Tuzkoy/ Cappadocia) has been considered a result of environmental exposure to erionite, which is found as a fibrous mineral in the local soil.[158] Dumortier et al.[159] evaluated BAL fluid from 16 subjects originating from Tuzkoy. The authors found ferruginous bodies in 12 subjects. Erionite was the central fiber of 95.7% of the ferruginous bodies while erionite fibers were found in the bronchoalveolar lavage fluid in all subjects. They concluded that the mean concentration of erionite fibers in lavage fluid was similar to that of tremolite fibers in Turks with environmental exposure to tremolite. These exposures illustrate an example of a nonasbestos, naturally occurring fibrous mineral that is considered as a causal agent for mesothelioma in man. Fibrous zeolites (erionite) occur in certain regions of the United States; however, these are mostly in areas with low population density. Recently, Kliment et al.[160] reported a mesothelioma case with appreciable erionite content in the lung tissue. The work history in the case indicated an approximate 2-year history of possible exposure to dust from floor tiles while working in "janitorial and maintenance services." The individual lived for 20–25 years in Mexico. There were no specific erionite exposures defined, although the implication is that the individual's exposure may have been from environmental sources in previous residencies, including in Mexico. The findings in this case included plaques and abundance of ferruginous bodies within lung tissue. The digested material contained elevated levels of ferruginous bodies and uncoated erionite structures. There were no "commercial or noncommercial" asbestos fibers reportedly found in the tissue.

De Vuyst et al.[161] evaluated BAL from six talc workers with pneumoconiosis. Two were defined as mainly exposed to American and Australian talc, and the other four were defined as exposed to French talc (Luzenac). The authors stated: "Talc particles and talc bodies were abundant, sometimes many years after the end of exposure. A qualitative difference was the presence of tremolite asbestos fibres in the two patients exposed to American and Australian talc and its absence in the four French talc workers. The presence of tremolite in lavage is attributed to a geological association of this mineral with the inhaled talc." The authors concluded that lavage "can confirm exposure to talc and provide information about the heterogeneity of inhaled dust."

In another study, the lavaged individuals worked in a cement manufacturing facility that used chrysotile and crocidolite as reflected in the content and type of uncoated asbestos fiber burden in their BAL fluid. A unique observation was obtained when analysis of lavage material was carried out by light and electron microscopic assessment from 15 brake lining workers considered to be only exposed to chrysotile and 44 asbestos cement workers exposed extensively to amphiboles.[162] As indicated by the authors, the literature is replete with references that chrysotile does not readily stimulate the formation of asbestos bodies (Figure 3.21).[162] However, analysis of BAL fluid indicated that an exposure to asbestos among brake lining factory workers occurred for longer fibers of chrysotile because 95.6% of the cores of asbestos bodies were chrysotile. This contrasted with 93.1% of cores of asbestos bodies that were formed on amphiboles analyzed from BAL fluid from

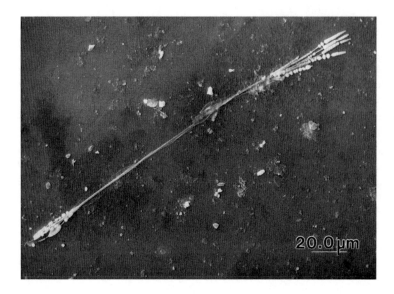

Figure 3.21   Although chrysotile cored ferruginous bodies are less common than those formed on amphibole cores, when longer fibers of chrysotile are inhaled the formation on such cores can occur as indicated in this micrograph. The beaded material representing the ferruginous coating is primarily located on the frayed ends of the fibers.

asbestos cement workers. A similar observation of chrysotile-cored ferruginous bodies in BAL fluid and lung tissue was found in our laboratory. Lung tissue evaluation from an individual with a unique asbestos exposure during work as a clutch rebuilder indicated the presence of longer fibers of chrysotile and the majority of asbestos bodies found in the lung tissue sample (77.2%) being formed on chrysotile asbestos cores.[163]

Recent publications[164–167] emphasized that brake dust contained predominately short chrysotile fibers, with most fibers being less than 5 µm. This suggests that exposure to brake dust would not be expected to result in asbestos body formation because, as previously stated, asbestos bodies form on longer fibers usually greater than 8 µm. However, disturbance of friction products during some activities can result in inhalation of longer fibers as verified by the presence of chrysotile-cored ferruginous bodies in lavage materials[162] and in tissue.[163]

The status of existing data regarding evaluation of BAL samples for the presence of asbestos provides the basis of the synopsis offered by Sartorelli et al.,[168] who stated that "fiber concentration in BALF can be considered as a reliable biomarker of past asbestos exposure, even many years after the end of exposure."

3.10 ASBESTOS BODY BURDEN IN EXPOSED AND GENERAL POPULATIONS

The asbestos body as a marker of past exposure to asbestos has been discussed in the context of its presence in tissue sections. A more sensitive method of assessing tissue samples for asbestos bodies is by sampling larger amounts of tissue via digestion techniques. The digested material is collected on a thin membrane (filter) and after being made transparent, as previously described, can be subjected to screening by light microscopy. The numbers of asbestos bodies found can be extrapolated to the numbers per gram of wet or dry tissue. Some earlier works combining light and electron microscopy for determining the numbers of asbestos bodies per gram of tissue and core identification were carried out by Churg and Warnock.[96,115,169–171] Their observations in tissues from individuals considered as representing the general population from larger cities led them to "arbitrarily consider 100 bodies to be the division between 'environmental' and 'occupational' exposure."[171] If one chooses to use a multiplier of 10 to approximate asbestos bodies per gram of dry weight, then the number would be 1000 per gram dry weight for nonoccupational exposures. These two numbers have been referenced as a "break point" that separates occupational from non-occupational levels of exposure to asbestos as defined by tissue burdens.[171,172] The report by the ERS Working Group[121] appropriately notes, "the dry to wet weight ratio varies from 5–20% and should be measured for each sample. The use of a mean conversion factor of 10 for the wet/dry ratio should be avoided." Data from our own experience indicate that the number of asbestos bodies in the non-occupationally exposed general population per gram of wet tissue is 0–20 asbestos bodies,[153,154,174] which is more in keeping with reference levels in general populations as reported by Breedin and Buss[175] and by Roggli et al.[176]

Churg and Warnock[169] analyzed core material of ferruginous bodies by ATEM in 23 autopsy and surgical patients, none of whom had occupational asbestos exposure. Of the 328 bodies examined, 264 (80%) had diffraction patterns consistent with amphibole asbestos whereas only 6 had chrysotile cores. In a separate study of 144 asbestos bodies isolated from 29 persons with fewer than 100 asbestos bodies per gram of wet lung tissue (below occupational levels)[170] ana-lyzed by electron diffraction, 143 were found to be formed on amphiboles whereas only 1 was formed on a chrysotile core. Chemical analysis by XEDA was used to further define the types of amphiboles. Twenty-one were determined to be formed on amosite or crocidolite cores, 13 on anthophyllite asbestos cores, and 1 on a tremolite asbestos core. Commercial amphiboles were the dominant cores of asbestos bodies in men (86%), whereas 57% of the asbestos bodies analyzed from women were formed on anthophyllite or tremolite cores. Cosmetic talc was sug-gested as the source of these "noncommercial" types of asbestos fibers in the women within the studies.[96,170]

Roggli et al.[176] studied asbestos body concentrations as related to types of asbestos-induced dis-eases. The highest numbers of asbestos bodies per gram of tissue were in individuals with asbestosis (≥2000 AB/g wet tissue). Intermediate levels were found in individuals with malignant mesotheli-oma and the lowest in patients with pleural plaques. As in other studies, the majority of the cores of asbestos bodies were on amphiboles. The explanation of why amphibole cores were most common is that amphiboles, being straight fibers, tend to be more readily inhaled in a longer form than chrys-otile. However, when longer fibers of chrysotile are readily available and inhaled, chrysotile cores of asbestos bodies are not uncommon. As stated previously, appreciable numbers of chrysotile-cored asbestos bodies were reported in BAL fluid from brake lining workers.[162]

Moulin et al.[177] analyzed cores of ferruginous bodies in 19 asbestos-exposed individuals and 25 nonexposed urban dwellers from the Belgium urban population. Of the 319 ferruginous bodies analyzed, 315 were formed on asbestos. The nonasbestos cores were on talc and crystalline silica. Eighty-two percent of the asbestos cores were commercial amphiboles (amosite/crocidolite) and 7% were formed on chrysotile cores. The remaining 3.8% were formed on noncommercial amphi-boles (anthophyllite/tremolite). In each study, some ferruginous bodies were totally coated and not capable of being analyzed by XEDA or selected area diffraction.

Holden and Churg[178] examined ferruginous body content from lungs of chrysotile miners and found that 64% of the cores were formed on chrysotile and 29% formed on amphiboles, although the amphiboles (tremolite and actinolite) constituted the majority of uncoated fibers in these cases. Levin et al.[179] reported a case of a clutch refabricator where 72% of the ferruginous bodies were formed on chrysotile asbestos cores (Figure 3.21).

An ideal model for determining tissue burden of asbestos fibers would be to develop a multiplier of the number of more easily seen ferruginous bodies (as determined by light microscopy) and extrapolate the concentration of uncoated asbestos fibers from this number. Such an effort is an exercise in futility as the ratio varies widely as does the efficiency for ferruginous body formation between individuals.[90,104,179–181]

For example, Srebro et al.[182] evaluated the tissue content of ferruginous bodies in 18 cases of mesothelioma compared with 19 "control" cases. The data, when combining uncoated asbestos burden, indicated that six mesothelioma cases might be asbestos-related despite asbestos body counts similar to those in the samples from the general population. A prudent recommendation was offered that "electron microscopic analysis of pulmonary mineral fibers may be required to differentiate asbestos-related mesotheliomas from nonasbestos-related cases when asbestos body counts are within the range of background values."

However, asbestos body burden is elevated in many occupationally exposed individuals, given that longer fibers reach the lower airways and thus provide a stimulus for coating as per the described data from our laboratory. In a group of 55 occupationally exposed asbestos individuals with mesothelioma, 46 had concentrations of asbestos bodies above 1000/g dry weight of lung tissue.[180] Of 841 ferruginous bodies analyzed, 781 (92.9%) were formed on amosite, 24 (2.9%) on crocidolite, 8 (1%) on tremolite, 3 (0.4%) on anthophyllite, 3 (0.4%) on actinolite, and 1 (0.1%) on chrysotile cores. Eleven (1.3%) of the ferruginous bodies were formed on nonasbestos cores and 10 (1.2%) were totally coated or successful analysis of the core material could not be achieved. Seven of 15 cases of women with mesotheliomas evaluated in another study had over 1000 asbestos bodies per gram.

Ferruginous body quantitation was carried out in 19 cases of individuals with a prior history of occupational asbestos exposure and lung cancer. The ferruginous body content in 11 cases was found to be over 1000 asbestos bodies per gram of dry tissue.[183] Three individuals lung tissue did not contain asbestos bodies (within limits of detectability of the study), and two were found to have concentrations at general population levels. One individual did not have detectable levels of asbestos fibers, although lung tissue from the remaining four contained asbestos fibers.

As mentioned earlier, asbestos bodies are not readily formed in some individuals although their lung tissue contains elevated numbers of longer asbestos fibers[182,184] suitable for iron–protein coating. The absence of detectable levels of ferruginous bodies implies little regarding the presence of chrysotile in the majority of samples. This suggests that the number of uncoated asbestos fibers found in tissue is independently important as an indicator of exposure/causation of asbestos-induced disease.[185]

Asbestos bodies have also been reported in colonic tissue from an insulation worker with asbestosis[186]; however, the question exists as to whether the fibers reached the area by ingestion of sputa, which contained the ferruginous bodies/asbestos fibers originally deposited within the lungs, or were relocated via some other route to the site of the tumor.

An excellent study was published recently that focused on the determination of the epigenetic profiles that distinguish pleural mesothelioma from normal pleura and predict lung asbestos burden and clinical outcome.[187] The authors conducted an elaborate investigation but took liberty to use their findings of asbestos bodies per gram as interchangeable with the overall asbestos burden. Although the increased numbers of ferruginous bodies may indeed be a predictor of mesothelioma, their presence only represents one small component of the overall asbestos burden in tissue. Asbestos bodies represent a selective population of the longer fibers (if the individual coats fibers) and tell us nothing regarding the number of shorter fibers (including most chrysotile in lung) and uncoated longer/thinner fibers that are less likely to coat. It thus remains for the uncoated asbestos burden to be defined before the story is complete.

3.11 UNCOATED ASBESTOS FIBERS IN OCCUPATIONALLY EXPOSED INDIVIDUALS AND IN LUNG TISSUE FROM THE GENERAL POPULATION

To evaluate uncoated asbestos fiber concentrations in tissue, it is imperative there is a clear understanding of what techniques were used to obtain asbestos concentration data. The resolution of the light microscope coupled with its lack of ability to distinguish fiber types greatly limits it usefulness in assessing fiber concentration in tissue. Even in the most ideal settings where tissue has been destroyed and there is minimal obstruction of fibers from view, only a small percent are detectable by light microscopic examination. Morgan and Holmes[188] reported that approximately one-half of uncoated fibers would have been detected by light microscopy. Ashcroft and Heppleston[113] reported that only 12%–30% of uncoated asbestos fibers from tissue samples in their study were visible by light microscopy. Rood and Streeter[189] compared the detection capabilities of light microscopy versus those of scanning and TEM for chrysotile fibers collected on a filter. All fibers (100%) would have been counted and analyzed by the transmission electron microscope, 60% by SEM, and only 25% of fibers greater than 5 µm long would have been identified with the light microscope (Figures 3.22 and 3.23). The data from our publications[101,179,180,183] generally agrees with the range for optically detectable fibers reported by Ashcroft and Heppleston[113] and by Rood and Streeter,[189] except when the population of asbestos fibers in a tissue sample is predominantly short and/or long, thin fibers.[54,104,136,190]

In such cases when the fiber burden is represented by chrysotile and crocidolite, the number of fibers detected by light microscopy is often 0%. Pooley and Ranson[191] correctly stated: "It is possible, using the electron microscope, to predict the asbestos fibre count that would be obtained by light microscopy, the reverse prediction cannot be made: it is impossible to determine the proportion of the various asbestos minerals types using the light microscope." A referral to our laboratory[192] further emphasizes the need to recognize what one "sees" with a given technique and at a given magnification with a specific instrument. A portion of a block of tissue was evaluated by SEM at relatively low magnification and the referring individual wanted to determine the findings via a high magnification evaluation by ATEM. The earlier assessment had evaluated fiber burden at 1000× and included only those fibers <5 µm in the count scheme. The individual had been reported to have had a work history that would have been expected to have specifically included chrysotile dust. One fiber that was considered to be chrysotile was found by SEM. The sheer numbers of short chrysotile fibers (>0.5 µm) and a count scheme at high magnification by ATEM that permitted their detection necessitated a modified count scheme consisting of a reduced count area from the total area we would usually review. Three very small chrysotile-cored ferruginous bodies were also found. Only three of the individual chrysotile fibers <5 µm were not in the form of fibrils. Only 7% of all lengths

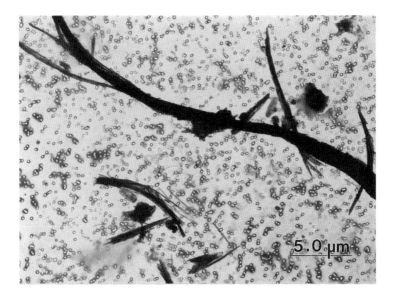

Figure 3.22 Bundles of chrysotile asbestos obtained from new brake components are shown in this field. The tendency is evident for the bundles to disassociate into smaller and smaller units, which indicate the potential that many of these units would be below the level of detection in the light microscope analysis of air samples.

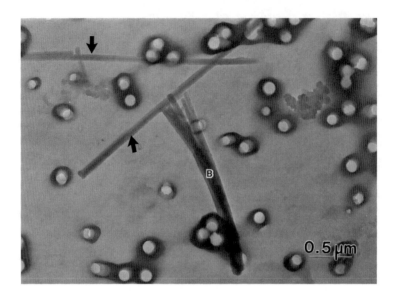

Figure 3.23   Neither the fibrils (arrows) of chrysotile asbestos seen in this field nor the bundle (B) would have been counted in a typical phase contrast light microscope counting scheme. The former because the fibrils are too thin to be detected in the light microscope and the latter in that the bundle is shorter than the 5-μm length included in 7400 count scheme of "fibers." This provides an example of the problems of interpreting environmental exposures or tissue burdens when large populations of fibers are excluded because of the limits of the count scheme or the magnification/resolution of the instrument of choice.

of chrysotile fibers were not fibrils (0.02–0.05 μm in diameter); thus, length is not the only determinate for detection of a fiber. This illustrates the importance of clearly understanding what is being used to evaluate a sample of fibers from tissue, air, or water and what is being included in a count as well as what is potentially there but not "seen" or included in the count scheme.[193]

In discussing uncoated fiber burden in tissue, it seems reasonable, on the basis of the aforementioned reasons, to compare data obtained by TEM to that generated via similar techniques. It is important to compare data generated at sufficient magnification and with a count scheme that includes "short" and long/thin asbestos fibers, as this population makes up the vast majority of asbestos fibers in lung tissue and extrapulmonary sites.[54,104,191–193]

Some of the earliest contributions using ATEM for analysis of tissue digestion from "control populations" were contributed from the research by Churg et al. In a study of individuals from the San Francisco area, Churg and Warnock[115] reported that "80% of uncoated fibers were chrysotile (mean: 130×10^3) with a range of 12×10^3 to 680×10^3 fibers per gram wet lung and 90% of chrysotile fibers less than 5 μm long." Total amphiboles had a mean of 25×10^3 and ranged from 1.3×10^3 to 75×10^3 fibers per gram wet lung tissue. Ninety-five percent were noncommercial amphiboles and two-thirds were less than 5 μm long. Approximately 20% of amosite, crocidolite, and anthophyllite fibers identified were longer than 10 μm. They concluded the following: (1) substantial amounts of asbestos, mainly chrysotile and noncommercial amphiboles, are present in the average lung in an urban environment; (2) most of these fibers are too small to form asbestos bodies or to be visible by light microscopy; (3) asbestos bodies may serve as some indication of exposure to long amphiboles but offer no information about the bulk of fibers present; and (4) it is probable that most of these fibers reflect general environmental contamination.

In a subsequent tissue study of individuals residing in Vancouver, British Columbia, Churg and Wiggs[16] reported the mean chrysotile burden to be "only" 0.2×10^6 g of dry lung when compared with approximately 1.0×10^6 g of dry lung in San Francisco. A possible difference was explained by known outcrops containing chrysotile asbestos in the San Francisco Bay area that might contribute to environmental exposures. However, the conclusion offered was that the majority of fiber types are "more or less the same in both cities."

Langer et al.,[194] in a study involving 28 individuals who resided in New York City, found chrysotile to be present in 24 cases with the other four being considered potentially "positive" by occurrence of background fibril contamination. Langer concluded that unaltered chrysotile is uncommonly found as the core in asbestos bodies removed from lung samples from general populations. The authors correctly stated that the vast majority of chrysotile structures in the lungs of the general population are "fibrillar units" and require ATEM for detection. The same is true from our experience for chrysotile structures isolated from lungs and extrapulmonary tissue from occupationally exposed individuals. In another study, Langer and Nolan[195] evaluated lung burden by ATEM of 126 autopsy cases of persons who died in New York City from 1966 through 1968. They considered 107 of the 126 cases to "probably" be nonoccupationally exposed. Their important observations were that "virtually all the chrysotile in nonoccupationally exposed persons was composed of short fibrils, most equal to or less than 1 μm in length, with the modal class between 0.2 and 0.5 μm." They further concluded that "analysis of selected fibers showed preservation of both chemistry and structure. It would appear, therefore, that in occupational exposure to chrysotile not only are doses higher, but the proportion of longer fibers is greater than in the chrysotile to which the general population is exposed."

Data from our own laboratory tend in many ways to agree with the early studies of Churg and Warnock.[115] The definition of a member of the general population used in our laboratory is that the individual has not been involved in a known asbestos-related work activity, has no disease conditions which may have been caused by asbestos, and has 20 or less (our general population number) asbestos bodies per gram of wet lung tissue. In a study by Dodson et al.,[153] 35% of uncoated asbestos fibers from 33 individuals considered as from the general population were chrysotile and 86% were <5 μm long.[153] Also, 83% of amphiboles in this study were noncommercial amphiboles and 73% of these were <5 μm long. The most commonly found asbestos fiber was chrysotile, which was observed in 14 cases, with anthophyllite being found in 12 cases. Of the 33 cases, 26 cases had no ferruginous bodies detected by light microscopy. Of the 33 individuals, 10 were not found to have asbestos fibers in their lung tissue (within the limit of detection in the procedure). The geometric mean of fiber length for each asbestos type found was less than 3 μm. An additional study of lung samples from 15 individuals considered as representing the general population[154] confirmed the findings from the earlier study. Only four individuals were found to contain asbestos bodies, and only two individuals' lung tissue contained an asbestos fiber in their lung digest (within limits of detection used in the study). In conclusion, our findings indicate that lung tissue from the general population contains low numbers of asbestos fibers. If detected, these fibers will likely be short chrysotile or noncommercial amphibole fibers. When commercial amphiboles are found, the fibers are short (<5 μm) and few in numbers. When a lung tissue sample contains appreciable numbers of asbestos fibers, long fibers, and/or commercial amphiboles (amosite or crocidolite), the suggestion is that the individual had an occupational or paraoccupational/bystander exposure to asbestos.

Additional data exist regarding asbestos burden in tissue from occupationally exposed individuals. As mentioned earlier, the chrysotile form of asbestos constituted 90%–95% of asbestos used in commercial applications in the United States. However, chrysotile veins have been reported to be "contaminated" with amphiboles, particularly actinolite, anthophyllite, tremolite, and more recently crocidolite.[196] Quebec chrysotile, which constituted the majority of chrysotile used in the United States, has been stated to have between 1% and 6.9% amphibole asbestos.[197,198] Tremolite has been suggested by McDonald et al.[199] as a "valid marker" for exposure to chrysotile asbestos. This same suggestion was made in a study by Churg[200] of nine chrysotile miners with "asbestos airway disease" (so-called "early asbestosis") but with no evidence of classic asbestosis (interstitial fibrosis) on pathological examination. The findings indicated a strong correlation between the amount of chrysotile and amphibole, suggesting that the amphibole (tremolite) component was a good measure of original (but no longer) chrysotile burden because of the more rapid clearance of the latter. In 1988, Churg[72] reviewed the literature on chrysotile, tremolite, and mesothelioma in man. Dr. Churg opined "induction of mesothelioma by chrysotile requires, on average, as great a lung fiber burden as induction of asbestosis by chrysotile, whereas amphibole (amosite or crocidolite)-induced mesotheliomas appear at several hundred fold smaller lung burden." In an additional study, Churg et al.[201] found that high tremolite fiber concentration was strongly associated with mesothelioma, airway fibrosis, and asbestosis in a study involving chrysotile miners and millers from Thetford Mines in Quebec. Pleural plaques and carcinoma of the lung were reported to show no relationship to tremolite burden.

Churg et al.[202] measured tissue burden by ATEM from 20 shipyard and insulation workers. The findings in this study indicated "amosite concentration, like chrysotile and tremolite concentration, is closely and directly related to fibrosis at the local lung level." The authors raised an important issue often ignored by those using counting schemes where only longer fibers (>5 µm) are counted, in the "possibility that short fibers may be more important than is commonly believed in the genesis of fibrosis in man." They also expressed their belief that an amosite fiber was more fibrogenic than a chrysotile or tremolite fiber and that tremolite was more fibrogenic than chrysotile.

McDonald et al.[203] concluded "that amphibole fibers could explain most mesothelioma cases in Canada and other inorganic fibers, including chrysotile, very few. Fibrous tremolite, contaminant of many industrial minerals including chrysotile, probably explained most cases in the Quebec (mesothelioma) mining and perhaps 20% elsewhere."

A study consisting of tissue evaluation of "young adults with mesothelioma" was reported by McDonald et al.[204] The project consisted of evaluating tissue from British mesothelioma cases where, because of the age group, "it was thought that most, but not all, work-related exposures would have been since 1970, when the importation of crocidolite, but not amosite, was virtually eliminated." The concentrations in the lung of "crocidolite and amosite fibers, which together could account for 80–90% of the cases, did not differ between occupational categories; those for amosite were appreciably higher than for crocidolite. Tremolite fibers were rarely found." "Contrary to expectation, however, some 90% of cases were in men who had started work before 1970."

Dufresne et al.[205] evaluated lung parenchymal samples by light microscopy and ATEM from 50 workers seeking compensation from the Workers' Compensation Board of Quebec for pleural or peritoneal mesothelioma. The group consisted of 12 from the Asbestos Township, 11 from Thetford Mines (mining and milling activities), and 27 from other types of industry (including asbestos factory, shipyard, and others). Data were compared with that obtained from a reference population. The fiber types in the three groups were different: "The lungs of workers from the Thetford Mines containing only chrysotile and tremolite; those from Asbestos Township containing chrysotile, tremolite, amosite, and crocidolite; and those from other industries containing largely amosite and crocidolite." They concluded that the "fiber types responsible for the tumors are probably different in the three different groups" and that "fiber analysis confirmed occupational asbestos exposure in every case."

An additional study from Churg's laboratory involved a cohort consisting of 144 shipyard workers and insulators from the Pacific Northwest. The major residual fiber type in the lungs from these individuals was amosite, and the lung tissue in most cases contained tremolite and chrysotile fibers.[206] Interestingly, the authors reported that "crocidolite fibers were found in only a very few cases, usually in quite small numbers, and have been excluded from all analysis." This indicates that the exposure to the second most commonly used form of "commercial amphibole," crocidolite, was minimal as reflected in the tissue burden of shipyard workers and insulators. The conclusion from the study was that mesothelioma occurred at much lower lung tissue amosite concentration than did asbestosis, which was in contrast to their conclusion for chrysotile-induced mesothelioma.

A study of lung tissue from former asbestos miners and millers from Thetford Mines and Asbestos regions was carried out by Nayebzadeh et al.[207] There were higher concentrations of tremolite asbestos in lung tissues from the Thetford Mines workers compared with workers from the Asbestos region. Fiber burden was categorized in three sizes: (1) those less than 5 μm long, (2) those greater than 5 μm and less than 10 μm long, and (3) those greater than 10 μm long. The conclusion from review of data was that "no consistent and biologically important difference was found for fiber dimension; therefore, fiber dimension does not seem to be a factor that accounts for the difference in incidence of respiratory diseases between the two groups." "The greater incidence of respiratory diseases among workers of Thetford Mines can be explained by the fact that they had greater exposure to fibers than did workers at the Asbestos region. Among the mineral fibers studied, retention of tremolite fibers was most apparent."

Langer and Nolan[208] reviewed lung tissue from 53 asbestos-exposed workers and one person with secondary exposure. They concluded that amosite was the most prevalent fiber, occurring in 74% of the specimens, with amosite always being found in the lungs of insulators and chrysotile found in only 50% of this group. Crocidolite was found in 24% of this group and increased to 40% of the workers with shipyard exposure. Langer and McCaughey[209] reported that the lung tissue from an individual with pleural mesothelioma and a work history of brake repair was found to contain chrysotile structures. Fibrils less than 1 μm and others longer than 5 μm were present. They noted that the findings were consistent with those of Pooley et al.[210] in that long fibrils have been frequently encountered in lung tissues from occupationally exposed workers[209] but not in persons with only environmental exposure. Ten percent of the fibrils were longer than 10 μm.

One early study from our laboratory emphasized the importance in some cases of assessing not only the asbestos body burden when defining past levels of asbestos exposure but also the uncoated asbestos fiber burden.[184] Analysis of lung tissue from 12 former amosite workers showed 10 with over 1000 ferruginous bodies per gram of dry tissue, whereas no ferruginous bodies were detected in the digest of the other two samples. This was an unexpected finding in that amosite can be readily inhaled in a longer form and is often found as the core of asbestos bodies in occupationally exposed individuals. The initial explanation was that individuals had relatively short exposure (0.5 and 3.3 months), although that exposure was known to be in very dusty occupations. Two samples from the individuals' tissue when analyzed by electron microscopy showed 1.2 and 2.1 million fibers per gram of tissue, respectively. Thus, even with the proper length (>8 μm) and considerable numbers of fibers being present in the lung, the individuals' lungs were apparently not efficient in coating the fibers. The importance of combining data for asbestos body content and uncoated asbestos fibers is further supported in the evaluation of an individual from a group of shipyard workers[104] who was not found to have chrysotile in his lung tissue. When tissue from his lymph node and pleural plaque was analyzed by ATEM, there were 21,000,000 chrysotile fibers per gram of dry tissue in the pleural plaque and 5,500,000 chrysotile fibers per gram of dry tissue in the lymph node. This finding suggests the efficiency of chrysotile clearance from lung tissue.

Amosite asbestos was found in lung tissue from 53 of 55 persons with mesothelioma whose tissue was evaluated by ATEM[180], with 39 patients having greater than 200,000 amosite fibers per gram dry weight of tissue. The geometric mean length of the amosite fibers was 13 μm, which contrasted with that found in lung tissue samples from the general population where amosite fibers are usually less than 5 μm. Forty-three percent of patients' lung tissue contained chrysotile asbestos and 40% contained crocidolite asbestos. Tremolite was the most commonly found of the "noncommercial" amphiboles (33 cases), whereas actinolite and anthophyllite were each found in 21 cases. There was no evidence chrysotile was the source of tremolite in that 11 of the patients had both, but 13 persons whose lungs contained tremolite had no detectable chrysotile. These findings contrast with the suggestion of Srebro and Roggli[211] that tremolite is "nearly ubiquitous and represents the most common amphibole fiber in the lungs of urbanites." The link, statistically, could be more easily made for chrysotile accounting for the amosite compared with the relationship of chrysotile to tremolite. Only a small percent of each type of asbestos would have been detected by light microscopy even of longer fibers of asbestos (based on diameter). In our mesothelioma study,[180] 26 of 55 patients did not have pathologic asbestosis, although most had appreciable ferruginous bodies and uncoated fiber burden.

Tissue from another group of mesothelioma cases from various regions in the United States was evaluated for the presence and numbers of ferruginous bodies and uncoated asbestos fibers.[212] The information generated was compared with that in the earlier 55 case study[180] that predominately consisted of individuals who had either worked in shipyards, related industries, or lived in adjacent areas to shipyard centers. There were 26 cases in this study that had over 1000 ferruginous bodies per gram of dry tissue. The most common form of asbestos found in this group (as in the 55 group study) was amosite (74%), which was less than the 94% positives in the earlier study. The second and third most common forms of asbestos were anthophyllite (61%) and tremolite (52%), whereas the other commercial forms of asbestos—crocidolite and chrysotile—were found in 43% and 50%, respectively.

There are reports that the presence of tremolite in the lungs of miners and millers "probably" reflects high burden in these cohorts[213] and that the tremolite component has been suggested to be an important contributor to the development of asbestos-related diseases in the mining region of Quebec.[199,214] Thus, much has been made as to the role tremolite has in inducing diseases among miners and millers in Canada.

A consideration of the impact of tremolite as a "contaminate" of chrysotile has been considered by Finkelstein[215] in an evaluation of data regarding chrysotile/amphibole burden in the lung tissue of brake mechanics as reported by Butnor et al.[164] The findings by Butnor et al.[164] essentially reported an appreciable amphibole (commercial amphibole in some cases) component in the lungs from these individuals whose work history was as brake mechanics (with friction products usually being manufactured with a chrysotile component). The assessment by Finkelstein[215] led him to conclude that the levels of tremolite in the lung tissue of brake mechanics could be explained from exposure to "dusts from friction products manufactured from Canadian chrysotile," which as previously noted contains appreciable tremolite (as per the studies of the lungs of chrysotile miners and millers).

Various agencies grapple with the definition of a "cleavage fragment" versus a fibrous form of the same mineral based, in part, on defining a "regulated fiber" under the asbestos regulations. There are clearly political, legal, and economic issues driving this discussion as clearly described in an article reviewing the chrysotile/tremolite relationship as written by a Canadian researcher, Dr. Bruce Case.[216,217] Ultimately, the question from a health effect perspective becomes not what is regulated but whether it causes disease in man when inhaled. The Canadian experience would strongly argue that the answer regarding tremolite is "yes." In fact, Dr. Case[216] stated that the relationship of chrysotile and tremolite in Canadian chrysotile products caused him at one point to favor a compound phrase "chrysotile/tremolite" to describe mined material and the products containing Canadian chrysotile. Dr. Case clearly defines the fact that the issue of tremolite fiber versus tremolite "cleavage fragment" is a distinction often defined by the mineralogists or regulators. The implication for all of those without a locked fixation on length, aspect ratio, and diameter of a structure being the predictor for risk of inducing disease overlooks the obvious question posed by Dr. Case if the reaction within a cell or a biosystem discriminates that the mineral form is a "cleavage fragment" from reactions with a fiber of the same general dimensions. His point is well taken in questioning if "potentially affected cells can distinguish between *asbestiform* and *nonasbestiform* fibres having equivalent dimensions."[217] In fact, the discussion in the United States has resulted in numerous industry sponsored "studies" or publications over the last several years focusing on the definition of a "nonasbestiform" entity and emphasizing it is not regulated as such under the Asbestos Standard as a "regulated fiber." In addition, an argument is often offered that exposures of cohorts to these "nonregulated" structures are not available for assessment of elevated occurrence of diseases. Realistically, exposure in the United States and in other parts of the world to "cleavage fragments" of minerals and the fibrous forms of the same minerals may occur simultaneously as well as exposures to other mixed dusts in the work place/environment. However, there does seem to be a concurrence in Canada among several researchers that tremolite is a major concern for causation of disease in chrysotile miners and millers, as previously discussed. The emphasis of a study by Williams-Jones et al.[218] described the relationship of chrysotile veins with other fibrous minerals, including tremolite, in the mining areas. They conducted evaluations of the Jeffrey mine in Asbestos, Quebec, and found the presence of amphibole group minerals: anthophyllite, cummingtonite, hornblend, and tremolite actinolite. "The bulk of the amphibole, however, was in the form of tremolite and actinolite, and was found mainly in sepentinite adjacent to or included within felsic dykes. Appreciable quantities of amphibole also are present in pyroxenite (tremolite) and slate (actinolite) in contact with serpentinite distal to the ore zones. Significantly, the chrysotile ores are essentially amphibole free. Most of the amphibole is fibrous, but a small proportion is asbestiform according to criteria established by the U.S. Occupational Safety and Health Administration." Therefore, if the exposure to tremolite is attributable to causing some/most/all the diseases in Canadian miners and millers, by this definition the tremolitic respirable dust would be considered by many as mineralogically definable as a nonasbestiform structure or "cleavage fragment."

We often evaluate the presence of tremolite and chrysotile in our studies simply on the basis of the previously mentioned issue of chrysotile being "contaminated" with tremolite within the mined product and contained as the minerals are processed during the mining/milling activity. However, in a study of 54 cases of mesothelioma from our laboratory,[212] there is more likelihood of tremolite occurring with anthophyllite (20 cases) than with chrysotile. There were 13 cases with both and 14 cases with chrysotile and no detectable tremolite. This is a common finding in all of our studies in that relationships between the finding of chrysotile in tissue with the expectation of finding tremolite do not occur. The common findings in observations within our reported mesothelioma studies[180,181,212] are the presence of various amounts of asbestos in most cases and with a composition often of mixed types of asbestos (commercial and noncommercial). Furthermore, there are some cases in these groups with lower levels of tissue burden.

Mesothelioma is a very rare tumor that occurs in men more than women. This has historically (and logically) been attributable to the higher potential for men to work in areas were occupational exposures to asbestos may occur. However, we evaluated tissue samples from a series of mesothelioma cases that occurred in women.[181] Some individuals were exposed to asbestos by secondary exposure via dust being brought home on the clothing of family members. The most commonly found asbestos in tissue from this series of 15 mesothelioma cases in women was amosite, and the second most commonly found fiber type was tremolite.[181] However, with the exception of the upper third of the study group, the tissue burden was much less than that found in the predominately male study groups. It should be noted that some tissue burdens in the lower group would not in any way be considered as reflective of past definitions for levels of occupationally exposed individuals. The common link in these cases with the larger study groups made up predominately of men[180,212] was that the fiber burden was often of mixed types of asbestos. The majority of fibers in all our mesothelioma publications were less than 5 μm in length, but a population of uncoated fibers within the lung samples were longer than 5 μm. The differences in the lung fiber characteristics (fiber type, concentration, and/or populations of longer fibers) in these mesothelioma cases offer a contrast with those same features reported from tissue analysis conducted on samples of tissue from the general population.

It would be helpful if a specific concentration of asbestos tissue burden could be linked to a specific disease. Some individuals have attempted to develop such a "threshold" concept for induction of disease such as mesothelioma. This usually begins with extracting data from a selected cohort, which may or may not equate with expected findings in another cohort. As pointed out by Warnock and Isenberg[219]: "Because large burdens of asbestos do not always cause pulmonary fibrosis, asbestosis may be a poor marker of fiber-related lung cancer." Indeed, in one of our studies, only 29 mesothelioma cases[180] out of 55 showed pathologic asbestosis. Compounding the issue further is that most reasonable people consider that mesothelioma is often a longer latency, lower dose-induced disease. The result historically is that many heavy dose-exposed individuals simply die from another asbestos-induced disease before living long enough after first exposure to develop mesothelioma. Another issue is that no one can define the vulnerability of an individual to a given asbestos exposure. Finally, mesothelioma can occur outside the lung, and little knowledge exists as to the relevance of the populations of fibers left in the lung over time with those that reach the extrapulmonary sites except as a confirmation of past exposure. As will be described in detail in the section on asbestos in extrapulmonary sites, it is evident that unique populations of asbestos fibers reach these sites.[220]

Further compounding the issue of extrapolating the meaning of fiber burden in the lung with events that induce mesothelioma is that at the time a lung sample is obtained, it is reflective of the dust concentration in the tissue at that time and does not indicate the number of fibers, particularly short fibers, that may have been in the lung and cleared via the mucociliary escalator and/or relocated to other sites within the body.[104] The question is why should these cleared fibers not have played a role in tissue response as well as creating the setting for permanent pathological changes to occur before their departure from the lung? This is particularly important relative to chrysotile or amphiboles, where repeated exposures would be expected to stimulate continued inflammatory responses and potential changes that could lead to pathological responses, including neoplasia, even if the clearance of chrysotile (more preferentially inhaled as shorter structures) is considered to occur more rapidly from the lung than do amphiboles.[73] Although smaller asbestos fibers would logically be more readily cleared from the lung, it is sometimes not adequately appreciated as to the effectiveness of the lung clearance for larger structures, including asbestos bodies as found in samples of sputa.[125,137,139–141] These clearly are very large particulates formed on a population of longer inhaled asbestos fibers. However, the question remains whether most chrysotile (or shorter amphiboles which also reach the lower airways in appreciable numbers) could be eliminated from lung tissue over time since first exposure until a lung sample is collected and yet still be present in appreciable numbers in extrapulmonary sites where they had been relocated from the lung and the clearance process is appreciably slower.[54,104,220]

3.12 EXPOSURE FROM ASBESTOS AS A COMPONENT OF OTHER MINERALS

There is potential asbestos exposure from products that are made from minerals that contain asbestos. This is often referred to as *contamination*, although contamination may not be the proper word to describe naturally occurring types of asbestos that occurs as a component of these minerals. Although many products are presented/assumed to not contain asbestos, the reality is that miners/millers and consumers have potential asbestos exposures from their use. Vermiculite, mined in Libby, Montana, is an example. This mineral has been distributed to numerous processing facilities in the United States and used in products ranging from garden products, for example, potting soil component, packing material, to insulation products. As early as 1986, McDonald et al.[221] stated that tremolite in vermiculite could cause asbestos-related diseases. Wright et al.[222] reported lung burdens of tremolite asbestos from exposure to asbestos-containing vermiculite of over 8,000,000 asbestos fibers per gram of dry lung in a person with brief exposure in a vermiculite expansion plant during a summer job 50 years prior. Sixty-eight percent of the fibers were tremolite asbestos. Compounding the issue further is that there are nonregulated fibrous amphiboles in the vermiculite vein, and debate rages on as to the implications of the role these nonregulated structures have as contributors in inducing disease.

Another widely used mineral that can contain asbestos is talc. Kleinfeld et al.[223] and Rohl et al.[224] reported that certain talc formations contained tremolite and anthophyllite asbestos. Thus, these asbestos fibers can occur in consumer talc products. Asbestos bodies and fibers have been reported in lung tissue from workers with asbestos-related diseases who worked in New York State talc mines.[225] The fibers in the lungs consisted of fibrous talc, tremolite, and related mineral series. A considerable burden of asbestos fibers and bodies were identified by Scancarello et al.[226] in individuals with respiratory diseases and bilateral pleural plaques after talc inhalation and as found in BAL fluid and tissue samples. These are a few examples where determining asbestos burden in tissue samples can offer potentially important information in settings where exposures occurred to products not thought to contain asbestos.

Roggli et al.[227] examined lung tissue from 312 mesothelioma cases for fiber burden. The majority of cases were reported to have exposure to dust from products containing asbestos. They concluded that "tremolite in lung tissue samples from mesothelioma victims derives from both talc and chrysotile and that tremolite accounts for a considerable fraction of the excess fiber burden in end-users of asbestos products."

3.13 ASBESTOS IN EXTRAPULMONARY SITES

The majority of the world's literature regarding asbestos in extrapulmonary sites is based on observations of a few asbestos bodies seen by light microscopy. These sites include the stomach,[228] the liver,[229] the kidney,[100,229] the spleen,[100,102,229] the lymph nodes,[54,103,104] and the pleural plaques.[230] The limited occurrence of such observations in pleural samples was noted in 1988 by Churg.[231] His conclusions were that "as a rule asbestos bodies are not seen in pleural plaques, although Rosen et al.[230] claim to have extracted a few bodies in some cases. As mentioned earlier, the asbestos content of plaques and pleurae appears to be quite different from that of the lung, and these sites are not useful for mineral analysis."[231] With respect to asbestos bodies, Dr. Churg was correct in that our laboratory has yet to find an asbestos body in digests of pleural plaques or parietal pleural (fibrotic) tissue. However, the presence of uncoated asbestos fibers in extrapulmonary sites, including pleura, is an important indicator of asbestos translocating from other sites. One cancer of greatest concern from exposure to asbestos is mesothelioma. This is a rare cancer of the serosal membranes of the body and is considered a marker of asbestos disease. Knudson[232] stated that "in the absence of asbestos, mesothelioma is so rare that it might never be studied."

Inhalation of asbestos can result in the occurrence of pathological responses in sites considerably removed from the lung (the original site of deposition).[106] Particulates can relocate through the lymphatic system to hilar lymph nodes and to more distant lymph nodes.[2] Schlesinger[59] described lymph nodes as "reservoirs of retained material." Gross and Detreville[8] stated that lymph nodes were "repositories for dust," and in heavy dust, exposures over time become "densely mineralized and stony hard." In cases of more toxic dust such as silica, lymph nodes may show necrosis, fibrosis, and calcification.[53] For those familiar with anatomy texts, a visit to Netter's[57] illustrated version of the respiratory system provides a refresher of not only the anatomy of the lymphatic drainage system in the chest cavity but also the designation as to which node drains what level of the lung. As proposed by Becklake[60] and Hillerdal,[61] the lymphatic route offers a mechanism for relocation of asbestos from the lung to other parts of the body. Knudson[232] stated that the "transport of the fibers to these surfaces (pleural and peritoneal) can lead to mesothelial proliferation, and after many years, to malignant mesotheliomas." Confirmation of relocation to extrapulmonary sites requires the application of the ATEM for identification of the type and size of asbestos fibers that reach extrapulmonary tissues.

A study in our laboratory was conducted to determine the content of lung and peritracheal lymph node tissue in 21 individuals who also conformed to the definition of general population.[233] Two lymph nodes were positive for at least one ferruginous body. There were no asbestos fibers detected in lymph nodes from eight cases. Five cases with asbestos fibers in lung tissue were not determined to have asbestos in lymph nodes. Nine cases had detectable levels of asbestos in lung and lymph nodes. The most common type of asbestos found in the lymph nodes was anthophyllite (nine cases), with the second most common type being tremolite (six cases). The composition of the asbestos burden (when present) from lymph nodes when compared with findings from samples of lung parenchyma from the general population is the predominance reflective of past exposures to short fibers (<5 μm) of noncommercial amphiboles or chrysotile (if asbestos fibers are detected at all).

Another recent publication from our laboratory further defines the analytical characterization of the asbestos burden in lung tissue versus the levels of lymph nodes that drain the lung.[54] The individuals had documented exposures to asbestos and died from various asbestos-related diseases. The article reviews the data regarding lymph drainage from the lung as well as experimental studies in animal models that have assessed particulate relocation. For purposes of brevity, only a few significant points will be made from the findings. The lymph nodes have some population of ferruginous bodies but not as elevated as in lung tissue. This is similar to findings in our earlier comparative study of lung burden with composition of lymph node and pleural plaques.[104] The asbestos types found in lymph nodes are consistent with types found in the lung; however, as in the earlier study,[104] the fiber size found in lymph nodes is appreciably shorter than those found in lung. Most fibers found in lymph nodes are a mixture of commercial and noncommercial amphiboles just as in lung tissue. The attempt to quantify the fiber numbers by light microscopy would be worthless because the vast majority would not be "seen" or counted in phase-contrast microscopy. The vast majority of fibers in all sites were <5 μm in length. ATEM is required to both detect and correctly analyze fiber burden in this study.

One of the first quantitative studies evaluating fiber burden in extrapulmonary sites and using ATEM was carried out by Sebastien et al.[220] He and his associates analyzed fiber content of lung samples and parietal pleural tissue from 29 cases sent to them for confirmation of diagnosis. The majority of patients had histories of asbestos exposure. In the study, 16 of 29 samples of parietal pleural tissue contained asbestos (within the detection limit of the study) and 27 lung tissue samples were positive. The pleural samples identified to have asbestos in them contained "almost all chrysotile." The reason light microscopic evaluation of extrapulmonary sites for asbestos is usually negative is evident by fiber size as reported by Sebastien et al.[220] The mean length of fiber in the lung was 4.9 μm, whereas the average length in the pleura was 2.3 μm. These asbestos fibers were not long enough to trigger asbestos body formation. Likewise, an assessment by light microscopy would not detect short or longer/thinner asbestos fibers from these tissues.

In a comparative study carried out by Dodson et al.[104] on samples of lung tissue, lymph nodes, and pleural plaques obtained from eight former shipyard workers from Italy, no asbestos bodies were found in the pleural plaques, whereas all but one sample of lymph node contained asbestos bodies. This suggests a relocation of mature bodies from the lungs to the lymph nodes, a selective segregation on the basis of the size of fibers that reach the two sites (a predictor of asbestos body formation), or differences in coating efficiency between these extrapulmonary sites. However, the population of longer fibers suitable for stimulation of coating in the lymph nodes constitutes a fraction of the total population when compared with the percent of longer fibers in total burden in lung tissue.

Amphiboles and chrysotile fibers were found at various concentrations in different sites with total concentrations often ranging into the millions of fibers per gram of dry tissue. The average length of chrysotile and amphibole asbestos fibers found in the lung was longer than lengths for the same type of fibers found in the lymph node and pleural plaques. Fibers in all three sites were represented by a majority that were less than 5 μm long with only 4% of the chrysotile in the lung being <10 μm and no chrysotile fiber >10 μm being detected in pleural plaques and lymph nodes. The amphibole content consisted of 80% being less than 10 μm in the lung with only 8% of the fibers in the pleural plaques and 2.5% in the lymph nodes being >10 μm. The importance of including short fibers in a count scheme is illustrated in one individual. The lung tissue from this individual was not determined to have chrysotile (within the limits of detectability). Thus, if this parameter alone was used, one could extrapolate this to mean no or low exposure. However, the pleural plaque tissue contained 21,000,000 fibers of chrysotile per gram of dry tissue and lymph node contained 5,500,000 fibers of chrysotile per gram of dry tissue. If only fibers longer than 5 μm were counted, only 3.1% of the total chrysotile from the plaques of this individual and none in the lymph nodes would have been counted (given sufficient magnification had been used to "see" the thin fibers). These findings indicated a past exposure to chrysotile and emphasized the lung's capability to clear short fibers after cessation of exposure, whereas extrapulmonary sites have less efficient mechanisms to rid their tissue of asbestos.

Suzuki and Yuen[234,235] analyzed asbestos content in lung and mesothelial tissue from individuals with mesothelioma. Using ATEM, Suzuki and Yuen[234,235] found that the majority of fibers in the lung and the mesothelial tumor tissue were less than 5 μm in length. They also found that the majority of short fibers were chrysotile. Only 4% of fibers fit the Stanton model for a more "pathogenically active" population of fiber (>8 μm long and thinner than 0.25 μm in diameter). They concluded that the majority of fibers in both lung and mesothelial tissues were <5 μm. A comparison made between the average length of asbestos fibers found in pleural tissue in studies by Sebastien et al.[220] and Dodson et al.[104] with those reported by Suzuki and Yuen [234,235] shows a striking similarity in that the fibers are very short. A more recent article by Suzuki et al.[236] evaluated lung and mesothelial tissues from 168 cases of human malignant mesothelioma. Their conclusions were as follows: "(1) long, thin asbestos fibers consistent with the Stanton hypothesis comprised only 2.3% of total fibers (247/10,575) in these tissues; (2) the majority (89.4%) of the fibers in the tissues examined were shorter than or equal to 5 μm in length (9,454 of 10,575), and generally (92.7%) smaller than or equal to 0.25 μm in width (9,808 of 10,575); and (3) among the asbestos types detected in the lung and mesothelial tissues, chrysotile was the most common asbestos type to be categorized as short, thin asbestos fibers." They concluded that "contrary to the Stanton hypothesis, short, thin, asbestos fibers appear to contribute to the causation of human malignant mesothelioma."

Of course the finding of short fibers as the primary component of lymph nodes that drain the lung and in pleural tissue does not bode well for the arguments supporting the "amphibole hypothesis"[237] for explaining most asbestos-induced diseases in extrapulmonary sites. The "amphibole hypothesis" is based, in part, on longer fibers being more pathogenically active (see discussion in section on fiber length and disease), and this, of course, skews risk for causation of cancer toward amphibole fibers, in part, because they are inhaled as longer fibers in the lung (because they tend to be straight) and thus are less readily cleared compared with the shorter chrysotile component that is found in lung tissue. There are some reasonable explanations that seem to support a greater potential for molecular interactions within tissue from interactions with amphiboles than chrysotile fibers. However, there are other models that indicate chrysotile is more reactive.[238] This subject will be covered in detail in the section on molecular biology-induced reactions with asbestos fibers.

It is obvious that the findings of predominately shorter asbestos in extrapulmonary sites leaves the "chrysophiles"[237] scrambling to explain how the predominate numbers of shorter asbestos fibers in extrapulmonary sites are noncontributors to carcinogenicity or to development of other asbestos-related changes in these sites.

It appeared initially that an excellent study by Boutin et al.[239] had uniquely linked the presence of amphiboles with concentrations of such fibers in areas within the parietal pleura in individuals apparently exposed to aerosols likely containing fossil fuel soot (coal dust). Apparently, the concept of finding black spots in the parietal pleura is rare in the United States (personal communication of Samuel Hammar, MD, who has been involved with thousands of autopsies). In such cases, areas within the parietal pleura contain parietal anthracosis described within "lymphatic vessels of the parietal pleura" and in this study are dubbed "black spots." The authors devised a study in which they looked at fiber burden content in lung and pleural tissue in 14 individuals. Eight individuals had defined asbestos exposure, and six were without defined asbestos exposure. In most subjects exposed to asbestos, "fiber concentrations in the lung and anthracotic pleural samples were >1 ×1 0⁶ fiber per gram, whereas there were practically no fibers in nonanthracotic pleural samples. In 5 of 11 patients, including all three mesothelioma patients, the concentration of fibers was even higher in black spots than in lung samples."

The conclusions from the study included the following: (1) fiber distribution is heterogeneous in the parietal pleura, (2) the fibers concentrate in black spots in high concentrations, and (3) this could explain why parietal pleura is the target organ for mesothelioma and plaques. The following is offered in able to better appreciate the findings that led to each of the conclusions and the issues to consider regarding their findings:

1. If asbestos is relocated from the lung tissue via the lymphatic drainage—which we have analytically confirmed,[54,104] then it is reasonable that the dust particles, including asbestos particles, could concentrate in the lymphatic-rich areas of the pleura.

2. The concentration of asbestos fibers in plaque areas has been previously shown[104,220,240,241]; however, most of the fibers in these studies have found chrysotile to often be the prevalent asbestos type, which is in contrast with the findings of only amphiboles in the study by Boutin et al.[239]

There are several interesting points regarding the study of Boutin et al.[239] that are sometimes overinterpreted as to significance. The first is that the study showed long amphiboles reached the parietal pleural where mesotheliomas develop. This observation is not unique and should be reviewed on the basis of two important findings in the report. First, 99% of the asbestos fibers in the lung were amphiboles, 95% were amphiboles in pleural black spots, and 61% were in nonanthracotic pleura. Thus, if one essentially has only amphiboles in the lung, then that constitutes the asbestos that is available to be translocated to extrapulmonary sites. Second, the issue of fiber length with the emphasis occasionally placed that "longer fibers of amphiboles reach the pleura" can be correct. However, what they said in detail was that in the "black spots" 22.5% of the fibers were 5 μm or longer and 10% were 8 μm or longer. These observations compare with LeBouffant's[240] report, where 7% of the amosite and 5% of the chrysotile in the parietal pleura were 5 μm or longer. Sebastien et al.[220] reported that 24% of the amphibole fibers and 14% of the chrysotile in the parietal pleura exceeded 4 μm in length. In our own study,[104] 10% of the amphiboles and 3.1% of the chrysotile were >5 μm. Thus, the findings in the study by Boutin et al.[239] appear to have shown the same as the previously stated studies in that the vast majority (in their study 77.5%) of the asbestos fibers (in their case amphiboles) in the pleura and in their cases within pleural "black spots" are <5 μm. The authors also offered a sound scientific explanation as to a potential reason that chrysotile was not detected stating: "From a technical point of view, short and thin chrysotile fibers could be less easily detected among a 'background' of particulates in anthracotic samples." For a review of this issue, the reader is referred to the section on tissue preparation and instrument selection previously discussed in this chapter.

3. The question of the anatomical concentration of asbestos in the "black spots" as defining regions with the potential for the development of mesothelioma and pleural plaques has been the subject of several additional European studies. Müller et al.[242] conducted a morphological evaluation of 12 "black spots" (four surgical and eight autopsy specimens) located in the parietal pleura. They concluded that "there were hints for an increased proliferation of mesothelial cells in some areas with black spots," but "our findings do not support the classification of black spots as an obligate early lesion in the development of malignant mesothelioma." They further stated "our results do not support the hypothesis whereby mesotheliomas develop 'preferentially' in the regions of preexisting black spots. In our collective of former miners of the Ruhr area we do not find asbestos fibers especially amphibole fibers directly located in black spots. But we found silicates, quartz and silicone as well as aluminum-rich minerals such as muscovite. There were no hints that black spots play a possible role in the development of mesotheliomas."

Mitchev et al.[243] evaluated the macroscopic appearance of "black spots" and possible relationships with pleural plaques in 150 consecutive necropsies of urban dwellers. Black spots were observed in 92.7% of cases and were noted mainly in the lower costal and diaphragmatic zones.

They reported "there was no relationship between the predominant locations of black spots and hyaline pleural plaques."

In summation, samples of the parietal pleura (specifically plaques) have been reported to contain asbestos fibers in occupationally exposed individuals. The majorities of these fibers are less than 5 μm in length and in most cases can only be detected at higher magnification by ATEM. Data derived from any other technical assessment of these tissues should be viewed with caution.

A theoretical review as to how fibers reach the extrapulmonary sites from the lung (site of original deposition) has been offered by Miserocchi et al.[244] Their discussion involves the mechanisms that permit inhaled fibers to pass the alveolar barrier. The proposed concepts include a "paracellular route down a mass water flow due to combined osmotic (active Na+ absorption) and hydraulic (interstitial pressure is subatmospheric) pressure gradient. Fibers can be dragged from the lung interstitium by pulmonary lymph flow (primary translocation) wherefrom they can reach the bloodstream and subsequently distribute to the whole body (secondary translocation)." Their conclusions regarding fiber size and as related to the likelihood for fiber relocation from the lung to extrapulmonary sites creates problems for the "longer fibers cause mesothelioma" concept. They do, however, reflect favorably on the actual findings regarding fiber size and relocation to extrapulmonary sites as previously described. Their specific point is that "ultrafine fibers (length <5 μm, diameter <0.25 μm) can travel larger distances due to low steric hindrance (in mesothelioma about 90% of fibers are ultrafine)."

Approximately 10%–15% of mesotheliomas occur in the peritoneal cavity. Recent investigations by Hasanoglu et al.[245] studied the effects of orally ingested asbestos in the lungs and pleura in a rat model. "Histopathological evaluation of lungs and pleura of rats after 6 months revealed significant mesothelial proliferation and asbestos bodies." They further suggested that the ingested asbestos traveled from the gastrointestinal system to the lungs, "likely via a lymphohematological route, leading to mesothelioma proliferation, which may lead to malignancies." Although this is an animal study, the observation is of importance in that the serosal tissues that give rise to peritoneal mesothelioma may receive fibers from the lymphatic drainage from the lungs to lymph system and/or be subjected to delivery of fibers that relocate from inside the gastrointestinal tract. Little is know about what population of asbestos fibers reach the parietal pleura and less regarding the composition of the fiber burden reaching the components of the peritoneal cavity.

Dodson et al.[101] conducted an analytical analysis of lung tissue, omentum, and mesentery (fatty lining tissue in the peritoneal cavity) from 20 mesothelioma cases. Asbestos bodies were found in lung tissue of 18 individuals and in five mesentery and two omentum samples. Uncoated asbestos fibers were found in lung tissue of 19 individuals with 17 individuals having fibers in at least one extrapulmonary site. Ten individuals had over 1.4 million asbestos fibers per gram of dry lung. Fourteen individuals had uncoated asbestos fibers in mesentery and omentum samples. The most common type of asbestos fiber found in omentum and mesentery was amosite, which was also the most prevalent asbestos fiber type found in lung tissue. The second most commonly found form of asbestos in the two sample sites was chrysotile. The fiber type and the concentration in the lung tissue were similar to that found in 55 mesothelioma cases reported in 1997[180] with regard to there being a mixture of asbestos types. Different asbestos fiber types were seen in omentum/mesentery in several individuals. The most common was amosite (consistent with the lung tissue); however, chrysotile was the second most common. Predictors from lung data for fiber presence in omentum and mesentery statistically included asbestos body concentration, amphibole concentration, fiber length, and aspect ratio. Obviously, this study showed asbestos fibers reached the peritoneal cavity in humans where peritoneal mesotheliomas develop.

A comparative study[154] of lung, mesentery, and omental tissue was conducted in tissue from 15 individuals who conformed to the definition of members of the general population (as used in our laboratory).[153] Four lung samples contained asbestos bodies, and two lung samples contained at least one asbestos fiber. The only asbestos fiber found in extrapulmonary sites consisted of one short chrysotile fiber (<3 μm) and one short tremolite fiber (<4 μm) in two samples of omentum.[154]

Monchaux et al.[246] found that translocation of fibers including UICC chrysotile A, UICC cro-cidolite, and JM 104 glass fibers occurred to various sites after intrapleural injection into rats. Ninety-day postexposure fibers were found in mediastinal lymph nodes, lung parenchyma, spleen, liver, kidneys, and brain. The concentration of fibers per gram of tissue was reported to be in the same range for all sites except in the thoracic lymph nodes where the concentration was reported as 10 to 100× greater. Interestingly, the findings included the observation that the "mean length of fibres observed in lung parenchyma increased with time." "After 210 days, the mean length of all three types of fibres was higher than the initial length; and after 380 days, the mean length of the fibres, and especially chrysotile fibres, was considerably higher than that of the injected fibres." The question was raised from the data as to whether the "hypothesis formulated by Lauweryns and Baert[247] that particles are removed from the pulmonary interstitium via the blood capillaries and the pulmonary lymphatics is correct, (thus) it can be assumed that only short fibres are cleared in this way, whereas long fibres are entrapped within the alveolar walls." Obviously, the findings from our studies support the concept that shorter fibers are the form that are most likely to reach extrapulmonary sites (see section on fiber burden in lymph nodes as well as section on fiber length and pathogenicity).

Uibu et al.[248] recently evaluated the asbestos fiber burden in para-aortic and mesenteric lymph nodes with that in lung tissue from 22 persons who underwent medicolegal autopsy. The individuals were suspected of having an asbestos-related cause of death. The findings indicated that some fibers >20 μm were found in lymph nodes, which they interpreted to mean that "macrophage migration is not the main transport mechanism for long asbestos fibers." They added "that asbestos fibers reach the parietal pleura with the fluid absorbed from the pleural space and pass along the lymph vessels into the subdiaphragmatic region. Depending on anatomical variations, some fibers accumulate in the PA (para-aortic lymph nodes) and other subdiaphragmatic lymph nodes and some are drained into the thoracic duct and venous systemic circulation." This would imply that macrophage "transport" requires the fiber be phagocytized within the macrophage. However, anyone who has evaluated samples of sputa would appreciate that multiple macrophages are associated with most ferruginous bodies cleared via the mucociliary route. Therefore, these structures are not within a macrophage but are being cleared with attached macrophages. If this association enhances clearance rate at least via the mucociliary escalatory or not remains an open question, but the fact that a directional flow occurs without the bodies being "internalized" within macrophages is factually correct. The authors further concluded that "even low level occupational exposure results in the presence of crocidolite, amosite, anthophyllite, tremolite, or chrysotile in these abdominal lymph nodes. Our results support the hypothesis of lymph drainage as an important translocation mechanism for asbestos in the human body."

3.14 FIBER LENGTHS AND THE RELATIONSHIP TO PATHOGENICITY

The discussion regarding fiber lengths and their relationships to pathogenicity have evolved into scientific discussions involving differences in opinions on one hand and polarized camps suggestive of representing vested interests on the other. The issue has evolved based in large part on the issue of fiber length versus pathogenicity. To be more specific, the focus of the discussion is often stimulated by economic/legal issues involving chrysotile. This is not a trivial issue because chrysotile was used in over 90+ percent of commercial asbestos products in the United States. The facts already described include the likelihood of chrysotile being aerosolized as a short and/or thin fiber that is not detectable by light microscopy (as acknowledged in the federal regulations), and furthermore, these are the exact size of chrysotile fibers that are found in human tissue. The often intense legal/political arena on the subject has varying levels of positioning. One approach is to simply disavow that chrysotile is harmful. Because most national and international health agencies take a different position, this is not usually a successful approach. Another approach is to simply use the phase contrast optical microscope (PCOM) to evaluate air samples with the full knowledge that chrysotile fibrils cannot be detected by phase-contrast microscopy,[65] so if the fibers cannot be seen, that portion of the aerosol certainly cannot be used to assess exposure levels.[80] The other strategy is to use an electron microscope with a count scheme (low magnification) that excludes short fibers (<5 μm) or long, thin fibers that are too thin to see at low magnification. In either case, the result is a conclusion that if the chrysotile is not seen it cannot be there. The other extreme is one in which a concept is offered that one fiber can cause cancer. This one is a total nonwinner for both sides. The issues used by the various players—defense and plaintiffs in the legal field—have been discussed in detail by Tweedle and McCullock.[237] The purpose of the following section will be to simply provide the reader with facts concerning what is known about fibers on the basis of their length as it influences counting schemes and as they interact with tissue. With this information, the reader is encouraged to formulate their own opinions as they read future articles. Thus, the intent is to provide the reader with the tools to ask the right questions in an attempt to determine the validity/completeness of the reported observations.

Aerosolized asbestos fibers assessed in the workplace are often counted via reproducible counting schemes by use of phase contrast light microscopy. This system is based on the definition of a "regulated fiber," which physically is sufficiently thick to be observed by light microscopy under the designated magnification. The count scheme includes fibers that are 5 μm or longer and the instrument cannot distinguish fiber type. This selection criterion was established to permit reproducibility between analysts and provides an inexpensive mode for determining the numbers of fibers in air sampled over a period of time and a certain volume of air. This formed the basis of the terms "action level," "permissible exposure limits," and "excursion levels," which have been used to establish levels of exposure for workers in asbestos-containing environments as defined by OSHA and/or EPA work practices. As Langer et al.[71] noted, the counting guidelines define the physical definition of a fiber to be included in a count, the aspect ratio for fibers to be included, and the definition of asbestos bundles and other structures as applicable to the count scheme. These selection criteria were based on "practicality and theoretical considerations" rather than having a target of a "more toxic" population of fibers. As already stated from our studies, it is evident that the predominance of asbestos fibers in tissue consist of short or longer/thin fibers that cannot be readily detected with the light microscope, just as in air samples.[65] These shorter fibers can be phagocytized within a cell such as shown in Figure 3.24 and can relocate to extrapulmonary sites.

What therefore is the scientific basis that long fibers are more likely to cause disease than short fibers? Simple logic indicates inhalation of longer fibers would result in less likelihood of rapid elimination via lung clearance mechanisms than an equivalent number of inhaled shorter fibers. However, it is unlikely that only long fibers are in the breathing zone; thus, there is a mixture of fiber sizes. There are unique occupational settings where the short fiber grades/types of chrysotile are used, and in these there are few fibers greater than 5 μm.

Many of the most important experimental studies regarding the inherent pathogenicity of fibrous particles on the basis of their morphology were conducted by Stanton et al.[249,250] in the United States and by Professor Fredrick Pott et al.[251–254] in Germany. The Stanton team used pleural implants of gelatin containing the fibers of interest, whereas the Pott team concentrated most of their studies using intraperitoneal exposures. Both the Stanton group and the Pott group chose models where the dust of interest could be placed directly into the target zone for determination of the level of response. Either technique permitted appreciable fibrous dusts to be given in the models. These animal exposures bypass the physiological route of fiber entry into these sites within the body because the lung and thus the previously described primary body defense systems in the respiratory system are a nonfactor. It is evident from our studies and others that a shorter population of fibers reach the extrapulmonary sites as compared with the burden in the lung. Thus, the concern for disease induction in the lung that has excellent clearance mechanisms may have variables for induction of

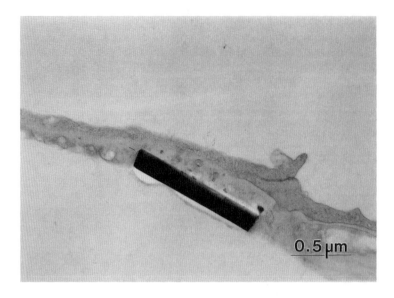

Figure 3.24 The short amosite fiber shown in this field is within the cytoplasm of a lining cell. Such "short" fibers in dividing cells create a physical challenge to proper cell division.

asbestos-related changes that are somewhat different on the basis of fiber characterizations than those for induction of changes in extrapulmonary sites.

However, the concept of fiber length and potential for causation of disease is often referenced in the United States on the basis of the innovative studies by Stanton et al.[249,250] The conclusions from his work using pleural implants in rats was that "the carcinogenicity of fibers depend on dimension and durability rather than on physicochemical properties."[250] As is evident from the chapter on the molecular mechanisms of asbestos-induced disease, the concept of physically based explanation of the pathogenicity of a fiber is only one factor that can induce pathogenic responses. The quote often attributed to Stanton's[250] observation is "the probability of pleural sarcoma correlated best with numbers of fibers that measured 0.25 μm or less in diameter and more than 8 μm in length." An advocacy that only long fibers induce cancer selects these dimensions as "Stanton Fibers." However, the sentence actually continued with the statement "but relative high correlations were noted with fibers in other size categories having diameters up to 1.5 μm and lengths greater than 4 μm."

Occasionally, the comparison of the population of fibers conforming to a "Stanton Fiber" is given for a particular analysis of tissue (for reference, the defined dimension of a "Stanton Fiber" is often included). In our own papers, the comparison is made with the full appreciation that the Stanton et al.[250] measurements were far from absolute as typified by the following quote taken from Stanton's article: "Of special interest are the data on the amphibole asbestoses: amosite, tremolite, and crocidolite, although estimates of the dimensions of the asbestoses are especially liable to error."

A dimension of a "Stanton Fiber" would seem to have particular importance in a discussion of the reduced relative potential of a chrysotile fiber to induce disease because most fibers of this type found in tissue are shorter than 8 μm. The "Stanton Fiber" is therefore freely used in discussions regarding the potential of this type of asbestos as a "lesser" causal agent of cancer when compared with amphiboles. However, specific data supporting a position that there is a lack of carcinogenicity of chrysotile are lacking when the argument is based on the specifics of the study by Stanton et al.[250] in that they did not use chrysotile as one of the tested fibers. The exact statement is[250] "chrysotile, although as carcinogenic as amphiboles at comparable dimensions, could not be included since it has proved difficult to be measured with any degree of precision." Obviously, this statement is not a good reference if one desires to present an argument that chrysotile is less carcinogenic than amphiboles.

The second series of studies on fiber length as related to pathogenicity was carried out by Pott et al.[251–254] Various sizes of fibrous dusts were injected intraperitoneally into rats to assess their tumorigenicity. Pott reported that asbestos fibers shorter than 10 μm in length could produce tumors.[254] In one experiment, milled "chrysotile A" consisting of 99.8% of fibers being less than 5 μm (few longer than 10 μm) produced tumors in 30% of the animals.

Fraire et al.[255] conducted a study to assess the cytopathological changes, if any, induced by the injection of short fiberglass (mean length of 2.2 μm and width of 0.15 μm) intrapleurally into rats. The histological changes, as graded by several pulmonary pathologists, included chronic inflammation, fibrosis, foreign body reaction, and more advanced proliferative/neoplastic changes of mesothelial hyperplasia and dysplasia. Surprisingly, the short fiber preparation resulted in mature mesotheliomas in three of 25 rats.

Goodglick and Kane[256] assessed the reactivity of long and short crocidolite asbestos fibers in an in vitro and in vivo experimental model. They found "both long and short crocidolite asbestos fibers were toxic to elicited macrophages in vitro. Similar to native crocidolite asbestos, long and short fibers stimulated the release of reactive oxygen metabolites from elicited macrophages in vitro." "In vivo, a single i.p. injection of long crocidolite fibers stimulates an intense inflammatory reaction, release of reactive oxygen metabolites near sites of fiber deposition, and cell death. In contrast, these events were minimal after a single injection of short fibers due to the removal of fibers from the peritoneal cavity. After five daily injections of short fibers, however, fibers were present on the surface of the mesothelium and provoked an inflammatory response. Cell death was observed on the surface of the mesothelium. Reactive oxygen metabolites were also produced near accumulations of short fibers." Their conclusions suggested "that both long and short crocidolite asbestos fibers are toxic to macrophages in vitro via an oxidant and iron-dependent mechanism. In vivo, short fibers are cytotoxic when the clearance of these fibers is prevented." This study illustrates the significance of considering the impact of cumulative exposures, which are the exposure scenarios that occur with most humans. Likewise, these determinations of intensity of the response is not simply defined by the physical features of a fiber.

Attempts have been made to extrapolate from tissue burden and animal studies the risk for developing specific asbestos-related diseases in humans. Lippmann[257] concluded that asbestosis was most correlated with the number of fibers longer than 2 μm and thicker than 0.15 μm, mesothelioma to the number of fibers longer than "about" 5 μm and thinner than "about" 0.1 μm, and lung cancer to the number of fibers longer than "about" 10 μm and thicker than "about" 0.15 μm. Churg and Vedal[206] concluded from tissue analysis of individuals heavily exposed to amosite and chrysotile that "except for pleural plaques, the association of fiber size and disease remains uncertain." They further concluded that "mesotheliomas are not associated with long fibers and in fact are probably associated with lower-aspect-ratio fibers than found in subjects without asbestos-related disease."

McDonald et al.[199] conducted fiber burden analysis in a series of individuals with mesothelioma who were 50 years or younger at time of diagnosis. They concluded that "shorter fibers were more abundant than longer fibers, and high concentrations of all fiber lengths tended to occur together." "Short, medium, and long fibers (of amphiboles) were all associated with mesothelioma risk: those longer than 10 μm had the greatest increment in risk per fiber, followed by medium [6–10 μm] and then by short [<6 μm]." Nayebzadeh et al.[207] observed that respiratory disease in a group of former Quebec chrysotile miners and millers was not related to fiber dimension but to the fiber burden in the tissue, a conclusion that we believe is more universally correct and has general applicability.

Some asbestos-induced changes in humans may be similar to changes induced by other causes. However, the disease that is specifically considered as a unique "asbestos marker disease" is mesothelioma. This tumor often occurs after a longer latency period from first exposure than other asbestos-induced diseases and can occur in individuals with lower level of exposures (such as secondary).

The development of mesothelioma as related to asbestos exposure is best summarized in the following statement from Robinson et al.:[258] "Mesothelioma owes its entire existence as a disease entity to its relation with asbestos." Chen et al.[259] noted that "mesothelioma is a rare fatal neoplasm that originates from cells lining the serosal cavities." They indicate that 90%–95% arise in the pleural cavity and 5%–10% in the peritoneal cavity. They stated that Hammar[260] acknowledged that the tumor has been reported rarely in the pericardium and tunica vaginalis. Mark and Yokoi[261] reviewed "background level of diffuse malignant mesothelioma" by retrospectively analyzing "the autopsy files of the Massachusetts General Hospital as well as the early literature on thoracic neoplasms." Their conclusions were "that the background level of diffuse malignant mesothelioma in Europe and in the United States prior to 1930 was extremely low. No case was detected at the Massachusetts General Hospital until 1946."

Nishikawa et al.[262] evaluated mortality from pleural mesothelioma from the perspective of a global assessment as correlated with patterns of asbestos use and international bans. They concluded that "observed disparities in global mesothelioma trends likely relate to country-to-country disparities in asbestos use trends."

The risks for the development of mesothelioma following occupational levels of exposure to asbestos are appreciated. The disease has the longest latency among asbestos-related diseases for occurrence from first exposure and occurs in lower dose settings. Thus, it has been the focus of several studies involving risks associated with nonoccupational exposures.

Magnani et al.[263] conducted a population-based case–control study in six areas from Italy, Spain, and Switzerland. Among the risk areas of concern were "cleaning asbestos-contaminated clothes, handling asbestos material and presence of asbestos material susceptible to damage. The estimated OR for high probability of environmental exposure (living within 2000 m of asbestos mines, asbestos cement plants, asbestos textiles, shipyards, or brake factories) was 11.5 (95% CI 3.5–38.2). Living between 2000 and 5000 m from asbestos industries or within 500 m of industries using asbestos could also be associated with an increased risk (of mesothelioma). A dose–response pattern appeared with intensity of both sources of exposure. It is suggested that low-dose exposure to asbestos at home or in the general environment carries a measurable risk of malignant pleural mesothelioma."

Kurumatani and Kumagal[264] assessed the impact of neighborhood exposures in a group of individuals who resided around a former large asbestos cement pipe plant in Amagasaki City, Japan. The time of potential exposure was between 1957 and 1975 when the plant used crocidolite and chrysotile asbestos. They identified 73 mesothelioma deaths (35 men and 38 women) among individuals with no occupational exposure to asbestos. "The regions with significantly elevated standardized mortality ratio reached 2200 m from the plant in the same direction in which the wind predominately blew." The authors concluded that "neighborhood exposure to asbestos can pose a serious risk to residents across a wide area."

Goldberg and Luce[265] evaluated epidemiological data to assess the risk for development of mesothelioma, lung cancer, and other respiratory diseases associated with nonoccupational exposure to asbestos. They concluded studies concerning exposure to naturally occurring asbestos "that begins at birth does not seem to affect the duration of the latency period, but the studies do not show whether early exposure increases susceptibility; they do not suggest that susceptibility differs according to sex. Solid evidence shows an increase risk of mesothelioma among people whose exposure comes from a paraoccupational or domestic source. The risk of mesothelioma associated with exposure as result of living near an industrial asbestos source (mines, mills, asbestos processing plants) is clearly confirmed." The authors further concluded that "nonoccupational exposures to asbestos may explain approximately 20% of the mesotheliomas in industrial countries."

Regulation of asbestos in occupational and bystander settings would be much simpler if only the longer/thicker fibers visible by light microscopy and scanning electron microscopy were the causative agent of all asbestos-related diseases. The accurate counting of fiber burdens would not require the more expensive, extensive preparative processes, and time consuming use of ATEM. There would be great liability relief provided to those who manufacture products whose dust consists of fibers that predominately can only be detected by ATEM. In reality, the majority of asbestos dust that makes up the predominate tissue burden found in the lung and extrapulmonary sites is represented by fibers shorter than 5 µm long and/or longer thin fibers not visible by light microscopy. In fact, the same can be said for many preparations and magnifications reported as used in studies involving scanning electron microscopy. The short fibers are the ones most readily cleared from the lung but are also the ones more readily translocated out of the lung to extrapulmonary sites. These are often misrepresented in some analyses of tissue samples by concluding that their absence or lack of detection means they had never been there, thus excluding them from possible participation in pathological mechanisms in the lung and other tissues. This ability for short chrysotile to be cleared over time from the lung might lead to the suggestion that occupational histories in some instances may be a better indicator of risk of lung cancer than fiber burden.[266]

An editorial in *Lancet*[267] correctly stated "asbestos has been linked with diseases such as asbestosis, mesothelioma, and lung cancer" and that "all forms of asbestos are carcinogenic." They note "that unlike carcinogens such as tobacco, the risk of developing mesothelioma increases over time, even after exposure to asbestos has been stopped." Furthermore, they noted "Canada is the only high-income country that still mines asbestos (in the form of chrysotile), and it is the second largest exporter of the toxin in the world (after Russia). Despite the country's claims that chrysotile poses a lower health risk than other types of asbestos, it acknowledges that chrysotile is a carcinogen and as such protects its own citizens by limiting its use within Canada; 98% of Canadian asbestos is exported to developing countries including India and Thailand." They conclude "the only way to eliminate asbestos-related illness is to stop the use of all types of asbestos, all over the world." This is a noble statement, but even if the utilization of asbestos is stopped in all countries, there will be years of exposure to degenerating asbestos in place and from demolition and abatement of the materials, particularly if incorrectly done, that will result in release of fibers in the workplace and environment.

3.15 CONCLUSION

The primary conclusions from the data presented in this chapter are that inhaled asbestos fibers cause asbestos-related diseases. The assumption that risks from asbestos exposure in the United States and induction of disease are going away in the near future are put in perspective by two recent articles. Attfield et al.[268] defined the trends in pneumoconiosis mortality and morbidity for the United States from 1968 to 2005 as related to indicators of the extent of exposure. They concluded that "asbestosis deaths from 1968–2005 closely followed the historical trend in asbestos consumption, and appear to be declining in most age groups." However, they noted "given appropriate exposure control, asbestosis could be eliminated by 2050." Obviously, prevention of exposure is critical if this "heavy dose" related disease is to essentially disappear. A CDC/MMWR report[269] in April 2009 reviewed the status and projections for cases of mesothelioma in the United States. The fundamental basis for concern is that this disease has an appreciable latency period from first exposure (often 30–40+ years). The best-case scenario would project the disease to peak in 2010. However, the "annual number of mesothelioma deaths is still increasing, and future cases will continue to reflect the extensive past use of asbestos. New cases also might result through occupational and environmental exposure to asbestos during remediation and demolition of existing asbestos in buildings if controls are insufficient to protect workers and the surrounding community."

A recent news release from the Office of the Surgeon General[270] offers a useful overview of asbestos exposure issues by stating: "In recent decades, because of concern about asbestos' health effects, production and use has declined substantially. Most individuals exposed to asbestos, whether in a home, in the workplace, or out-of-doors will not develop disease-but there is no level of asbestos exposure that is known to be safe and minimizing your exposure will minimize your risk of developing asbestos-related diseases."

The tissue burden in individuals with asbestos-induced diseases consists most frequently of mixtures of asbestos types and sizes reflecting the features of many occupational exposures. Data from any tissue analysis for asbestos must be judged on what is included in the observations and what is realistically or potentially excluded. This requires an understanding of the preparative techniques, the capabilities/magnification of the selected instruments used in obtaining the information, and the parameters defining the count scheme used in a given study of human material.

Conflict-of-Interest Statement: Dr. Dodson has served as an expert in medical legal cases involving asbestos induced diseases for both plaintiff and defense. He has also appeared before courts charged with reviewing the general issues related to asbestos exposure and the potential for development of disease.

REFERENCES

1. Robertson B. Basic morphology of the pulmonary defense system. *Eur J Respir Dis* 1980;61:21–40.
2. Lippmann M, Yeates DB, Albert RE. Deposition, retention, and clearance of inhaled particles. *Br J Ind Med* 1980;37:337–62.
3. Witschi H. Proliferation of type II alveolar cells: A review of common responses in toxic lung injury. *Toxicology* 1976;5:267–77.
4. Burri PH. Morphology and respiratory function of the alveolar unit. *Int Arch Allergy Appl Immunol* 1985;76:2–12.
5. Ochs M, Nyengaard JR, Jung A, Knudsen M, Wahlers T, Richter J, Gundersen HJG. The number of alveoli in the human lung. *Am J Respir Crit Care Med* 2004;169:120–4.
6. Weibel ER. How does lung structure affect gas exchange? *Chest* 1983;83:657–665.
7. Turino GM. The lung parenchyma—A dynamic matrix. *Am Rev Respir Dis* 1985;132:1324–34.
8. Gross P, Detreville RT. The lung as an embattled domain against inanimate pollutants. *Am Rev Respir Dis* 1972;106:684–691.
9. Breeze R, Turk M. Cellular structure, function and organization in the lower respiratory tract. *Environ Health Perspect* 1984;55:3–24.
10. Mason RJ, Dobbs LG, Greenleaf RD, Williams MC. Alveolar type II cells. *Fed Proc* 1977;36:2697–702.
11. Rubins JB. Alveolar macrophages. *Am J Respir Crit Care Med* 2003;167:103–4.
12. Werb Z. How the macrophage regulates its extracellular environment. *Am J Anat* 1983;166:237–56.
13. Camner P, Anderson M, Philipson K, Bailey A, Hashish A, Jarvis N, et al. Human bronchiolar deposition and retention of 6-, 8-, and 10-mm particles. *Exp Lung Res* 1997;23:517–35.
14. McFadden D, Wright JL, Wiggs B, Churg A. Smoking inhibits asbestos clearance. *Am Rev Respir Dis* 1986;133:372–4.
15. Churg A, Thon V, Wright JL. Effects of cigarette smoke exposure on retention of asbestos fibers in various morphological compartments of the guinea pig lung. *Am J Pathol* 1987;129:385–93.
16. Churg A, Wiggs B. Mineral particles, mineral fibers, and lung cancer. *Environ Res* 1985;37:364–72.
17. Albin M, Pooley FD, Stromberg U, Attewell R, Mitha R, Johansson L, et al. Retention patterns of asbestos fibres in lung tissue among asbestos cement workers. *Occup Environ Med* 1994;51:205–11.
18. Churg A, Stevens B. Enhanced retention of asbestos fibers in the airways of human smokers. *Am J Respir Crit Care Med* 1995;151:1409–13.
19. Oberdorster G. Lung particle overload: Implications for occupational exposures to particles. *Regul Toxicol Pharmacol* 1995;27:123–35.

20. Morrow PE. Possible mechanisms to explain dust overloading of the lungs. *Fundam Appl Toxicol* 1988;10:369–84.

21. Pritchard JN. Dust overloading causes impairment of pulmonary clearance: Evidence from rats and humans. *Exp Pathol* 1989;37:39–42.

22. Stober W, Morrow PE, Hoover MD. Compartment modeling of the long-term retention of insoluble particles deposited in the alveolar region of the lung. *Fundam Appl Toxicol* 1989;13:823–42.

23. Castranova V, Driscoll K, Harkema J, Jarabek A, Morgan D, Nauss K, et al. The relevance of the rat lung response to particle overload for human risk assessment: A workshop consensus report. *Inhal Toxicol* 2000;12:1–17.

24. Coin PG, Osornio-Vargas AR, Roggli VL, Brody AR. Pulmonary fiberogenesis after three consecutive inhalation exposures to chrysotile asbestos. *Am J Resp Crit Care Med* 1996;154:1511–9.

25. Dodson RF, Ford JO. Tissue reaction following a second exposure to amosite asbestos. *Cytobios* 1991;68:53–62.

26. Pinkerton KE, Pratt PC, Brody AR, Crapo JD. Fiber localization and its relationship to lung reaction in rats after chronic inhalation of chrysotile asbestos. *Am J Pathol* 1984;117:484–98.

27. Reeves AL, Puro HE, Smith RG, Vorwald AJ. Experimental asbestos carcinogenesis. *Environ Res* 1971;4:496–511.

28. Kimizuka G, Shinozaki K, Hayashi, Y. Comparison of the pulmonary responses to chrysotile and amosite asbestos administrated intratracheally. *Acta Pathol Jpn* 1992;42(10):707–11.

29. Hesterberg TW, Hart GA, Chevalier J, et al. The importance of fiber biopersistence and lung dose in determining the chronic inhalation effects of X607, RCF1, and chrysotile asbestos in rats. *Toxicol Appl Pharmacol* 1998;153:68–82.

30. Rodelsperger K. Extrapolation of the carcinogenic potential of fibers from rats to humans. *Inhal Toxicol* 2004;16:801–7.

31. Brody AR. Whither goes the alveolar macrophage? Another small chapter is written on the localized response of this crucial cell. *J Lab Clin Med* 1998;131:391–2.

32. Dodson RF, Williams MG, Hurst GA. Acute lung response to amosite asbestos: A morphological study. *Environ Res* 1983;32:80–90.

33. Hasselbacher P. Binding of immunoglobulin and activation of complement by asbestos fibers. *J Allergy Clin Immunol* 1979;64:294–8.

34. Johnson RB Jr, Godzik CA, Cohn ZA. Increased superoxide anion production by immunologically activated and chemically elicited macrophages. *J Exp Med* 1978;148:127.

35. Hoidal JR, Beall GD, Repine JE. Production of hydroxyl radical by human alveolar macrophages. *Infect Immun* 1979;26:1088–94.

36. Hunninghake GW, Gadek JE, Fales HM, Crystal RG. Human alveolar macrophage-derived chemotactic factor for neutrophils. *J Clin Invest* 1980;66:473–83.

37. Rennard SI, Hunninghake GW, Bitterman PB, Crystal RG. Production of fibronectin by the human alveolar macrophage: Mechanism for recruitment of fibroblasts to sites of tissue injury in interstitial lung diseases. *Proc Natl Acad Sci U S A* 1981;78:7147–51.

38. Werb Z, Gordon S. Secretion of a specific collagenase by stimulated macrophages. *J Exp Med* 1975;142:346–60.

39. Werb Z, Gordon S. Elastase secretion by stimulated macrophages. *J Exp Med* 1975;142:361–77.

40. Henke C, Marineili W, Jessurun J, Fox J, Harms D, Peterson M, et al. Macrophage production of basic fibroblast growth factor in the fibroproliferative disorder of alveoli fibrosis after lung injury. *Am J Pathol* 1993;143:1189–99.

41. Bitterman PB, Rennard SI, Hunninghake GW, Crystal RG. Human alveolar macrophage growth factor for fibroblasts: regulation and partial characterization. *J Clin Invest* 1982;70:806–22.

42. Bitterman PB, Rennard SI, Adelberg S, Crystal RG. Role of fibronectin as a growth factor for fibroblasts. *J Cell Biol* 1983;97:1925–32.

43. Bowden DH. Macrophages, dust, and pulmonary diseases. *Exp Lung Res* 1987;12:89–107.

44. Bowden DH. The alveolar macrophage. *Environ Health Perspect* 1984;55:327–41.

45. Brain JD. Macrophage damage in relation to the pathogenesis of lung diseases. *Environ Health Perspect* 1980;35:21–8.

46. Corry D, Kulkarni P, Lipscomb MF. The migration of bronchoalveolar macrophages into hilar lymph nodes. *Am J Pathol* 1984;225:321–8.

47. Snipes MB. Long-term retention and clearance of particles inhaled by mammalian species. *Crit Rev Toxicol* 1989;20:175–211.

48. Ferin J, Feldstein ML. Pulmonary clearance and hilar lymph node content in rats after particle exposure. *Environ Res* 1978;16:342–52.

49. Lauweryns JM. The juxta-alveolar lymphatics in the human adult lung: Histologic studies in 15 cases of drowning. *Am Rev Respir Dis* 1970;102:877–85.

50. Lauweryns JM, Baert JH. The role of the pulmonary lymphatics in the defenses of the distal lung: morphological and experimental studies of the transport mechanisms of intratracheally instilled particles. *Ann N Y Acad Sci* 1974;221:244–75.

51. Camner P. Alveolar clearance. *Eur J Respir Dis* 1980;61:59–72.

52. Tosi P, Franzinelli A, Miracco C, Leoncini L, Minacci C, Baldelli C, et al. Silicotic lymph node lesions in non occupationally exposed lung carcinoma patients. *Eur J Respir Dis* 1988;68:362–9.

53. Craighead JE, Kleinerman J, Abraham JL, Gibbs AR, Green FHY, Harley RA, et al. Diseases associated with exposure to silica and nonfibrous silicate minerals. *Arch Pathol Lab Med* 1988;112:673–720.

54. Dodson RF, Shepherd S, Levin J, Hammar SP. Characteristics of the asbestos concentration in various levels of lymph nodes that collect drainage from the lung. *Ultrastruct Pathol* 2007;31:95–153.

55. Oberdorster G, Morrow PE, Spurny K. Size dependent lymphatic short-term clearance of amosite fibres in the lung. *Ann Occup Hyg* 1988;32(Suppl 1):149–56.

56. Hammar SP. Common neoplasms. In: Dail DH, Hammar SP, editors. *Pulmonary Pathology*. New York: Springer-Verlag; 1994, pp. 1123–1278.

57. Netter, FH. Respiratory system. In: Divertie MB, Brass A, editors. *The Ciba Collection of Medical Illustrations*. New Jersey: Ciba Pharmaceutical; 1979, pp. 32–33.

58. Cullen RT, Tran CL, Buchanan D, Davis JMG, Searl A, Jones AD. Inhalation of poorly soluble particles: I. Differences in inflammatory response and clearance during exposure. *Inhal Toxicol* 2000;12:1089–111.

59. Schlesinger RB. Clearance from the respiratory tract. *Fundam Appl Toxicol* 1985;5:435–50.

60. Becklake MR. Asbestos-related diseases of the lung and other organs: Their epidemiology and implications for clinical practice. *Am Rev Respir Dis* 1976;114:187–227.

61. Hillerdal G. The pathogenesis of pleural plaques and pulmonary asbestosis: Possibilities and impossibilities. *Eur J Respir Dis* 1980;61:129–38.

62. Davis JMG, Jones AD, Miller BG. Experimental studies in rats on the effects of asbestos inhalation coupled with the inhalation of titanium dioxide or quartz. *Int J Exp Path* 1991;72:501–25.

63. Pintos J, Paren M-E, Case BW, Rousseau M-C, Siemiatycki J. Risk of mesothelioma and exposure to asbestos and man-made vitreous fibers: Evidence from two case–control studies in Montreal, Canada. *J Occup Environ Med* 2009;51:1177–84.

64. Craighead JE, Mossman BT. The pathogenesis of asbestos-associated diseases. *N Engl J Med* 1982;306:1446–55.

65. Upton AC, Barrett JC, Becklake MR, Burdett G, Chatfield E, Davis JMG, et al. *Health Effects Institute–Asbestos Research: Asbestos in Public and Commercial Buildings*. A Literature Review and Synthesis of Current Knowledge. Cambridge: Health Effects Institute; 1991.

66. Bowles O. *Asbestos: The Silk of the Mineral Kingdom*. New York: The Ruberoid Co.; 1946.

67. Syracuse Research Corporation Under Contract No. 205-1999-00024. Toxicological profile for asbestos (update). Atlanta (GA): Agency for Toxic Substances and Disease Registry; 2001; p. 1.

68. Hendry NW. The geology occurrences and major user of asbestos. In: Boland B, editor. *Annals of the New York Academy of Sciences*. New York: New York Academy of Sciences; 1965, p. 12.

69. Clifton RA. Asbestos. In: Bureau of Mines, editor. *Bureau of Mines Minerals Yearbook*. Washington (DC): United States Department of the Interior; 1973, pp. 1–5.

70. Anonymous. Non-occupational exposure to mineral fibres. IARC Scientific Publication No. 90. Lyon (France): World Health Organization International Agency for Research on Cancer; 1989, p. 330.

71. Langer AM, Nolan RP, Addison J. Distinguishing between amphibole asbestos fibers and elongate cleavage fragments of their non-asbestos analogues. In: Brown RC, et al., editors. *Mechanisms in Fibre Carcinogenisis*. New York: Plenum Press; 1991, pp. 253–67.

72. Churg A. Chrysotile, tremolite, and malignant mesothelioma in man. *Chest* 1988;93:621–8.

73. Bernstein DM, Chevlier J, Smith P. Comparison of calidria chrysotile asbestos to pure tremolite: inhalation biopersistence and histopathology following short-term exposure. *Inhal Toxicol* 2003;15:1387–419.

74. Pezerat H. Chrysotile biopersistence. *Int J Occup Environ Health* 2009;15:102–6.
75. Hamilton JA. Asbestos fibers, plasma and inflammation. *Environ Health Perspect* 1983;51:281–5.
76. Valerio F, Balducci D, Lazzarotto A. Adsorption of proteins by chrysotile and crocidolite: Role of molecular weight and charge density. *Environ Res* 1987;44:312–20.
77. Xu A, Zhou H, Yu D, Hei T. Mechanisms of the genotoxicity of crocidolite asbestos in mammalian cells: implication from mutation patterns induced by reactive oxygen species. *Environ Health Perspect* 2002;110:1003–8.
78. MacCorkle RA, Slattery SD, Nash DR, Brinkley BR. Intracellular protein binding to asbestos induces aneuploidy in human lung fibroblasts. *Cell Motil Cytoskeleton* 2006;63:646–57.
79. Lee KP, Lung response to particulates with emphasis on asbestos and other fibrous dusts. *CRC Crit Rev Toxicol* 1985;14:33–86.
80. Anonymous. Task group on lung dynamics: deposition and retention models for internal dosimetry of the human respiratory tract. *Health Phys* 1966;12:173–207.
81. Dodson RF, Atkinson MAL, Levin JL. Asbestos fiber length as related to potential pathogenicity: A critical review. *Am J Ind Med* 2003;44:291–7.
82. Timbrell V, Ashcroft T, Goldstein B, et al. Relationships between retained amphiboles fibres and fibrosis in human lung tissue specimens. *Ann Occup Hyg* 1988;32(Suppl 1):323–40.
83. Marchand F. Uber eigentumliche pigmentkristalle in den lungen. *Verh Dtsch Ges Pathol* 1906;17:223–8.
84. Cooke WE. Asbestos dust and the curious bodies found in pulmonary asbestosis. *Br Med J* 1929;2:578–80.
85. Gloyne SR. The formation of the asbestos body in the lung. *Tubercle* 1931;12:399–401.
86. Gloyne SR. The morbid anatomy and histology of asbestosis. *Tubercle* 1933;14:550–8.
87. Davis JMG. Further observations on the ultrastructure and chemistry of the formation of asbestos bodies. *Exp Mol Pathol* 1970;13:346–58.
88. Governa M, Rosanda C. A histochemical study of the asbestos body coating. *Br J Ind Med* 1972;29:154–9.
89. Dodson RF, O'Sullivan MF, Williams MG, Hurst GA. Analysis of cores of ferruginous bodies from former asbestos workers. *Environ Res* 1982;28:171–8.
90. Dodson RF, O'Sullivan M, Corn CJ. Relationships between ferruginous bodies and uncoated asbestos fibers in lung tissue. *Arch Environ Health* 1996;16:637–47.
91. Churg A. The diagnosis of asbestosis. *Hum Pathol* 1989;20:97–9.
92. Dodson RF, Williams MG, Hurst GA. Method for removing the ferruginous coating from asbestos bodies. *J Toxicol Environ Health* 1983;11:959–66.
93. Gross P, Tuma J, Detreville RTP. Unusual ferruginous bodies. *Arch Environ Health* 1971;22:534–7.
94. Gross P, Detreville RTP, Cralley LJ, Davis JMG. Pulmonary ferruginous bodies. *Arch Pathol* 1968;85:539–46.
95. Holmes A, Morgan A, Davison W. Formation of pseudo-asbestos bodies on sized glass fibres in the hamster lung. *Ann Occup Hyg* 1983;27:301–13.
96. Churg A, Warnock ML. Asbestos and other ferruginous bodies. *Am J Pathol* 1981;102:447–56.
97. Dodson RF, O'Sullivan MF, Corn C, Williams MG, Hurst GA. Ferruginous body formation on a nonasbestos mineral. *Arch Pathol Lab Med* 1985;109:849–52.
98. Dodson RF, O'Sullivan M, Corn CJ, Garcia JGN, Stocks JM, Griffith DE. Analysis of ferruginous bodies in bronchoalveolar lavage from foundry workers. *Br J Ind Med* 1993;50:1032–38.
99. Dodson RF, O'Sullivan MF, Corn CJ, Hammar SP. Quantitative comparison of asbestos and talc bodies in an individual with mixed exposure. *Am J Ind Med* 1995;27:207–15.
100. Auerbach O, Conston AS, Garfinkel L, Parks VR, Kaslow HD, Hammond EC. Presence of asbestos bodies in organs other than the lung. *Chest* 1980;77:133–7.
101. Dodson RF, O'Sullivan M, Huang J, Holiday DB, Hammar SP. Asbestos in extrapulmonary sites: Omentum and mesentery. *Chest* 2000;117:486–93.
102. Godwin MC, Jagatic JJ. Asbestos and mesotheliomas. *Environ Res* 1970;3:391–416.
103. Roggli VL, Benning TL. Asbestos bodies in pulmonary hilar lymph nodes. *Mod Pathol* 1990;3:513–7.
104. Dodson RF, Williams MG, Corn CJ, Brollo A, Bianchi C. Asbestos content of lung tissue, lymph nodes and pleural plaques from former shipyard workers. *Am Rev Respir Dis* 1990;142:843–7.

105. Williams MG, Dodson RF, Dickson EW, Fraire AE. An assessment of asbestos body formation in extra-pulmonary sites: Liver and spleen. *Toxicol Ind Health* 2001;17:1–6.
106. Craighead JE, Abraham JL, Churg A, Green HY, Kleinerman J, Pratt PC, et al. The pathology of asbestos-associated diseases of the lungs and pleural cavities: Diagnostic criteria and proposed grading schema. *Arch Pathol Lab Med* 1982;106:544–96.
107. Crouch E, Churg A. Ferruginous bodies and the histological evaluation of dust exposure. *Am J Surg Pathol* 1984;8:109–16.
108. Millette JR, Twyman JD, Hansen EC, Clark PJ, Pansing MF. Chrysotile, palygorskite, and halloysite in drinking water. *Scan Electron Microsc* 1979;1:579–86.
109. Berkley C, Churg J, Selikoff IJ, Smith WE. The detection and localization of mineral fibers in tissue. In: Boland B, Hitchcock J, Kates S, editors. *Biological Effects of Asbestos*. New York: New York Academy of Sciences; 1965, pp. 48–63.
110. Carter RE, Taylor WF. Identification of particular amphibole asbestos fiber in tissue of persons exposed to a high oral intake of the mineral. *Environ Res* 1980;21:85–93.
111. Chatfield EJ. Preparation and analysis of particulate samples by electron microscopy, with special reference to asbestos. *Scan Electron Microsc* 1979;1:563–78.
112. Chatfield EJ, Dillon MJ. Some aspects of specimen preparation and limitations of precision in particulate analysis by SEM and TEM. *Scan Electron Microsc* 1978;1:487–96.
113. Ashcroft T, Heppleston AG. The optical and electron microscopic determination of pulmonary asbestos fiber concentration and its relation to the human pathological reaction *J Clin Pathol* 1973;26:224–34.
114. Langer AM, Rubin IB, Selikoff IJ. Chemical characterization of asbestos body cores by electron micro-probe analysis. *J Histochem Cytochem* 1972;20:723–34.
115. Churg A, Warnock ML. Asbestos fibers in the general population. *Am Rev Respir Dis* 1980;122:669–78.
116. Stasny JT, Husach C, Albright FR, Schumacher DV, Sweigart DW, Boyer K. Development of methods to isolate asbestos from spiked beverages and foods for SEM characterization. *Scan Electron Microsc* 1979;1:587–95.
117. Sundius N, Bygden A. Isolation of the mineral dust in lungs and sputum. *J Ind Hyg Toxicol* 1938;20:351–9.
118. Vallyathan V, Green FHY. The role of analytical techniques in the diagnosis of asbestos-associated disease. *CRC Crit Rev Clin Lab Sci* 1985;22:1–42.
119. Gylseth B, Baunan RH, Bruun R. Analysis of inorganic fibre concentrations in biological samples by scanning electron microscopy. *Scand J Work Environ Health* 1981;7:101–8.
120. Gylseth B, Baunan RH. Topographic and size distribution of asbestos bodies in exposed human lungs. *Scand J Work Environ Health* 1981;7:190–5.
121. De Vuyst P, Karjalainen A, Dumortier P, et al. Guidelines for mineral fibre analysis in biological samples: Report of the ERS Working Group. *Eur Respir J* 1998;11:1416–26.
122. Dement JM. Overview on fiber toxicology research needs. *Environ Health Perspect* 1990;88:261–268.
123. Williams MG, Dodson RF, Corn C, Hurst GA. A procedure for the isolation of amosite asbestos and ferruginous bodies from lung tissue and sputum. *J Toxicol Environ Health* 1982;10:627–38.
124. Smith MJ, Naylor B. A method of extracting ferruginous bodies from sputum and pulmonary tissue. *Am J Clin Pathol* 1972;58:250–4.
125. Dodson RF, Williams MG, McLarty JW, Hurst GA. Asbestos bodies and particulate matter in sputum from former asbestos workers. *Acta Cytol* 1983;27:635–40.
126 Dodson RF, Garcia JGN, O'Sullivan M, Corn C, Levin JL, Griffith DE, Kronenberg RS. The usefulness of bronchoalveolar lavage in identifying past occupational exposure to asbestos: A light and electron microscopy study. *Am J Ind Med* 1991;19:619–28.
127 O'Sullivan MF, Corn CJ, Dodson RF. Comparative efficiency of Nuclepore filters of various pore sizes as used in digestion studies of tissue. *Environ Res* 1987;43:97–103.
128. Webber JS, Czuhanich AG, Carhart LJ. Performance of membrane filters used for TEM analysis of asbestos. *J Occup Environ Hyg* 2007;4:780–9.
129. Middleton AP, Jackson EA. A procedure for the estimation of asbestos collected on membrane filters using transmission electron microscopy (TEM). *Ann Occup Hyg* 1982;25:381–91.
130. Middleton AP. Visibility of fine fibres of asbestos during routine electron microscopical analysis. *Ann Occup Hyg* 1982;25:53–62.

131. Small JA. *Proceeding of the Asbestos Fibers Measurements in Building Atmospheres*. Mississauga (Ontario, Canada): Ontario Research Foundation; 1982, p. 69.

132. Teichert U. *Proceedings of the Fourth International Colloquium on Dust Measuring Techniques and Strategies*, Edinburgh, Scotland, September 20–23, 1982. London (UK): Asbestos International Association; 1982, p. 130.

133. Small JA, Newbury DE, Myklebust RL. *Proceedings of the 18th Annual Conference of the Microbeam Analysis Society*. San Francisco (CA): San Francisco Press; 1983.

134. Lee RJ. *Basic Concepts of Electron Diffraction and Asbestos Identification Using Selected Area Diffraction*. O'Hare (IL): SEM; 1978.

135. Ruud CD, Russell PA, Clark RL. Selected area electron diffraction and energy dispersive x-ray analysis for the identification of asbestos fibers, a comparison. *Micron* 1976;7:115–32.

136. Dodson RF, O'Sullivan MF, Corn CJ. Technique dependent variations in asbestos burden as illustrated in a case of nonoccupational exposed mesothelioma. *Am J Ind Med* 1993;24:235–40.

137. Greenberg SD, Hurst GA, Matlage WT, Christianson C, Hurst IJ, Mabry LC. Sputum cytopathological findings in former asbestos workers. *Tex Med* 1976;72:39–43.

138. Bignon J, Sebastien P, Jaurand MC, Hem H. Microfiltration method for quantitative study of fibrous particles in biological specimens. *Environ Health Perspect* 1974;9:155–60.

139. McLarty JW, Greenberg SD, Hurst GA, Spivey CG, Seitzman JW, Hieger LR, et al. The clinical significance of ferruginous bodies in sputa. *J Occup Med* 1980;22:92–6.

140. Modin BE, Greenberg SD, Buffler PA, Lockhart JA, Seitzman LH, Awe RJ. Asbestos bodies in a general hospital/clinic population. *Acta Cytol* 1982;26:667–70.

141. Paris C, Galateau-Salle F, Creveuil C, Morello R, Raffaelli C, Gillon MA, et al. Asbestos bodies in sputum of asbestos workers: correlation with occupational exposure. *Eur Respir J* 2002;20:1167–73.

142. Sebastien P, Armstrong B, Case BW, Barwick H, Keskula H, McDonald JC. Estimation of amphibole exposure from asbestos body and macrophage counts in sputum: a survey in vermiculite miners. *Ann Occup Hyg* 1988;32(Suppl 1):195–201.

143. Dodson RF, Williams MG, Corn CJ, Idell S, McLarty JW. Usefulness of combined light and electron microscopy evaluation of sputum samples for asbestos to determine past occupational exposure. *Mod Pathol* 1989;2:320–2.

144. Goldstein RA, Rohatgi PK, Bergofsky EH, et al. Clinical role of bronchoalveolar lavage in adults with pulmonary disease. *Am Rev Respir Dis* 1990;142:481–6.

145. Begin RO. Bronchoalveolar lavage in the pneumoconioses. *Chest* 1988;94:454.

146. De Vuyst P, Dumortier P, Moulin E, Yourassowsky N, Yernault JC. Diagnostic value of asbestos bodies in bronchoalveolar lavage fluid. *Am Rev Respir Dis* 1987;136:1219–24.

147. De Vuyst P, Jedwab J, Dumortier P, Vandermoten G, Vande Weyer R, Yernault JC. Asbestos bodies in bronchoalveolar lavage. *Am Rev Respir Dis* 1982;126:972–6.

148. De Vuyst P, Dumortier P, Moulin E, Yourassowsky N, Roomans P, deFrancquen P, Yernault JC. Asbestos bodies in bronchoalveolar lavage reflect lung asbestos body concentration. *Eur Respir J* 1988;1:362–367.

149. Dumortier P, Coplu L, de Maertelaer V, Emri S, Baris YI, De Vuyst P. Assessment of environmental asbestos exposure in Turkey by bronchoalveolar lavage. *Am J Respir Crit Care Med* 1998;158:1815–24.

150. Sebastien P, Armstrong B, Monchaux G, Bignon J. Asbestos bodies in bronchoalveolar lavage fluid and in lung parenchyma. *Am Rev Respir Dis* 1988;137:75–8.

151. Schwartz, DA, Galvin, JR, Burmeister, LF, Merchant, RK, Dayton, CS, Merchant, JA, Hunninghake, GW. The clinical utility and reliability of asbestos bodies in bronchoalveolar fluid. *Am Rev Respir Dis* 1991;144:684–8.

152. Oriowski E, Pairon JC, Ameille J, Janson X, Iwatsubo Y, Dufour G, et al. Pleural plaques, asbestos exposure, and asbestos bodies in bronchoalveolar lavage fluid. *Am J Ind Med* 1994;26:349–58.

153. Dodson RF, Williams G, Huang J, Bruce JR. Tissue burden of asbestos in nonoccupationally exposed individuals from East Texas. *Am J Ind Med* 1999;35:281–6.

154. Dodson RF, O'Sullivan M, Brooks DR, Bruce JR. Asbestos content of omentum and mesentery in nonoccupationally exposed individuals. *Toxicol Ind Health* 2001;17:138–43.

155. Gellert AR, Kitajewska JY, Uthayakumar S, Kirkham JB, Rudd RM. Asbestos fibres in bronchoalveolar lavage fluid from asbestos workers: examination by electron microscopy. *Br J Ind Med* 1986;43:170–6.

156. De Vuyst P, Dumortier P, Gevenois PA. Analysis of asbestos bodies in BAL from subjects with particular exposures. *Am J Ind Med* 1997;31:699–704.

157. Dodson RF, O'Sullivan M, Brooks DR, Levin JL. The sensitivity of lavage analysis by light and analytical electron microscopy in correlating the types of asbestos from a known exposure setting. *Inhal Toxicol* 2003;15:461–71.

158. Artivinli M, Baris YI. Environmental fiber-induced pleuro-pulmonary diseases in an Antolian Village: An epidemiology study. *Arch Environ Health* 1982;37:177–81.

159. Dumortier P, Coplu L, Broucke I, Emir S, Selcuk T, Maertelaer V, De Vuyst P, Baris I. Erionite bodies and fibres in bronchoalveolar lavage fluid (BALF) of residents from Tuzkoy, Cappadocia, Turkey. *Occup Environ Med* 2001;58:261–6.

160. Kliment CR, Clemens K, Ory TD. North American erionite-associated mesothelioma with pleural plaques and pleural fibrosis: a case report. *Int J Clin Exp Pathol* 2009;2:407–10.

161. De Vuyst P, Dumortier P, Leophonte P, Vande Weyer R, Yernault, JC. Mineralogical analysis of bronchoalveolar lavage in talc pneumoconiosis. *Eur J Respir Dis* 1987;70:150–6.

162. Dumortier P, De Vuyst P, Strauss P, Yernault, JC. Asbestos bodies in bronchoalveolar lavage fluids of brake lining and asbestos cement workers. *Br J Ind Med* 1990;47:91–8.

163. Levin JL, O'Sullivan MF, Corn CJ, Dodson RF. An individual with a majority of ferruginous bodies formed on chrysotile cores. *Arch Environ Health* 1995;50:462–5.

164. Butnor K, Sporn T, Roggli VL. Exposure to brake dust and malignant mesothelioma: A study of 10 cases with mineral fiber analysis. *Ann Occup Hyg* 2003;47:325–30.

165. Paustenbach D, Richter R, Finley B, Sheehan P. An evaluation of the historical exposures of mechanics to asbestos in brake dust. *Appl Occup Environ Hyg* 2003;18:786–804.

166. Weir F, Meraz L. Morphological characteristics of asbestos fibers released during grinding and drilling of friction products. *Appl Occup Environ Hyg* 2001;16:1147–9.

167. Weir F, Tolar G, Meraz L. Characterization of vehicular brake service personnel exposure to airborne asbestos and particulate. *Appl Occup Environ Hyg* 2001;16:1139–46.

168. Sartorelli P, Scancarello G, Romeo R, Marciano G, Rottoli P, Arcangeli G, Palmi S. Asbestos exposure assessment by mineralogical analysis of bronchoalveolar lavage fluid. *J Occup Environ Med* 2001;43:872–81.

169. Churg A, Warnock ML. Analysis of the cores of ferruginous (asbestos) bodies from the general population: I. Patients with and without lung cancer. *Lab Invest* 1977;37:280–6.

170. Churg, A., Warnock, ML. Analysis of the cores of ferruginous (asbestos) bodies from the general population: III. Patients with environmental exposure. *Lab Invest* 1979;40:622–6.

171. Churg A, Warnock ML. Correlation of quantitative asbestos body counts and occupation in urban patients. *Arch Pathol Lab Med* 1977;101:629–34.

172. Mollo F, Magnani C, Bo P, Burlo P, Cravello M. The attribution of lung cancers to asbestos exposure: A pathological study of 924 unselected cases. *Anatom Pathol* 2002;117:90–5.

173. De Vuyst P, Karjalainen A, Dumortier P, Pairon E, Brochard P, Teschler H, et al. Guidelines for mineral fibre analyses in biological samples: Report of the ERS Working Group. *Eur Respir J* 1998;11:1416–26.

174. Dodson RF, Greenberg SD, Williams MG, Corn CJ, O'Sullivan MF, Hurst GA. Asbestos content in lungs of occupationally and nonoccupationally exposed individuals. *JAMA* 1984;252:68–71.

175. Breedin PH, Buss DH. Ferruginous (asbestos) bodies in the lungs of rural dwellers, urban dwellers and patients with pulmonary neoplasms. *South Med J* 1976;69:401–4.

176. Roggli VL, Pratt PC, Brody AR. Asbestos content of lung tissue in asbestos associated diseases: A study of 110 cases. *Br J Ind Med* 1986;43:18–28.

177. Moulin E, Yourassowsky N, Dumortier P, De Vuyst P, Yernault JC. Electron microscopic analysis of asbestos body cores from the Belgian urban population. *Eur Respir J* 1988;1:818–22.

178. Holden J, Churg A. Asbestos bodies and the diagnosis of asbestosis in chrysotile workers. *Environ Res* 1986;39:232–6.

179. Levin J, O'Sullivan M, Corn C, Williams MG, Dodson RF. Asbestosis and small cell lung cancer in a clutch refabricator. *Occup Environ Med* 1999;56:602–5.

180. Dodson RF, O'Sullivan M, Corn C, McLarty JW, Hammar SP. Analysis of asbestos fiber burden in lung tissue from mesothelioma patients. *Ultrastruct Pathol* 1997;21:321–36.

181. Dodson RF, O'Sullivan M, Brooks DR, Hammar SP. Quantitative analysis of asbestos burden in women with mesothelioma. *Am J Ind Med* 2002;43:188–95.

182. Srebro SH, Roggli VL, Samsa GP. Malignant mesothelioma associated with low pulmonary tissue asbestos burdens: a light and scanning electron microscopic analysis of 18 cases. *Mod Path* 1995;8(6):614–21.

183. Dodson RF, Brooks DR, O'Sullivan M. Quantitative analysis of asbestos burden in a series of individuals with lung cancer and a history of exposure to asbestos. *Inhal Toxicol* 2004;16:637–47.

184. Dodson RF, Williams MG, O'Sullivan MF, Corn CJ, Greenberg SD, Hurst GA. A comparison of the ferruginous body and uncoated fiber content in the lungs of former asbestos workers. *Am Rev Respir Dis* 1985;132:143–7.

185. Warnock ML, Wolery G. Asbestos bodies or fibers and the diagnosis of asbestosis. *Environ Res* 1987;44:29–44.

186. Ehrlich A, Rohl AN, Holstein EC. Asbestos bodies in carcinoma of colon in an insulation worker with asbestosis. *JAMA* 1985;254(20):2932–3.

187. Christensen BC, Houseman EA, Godleski JJ, et al. Epigentic profiles distinguish pleural mesothelioma from normal pleura and predict lung asbestos burden and clinical outcome. *Cancer Res* 2009;69:227–33.

188. Morgan A, Holmes A. The distribution and characteristics of asbestos fibers in the lungs of Finnish anthophyllite mine-workers. *Environ Res* 1984;33:62–75.

189. Rood AP, Streeter RR. Size distributions of occupational airborne asbestos textile fibres as determined by transmission electron microscopy. *Ann Occup Hyg* 1984;28:333–95.

190. Dodson RF, Williams MG, Satterley JD. Asbestos burden in two cases of mesothelioma where the work history included manufacturing of cigarette filters. *J Toxicol Environ Health* 2002;65:1109–20.

191. Pooley FD, Ranson DL. Comparison of the results of asbestos fibre dust counts in lung tissue obtained by analytical electron microscopy and light microscopy. *J Clin Pathol* 1986;39:313–7.

192. Dodson RF, Hammar SP, Poye LW. A technical comparison of evaluating asbestos concentration by phase-contrast microscopy (PCM), scanning electron microscopy (SEM), and analytical transmission electron microscopy (ATEM) as illustrated from data generated from a case report. *Inhal Toxicol* 2008;20:723–2.

193. Dodson RF, Atkinson MAL. Measurements of asbestos burden in tissues. *Ann N Y Acad Sci* 2006;1076:281–91.

194. Langer AM. Chrysotile asbestos in the lungs of persons in New York City. *Arch Environ Health* 1971;22:348–61.

195. Langer AM, Nolan RP. Chrysotile biopersistence in the lungs of persons in the general population and exposed workers. *Environ Health Perspect* 1994;102(Suppl 5):235–9.

196. Egilman D, Fehnel C, Bohme S. Exposing the "myth" of ABC, "anything but chrysotile": A critique of the Canadian Asbestos Mining Industry and McGill University Chrysotile Studies. *Am J Ind Med* 2003;44:540–57.

197. Lindell FDK. Magic, menace, myth and malice. *Ann Occup Hyg* 1997;41:3–12.

198. Addison J, Davies LST. Analysis of amphibole asbestos in chrysotile and other minerals. *Ann Occup Hyg* 1990;34:159–75.

199. McDonald JC, Armstrong BG, Edwards CW, Gibbs AR, Lloyd HM, Pooley FD, et al. Case referent survey of young adults with mesothelioma: I. Lung fibre analysis. *Ann Occup Hyg* 2001;45:513–8.

200. Churg A. Asbestos fiber content of the lungs in patients with and without asbestos airways disease. *Am Rev Respir Dis* 1983;127:470–3.

201. Churg A, Wright JL, Vedal S. Fiber burden and patterns of asbestos-related disease in chrysotile miners and millers. *Am Rev Respir Dis* 1993;148:25–31.

202. Churg A, Wright J, Wiggs B, Depaoli L. Mineralogic parameters related to amosite asbestos-induced fibrosis in humans. *Am Rev Respir Dis* 1990;142:1331–6.

203. McDonald JC, Armstrong B, Case B, et al. Mesothelioma and asbestos fiber type—Evidence from lung tissue analysis. *Cancer* 1989;63:1544–7.

204. McDonald JC, Edwards CW, Gibbs AR, et al. Case-referent survey of young adults with mesothelioma: II Occupational analysis. *Ann Occup Hyg* 2001;45(7):519–23.

205. Dufresne A, Begin R, Churg A, Masse S. Mineral fiber content of lungs in patients with mesothelioma seeking compensation in Quebec. *Am J Respir Crit Care Med* 1996;153:711–8.

206. Churg A, Vedal S. Fiber burden and patterns of asbestos-related disease in workers with heavy mixed amosite and chrysotile exposure. *Am J Respir Crit Care Med* 1994;150:663–9.

207. Nayebzadeh A, Dufresne A, Case B, Vali H, Williams-Jones AE, Martin R, et al. Lung mineral fibers of former miners and millers from Thetford-Mines and asbestos regions: A comparative study of fiber concentration and dimension. *Arch Environ Health* 2001;56:65–76.

208. Langer AM, Nolan RP. Non-occupational exposure to mineral fibres, fibre type and burden in paren-chymal tissues of workers occupationally exposed to asbestos in the United States. *IARC Sci Publ* 1989;90:330–5.

209. Langer AM, McCaughey WTE. Mesothelioma in a brake repair worker. *Lancet* 1982;2:1101–3.

210. Pooley FD, Oldham FD, Chang-Hyum UM, Wagner JC. The detection of asbestos in tissues. In: Shirpio HA, editor. *Pnuemonoconiosis: Proceeding of the 2nd International Conference (Johannesburg)*. London: Oxford University Press; 1970, pp. 108–16.

211. Srebro SH, Roggli VL. Asbestos-related disease associated with exposure to asbestiform tremolite. *Am J Ind Med* 1994;26:809–19.

212. Dodson RF, Graef R, Shepherd S, O'Sullivan M, Levin JL. Asbestos burden in cases of mesothelioma from individuals from various regions of the United States. *Ultrast Pathol* 2005;29:415–33.

213. Churg A, Wright JL, Vedal S. Fiber burden and patterns of asbestos-related disease in chrysotile miners and millers. *Am Rev Respir Dis* 1993;148:25–31.

214. McDonald JC, McDonald AD. Chrysotile, tremolite and mesothelioma: Letter published in *Science* 1995;267:775–6.

215. Finkelstein MM. Asbestos fibre concentrations in the lungs of brake workers: Another look. *Ann Occup Hyg* 2008;52:455–61.

216. Case BW. Health effects of tremolite. The third wave of asbestos disease: Exposure to asbestos in place-public health control. *Ann N Y Acad Sci* 1991;643:491–504.

217. Case BW. On talc, tremolite, and tergiversation. *Br J Ind Med* 1991;48:357–60.

218. Williams-Jones AE, Normand C, Clark JR, Vali H, Martin RF, Dufresne A, Nayebzadeh A. Controls of amphibole formation in chrysotile deposits; evidence from the Jeffrey mine, Asbestos, Quebec; the health effects of chrysotile asbestos: contribution of science to risk-management decisions. *Can Mineral* 2001;5:89–194 [special issue].

219. Warnock ML, Isenberg W. Asbestos burden and the pathology of lung cancer. *Chest* 1986;89:20–6.

220. Sebastien P, Jason X, Gaudichet A, Hirsch A, Bignon J. Asbestos retention in human respiratory tissues: Comparative measurements in lung parenchyma and in parietal pleura. In: Wagner JC, editor. *Biological Effects of Mineral Fibers*. Lyon: IARC; 1980, pp. 237–46.

221. McDonald JC, McDonald AD, Armstrong B, Sebastien P. Cohort study of mortality of vermiculite min-ers exposed to tremolite. *Br J Ind Med* 1986;43:436–44.

222. Wright RS, Abraham JL, Harber P, Burnett BR, Morris P, West P. Fatal asbestosis 50 years after brief high intensity exposure in a vermiculite expansion plant. *Am J Respir Crit Care Med* 2002;165:1145–9.

223. Kleinfeld M, Messite J, Langer M. A study of workers exposed to asbestiform minerals in commercial talc manufacture. *Environ Res* 1973;6:132–143.

224. Rohl AN, Langer AM, Selikoff I, et al. Consumer talcums and powders: mineral and chemical character-ization. *J Toxicol Environ Health* 1976;2:255–84.

225. Hull MJ, Abraham JL, Case BW. Mesothelioma among workers in asbestos fiber-bearing mines in New York State. *Ann Occup Hyg* 2002;1:132–135.

226. Scancarello G, Romeo R, Sartorelli E. Respiratory disease as a result of talc inhalation. *J Occup Environ Med* 1996;38: 610–4.

227. Roggli VL, Vollmer RT, Butnor KJ, Sporn TA. Tremolite and mesothelioma. *Ann Occup Hyg* 2002;46:447–53.

228. Telischi M, Rubenstone AI. Pulmonary asbestosis. *Arch Pathol* 1961;72:116–25.

229. Langer AM. Inorganic particles in human tissues and their association with neoplastic disease. *Environ Health Perspect* 1974;9:229–33.

230. Rosen P, Gordon P, Savino A, Melamed M. Ferruginous bodies in benign fibrous pleural plaques. *Am J Clin Pathol* 1980;60:608–17.

231. Churg A, Green FHY. Quantitative assessment of asbestos bodies from lung tissue. In: Churg A, Green FHY, editors. *Pathology of Occupational Lung Disease*. New York: Igaku-Shoin; 1988, pp. 385–6.

232. Knudson A. Asbestos and mesothelioma: genetic lessons from a tragedy. *Proc Natl Acad Sci U S A* 1995;92:10819–20.

233. Dodson RF, Huang J, Bruce JR. Asbestos content in the lymph nodes of nonoccupationally exposed individuals. *Am J Ind Med* 2000;37:169–74.

234. Suzuki Y, Yuen SR. Asbestos tissue burden study on human malignant mesothelioma. *Ind Health* 2001;39:150–60.

235. Suzuki Y, Yuen SR. Asbestos fibers contributing to the induction of human malignant mesothelioma. *Ann N Y Acad Sci* 2002;1: 1–14.

236. Suzuki Y, Yuen SR, Ashley R. Short, thin asbestos fibers contribute to the development of human malignant mesothelioma: Pathological evidence. *Int J Hyg Environ Health* 2005;208:201–10.

237. Tweedale G, McCulloch J. Chrysotile versus chrysophobes—The white asbestos controversy, 1950–2004. *Isis* 2004;95:239–59.

238. Kamp DW, Weitzman SA. The molecular basis of asbestos induced lung injury. *Thorax* 1999;54:638–52.

239. Boutin C, Dumortier RF, Viallat JR, De Vuyst P. Black spots concentrate oncogenic asbestos fibers in the parietal pleural. Thoracoscopic and mineral study. *Am J Respir Crit Care Med* 1996;153:444–9.

240. LeBouffant L. Physics and chemistry of asbestos dust. In: Wagner JC, editor. *Biological Effects of Mineral Fibres*. Lyon (France): IARC Scientific Publications; 1980, pp. 15–33.

241. Kohyama N, Suzuki Y. Analysis of asbestos fibers in lung parenchyma, pleural plaques, and mesothelioma tissues of North American insulation workers. *Ann N Y Acad Sci* 1991;643:27–52.

242. Muller K-M, Schmitz I, Konstantinidis, K. Black spots of the parietal pleura: morphology and formal pathogenesis. *Respiration* 2002;69:261–7.

243. Mitchev K, Dumortier P, De Vuyst P. "Black spots" and hyaline pleural plaques on the parietal pleura of 150 urban necropsy cases. *Am J Surg Pathol* 2002;25:1198–206.

244. Miserocchi G, Sancini G, Mantegazza F, Chiappino G. Translocation pathways for inhaled asbestos fibers—A review. *Environ Health* 2008;7:4.

245. Hasanoglu HC, Bayram E, Hasanoglu A, Demirag F. Orally ingested chrysotile asbestos affects rat lungs and pleura. *Arch Environ Occup Health* 2008;63(2):71–5.

246. Monchaux G, Bignon J, Hirsch A, Sebastien P. Translocation of mineral fibres through the respiratory system after injection into the pleural cavity of rats. *Ann Occup Hyg* 1982;26:309–18.

247. Lauweryns JM, Baert JH. State of the art. Alveolar clearance and the role of the pulmonary lymphatics. *Am Rev Respir Dis* 1977;115:625–83.

248. Uibu T, Vanhala E, Sajantila A, et al. Asbestos fibers in para-aortic and mesenteric lymph nodes. *Am J Ind Med* 2009;52:464–70.

249. Stanton MF, Wrench C. Mechanisms of mesothelioma induction with asbestos and fibrous glass. *J Natl Cancer Inst* 1972;48:797–821.

250. Stanton MF, Layard M, Tegeris E, Miller E, May M, Morgan E, Smith A. Relation of particle dimension to carcinogenicity in amphibole asbestoses and other fibrous minerals. *J Natl Cancer Inst* 1981;67:965.

251. Pott F. Problems in defining carcinogenic fibres. *Ann Occup Hyg* 1987;31:799–802.

252. Pott F, Ziem U, Reiffer FJ, Huth F, Ernst H, Mohr U. Carcinogenicity studies on fibres, metal compounds, and some other dusts in rats. *Exp Pathol* 1987;32:129–52.

253. Pott F, Roller M, Ziem U, Reiffer F-J, Bellman B, Rosenbruch M, Huth F. Carcinogenicity studies on natural and man-made fibres with the intraperitoneal test in rats. *Symposium on Mineral Fibres in the Non-occupational Environment*, Lyon, September 8–10, 1987, Lyon, 1–4, 1988.

254. Pott F, Huth F, Friedrichs KH. Tumorigenic effect of fibrous dusts in experimental animals. *Environ Health Perspect* 1974;9:313–5.

255. Fraire AE, Greenberg SD, Spjut HJ, Roggli VL, Dodson RF, Cartwright J, et al. Effect of fibrous glass on rat pleural mesothelium. *Am J Respir Crit Care Med* 1994;1509:521–7.

256. Goodglick LA, Kane AB. Cytotoxicity of long and short crocidolite asbestos fibers in vitro and in vivo. *Cancer Res* 1990;50:5153–63.

257. Lippmann M. Review: asbestos exposure indices. *Environ Res* 1988;46:86–106.

258. Robinson BWS, Musk AW, Lake RA. Seminar—Malignant mesothelioma. *Lancet* 2005;366:397–408.

259. Chen HC, Tsai KB, Wang CS, Hsieh TJ, Hsu JS. Duodenal metastasis of malignant pleural mesothelioma. *J Formos Med Assoc* 2008;107:961–4.

260. Hammar SP. Macroscopic, histological, histochemical, immunohistochemical, and ultrastructual features of mesothelioma. *Ultrastruct Pathol* 2006;30:3–17.

261. Mark EJ, Yokoi T. Absence of evidence for a significant background incidence of diffuse malignant mesothelioma apart from asbestos exposure: Part 8. The neoplasms of asbestos exposure; the third wave of asbestos diseases: exposure to asbestos in place-public health control. *N Y Acad Sci* 1991;643:196–204.

262. Nishikawa K, Takahashi K, Karjalainen A, et al. Recent mortality from pleural mesothelioma, historical patterns of asbestos use, and adoption of bans: A global assessment. *Environ Health Perspect* 2008;116:1675–80.

263. Magnani C, Agudo A, Gonzalez CA, et al. Multicentric study on malignant pleural mesothelioma and non-occupational exposure to asbestos. *Br J Cancer* 2000;83:104–11.

264. Kurumatani N, Kumagal S. Mapping the risk of mesothelioma due to neighborhood asbestos exposure. *Am J Respir Crit Care Med* 2008;178:624–9.

265. Goldberg M, Luce D. The health impact of nonoccupational exposure to asbestos: What do we know? *Eur J Cancer Prev* 2009;18:489–503.

266. Henderson D, Rantanen J, Barhart S, et al. Asbestos, asbestosis, and cancer: The Helsinki criteria for diagnosis and attribution. *Scand J Work Environ Health* 1997;23:311–6.

267. Asbestos-related disease—A preventable burden [editorial]. *Lancet* 2009;371:1927.

268. Attfield MD, Bang KM, Petsonk EL, Schleiff PL, Mazurek JM. Trends in pneumoconiosis mortality and morbidity for the United States, 1968–2005, and relationship with indicators of extent of exposure, inhaled particulates X. *J Phys Conf Ser* 2009;151.

269. Anonymous. Malignant Mesothelioma Mortality—United States, 1990–2005. *Morbidity and Mortality Weekly Report*; April 24, 2009. Centers for Disease Control Report No. 15.

270. Galson SK. Statement from Acting Surgeon General Steven K. Galson about National Asbestos Week. Office of the Surgeon General; April 1, 2009.

CHAPTER 4

The Molecular Pathogenesis of Asbestos-Related Disorders

Sonja Klebe and Douglas W. Henderson

CONTENTS

4.1 INTRODUCTION

Asbestos fibers initiate variable effects in mesothelial cells and lung mesenchymal and epithelial cells, the target cells of malignant mesothelioma, asbestosis, and lung cancer.[1,2] The effects mediated by the different types of asbestos are dependent on fiber shape (and size) as well as the chemistry of the fibers. Especially, the surface composition of fibers plays an important role, with many effects mediated by iron either as an integral part of the fiber or as an impurity on its surface. Some effects are purely mechanical, whereas others are mediated via direct interactions of asbestos fibers with cell components, such as receptors, and via generation of reactive oxygen species (ROS). All result in the alteration of cell signaling pathways that regulate gene expression or regulatory pathways involved in apoptosis. Although the end result may be different, the initial disruption of a number of cellular *pathways* is a recurrent event (Figure 4.1). Therefore, it may be useful to think of asbestos-related disorders as unified by similar initial events and with disruption of certain cell pathways. We shall concentrate on those pathways and their potential effects for the specific disorder rather than discussing each cytokine, transcription factor, and disorder separately. This also means that the discussion will be limited to those pathways that are affected in fibrotic and malignant asbestos-related disorders.

One important development over the last few years is renewed interest in, and confirmation of, Virchow's original 1860s hypothesis that "the sites of chronic inflammation reflect the origin of cancer."* In the case of asbestos-mediated disorders, inflammation may play some role in the development of malignant conditions, with recent experimental evidence providing some linking pathways, for example, in the form of tumor necrosis factor α (TNF-α) and nuclear factor κB (NF-κB) activation (reviewed in the following sections).[3]

Another important piece of evidence concerns the role of bone marrow–derived nonhematogenous stem cells in the development of asbestos-related disorders. Evidence for the relevance of this mechanism is provided in the work of Spees et al.,[4] who demonstrated specific migration and engraftment of bone marrow–derived nonhematopoietic stem cells to the lungs of female rats that had been lethally irradiated, rescued by bone marrow transplant with Green fluorescent protein (GFP)-positive male cells and then exposed to chrysotile asbestos aerosol at 10 mg/m³ for 5 h on three consecutive days. One day and 2.5 weeks after exposure, significant numbers of GFP-labeled male cells had preferentially migrated to the bronchiolar-alveolar duct bifurcations, the anatomic site at which asbestos appears to produce its initial effects. The data suggest that bone marrow–derived stem cells may play a crucial role rather than or in addition to preexisting local epithelial and stromal cells. Not surprisingly, GFP-positive cells were also present at the lesions as an inflammatory component consisting of monocytes and macrophages as well as fibroblasts and myofibroblasts or smooth muscle cells. Lack of apoptosis was also demonstrated. These studies confirm a role for bone marrow–derived nonhematopoietic cells in the development of asbestos-related disorders.

4.2 THE LIMITATIONS OF EXPERIMENTAL MODELS AND THEIR APPLICABILITY TO HUMAN EXPOSURES

It is worth noting at this point that much of the data described in the following sections is the result of in vitro or animal models. Many cell lines used in such experiments have been immortalized and hence carry preexisting (albeit usually well-characterized) cytogenetic and molecular modulations that may facilitate carcinogenesis.[5,6] One might even argue that an immortalized cell line has in fact already acquired one of the key features of malignant cells—that is, the capacity to proliferate indefinitely. In the case of mesothelial cells, the standard "normal human mesothelial" ATCC cell line Met-5A (www.atcc.org) comprises nonneoplastic human mesothelial cells that have been immortalized by transfection with a plasmid containing the SV40 early region DNA. This is of particular interest because a potential role for SV40 in the induction of malignant mesothelioma has been suggested by some authors in the past, and there is no doubt that SV40 can be oncogenic under

---

* In the sense of the molecular changes resulting from the interaction between asbestos fibers and cells such as lung macrophages: There are some shared initial events and alteration of the same molecular pathways, which may have both inflammatory and neoplastic potential. Recent experimental findings confirm a close relationship between inflammation (in the sense of the reactions of irritated nonneoplastic cells that retain vitality)/fibrosis/tissue remodeling and neoplastic disease at a molecular level by identifying common pathways that may influence either process. This does not mean that evidence of fibrosis or tissue remodeling is a prerequisite for asbestos-induced malignancy; rather, the molecular events that follow interaction between asbestos fibers and cells such as macrophages or epithelial or mesothelial cells can follow a pathway that leads to inflammation/fibrosis or neoplasia, without an obligate linkage between overt inflammation/fibrosis and the process of neoplasia (see Chapter 6 and Figure 4.1).

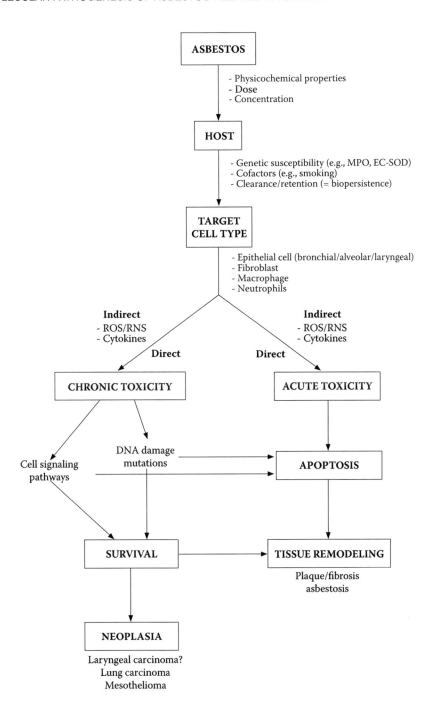

Figure 4.1 *Asbestos and host response.* An individual's response to asbestos depends first on the type and quantity of asbestos inhaled and second on host factors such as genetic susceptibility or preexisting cofactors such as smoking or environmental pollution. Different target cell types may also show different responses, mediating their effects either directly or indirectly via ROS. There will be either acute or chronic toxic effects or a mixture of chronic and acute effects. One possible outcome of acute toxicity may be apoptosis, but chronic inflammation may also still result in apoptosis. If the affected cells survive the toxic insult, they will show altered cell signaling and may also contain genetic alterations resulting in tissue remodeling, neoplasia, or both.

certain conditions. For example, if this DNA virus is injected into the heart or pleura of hamsters, it has been shown to induce mesotheliomas.[7] The polyomavirus SV40 was discovered as a contaminant in the monkey kidney cells that were used to produce poliomyelitis vaccines between 1955 and 1963, and the vaccine has been invoked as a potential source for SV40 DNA.[8] Although it appears certain that SV40 can induce tumors in animal models and in vitro, there is to date no convincing data that it contributes to mesothelioma carcinogenesis in humans.[9] In fact, recent evidence suggests that many of the earlier results demonstrating SV40 may be false-positive results because of preexisting laboratory contamination by common laboratory plasmids containing SV40 sequences.[10]

Animal models for asbestos-induced diseases include mice, rats, guinea pigs, hamsters, gerbils, rabbits, sheep, cats, baboons, and vervet monkeys, but no animal model can exactly reflect the situation in humans.[11–17] It should be noted that these animal models, in general, did not aim to establish carcinogenicity of asbestos (already established by epidemiological studies in human subjects) but aimed to investigate the *mechanisms* of asbestos-induced toxicity. Currently, most researchers use rats and mice. However, it is obvious from histologic examination that there are crucial differences in the host response that may affect the interpretation of results; humans commonly produce asbestos bodies, as do mice, guinea pigs, hamsters, and monkeys, but rats usually do not.[11] Some models inject asbestos directly into body cavities, whereas others practice inhalation exposure.[18] However, it is difficult to induce mesothelioma in rats by inhalation studies, whereas injection of the same type of asbestos will often readily produce tumors.[19] Each approach has some merits but also limitations. For example, rodents must breathe through the nose, so there is no exposure of the pharynx as there would be in humans. Rodents also have very effective mucociliary defenses, and one would expect a large proportion of (especially larger fibers) to be expelled (and possibly swallowed, although there are currently no studies investigating this). The long latency of the asbestos-mediated effect that is seen in humans also applies to animal models. Even considering the shorter life span of small animals and rodents in particular, delays of 15 months between exposure and development of tumor are common.

The different susceptibilities of different species to the same toxin further complicate the situation. For example, hamsters appear to be more susceptible to the development of mesothelioma than rats following inhalational exposure but do not seem to develop lung cancers as readily after the same pattern of exposure.[20] Because of different physicochemical properties, asbestos samples from different sites will have different carcinogenic effects, further complicating interpretation and comparison between studies and experiments.[21] There also are difficulties in comparing the doses given with experimental animals—some researchers measure the amount of inhaled asbestos by weight (gravimetric), whereas others use fiber counts per milliliter (or deciliter or cubic meter) of air. No universally agreed method for conversion of one to the other is available, although several studies have been conducted.[22–24] In 1978, Davis et al.[25] concluded "neither a single mass standard, nor the present fiber-number standards are satisfactory." Finally, how do these doses relatively compare with those inhaled by humans? Rats have been exposed to large amounts of chrysotile asbestos (10 mg/m³) using nose-only inhalation chambers, 6 h/day 5 days/week for up to 24 months, whereas young Syrian golden hamsters were exposed via nose-only inhalation for 6 h/day 5 days/week for 78 weeks to amosite asbestos at 250–300 WHO fibers per cubic meter.[26–28] At the end of the 2 years of exposure to asbestos, the rats had pulmonary fibrosis, 1 (1.4%) of 69 rats had mesothelioma, and 13 (19%) had lung tumors (both adenomas and carcinomas were counted as tumors). In the Syrian hamster model, 20% of the animals developed mesotheliomas, but there were no lung tumors. All the animals developed pulmonary fibrosis. In another study, Syrian hamsters exposed to chrysotile asbestos at 10 mg/m³ for 18 months developed only pulmonary fibrosis.[29,*]

---

* These experiments also emphasize that although there may be shared pathways, there is no obligatory link between fibrosis/asbestosis and neoplasia because, in some experiments, animals most susceptible to pulmonary fibrosis were quite resistant to developing neoplasms.

Such studies also indicate that rabbits develop reactive effusions but are relatively resistant to tumor development of any kind, that guinea pigs readily develop pulmonary fibrosis after inhalation of asbestos, and that rats are more sensitive to development of pulmonary intraparenchymal tumors after asbestos exposure than are Syrian hamsters.[12,21] The previous studies also indicate that chrysotile is less potent than amphiboles. Interestingly, in none of the species reviewed did chronic asbestos exposures by inhalation lead to tumors in the oropharynx—perhaps explicable by the abovementioned mode of breathing in rodents. However, there were also no tumors of the larynx, whereas a causal relationship in humans is recognized by some authors, although this is still the subject of some disagreement (discussed in Chapter 8). [30]

The interspecies variability in response to certain toxins is now well recognized to hamper all animal studies—aspirin is highly toxic to cats but quite safe for humans, and thalidomide is harmless for pregnant rats but not for women: the list of examples highlighting those differences is extensive. The link between cigarette smoking and lung cancer was well established in 1963 by prospective and retrospective studies in human patients, but most animal experiments to produce lung cancer using cigarette smoke had failed.[31] At that time, one cancer animal researcher, Clarence Little, wrote: "The failure of many investigators to induce experimental cancers, except in a handful of cases, during fifty years of trying, casts serious doubt on the validity of the cigarette-lung cancer theory."[32] In addition to the highly variable interspecies susceptibility, different strains of the same species may demonstrate very different susceptibilities to the same toxin: for example, the 129J strain of mice is resistant to asbestos-induced pulmonary fibrosis, whereas C57BL/6 mice are highly susceptible.[33] The basis for the difference is not yet fully understood, but that difference makes it difficult to compare studies using different species, or even different strains of the same species.

Genetic, molecular, and immunological differences between humans and other animals make it impossible for data to be directly extrapolated to the human situation. Finally, humans are often exposed to a variety of toxins including tobacco smoke, air pollution, and mixed dust exposures that are highly individualized and difficult to mimic in the laboratory—and as we have just seen, although rats may develop lung cancer after inhalational exposure to asbestos, they are not very susceptible to cigarette smoke. Nonetheless, much information has been gathered from animal work, and in particular, recently developed mouse knockout models have provided important new *in principle* evidence for certain pathogenetic pathways. This work has greatly furthered our understanding, but the limitations of all of these models in their applicability to the human situation need to be remembered.

4.3 APOPTOSIS: FRIEND OR FOE?

One of the immediate and direct effects of asbestos in vitro is the initiation of apoptosis. Apoptosis—"orderly and programmed cell death"—is essentially a highly regulated mechanism that eliminates cells damaged beyond repair and as such is considered protective of neoplasia. Apoptosis after exposure to asbestos has been demonstrated in cultured normal mesothelial cells as well as alveolar epithelial cells and alveolar macrophages.[34–41] This raises one important question: how can asbestos induce a plethora of effects ranging from fibrosis and pleural effusions to lung cancer and mesothelioma if the cells affected initially die? This highlights the limitations of models because, in vivo, asbestos fails to initiate comprehensive apoptosis as a protective mechanism. However, even when some apoptosis occurs in vivo, factors released from the damaged cell can also affect nearby cells, initiating proliferation and inflammation. Also, asbestos appears to simultaneously stimulate compensatory (and eventually excessive) cell proliferation directly, which may then be associated with fibrosis or malignancy. In malignancies, it is usually loss of regulation of apoptosis that contributes to unrestrained growth of tumors. These current findings suggest that apoptosis plays a role in all asbestos-related diseases. This raises the second question: how can exposure to the same toxin result in such varied outcomes? Again, genetic variability between individuals resulting in disparities in effector proteins may hold some of the answers. In addition, the distribution of asbestos fibers (from bronchial walls, to bronchiolar-alveolar bifurcations, to parietal pleura) and the timing of cellular events may account for some of these differences, but to date, these questions have not yet been fully answered. Nonetheless, recent years have witnessed significant advances in an understanding of the molecular mechanisms of asbestos-related diseases, which shed light onto some of these questions as well as suggesting ways to devise more effective and targeted therapies.

4.3.1 The Role of Apoptosis in the Development of Fibrosis and Malignancies

Apoptosis is a normal regulatory mechanism that removes damaged cells, but it is a complex process, and the controlled removal of damaged cells may be accompanied by a compensatory increase in cell proliferation. If excessive, this may lead to fibrosis.

Gene profiles performed on normal bronchial epithelial cells in cultures exposed to chrysotile showed, among other findings, alteration of profiles correlated with apoptosis. There was concurrent up-regulation of proinflammatory cytokines, chemokines, and growth factors, highlighting the interconnection of effects of chrysotile on apoptosis, inflammation, cell proliferation, and, in some instances, fibrosis.[11] There is good evidence that apoptosis of alveolar epithelial cells and mesothelial cells is an early event in asbestos-induced lung injury, and in a model of bleomycin-induced fibrosis, apoptosis is maintained during the development of fibrosis (for a more detailed review, see original article[42]).

The exact mechanisms for apoptosis in alveolar epithelial cells are not well understood. However, a functional role for protein kinase C δ (PKC-δ) in the induction of apoptosis and inflammatory processes by crocidolite has been suggested. Asbestos increased the kinase activity of PKC-δ in alveolar type II epithelial cells, whereas pretreatment with a PKC-δ selective inhibitor, before the addition of asbestos, prevented apoptosis. Direct activation of PKC-δ by hydrogen peroxide, an ROS, was demonstrated.[39] In in vivo experiments, PKC-δ knockout mice were protected from asbestos-induced epithelial proliferation and of inflammatory cytokines, including TNF-α, transforming growth factor α (TGF-α), TGF-β, platelet-derived growth factor, and interleukin-1 (IL-1). Cytokine profiles in bronchoalveolar lavage fluids showed increases in IL-1β, IL-4, IL-6, and IL-13. PKC-δ knockout mice also exhibited decreased lung infiltration of polymorphonuclear cells, natural killer cells, and macrophages in bronchoalveolar lavage fluid and lung. These data show that modulation of PKC-δ-mediated apoptosis exhibits effects on peribronchiolar cell proliferation as well as proinflammatory and profibrotic cytokine expression and immune cell profiles in lung.[43]

4.3.2 The Role of Apoptosis: Malignant Neoplasia

Malignant cells are commonly resistant to apoptosis via normal pathways, and mesothelioma and asbestos-induced lung cancer are no exception. Mesothelioma cell lines have been shown to be highly resistant to oxidant (asbestos and ROS) and nonoxidant-induced apoptosis. This effect is not related to up-regulation of expression of Bcl-2, an important antiapoptotic regulator of apoptosis, which is mutated in many tumors. The mechanism underlying this resistance is currently not fully understood[44]; however, recent evidence suggests the disruption of multiple pathways and effector proteins (Figure 4.2).[45,46]

The overexpression of coatomer protein complex subunit alpha in some mesothelioma cell lines has received particular attention recently because coatomer protein complex subunit alpha knockdown via a genome-wide small interfering RNA library induced apoptosis and suppressed tumor growth in a mesothelioma mouse model.[47] Similarly, in lung cancer, disruption of apoptotic pathways and resistance to apoptosis has been demonstrated.[48,49]

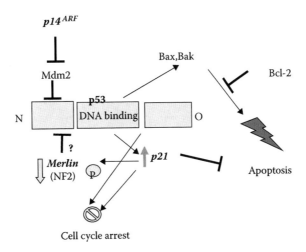

Cell cycle arrest

Figure 4.2 (See color insert.) *Alternative pathways of regulation of apoptosis.* Apoptosis is a normal process that allows deletion of damaged and potentially dangerous cells, such as cells that contain
irreparable DNA damage. There are several potential pathways that may lead to apoptosis, and
the tumor suppressor p53 plays a central role. Mesotheliomas often express normal p53, but the
p53 pathway is still commonly affected in mesotheliomas. Activated p53 may arrest the cell cycle
via up-regulation of p21, a cyclin-dependent kinase, which has been found to be altered in some
mesotheliomas. Depending on the cell type, p21 may not only induce cell cycle arrest but also
initiate apoptosis directly. In addition, p21 phosphorylates merlin. Merlin is the gene product of
the NF2 gene at chromosome 22 and has been found to be mutated in many mesotheliomas.
Phosphorylation decreases function of merlin, which is thought to act as a tumor suppressor gene.
Alternative pathways to apoptosis lead via the mitochondrial-bound proteins Bax and Bak, which
are opposed by the antiapoptotic protein Bcl-2. This pathway is commonly affected in malignant
tumors and also mediates apoptosis in alveolar epithelial cells exposed to asbestos.[40] (With kind
permission of Springer Science + Business Media: From Hammar SP, Henderson DW, Klebe S,
Dodson RF. Neoplasms of the pleura, in J.F. Tomashefski, Jr. et al. (eds.), *Dail and Hammar's
Pulmonary Pathology*, 3rd ed., vol. 2, p. 591, 2008.)

The "guardian of the genome," p53, is a tumor suppressor gene that is commonly altered in malignancies, but mesotheliomas often express wild-type p53. Nonetheless, the p53 pathway is still affected
in mesotheliomas. For example, activated p53 may arrest the cell cycle via up-regulation of p21, a
cyclin-dependent kinase, which has been found to be altered in some mesotheliomas. Depending on the
cell type, p21 may not only induce cell cycle arrest but also initiate apoptosis directly. In addition, p21
phosphorylates merlin, the gene product of the NF2 gene at chromosome 22, which has been found to
be mutated in a significant number of mesotheliomas. Phosphorylation decreases function of merlin,
which is thought to act as a tumor suppressor gene, although the exact mechanism is not well understood.[40] Message levels of the p53-induced molecular switch p21[CIP/WAF1] and KLF4 have been shown
to be up-regulated in crocidolite-treated cells. Together, these two products can have an antiapoptotic
effect, which impacts on the p53–protein pathway without necessitating mutations in p53 itself.

In addition, there are alternative pathways to apoptosis via the mitochondrion-bound proteins
Bax and Bak, which are opposed by the antiapoptotic protein Bcl-2. This pathway is commonly
affected in malignant tumors, including lung cancers, but there is currently insufficient evidence to
suggest it plays a major role in the development of mesothelioma.

4.4 DIRECT CELLULAR EVENTS AFTER INHALATION OF ASBESTOS

After inhalation of asbestos, the fibers must first pass bronchiolar-alveolar bifurcations, where
some of the acute changes appear to take place. Phagocytosis may be mediated by a number of cell

types and results in the generation of phagolysosomes containing the asbestos fibers. Epithelial cells, interstitial cells, and alveolar macrophages are all involved in this process at various stages. Increased numbers of alveolar macrophages are considered an early indicator of asbestos inhalation,[1] and uptake of asbestos fibers into alveolar epithelial cells is mediated via avb5 integrin receptor-mediated endocytosis.[41] Fibers will migrate from the lung to the pleural space where they cluster in the parietal pleura. Fiber dimensions influence the extent and rate of fiber deposition as well as biopersistence and have been linked mechanistically with persistent inflammation in a variety of toxicologic studies as reviewed in the article by Bernstein et al.[50] These factors also affect fiber movement to the pleura. Long, thin asbestos fibers are more easily trapped at the level of the terminal/respiratory bronchioles or are deposited in the alveolar spaces. Long fibers are also less efficiently phagocytosed by alveolar macrophages and are more likely to stimulate persistent production of proinflammatory mediators such as ROS, cytokines, and growth factors. Partial phagocytosis results in increased ROS levels and impairs macrophage motility. If fibers cannot be cleared effectively, they may move to the lung interstitium, the pleura, or the peritoneum. Regardless of the site, the persistence of fibers can cause chronic macrophage activation and ongoing epithelial/mesothelial cell injury, release of ROS, inflammation, and compensatory repair, accompanied by cell proliferation.

4.4.1 Reactive Oxygen Species

Regardless of cell type, uptake of asbestos fibers results in accumulation of ROS and reactive nitrogen species, which act as second messengers of asbestos-mediated toxicity. ROS can cause peroxidation of phospholipids such as those present in cell membranes; mediate breakage of DNA as well as modify cellular proteins (including those enzymes involved in signaling cascades); and initiate cytokine release, especially TNF-α (see next section).[51]

All types of asbestos contain iron cations, either as part of their crystalline lattice structure (crocidolite and amosite, and amounting to as much as up to 27% by weight in crocidolite) or as a surface impurity (chrysotile). ROS may be generated at the surface of asbestos fibers by chemical reactions catalyzed by the iron component of the fibers, or they may be the result of frustrated phagocytosis of asbestos fibers by alveolar macrophages and neutrophils.[2] Consequently, the iron content of the different types of asbestos fibers has been implicated in their relative toxicities.

Briefly, the Fenton reaction is the primary reaction involved in free radical (OH$^-$) formation, but free radicals may be produced by the Haber–Weiss reaction in the presence of iron, resulting in generation of hydrogen peroxide (H_2O_2).

1. $Fe^{2+} + H_2O_2 \rightarrow Fe^{3+} + OH^- + OH^-$ (Fenton reaction)
2. $Fe^{3+} + O_2^- \leftrightarrow Fe^{2+} + O_2$
3. $2O_2^- + 2H^+ \rightarrow H_2O_2 + O_2^-$
4. $H_2O_2 + Fe^{2+} \rightarrow OH^- + OH^- + Fe^{3+}$ (iron-catalyzed Haber–Weiss reaction)

This process is reviewed by Kamp and Weitzman.[52]

However, ROS have an extremely short half-life; therefore, physical proximity of DNA and cell membranes or other structures susceptible to the damage by ROS is a prerequisite for damage to occur. It is likely that a significant proportion of the cell damage in vivo is actually induced by oxidoreduction secondary to inflammatory cellular processes and phagocytosis in particular. Some of the damage may be transmitted via secondary molecules that are more stable than ROS. When incubated with neutrophils in vitro, crocidolite, amosite and chrysotile fibers induce greater release of lactate dehydrogenase than rock wool, glass wool, or ceramic fibers. Experimental studies have also shown that crocidolite, amosite, and chrysotile fibers appear to produce significantly greater amounts of free radicals from mixtures of neutrophils and asbestos fibers than from mixtures of such cells and man-made fibers such as rock wool, glass wool, and ceramic fibers; it appears that asbestos fibers are more efficient for stimulation of ROS from phagocytic cells than nonfibrous mineral dusts.[53] The neutrophil-derived enzyme myeloperoxidase (MPO) originates from lysosomes and is found in high concentrations in human lung because of recruitment of neutrophils. MPO activates benzo[a]pyrene as well as aromatic amines in tobacco smoke and generates carcinogenic free radicals. Mutations that confer low enzyme activity have been found to be associated with decreased lung cancer risk.[54] In a mouse model, asbestos-exposed MPO knockout mice exhibited a significant decrease in asbestos-associated lung inflammation compared with normal mice. This was associated with increased expression of the proliferation markers Ki-67 and cyclin D1 in the distal bronchiolar epithelium. These findings suggest that MPO status influences early asbestos-induced oxidative stress by mediating inflammation and epithelial cell proliferation.[55] With regard to fibrosis, decreased MPO levels were seen in proteoglycan-treated hamsters in a bleomycin model of pulmonary fibrosis compared with bleomycin-treated hamsters that did not receive the proteoglycan and did develop significant fibrosis.[56]

4.5 OXIDATIVE STRESS AND INFLAMMATORY RESPONSES

4.5.1 Antioxidants and the Role of the Extracellular Matrix

The breakdown of antioxidant defenses of the lung plays a significant role in the mediation of the effects of oxidative stress. Antioxidant enzymes that have been investigated in the lung and pleura include catalase and superoxide dismutase (SOD); antioxidant peptides include glutathione and thiol proteins; and nutritional antioxidants include vitamins A, C, and E.[57–62] The data for nutritional supplements are, however, contradictory with some studies showing reduction of oxidative damage in smokers taking antioxidant supplements and others failing to demonstrate any correlation between antioxidant levels and markers of oxidative stress.[63–65] At least in vitro, a protective effect has been demonstrated convincingly for SOD and catalase[66] as well as for glutathione, both in alveolar epithelial cells and in cultured normal mesothelial[67] and mesothelioma cells.[68] The antioxidant enzyme extracellular superoxide dismutase (EC-SOD) has been found to be instrumental in animal models of interstitial lung injury.[69–73] Its importance in human lungs is evident in the demonstrated lack of expression in lung tissue with interstitial pneumonias, where lack of expression has been mapped to areas of fibrosis in other types of interstitial pneumonia.[74] For example, in a mouse model of crocidolite-induced interstitial fibrosis, intratracheal instillation of crocidolite resulted in decreased EC-SOD activity within the lung tissue of these mice, whereas increased activity was found in the bronchiolar-alveolar lavage fluid of the mice. The redistribution of the protective enzyme correlated with the development of fibrosis 14 days later, suggesting that lack of expression of EC-SOD in the lung is associated with an increased risk of fibrosis.[75] This is supported by the fact that mice deficient in the enzyme are more sensitive to asbestos-induced oxidative damage, whereas mice overexpressing the enzyme are somewhat protected from radiation-induced fibrosis, a comparable model because radiation damage is also induced via oxidative stress.[76,77] The effects of EC-SOD are mediated via a number of pathways, which appear to be largely related to the protection of the extracellular matrix (ECM) components from degradation and shedding. ECM molecules include glycosaminoglycans such as heparan sulfate, which were described previously as "ground substances" and thought to simply fill the space necessary for organization of the ECM, but their role in growth factor and chemokine activation is now widely acknowledged.[78,79] Heparan sulfate is a glycosaminoglycan that is abundant in lung and enables growth factor function and modifies enzyme functions. Heparan sulfate also interacts with cytokines and chemokines and participates in leukocyte selectin binding to promote the recruitment of leukocytes. Heparan sulfate is tightly bound to EC-SOD and hence protected from oxidative fragmentation. In EC-SOD knockout mice, ROS induced fragmentation of heparan sulfate resulting in neutrophil chemotaxis and hence further inflammation—as well as further increase in ROS. In vivo, bronchiolar-alveolar lavage fluid from EC-SOD knockout mice at 1, 14, and 28 days after asbestos exposure showed increased heparan sulfate shedding from the lung parenchyma. This effect could be inhibited by the presence of EC-SOD. The neutrophil chemotaxis in response to oxidatively fragmented heparin is mediated by Toll-like receptor-4.[59,79]

Additional molecules protected by EC-SOD include hyaluronan, which in its fragmented form has been shown to activate macrophages and up-regulate inflammatory pathways[80] as well as syndecan-1,[81] a transmembrane proteoglycan that mediates cell binding and cell signaling. Syndecan-1 ectodomain induces neutrophil chemotaxis, inhibits alveolar epithelial wound healing, and promotes fibrosis. Syndecan-1 has been shown to be significantly elevated in the lavage fluid of EC-SOD knockout mice after exposure to asbestos (or bleomycin), and increased syndecan-1 staining as assessed by immunohistochemistry is seen within fibrotic areas of both human and mouse lungs, regardless of the cause of fibrosis. Apart from local factors such as asbestos, a decrease in EC-SOD may also be systemically mediated, for example, in systemic inflammatory states, as demonstrated in the mouse endotoxin model of systemic inflammation, resulting in similar molecular signatures to the local effectors described earlier.[82] It may be that the effects of an inhaled toxin would be more pronounced if exposure occurred during a time of systemic inflammation with decreased EC-SOD levels. For example, these findings suggest that an individual's response to inhaled asbestos may depend on the systemic immune response/inflammatory state at that time, but there are currently no studies investigating this, and it would be difficult to collect data retrospectively.

In summary, it appears that the proteolytic breakdown of EC-SOD results in oxidative shedding of several proteoglycan components of the ECM, including heparan sulfate, hyaluronan, and syndecan-1, which induce neutrophil chemotaxis as well as aberrant wound healing, all of which are known factors that may contribute to pulmonary fibrosis.

But does this breakdown of specific antioxidant defenses with release of ECM components also contribute to the development of asbestos-related malignancies? A causative role for EC-SOD in the induction of malignant conditions has not yet been established, but decreased levels of SOD have been demonstrated in pulmonary squamous cell carcinomas and adenocarcinomas by immunohistochemistry, Western blot, and functional assays when compared with normal human lung tissue samples.[83,84] Although a direct effect of EC-SOD on early lung tumor induction has not been shown experimentally, it is likely that low expression of EC-SOD has fundamental effects on the extracellular redox state of lung tumors, which in turn may affect tumor behavior. Because EC-SOD is located in the extracellular space, low expression in lung cancer may have fundamental importance for tumor invasion, which is regulated by the cellular redox state. This role in altering tumor behavior potential seems related to the release of heparanase.[85,86] In prostate cancer, increase in the expression of EC-SOD reduced the cells' capacity for invasion. In a mouse metastasis model, inoculation of genetically modified EC-SOD-secreting fibroblasts suppressed both artificial and spontaneous metastatic lung nodules. These data indicate a role for low EC-SOD expression in tumor progression and establishment of metastatic disease, and suggest that antimetastatic gene therapy using the EC-SOD gene may be feasible in the future.[87]

It is worth noting at this point that there is a known functional polymorphic variant of EC-SOD (3%–6% in various populations), which decreases the ability of EC-SOD to anchor to the negatively charged polysaccharides in the ECM where this enzyme is mainly located.[88] This may explain, at least in part, a genetic susceptibility to asbestos-induced pathology. However, to date, there are no studies on this polymorphism in individuals with interstitial or malignant lung diseases, with or without exposure to asbestos. However, a role in the susceptibility to development of COPD (also related to the oxidative stress caused by smoking) has been established.[89]

But how does this relate to the pleura? There is no doubt about the importance of oxidative stress in the development of malignant mesothelioma. Some antioxidant-enzymes have been mapped to pleura and mesothelial cells in vitro, but no targeted studies are available investigating the specific role of EC-SOD.[57] A role for antioxidant enzymes has been established in principle, but the role of EC-SOD has not been further investigated at this stage.[90]

4.5.2 Activation of Transcription Pathways

The release of ROS or reactive nitrogen species triggers activation of a number of genes involved in cell proliferation and apoptosis, including cytokines, growth factors, and adhesion molecules as well as proto-oncogenes such as *c-myc*. ROS also induce expression of the AP1 transcription factors c-*fos* and c-*jun* amino-terminal kinase, both of which are also proto-oncogenes[91] implicated in malignant transformation. However, recent experiments investigating protein expression and phosphorylation status (activity) of the extracellular-regulated kinase, the c-*jun*, and the high-osmolarity glycerol response kinase (p38)—in fresh frozen reactive mesothelium and mesothelioma specimens—did not detect significant differences between reactive mesothelium and mesothelioma.[92] Although there is undoubtedly up-regulation of these genes, there is still insufficient experimental evidence at present to conclude that mitogen-activated protein kinase (MAPK) activation contributes significantly to malignant transformation.

4.5.3 Activation of Growth Factors and the Role of TNF-α

As mentioned earlier, another effect of ROS is the induction of release of TNF-α as well as up-regulation of TNF-α messenger RNA. This effect has been demonstrated in vitro and in vivo in a variety of laboratory models as well as in patients with asbestosis.[51,93–96] The secretion of TNF-α is also linked with the apoptosis paradox. As mentioned before, crocidolite asbestos is cytotoxic and, in isolation, fails to transform primary human mesothelial cells in culture, thus causing extensive cell death instead. In in vitro experiments, treatment with TNF-α significantly reduced crocidolite cytotoxicity and instead promoted cell survival, thus increasing the pool of asbestos-damaged cells susceptible to malignant transformation.[97] In vivo, multiple cell types and mechanisms may contribute to this net increase in TNF. For example, in the alveolar space, macrophages may directly release TNF-α.[93] The level of secretion of TNF-α has been linked with fiber length, with longer and more carcinogenic fibers inducing higher levels of secretion.[93,97]

TNF-α is firstly a potent proinflammatory cytokine that may induce fibrosis directly by activation of extracellular-regulated kinase–specific pathways, resulting in stabilization of TGF-β1 messenger RNA and increased expression of TGF-β1, which plays a major role in promoting pulmonary fibrosis (reviewed in the next section).[98] TNF-α can elicit its effects via three main pathways: (i) activation of NF-κ pathways; (ii) activation of the MAPK pathways; and (iii) induction of apoptosis via death-receptor signaling and caspase-8 activity (Figure 4.2). However, the proapoptotic effect is usually minor compared with the proliferative effect initiated by NF-κB signaling.

TNF signaling plays a major role both in reactive/fibrotic and neoplastic asbestos-induced conditions in the lung. A role for TNF-α in the induction of fibrosis has been demonstrated in several animal models.[95,96,99–101] There is good experimental evidence that pulmonary inflammation (and the end-result, interstitial pulmonary fibrosis) is at least in part mediated via TNF-α signaling, in close association with TGF-β pathways. Using a transgenic mouse model overexpressing TGF-β, Yamasaki et al.[102] showed that TGF-β induced the cyclin-dependent kinase inhibitor p21 via a TNF-α-signaling pathway and that p21 is a negative modulator of TGF-β-induced TNF-α expression. (The role of p21 in modulating p53-pathway apoptosis was discussed earlier and provides another example of the close interconnection between inflammatory and apoptotic pathways.) This effect had been previously seen by other authors.[103] Yamasaki et al.[102] demonstrated that p21 regulates TGF-β-induced apoptosis, inflammation, fibrosis, and alveolar remodeling by interacting with TNF-α-signaling pathways. Others have shown the development of fibrosis correlates directly with TNF-α levels.[103]

Compelling proof of principle for the role of TNF-α in pulmonary fibrogenic conditions is also provided by the rodent bleomycin and silica models of pulmonary injury and fibrosis, where instillation of soluble TNF-α receptor that bound free TNF prevented fibrosis.[104] Transgenic mice overexpressing TNF-α in type II alveolar epithelial cells spontaneously develop fibrotic lesions similar to those observed in asbestosis.[105] Finally, TNF-α receptor knockout mice fail to develop the fibrosis seen in wild-type mice after chrysotile asbestos exposure.[106]

The role of TNF-α extends to malignant conditions where a crucial effect in tumor promotion and malignant cell transformation has been demonstrated because TNF-α induces NF-κB, which is involved in promoting oncogenesis.[3,107,108] Using models of inflammatory-induced cancers, these studies demonstrate that NF-κB provides a link between inflammation and cancer (for an extensive review, see Greten and Karin[108]). As discussed earlier, NF-κB signaling may activate proinflammatory cytokines, but NF-κB-dependent genes also include the proto-oncogene c-*myc* as well as the antiapoptotic/prosurvival genes c-*jun* amino-terminal kinase and c-IAP1 and c-IAP2.[109,110] The results of these studies suggest that NF-κB has both direct oncogenic effects on cells and also affects the microenvironment surrounding the tumor, thus stimulating the release of inflammatory mediators from activated macrophages. This is, of course, of particular interest in the case of asbestos-related malignancies where macrophages abound in the early stages of the physiological response to asbestos inhalation. In fact, independent studies have demonstrated activation of the NF-κB pathway by TNF-α in rat mesothelial cells exposed to oxidative stressors.[111] In rats inhaling crocidolite, NF-κB, p65 nuclear translocation in both lung epithelial cells and mesothelial cells was increased, and activation of c-*jun* and c-*fos* signaling has been demonstrated.[91,109,112] These findings provide evidence for a role of the TNF-α-mediated NF-κB factor activation for both lung cancer and mesothelioma.

Apart from being involved in tumor initiation, a role for TNF-α in promoting tumor progression and metastasis has also been established.[113,114]

The induction of TNF-α may also initiate apoptosis in some cell types, but many cells, including alveolar epithelial cells, survive increased TNF-α levels because of activation of the NF-κB pathway.[115] In human mesothelial cells, TNF-α signaling promotes cell survival via an NF-κB-dependent pathway that allows mesothelial cells damaged by asbestos cytotoxicity to escape from apoptosis (Figure 4.3).[97]

As always, however, "it is the dose that makes the poison." The data discussed provide critical evidence to support the link between increased TNF-α expression and fibrosis as well as chronic, low-level TNF-α expression and the malignant transformation of cells and also tumor progression and metastasis. However, it is worth remembering in the context of this discussion that high-dose TNF has also been used successfully as a cytotoxic agent.[116] It appears that TNF-α plays a crucial role in the interaction of stromal and inflammatory cells and in premalignant and malignant tumor cells. Better understanding of the multiple roles of TNF-α in pulmonary fibrosis and in pleural and lung malignancies may aid the development of targeted therapy.

4.5.4 TGF-β and Asbestos-Related Diseases

TGF-β is a peptide that inhibits epithelial and mesenchymal cell proliferation and stimulates synthesis of ECM components, potentially contributing to fibrosis. The interrelationship between TNF-α and TGF-β has been discussed earlier in detail. The role of TGF-β in pulmonary fibrosis has long been appreciated. Sheep exposed to chrysotile asbestos intratracheally developed asbestosis, and all three TGF-β isoforms were found in fibrotic areas. As the lesions developed, increased immunohistochemical labeling was seen in bronchial and bronchiolar epithelium, macrophages, and bronchial and vascular smooth muscle when compared with control lungs.[17] Similar features and patterns of distribution were seen in the fibrotic lesions of asbestosis and pleural fibrosis in the lungs of 16 asbestos miners and millers from Quebec, Canada.[117] The up-regulation of TGF-β has also been shown in other types of pulmonary fibrosis.[118] TGF-β is released as a biologically inactive

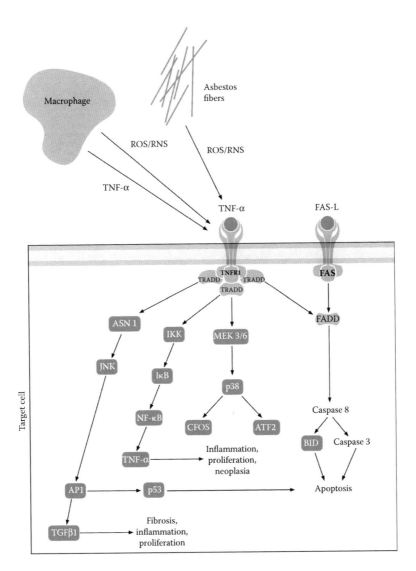

Figure 4.3 *The TNF-α and NF-κB pathways.* In epithelial tissues, TNF-α binds to TNF-R1. Upon contact with their ligand, TNF receptors form trimers, and this is followed by dissociation of the adaptor protein TRADD to bind to the death domain, serving as a platform for subsequent protein binding. After TRADD binding, three pathways can be initiated. *Activation of NF-κB*: TRADD recruits the multicomponent protein kinase IKK. An inhibitory protein, IκB, that normally binds to NF-κB and inhibits its translocation is phosphorylated by IKK and subsequently degraded, releasing NF-κB. NF-κB translocates to the nucleus and mediates transcription of proteins involved in cell survival and proliferation, inflammatory response, and antiapoptotic factors. *Activation of the MAPK pathways*: Of the three major MAPK cascades, TNF induces a strong activation of the stress-related JNK group. (MAPK was originally called microtubule-associated protein kinase and then renamed mitogen-activated kinase. These pathways couple intracellular responses and cascade to extracellular ligand binding via signal transduction pathways.) JNK translocates to the nucleus and activates transcription factors such as c-Jun and ATF2. The JNK pathway is involved in cell differentiation, proliferation, and inflammation but may be proapoptotic at the level of AP1. Once release of TGF-β has taken place, the balance shifts toward proinflammatory effects. *Induction of death signaling*: TRADD binds FADD, which then recruits the cysteine protease caspase-8. Caspase-8 induces cleaving of effector caspases, leading to cell apoptosis. However, TNF-induced cell death plays only a minor role compared with the activation of the inflammatory process. In particular, the proapoptotic effect is countered by the antiapoptotic effects of NF-κB.

complex bound to a latent-associated peptide; disassociation of this complex regulates TGF-β activity. A number of mechanisms have been shown to activate TGF, and direct activation of human latent TGF-β in a cell-free system by ROS derived from asbestos has been demonstrated.[119] Ongoing apoptosis-independent secretion of TGF-β by alveolar macrophages has been seen after low-dose exposure to chrysotile.[120]

4.6 SYNERGISTIC EFFECTS WITH OTHER TOXINS

Factors that may influence the extent of oxidative damage to the lung include environmental factors, including inhalation of tobacco smoke (active and passive smoking), air pollution, and inhalation of other dusts. Epidemiologic studies have established that exposure to asbestos fibers increases the risk of lung cancer, particularly in cigarette smokers (reviewed in detail elsewhere in this book and by Erren et al.[121]). There are multiple indirect mechanisms that may contribute to the synergistic interaction between smoking and asbestos. For example, smoking alters the mucociliary functions and thus may delay or impair clearance of fibers from the bronchi and alveoli, and enhanced alveolar penetration may also play a role.[122,123] In rat tracheal explants and in vivo in guinea pigs, cigarette smoke enhanced penetration of asbestos fibers into airway epithelium and exacerbated epithelial hyperplasia and small-airway disease.[124] Apart from mechanistic synergies, it has also been suggested that asbestos enhances the delivery of mutagenic polyaromatic hydrocarbons to the respiratory epithelium and directly enhances the carcinogenicity of toxins in tobacco smoke.[125,126] This work showed that the delivery of cigarette smoke condensate to cells was improved by adhesion on asbestos fibers before exposure (see Chapter 6).

4.7 OTHER FACTORS OF INTEREST

4.7.1 Mutations

The Kirsten rat sarcoma viral oncogene homologue (k-*ras*) acts as an early player in mutations in many signal transduction pathways. A single amino acid substitution is responsible for an activating mutation. Presence of this mutation in patients with lung adenocarcinoma is common, and some studies have suggested that asbestos exposure is also associated with a high incidence of k-*ras* mutations in adenocarcinoma of the lung.[127] Nelson et al.[128] showed that in a study involving 84 patients newly diagnosed with lung cancer, the prevalence of k-*ras* mutations was higher among those with a history of occupational asbestos exposure (crude odds ratio [OR] = 4.8) compared with those without asbestos exposure, and this association remained after adjustment for age and pack-years smoked (adjusted OR = 6.9). An index score weighing both the dates of exposure and the estimated intensity of exposure indicated that those with k-*ras* mutations had significantly greater asbestos exposures than those without mutations ($p < 0.01$). Analysis of the descriptive components of exposure indicated it was not the duration of exposure that was associated with k-*ras* mutation. Instead, the time since initial exposure was significantly associated with mutation status. Importantly, k-*ras* mutations were present in asbestos-exposed individuals who did not have asbestosis, affirming that asbestosis was not a necessary prerequisite for the development of lung cancer. This suggests the hypothesis that "lung cancer risk is elevated only in humans exposed to asbestos when there is asbestosis"[129] is likely false (see Chapter 6).

4.7.2 Host Factors

It is not clear why some individuals develop pleural effusions or plaques and some experience asbestosis, whereas others will develop lung cancer or mesothelioma—or a combination of two or more of the above. There is some experimental evidence that different cell types are variably effective in dealing with asbestos-mediated cellular damage, suggesting that the initial site of contact with the toxin may play a role.[130]

In addition, some genetic disparities which may be associated with increased risk for asbestos-related disorders have recently been discovered and this may explain at least some of these individual differences. The genes affected include the effector proteins in oxidative damage pathways commonly affected by exposure to asbestos such as SOD, discussed in some detail below.[54,88,131–133] Another enzyme involved in oxidative damage control is glutathione S transferase 1 (GSTM1), which detoxifies electrophilic compounds, including products of oxidative stress, by conjugation with glutathione. The genes encoding the GSTM1 are organized in a gene cluster on chromosome 1p13.3 and are known to be highly polymorphic. These genetic variations can influence an individual's susceptibility to various carcinogens, and an increased risk has been identified for all asbestos-related diseases for individuals with the null genotype in the majority of studies.[132–137] Importantly, this also increased the risk for smoking-associated morbidity, possibly explaining in part the synergistic effects of smoking and asbestos exposure.[134,136] For patients with malignant mesothelioma, both GSTM1-null genotype and two variant alleles of the DNA repair genes XRCC1 and XRCC3 were associated with slightly increased risks.[138]

Some interesting results have come from a study investigating the effects of α-1-antitrypsin polymorphism in asbestosis.[139] Alpha-1-antitrypsin protects alveolar walls against the effects of the proteolytic enzyme elastase, which is secreted by neutrophils and macrophages. An association between α-1-antitrypsin deficiency states and increased susceptibility to smoke-associated toxicity is well recognized. With regard to asbestos, the study group consisted of 100 patients with asbestosis, 94 asbestos workers without asbestosis, and 121 hospital controls. Those heterozygotes who carried the PI*Z allele were at higher risk for asbestosis than PI*S homozygotes (because of the rarity of the PI*Z allele, no homozygotes were included in the study). There is also good evidence for the role of MPO in asbestos-related and smoking-related lung cancer.[54,55,131] N-acetyltransferase 2 (NAT2) is an enzyme involved in the metabolism of xenobiotics, including potential carcinogens. Allelic variants of the NAT2 gene are determined by a pattern of single nucleotide polymorphisms resulting in slow, intermediate, or rapid acetylator phenotypes and therefore causing individual differences in the NAT2 metabolic capacity. Initial Finnish and Italian studies gave conflicting results, but a recent large Italian study involving 252 mesothelioma patients and 262 controls who had heavy asbestos exposure but no mesothelioma showed that NAT2 fast acetylator genotypes showed an increased OR—but this was not statistically significant.[140]

With regard to other pathways, TGF-β promotes fibrosis, including lung fibrosis, and acts as a tumor suppressor in normal cells. Two genetic polymorphisms exist which are associated with different TGF-β protein production. A significant association was found for the proline allele when comparing patients with asbestosis (OR = 3.72) with patients with asbestos-induced lung cancer, thus confirming the hypothesis that TGF-β1 polymorphisms are associated with pulmonary fibrosis and asbestos-induced fibrosis.[141]

The fragile histidine triad (FHIT) tumor suppressor gene is located at 3p14.2 and represents a site of genomic fragility relevant to pathogenesis of both lung cancer and mesothelioma.[142–144] FHIT protein is expressed in most nonneoplastic tissues, and the highest levels of expression occur in epithelial cells. Apoptosis induced by FHIT depends on the expression level and status of FHIT, and the FHIT gene can alter the cell cycling properties. Importantly, the apoptotic process induced by FHIT has no relation to the p53 gene. FHIT appears to be subject to deletion or loss of heterozygosity, mediated both by cigarette smoke and asbestos.[142–145] Diminished expression of FHIT has been recorded in up to 80% of cigarette smoke-associated lung cancers,[145] in asbestos-associated lung cancers (~69%) and nonexposed cases (~59%) in one study,[143] and in ~54% of mesotheliomas.[144] In addition, altered FHIT expression has been demonstrated in idiopathic pulmonary fibrosis, in some cases mapped to metaplastic or atypical foci. There are currently no data for expression of FHIT in asbestosis. Nonetheless, the data available support the significance of FHIT inactivation in development of both lung cancer and mesothelioma, with some evidence for a possible role in pulmonary fibrosis.

Although these data provide insights into possible reasons for individual susceptibility to asbestos-nduced disease, it must be remembered that much of the data require validation in further studies because the reliability of most of the cited studies is limited by the overall small size of the study groups.

4.8 SUMMARY

Asbestos can induce a plethora of biologically diverse effects in multiple tissues at various sites, including the lung, pleura, and peritoneum. These include inflammatory disorders such as pleural effusions, benign fibrotic conditions such as pleural plaques, and disorders such as pulmonary fibrosis/asbestosis which, although not cancerous, may be lethal. Some pathogenetic similarities between neoplastic disorders and idiopathic pulmonary fibrosis have been recognized, and a similar concept may be applied to enhance an understanding of asbestosis.[146] Finally, asbestos may induce malignant disorders such as malignant mesothelioma and lung carcinomas. These disorders may occur independently, coexist in the same patient, or occur sequentially. Importantly, the existence of one of these disorders is not a prerequisite for the development or diagnosis of any of the others. The molecular pathways that propagate either disease may use the same basic processes that include genetic alterations, changed response to growth proliferative and inhibitory signals, development of resistance to apoptosis, altered intercellular signaling, and changes in intracellular signaling pathways. These are features of both benign and malignant asbestos-induced disorders. Current findings have demonstrated that in some instances the same initial pathway may be affected, and it is not yet understood why in some individuals the process branches off and develops preferentially toward the inflammatory pathways while others will preferentially develop malignancies, yet others will develop a combination of disorders. On the basis of the data available, it appears that a combination of external and host factors are involved. However, it appears there are fundamentally shared biological pathogenic mechanisms leading to fibrotic/reactive and/or neoplastic disorders. This understanding may, in time, allow the development of new treatment options that interfere with the early stages of the abovementioned pathways.

REFERENCES

1. Heintz NH, Janssen-Heininger YM, Mossman BT. Asbestos, lung cancers, and mesotheliomas: From molecular approaches to targeting tumor survival pathways. *Am J Respir Cell Mol Biol* 2010;42(2):133–9.
2. Shukla A, Gulumian M, Hei TK, Kamp D, Rahman Q, Mossman BT. Multiple roles of oxidants in the pathogenesis of asbestos-induced diseases. *Free Radic Biol Med* 2003;34(9):1117–29.
3. Ditsworth D, Zong WX. NF-kappaB: Key mediator of inflammation-associated cancer. *Cancer Biol Ther* 2004;3(12):1214–6.
4. Spees JL, Pociask DA, Sullivan DE, et al. Engraftment of bone marrow progenitor cells in a rat model of asbestos-induced pulmonary fibrosis. *Am J Respir Crit Care Med* 2007;176(4):385–94.
5. Hei TK, Wu LJ, Piao CQ. Malignant transformation of immortalized human bronchial epithelial cells by asbestos fibers. *Environ Health Perspect* 1997;105(Suppl 5):1085–8.
6. Hesterberg TW, Barrett JC. Dependence of asbestos- and mineral dust-induced transformation of mammalian cells in culture on fiber dimension. *Cancer Res* 1984;44:2170–80.
7. Cicala C, Pompetti F, Carbone M. SV40 induces mesotheliomas in hamsters. *Am J Pathol* 1993;142(5):1524–33.
8. Strickler HD, Rosenberg PS, Devesa SS, Hertel J, Fraumeni JF, Jr, Goedert JJ. Contamination of poliovirus vaccines with simian virus 40 (1955–1963) and subsequent cancer rates. *JAMA* 1998;279(4):292–5.
9. Shah KV. SV40 and human cancer: A review of recent data. *Int J Cancer* 2007;120(2):215–23.

10. Lopez-Rios F, Illei PB, Rusch V, Ladanyi M. Evidence against a role for SV40 infection in human meso-theliomas and high risk of false-positive PCR results owing to presence of SV40 sequences in common laboratory plasmids. *Lancet* 2004;364(9440):1157–66.

11. Davis JMG. The use of animal models for studies on asbestos bioeffects. *Ann N Y Acad Sci* 1979;79:795–8.

12. Shore BL, Daughaday CC, Spilberg I. Benign asbestos pleurisy in the rabbit: a model for the study of pathogenesis. *Am Rev Respir Dis* 1983;128(3):481–5.

13. Kane AB. Animal models of malignant mesothelioma. *Inhal Toxicol* 2006;18(12):1001–4.

14. Nakataki E, Yano S, Matsumori Y, Goto H, Kakiuchi S, Muguruma H, et al. Novel orthotopic implanta-tion model of human malignant pleural mesothelioma (EHMES-10 cells) highly expressing vascular endothelial growth factor and its receptor. *Cancer Sci* 2006;97(3):183–91.

15. Schepers GW. Chronology of asbestos cancer discoveries: Experimental studies of the Saranac Laboratory [see comments]. *Am J Ind Med* 1995;27(4):593–606.

16. Gardner LV. Chrysotile asbestos as an indicator of subtle differences in animal tissues. *Am Rev Tuberc* 1942;45:762.

17. Lee TC, Gold LI, Reibman J, Aston C, Begin R, Rom WN, Jagirdar J. Immunohistochemical localization of transforming growth factor-beta and insulin-like growth factor-I in asbestosis in the sheep model. *Int Arch Occup Environ Health* 1997;69(3):157–64.

18. Wagner JC, Berry G, Skidmore JW, Pooley FD. The comparative effects of three chrysotiles by injection and inhalation in rats. *IARC Sci Publ* 1980(30):363–72.

19. Davis JMG, Addison J, Bolton RE, Donaldson K, Jones AD. Inhalation and injection studies in rats using dust samples from chrysotile asbestos prepared by a wet dispersion process. *Br J Exp Pathol* 1986;67:113–29.

20. Hesterberg TW, Axten C, McConnell EE, Oberdorster G, Everitt J, Miiller WC, et al. Chronic inhalation study of fiber glass and amosite asbestos in hamsters: Twelve-month preliminary results. *Environ Health Perspect* 1997;105(Suppl 5):1223–9.

21. Davis JM, Addison J, McIntosh C, Miller BG, Niven K. Variations in the carcinogenicity of tremolite dust samples of differing morphology. *Ann N Y Acad Sci* 1991;643:473–90.

22. Puledda S, Marconi A. Study of the count-to-mass conversion factor for asbestos fibres in samples col-lected at the emissions of three industrial plants. *Ann Occup Hyg* 1991;35(5):517–24.

23. Dodic-Fikfak M. An experiment to develop conversion factors to standardise measurements of airborne asbestos. *Arh Hig Rada Toksikol* 2007;58(2):179–85.

24. Huang JQ. A study of conversion of gravimetric to fibre counting concentration of airborne asbestos dust in a chrysotile product factory. *Zhonghua Yu Fang Yi Xue Za Zhi* 1986;20(5):276–9.

25. Davis JMG, Beckett ST, Bolton RE, Collings P, Middleton AP. Mass and number of fibres in the patho-genesis of asbestos related lung diseases in rats. *Br J Cancer* 1978;37:673–88.

26. Hesterberg TW, Miiller WC, McConnell EE, Chevalier J, Hadley JG, Bernstein DM, et al. Chronic inhala-tion toxicity of size-separated glass fibers in Fischer 344 rats. *Fundam Appl Toxicol* 1993;20(4):464–76.

27. Hesterberg TW, Axten C, McConnell EE, Hart GA, Miiller W, Chevalier J, et al. Studies on the inhala-tion toxicology of two fiberglasses and amosite asbestos in the Syrian golden hamster: part I. Results of a subchronic study and dose selection for a chronic study. *Inhal Toxicol* 1999;11(9):747–84.

28. McConnell EE, Axten C, Hesterberg TW, Chevalier J, Miiller WC, Everitt J, et al. Studies on the inhala-tion toxicology of two fiberglasses and amosite asbestos in the Syrian golden hamster: Part II. Results of chronic exposure. *Inhal Toxicol* 1999;11(9):785–835.

29. McConnell EE. Synthetic vitreous fibers—Inhalation studies. *Regul Toxicol Pharmacol* 1994;20(3 Pt 2):S22–34.

30. Purdue MP, Jarvholm B, Bergdahl IA, Hayes RB, Baris D. Occupational exposures and head and neck cancers among Swedish construction workers. *Scand J Work Environ Health* 2006;32(4):270–5.

31. Doll R, Hill AB. The mortality of doctors in relation to their smoking habits: A preliminary report. *Br Med J* 1954;1(4877):1451–5.

32. Northrup E. Men, mice and smoking. In: *Science Looks at Smoking*. New York: Coward-McCann; 1957, p. 133.

33. Warshamana GS, Pociask DA, Sime P, Schwartz DA, Brody AR. Susceptibility to asbestos-induced and transforming growth factor-beta1-induced fibroproliferative lung disease in two strains of mice. *Am J Respir Cell Mol Biol* 2002;27(6):705–13.

34. Broaddus VC. Asbestos, the mesothelial cell and malignancy: A matter of life or death [editorial, com-ment]. *Am J Respir Cell Mol Biol* 1997;17(6):657–9.

35. Broaddus VC. Apoptosis and asbestos-induced disease: Is there a connection? *J Lab Clin Med* 2001;137(5):314–5.

36. Kahlos K, Soini Y, Paakko P, Saily M, Linnainmaa K, Kinnula VL. Proliferation, apoptosis, and manganese superoxide dismutase in malignant mesothelioma. *Int J Cancer* 2000;88(1):37–43.

37. Kamp DW, Panduri V, Weitzman SA, Chandel N. Asbestos-induced alveolar epithelial cell apoptosis: role of mitochondrial dysfunction caused by iron-derived free radicals. *Mol Cell Biochem* 2002;234–235(1–2):153–60.

38. Shukla A, Jung M, Stern M, Fukagawa NK, Taatjes DJ, Sawyer D, et al. Asbestos induces mitochondrial DNA damage and dysfunction linked to the development of apoptosis. *Am J Physiol* 2003;285(5):L1018–25.

39. Shukla A, Stern M, Lounsbury KM, Flanders T, Mossman BT. Asbestos-induced apoptosis is protein kinase C delta-dependent. *Am J Respir Cell Mol Biol* 2003;29(2):198–205.

40. Panduri V, Surapureddi S, Soberanes S, Weitzman SA, Chandel N, Kamp DW. P53 mediates amosite asbestos-induced alveolar epithelial cell mitochondria-regulated apoptosis. *Am J Respir Cell Mol Biol* 2006;34(4):443–52.

41. Liu W, Ernst JD, Broaddus VC. Phagocytosis of crocidolite asbestos induces oxidative stress, DNA damage, and apoptosis in mesothelial cells. *Am J Respir Cell Mol Biol* 2000;23(3):371–8.

42. Robledo R, Mossman B. Cellular and molecular mechanisms of asbestos-induced fibrosis. *J Cell Physiol* 1999;180(2):158–66.

43. Shukla A, Lounsbury KM, Barrett TF, Gell J, Rincon M, Butnor KJ, et al. Asbestos-induced peribronchiolar cell proliferation and cytokine production are attenuated in lungs of protein kinase C-delta knockout mice. *Am J Pathol* 2007;170(1):140–51.

44. Narasimhan SR, Yang L, Gerwin BI, Broaddus VC. Resistance of pleural mesothelioma cell lines to apoptosis: relation to expression of Bcl-2 and Bax. *Am J Physiol* 1998;275(1 Pt 1):L165–71.

45. Fennell DA, Rudd RM. Defective core-apoptosis signalling in diffuse malignant pleural mesothelioma: opportunities for effective drug development. *Lancet Oncol* 2004;5(6):354–62.

46. Villanova F, Procopio A, Rippo MR. Malignant mesothelioma resistance to apoptosis: Recent discoveries and their implication for effective therapeutic strategies. *Curr Med Chem* 2008;15(7):631–41.

47. Sudo H, Tsuji AB, Sugyo A, Kohda M, Sogawa C, Yoshida C, et al. Knockdown of COPA, identified by loss-of-function screen, induces apoptosis and suppresses tumor growth in mesothelioma mouse model. *Genomics* 2010;95(4):210–6.

48. Nymark P, Wikman H, Hienonen-Kempas T, Anttila S. Molecular and genetic changes in asbestos-related lung cancer. *Cancer Lett* 2008;265(1):1–15.

49. Ruosaari S, Hienonen-Kempas T, Puustinen A, Sarhadi VK, Hollmen J, Knuutila S, et al. Pathways affected by asbestos exposure in normal and tumour tissue of lung cancer patients. *BMC Med Genomics* 2008;1:55.

50. Bernstein D, Rogers R, Smith P. The biopersistence of Canadian chrysotile asbestos following inhalation: Final results through 1 year after cessation of exposure. *Inhal Toxicol* 2005;17(1):1–14.

51. Gossart S, Cambon C, Orfila C, Seguelas MH, Lepert JC, Rami J, et al. Reactive oxygen intermediates as regulators of TNF-alpha production in rat lung inflammation induced by silica. *J Immunol* 1996;156(4):1540–8.

52. Kamp DW, Weitzman SA. The molecular basis of asbestos induced lung injury. *Thorax* 1999;54(7):638–52.

53. Ruotsalainen M, Hirvonen MR, Luoto K, Savolainen KM. Production of reactive oxygen species by man-made vitreous fibres in human polymorphonuclear leukocytes. *Hum Exp Toxicol* 1999;18(6):354–62.

54. London SJ, Lehman TA, Taylor JA. Myeloperoxidase genetic polymorphism and lung cancer risk. *Cancer Res* 1997;57(22):5001–3.

55. Haegens A, van der Vliet A, Butnor KJ, Heintz N, Taatjes D, Hemenway D, et al. Asbestos-induced lung inflammation and epithelial cell proliferation are altered in myeloperoxidase-null mice. *Cancer Res* 2005;65(21):9670–7.

56. Giri SN, Hyde DM, Braun RK, Gaarde W, Harper JR, Pierschbacher MD. Antifibrotic effect of decorin in a bleomycin hamster model of lung fibrosis. *Biochem Pharmacol* 1997;54(11):1205–16.

57. Kinnula VL, Paakko P, Soini Y. Antioxidant enzymes and redox regulating thiol proteins in malignancies of human lung. *FEBS Lett* 2004;569(1–3):1–6.

58. Shvedova AA, Kisin ER, Murray AR, Gorelik O, Arepalli S, Castranova V, et al. Vitamin E deficiency enhances pulmonary inflammatory response and oxidative stress induced by single-walled carbon nanotubes in C57BL/6 mice. *Toxicol Appl Pharmacol* 2007;221(3):339–48.

59. Kliment CR, Tobolewski JM, Manni ML, Tan RJ, Enghild J, Oury TD. Extracellular superoxide dismutase protects against matrix degradation of heparan sulfate in the lung. *Antioxid Redox Signal* 2008;10(2):261–8.

60. Kinnula VL, Crapo JD. Superoxide dismutases in the lung and human lung diseases. *Am J Respir Crit Care Med* 2003;167(12):1600–19.

61. Kinnula VL, Everitt JI, Mangum JB, Chang LY, Crapo JD. Antioxidant defense mechanisms in cultured pleural mesothelial cells. *Am J Respir Cell Mol Biol* 1992;7(1):95–103.

62. Marklund SL, Westman NG, Lundgren E, Roos G. Copper- and zinc-containing superoxide dismutase, manganese-containing superoxide dismutase, catalase, and glutathione peroxidase in normal and neoplastic human cell lines and normal human tissues. *Cancer Res* 1982;42(5):1955–61.

63. Singh R, Sram RJ, Binkova B, Kalina I, Popov TA, Georgieva T, et al. The relationship between biomarkers of oxidative DNA damage, polycyclic aromatic hydrocarbon DNA adducts, antioxidant status and genetic susceptibility following exposure to environmental air pollution in humans. *Mutat Res* 2007;620(1–2):83–92.

64. Brown KM, Morrice PC, Arthur JR, Duthie GG. Effects of vitamin E supplementation on erythrocyte antioxidant defence mechanisms of smoking and non-smoking men. *Clin Sci (Lond)* 1996;91(1):107–11.

65. Duthie SJ, Ma A, Ross MA, Collins AR. Antioxidant supplementation decreases oxidative DNA damage in human lymphocytes. *Cancer Res* 1996;56(6):1291–5.

66. Hei TK, He ZY, Suzuki K. Effects of antioxidants on fiber mutagenesis. *Carcinogenesis* 1995;16(7):1573–8.

67. Puhakka A, Ollikainen T, Soini Y, Kahlos K, Saily M, Koistinen P, et al. Modulation of DNA single-strand breaks by intracellular glutathione in human lung cells exposed to asbestos fibers. *Mutat Res* 2002;514(1–2):7–17.

68. Sandstrom BE, Marklund SL. Effects of variation in glutathione peroxidase activity on DNA damage and cell survival in human cells exposed to hydrogen peroxide and t-butyl hydroperoxide. *Biochem J* 1990;271(1):17–23.

69. Fattman CL, Chang LY, Termin TA, Petersen L, Enghild JJ, Oury TD. Enhanced bleomycin-induced pulmonary damage in mice lacking extracellular superoxide dismutase. *Free Radic Biol Med* 2003;35(7):763–71.

70. Bowler RP, Crapo JD. Oxidative stress in airways: Is there a role for extracellular superoxide dismutase? *Am J Respir Crit Care Med* 2002;166(12 Pt 2):S38–43.

71. Sentman ML, Brannstrom T, Marklund SL. EC-SOD and the response to inflammatory reactions and aging in mouse lung. *Free Radic Biol Med* 2002;32(10):975–81.

72. Bowler RP, Nicks M, Warnick K, Crapo JD. Role of extracellular superoxide dismutase in bleomycin-induced pulmonary fibrosis. *Am J Physiol* 2002;282(4):L719–26.

73. Fattman CL, Chu CT, Kulich SM, Enghild JJ, Oury TD. Altered expression of extracellular superoxide dismutase in mouse lung after bleomycin treatment. *Free Radic Biol Med* 2001;31(10):1198–207.

74. Kinnula VL, Hodgson UA, Lakari EK, Tan RJ, Sormunen RT, Soini YM, et al. Extracellular superoxide dismutase has a highly specific localization in idiopathic pulmonary fibrosis/usual interstitial pneumonia. *Histopathology* 2006;49(1):66–74.

75. Tan RJ, Fattman CL, Watkins SC, Oury TD. Redistribution of pulmonary EC-SOD after exposure to asbestos. *J Appl Physiol* 2004;97(5):2006–13.

76. Fattman CL, Tan RJ, Tobolewski JM, Oury TD. Increased sensitivity to asbestos-induced lung injury in mice lacking extracellular superoxide dismutase. *Free Radic Biol Med* 2006;40(4):601–7.

77. Kang SK, Rabbani ZN, Folz RJ, Golson ML, Huang H, Yu D, et al. Overexpression of extracellular superoxide dismutase protects mice from radiation-induced lung injury. *Int J Radiat Oncol Biol Phys* 2003;57(4):1056–66.

78. Taylor KR, Gallo RL. Glycosaminoglycans and their proteoglycans: Host-associated molecular patterns for initiation and modulation of inflammation. *FASEB J* 2006;20(1):9–22.

79. Taylor KR, Trowbridge JM, Rudisill JA, Termeer CC, Simon JC, Gallo RL. Hyaluronan fragments stimulate endothelial recognition of injury through TLR4. *J Biol Chem* 2004;279(17):17079–84.

80. Gao F, Koenitzer JR, Tobolewski JM, Jiang D, Liang J, Noble PW, et al. Extracellular superoxide dismutase inhibits inflammation by preventing oxidative fragmentation of hyaluronan. *J Biol Chem* 2008;283(10):6058–66.

81. Kliment CR, Englert JM, Gochuico BR, et al. Oxidative stress alters syndecan-1 distribution in lungs with pulmonary fibrosis. *J Biol Chem* 2009;284(6):3537–45.

82. Ueda J, Starr ME, Takahashi H, et al. Decreased pulmonary extracellular superoxide dismutase during systemic inflammation. *Free Radic Biol Med* 2008;45(6):897–904.

83. Svensk AM, Soini Y, Paakko P, Hiravikoski P, Kinnula VL. Differential expression of superoxide dismutases in lung cancer. *Am J Clin Pathol* 2004;122(3):395–404.

84. Yoo DG, Song YJ, Cho EJ, Lee SK, Park JB, Yu JH, et al. Alteration of APE1/ref-1 expression in non-small cell lung cancer: The implications of impaired extracellular superoxide dismutase and catalase antioxidant systems. *Lung Cancer (Amsterdam, Netherlands)* 2008;60(2):277–84.

85. Nadir Y, Brenner B. Heparanase coagulation and cancer progression. *Best Pract Res Clin Haematol* 2009;22(1):85–92.

86. Vlodavsky I, Ilan N, Nadir Y, Brenner B, Katz BZ, Naggi A, et al. Heparanase, heparin and the coagulation system in cancer progression. *Thromb Res* 2007;120(Suppl 2):S112–20.

87. Tanaka M, Kogawa K, Nakamura K, Nishihori Y, Kuribayashi K, Hagiwara S, et al. Anti-metastatic gene therapy utilizing subcutaneous inoculation of EC-SOD gene transduced autologous fibroblast suppressed lung metastasis of Meth-A cells and 3LL cells in mice. *Gene Ther* 2001;8(2):149–56.

88. Sandstrom J, Nilsson P, Karlsson K, Marklund SL. 10-Fold increase in human plasma extracellular superoxide dismutase content caused by a mutation in heparin-binding domain. *J Biol Chem* 1994;269(29):19163–6.

89. Oberley-Deegan RE, Regan EA, Kinnula VL, Crapo JD. Extracellular superoxide dismutase and risk of COPD. *COPD* 2009;6(4):307–12.

90. Broaddus VC, Yang L, Scavo LM, Ernst JD, Boylan AM. Crocidolite asbestos induces apoptosis of pleural mesothelial cells: role of reactive oxygen species and poly(ADP-ribosyl) polymerase. *Environ Health Perspect* 1997;105(Suppl 5):1147–52.

91. Janssen Y, Marsh J, Quinlan T, Timblin C, Bérubé K, Jimenez L, et al. Activation of early cellular responses by asbestos: Induction of *c-FOS* and *c-JUN* protooncogene expression in rat pleural mesothelial cells. In: Davis JMG, Jaurand M-C, editors. *Cellular and Molecular Effects of Mineral and Synthetic Dusts and Fibres,* NATO ASI Series, H85. Berlin: Springer-Verlag; 1994, pp. 205–13.

92. Vintman L, Nielsen S, Berner A, Reich R, Davidson B. Mitogen-activated protein kinase expression and activation does not differentiate benign from malignant mesothelial cells. *Cancer* 2005;103(11):2427–33.

93. Donaldson K, Li XY, Dogra S, Miller BG, Brown GM. Asbestos-stimulated tumour necrosis factor release from alveolar macrophages depends on fibre length and opsonization. *J Pathol* 1992;168:243–8.

94. Fubini B, Hubbard A. Reactive oxygen species (ROS) and reactive nitrogen species (RNS) generation by silica in inflammation and fibrosis. *Free Radic Biol Med* 2003;34(12):1507–16.

95. Murthy S, Adamcakova-Dodd A, Perry SS, Tephly LA, Keller RM, Metwali N, et al. Modulation of reactive oxygen species by Rac1 or catalase prevents asbestos-induced pulmonary fibrosis. *Am J Physiol* 2009;297(5):L846–55.

96. Tephly LA, Carter AB. Asbestos-induced MKP-3 expression augments TNF-alpha gene expression in human monocytes. *Am J Respir Cell Mol Biol* 2008;39(1):113–23.

97. Yang H, Bocchetta M, Kroczynska B, Elmishad AG, Chen Y, Liu Z, et al. TNF-alpha inhibits asbestos-induced cytotoxicity via a NF-kappaB-dependent pathway, a possible mechanism for asbestos-induced oncogenesis. Proceedings of the National Academy of Sciences of the United States of America 2006. Available at: www.pnas.org/cgi/doi/10.1073/pnas.0604008103.

98. Sullivan DE, Ferris M, Nguyen H, Abboud E, Brody AR. TNF-alpha induces TGF-beta1 expression in lung fibroblasts at the transcriptional level via AP-1 activation. *J Cell Mol Med* 2009;13(8B):1866–76.

99. Piguet PF. Is "tumor necrosis factor" the major effector of pulmonary fibrosis? *Eur Cytokine Netw* 1990;1(4):257–8.

100. Piguet PF, Collart MA, Grau GE, Sappino AP, Vassalli P. Requirement of tumour necrosis factor for development of silica-induced pulmonary fibrosis. *Nature* 1990;344(6263):245–7.

101. Piguet PF, Vesin C. Treatment by human recombinant soluble TNF receptor of pulmonary fibrosis induced by bleomycin or silica in mice. *Eur Respir J* 1994;7(3):515–8.

102. Yamasaki M, Kang HR, Homer RJ, Chapoval SP, Cho SJ, Lee BJ, et al. P21 regulates TGF-beta1-induced pulmonary responses via a TNF-alpha-signaling pathway. *Am J Respir Cell Mol Biol* 2008;38(3):346–53.

103. Lemaire I, Ouellet S. Distinctive profile of alveolar macrophage-derived cytokine release induced by fibrogenic and nonfibrogenic mineral dusts. *J Toxicol Environ Health* 1996;47(5):465–78.

104. Picklesimer AH, Zanagnolo V, Niemann TH, Eaton LA, Copeland LJ. Case report: Malignant peritoneal mesothelioma in two siblings. *Gynecol Oncol* 2005;99(2):512–6.

105. Miyazaki Y, Araki K, Vesin C, Garcia I, Kapanci Y, Whitsett JA, et al. Expression of a tumor necrosis factor-alpha transgene in murine lung causes lymphocytic and fibrosing alveolitis. A mouse model of progressive pulmonary fibrosis. *J Clin Invest* 1995;96(1):250–9.

106. Liu JY, Brass DM, Hoyle GW, Brody AR. TNF-alpha receptor knockout mice are protected from the fibroproliferative effects of inhaled asbestos fibers. *Am J Pathol* 1998;153(6):1839–47.
107. Pikarsky E, Porat RM, Stein I, Abramovitch R, Amit S, Kasem S, et al. NF-kappaB functions as a tumour promoter in inflammation-associated cancer. *Nature* 2004;431(7007):461–6.
108. Greten FR, Karin M. The IKK/NF-kappaB activation pathway—A target for prevention and treatment of cancer. *Cancer Lett* 2004;206(2):193–9.
109. Janssen YM, Barchowsky A, Treadwell M, Driscoll KE, Mossman BT. Asbestos induces nuclear factor kappa B (NF-kappa B) DNA-binding activity and NF-kappa B-dependent gene expression in tracheal epithelial cells. *Proc Natl Acad Sci U S A* 1995;92(18):8458–62.
110. Timblin CR, Janssen YW, Mossman BT. Transcriptional activation of the proto-oncogene c-*jun* by asbestos and H_2O_2 is directly related to increased proliferation and transformation of tracheal epithelial cells. *Cancer Res* 1995;55(13):2723–6.
111. Milligan SA, Owens MW, Grisham MB. Differential regulation of extracellular signal-regulated kinase and nuclear factor-kappa B signal transduction pathways by hydrogen peroxide and tumor necrosis factor. *Arch Biochem Biophys* 1998;352(2):255–62.
112. Janssen YM, Driscoll KE, Howard B, Quinlan TR, Treadwell M, Barchowsky A, et al. Asbestos causes translocation of p65 protein and increases NF-kappa B DNA binding activity in rat lung epithelial and pleural mesothelial cells. *Am J Pathol* 1997;151(2):389–401.
113. Malik ST, Naylor MS, East N, Oliff A, Balkwill FR. Cells secreting tumour necrosis factor show enhanced metastasis in nude mice. *Eur J Cancer* 1990;26(10):1031–4.
114. Balkwill F. TNF-alpha in promotion and progression of cancer. *Cancer Metastasis Rev* 2006;25(3):409–16.
115. Ashkenazi A, Dixit VM. Death receptors: Signaling and modulation. *Science (New York)* m1998;281(5381):1305–8.
116. Szlosarek P, Charles KA, Balkwill FR. Tumour necrosis factor-alpha as a tumour promoter. *Eur J Cancer* 2006;42(6):745–50.
117. Jagirdar J, Lee TC, Reibman J, Gold LI, Aston C, Begin R, et al. Immunohistochemical localization of transforming growth factor beta isoforms in asbestos-related diseases. *Environ Health Perspect* 1997;105(Suppl 5):1197–203.
118. Mastruzzo C, Crimi N, Vancheri C. Role of oxidative stress in pulmonary fibrosis. *Monaldi Arch Chest Dis* 2002;57(3–4):173–6.
119. Pociask DA, Sime PJ, Brody AR. Asbestos-derived reactive oxygen species activate TGF-beta1. *Lab Invest* 2004;84(8):1013–23.
120. Nishimura Y, Nishiike-Wada T, Wada Y, Miura Y, Otsuki T, Iguchi H. Long-lasting production of TGF-beta1 by alveolar macrophages exposed to low doses of asbestos without apoptosis. *Int J Immunopathol Pharmacol* 2007;20(4):661–71.
121. Erren TC, Jacobsen M, Piekarski C. Synergy between asbestos and smoking on lung cancer risks. *Epidemiology* 1999;10(4):405–11.
122. McFadden D, Wright J, Wiggs B, Churg A. Smoking increases the penetration of asbestos fibers into airway walls. *Am J Pathol* 1986;123:95–9.
123. McFadden D, Wright JL, Wiggs B, Churg A. Smoking inhibits asbestos clearance. *Am Rev Respir Dis* 1986;133:372–4.
124. Hobson J, Gilks B, Wright J, Churg A. Direct enhancement by cigarette smoke of asbestos fiber penetration and asbestos-induced epithelial proliferation in rat tracheal explants. *J Natl Cancer Inst* 1988;80(7):518–21.
125. Gerde P, Scholander P. Adsorption of benzo(a)pyrene on to asbestos and manmade mineral fibres in an aqueous solution and in a biological model solution. *Br J Ind Med* 1988;45(10):682–8.
126. Nelson HH, Kelsey KT. The molecular epidemiology of asbestos and tobacco in lung cancer. *Oncogene* 2002;21(48):7284–8.
127. Tam IY, Chung LP, Suen WS, Wang E, Wong MC, Ho KK, et al. Distinct epidermal growth factor receptor and KRAS mutation patterns in non-small cell lung cancer patients with different tobacco exposure and clinicopathologic features. *Clin Cancer Res* 2006;12(5):1647–53.
128. Nelson HH, Christiani DC, Wiencke JK, Mark EJ, Wain JC, Kelsey KT. k-*ras* mutation and occupational asbestos exposure in lung adenocarcinoma: Asbestos-related cancer without asbestosis. *Cancer Res* 1999;59(18):4570–3.

129. Weiss W. Asbestosis: a marker for the increased risk of lung cancer among workers exposed to asbestos [review]. *Chest* 1999;115(2):536–49. Published erratum appears in *Chest* 1999;115(5):1485.
130. Nygren J, Suhonen S, Norppa H, Linnainmaa K. DNA damage in bronchial epithelial and mesothelial cells with and without associated crocidolite asbestos fibers. *Environ Mol Mutagen* 2004;44(5):477–82.
131. Schabath MB, Spitz MR, Delclos GL, Gunn GB, Whitehead LW, Wu X. Association between asbestos exposure, cigarette smoking, myeloperoxidase (MPO) genotypes, and lung cancer risk. *Am J Ind Med* 2002;42(1):29–37.
132. Landi S, Gemignani F, Neri M, Barale R, Bonassi S, Bottari F, et al. Polymorphisms of glutathione-*S*-transferase M1 and manganese superoxide dismutase are associated with the risk of malignant pleural mesothelioma. *Int J Cancer* 2007;120(12):2739–43.
133. Neri M, Ugolini D, Dianzani I, Gemignani F, Landi S, Cesario A, et al. Genetic susceptibility to malignant pleural mesothelioma and other asbestos-associated diseases. *Mutat Res* 2008;659(1–2):126–36.
134. London SJ, Daly AK, Cooper J, Navidi WC, Carpenter CL, Idle JR. Polymorphism of glutathione *S*-transferase M1 and lung cancer risk among African-Americans and Caucasians in Los Angeles County, California. *J Natl Cancer Inst* 1995;87(16):1246–53.
135. Hirvonen A, Saarikoski ST, Linnainmaa K, Koskinen K, Husgafvel-Pursiainen K, Mattson K, et al. Glutathione *S*-transferase and *N*-acetyltransferase genotypes and asbestos-associated pulmonary disorders. *J Natl Cancer Inst* 1996;88(24):1853–6.
136. Anttila S, Luostarinen L, Hirvonen A, Elovaara E, Karjalainen A, Nurminen T, et al. Pulmonary expression of glutathione *S*-transferase M3 in lung cancer patients: Association with GSTM1 polymorphism, smoking, and asbestos exposure. *Cancer Res* 1995;55(15):3305–9.
137. Kelsey KT, Nelson HH, Wiencke JK, Smith CM, Levin S. The glutathione *S*-transferase theta and mu deletion polymorphisms in asbestosis. *Am J Ind Med* 1997;31(3):274–9.
138. Dianzani I, Gibello L, Biava A, Giordano M, Bertolotti M, Betti M, et al. Polymorphisms in DNA repair genes as risk factors for asbestos-related malignant mesothelioma in a general population study. *Mutat Res* 2006;599(1–2):124–34.
139. Lafuente MJ, Casterad X, Laso N, Mas S, Panades R, Calleja A, et al. Pi*S and Pi*Z alpha 1 antitrypsin polymorphism and the risk for asbestosis in occupational exposure to asbestos. *Toxicol Lett* 2002;136(1):9–17.
140. Betti M, Neri M, Ferrante D, Landi S, Biava A, Gemignani F, et al. Pooled analysis of NAT2 genotypes as risk factors for asbestos-related malignant mesothelioma. *Int J Hyg Environ Health* 2009;212(3):322–9.
141. Helmig S, Belwe A, Schneider J. Association of transforming growth factor beta1 gene polymorphisms and asbestos-induced fibrosis and tumors. *J Investig Med* 2009;57(5):655–61.
142. Nelson HH, Wiencke JK, Gunn L, Wain JC, Christiani DC, Kelsey KT. Chromosome 3p14 alterations in lung cancer: evidence that FHIT exon deletion is a target of tobacco carcinogens and asbestos. *Cancer Res* 1998;58(9):1804–7.
143. Pylkkanen L, Wolff H, Stjernvall T, Tuominen P, Sioris T, Karjalainen A, et al. Reduced Fhit protein expression and loss of heterozygosity at FHIT gene in tumours from smoking and asbestos-exposed lung cancer patients. *Int J Oncol* 2002;20(2):285–90.
144. Pylkkänen L, Wolff H, Stjernvall T, Knuuttila A, Anttila S, Husgafvel-Pursiainen K. Reduced Fhit protein expression in human malignant mesothelioma. *Virchows Arch* 2004;444:43–8.
145. Sozzi G, Sard L, De Gregorio L, Marchetti A, Musso K, Buttitta F, et al. Association between cigarette smoking and FHIT gene alterations in lung cancer. *Cancer Res* 1997;57(11):2121–3.
146. Vancheri C, Failla M, Crimi N, Raghu G. Idiopathic pulmonary fibrosis: A disease with similarities and links to cancer biology. *Eur Respir J* 2010;35(3):496–504.

Epidemiology of Asbestos-Related Diseases and the Knowledge That Led to What Is Known Today

Richard A. Lemen

CONTENTS

5.1 INTRODUCTION

"Asbestos is one of the most marvelous productions of inorganic nature. It is a physical paradox, a mineralogical vegetable, both fibrous and crystalline, elastic and brittle; a floating stone, as capable of being carded, spun, and woven, as wool, flax, or silk. Occupying the apparent position of a connecting link between the mineral and vegetable kingdom, it would appear to possess some of the characteristics of both, while being altogether different from either."[1]

5.1.1 History and Usage of Asbestos

The use of asbestos* dates back to thousands of years when asbestos fibers were being incorporated into pottery.[2,3] Agricola attributes Theophrastus (d. 287 BCE) with the earliest reference to asbestos when he wrote: "There is also found in the mines of Scaptesylae a stone, in its external

---

* The term dates back as a noun to 1607 as *asbest* and to 1658 *asbestos*, mineral that does not burn, which was borrowed from Latin asbestos, replacing abeston applied to quicklime (before 1387, and still earlier *abestus* before 1100. The term borrowed from Old French *abeste*, *abeston*, and *asbeston* and Medieval Latin *albeston*, from Latin asbestos, from Greek asbestos unquenchable (a- not + *sbestós*, verbal adjective of *shennýnai* to quench). The Latin word was

appearance somewhat resembling wood, on which, if oil be poured, it burns; but when the oil is burnt away, the burning of the stone ceases, as if it were in itself not liable to such accidents." Sotacus, the Greek author of the third century BCE, is mentioned by Pliny as a foreign writer on stones that has one of the fullest accounts of asbestos. In the following account from the *Histories Commentitiae*, also in the third century BCE and attributed to Apollonius Dyscolus, it was stated: "The Carystain stone has wolly and colored appendages, which are spun and woven into napkins. The substance is also twisted into wicks, which, when burnt, are bright, but do not consume. The napkins, when dirty, are not washed with water, but a fire is made of sticks, and then the napkin is put into it. The dirt disappears, and the napkin is rendered white and pure by the fire, and is applicable to the same purposes as before. The wicks remain burning with oil continually without being consumed. This stone is produced in Carystus, from which it has its name, and in great abundance in Cyprus under rocks to the left of Elmseum, as you go from Gerandros to Soli."[4]

Greek sculptor Callimachus (436 BCE) found asbestos worked well as a lamp wick and used it in a golden lamp he made and kept perpetually lit in the temple of Pallas Athene.[5]

Roman scholar Varro (116–27 BCE) discusses asbestos cloth as a Greek invention in *De Lingun Lat. L.* v. p. 134. Ed. Spengel.[4]

Strabo (d. 23? CE) stated about asbestos that "At Carystus [Greek city] there is found in the earth a stone which is combed like wool, and woven, so that napkins are made of this substance, which when soiled, are thrown into the fire and cleaned, as in the washing of linen."[2] (Pedanius) Dioscorides (40–90 CE) is also said to have mentioned asbestos in his writings.[2]

Pliny the Elder (23–79 CE) described amiantus (chrysotile asbestos) to look like alum and that it was quite indestructible by fire and that it provided protection against spells, especially those of the Magi.[6] Additionally, Gilroy stated that if we can rely on Pliny's testimony as given in the existing editions of his works that asbestos was obtained in both Arcadia and India and described it as follows: "A kind of flax has been discovered which is incombustible by fire. It is called live flax; and we have seen napkins of it burning upon the hearth at entertainments, and, when thus deprived of their dirt, more resplendent through the agency of fire than they could have been by the use of water. The funeral shirts make of it for kings preserve the ashes of the body separate from those of the rest of the pile. It is produced in deserts and in tracts scorched by the Indian sun where there are no showers, and among dire serpents, and thus it is inured to live even when it is burnt. It is rare, and woven with difficulty on account of the shortness of its fibres. That variety which is of a red color becomes resplendent in the fire. When it has been found it equals the prices of excellent pearls. It is called by the Greeks asbestine flax, on account of its nature. Anaxilaus [*sic*] relates that if a tree surrounded with cloth made of it be beaten, the strokes are not heard. On account of these properties, this flax is the first in the world. The next in value is that made by byseus [*sic*], which is produced about Elis in Achain and used principally for fine female ornaments. I find that a scruple of this flax as also of gold was formerly sold for four denarii [1 denarius is @ $20].[*] The nap of linen cloths, obtained chiefly from the sails of ships, is of great use in surgery, and their ashes have the same effect as spodium. There is a certain kind of poppy the use of which imparts the highest degree of whiteness to linen cloths."[4]

Vesuvius erupted in 79 CE and upon later evacuation there were found pieces of asbestos cloth thought to be used for dressing the dead and later referred to as the funeral dress of kings.[5]

Plutarch (Mestrius Plutarchus, 46–120 CE), the Greek philosopher–historian, mentioned napkins, nets, and headdresses made of the Carystian stone; however, it was rarely found in his time except only in thin veins, like hairs found in rock.[4]

Pausanias (flourished CE 143–176), the Greek geographer, discussed the wick of the golden lamp kept burning night and day in the temple of Minerva Polias at Athens and was made of Carpasian

---

mistakenly applied by Pliny to quicklime (the "unquenchable" stone). From *The Barnhart Concise Dictionary of Etymology*, by Robert K. Barnhart, 1995, first edition, H.W. Wilson Company.

[*] That is, 18 grains of this flax were worth 2s. 10d. stg., being equal in value to its weight in gold (Gilroy, 1945; http:// dougsmith.ancients.info/worth.html).

flax, the only indestructible type of flax which was asbestos found in the vicinity of Carpasus in the town Carpas near the north-east corner of Cyprus. Dioscorides (40–90 CE), the Greek physician, had previously given a similar account of the uses of Amiantus (asbestos) and pointed out it was produced in Cyprus.[4]

The historian Hierocles (flourished c. 430 CE), as quoted by Stephanus Byzantinus, the Greek sixth-century author of a geographical dictionary called Ethnica, reported of asbestos in India as "The Brachmans use cloth made of a kind of flax, which is obtained from rocks. Webs are produced from it, which are neither subject to be consumed by fire nor cleaned by water, but which, after they have become full of dirt and stains, are rendered clear and white by being thrown into the fire"[4] (Gilroy,1845; http://www.1911encyclopedia.org/Stephanus_Byzantinus).

In 1633 Italy, Pliny's earlier account of the use of asbestos for wrapping corpses was validated by the finding of pieces of asbestine (asbestos) cloth in tombs, that is, from a tomb in Puzzuolo and then preserved in the Barberini gallery in Rome (National Gallery of Ancient Art of Barberini Palaces)[4] (Gilroy, 1845; http://www.galleriaborghese.it/barberini/en/einfo.htm).

Deposits of asbestos were discovered in 1712 in the Ural Mountains in Russia.[5] In a vineyard in 1760, a marble sarcophagus was found to contain a cloth, about 5 ft. wide and 6.5 ft. long, which contained a skull and other burnt bones of a deceased man apparently of high rank and having lived around the time of Constantine. This relic is preserved in the Vatican Library, and as described by J. E. Smith who saw it there, "It is coarsely spun, but as soft and pliant as silk. Our guide set fire to one corner of it, and the very same part burnt repeatedly with great rapidity and brightness without being at all injured."[4,7]

5.1.1.1 Premodern and Unique Uses

Asbestos is often referred to as the "magic mineral," having 3000 or more uses, including such uses as being woven into cloth with vegetable fibers; to still the sound of falling trees during construction projects within the Roman empire; for wrapping corpses, referred to by Pliny as the funeral dress of kings, before cremation to help collect the deceased ashes; and in making clay pots some 4000 years ago; it was even mentioned by Marco Polo during his travels to the far east about 1250 CE, where he found the people told him the cloth that resisted fire was made from salamander skin. Polo was far to "wary a traveler" to be fooled by such a fable and found it was mined from the mountains, extracted, then crushed by subjects of the Great Khan into a fibrous-like wool that was then spun and made into cloth, of which some were used for table cloths that, when soiled, were thrown into the fire and came out "white as snow and without a stain" for use again. He found the material to be called "amianto." A napkin made of this material was sent by "a certayne King of the Tartars" to the Bishop of Rome, in which cloth he keeps the "Sudarium [handkerchief] of our Lord."[1] Also, Pope Clement the Eleventh ordered an intact shroud of considerable length, in good condition and as pliant as silk, found in a sarcophagus by the Via Praenestina in 1702, a road to the very ancient city of Latium, lying 23 miles east of Rome, placed in the Vatican library where it can still be seen.[1] Strabo and Plutarch both mentioned the use of asbestos for wicks used in the lamps of the Vestal Virgins as well as being used for sacred fires in the Temples, being referred to as perpetual because the flames do not consume the wicks or the asbestos placed in the fires.[1] Charlemagne used the "amianthine" (asbestos) table cloths to astonish his rude warrior guests, throwing them into the fire then withdrawing it cleansed and unconsumed.[1] At the Royal College of Surgeons in England, the oldest mummy in the world, upwards of 6000 years old, was unwrapped by a Professor Stewart who found the body wrapped in gauze-like material and the cavities of the body stuffed with the same type material, which later was identified as a linen-like material thought to be made of asbestos fibers.[1] Tribes of Indians were known to have made dresses of asbestos, "which they cleanse by throwing them into fire."[1] Benjamin Franklin even bought a purse from the "northern part of America" made from woven tremolite asbestos, a picture of which can be found in the book by Selikoff and Lee.[8–10]

Giuseppe della Corona, a Florentine priest, is credited with the introduction of asbestos millboard in the mid-1800s.[1] A unique use can be found in John Baxter's book *A Pound of Paper*, in which he discussed the use of Johns-Manville Quintera, a form of asbestos, to cover a limited edition of author Ray Bradbury's book Fahrenheit 451, published in 1953.[11] The manufacture of asbestos paper dates back to around 1700, when it was made in Norway, and for printing banknotes and other securities in Italy in the mid-1800s.[1] In Cincinnati, Ohio, baby incubators were lined with asbestos to prevent the effect of radiating heat and to make it airtight. Asbestos was found in soap, cigarette papers, knitting yarns, jewelers' molds, mail bags, firemen's and stokers' aprons, paints, food filters, and tobacco pipes. Far more in-depth descriptions of the uses of asbestos can be found in the tenth chapter of *Asbestos and Asbestic: Their Properties, Occurrences and Use* written by Robert H. Jones, a mineralogist, published in 1897, and in discussions of the *Magic Mineral* by Paul Brodeur.[1,12,13]

The book *Asbestos & Fire* by Rachel Maines[14] discusses the advantages of asbestos and why the substance came into such widespread usage. According to the author,[14] the book was suggested by the Winthrop Group, "... a boutique consultancy of experienced executives who drive growth for Fortune 1000 and emerging companies" (http://www.winthropgrp.com/). Although the book downplays the overwhelming health risks, it does discuss the plethora of uses of asbestos through history.

5.1.1.2 Modern Industry

In 1824, asbestos was discovered in the United States near Lowell, Vermont, but not much interest was shown until the 1890s.[15] In 1879, a Canadian chrysotile mine opened in the Province of Quebec.[1] The modern industry dates from 1880, when asbestos was used to make heat- and acid-resistant fabrics.[16–18] In Osaka, the first Japanese asbestos factory opened in 1886 making packing and other insulation products.[19] In South Africa, the first discovery of asbestos was made by Liehtenstein between 1803 and 1806, where he collected a heavy blue mineral near the Orange River valley near Prieska. It was first named "Blau-Eisenstein" but was renamed in 1831 to Asbestiform crocidolite, which means "woolly stone." Crocidolite was not actively mined until the demands of the Second World War.[21–24] Chrysotile was discovered in South Africa in 1905 and prospecting in Havelock in Northern Swaziland began in 1928.[20] A patent was awarded in England in 1895 for railroad brake linings containing asbestos, and by 1903 friction brake products were sold in the United States.[25]

Commencement of mining of the amphibole asbestos anthophyllite began in Finland in 1890 (http://www.active-asbestos.co.uk/frame_centre_about_history.html). During 1904, a second deposit of asbestos was found in South Africa, in northeast Transvall, and in 1918 it was named amosite, from the village Amosa, which was the acronym for the term Asbestos Mines of South Africa. Production began in the mid-1920s by Cape Asbestos Company, the same company already mining and producing crocidolite.[24,26] The commercial importance of asbestos was well recognized when, on January 13, 1906, Johns-Manville* ran full page advertisements in the Saturday Evening Post© saying (asbestos) "serves more people in more ways than any institution of its kind in the world." Products for the home-builder, the industrial and commercial builder, and the automobilists were included in this ad. Asbestos was being used by American steel companies for insulation of large furnaces.[27]

Upon its introduction in Canada, asbestos was looked upon with some degree of suspicion and only 300 tons were mined during the first year, which realized no more than $19,500. As it became better known, the rapidity of its progress was prodigious. By 1890, the output had grown to 9860 tons and its saleable value reached $1,260,240. This was a grand time for mine owners who, under the stimulus of daily advancing prices, were unable to supply the demands of the manufacturers. No

---

* That is, 18 grains of this flax were worth 2s. 10d. stg., being equal in value to its weight in gold (Gilroy, 1945; http://dougsmith.ancients.info/worth.html).

forward contracts could be made, and it was impossible to foretell how high prices would eventually reach.[1]

Some of the highlights of the modern uses of asbestos included asbestos used as a heat insulation beginning in 1866[28] and then mixed with cement as a boiler covering in 1870.[29] The first asbestos factory was opened in 1871 in Great Britain.[30] The commercial production of asbestos insulation materials began in 1874.[29] In 1890, the first processing of Canadian asbestos into textile began in the United States.[31] By the turn of the twentieth century, the asbestos cement pipe industry had its origins in Italy.[32] By 1903, asbestos cement production started in the United States, but the pipe-making machines were not imported into the United States until 1928.[31] Cement-based flat asbestos cement board, now a major building product of the third world, was first produced in the United States in 1904.[33] Brake linings containing asbestos were first used in 1906.[30] Asbestos spraying of deck heads and bulkheads began in 1944 for British navy ships and was discontinued in 1963.[34,35]

By 1910, asbestos was being used by American steel companies for insulation of large furnaces.[27]

The August 1, 1916, issue of the Scientific American published an article on asbestos stating that because of restriction on the shipment of asbestos from Canada to the United States, attention was being given by the U.S. Geological Survey to the possibility of using asbestos deposits in the United States to an increased extent. In 1915, the production of high-grade asbestos increased in Arizona. This increase came about because of more demand for asbestos' "protective purposes in the furnace of the industrial safety movement."[36,37]

According to the U.S. Bureau of Foreign and Domestic Commerce in 1916, "Although there are extensive deposits of asbestos in many parts of British South Africa, little interest has been taken in the possibilities of mining it. Many who owned land having such deposits upon it refused to engage to any extent in operations for its recovery, preferring to wait until a suitable market was permanently established. The industry now has a more hopeful future, as many asbestos merchants are endeavoring to establish and maintain foreign markets. Ine [sic] principal markets in the past have been in England and on the Continent, but the war has affected the conditions. During the years 1909 to 1911, a larger quantity of asbestos was shipped from South Africa to the Continent than to the United Kingdom, while in 1913 and 1914 the reverse was the case. Now shipments to parts of the Continent have ceased. Exporters Now Looking to the United States."[38]

Hoffman stated that because of the fire-resistant properties of asbestos, this led to extensive employment for covering pipe, furnaces, and so forth, and as use in wall plaster and roofing materials, and because of its nonconducting properties, asbestos has been used by electricians and in the storage rooms of refrigerating plants.[37]

Asbestos forms about 15% of the insulation, which acts as a binder for the more important insulation material of magnesia and carbonate. As the percentage of asbestos increases, the product becomes heavier and the less effective the insulating properties become. Eighty-five percent magnesia claims a crushing strength of 100 lb/sq in., which means gradually applied and without shock.[39]

By 1928, cement pipe was being used in the United States for the transport of water under pressure.[5] In 1929, Oliver described the manufacture of mattresses in a British textile factory that were used to cover and protect the internal machinery of automobiles.[40]

5.1.1.3 Asbestosis

The evolution of epidemiologic knowledge of exposure to asbestos spans the millennium of human history. Although the first writings of human history lead to clues of worker diseases, they do not illuminate the nature of nor the degree of the epidemic during the twentieth century. In her historical sketch, Adelaide M. Anderson tells of such early millennial knowledge stating: "In the

great civilizations of antiquity, whether in the East, West, or in Europe generally, there was sufficient concentration of the forces of labour to produce the intensest forms of the maladies classed
by Pliny as the 'diseases of slaves'. Some of the most injurious processes known to us now are
extremely ancient. To mention but a few: ... weaving asbestos and flax."[41]

Miss Lucy Dean, predecessor to Anderson as Women Inspector of Factories, wrote in the 1899
Annual Report on the Health of Workers for 1898 that "[T]he evil effects of asbestos dust have
instigated a microscopic examination of the mineral dust [asbestos] by HM Medical Inspector
... , the effects have been found to be injurious as might have been expected." She further stated
that "the worker can continue for a very long time apparently unaffected, before the symptoms of
the evil become marked."[42] The Woman Inspector of Factories Lucy Dean stated: "Among other
dusty processes which engaged the attention of Miss Paterson and myself in 1899 were those in
works for the manufacture of nonconducting jacketing for pipes, involving use of asbestos (the
injuriousness of which substance was demonstrated in last year's report), and certain hempen-
rope and sail-cloth works. In both sets of factories, the action necessary to secure exhaust ventilation required for the removal of dust from the point at which it is generated has extended into the
present year. In the latter class of work, we found a curious, unnecessary, and most undesirable
mode of employment of little girls, whose duty it was to pack refuse of flax and hemp into large
bags or sacks. To pack the material tightly, they got inside the sacks and vigorously tramped it
down. Apart from other objections, the necessary inhalation of excessive quantities of the dangerous dust and the absorption of it in their clothes made it most desirable to put an end to the
practice."[42]

Three years later, Adelaide Anderson, now Lady Inspector of Factories, included asbestos among
the dusts known to cause injury to man in a publication on dangerous industries in England.[41] The
first recorded case of "asbestosis" was reported in London by Dr. Murray, a Charing Cross Hospital
Physician, in 1907. The case involved a 33-year-old man who worked in an asbestos textile plant for
14 years.[43] Numerous deaths (50) were also reported in a French asbestos textile factory.[44] Italian
physicians reviewed the cases of 30 asbestos workers seen in a Turin clinic between 1894 and 1906
as having a serious pulmonary disease thought to be tuberculosis; however, it was extremely progressive and unlike the typical tuberculosis case. This was the first indication of the progressive
nature to the asbestos-induced lung disease, a finding later confirmed through epidemiological studies of asbestos workers conducted during the 1930s.[45]

Animal studies had also begun around the turn of the twentieth century, and it was reported in
the Annual Report of HM Chief Inspector of Factories for 1910 that Prof. J. M. Beattie of Sheffield
University in the United Kingdom had found a mild degree of fibrosis in experimental animals
after inhalation of asbestos-containing dust and that five deaths of persons with phthisis occurred
among a workforce of 40 years and younger in the production of woven asbestos. This led to the
industrial practice, later emphasized by Merewether and Price,[46] for dust suppression as a prevention tool that could be obtained through ventilation to protect workers from asbestos-induced lung
disease.[47]

Around the same time, the American Association for Labor Legislation and the government of
Canada's Department of Labour included asbestos-related diseases as an industrial disease.[33,48]

A couple of years later in Germany, the report of a woman who worked in a German asbestos
factory and who died of an acute lung illness resembling pleural pneumonia, on autopsy, was found
to have a "... large number of crystals of a peculiar nature," which was presented to the medical
society of Hamburg and was later recognized as a case of asbestosis.[49] In 1918, it was reported in the
Bulletin of US Labor Statistics that American and Canadian insurance companies would not insure
asbestos workers because of the unhealthy conditions in the industry.[37]

With the discovery by Wilhelm C. Roentgen of the x-ray on November 8, 1895, the imaging
of the respiratory system developed quite rapidly. The first description of radiographic changes in
15 individuals exposed to asbestos was reported in 1918.[50] Pancoast and Pendergrass[51] published a

review on pneumoconiosis,[*] including asbestosis, in 1925 in the *American Journal of Roentgenology and Radium Therapy.*

Clinical descriptions of asbestosis were becoming more common in the medical literature. The case of Nellie Kershaw, a 33-year-old asbestos factory worker who worked since age 13 years in the textile factories in England, was the sentinel case accounting for the naming of asbestosis as a distinct pneumoconiosis and for giving the first discussions on asbestos bodies. In 1922, Mrs. Kershaw consulted her local physician, Dr. Walter Joss, who concluded she suffered from "asbestos poisoning." Five years before her final illness and due to failing health, she worked intermittently. Mrs. Kershaw died on March 15, 1924, and was buried in an unmarked grave. She received only 7s per week for 7 months in the final year of her life from the National Health Insurance. Her employer, Turner Brothers, paid nothing.[52] Cooke's presentation of this case in 1924 gave the best and most complete description of the effects of asbestos on the lungs. This case presented with pleural thickening over the entire surface of the lung and dense adhesions on the chest wall and pericardium. The right lung showed extensive fibrosis, caseous foci, and cavities having thick fibrous walls. Numerous giant cells were found around the caseous areas, and tuberculosis lesions were present.[54]

In 1927, Cooke and Hill[55] reported that although the asbestos industry dates back some 2000 years, the industry was to "… have been devoid of appliances for the prevention and extraction of dust." The fibers found in the lung tissue of Mrs. Kershaw varied from 3 to 360 µm in length and appeared to be "… the heavy, brittle, iron-containing fragments of the asbestos fibre." In comparing the two sources of asbestos used in the textile factories where Mrs. Kershaw worked, Cooke reported the only significant difference between the Italian fiber and the Canadian Chrysotile was that the Italian fiber had less iron in the form of ferrous oxide (0.87% vs. 2.81% in the Canadian Chrysotile) and the Italian fiber had more Alumina (2.27% vs. 0.90% than that in the Canadian Chrysotile). Because ferrous oxide fibers are heavy, Cooke felt this explained the greater amount of fibrosis in the right lung due to the ease of the particles to pass "… more easily down the more vertical right bronchus than the horizontal left bronchus." During the carding process, the collected dust, as analyzed by Byrom, contained 18.4% ferrous oxide compared with 2.8% found in raw material, thus indicating the removal of much of the iron content during this process. The finished product contained only 0.1% iron. Dr. Cooke gave the first detailed description of "curious bodies" having "discoid arrangement and globular ends" within a phagocytic cell. Dr. Cooke referred to the case described by Murray[43] of the man who died of pulmonary fibrosis, as having "spicules of asbestos" as the first and only recorded case of death due to asbestos before his 1924 report concerning Nellie Kershaw.

McDonald,[56] Cooke and Hill,[55] and Cooke[57] continued to describe curious bodies in the lungs now known as asbestos bodies. It has been shown that asbestos bodies can form in extrapulmonary sites such as the liver and spleen.[58] McDonald confined his comments as to the histological appearance of the bodies, which are found both in alveoli and interstitial substances of the lungs. In addition to the case described by Cooke,[59] he examined a second case obtained from a physician in Leeds, UK. Some asbestos bodies were free, whereas others were phagocytized by large mononuclear cells found in the alveoli. Some were small and easily phagocytized, but the majority were between 20 and 70 µm and more. All had a distinct yellowish-brown color, which he suggested was a blood pigment, and some had club-like extremities at one or both ends. Those bodies too large for the phagocytes were then surrounded by plasmodial masses. McDonald had the bodies examined by experts in zoology and botany, both of whom said they were neither of animal nor of vegetable nature. He further explained that the fiber type of the second patient was Canadian serpentine (chrysotile), which had about equal parts silica and magnesium salt (40%), 3% ferrous oxide, 1% alumina, and water. Although tuberculosis was present in both cases, it was Dr. McDonald's opinion that it was a superadded infection because there was a considerable degree of fibrosis without the tuberculosis infection in the second case he examined. Cooke[57] felt that when curious bodies were

---

[*] A term meaning dust affecting the lung, taken from Zenker's original term pneumonokoniosis.

found "in any numbers," they would be "pathognomonic of pulmonary asbestosis." Today they are thought to be the histologic hallmark of exposure to asbestos and their presence not necessarily a marker of disease.[60–62] Some studies have shown a correlation between the number of asbestos bodies (ferruginous bodies) in the sputa and radiographic finding of interstitial pulmonary disease and pleural thickening as well as with spirometric findings of a restrictive lung disease.[63] Sporn and Roggli[64] claim "… the identification of asbestos bodies within tissue sections remains the diagnostic *sine qua non* in view of the non-specificity of interstitial fibrosis as a response to diffuse lung injury, and the large number of disorder that may cause scarring in the lung."

In May 1928, four cases of asbestosis were reported, one case having only 2 years of exposure to asbestos and having no histological evidence of tuberculosis. The report[65] stated it had been known for some time that workers exposed to asbestos materials suffered from pulmonary disabilities. One case, a South African asbestos mill worker, was only exposed for 12 months, died of rapid TB, and on autopsy was found to have moderate fibrosis. Simson[65] reported that asbestos dust was much more rapid than fibrosis produced by silica. In examination of the lungs of a guinea pig supplied by Dr. Mavrogordato of the same Institute as Simson, the presence of golden-yellow bodies similar to those found in human lungs with asbestosis were identified. The lungs of the guinea pig had been exposed to Southern Rhodesian chrysotile for 2 h per day for 50 days. As more case reports of asbestosis appeared in the literature, the *Journal of the American Medical Association* (*JAMA*) ran an editorial on pulmonary asbestosis in January 1928 because of the continuing presence of asbestosis in the medical literature and because of the dangers of asbestosis and its unique pathologic features.[66] In December 1928, a case report of fibrosis in a 40-year-old man who worked in the asbestos industry for 22 years was published in which all other potential causes were excluded, including tuberculosis.[67] Cooke[57] and Gloyne[68] further described the presence of curious bodies in pulmonary asbestosis. Gloyne[68] suggested these curious bodies be called asbestos bodies, as this more adequately described their origin. In 1929, Stewart,[69] at the University of Leeds, described how to examine sputum for asbestos bodies and stated that "as a rule they are present in very small numbers, perhaps only one or two in the whole film. In the case of some of the older workers, however, numerous bodies up to one or two per field in certain portions of the film have been found" (see in-depth reference to all of Professor Matthew Stewart's work in Greenberg M, 1997).[70] Stewart and Haddow[71] demonstrated asbestos bodies could be found in the lung, in lung juices, and in sputum of asbestos workers. Reports of curious bodies, asbestos bodies, and ferruginous bodies would continue to be discussed in the literature and their relationship to the etiology of asbestos-related disease would continue.

Wood[72] provided a good description of 16 cases of radiological changes in the chests of asbestos workers as seen in skiagrams.* Wood concluded that, with reference to the radiograms, "… in general the density and extent of the lung shadows is proportional to the duration of the exposure to the dust." An article in the *British Medical Journal* reviewed occupational-induced dust diseases, including asbestos-related disease, and stated, "Prevention does not, in the case of disease produced by occupational dusts, rest with the medical profession, although we may be able to assist. The sure and only certain way of preventing dust affecting the worker is to prevent its formation, or, if this is impossible, to secure its removal before reaching the workers."[73] Klokov[74] found it is necessary to do pulmonary function testing for early diagnosis because pulmonary changes appeared before radiological changes.

In the 1930s, the first epidemiological study was conducted of persons exposed to asbestos. The cohort was of asbestos textile workers, which supported the general causal relationship between exposure to asbestos and the lung disease asbestosis. This study showed that asbestosis was clearly a preventable industrial disease. The 1930s were very productive in our growth of knowledge about

---

* Skiagram: A photographic image produced on a radiosensitive surface by radiation other than visible light (especially by x-rays or gamma rays) (http://www.wordwebonline.com/en/SKIAGRAM).

asbestos-related diseases. Pleural adhesions were first reported on autopsy showing the pleural surfaces had fused; asbestos fibers were reported to pass into the lymphatic system; asbestosis was found to be a progressive disease, even in the absence of further exposures; and the suspicion that cancer of the lung was an asbestos-related disease because of its occurrence in persons living with asbestosis arose.

The book *Recent Advances in Preventive Medicine* by J. F. C. Haslm and S. J. Cowell, published in 1930[75] had 10 pages devoted to the knowledge gained through 1929 on the hazards associated with asbestos exposure. In the section on pulmonary asbestosis, the authors pointed out that "several of the processes to which crude asbestos is submitted in course of manufacture into articles of commerce produce large quantities of dust," and that "medical men practicing among asbestos workers have long suspected that this dust caused bronchial and pulmonary trouble, but until lately nothing at all definite was known about a pneumonoconiosis due to asbestos, and factories manufacturing asbestos products were often without special precautions against dust inhalation long after silicosis had been recognized and guarded against." The book goes on to review the case-reports from Murray in 1907 through Haddow in 1929. Unlike silicosis, the book points out the absence of confounding tuberculosis with asbestosis.[75]

Asbestos, a trade journal for the asbestos industry, made reference to asbestosis in their March 1930 issue citing the U.S. Bureau of Labor Statistics of the Department of Labor. The journal stated that pulmonary asbestosis was a disease related to asbestos dust, and the Bureau urged the suppression of asbestos dust. The trade journal stated the disease consisted of pulmonary fibrosis attacking the bases of the lungs and, like silicosis, was frequently complicated with tuberculosis. The part about tuberculosis was, however, incorrect as it had not been found as frequent as with silica as case-reports have observed.[76]

This first epidemiology study of asbestos textile workers published on March 14, 1930, by E. R. A. Merewether and C. W. Price[78] along with the U.K. Government Home Office established general causation between asbestos exposure and the lung disease asbestosis. This study is of monumental significance in the developing history of asbestos disease knowledge. The results of this study of 363 asbestos workers or approximately 16.5% of the then suspected 2200 asbestos workers in the United Kingdom stated: "There is no doubt that fibrosis of the type produced by asbestos can of itself lead to complete disablement and to a fatal termination, and this, in the absence of a super-added tuberculous infection. To sum up, therefore, it appears probable that concentration of dust and length of exposure as factors in the production of fibrosis are interdependent within certain limits. Although it seems necessary for the production of generalized fibrosis of the lungs that a definite minimal quantity of dust must be inhaled, the lower the concentration of dust in the air breathed the longer the lapse of time before the fibrosis is fully developed, and within a certain limit, the higher concentration of dust, the sooner the fibrosis becomes fully developed and the more intense the involvement of the lung tissue. This demonstration of a dose–response relationship is important as it implies that dust reduction will be a useful prevention method." The authors, concerned that the number of workers less than 5 years of employment was so great, tried to select their population for study to include a larger proportion of those employed more than 5 years. As a result, they were able to get a better idea of the effects to longer-term workers. Although the authors stated they had selected 363 workers, they actually examined 374 workers of both sexes and 105 were found to have diffuse fibrosis of the lungs attributable to the inhalation of dust, but 11 of these were excluded from further consideration because of previous work in other dusty occupations. As a result, 95 (26.2%) of the 363 showed fibrosis because of inhalation of asbestos dust. One-hundred thirty-three were radiographed and 62 had signs of diffuse fibrosis and another 25 had suggestive changes. The authors stated sex had no effect on the results, age had a negligible effect, and although years of employment were most significant as they increased, so did fibrosis. It found that the incidence of disease was greatest in those operations that were the dustiest. The authors indicated this was hard to evaluate because of the practice of the textile industry to house many processes in one room, allowing cross contamination between processes. The dust found in the plant varied from continuous exposure to short bursts to insignificant. The authors showed that wetting the asbestos was much more effective than local exhaust ventilation in reducing airborne dust. No evidence was found to indicate any difference between the effects of chrysotile, crocidolite, or amosite, the three fiber types used in the factory. Dustiness was measured using the Owens' Jet Apparatus at the breathing zone level. Although the authors did not state the actual measurement count, it was probably expressed as per cubic centimeter of air, as this appears to be the normal count measurement using the Owens' Jet Apparatus.[77] The small number of measurements taken shows the effectiveness of various methods of control compared with no control. The authors gave only 11 sample results from five different operations. Without dust controls, the measurements were from one particle per cubic centimeter of air in spinning to 2.34 in opening and handling fiber. When local exhaust was applied, the measurements went down some, but with damp methods, the counts were halved except in the smaller product operation of band cutting where local exhaust ventilation was actually better than the damp methodology. However, the authors stated the damp method measurement was not "... accurate since the figure was raised by dust from a neighbouring [sic] dry cloth loom." This observation is important as it shows the ability of fibers to drift from one area to another within the plant, thus contaminating other operations.*

The authors show the limits of their study when they remind us that only current workers were surveyed and that others with fibrosis who left the factory would be missed. In fact, they found information that a number of persons previously employed were either at home or in a sanatorium suffering from chest complaints. Finally, this study did not find a connection between tuberculosis and asbestosis, as was the case with silicosis. The authors felt that dust suppression would reduce the risk of disease in the future.

Besides the confirmation that asbestos exposure was causally related to the disease asbestosis, this study outlined a hierarchy of preventive measures, which are still used today. Additionally, they divided the asbestos industry into seven main groups: textiles, nontextiles, millboard, paper, cement sheets, tiles and other building materials, insulation, brake and clutch linings, packing and jointings, asbestos-covered electric products, and miscellaneous goods. In each of these groups, they gave methods for controlling dust. These methods included substitution and elimination of certain dust-producing appliances, application of efficient localized exhaust ventilation, substitution of enclosed mechanical methods for hand conveyance or for dusty hand work, substitution of wet methods for dry, abandonment of settling chambers in manufacturing processes, separation of processes to prevent unnecessary exposures, use of vacuum methods for cleaning, education of workers, and finally, as a last or emergency measure, the use of respirators. The authors warned that respirators give only partial protection, that their use can give a false sense of security, and that the discomfort and difficulty in speech render workers very unwilling to use respirators. They advised that most particles were of the order of 2 μm with many being 0.5 μm and that although respirators would remove the larger particles, they were not valueless. However, primary suppression of dust at its origin remained the best line of disease prevention.[78]

On April 4, 1930, *The Engineer* reported on the Merewether and Price report concerning the danger to employees in the asbestos industry caused by inhalation of dust and emphasized, as preventive measures, "the education of the individual, as in other dangerous trades, to a sane appreciation of the risk, and to his personal responsibility in the prevention and suppression of dust." The protection afforded by respirators was, it is said, only partial, and there was a real danger that the use of them might give a sense of false security.[79]

On April 19, 1930, the *Lancet*, a joint American and British medical journal, published an article titled Pulmonary Asbestosis in which they outlined the premodern use of asbestos and highlighted

---

* This may actually be the first observation of fiber drift in the literature and as such points to the inaccuracy of using job title as a surrogate for exposure measurement.

the British Government study of Merewether and Price. The *Lancet* stated the significance of this epidemiologic study lied in its finding and documentation of an irreversible and fatal lung disease among a group of asbestos factory workers, which up to this time only case reports had documented cases of asbestosis.[80]

The 1930 May issue of the *Journal of Industrial Hygiene* published a report by Dr. E. R. A. Merewether on "The occurrence of pulmonary fibrosis and other pulmonary affections in asbestos workers."[81] This journal was published by The Harvard School of Public Health in the United States. Dr. Merewether stated that before the initiation of his study in February 1928, only two deaths, for which there was expert opinion that asbestos dust played a roll, had been brought to the attention of the Factory Inspectorate. Then in February 1928, Dr. MacGregor, the Medical Officer of Health for Glasgow, England, brought attention to another asbestos worker receiving treatment. This case was reported by Seiler in the December 1928 issue of the *British Medical Journal*.[82] With this case, the Factory Department recognized four essential conditions necessary to establish a relationship between the inhalation of asbestos dust and the development of fibrosis: (1) work involving exposure to asbestos dust; (2) the existence, demonstrable clinically and radiologically, of a definite pulmonary fibrosis; (3) the absence of previous or present infections known to cause pulmonary fibrosis—for example, tuberculosis, influenza, or pneumonia; and (4) the absence of previous or present work involving exposure to other dusts which might cause pulmonary fibrosis. Dr. Merewether then stated: "These conditions being fulfilled, a relationship between the inhalation of asbestos dust and the development of the pulmonary fibrosis may be presumed." Because of this, Dr. Merewether concluded that "... steps were taken, forthwith, to obtain *prima facie* evidence in proof, or disproof, of the existence of such a risk." Besides the three cases known to the Factory Department by 1928, in 1914 the Royal Commission on Metalliferous Mines and Quarries had reported ... "we do not know whether other dusts besides those containing free crystalline silica induce a pathological condition in the lungs although the experiments of Professor Beattie in animals suggest that this may occur."

Out of 775 workers, Dr. Merewether selected 363 workers in the asbestos industry for an in-depth investigation to access their fibrotic status. Merewether decided to select primarily those with the longest employment and to obtain information on length of exposure and to the particular process in which they were engaged. There was an enormous preponderance of workers employed for less than 5 years. By segregating those by longest employed and by process, a greater proportion of the total number could be seen as the 5-year employment groups' increased. In other words, of the 775, 62.3% were employed less than 5 years, but when selection occurred by Dr. Merewethers' process, only 23.5% were employed less than 5 years, allowing his selected cohort to capture a greater number in each progressive 5-year employment category. All but one of those examined were present at work on the day of the examination. Merewether pointed out that all those examined were volunteers and the examinations were therefore dependent upon both the employers and the employees' cooperation. As symptoms may increase from other causes during winter months, every effort was made to complete the examinations before the onset of winter. Among those with fibrosis, 59.3% had cough, 55.9% had cyanosis, 51.6% had dyspnea, 34.1% had expectoration, and 10.6% had pain. Ninety-five of the 363 examined had fibrosis by clinical examination and 52 of 133 examined radiographically had fibrosis, which equates to 26.2% clinically and 39.1% radiographically. Twenty-one (5.8%) of the 363 were additionally classified with prefibrosis on clinical examination. Specific case descriptions are given for 14 of the cases.[81]

Engineering Magazine reported in their May 2, 1930, issue on the dangers of asbestos in an article on *Mineral Dust in Factories*. The article described the findings of Dr. E. R. A. Merewether and Mr. C. W. Price recently released by the Home Office on March 14th. The article stated: "While the effect of the report is not such as to cause panic, and in Dr. Merewether's opinion the outlook for preventive measures is such that in 10 years or so their energetic application should produce a great reduction in the incidence of the disease, the results recorded seem to leave no doubt that, as Sir

Gerald Bellhouse, of the Home Office, observes in submitting the report, the disease itself is serious and the necessity for suppressing the dust from which it arises has only recently been appreciate." "The time is, therefore, opportune for considering what measures are necessary to enable this valuable industry to be carried on without adding to the number of those who suffer from occupational diseases." As the report points out, because the dust is so fine and floats in the air in sizes no larger than a 500th of a millimeter with many smaller than 2000th of a millimeter, respirators, although difficult to get workers to wear for extended periods, are unable to protect adequately from these finer particles of dust and should only be used as a second line of defense. Although the article points out that local exhaust is the best line of defense, "each industry knows its own difficulties and probably knows them better than they are known to factory inspectors."[83]

Ralph G. Mills, a local physician in Fond du Lac, Wisconsin, reported the first case of asbestosis in the United States in a 58-year-old man, who "as a boy he had traveled the seven seas with his grandfather, who was a sea captain." The man died after 2 days in the hospital and upon postmortem examination, lung fibrosis was identified. Dr. Mills' curiosity led him to contact one of the man's business partners to ask if he knew of any contact the man may have had with asbestos. After 8 months, the partner wrote back to say "... he had ascertained that the deceased had, as a young man, worked in asbestos mine in South America." Sometime later, another business associate wrote that "while the patient had been in South America he had drilled asbestos bearing rock. The shot holes were cleaned by air. This had been around 1898 ... at least thirty-two years before his death."[84,*]

The July 28, 1930, issue of the JAMA[85] published statistical highlights of asbestosis as reported in the United Kingdom and other knowledge of asbestosis, including the case report by Dr. Ralph G. Mills[84] in the United States. The JAMA[5] stated: "Concerning the relation of physicians of the United States to this industry, Mills pointed out that asbestos is mined and manufactured in many parts of this country and that pulmonary asbestosis surely will be encountered." The JAMA also reported: "In England the workmen's compensation act has recently been extended to include this condition" (asbestosis).[85] By 1920, the JAMA was mailed to 48% of U.S. doctors but was estimated to be read by 80% of U.S. physicians.[86]

Three additional early reports led many investigators to conclude that people exposed to asbestos dust, including during manufacturing, developed the disease "asbestosis."[87–89] Wood and Page[87] evaluated the case of a 21-year-old woman with rapid development of tuberculosis who was exposed to asbestos. Asbestos bodies were stated to have developed within 2 years from first exposure, and asbestos fibers were found in the lungs on postmortem examination. Wood and Gloyne[88] summarized 37 cases, including four asbestos workers with doubtful diagnosis together with four records of postmortem findings. They discussed a suggested classification of stages of pulmonary asbestosis and stated pulmonary asbestosis would fall into group B [1] of occupational diseases of Bridges' classification. Wood and Gloyne[88] stated three stages could be defined for asbestosis: (1) the presence of asbestos fibers in nasal secretion or in the mouth, merely indicating exposure but not necessarily disease; (2) the presence of asbestos bodies, which is a sign of a tissue response to the infecting dust; and (3) the typical symptoms, sign, and radiographic appearances, which are clear evidence of the disease irrespective of the finding of asbestos bodies. They concluded that "obviously (1) is no evidence of disease; but we can accept (2) as a sign that disease is present. In the absence of sputum diagnosis must be made on (3) alone." Finally, they[88] concluded that by raising the question of pulmonary tuberculosis as a complication for which they concluded it was currently

---

* This case may well reflect the power of publishing studies in the medical literature. The Merewether and Price report spread so fast outside of the United Kingdom that an astute physician like Dr. Mills, a practitioner from Fond duc, Wisconsin, who had sent the man to the Mayo Clinic in Minnesota, where he died, was aware of the reports of pulmonary asbestosis from the medical journals. Like many discoveries, Dr. Mills' astute observation and follow-up that led to this finding and the issuance of the first case report on asbestosis to appear in an American medical journal *Minnesota Medicine* in July of 1930, just 2 months after the American/U.K. journal the *Lancet* had published the findings of the Merewether and Price study released in April 1930.

impossible to decide this question, that if it does occur with pulmonary asbestosis, it is liable to be of an anomalous type. Soper[89] reported the case of a 30-year-old man who began work in an asbestos plant at age 17 years. In this case report, Soper[89] stated that the most common symptom in pulmonary asbestosis was dyspnea and that lung fibrosis was a progressive disease with fibrosis of both lungs and basal pleurisy.

In 1930, Merewether[81] also described pulmonary fibrosis as affecting the basal region of both lungs and discussed the differences between silicosis and asbestosis and the progressive nature of the disease.

The International Labour Office (ILO) released their Encyclopedia of Hygiene, Pathology and Social Welfare for 1930[90] in which they described the general properties of asbestos, technology, industrial uses, dangers and hygiene, and legislation. In the Dangers and Hygiene section, they discussed many of the case reports up to 1930, one of the highlights of which included the discussion of how women working next to mattress beaters were at risk from fiber drift to their work area. They also reported the case of 40 deaths occurring among the spinning and weaving factory in Calavos between 1890 and 1895 and mentioned that a local Canadian doctor reported a frequent number of respiratory and tuberculosis diseases among asbestos workers. The risk of lead poisoning was also reported by Rambousek when the weaving of asbestos included a thread of lead added to the welt. Chronic conjunctivitis with hypertrophy of the rims of the pupils was reported among asbestos workers of the Island Cyprus who were engaged in grinding, screening, and packing asbestos in sacks. Referring to the Hoffman report of 1918, they reiterated the practice of American and Canadian life insurance companies generally refusing asbestos workers because of the deleterious conditions in the industry. Finally, under legislation, they pointed out that, in Italy, boys younger than 15 years and girls younger than 21 years were excluded from working in shops where asbestos was woven "... unless effective means are taken to prevent the diffusion of dusts throughout the atmosphere."[90]

Pedley,[91] who predicted that the literature on asbestos would "grow very much larger as time goes on," did not see asbestosis as being of much public health importance either from the standpoint of morbidity or mortality. However, as Greenberg[70] pointed out, the actuaries knew better.[37,93] Pedley[91] stated that although most of the cases of asbestosis were reported in the manufacture of asbestos, other cases had probably gone unrecognized because they were not in large cities where factories were located but rather in the mines located in rural areas where autopsies were less likely to be performed than that in larger cities.

In 1931, Lynch and Smith[94] reported on 172 cases of pulmonary asbestosis up to the time of their case report. Twenty-seven were confirmed to have asbestos bodies in sputum. Necropsy was performed on 18 cases, 3 having complications from pulmonary tuberculosis, 3 with lobar pneumonia, 3 with bronchopneumonia, and 1 being a traumatic death. In the case of a 46-year-old white man in 1925 diagnosed with pulmonary tuberculosis and having worked about 11½ years as a carder in an asbestos factory, no asbestos bodies were found in the sputum. From this case, the authors concluded that "[O]n account of the extreme fibrosis and the fixed condition of the lungs it is likely that there was very little expulsion of material from alveoli in the bronchial tract." This finding led the authors to suggest that asbestos bodies may not appear in the sputum of late stage cases of asbestosis. Asbestos bodies were, however, found on postmortem examination. Although the patient had been diagnosed with tuberculosis and confined to a sanatorium for 3 months, his sputum tests were negative for tubercle bacilli after the finding of asbestosis, which suggests the misdiagnosis of dust-induced diseases like asbestosis.[94] More importantly, this finding pointed to the need, as first suggested by Bernardio Ramazzini in the 1700s, that "I may venture to add one more question: What occupation does he follow?" Ramazzini recommended this be added to those questions suggested by Hippocrates in his work *Affections* after he had observed that "In medical practice, however, I find that attention is hardly ever paid to this matter, or if the doctor in attendance know it without asking, he give little heed to it, through for effective treatment evidence of this sort has the utmost weight."[95,96]

Asbestos-induced discrete pleural thickening (pleural plaques) were first reported by Sparks in 1931.[97] He described small irregular calcareous deposits in the lower parts of the lung. Sparks concluded that because all his patients came for examination voluntarily once symptoms appeared, examination of a group of workers from an asbestos factory was unlikely to discover gross changes, thus questioning the value of cross-sectional screening of the active workforce at one point in time compared with continued follow-up of an active workforce.

Humans were not the only victims to be affected by asbestos. Take the case report of asbestosis in a 10-year-old rough-haired terrier used as a ratter in an asbestos factory.[98] The dog lived most of its life in the factory, which used all three commercial types of asbestos (chrysotile, amosite, and crocidolite). The dog suffered for 2 years from cough and dyspnea before the condition progressed to the point that the dog was euthanized. The dog's lungs showed asbestos fibers in large numbers throughout all parts of the lung and ranged in length between 8 and 60 μm, appearing as long, fine, bright lines under the microscope with fewer slightly cured, and appeared as asbestos after it had been crushed up. Schuster[98] considered this case to provide as good a specimen of uncomplicated asbestosis as will ever be seen, apart from experimental cases. Although the case mimicked that found in humans, two important differences were observed. First, the absence of septic infection and acute lamination, and second, the absence of asbestos bodies in the dog. Schuster suggested this might mean that the bodies might be a concentration of organic material around a fiber and that these would be more profuse when active inflammation was present. Schuster concluded there was no causal relationship between asbestos bodies and inflammation and that whatever "juices" took part in asbestos body formation were produced during normal metabolism. Schuster's conclusion came from the findings to date that asbestos bodies may occur in active inflammation in the lung, as seen in humans, or without, as seen in guinea-pigs, but may be absent when active inflammation is present, as seen in rats, or when there is none, as in the terrier in this study. Alternatively, Schuster reported that Gardner suggested that asbestos bodies were mainly composed of altered asbestos and the host merely supplied a suitable reagent or physical condition, and because of their lack in the dog, asbestos bodies were not present in the dog. The finding in the case of the dog supports pulmonary fibrosis as the result of diffuse distribution of asbestos in the lung, either from trauma of the fibers or from a toxic effect of the silicate. Although silicosis and asbestosis are not the same, they both have a similar finding in that the sharpness of the silica particle is not responsible for the reactions of silicosis and there is no such evidence that asbestos spicules do mechanical damage to tissue. Schuster concluded these were based on the findings of Gye and Purdy,[99] showing the toxic action of finely divided silica; Mavrogordato's[100] finding that silica is soluble to a certain extent in body fluids; and finally Gloyne's experiments showing that asbestos is a benign irritant with regards to the production of granulation tissue. Finally, Schuster concluded that asbestos bodies do not alter the course or nature of asbestosis.[98]

In 1932, the *Lancet*[101] published an editorial on the German work on pulmonary asbestosis beginning before World War I. It described Buttner-Wobst and Trillitzsch's (1931) eight cases from two factories near Dresden.[102] They found disease via radiograms occurring in the early stages, mainly in the lower lobes, and as disease progressed, so did the shadows. They pointed out that it can be difficult to exclude the possibility of tuberculosis and observed that after removal from exposure to asbestos, the disease did not necessarily get worse, which differed from the findings of W. Burton Wood, which showed progression even after removal from exposure. The Germans also raised "… the question whether the different types of asbestos may show different harmful effects, as in silicosis." The article[102] commented on the study of Krüger et al. (1931) of 18 men and 34 women, in which 8 of 28 cases tested had asbestos bodies and that there was a fall in hemoglobin. The radiograms in the study showed three stages: (1) an increase of normal lung striation, (2) a thicker network with delicate sharply defined opaque spots, and (3) intensification of this network forming a shadowy veil covering the lung with the signs most prominent in the mid and lower lobes. A study by Gerbis and Ucko[103] in 1931 found that after 10 years, asbestosis could be seen radiologically. They went on to say that even the most severe cases did not give as "pronounced" a picture as did silicosis, radiologically. They theorized that "... in asbestosis, the silicic acid acts as a chemical irritant which leads to fibrosis." Lastly, the editorial discussed Timmermans'[104] finding of two types of asbestos bodies: the "handle-form," having a knob on both ends like a dumbbell, and the "carrot-form," having a tapered end, which he attributed to differences in formation with the "handle-form" forming in places where there is no lung movement and the "carrot-form" forming where the tissue fluid is in motion.

Asbestos regulations, including identification and control, went into effect in the United Kingdom in 1931.[105] The British Government concluded that asbestosis was a disease caused by the inhalation of asbestos dust for several years. They concluded that once the fibrous tissues developed in the lung, the disease became progressive. The report stated that, in addition to manufacturing of asbestos material, the mixing, breaking, crushing, disintegrating, opening, and grinding of asbestos can be dangerous. The United Kingdom report identified sawing, grinding, and turning of dry particles composed wholly or partially of asbestos, that is, motor car brakes and clutch linings, electric conductors, and packing and jointings as dangerous. Dust suppression, including using wet methods and enclosing dusty operations and exhausts, was recommended to reduce the concentrations.

Dr. Albert Russell with the U.S. Public Health Service presented a paper to a conference of the Industrial Commission of Wisconsin in Chicago in November 1932 concerning the effects of dusts.[106] His presentation showed different radiological patterns of various pneumoconiosis, including one of an asbestotic who worked for 6 years as a cleaner and restorer of asbestos on pipes. His x-ray showed fibrosis of both lungs. Dr. Russell pointed out that the fibrosis produced by asbestos is quite different from that of granite workers exposed to silica dust. Dr. Russell mentioned the government compensated this man for his asbestos-related disease. This paper shows one of the first cases of asbestosis linked to a user of an asbestos-containing end product—pipe covering.[106]

In 1933, Dr. Philip Ellman[107] reported seven asbestosis cases among production workers and described the slow development of the disease with the patient often free of symptoms for several years, thus describing a latency period as a part of the etiology of asbestosis. Finger clubbing was discussed, as were asbestos corns. Case 1 was a 22-year-old female mattress maker with 4 years exposure. Case 2 was a 35-year-old female asbestos factory worker with 5 years exposure. Case 3 was a 26-year-old card room worker with progressive spread of fibrosis in both lungs within less than 9 months who had 6 years of exposure. Case 4 was a 31-year-old female asbestos factory worker making mattresses for 3 years. Case 5 was a 34-year-old female asbestos factory worker for 6 years who was seen 13 years later with progressive cough and dyspnea and with asbestos corns on her hand and elbow. Case 6 was a 43-year-old man who was superintendent of the card room for 9 years who first developed mild dyspnea on exertion and a dry cough after 4 years, which worsened to the extent he was forced to quit 5 years later and was confined to bed because of a right pleural effusion. He had marked clubbing of the fingers and died 3 years later. Case 7 was a 10-year-old rough-haired terrier dog used as a ratter in an asbestos factory who developed asbestosis. This case was described earlier in 1931 by Dr. Norah Schuster.[98] Ellman[107] concluded that pulmonary asbestosis may be complicated with tuberculosis, that the presence of asbestos bodies was merely indicative of past exposure and not necessarily of clinical significance, that the average length of employment in fatal cases was only one-half that of silicosis, and that pulmonary asbestosis was a progressive disease with a bad prognosis and its treatment only palliative.*,† Unlike silica, which damages

---

* These studies and others describe both the latent period for disease development and the longer the duration of exposure, the greater the risk of developing disease. In other words, a dose–response relationship.

† **Notes on asbestosis in field animals:** Asbestosis is not specific to humans and has occurred in animals other than under experimental situations. Besides the terrier described above by Ellman (1933) and Schuster (1931), Webster (1963) described asbestosis in donkeys hauling asbestos ore. Environmentally induced asbestosis has also been found in field rats living in and around an asbestos mill and also in baboons living near an asbestos mill.[110] Animals can serve as sentinel species for use in risk assessment when they are exposed in habitats shared with humans and at similar concentrations. However, no animal species can be expected to respond in exactly the same way as humans and one must take

pulmonary macrophages, we now know asbestos does not appear to do the same. Thus, tuberculosis does not appear to be increased in connection with asbestosis as it is with silicosis.[108] In a second paper in 1933, Ellman[112] discussed a case of asbestosis in a 33-year-old woman exposed to asbestos dust for 5 years and showing symptoms beginning 3 years after first employment. Examination by Dr. Schuster found asbestos bodies. The diaphragmatic movements were poor and there was evidence of basal pleurisy. The skiagram of the chest showed infiltration of both lungs, which appeared indicative of this condition. Ellman reported: "It has not been recognized until comparatively recently that pneumoconiosis may result from the inhalation of asbestos dust, and asbestos factories have taken little precaution against it." The adventitious sounds of the lungs are described as dry and crackling, probably because of friction from the accompanying basal pleurisy. The radiology shows a progressive, fine, diffuse fibrosis affecting the lower and middle zones. Ellman stated: "When there is persistent absence of tubercle bacilli and a history of prolonged exposure to the dust, when [sic] sign and symptoms already outlined, a diagnosis of pulmonary asbestosis can be made." Ellman described two more cases of pulmonary asbestosis—one a woman aged 28 years with a 5-year history of making asbestos mats, and the second in a woman aged 32 with a 6-year history of working in an asbestos factory previously who then began working in the factory 18 years later when symptoms of a slight cough began about 9 months later. Asbestos corns were discussed as being common among asbestos-exposed workers and were apparently hyperkeratoses.

In 1933, S. Roodhouse Gloyne[114] discussed *The Morbid Anatomy and Histology of Asbestosis* in which he stated: "The history of the discovery of the asbestosis [asbestos] body itself and the study of the disease is now so well documented that further reference to it is unnecessary." Gloyne discussed workers whose asbestos exposure had been inconspicuous or even unrecognized where lesions of pulmonary asbestosis, although generally slight, were often detected by accident and, because of migration from industry to industry, might make determining the association with asbestos difficult. In describing the morbid effects on the pleura, Gloyne stated the picture of asbestosis superimposed upon a lung already affected with some degree of "anthracosis" because of the workers usually living in urban areas.* The adhesions tend to be the most marked over the lower lobes, between lungs, pericardium, and diaphragms, meaning the lower parts or the sacs become obliterated first. As the disease progresses, the pleura becomes thicker.† Lesions can appear in one side of the lung and be absent in the other and are nearly always attached, fusing the affected portions of the two layers of the pleura together into one fibrous sheet. Fibers passing into the lymphatic system are picked up by the phagocytes. In part III of his paper, Gloyne described these phagocytic cells stating: "The phagocytic dust cells can be found in the terminal portions of the bronchioles, and in the air sacs, surrounding the fibre and attempting to engulf it. Frequently the fibre is too long to be completely engulfed and looks as although it was sticking into the cell with one end protruding, like a pin in a pincushion." Gloyne[114] described the asbestosis lung as having five different particles, including: (1) carbon pigment, common to all town dwellers; (2) amorphous brown pigment, presumably blood; (3) sharp jagged particles, probably carbonaceous; (4) asbestos fiber; and (5) asbestos body. In 1930, Lynch and Smith[113] found asbestos bodies in the thrombi of veins in a male asbestos worker after 4.5 years working in an asbestos mill. In describing the tissue reaction to asbestos fibers, Gloyne stated there was thickening of the fiber with the formation of the asbestos body, the accumulation of large phagocytic dust cells and asbestosis giant cells, and then fibrosis. The giant cell was not a cell at all according to Gloyne,[114] but a minute collection of phagocytes.

---

into consideration when using such data in risk assessment several things, including toxic properties of the substance, physiology of the specific animal species and their relationship to potential human exposures.[111]

* Although this is an observation made in highly polluted urban areas of the United Kingdom 65 years ago, it could well apply to urban pollution even seen in more recent times by adding to the total lung burden of air pollutants including asbestos.

† This is the first reference I have found that discusses pleural involvement from exposure to asbestos and is an indicator that the fibers are leaving the lung and causing damage in other areas of the body and later be responsible for the malignant tumor mesothelioma.

Merewether[115] stated that "[A]ny manipulation of asbestos, therefore, produces dust, which is easily projected into the air." Merewether found that exposure to asbestos for a period of less than 5 years can cause asbestosis, which can result in death, but generally, most cases occur after more years. There was a clear latency period demonstrated in the 1512 workers examined. Merewether emphasized that to prevent asbestosis, it was necessary to reduce the concentration of asbestos dust. Merewether believed there was a concentration below which "development of a disabling degree of asbestosis will not occur within the space of an average working lifetime." The shortest length of exposure resulting in death was 4.4 years in his study. On the basis of his studies, the concentration "that to prevent the full development of the disease among asbestos workers within the space of an average working life-time, it is necessary to reduce the concentration of dust in the air of the workrooms to a figure below that pertaining to spinning at the time over which these cases were exposed." Merewether referred to this concentration as the "dust datum," although he stated examination of the average length of employment of cases of asbestosis, of the radiograms, and of the particulars of the recorded fatal cases also indicated that not only were "spinners" less likely to develop asbestosis, but when they did, it took longer to develop; in other words, in "spinners" the maturation period of the fibrosis was longer than that in workers in the more dusty processes. Therefore, his safe concentration may not have been safe.

Merewether thought the disease risk for asbestosis was less than that for silicosis. He found that tuberculosis occurred less in those with asbestosis compared with those with silicosis, for example, 35.7% versus 59.4%, respectively. The inhalation of asbestos dust did not appear to affect old inactive pulmonary tuberculosis or to modify the end result of coincidental tuberculosis infection. This study showed that because spinners had the lowest risk of developing asbestosis, their latency period was extended when compared with those more likely to develop disease. It is interesting that although Merewether found what he thought to be a "dust datum" as described above for safe working conditions for preventing asbestosis, he also made the following statement: "If only the slightest exposure to the dust results ultimately in death, then the scope of the necessary preventive measures is summed up in one word—prohibition ..." At this time, Merewether and others were not aware of asbestos and its association with cancer.

Dr. J. Donnelly[116] found that asbestosis occurred even after short periods of exposure (18 months in this group) and that radiographic changes occurred in workers exposed less than 5 years as described among the three cases he reported. Dr. Donnelly stated: "The 'dusty trades' for a long time have been considered 'inimical' [hostile] to the health of employees." "The conditions surrounding the greater proportion of the employees constitute a distinct and serious industrial hazard, and often sufficient devices for protection have not been provided. It is doubtful if any single employee in certain departments of this mill can possibly escape some damage to his respiratory system because of the unavoidable inhalation of asbestos dust." Further, asbestosis, once acquired, is definitely a serious industrial hazard which is permanent and more or less rapidly progressive. The consensus among researchers and asbestos workers is that the protective devices now in use for many plants are most inadequate. The paper further described the 1931 Asbestos Industry Regulations in England to require substitution of wet methods for dry, enclosing dust-producing machines, using mechanical methods in lieu of hand conveyance and handwork generally, the installation of exhaust drafts at dust producing points, and that workers in asbestos plants appear for periodic medical examinations. Finally, "the fact that efficient protective devices in this industry, in spite of the added expense, will effect a substantial financial saving is becoming more apparent. The workers themselves are becoming informed of the danger to health, and many civil suits for damages against factory owners are the result."[116]

Robert Page[117] stated that since so much had been written on pulmonary asbestosis by 1933, he would only briefly mention the disease except to say the shortness of exposure it takes to result in asbestosis after a longer interval of time had elapsed such as 7 years as mentioned by Merewether (1933–1934).[115] Exposures as short as 18 months, provided exposure had been sufficiently high, might result in disease. What Page did discuss in detail were asbestos bodies, the two chief varieties being (1) the spindle-shaped elongated form, slender in the center and growing bigger toward the ends, and (2) the beaded form, with the smallest elements in the center and gradually increasing in size to the terminal knobs.[*] These bodies range in size from a few to several hundred microns. In 1928, Simson[65] found asbestos bodies in the lung of a patient with only 2 months of exposure. In 1933, Ellman[107] found asbestos bodies after only 10 weeks of exposure. The presence of clumps of asbestos bodies means disintegration of the lung tissue with lung destruction and can be virtually diagnostic of underlying asbestosis. However, their absence does not mean the absence of asbestosis. Also, the larger the size of the asbestos bodies, the longer the interval between onset of exposure. Thus, the number of fibers is not as important as their sizes or if they appear in clumps. Young bodies are also encountered in the sputum in persons who have not inhaled asbestos in years. In other words, the asbestos bodies continue to develop even in fibers having long residence times in the lung.[117]

Demonstrating the increasing nature and awareness of asbestos-related disease, Stock[118] described a fatal case of pneumoconiosis without tuberculosis in a textile operator working in the asbestos textile industry who had previously been a seamen in the U.S. Navy for 2 years; however, no discussion of asbestos exposures were mentioned from his Navy experience.[†] Necropsy showed that the left visceral pleura was adherent over the lower half of the lower lobe anteriorly, laterally, and posteriorly and contained clear straw-colored fluid. The adhesions were of moderate density and separated readily. There were no adhesions in the right pleura and no fluid was found. The interesting feature of this case was the unusual characteristics of the asbestos bodies. They were found of various appearances: some like animal or vegetable hairs and others spheric. They had stalks on the end on which three or four small spherules were clustered. Others were club-like and were from 10 to about 100 μm in size. Gloyne[114] observed similar pleural findings indicating the spread of the disease outside the lung and into the pleural space.

Wood and Gloyne[119] concluded that whether or not tuberculosis was associated with asbestosis, it was certainly less than that found with silicosis.

It is interesting to note that Dr. Roscoe N. Gray, Surgical Director of Aetna Life Insurance Company, published a book in 1934 titled the *Attorneys' Textbook of Medicine*[120] in which he outlined the diseases associated with asbestos, especially asbestosis. In the book he stated: "[A]sbestos particles inhaled into the lung produce an exceedingly severe and perhaps fatal inflammation." Furthermore, all processing of asbestos is "accompanied by a tremendous volume of very fine dust." These particles are mixed with other larger particles, but it is the inhaled fibers that cause the lung problems. These consist of very thin spicules 1–360 μm or one-tenth of an inch. The inhalation of these spinicles causes the bronchiole to become plugged, no longer letting air pass, and the lung dies in this area or becomes abscessed or replaced with scar tissue. The authors concluded that in textile manufacturing, dust concentrations in the spinning room were safe because relatively little dust occurred. This is in contrast to Merewether[81] who put the counts at 13,500,000 per cubic foot compared with dustier departments with counts as high as 170,748,000 per cubic foot.

Gray[120] tells the attorney that "[I]nvestigation must be thoroughly conducted along three lines: duration and intensity of exposure, and the true cause of the disability." In writing for the insurer's benefit, Gray states that "very few men have continued to work this long for a single assured, and but rarely is the same carrier on the risk throughout the entire exposure the patient has had." Gray prorates the exposures accordingly so that "Justice must be done to both the patient and the Company."

---

[*] Recall Timmermans described asbestos bodies as of two types: the "handle form" having a knob on both ends, like a dumbbell, and the "carrot-form" having a tapered end.[104]
[†] Although some asbestos was used in ships previously, it was not until around 1934 that international experts in marine construction recommended asbestos as a fire protection on ships. The fire on the *Morro Castle* in September 1934 as well as other shipboard fires and explosion disasters prompted the widespread use of asbestos on ships. See *Asbestos & Fire—Technological Trade-offs and the Body at Risk*, by Rachel Maines, 2005, Rutgers University Press, p. 76.

The book ends the asbestos discussion presuming there will be a trial as it gives references to the attorney stating that "[T]he following authorities may be of value during study and trial."

Fulton et al.[121] reported linking asbestos exposures with asbestosis and discussed findings of a survey conducted by the state of Pennsylvania starting in 1933. The Pennsylvania Department of Labor and Industry was concerned with a lack of information in their state about asbestos and asked the asbestos industry in the state to help survey the hazard as it pertained to dustiness and physical condition of the workers. They found that when counting all particles, those particles less than 10 μm in diameter averaged 95% of the total and that the length of the crude fiber was less than 5 μm in more than 95% of the total samples. Crude fibers were used in the cheaper grades of textile and in asbestos shingles, paper, plaster, and cement. The milled fibers were less than 5 μm in length in 97% of those counted. The best grades of crude asbestos fiber were used in manufacturing asbestos textiles. Preparation of asbestos for making it into a thread had the highest airborne concentrations (up to and more than 100 million particles per cubic foot (mppcf), averaging 44.26 in preparation and carding; 16.37 mppcf in weaving and mule spinning; and 4.61 in other operations such as gasket making, etc.). Milled asbestos fiber gave rise to higher concentrations of crude fiber. Wet methods significantly reduced counts. Of the 64 workers examined and of the 57 with exposures to asbestos, 14 (25%) had asbestosis and 43 were negative. The most common symptoms were cough and dyspnea, and pleural thickening was found in some.[121]

In the 1935 study by Lanza et al.[122] of asbestos textile workers, they found 43% had fibrosis (lung scarring), 58% of workers with 10–15 years exposure had fibrosis, and 87% of workers with more than 15 years exposure had radiographic changes. Cases of cardiac enlargement were frequently found (later described as Cor-pulmonale). No predisposition to tuberculosis due to asbestos exposure was found. The authors suggested workers undergo physical examination at least every 2 years, including radiographic examination of the chest. The authors found that the dustiness was greatest in the preparation areas of the five plants studied, that engineering controls reduced the dust by 50%, and that with further alterations they could reduce the dust by 75%, although it was cost prohibitive to install equipment that would make the environment dust free.[122] In 1938, Lanza expanded his thoughts on asbestos in a book titled *Silicosis and Asbestosis*.[137]

Shull[123] examined 71 chests of workers dismissed from local asbestos plants. He was not convinced that asbestosis was primarily progressive as was the case with silicosis. However, in asbestotics, he found a definite tendency toward pleural and pericardial involvement, which is absent in silicosis. Shull found that even after 10 months of exposure in an asbestos mill, only one patient had asbestosis.

By 1936, many in the asbestos industry were concerned with occupationally associated diseases, including dust-induced lung disease. Thus, the Air Hygiene Foundation (1936–1941) was founded under the auspices of the Mellon Institute.[124] Its membership was composed of a cross section of large industrial companies. The Industrial Hygiene Foundation (IHF) conducted medical and industrial hygiene surveys and produced a digest—the *Industrial Hygiene Digest* (IHD), which provided health and safety information to members. The IHF meetings were covered by various news and wire services such as the *Wall Street Journal*, the *New York Times*, the Associated Press, and United Press International. The IHF was labeled by at least one person, Vandiver Brown of the Johns Manville Company, who in describing it to C. J. Stover, the publisher of *Asbestos* in the December 4, 1936, edition, that it [IHF] was "the creature of industry and the one institution upon which employers can rely completely for a sympathetic appreciation of their viewpoint."[125]

The *JAMA* carried an article by Dr. Lanza of the Metropolitan Insurance Company describing asbestosis and its history and stated about 10,000 people were exposed to asbestos at work in 1936.[126] Other studies continued to appear in the literature concerning asbestosis (Donnelly, 1936; Egbert and Geiger, 1936; McPheeters, 1936) describing the continued exposure to asbestos could increase the fibrosis in existing asbestotics, reporting some evidence that asbestosis develops more rapidly in younger persons, stating that no connection to tuberculosis could be found, and that reducing asbestos dust should significantly reduce the incidence of asbestosis.[127–129]

Drinker and Hatch[130] in their 1936 book *Industrial Dust—Hygienic Significance, Measurement and Control* included asbestos dust as a cause of asbestosis, which they described as a diffuse fibrosis, and with pathology different from that of silicosis. They stated asbestos fibers grouped about the neck of an alveolus and shut it off, causing what is known as atelectasis. They did not believe there was definite migration or transportation of the dust particles to lymph nodes. They quoted Wood and Gloyne as seeing patients with asbestosis "whose condition appears to have remained stationary since stopping work in the factory" but say Merewether and Lanza were less certain about this point. Drinker and Hatch described asbestos bodies in the lungs characteristic of asbestosis and stated that Stewart gave considerable diagnostic weight to their presence. In describing asbestos they stated: "[A]sbestos is not a true mineral but a general name for any mineral separable into more or less flexible fibers. The commonest variety, the mineral chrysotile, $H_4Mg_3Si_2O_9$, is mined extensively in Canada and is used in making special fabric-like materials, brake linings, special insulation, and the like. It is now believed that at any stage of its processing, sufficient exposure to asbestos dust can cause a definite pulmonary disability, asbestosis, with characteristic symptoms and chest x-rays."[130]

A U.S. Public Service Health study of 541 men and women in three asbestos textile factories found asbestosis was dose–response related and later used their findings for setting a guidance limit for occupational exposure to asbestos of 5 mppcf.[131]

In the February 17, 1940, issue of the *JAMA*, Dr. Leroy Gardner, Director of the Saranac Laboratories, wrote on pneumoconiosis.[132] He suggested the effect of asbestos bodies may well be mechanical and not chemical and reported on the dose–response nature of disease. He found that in the dozen or more cases without a history of asbestos exposure, asbestos bodies were identified in the lungs. He speculated that if the effects of asbestos bodies were indeed mechanical, then there should be no progression because of the rounded nature of the bodies as compared with the rough edges of asbestos fibers, which are freshly inhaled.[132]

Rutherford T. Johnstone's 1941 book *Occupational Diseases: Diagnosis, Medicolegal Aspects and Treatment*[133] discusses asbestosis by concluding that irritation by asbestos fibers may be the cause of the disease and not the chemical composition of the fiber. He concluded the disease *asbestosis* was progressive even after the cessation of exposure. He stated that the allowable concentration was 10 mppcf for fibers between 0.5 and 5 μm.*

The U.S. Navy recognized the need for constant vigilance for the detection of asbestos disease since asbestos was used in insulation that covers flanges, valves, and high-temperature steam turbines. In their initial survey of a pipe shop in a New York Naval Yard, no asbestos diseases were detected; however, the material was wetted and localized exhaust was used, while respirators were used for the dustiest aspects of the jobs.[134] Philip Drinker, a health consultant to the U.S. Maritime Commission, stated: "The pressure to turn out ships is great—it should be, for the need is urgent— and often we must condone practices that we would not accept in peacetime."[135]

On November 16, 1944, the Asbestos Textile Institute was established at a meeting of the University Club in New York City for the purposes of the following: (1) to promote ethical business standards, (2) to develop standards for the quality of the industry's products, etc., (3) to lawfully promote and foster industry policies, and (4) to act as a clearing house with respect to industry manufacturing and other such information.[136]

Asbestosis was identified among three pipe coverers at four naval shipyards—two were contract yards and two were operated by the Navy.[138] From these results, the authors[138] concluded: "Since each of the 2 cases of asbestosis had worked at asbestos pipe covering in shipyards for more than 20 years, it may be concluded that such pipe covering is not a dangerous occupation." The authors identified 1683 total pipe coverers of which they x-rayed 1074 to identify asbestosis. They were

---

* This concentration of 10,000,000 particles per cubic foot of air, of a size between 0.5 and 5 μm is not mentioned anywhere else and is inconsistent with the U.S. Public Health Service and the ACGIH guidelines of 1938 and 1946, respectively.

further able to determine the number of years employed by the shipyards in 1124 cases. The three asbestosis cases were long-term pipe coverers who had exposure to asbestos during preshipyard employment. Of the 1124 whose duration of employment was known, 84% had less than 5 years doing pipe covering. Because this was a cross-sectional medical surveillance study, only active workers were studied. The authors claimed this to be a very low incidence of asbestosis among those x-rayed (0.29% of the 1074); however, what was known at the time was that there was generally a latency for development of asbestosis and, given that the majority of workers were exposed less than 5 years, the risk of developing asbestosis among this population would be quite low. In fact, all the asbestosis cases developed in those pipe coverers with more than 10 years of exposure, which brought the percentage of cases in this group of 51 workers with 10 or more years exposure to 5% with asbestosis, a number much higher than 0.29% if all those x-rayed were considered to be of equal risk, which was not the case. Also, it is interesting that 609 of the total pipe coverers were not included in the study for which we know very little about. Apparently 50 of these missing 609 were included in the authors' calculations of duration of time as a pipe coverer. Additionally, many of the controls recommended for dust suppression were used by the yards, further reducing exposures. Overall, this study was of a population with minimal risk. However, I have found no reviews of the study at the time it was published; thus, the results were not questioned for some 20 years.[138]

In some countries asbestosis was not often observed. In Scandinavia in 1947, only 5 cases were known to have been published from Norway.* In Finland, where the asbestos industry had been around for a couple of decades, researchers were beginning to see asbestosis occurring in appreciable extent. Carl Wegelius[139] decided to publish a series of 126 cases he observed in Finland of what he called "... this serious highly disabling and even mortal disease ..." Wegelius commented that until his publication there were about 100 deaths from asbestosis. The author's 126 cases came from 476 workers employed by the firm of Finska Mineral A. R. Thirty-four of the asbestosis cases were from the company's dressing works at the mine in Paakkila, whereas the rest were working in the factory for finishing the product near Helsingfors. Wegelius did not find a single case of tuberculosis in conjunction with asbestosis nor any other cancer. Among the 126 cases, 79 were mild, 15 were mild-medium, 19 were medium, 4 were medium-advanced, and 9 were advanced stages of asbestosis. The most common complications were pleural and pericardial thickening, which ranged from 18% in the mild stages to 100% in the advanced stages.[139]

In a study of 1561 employees of an asbestos company to examine nonoccupational respiratory disease, 45% of the claims occurred among those working in dusty conditions. This cross-sectional study in a subset of 708 employees found seven cases of asbestosis. The author[140] accepted that the fibrosis was due to mechanical action of the fibers and not their chemical composition. As the author stated: "Physiologically, asbestosis is the problem of the 'tight' lung. Expansion of the lung is difficult, and there is impaired gas transfer through the lung. Diffuse, obstructive emphysema is not common."[140] The radiological findings of asbestosis, unlike silicosis, are related to the severity of symptoms with the greater the severity, the greater the expected findings on x-ray. The most common symptoms were affirmed: shortness of breath or dyspnea followed by tightness of the chest with pain, lack of energy, and tiredness.[141]

Many case reports of asbestosis continued throughout the 1940s, 1950s, and 1960s up to the passage in the United States of the Occupational Safety and Health Act (OSHA) of 1970 and the birth of the Environmental Protection Agency (EPA) on December 2, 1970. These reports included cases from a variety of occupational groups, such as the construction sector, the shipyard sector, and the asbestos manufacturing sector, and so forth. In the section on occupations, I will go through those that have been studied as they apply to the job areas or occupational sectors studied. Today, asbestosis cases are still commonly reported, but as all worksites apply preventive measures required by

---

* See Wolff, *Nordiak Medicin* 1940;5:555; Schrumppf, *Nordiak Medicin* 1940;9:709; and Schiötz, *Nordiak Medicin* 1941;12:3349.

OSHA, EPA, HSE, and so forth, this disease can be eradicated as has the infectious disease small-pox 30 years ago (http://www.cdc.gov/features/smallpoxeradication).

5.1.2 Latency, Progression, and Asbestosis

Merewether[115] concluded exposure to asbestos for a period of less than 5 years can cause asbestosis, which can result in death. He emphasized the prevention of asbestosis was to reduce the concentration of dust. The "dusty trades" have been considered "inimical" [hostile] to the health of employees for a long time and asbestosis, once acquired, is a definite and serious industrial hazard which is permanent and more or less rapidly progressive.[116] Wood and Gloyne[119] concluded that whether or not tuberculosis was associated with asbestosis, it was certainly less than that found with silicosis.

In the study by Lanza et al.[122] of asbestos textile workers, they found 43% overall had fibrosis (lung scarring) in 58% of workers with 10–15 years exposure and in 87% of workers with more than 15 years of exposure.

McPheeters[129] described continued exposure to asbestos could increase the fibrosis in existing asbestotics and reported some evidence that asbestosis develops more rapidly in younger persons. No connection to tuberculosis was found, and reduction of asbestos dust should significantly reduce the incidence of asbestosis.

Shull[123] found one case of asbestosis after 16 months of exposure. Shull found that asbestosis differs for silicosis clinically, pathologically, and roentgenologically and that asbestosis did not pre-dispose one to tuberculosis, although he did not observe asbestosis as primarily a progressive dis-ease. The U.S. Public Service Health study of 541 men and women in three asbestos textile factories found asbestosis to be dose–response related and thus used this finding for setting guidance limits for occupational exposure to asbestos at 5 mppcf.[131] Asbestosis was described as a latent disease with radiographic changes occurring early to the lower lobes of the lung, that improved dust controls would reduce the disease, and that asbestosis was a preventable disease.[142]

5.1.3 Pleural Plaques and Asbestosis

Asbestos-induced discrete pleural thickening (pleural plaques) was first reported by Sparks.[97] He also described small irregular calcareous deposits in the lower parts of the lung.

The first description of typical pleural plaques was by Porro et al.[143] from a survey of 15 cases in the talc industry. Other reports followed, including Siegal et al.[144] of pleural plaques in talc workers exposed to talc dusts containing tremolite asbestos. Siegal et al. noted that it was reported at the 57th Annual Medical Report of the Trudeau Sanatorium that experimental production of intrapleural adhesions was produced in exposed animals. In the 1950s, other reports of pleural calcification and pleural activity were reported in asbestos workers: Smith[145]—tremolite talc; Jacob and Bohlig[146]—pleural thickening among a cohort of 343 cases in Dresden Germany; Fehre,[147] who observed pleural calcifications thought to be due to inhalation of silica (however, the author concluded they were similar to those observed in persons exposed to asbestos dust); and Frost et al.,[148] who observed 22 cases of radiographic changes in 31 lagers surveyed from a trade union in Denmark, 19 having had pleural abnormalities, including pleural thickening and calcifications. In a review from China of six studies on the complications of pleu-ral plaques in asbestosis patients, pleural plaques ranged from 34.2% to 100%. In another six studies of asbestos workers, the prevalence of pleural plaques ranged from 1.3% to 29.8%.[149]

Calcifications resulting from fibrous dust generally are bilateral and situated on the parietal pleura and probably very small amounts of dust are capable of causing pleural calcifications, which appear to be due to mechanical irritation.[150] Plaques are progressive and cause adverse respiratory symptoms such as dyspnea (breathlessness) and decrements in pulmonary function, although it is more likely that diffuse pleural thickening will cause functional impairment.[151–154] There is some evidence that reduction in forced expiratory volume in one second and forced vital capacity (FVC) of 200 and 300 mL, respectively, can be attributed to isolated pleural plaques.[155] Pleural thickening is considered a marker of past exposures.[156] There is evidence that persons with pleural plaques are more likely to develop asbestos-induced parenchymal fibrosis than those without plaques.[157] Furthermore, it has been found that in occupationally exposed persons, appreciable amounts of fibers were found in their thoracic lymph nodes as well as in pleural plaques.[158,159] Asbestos-induced pleural plaques are the most common of the asbestos-related abnormalities.[160] Asbestos and erionite fibers appear to be the only causative agents for typical pleural plaques with the latency normally being several decades. Also, they can result from low exposures that are not an important risk factor for asbestos-induced lung cancer.[160] Others believe there is evidence that individuals with asbestos-induced pleural plaques are at a marked increased risk of developing and dying of lung cancer or malignant mesothelioma.

Fletcher[161] reported that asbestos-exposed shipyard workers diagnosed with pleural plaques were at a 137% greater risk from dying of lung cancer (16 observed vs. 6.74 expected; $p < .005$; calculated relative risk [RR] = 2.37; 95% confidence interval [CI] = 1.36–3.86), none of which had radiological evidence of asbestosis, at a 2900% increased risk of dying from mesothelioma (3 observed vs. 0.10 expected; $p < .001$; calculated RR = 30, 95% CI = 6.19–87.67), and at a 55% increased risk of dying from other cancers when compared with the general population of the same age who were not exposed to asbestos. The risks were insignificant among those without pleural plaques. The workers included a variety of crafts workers. In another study of shipyard workers, Edge[162] reported that workers with mixed asbestos exposures and pleural plaques (without evidence of pulmonary fibrosis) had a 2.5 times greater risk of developing carcinoma of the bronchus when compared with the matched controls without plaques who had a 1.2 times greater risk. Also, Edge observed three mesotheliomas in those with plaques while none occurred in those without plaques. Edge,[163] in a later study of shipyard workers, found that out of 156 workers with asbestos-induced pleural plaques but with no other radiographic evidence of pulmonary fibrosis, there were eight deaths from lung cancer compared with three deaths in those without pleural plaques, a twofold increase, and that smoking could not explain the increase in lung cancer in these workers. Edge found 13 mesotheliomas among those with plaques and two in those without plaques, a sixfold increase. Edge observed that if he removed the one mesothelioma occurring within the first 2 years of observation, seven cases occurred in 2637 man-years of observation for an incidence of 1/377 per year.

Hillerdal[164] gave several facts concerning pleural plaques. First, plaques are always more widespread on autopsy than x-ray. Second, in populations without endemic plaques, 80%–90% of the strictly defined plaques are due to occupational exposure and can be found in persons with low-level exposure. Third, asbestos bodies are more prevalent in persons with pleural plaques. Fourth, pleural plaques are related to time after exposure to asbestos rather than to dose. Fifth, in industrially developed countries, 2%–4% of all men older than 40 years usually have plaques. Sixth, plaques themselves are usually harmless but are indicators of sufficient latency for asbestos-induced cancers. For example, persons with pleural plaques are twice as likely to develop lung cancer as those without such plaques, and those with plaques are more at risk of mesothelioma. Seventh, those with pleural plaques, in general, have lower lung function. Finally, persons having high rates of pleural plaques from living in areas of local deposits of asbestos such as tremolite, amosite, and crocidolite have a high risk of mesothelioma, whereas those living in areas of anthophyllite do not. In residents of Da-yao, China, with environmental exposure to crocidolite, pleural plaques were prevalent in 11% of those older than 20 years and in 20% in those older than 40 years.[165]

Pleural effusions, diffuse pleural thickening, and rounded atelectasis are also caused by exposure to asbestos.[166] Becklake et al.,[155] in their state-of-the-art review, stated that many with circumscribed pleural plaques had normal lung function at rest but not upon exercise when they experienced shortness of breath. However, there is controversy as to whether pleural plaques are associated with ventilatory dysfunction. Pleural thickening usually leads to significantly reduced vital capacity and diffusing capacity.

5.1.4 Lung Cancer

In early studies, asbestosis was frequently found in conjunction with lung cancer among workers exposed to asbestos.[167–169] The first case reports of lung cancer were from Gloyne (1935)[170] and from Lynch and Smith (1935)[171] in which all cases had asbestosis. This led some to speculate that asbestosis was necessary and somehow associated in the etiology of lung cancer among those exposed to asbestos, some attributing this association to the "scar" theory of carcinogenesis. This is not strongly supported for all asbestos-associated lung cancers according to Hillerdal,[172] who observed that a majority of tumors were squamous cell cancers and not adenocarcinomas. Adenocarcinomas were found most commonly among patients with asbestosis and in the lower lobes of the lung where asbestosis is most prevalent.[173] It is true, however, that in some cases of advanced asbestosis, scar carcinomas may develop as an outgrowth of uncontrolled fibrogenesis just like they do with usual interstitial pneumonitis, the typical pathologic lesion in asbestosis.[175] Asbestos exposure appears to increase the risk for all histological types of lung cancer.[173] Those individuals with asbestos exposure and those with asbestosis have higher risks of lung cancer than those found in the nonexposed general population.[175] It is more likely that asbestosis is not a precursor to lung cancer but rather that both are independent diseases associated with a dose–response relationship from exposure to asbestos and that cancer of the lung can and does occur in the absence of asbestos.[172,174,176–178] McDonald et al.[179] have presented epidemiological data showing the increased risk of lung cancer in occupations with exposure to asbestos in the absence of radiological evidence of pulmonary fibrosis. Hillerdal,[172] in a well-designed study having sufficient statistical power, found lung cancer to occur in patients with bilateral parietal pleural plaques but without radiological evidence of asbestosis. Lung cancer continues to be statistically elevated among asbestos workers under surveillance (standard incidence ratio [SIR] 1.14, 95% CI = 1.01–1.26).[180] In a Chinese study of eight asbestos factory cohorts and three mining cohorts, the complication rate of lung cancer among asbestotics ranged from 3.5% to 26.9%.[149] That exposure levels for carcinogens were safe (including asbestos) is brought into question by the findings that the lungs may accumulate massively more cancer-causing airborne particles than previously thought. The bifurcations within the lung may allow high concentrations of particles to build up as much as 100 times as in other parts of the lung.[181] In fact, by some estimates uncoated asbestos fibers exceed the number of asbestos bodies by 5000 to 10,000 times.[155]

5.1.5 Smoking and Risk

Increases of lung cancer in smokers are more than just additive but are multiplicative in nature. Both asbestos and smoking are independently capable of increasing the risk of lung cancer. One of the largest cohorts of asbestos workers to demonstrate this is that of North American insulators studied by Dr. Selikoff. His coinvestigator, Cyler Hammond of the American Cancer Society (ACS), reported that among 12,051 insulation workers with more than 20 years of work experience when compared with a control population from the ACS of 73,763 men, both of whose smoking history was known, the RR went up to 53.24 for smoking asbestos insulation workers compared with nonsmoking asbestos workers, which was only 5.17, and smoking non-asbestos-exposed workers (as controls) was 10.85.[182] A study of 912 smokers out of 1479 asbestos-exposed workers among the industries of Barcelona, Spain found that the incidence of asbestosis was significantly higher in smokers (161; 17.65%) versus (44; 11.39%) nonsmokers, as were the clinical symptoms (cough, expectoration, and dyspnea)—72.58% versus 55.18%, respectively. Nonsmokers with asbestosis had more restrictive disease or mixed-type syndromes than did smokers with asbestosis. A linear relationship between asbestosis and duration of exposure was found in 1% of those having less than 5 years exposure up to 65% among those with 30+ years of exposure.[183] Another summary combining smoking and asbestos exposure reported the RR for three additional studies to be 8.2, 32.7, and 25.7.[184] Asbestosis patients had a standard mortality ratio (SMR) of 15.47 (95% CI = 11.2–20.8) for lung cancer.[185] An analysis of 23 studies on asbestos exposure and smoking showed that asbestos multiplied the risk of lung cancer in nonsmokers and smokers by a similar factor and that the combined relationship of exposure to asbestos and smoking can be best described by a multiplicative rather than an additive model.[186] Berry and Liddell estimated the RR to be about three times higher in nonsmokers than smokers and that the RR was highest for the interaction of asbestos and smoking in the very light smoker and nonsmoker when compared with the light or heavy smoker. They concluded that if the populations studied included smokers and nonsmokers, then the calculated RR from the epidemiology study applied to that of the smokers.[187]

In one animal study looking at the penetration of asbestos fibers into airway walls using guinea pigs, the authors[188] found the burden of fibers in the walls of respiratory bronchioles increased with time in both smoke-exposed and non-smoke-exposed animals despite the fact that only a single dose of asbestos was administered at a single point in time. The authors[188] suggested that this continuing fiber transport from the airspace to the interstitium after cessation of exposure may be the factor that produces continuing fibrosis and that smoking increases the number of fibers which penetrate into the walls of the respiratory bronchioles. The authors[188] believe this may be the reason for increased asbestos-related disease in smokers exposed to asbestos.

Liddell and Armstrong[189] looked at the combined effects of smoking and lung cancer in miners and millers of Quebec. In their study involving 7279 men, lung cancer caused 533 deaths when 405.23 were expected (SMR = 1.32, calculated 95% CI = 2.47–3.32). The analysis found that smoking and exposure to chrysotile asbestos appeared to have acted independently in causing lung cancer. Those smoking 10 cigarettes a day would have roughly the effect of exposure to 700 mppcf-years. They found the additive model fitted their data best and that the fit for each multiplicative model was not supported. They[189] stated that refutation of the multiplicative hypothesis in their data and because the additive hypothesis was not generally applicable, there was no reason to believe that interactions conformed to any simple theory.

A population-based case-referent study investigating lung cancer and occupational exposures to asbestos and the interaction with tobacco smoking was undertaken in Sweden.[190] This study focused on low-dose concentrations. Questionnaires were given with 87% (1038) cases and 85% (2359) referents responding. The results confirmed that lung cancers were dose–response related and increased with cumulative dose. It is interesting that they found the risk per fiber-year observed, on the basis of a population in which the level of exposure was low, was actually much higher than when linearly extrapolating dose down from highly exposed cohorts. Thus, linear-dose extrapolation may underestimate the risks of lung cancer at low doses. Their finding of the relationship between smoking and exposure to asbestos was less than multiplicative and not much in excess than predicted when using an additive model, which is consistent with recent studies. They found that lung cancer was increased in both asbestos-exposed smokers as well as asbestos-exposed lifelong nonsmokers.[190]

Reid et al.,[191] in looking at 2935 former crocidolite miners and millers from Wittenoom, Australia, found that those who had ceased smoking for 20 or more years by the end of the study follow-up period had reverted their risk of lung cancer back to that of never smokers. However, those who had only quit for 6 years or less had a 22 times greater risk than did never smokers, but after 6 years the risks began going down. Interestingly, those who smoked 20 cigarettes per day had twice the risk of those who smoked less than 20 cigarettes per day. In general, smokers had a higher risk than never smokers, but the asbestos effect found the RR was higher in never smokers and ex-smokers (>20 years) than that in current smokers. This study also found the interaction between smoking and asbestos exposure to be less than multiplicative, something found in other studies discussed above.

5.1.6 Relative Risk

The RR for lung cancer has varied from 1.0[192] to 17.6[193] with an average of 9.8. The prognosis and treatment of asbestos-induced lung cancer is no different than lung cancer having another etiology. It appears that all cell types of lung cancer occur in asbestos workers and that the presence or absence of one cell type cannot be used to prove or disprove an association between asbestos exposure and lung cancer.[194] Since 1997, asbestos has been the leading cause of occupational lung cancer in Japan.[195] Most studies of asbestos workers have been among white men; however, when race is considered, black men are at a higher risk when exposed to asbestos. One study reported an odds ratio (OR) of 1.8 (95% CI = 1.03–3.1) for lung cancer in black men; however, when using Surveillance, Epidemiology, and End Results (SEER) data from 1988 to 1992, mesothelioma was higher in white men than black men (1.7 vs. 0.9/100,000).[196] In a survey of Hungarian workers exposed to asbestos with lung tumors, 72 (24%) of 297 patients had cumulative occupational asbestos exposures assessed below 25 fiber-years (between 0.01 and 23.9 fiber-years).[197] In West Germany, a case–control study reported by Pohlabeln et al.[198] supported a doubling of the lung cancer risk with 25 fiber-years of exposure, and when using a two-phase logistic regression model, the OR increased from 0 to ≤1 fiber-years (0.86; 95% CI = 0.55–1.33), from 1 to ≤10 fiber-years (1.33; 95% CI = 0.80–2.33), and from 10+ fiber-years (1.94; 95% CI = 1.10–3.43), which are similar to those found by Stayner et al.[199] and by Dement and Brown.[200] A case-referent study of Swedish lung cancer patients[190] found clear evidence for the risk of lung cancer at low-dose levels and that linear extrapolation from high exposure levels may underestimate the risks for low doses. Never smokers exposed at 1–2.49 fiber-years had an RR of 2.7 (95% CI = 0.7–9.5) and for those smoking >20 cigarettes/day an RR of 80.6 (95% CI = 20.2–322.0).

There is evidence of an increased number of multiple primary cancers at the same time among those exposed to asbestos compared with the general population.[201]

5.1.7 Mesothelioma

Mesothelioma is a cancer of the mesothelium, the thin layer of cells derived from the mesoderm, the lining that covers the major internal organs of the body. The rarity and the fact that this type of tumor is strongly associated with asbestos exposure makes it a "signal tumor." This means that it is considered an epidemiological marker for asbestos exposure.[60,202] Wagner was the first to recognize and report primary pleural tumors in 1870.[203] Credit was given to Adami for the term *mesothelioma* in 1909.[204] The modern concepts concerning the pathology and diagnosis of mesothelioma were set forth in 1931 by Klemperer and Rabin.[205] Gloyne[114] described the migration of fibers to the lymph stream and especially into the mediastinal glands in a person with asbestosis. Becklake et al.[155] explained that fibers less than 3 μm are phagocytized by activated macrophages, which then drain through the lymphatics into the pleural surface and then into the pleural space. It is interesting to note that Hesychius the lexicographer defined asbestosis as stuccoing or plastering and Cooke gave the name asbestosis which now, in addition to asbestosis, "may indeed stucco the pleura or the peritoneum" as well as other organs having mesothelial linings.[206] The first asbestos-associated case of mesothelioma was described in an asbestosis case by Wedler in Germany in 1943.[207] Mathew Stewart actually made the association between mesothelioma and asbestos in 1927; however, this was not published until 1955.[208] Including Wedler's report, other reports of mesothelioma associated with asbestos exposure appeared in 1943 and again in 1946.[209]

Mesothelioma of the pleura with asbestosis was found on pathologic examination in a 37-year-old insulation worker with a history of cutting asbestos-containing insulation board. The author,[210] however, did not connect asbestosis with mesothelioma. Further reports of mesothelioma in association with asbestos exposure continued.[211,167,212] Cases of pleural mesothelioma without asbestosis were discussed by Smith[213] and Cartier[214] in 1952. Cartier published a case of both pleural and peritoneal mesothelioma in chrysotile miners in Quebec.

Peritoneal mesothelioma occurred in a 53-year-old asbestos factory worker who was a yarn spinner. This worker also had asbestosis after 26 years of exposure.[215] Peritoneal cancers in one male and three female asbestos textile workers were found at postmortem examination, all of which were anaplastic carcinomas without any other primary site identified. Two were adenocarcinomas of the pleura—one disseminating and one not. Bonser et al.[208] found that all combined cancers and asbestosis developed in only those exposed before 1931 regulations; however, five cases of just fibrosis occurred in persons exposed after 1931, thus indicating the 1931 regulations were insufficient to eliminate fibrosis and raising the question of how will the lower exposures affect the latency period for cancer, if at all. In this report, the latency period would have only reached 23 years maximum, although mesothelioma has an average latency period of more than 30 years. Van der Schoot[216] reported pleural and peritoneal mesothelioma in insulation workers in Holland. In 1960, Konig[217] reported four pleural and three peritoneal mesotheliomas.

In a series of asbestosis cases, it was found that 9 of 15 deaths in women were associated with ovarian or peritoneal cancer, giving an incidence, according to the author,[218] of 60%, and there was one death in 15 men with asbestosis. The women's latency from first exposure ranged from 21 to 46 years with duration of exposure ranging from 1 to 21 years, whereas the one male's latency was 26 years with duration of exposure of 23 years.[218]

The study of Wagner et al.[20,219] of miners, millers, and transporters of asbestos and of nonmining residents looked at 33 (22 men and 11 women) cases of mesothelioma occurring between 1956 and 1960. These cases occurred in one part of South Africa, the northwestern portion of the Cape Province known to have many asbestos mines. The mining in this area was mainly crocidolite asbestos; however, small deposits of amosite were present. The first case was in a 36-year-old Bantu man who was born on the asbestos fields but worked as a shower attendant at a Witwatersrand gold mine and had asbestos bodies confirmed histologically but no evidence of fibrosis. Another case was in a 55-year-old woman, the daughter of a dentist, who lived from age 1 to 6 years in one of the asbestos mining villages. The fact that residential exposures also occurred have been attributed to the fact that low-level, nonoccupational exposures to asbestos can be hazardous. The 1960 report was attributed to confirming a causal association between exposure to asbestos and mesothelioma. Further discussion of this paper can be found in the section on crocidolite asbestos.[20,219]

The first study in the United States to associate mesothelioma with asbestos exposure was reported in 1963 by Mancuso and Coulter.[220] This was followed by the landmark study of Dr. I. J. Selikoff and colleagues of end-product uses of asbestos-containing products and members of the asbestos workers union where mesothelioma was confirmed in these workers.[221,222]

Mesothelioma is now reported in almost every major study of persons exposed to asbestos. Some have estimated that pleural mesothelioma occurs with an incidence of one for every two lung cancers; however, these estimates have generally been related to the overall mortality within specific cohorts of asbestos workers and, in some, on the basis of cumulative asbestos exposure of 25 or more fiber-years, which can be misleading either as overestimates or vice versa.[197] In one analysis by McDonald and McDonald,[223] the authors, after having thrown out the three highest and the three lowest ratios, reported a range of ratios for mesothelioma to lung cancer from 1.0 to 5.2; however, they actually threw out the four lowest, so the range was really 0.5–5.2 (median = 2.4). If they had looked at the entire range, it would have been from 0.3 to 18.5 (median = 3.67).[223] Thus, the actual ratio varies between studies and any reflection on just the median ratio is misleading. Pleural mesothelioma incidence has been increasing in all asbestos-using countries despite control measures put in place since the 1970s.[224] Jarvholm et al.[225] reported that the annual incidence of pleural mesothelioma attributable to occupational exposures was larger than all fatal occupational accidents in Sweden and that prevention measures had not yet been evident in decreasing the risk. The dose–response relationship for mesothelioma was first shown among textile workers exposed to asbestos and then among gas mask workers, miners and millers, and shipyard workers.[226–229]

Using the SEER data of the National Cancer Institute, which covers nine geographic areas and represents about 10% of the U.S. population, 542 incident cases of mesothelioma were reported between 1998 and 1999 and 447 cases between 1999 and 2000. Pinherio et al.[230] concluded these nine areas were generally representative of the entire United States and that using the ICD 10 coding which went into effect in 1999, the accuracy for reporting mesothelioma was now about 80% effective. This would mean that in the United States there are more than 6000 cases of mesothelioma per year if the mortality and incidence ratios averaged about 80%–85%. They noted that before the implementation of the ICD 10 code, previous codes did not permit analysis of specific data for mesotheliomas. For example, in Minnesota only, one of eight cases of pleural mesothelioma was coded correctly using previous ICD codes. Because of this inaccuracy of reporting and because of the absence of an appropriate ICD code until the implementation of the new ICD 10 coding system, the projections of mesothelioma in the United States were based on insufficient data to obtain an accurate picture of the U.S. mesothelioma trends. Unfortunately, the new ICD 10 code has only been in existence for the past 11 years, and any trends on the basis of these data are unwarranted. Thus, it will be many years until an accurate picture can be seen as to the real mesothelioma trends within the United States. What is clear, however, is that the projections using SEER data before the implementation of the ICD 10 codes are most likely inaccurate and most likely underestimate the true incidence of mesothelioma in the United States. Thus, studies using the pre-ICD-10 codes for concluding the risk of mesothelioma in the United States is on the decline may well be in error.[231,232] Trends in mesothelioma are on the rise in many countries and a large multicentric study[233] on malignant pleural mesothelioma and nonoccupational exposures to asbestos projects that low doses from the home and general environment may carry a measurable risk of mesothelioma over the next few decades.[180,234–238] The new ICD 10 codes for mesothelioma are C45.0 for pleural and C45.1 for peritoneal (ICD 10, 1994). As the incidence of mesothelioma in women is much less associated with asbestos exposure, Steenland et al.[239] suggested that if take-home asbestos exposure were considered, the attributable risks would rise to around 90%. Price and Ware[232] suggested that because the female lifetime mesothelioma risk across birth cohorts has remained constant, this supports a threshold exposure for mesothelioma which has yet to be shown, and no epidemiological study to date has been able to demonstrate such a threshold. As the bans on asbestos take effect in many countries, the incidence of mesothelioma should begin to decrease several decades into the future. We are starting to see this in the United Kingdom, which now has one of the highest mesothelioma death rates in the world. Although the mesothelioma death rate is still increasing in those older than 60 years, it is now falling in those aged 35–49 years. This is probably an indication of the reduction of asbestos use in the United Kingdom since the mid-1970s.[240] A recent report from the Health and Safety Executive (HSE) of the United Kingdom indicates an increasing trend in female mesothelioma rates in the United Kingdom. In comparison to the United States, the U.K. female mesothelioma death rate by age 70 years is now more than three times higher in the United Kingdom (0.037%) than that in the United States (0.012%). The threefold mesothelioma death rate in the U.K. women implies at least 30% of the female cases are causal by either environmental or by occasional or ambient asbestos exposure in occupational settings considered as low risk. The report suggests that the apparently so-called spontaneous mesotheliomas are likely due to increases in ambient asbestos exposures concurrent with the widespread uses of asbestos in the 1960s and 1970s.[241]

Peritoneal mesothelioma is a much rarer tumor than pleural mesothelioma. For example, in Sweden, the male incidence is 10-fold less than for pleural tumors, but in women it is somewhat higher or about half that of pleural tumors. Swedish men have shown no increase in peritoneal mesothelioma since 1985, but in women peritoneal mesothelioma has been steadily increasing and has surpassed the rate of pleural mesothelioma (0.16/100,000).[224] The report of Neumann et al.[242] from the German mesothelioma registry stated peritoneal mesothelioma was associated with higher lung burden than pleural mesothelioma. Suzuki[243] reported peritoneal mesothelioma was more commonly found in his group of 1517 mesothelioma cases among asbestos insulation workers. The overall mesothelioma ratio between pleural and peritoneal mesothelioma in Suzuki's group was approximately 3:1, but this was reversed when only insulation workers were evaluated (1:2.6). Israeli researchers found the incidence by anatomical site to be 74.1% for pleural compared with 24.6 for peritoneal among 317 cases reported between 1960 and 1996.[244]

The National Institute for Occupational Safety and Health (NIOSH) in conjunction with the National Center for Health Statistics reported that between 1987 and 1996, various work groups had extremely elevated proportional mortality ratios (PMRs) for pleural malignancies, including insulation workers at 23.08 (95% CI = 10.59–43.80); boilermakers at 15.37 (95% CI = 7.68–27.50); plasterers at 11.61 (95% CI = 3.76–27.13); sheet metal workers at 10.35 (95% CI = 6.55–15.54); plumbers, pipefitters, and steamfitters at 7.02 (95% CI = 5.12–9.40); and 13 other specific occupations with PMRs of 2 or greater.[245] They reported these occupations taking place in several industries, including ship/boat building and repairing with a PMR for pleural tumors of 12.60 (95% CI = 8.75–17.52) and petroleum refining with a PMR of 5.76 (95% CI = 3.29–9.35). Another 15 industries had PMRs more than 2 with all 95% CIs that did not include one. The latest data from NIOSH[246] through 1999 showed that the top 5 industry sectors with the greatest PMRs included ship/boat building and repair with a PMR of 6.0 (7 deaths; 95% CI = 2.4–12.3), industrial and miscellaneous chemicals with a PMR of 4.8 (19 deaths; 95% CI = 2.9–7.5), petroleum refining with a PMR of 3.8 (5 deaths; 95% CI = 1.2–8.9), electrical light and power with a PMR of 3.1 (10 deaths; 95% CI = 1.5–5.7), and construction with a PMR of 1.6 (77 deaths; 95% CI = 1.2–1.9). The top 4 PMRs were as follows: plumbers, pipefitters, and steam fitters with a PMR of 4.8 (18 deaths; 95% CI = 2.8–7.5); mechanical engineers with a PMR of 3.0 (6 deaths; 95% CI = 1.1–6.6); electricians with a PMR of 2.4 (12 deaths; 95% CI = 1.3–4.2); and elementary school teachers with a PMR of 2.1 (13 deaths, 95% CI = 1.1–3.6). These statistics were from 19 selected states with a total of 541 mesothelioma deaths.* The finding of such a high PMR for ship/boat building and repair is consistent with the study of Tagnon et al.[247] of the shipbuilding in coastal Virginia, which found 61 cases of mesothelioma among white men with an RR of 15.7 for the shipyard employees reporting exposure to asbestos compared with 4.9 for shipyard employees who did not report exposure to asbestos. Statistics from the latest SEER data pointed out the highest incidence for mesothelioma occurred in major shipbuilding areas such as Seattle (Puget Sound), Washington, and San Francisco–Oakland, California.[230]

The ratio of occurrence for pleural mesothelioma compared with peritoneal mesothelioma appears to be associated with the degree of exposure.[248] Among the large occupationally exposed groups studied, approximately 5%–10% of deaths were due to mesothelioma except in the small cohort of 33 cigarette-filter workers using crocidolite where it was 15% (five mesotheliomas).[249–252] In Scotland, only 5% of mesothelioma cases gave no history of asbestos exposure, whereas in Canada this lack of association was higher. The Canadian survey gave the annual incidence of about one per million.[253] Other studies have shown the ranges higher (up to 23%).[254] Another estimate projected that as many as 11% of all asbestos worker deaths in England will be from mesothelioma.[226] RR ranged between 2.3 and 7.0, with a mean of 4.6 for studies published between 1965 and 1975.[255–263] The association between mesothelioma and asbestos exposure has generally been very high (generally more than 80%), and in those who had not reported such exposures, when followed up they actually did show exposure.[264] Dodson et al.[265] have shown that 10%–15% of mesotheliomas arise in the peritoneal area and that fibers reach the mesentery and omentum in the peritoneal region.

In a 1960 report of abdominal cancers, eight cases of peritoneal cancers were reported in women, four of which were suggested to be primary from the ovary and four from the peritoneum. All had asbestosis. One case was reported in the same series in a male ventilator cleaner with asbestosis.[218] Previously, a case of peritoneal cancer was reported in a 53-year-old asbestos worker with asbestosis and asbestos fibers were found in the tumor tissue.[215] Three cases of peritoneal mesothelioma were reported among 36 asbestosis cases, and another case of peritoneal mesothelioma was reported in an insulator.[216,217] In another series of 72 asbestosis cases, four peritoneal cancers were reported (one in men and three in women), two of which were thought to be primary ovarian cancers.[266] Eleven

---

* The selection of these 19 states was based on the National Center for Health Statistics Quality Criteria for adequate industrial and occupational codes from death certificates and is not necessarily representative of the entire United States. What this tells us is that we still have inadequate and spotty reporting of mesothelioma in the United States.

cases of peritoneal mesothelioma were reported among eight men and three women between the ages of 38 and 78 years, with latency periods of 20–46 years and exposures between 10 months and 32 years. The authors reported that a "remarkable feature" of the cases was the minimal degree of fibrosis in the lungs.[267] Peritoneal mesotheliomas continued to be reported among various occupations with exposure to asbestos, including a 47-year-old insulator and a 46-year-old insulator,[268,269] three cases among radiologically confirmed asbestotics,[270] four among asbestos textile workers,[221] 17 cases with known asbestos exposures,[271] a 60-year-old former shipyard insulator,[272] three cases among asbestos textile workers,[273] and four cases among asbestos textile workers.[274] Newhouse and Thompson[256] reported 27 peritoneal mesotheliomas in London with occupational and domestic exposures.

Other sites of mesothelioma have been reported but not with the same incidence as pleural or peritoneal and their relationship to asbestos exposure needs further analysis. Pericardial mesothelioma has been reported, although it has a very low incidence (less than 0.0022%) as reported in one large autopsy study and, by some estimates, represents about 6% of all mesotheliomas.[275] Dusting of the pericardium with mixed dusts, including asbestos, was reported in an individual when treated for angina pectoris 15 years earlier.[276] Congenital malignant peritoneal mesothelioma has been observed, albeit very rarely, with only three cases documented and their association with asbestos unclear.[277]

5.2 PRODUCT USAGE AND DISEASE

Products containing asbestos have been found in the shipyard industry, the construction industry, the brake repair and transportation industry, the electronic and electrical industries, the paint industry, the optical goods industry, the plumbing industry, and other general industry manufacturing sectors.[278–280] Hundreds of buildings were reported to contain "asbestosis" (asbestos) in New York as early as 1897.[1] Exposures in the construction industry in New York varied as shown in the study by Reitze et al.[281] when they measured fiber counts from spraying asbestos onto buildings. They found 70 fibers/mL 10 ft. from the nozzle of the spray gun and 3 fibers/mL at 25 ft. from the nozzle. This indicates that not only were the spray operators at risk of exposure but also the auxiliary workers such as carpenters, pipefitters, welders, electricians, plumbers, and so forth.[281]

Diseases occur in nonoccupationally exposed persons living near industrial sources of asbestos, and familial exposure to asbestos occurs when a worker brings home asbestos-containing material from the worksite or when the worker does not shower or wears the same clothes home that had been worn during the work process.[219,256,283–286] Domestic exposures have been associated with household repairs and do-it-yourself construction using products containing asbestos or when disturbing products containing asbestos.[287] Pets of owners with asbestos-related occupations or hobbies that expose them to asbestos-containing materials have lead to their pets developing mesothelioma.[288]

In the first radiological description of asbestos-induced fibrosis, one of the cases reported was in a marine fireman.[289] The disease *asbestosis* was causally linked with end-product usage in the United States as early as 1932 when a maintenance employee who was cleaning and restoring asbestos insulation on pipes in a government-run hospital developed the disease. A workers' compensation claim was awarded in this case without any medical challenge.[106] Concerns were raised by the British Government of the health risks from the sawing, grinding, and turning in the dry state of materials partly or wholly composed of asbestos. Examples included such products as motor car brakes and clutches, electric conductors, and packing and jointing materials, thus demonstrating the ability of asbestos exposures from doing jobs outside the manufacturing sector.[290] Asbestos use and disease in the railroad industry was reported by the American Railway Association's Medical and Surgical Section, and the term *asbestosis* was specifically referred to in 1935.[291,292] The insulation industry was also singled out early as to health problems as discussed by Ellman[293] and previously reported by Russell,[106] including other cases of asbestos insulation used on lead pipes. Specific examples of other asbestos end-product uses by worker category can be found within the sections on worker exposures by trade discussed later in this chapter. As a result of these reports, the American Medical Association Council on Occupational Health published a whole thesis titled "The Pneumoconioses" in *the Archives of Environmental Health* in August 1963 in which asbestosis was discussed.[294] The intent of this document was to alert physicians throughout the country to the hazards of dust exposures and disease and how to recognize and treat them. The report was reprinted by the American Medical Association and circulated widely. By 1964, close to 50 medical articles were published, the majority in English, describing more than 150 cases of noncancerous lung disease (asbestosis) among end-product users of asbestos-containing products. Many of these products were used in construction of buildings and, as with any building, through periodic maintenance when asbestos is disturbed and released.

In 1942, Holleb and Angrist[295] first reported cancer in end-product users when lung cancer was reported in insulators. In 1947, Mallory et al.[210] reported mesothelioma in a 37-year-old Swedish insulator. Mesotheliomas have also been observed in pets. In one study of 18 dogs diagnosed with mesothelioma,[288] the owners for 16 were identified and 12 were able to identify possible sources of asbestos exposure. Nine of the dogs' owners had asbestos-related occupations or hobbies, five had remodeled their homes, five had residential proximity to an industrial source of asbestos, and five used flea powders known to contain asbestos-contaminated talc.

Other cancers also appeared in the scientific literature when Selikoff et al.[222] reported stomach cancer, colon cancer, rectal cancer, lung cancer, and pleural and peritoneal mesothelioma in insulators. In October 1964, a watershed event occurred that brought broader international attention to the hazards of working with asbestos and to products containing asbestos when the New York Academy of Sciences held a conference on the "Biological Effects of Asbestos." Presentations by more than 80 of the world's leading researchers on asbestos were given. This conference was widely covered by the news media, and the proceedings were published in 1965 in a 766-page annal.[296] Although this conference reported on the known health effects of exposure to asbestos (asbestosis and cancers), a major theme was the emphasis placed on the areas of prevention, including dust control techniques, community and other indirect exposures, and the significance of air pollution control.

5.2.1 Other Diseases Reported in Asbestos-Exposed Workers

Other diseases reported among persons exposed to asbestos include oropharyngeal cancer;[297] multiple primary cancer;[298] suicides;[299,300] ovarian cancer;[301–304] renal cancer;[305,306] penile cancer;[307] bladder cancer;[308] breast cancer;[309] leukemia, multiple myeloma, and Waldenstrom's macroglobulinemia;[302,310–312] and prostate cancer.[180] Whether these diseases are causally associated with exposures to asbestos have not necessarily been established except for ovarian cancer, which is discussed in Chapter 8. At the time this chapter was written, these are clearly associations only and should not be deemed as established. However, as research on asbestos continues, these diseases may or may not be determined as causally associated with asbestos exposures.

5.3 OCCUPATIONAL REGULATIONS AND PREVENTION FOR ASBESTOS-RELATED DISEASES

5.3.1 Dust and Dust Control

The term dust, as described by Cox in 1857, is "solid mechanical impurities floating in a minute state of division" … "impalpable powder." An International Conference of Experts, when defining pneumoconiosis, defined "The term 'dust' as particulate matter in the solid phase but excluding living organisms."[313] The measurement of dust is usually expressed in microns. For example, 1 in. is about 25,000 μm, the human hair about 100 μm, cement dust 2–100 μm, bacteria 0.2–15 μm, and tobacco smoke 0.01–0.5 μm.[314] Dusts are found in every part of the world, most not being noxious whereas a few are toxic. The body's defenses protect us from most of these, but the body may inhale more of these dust particles in just a few seconds or minutes, like those of asbestos, even when the dust cannot be seen. In other words, asbestos-containing dusts can be an invisible hazard, and hazardous levels may be present even in the absence of visible dust. Support for this opinion dates back to many years. Dr. E. R. A. Merewether in his scientific publication "Dusts and the Lungs with Particular Reference to Silicosis and Asbestosis" in *Industrial Medicine*, Symposium No. 3, in 1938 stated: "The majority of the particles, however, which get into and stay in the lungs are much smaller in each case—up to 5 μm in the case of silica dust and up to about 50 μm in the case of asbestos. That is to say that, the dust particles which are invisible to the naked eye are the important ones: this leads us to the practical point that if silica or an asbestos process produces visible dust in the air, then the invisible dust is certainly in dangerous concentrations:"[315] An industrial hygienist, Warren A. Cook,[316] Director, Division of Industrial Hygiene and Engineering Research Zurick General Accident and Liability Insurance Company, Ltd., Chicago, stated: "In the case of the asbestos dust condition, our evaluation of the exposure should be based on the knowledge that the present toxic limit for asbestos is five million particles of dust per cubic foot of air. This is a very small concentration, so small in fact that the condition may look good even to a critical eye and still present an exposure greater than this low limit." Although these statements are based on the judgment of both Dr. Merewether and Mr. Cook, the visibility of dust has been quantified by W. C. L. Hemeon,[317] Engineering Director, IHF of America, Inc., of the Mellon Institute of Pittsburgh, Pennsylvania, who found that in "Bright daylight 'north' illumination (i.e., interior but no direct sun) that the visible concentrations range from 10 to 20 million particles per cubic feet; at distances of less than 10 to 15 ft. and in 'low-intensity daylight' 20–40 million particles per cubic feet."

It has long been known that suppression of dust was the best method to control diseases associated with exposures to dusts as was described by Ramazzini[95] and by Oliver.[318] In the United Kingdom, the Chief Inspector of Factories in London recommended to one factory that exhaust ventilation and annual medical examinations be instituted after having experienced five deaths due to phthisis (asthma-like disease).[319] Merewether and Price[46] were among the very first to set forth very specific recommendations for dust suppression in the asbestos industry, which included the following: (1) application of efficient localized exhaust ventilation at dust-producing points; (2) substitution of enclosed mechanical methods for hand conveyance and for dusty hand work; (3) effective enclosure of dust-producing machines; (4) substitution of wet methods instead of dry material handling; (5) elimination of certain dust-producing appliances; (6) abandonment of settling chambers in manufacturing processes, to the utmost extent; (7) effectual separation of processes to prevent unnecessary exposure to dust; (8) wide spacing of dust-producing machines in new factories and, as far as practicable, in existing works; (9) use of sacks of close texture material for internal work; (10) efficient cleaning systems with wide use of vacuum methods; (11) storage of asbestos and other goods outside workrooms; and (12) exclusion of young persons from especially dusty work.

Safety Engineering magazine ran an article in 1931 on "The Very Least an Employer Should Know about Dust and Fume Diseases," warning that dust, including asbestos containing dust, could be seriously harmful and that controlling the dust was necessary.[320] McPheeters[129] suggested implementing dust controls methods in 1936 for the prevention of asbestosis. Many others have also given methods for preventive actions from hazardous dusts, including the classic work in the 1930s of the U.S. Public Health Service.[131,321] For asbestos disease control, Lanza et al.[122] described the serious hazards of dust faced by the industry in 1935 and recommended studies on its control as related to disease prevention. However, not much attention was given to hygiene in the early history of exposure to asbestos.[322]

As early as 1942, The Assistant Director and Principal Pathologist of the Warner Institute for Therapeutic Research in New York City, W. C. Hueper, in his historic book *Occupational Tumors*

and Allied Diseases, recommended controlling asbestos by methods of wetting, closed production, ventilation, or other engineering controls as well as use of personal protective devices (i.e.,
respirators).[17] Fleischer et al.[323] expanded this advice in 1946 and gave even more extensive guidance
for dust control to end-product users of asbestos-containing materials, recommending wetting the
material, exhausting the dust where possible, employing respirator usage by workers, isolating dusty
operations to protect other workers not directly working with asbestos, and providing room ventilation. Fleischer et al.[323] concluded: "There are no established figures for permissible or safe dustiness
in pipe covering operations" They stated: "During the handling, unwrapping and unrolling of the
asbestos [material], considerable dust arises, but appears to settle readily. A very fine water spray
should be used for wetting down the material as a high velocity spray stirs up dust." Pertaining to
the use of saws used to cut the end product, Fleischer et al.[323] recommend that "... the band saw
should be enclosed in a room by itself and should be equipped with adequate local exhaust ventilation both above and below the saw table." Further, Fleischer et al. pointed out those end-product
users such as "... asbestos pipe covering differs markedly from the asbestos textile industry where
dust concentrations for an operation do not fluctuate widely and where a worker will usually remain
at a specific job for some years." Finally, the Fleischer et al.[323] recommendations were some of the
most extensive on pipefitting ever made and were published in a prominent professional journal of
that time, the *Journal of Industrial Hygiene and Toxicology*, which was read by occupational health
specialists and gave warning to the extreme importance of reducing dust in the use of asbestos-
containing thermal pipe insulation. It was not a paper implying that the use of asbestos thermal
pipe insulation work was safe unless adequate dust control was practiced to eliminate exposure to
asbestos-containing dust.

5.3.2 Asbestosis and Cancers below Guidance Limits

Since 1935, several studies have shown asbestosis occurring in workers at concentrations
below 5 mppcf.[121,131,323–327] Today, the quest for safe exposure concentrations is still ongoing and
has unsettled answers. The only tools for use in epidemiology with which to make such assessments are confined to either exposure concentration analysis or tissue burden analysis. First,
asbestos measurement techniques have evolved with time, which makes it difficult to compare
one another. Second, because of the differences in biopersistence of fibers and their clearance
from the lung, such analysis also presents problems. Third, the presence of asbestos bodies is
sometimes used as a surrogate for exposure analysis but is not very accurate because lung samples
from occupationally exposed persons have significant variation between the ratio of uncoated
fibers and the asbestos bodies, and chrysotile short fibers are rarely found as core material of
asbestos bodies.[328] When exposure data have existed and have been used to determine the risk of
disease, such determinations have been based on a calculation of fiber-years of exposure (fibers/
cm^3 × years of exposure). Such calculations have led to few conclusions as have lung-burden studies and analysis of asbestos body counts. Pleural plaques have also been used as an indicator of
asbestos exposure.

Fiber-year analysis has resulted in the estimation that, for lung cancer, the RR is increased from
0.5% to 4% for each fiber year, indicating that at 25 fiber-years, a twofold risk for lung cancer exists.[166]
Epidemiologic findings have observed cumulative exposure below 25 fiber-years support even lower
cumulative exposures resulting in elevated SMRs for lung cancer: at 2.7–6.8 fiber-years, the SMR =
2.1 (95% CI = 1.1–3.8), and at 6.8–27.4 fiber-years, the SMR = 1.8 (95% CI = 1.0–3.35).[329] A study of
297 Hungarian lung cancer patients reported 63% with no exposure to asbestos and 30% with <25
fiber-years but only 5.5% with >25 fiber-years.[197] For lung fibrosis, the OR at <0.1 fiber-years was
1.0, whereas between 0.1 and 5.0 it increased to 2.5; at 5.1–25.0 fiber-years it increased to 3.8; and
at >25 fiber-years it increased to 24.9. Analysis of fiber concentrations measured at the Uralasbestos
Company Mine in Russia found background levels in the quarries to be around 0.08 fibers/cm^3

(range = 0.01–0.27), which is similar to that found in Zimbabwe and Indian chrysotile mining. Also, because chrysotile ore is not very dusty, it takes much effort to create fiber levels above 1 fiber/cm^3.[330] These findings bring into question the fiber concentrations stated for the Canadian cohort studies of Canadian miners and millers, which may well be overestimated. This may also explain the differences between the Canadian studies and those of the textile mill studied by Dement. When lung burden data were included in the analysis, the ORs increased to 2.5 for 0.1–5.0 cumulative fiber-years exposure, to 13.3 at 5.1–25.0 fiber-years, and to 46.2 at greater than 25.0 fiber-years.[329] Because chrysotile fibers clear from the lung more rapidly compared with the amphibole forms of asbestos, determination of causation from lung burden studies may not be reliable.[331–333] Rodelsperger et al.[334] reported mesothelioma as having a distinct dose–response relationship at levels of exposure below 1 fiber-year. As a result of both animal and human studies, the identification of a safe concentration below which disease will not occur, especially for mesothelioma, has eluded researchers.[330,335–337] The study by Iwatsubo et al.[338] has shown a dose–response effect even at low exposures. Iwatsubo et al. calculated that with a latency period of 20 years and at cumulative asbestos exposures for all 3498 job periods among 11 different occupational groups between 0.5 and 0.99 fibers/mL-years, the OR of mesothelioma rises to 4.2 (95% CI = 2.0–8.8). These findings are significant for interpreting a risk of exposure sufficient to induce mesothelioma in persons having lower doses of exposure such as ancillary workers not directly working with asbestos full time. Although there is no doubt that all forms of asbestos can cause lung cancer and mesothelioma, Valic[339] opined: "The practical application of unit risks of such uncertainty lead to unachievable exposure limits." In addition, Valic projects: "It cannot be predicted with any degree of certainty what will the consequences of the current, incomparably lower exposure levels be in the future. Yet, there is no doubt that it is advisable to replace any potential carcinogenic material whenever possible."

5.3.3 Effectiveness of Guidance Concentrations in Preventing Disease

Commenting on the effectiveness of such guidance concentrations, S. A. Roach of the University of London stated that "… 5 million particles per cubic feet, are simply standards, although I hope I did not use the word 'safe.' These are standards which are actually used, although they are not ever expressed as being safe standards."[340] Roach further stated that even if this was dropped to 2 mppcf, this would not necessarily be a "perfectly safe level of dust." It is interesting to note that a worker would not be able to see this concentration of dust in the ambient air and would not see any dust until a concentration between 20 and 40 mppcf was reached.[317] Warren Cook, Director, Industrial Hygiene and Engineering Research of the Zurich General Accident and Liability Insurance Company in Chicago, in 1942 stated: "This [5 mppcf] is a very small concentration, so small in fact that the condition may look good even to a critical eye and still present an exposure greater than this low limit."[316] The 5 mppcf guidance concentration remained in effect until the 1960s.[341] Cooper[342] stated that the 5 mppcf recommendation for protection from asbestos exposure proposed by the American Conference of Governmental Industrial Hygienists (ACGIH) since 1946 rests on shakier evidence compared with other such recommendations.

5.3.4 Asbestos Counting and Fiber Size Implications

The British adopted a new counting method for asbestos that counted actual fibers instead of using a concentration based on total dust particles.[343] The method became the choice for regulatory purposes, however, using the phase-contrast microscope (PCM) method, only fibers greater than 5 μm in length with an aspect ratio of 3:1 were counted because of limitations with statistical accuracy. Thus, epidemiology studies that compared dose within their cohorts and that relied upon the total dust count before the PCM method came along now had to develop a way to compare the earlier doses of total dust with the new fiber counting method. One such comparison was developed by Ayer et al.[344] in which they estimated that 1 mppcf was roughly equal to 6 fibers/cm^3. Because only fibers longer than 5 μm in length were counted and only those impacted on a membrane filter, other variables needed to be evaluated that might affect the airborne fiber counts. Peck and Serocki,[345] at the OSHA laboratory in Salt Lake City, Utah, reported a source of "random error" in the P&CAM-239 method because of the presence of electrostatic charges generated within the plastic filter cassettes used. This OSHA laboratory finding indicated that their finding could result in sampling errors from nondetectable up to seven times those actually reported and thus result in airborne asbestos measurements that could underestimate fiber count. The authors suggested that if antistatic spray was used on the cassette surface, this effect might be neutralized. However, the implications of this could indicate that any samples taken before 1985 using this membrane method and without correcting for the static effect may well have underestimated the actual exposures to fibers. In 2009, Loomis et al.[346] reported that comparing total dust counts from the impinger results varied in conversion from 1.60 to 8.04 fibers/mL using the phase-contrast counting scheme. This finding demonstrated the difficulty of using one universal conversion factor to compare impinger results to PCM fiber counts.

It must be noted that the PCM analytical method was chosen on the basis of its ability to count fibers and not on a health effect basis.[*] Although PCM has been the international regulatory method for analysis, it is not able to detect thin diameter fibers (<0.2 μm in diameter). Therefore, use of the PCM method not only misses fibers shorter than 5 μm in length (based on the definition of length for inclusion of fibers) but also, because the limit of detection based on diameters resolved results in the exclusion of those fibers such as chrysotile "fibrils" and thinner amphiboles, which are between 0.02 and 0.2 μm in diameter. Thus, in the case of chrysotile where the individual units are from 0.02 to 0.05 μm in diameter, one would in such a count scheme only detect chrysotile bundles (multiple aligned "fibrils"). The implication is that chrysotile fibers will be underestimated compared with amphibole fibers and, because of this, it has been suggested that transmission electron microscopy (TEM) should be an adjunct to PCM. Tissue analysis is discussed in other chapters of this book; however, for the epidemiologist, it is important to know that using the light microscope to detect uncoated fibers in tissue sections of the lung, as stated by Dodson and Atkinson, is "... an exercise in futility." "In addition, the counting scheme counts any 'fiber' and does not distinguish the type of fiber." Thus, the analytical methods of most accuracy are the electronic microscope, but the scanning electron microscope (SEM) is less desirable than the TEM. This is because the TEM will (1) detect the smallest fiber, (2) identify the mineral type of fiber, and (3) be able to detect all fiber types equally, including chrysotile. Using an analytical transmission electronic microscope at very low magnification will miss many fibers due to their lack of visibility. Therefore, the epidemiologist should determine the physical limits and the resolvability of the analytical method used before concluding the validity of the fiber analysis results. Dodson and Atkins[347] stated that the data from their own laboratory found most uncoated fibers in tissue are less than 5 μm, and even when long fibers are present, the fibers are below the limit of detection due to their thin diameter. Thus, the limits of the light microscope preclude its accuracy or reliability to determine fiber size and type.

---

[*] "The first decision made concerned that part of the dust spectrum which should be counted and it was agreed that only fibers or fiber bundles having a minimum length of 5 μm and a maximum of 100 μm should be counted, the definition of a fiber being arbitrarily taken as a particle whose length was at least three times its diameter. This decision was taken in the light of evidence to the effect that the particle size distribution or spectrum of an asbestos dust cloud was reasonably constant over a wide range of textile processes, although later work has suggested that this might not be strictly true." This decision represent the conclusions made for use of the Thermal Precipitator Method in collecting asbestos-containing dust and when the membrane filter technique came into use, the basis for the method referred to as PCM method, it was determined that the 5 μm in length would remain the standard as "The filter on the other hand, having a pore size in the region of 0.145 μm, would appear to be quite adequate for trapping fibers in the length range 5–100 microns." Although it was thought the Membrane Filter Technique would be more representative in assessing the "true health hazard to which an operative is subjected," it did not rely upon knowledge that fibers less than 5 μm in length had been shown harmless. (Holmes S. Developments in dust sampling and counting techniques in the asbestos industry. *Ann N Y Acad Sci* 1965;132:288–97.

5.3.5 Short Fiber Toxicity

To assume that shorter fibers do not cause disease is not scientifically justified from the epidemiology or the toxicology studies. Unfortunately, the role of short asbestos fibers has mostly been ignored. What studies that have been done such as Stanton and Wrench[348] and Stanton et al.[349] found that longer, thinner fibers were more carcinogenic but could not identify a precise fiber length that did not demonstrate biological activity. In fact, Dr. Stanton has never said long fibers are bad and short fibers are good and appreciated that a large number of short fibers individually of low tumorigenic probability might be more hazardous than fewer long fibers individually of high probability.[350] It has been shown that it is not just the size and shape of the various asbestos fibers that are important in the fiber's ability to produce disease, but other factors may also play a role in the carcinogenicity of the mineral fiber.[351,352]

Dement and Wallingford[353] found that in typical occupational environments, fibers shorter than 5 μm outnumber the longer fibers by a factor of 10 or more. Studies looking at human tissues have also found that the majority of asbestos fibers in mesothelial tissues were shorter than 5 μm in length, thus indicating the ability of the shorter fibers to reach the tumor site, remain there, and therefore their role in the etiology of disease is implicated.[265,332,354] Shorter fibers must be studied in more depth and should not be disregarded, especially when clearance is retarded.[355] That chrysotile fibers tend to split longitudinally and partially dissolve, resulting in shorter fibers within the lung, was reported in a review of several articles.[356] Additionally, Fubini[357] argued that because all asbestos types appear nearly equally potent, length and fiber form does not appear influential on the outcome of disease. Fubini makes this conclusion based on the work of Boffetta,[358] which concludes that the specific type of asbestos is not correlated with lung cancer risk but that industry-specific exposure appears to fit the linear slope best, a finding also supported by Dement and Brown.[356] For mesothelioma, induction was related to the time since first exposure and potency with both industry type and asbestos type.[358] Although longer fibers tend to be retained in the human lung parenchyma, those found in the pleural tissues show a predominance of shorter fibers, mostly chrysotile, with only 2% of the fibers in the pleura being longer than 8 μm in length compared with 15% in the lung parenchyma and mostly amphiboles.[359] These findings found no relationship between fiber counts from lung parenchyma versus parietal pleura. Fibers found in bronchoalveolar lavage fluid were shorter than those found from digestion studies of the lung parenchyma, indicating the ability of longer fibers to penetrate and stay within the alveolar tissue. The fibers found in the parietal pleura did not show uniform distribution, although studies using radioactive particles have shown uniform distribution within the lung parenchyma appearing more conducive in the development of lung cancers[360]; however, such a pattern within the parietal pleura has not been shown.

The fact that short fibers (<5 μm) have been shown to produce toxic effects in macrophages in vitro and to be fibrogenic and tumorigenic in animals in vivo[361] and that they reach the site of mesothelioma development[265,332,362] supports the inappropriateness of discounting their role in asbestos-related diseases. By doing this, EPA contractors Berman and Crump have invalidated their risk assessment index.[363] The data to date strengthen the role of short fibers in the etiology of asbestos-related diseases. There remains a need to change the analytical methodology to include short fibers and a reevaluation of the current OSHA standard to include short fibers in addition to those greater than 5 μm in length.

5.3.6 Guidance Limits and Regulations for Worker Exposures to Asbestos in the United States

"No industry can proceed at full speed unless its individual human units have a fair degree of the personal (physical and mental) health so vital to the quantity, quality, and continuity of production. One skilled worker absent because of preventable illness can greatly disturb the smooth functioning of the production line and cause losses out of all proportion to expectation, because of the disruption of teamwork."[364] The first regulations were jointly prepared by the British government and the industry being regulated.[105] "The idea of adopting standards of permissible dustiness for each harmful dust has a medicolegal appeal that is not at all justified by the data available today."[130] The U.S. Public Health Service introduced guidance limit of 5 mppcf as a guide for the control of asbestos dust although they found three cases of asbestosis below this recommended guideline.[131] Fulton et al.[121] reported 2 of 20 workers exposed to an average asbestos dust concentration of 4.64 mppcf for greater than 5 years to have both clinical and radiographic evidence of asbestosis. This recommended guidance concentration for exposure to asbestos of 5 mppcf was later adopted by the newly organized ACGIH in the United States.[365] In 1952, the U.S. Government set occupational standards for workers including a specific asbestos standard for contractors performing Federal Supply Contracts under the Walsh–Healey Public Contracts Act of 5 mppcf.[366] In 1960, the U.S. Department of Labor set standards for employers under the Longshoremen's Act for asbestos of 5 mppcf.[341] On April 26, 1964, revised safety and health regulations went into effect for ship repairing, inducing the 5 mppcf for asbestos exposure.[367] On November 9, 1967, the regulations for ship repairing were again updated to include the TLVs of the ACGIH were adopted as standards under the Longshoreman's and Harbor Workers' Compensation Act.[368]

In 1968, the ACGIH proposed a new guidance limit of 12 fibers/mL or 2 mppcf.[369] Then the U.S. Department of Labor adopted a new standard for asbestos in 1969 of 12 fibers/mL or 2 mppcf under the Walsh–Healey Act.[370] The ACGIH recommended a change in their guidance limit of 5 fibers/mL for asbestos in April 1971.[371]

A major event occurred on April 28, 1971, when the OSHA of 1970 became effective.[372] The very next month, the OSHA adopted the ACGIH recommendation of 12 fibers/mL or 2 mppcf as a legal standard under the provisions of the new OSHAct for adopting existing consensus recommendations, on a one-time basis, as initial start-up standards, after which they would develop their own official standards using the OSHAct promulgation procedures.[373] Then, on November 17, 1971, the newly created NIOSH Director Dr. Marcus Key sent a letter to OSHA recommending a reduction of the current OSHA asbestos standard from 12 to 5 fibers/cm^3.[374] In response to this, on December 7, 1971, OSHA set an emergency legal standard of 5 fibers/mL, and on January 12, 1972, OSHA issued an additional emergency standard covering the ship repairing, shipbuilding, shipbreaking, and longshoring industries. This emergency standard held the same requirements as the December 7, 1971, emergency legal standard.[375] At the same time, OSHA proposed to modify their existing 12 fiber/cm^3 or 2 mppcf standard to 5 fibers/cm^3.[375]

On February 25, 1972, NIOSH sent OSHA its first criteria document on asbestos recommending that OSHA promulgate a standard for asbestos of 2 fibers/cm^3 on the basis of a count of fibers greater than 5 μm in length and an aspect ratio (length to width) of 3:1.[374] Following this, on June 7, 1972, OSHA promulgated a new standard (permissible exposure limit—PEL) for asbestos of 5 fibers/cm^3, intended to prevent asbestosis and provide some degree of protection against asbestos-induced cancers and that in July 1976 this standard would be lowered to 2 fibers/cm^3.[375]

In October 1975, OSHA proposed to revise its asbestos standard to 0.5 fibers/cm^3 and to designate asbestos as a carcinogen.[376] In December, NIOSH sent OSHA a revised recommended asbestos standard recommending OSHA promulgate a new standard for asbestos of 0.1 fibers/cm^3 on the basis of its carcinogenicity and the available technology of the PCM to only measure fibers accurately down to this concentration. NIOSH stated this recommendation was intended (1) to protect against the noncarcinogenic effects of asbestos and (2) to materially reduce the risk of asbestos-induced cancer and that only a ban on asbestos could assure protection against the carcinogenic effects of asbestos.[377]

In April 1980, the NIOSH/OSHA Working Group on Asbestos recommended that there was no safe level of exposure to asbestos and discussed the inadequacy of the current OSHA standard of 2 fibers/cm^3, thus recommending an immediate reduction to 0.1 fibers/cm^3.[378] On November 4, 1983, OSHA published the Emergency Temporary Standard for asbestos of 0.05 fibers/cm^3 [*sic*].[379]

The following year, on March 7, 1984, the OSHA Emergency Temporary Standard for asbestos was invalidated by the U.S. Circuit Court of Appeals for the Fifth Circuit.[380]

Following this invalidation, on June 20, 1986, OSHA issued two revised standards for asbestos—one for general industry and a second for the construction industry—at 0.2 fibers/cm^3.[381] On September 14, 1992, OSHA added a 30-min excursion limit of 1 fiber/cm^3.[382] In 1992, OSHA again revised this standard by deleting nonasbestiform, tremolite, anthophyllite, and actinolite.[383] This action was in direct contrast to the recommendations of NIOSH, who indicated all fibrous asbestos material should be regulated whether or not they occurred just in the asbestiform asbestos minerals.[384] The current standard of asbestos was promulgated on August 10, 1994, setting the PEL at 0.1 fibers/cm^3,[385] the number recommended by NIOSH in 1976.[377]

5.3.7 Risk of Asbestos-Related Diseases from Exposure at the Current OSHA Standard

Asbestos-containing materials are regulated if they contain more than 1% asbestos.[386] Higher exposures to asbestos result in higher risks and lower exposures to asbestos result in lower risks of developing asbestos-related diseases. Humans breathe 12 cm^3 of air per day and at the current OSHA standard of 0.1 fibers/cm^3, this would equate to the inhalation of 1,200,000 fibers/day. The exposure–response relationship for lung cancer is linear.[387] At the current OSHA standard, the risk of death is 3.4 per 1000 at 0.1 fibers/cm^3.[381] A study by Gustavsson et al.,[190] which was discussed under the risk section for lung cancer, suggested that the use of linear extrapolation from high-exposure levels may underestimate the risks at low doses. Gustavsson et al. stated their study had indirect support[388–391]; however, at least one study did not give such support.[392] Even at the current OSHA limit, it can clearly be seen that the risk of dying from cancer is not zero nor does it even approach it. Dement and Brown[356] reported statistically significant excess for lung cancer at exposures as low as less than 3 fiber/years. The WHO[393] stated: "[T]he human evidence has not demonstrated that there is a threshold exposure level for lung cancer or mesothelioma, below which exposure to asbestos dust would not be free of hazard to health." The International Programme for Chemical Safety reiterated this position.[335]

These conclusions continue to support what the industry representatives said in 1965; namely, that the only safe level to prevent disease is zero. It also supports the finding that nonmalignant respiratory diseases (NMRDs) need not be present before cancer of the lung or mesothelioma can develop. In 1965, Addingley,[394] of the British Belting and Asbestos Ltd. Industry, stated: "We do not believe there is any safe limit. ... Therefore, I would like it to be clearly understood that we do not accept 4 fibers/mL as a safe maximum limit in the asbestos industry." At the same conference, Wells,[395] of the American Asbestos industry U.S. Rubber Co., stated: "Our own conclusion, as we began seeing what was happening in our own process, was that the only safe amount of asbestos dust exposure was zero and that the efforts in terms of achieving that lay basically in engineering, and, secondly, in education." NIOSH, created with the passage of the OSHA of 1970, also concluded that for the complete elimination of the carcinogenic and preventable asbestos-related diseases "... (only a ban can assure protection against carcinogenic effects of asbestos). ..."[337] For the first time, the U.S. Government concluded, as did industry representatives by 1965, that the elimination of all asbestos from the workplace was the only solution to the eradication of asbestos-induced cancer from the workplace.

Multiple studies and scientists have concluded that both asbestosis and lung cancer are independent diseases related both with a dose–response from exposure to asbestos and that cancer of the lung can and does occur in the absence of asbestosis.[172–173,396–397] Thus, these conclusions support that any standard aimed at the prevention of asbestosis will not necessarily protect against the more long-term effects of asbestos exposure that result in cancers.

As discussed in the section on smoking and lung cancer, there is a marked enhancement of the risk of lung cancer in workers exposed to asbestos who also smoke cigarettes.[182,249,396–397] Data from

Hammond et al.[182] and Weiss[398] suggest that cigarette smoking may also contribute to the risk of asbestosis. Smoking, however, has not been found to be associated with an increased risk of pleural or peritoneal mesothelioma. OSHA attributes asbestos exposure with 79.4% of the lung cancer deaths among asbestos-exposed workers who smoke and 77.2% of lung cancer deaths among nonsmokers.[381] Berry and Liddell[187] estimated the RR to be about three times higher for lung cancer in nonsmokers versus smokers. This supports that nonsmoking asbestos workers face elevated risks of lung cancer. As discussed in the section on smoking and risk, more recent studies suggest the smoking and asbestos exposure relationship may be more additive than multiplicative.[189–191]

5.4 FINDINGS SPECIFIC TO OCCUPATIONS

Specific occupations have been identified and some studied to better define their risk of asbestos-related diseases. Specific occupations do not need to be studied nor do epidemiological studies need to be performed to show risk of disease before prevention actions are taken or causal connections concluded. To wait for epidemiology studies of each occupational group is not warranted but has been taken by many in the medico-legal profession as necessary to prove causation by occupation. Such misconceived thinking has been very harmful to the future prevention of asbestos-related diseases because it is not the job that causes disease but it is the exposure to and the inhalation of asbestos fibers that increase the risk of disease. This section will show what has been shown, what is known, what job categories have been studied, and which asbestos-related diseases have been reported. This section is not intended to stifle prevention of asbestos-related diseases, which must proceed even in the absence of studies or reports on a particular occupational category or job classification and is not necessarily all inclusive of each occupational category or job reported in this section. Asbestos-related diseases do not occur in just those occupations that have been studied, and to conclude such, until studies of each and every occupation or job categories are conducted or from which cases are reported, is to ignore the established fact that it is exposure to asbestos, not the occupation or the specific job, that is responsible for asbestos-related diseases. Physicians, however, can further help clarify specific occupations and jobs where disease occurs by what Ramazzini suggested some 300 years ago in his classic works on *Diseases of Workers* stating: "[T]here are many things that a doctor, on his first visit to a patient, ought to find out either from the patient or from those present. For so runs the oracle of our inspired teacher: when you come to a patient's house, you should ask him what sort of pains he has, what caused them, how many days he has been ill, whether the bowels are working and what sort of food he eats." So says Hippocrates in his work *Affections*. "I may venture to add one more question: What occupation does he follow?"[95]

The following occupations and jobs have been studied or have had reported cases of asbestos-related diseases. The reports cited here are not meant to be all inclusive but rather to show that certain occupational groups or job titles have been studied to determine the overall risk to occupation-related asbestos diseases in their group as a whole. It should not be construed that because an occupation or job title does not appear in this section there is no risk to that occupation or job title. According to NIOSH, in their latest survey, there are more than 522 major industry types and 377 occupational categories, and more than 75 of these occupational groups have known exposures to asbestos, and there are multiple job titles within each group of which only a few have ever been studied (www.cdc.gov/noes). The real issue remains that it is the exposure to asbestos and the individual not the occupation or job title that causes or puts one at risk of developing an asbestos-related disease. The Report of the Advisory Committee to the Surgeon General of the Public Health Service[399] emphasized this same point when in 1964 they told the U.S. Surgeon General that "The situation of smoking in relation to the health of mankind includes a host (variable man) and a complex agent (tobacco and its products …" It is not hard to see asbestos and its products in place of tobacco and its products. When the committee uses the word "variable" man, they recognize the effect of the agent can vary with the man. They go further stating: "It is recognized that often the coexistence of several factors is required for the occurrence of a disease, and that one of the factors may play a determinant role, that is. without it the other factors (as genetic susceptibility) are impotent." Thus, they are saying all of the right conditions must be met or exposure to the agent (asbestos is this case) is impotent unless the variable man has other characteristics within that allow "... the multiple etiology of biological processes" to take place before the disease manifests itself. For these reasons, why do not all individuals under similar conditions (of exposure to asbestos) develop asbestos-related diseases? It is also true why groups exposed to relatively low concentrations of asbestos may show no excess of disease overall, although individuals within the group, under these same exposure conditions or due to unusually higher exposure conditions even within the low exposure cohort, may develop disease. Thus, the multiplicity of the biological process as well as the individual exposure scenario must be considered in making cause-specific conclusions for persons when they suffer from known asbestos-related diseases such as asbestosis and mesothelioma and not solely on the cohort of workers studied in this section. This section does have the advantage of showing occupational and job categories that have been studied and in some case with high risks of asbestos-related diseases, but this section or the absence of a study should not be used to disavow individuals within other occupations or jobs or with overall low risk not to have experienced an asbestos-related disease.

5.4.1 Boilermakers (Also See Section 5.4.3.12)

Breslow et al.[400] were one of the first to show that certain occupational groups, in conjunction with cigarette smoking, have higher lung cancer risks. When categorizing persons by occupational groupings, they observed steamfitters, boilermakers, and asbestos workers who worked in these occupational groups experienced ten lung cancers compared with one in controls. Mesothelioma has been reported in laggers, pipe fitters, and boilermakers.[401] Oels et al.[402] reported two pleural mesotheliomas from a review of 37 cases at the Mayo Clinic since 1967. In an epidemiological survey between 1945 and 1972, 36 cases of mesothelioma were identified of which one was a boilermaker in a local shipyard.[403] While surveying the area around Plymouth, England, 108 mesothelioma deaths were reported, of which 6 were boilermakers at the Devonport dockyard.[404] This resulted in an above average rate of mesothelioma or a rate of 161/100,000, just under the rate for laggers and sprayers. Boilermakers tended to have more consistently concentrated exposures because they do not move around the other parts of the ship. Boilermakers made up 10.6% of the identified mesothelioma cases in the Australian Mesothelioma Registry between 1980 and 1985.[405] The prevalence ratio for pleural plaques greater than 4.0 for boilermakers and workers in high-exposure shops who were smokers were found to have the highest prevalence of pleural plaques.[406] Canadian boilermakers exposed to both asbestos and welding fumes showed 20% had radiographic changes; 8% were circumscribed and 9% with diffuse pleural thickening. Boilermakers with the longest service had more pulmonary function changes when compared with those working as welders. The authors stated that these findings were in support of and consistent with past studies, which have shown boilermakers having an increase in mortality from lung cancers, radiographic changes, and asbestosis.[407] Studies among pattern makers in the Italian auto industry found three cases of colon cancer among pipefitters and boilermakers when only one was found in the control population for an OR of 10.7 (95% CI = 1.07–103).[408] Members of the Michigan Boilermakers Union were studied, and it was found that interstitial fibrosis and pleural plaques were related to 10 or more years in the trade with 25% showing at least a 1/0 profusion and 30% with bilateral pleural abnormalities.[409] Boilermakers in the petro-refinery industry were shown to have an excess of mesothelioma.[410] NIOSH scientists reported at the 131st meeting of the American Public Health Association in November 2003 that boilermakers had the second highest PMR of 20.3 for asbestosis.[411] In another NIOSH study by Bang et al.,[412] boilermakers were found to have jobs with significantly elevated pleural neoplasms.

5.4.2 Bakers

Eight malignant pleural mesotheliomas were reported among bakers and pastry cooks in the Rome and Orbassano/Turin Italy area, none of which had radiological evidence of asbestosis.[413] Three cases were among sisters, suggesting a possible genetic role in their etiology. The other four had no familial connections. It has been found that asbestos was used in and around the ovens and other asbestos-containing products during the 1980s and up through the 1990s.[414] Five additional cases of pleural mesothelioma were reported in Italy among bakery workers; however, two may have had other exposures in addition to their bakery work.[415]

5.4.3 Brake Repair and Installation Workers

Mesothelioma has been reported among brake mechanics, their wives and children.[256,258,414,416–420] Huncharek et al.[419] described a 47-year-old lifetime nonsmoking man with pleural mesothelioma whose only known exposure to asbestos occurred while he was a brake mechanic from age 30 to 41 years, with a latency of 17 years. Langer and McCaughey[416] reported only chrysotile fibrils in the lung parenchyma tissue of a 55-year-old brake repair worker of which 10% were longer than 10 μm. They further described that "... besides this submicroscopic chrysotile fiber in brake drum housing there is a more significant source of free, unaltered fiber in the bevelling, refurbishing, and refitting of brake pads. There is thus ample opportunity, during brake maintenance and repair, for contact with chrysotile fibre both in drum debris (where it will usually be in a transformed state) and as long and predominantly unaltered fibres liberated by machining." Langer and McCaughey also reported that pathologic diagnosis of asbestos-related diseases in people exposed to chrysotile is complicated because asbestos-bodies do not form readily. Vianna and Polan[421] reported three mesotheliomas in women having exposure to brake linings. Godwin and Jagatic[422] reported a case of peritoneal meso-thelioma in a 43-year-old man who spent 3 years weaving brake linings made of chrysotile asbestos.

The EPA, in a study by Falgout,[423] clearly shows asbestos fibers are released when asbestos-containing brakes are ground and that they are in sufficient amounts to exceed the 1985 OSHA 15-minute ceiling of 10 fibers/mL as well as the current excursion limit of 1 fiber/mL more than a 30-min time period. In addition to looking at the short-term exposure concentrations in evaluating the risk potential for brake repair and service workers, the range of exposure is crucial because this indicates some workers may be exposed to much higher exposures than the mean or average found. Take for example the results reported by Paustenbach et al.[424] where they reported the mean time-weighted average (TWA) for automobile brake workers at 0.04 fibers/mL, but the high end of the range was 0.68 or six times the current occupational exposure limit, and for truck workers, the mean TWA was 0.2 fibers/mL, with the upper concentration at 1.75 or 175 times greater than the current OSHA standard.

Epidemiological studies have been equivocal. For example, Rushton et al.[425] concluded that their study, although negative, suffered from small numbers of men and that follow-up time would be required to determine any definite causal mortality patterns. Teta et al.[426] reported an RR of 0.65 (calculated 95% CI = 0.08–5.53) for automobile repair and related services when they observed six of 220 cases of mesothelioma found in the Connecticut Tumor Registry from 1955 to 1977. They[426] concluded that difficulties in ascertaining occupational histories in their study population indicated a better need for record keeping and that lack of detailed information regarding the residual cases might obscure the true number of occupationally exposed cases.

Rodelsperger et al.[427] reported that approximately 300,000 mechanics in automotive service stations in Germany are exposed to asbestos. In their clinic, they observed four cases of mesothelioma. The observation of four mesotheliomas from one clinic is clearly not representative of the overall incidence of mesothelioma among brake mechanics in Germany, but it is an indication of risk in this job category. Wong[428] reported that the three cases (actually four) observed by Rodelsperger et al.[427] were not above background. Given there might exist a background level of mesothelioma occurring in the absence of exposure to asbestos, although there is no proof of this, the "natural level" is probably much lower than the 1–2/million/year that has often been cited[237]; therefore, if such a background level is presumed, then 4 of some 300,000 auto repair workers is clearly above background. Jarvholm and Brisman[429] reported no excess of mesothelioma, but a slight increase in lung cancer, among car mechanics. In their cancer linkage study using Swedish census and death registry data, they[429] concluded that because other exposures could not be ruled out, such a study methodology could not answer the question concerning cancers among car mechanics. Hansen[430] reported increases in pleural mesothelioma in Danish auto mechanics. In their study[430] of malignant mesothelioma, and relying on interviews of next of kin, they found a slight excess of mesothelioma among those performing brake lining work or repair, although it was statistically insignificant. They[430] found that 90% of the incidences of pleural mesothelioma among men were directly attributable to past exposures to asbestos. The authors[430] concluded that next-of-kin interviews may have resulted in biased responses. Spirtas et al.[431] reported 33 cases of mesothelioma in persons with a history of performing brake repair work. One of the confounding factors preventing Spirtas et al.[431] from calculating an RR for brake work was that an overwhelming majority of those workers had also been exposed to asbestos as insulators or shipbuilders.

In a study of mesothelioma among car mechanics in Germany, Woitowitz and Rodelsperger[432] found no evidence of an increased risk of mesothelioma but concluded that if there was a mesothelioma risk and, if it was small, it would not be detected and that the absence of fibers in the lung tissue of one of the cases did not exclude the possibility that, decades before, chrysotile fibers were active at the target cells. Teschke et al.[433] did not find an excess of mesothelioma among vehicle mechanics, but because their findings were based on small numbers, judgments about any causal associations would be speculative according to the authors. However, they[433] concluded that most of the mesotheliomas were explainable by exposure to asbestos.

Iwatsubo et al.,[338] in a dose–response study with low levels of asbestos exposure in a French-based case–control study, found that 82% of motor vehicle mechanics had frequent exposure. The authors[338] found a clear dose–response relationship between cumulative exposures and pleural mesothelioma and that a significant excess of mesotheliomas was observed at levels that were probably below the limits adopted in most industrial countries. Henderson[434] reported that 58 mesotheliomas were identified among Australian brake mechanics having no other exposures to asbestos and that only a small fraction of the total 82,827 mechanics in Australia worked with brake blocks or brake linings. Thus, Henderson concluded that these 58 cases represented 1,062,946 person-years and that if one rounds off the total mechanics to 100,000 mechanics, this represents 45 mesotheliomas per million person-years, and if one doubles this number to 200,000 mechanics to include retirees and other workers who moved to other occupations, then the mesothelioma rate becomes 22.6 per million person-years, a rate substantially above the upper limit of the estimated background rate of one to two mesotheliomas per million person-years, or around a 10-fold excess. (There has been litigation testimony refuting some of the findings reported from the Australian Registry; however, the risk of disease among brake mechanics, while reputedly reduced according to this more recent testimony, has never shown or claimed that the risk is eliminated.)

In a reanalysis of the data on lung content for asbestos by Butnor et al. (2003),[436] Roggli et al.[437] and Finkelstein[438] believed that a different interpretation is appropriate. Finkelstein used three tools for comparison of the fiber concentration in the lungs of cases and controls: the t-test, the bootstrap method, and the interval-censored survival analysis. Originally, Butnor et al. wrote "lung burden analysis in automotive brake repair workers with malignant mesothelioma in our series reflect asbestos content within the normal range or elevated commercial amphiboles." Finkelstein found both the mean concentrations for chrysotile and tremolite higher among brake workers than the controls. The three methods of comparison used by Finkelstein were all in agreement with his reanalysis that tremolite but not chrysotile's mean of the log (concentrations) was significantly higher in the lungs of the cases than the controls. It is interesting that Butnor and Roggli classified the noncommercial amphiboles as TAA with no explanation; however, upon examination, Finkelstein concluded the vast majority of the TAA were of the "chemical signature for tremolite." Finkelstein asked, "how could it be possible for the concentrations of a minor contaminant[*] to be higher than the concentrations of the principal commercial fibre?" and "does this exonerate occupational exposure to brake dust as the source of the fibres?" Referring to a paper he and Dufresne[439] wrote, they concluded that tremolite fibers persisted in the lung tissue while chrysotile fibers were cleared more quickly with half-life's varying inversely with fiber length of the chrysotile fibers (the longer >10 μm in length having clearance half-life estimated at ~8 years and ~6 years for fibers 5–10 μm in length). When comparing their reanalyses findings with those for the Quebec chrysotile miners, the results were similar and, because the majority of chrysotile fibers for the brakes came from the Quebec chrysotile mines, that tremolite served as a better marker of exposure to the Quebec chrysotile than the chrysotile itself. Different from the interpretation of Butnor and Roggli, Finkelstein believes the data show automotive mechanics have elevated concentrations of asbestos fibers in their lungs consistent with occupational exposure to commercial chrysotile. Although acknowledging that the asbestos exposures to the miners and millers would have been greater than to the automotive mechanics, however, when it is estimated that 1 million American workers are involved in installing and repairing clutch facings and brake shoes, even a mild increase in risk might have produced cases of asbestos-associated cancers among automotive mechanics.

In another reanalysis of an earlier paper by Spirtas et al.,[431] Hessel et al.[440] performed a case–control study of mesothelioma cases. In their analysis, 147 cases met their selection criteria as being white men with highly or generally reliable work histories and nonmissing response for brake work. Of these, 33 cases and 171 controls were not exposed to any of eight listed activities (furnace or boiler installation or repair, building demolition, plumbing or heating repair, installation or repair, production of textiles, and production of paper products). From this, they[440] identified 12 with occupational exposures that included brake work. In their segregated group without any connection to the eight occupational activities, only one case of mesothelioma was identified with only exposure to brake work and no other occupational exposure out of the original 203 beginning cases of men with mesothelioma. When they compared this one case with the nine controls, the OR for occupational brake work was 0.62 (95% CI = 0.01–4.71) showing no association. Other approaches were also conducted with similar results when controlled for exposures in occupations with known risk of mesothelioma. It was clear to the authors that "the study was limited by the relatively small numbers of brake workers, especially in the analyses that excluded those with other potential asbestos exposures." Very little can be derived from this study because of the limited number of brake workers overall.

There have been at least five papers since 2007 that have reanalyzed brake exposures from historical data as well as collecting some recent data on brake and clutch worker exposures.[441–445] These, all sponsored by the various brake or clutch manufacturers, have findings consistently below the 8 h OSHA TWA of 0.1 fibers/mL >5 μm in length. However, there are other papers before this series that have shown much higher asbestos fiber releases as well as TWAs in excess of the OSHA standard. They also document asbestos exposures away from the brake mechanic to bystanders at distances of 25 to 30 meters from a mechanic when blowing dust from the brakes with compressed air. It has generally taken 15 to 20 min for the asbestos-containing dust to settle until the background concentration of 0.1 fibers/mL is reached.[420,446] During grinding of new brake linings, similar findings have reported high releases of asbestos-containing dust to the worker, even in areas up to 10 meters away from the actual grinding.[420]

What do these multiple studies mean? From preventing asbestos-related disease especially mesothelioma from which there has been no known safe exposure limit, that use of brake and

---

[*] It is estimated that tremolite is a contaminate of chrysotile being around 1% within the asbestos containing dusts, see discussion in the chrysotile and cancer section of this chapter.

clutch materials containing asbestos can release asbestos fibers and put exposed workers at risk. As known from the NIOSH 1976 criteria document,[337] the current OSHA standard of 0.1 fibers/mL as a TWA is not a health-based standard but one based on the reliability of detection at that concentration by the PCM method recommended by OSHA. The OSHA-recommended analytical method using the PCM is also incapable of detecting small asbestos fibers that are nevertheless potentially capable of causing disease.[447] Brake repair workers as a whole have much lower risks of developing an asbestos-related disease as reported by Nicholson[448] in that the probability of an auto maintenance worker's risk of developing an asbestos-related cancer is more than 10 times less than when compared with either asbestos-exposed insulation or manufacturing workers. Therefore, it is not the brake or clutch or the title brake mechanic that is the indicator of risk, but the asbestos exposure resulting from the use of the brake or the clutch by the brake mechanic that results in the risk. Because it is clear that the overall risk is not significant to this group as a whole (brake mechanics), it can still be a significant risk for an individual (brake mechanic) who experiences elevated exposures to asbestos and who may, for reasons we cannot yet define, be more susceptible to developing an asbestos-related disease such as mesothelioma. It should be noted that even in the highest risk categories such as insulators or textile workers exposed to heavy concentrations of asbestos, no more than 10% develop mesothelioma. As stated at the beginning of this section, one cannot determine a worker's risk of an asbestos-related disease by job title or occupational group because it is the individual's own exposure to asbestos within the job or occupational group that determines the risk.

Although the results of these reports and epidemiological studies are equivocal, they by no means exonerate the brake mechanic from being susceptible to a causal relationship between asbestos exposure and mesothelioma. The presence of any asbestos and the fact that asbestos fibers are released during brake repair or installation in this industry is further evidence of this risk (for a more detailed analysis of the totality of evidence that brake repair workers are at risk of asbestos-induced cancers, see Lemen[435]).

5.4.4 Bricklayers and Masons

Brick masons were found to have statistically elevated cancer risks for lung cancer among male construction workers in North Carolina who resided and died in North Carolina during the period 1988–1994.[449] In a survey of unrecognized sources of asbestos exposure in British Columbia, the incidence of mesothelioma in bricklayers resulted in an OR of 3.5 with a 95% CI of 0.9–14 and, although statistically insignificant, the OR was elevated.[433] Swedish bricklayers had an overall SIR of 2.23 (95% CI = 1.34–3.49) for pleural mesothelioma when followed from 1961 to 1998.[224] A national study of 10,400 members of the International Union of Bricklayers and Allied Craftsmen between 1986 and 1991 found proportionate mortality ratios (PMRs) for malignant neoplasms of the trachea, bronchus, and lung with a PMR of 1.37 and asbestosis with a PMR of 5.50.[450]

5.4.5 Carpenters

In a study that identified mesothelioma patients younger than 50 years exposed predominantly to amosite, construction workers predominated with carpenters and three other job titles dominating among these young patients with mesothelioma.[451] In a proportionate mortality study in North Carolina, construction workers and carpenters were found to have an elevated risk of lung cancer.[449] The Connecticut Tumor Registry between 1955 and 1977 found an RR for carpenters and cabinetmakers of 2.25 with a p value of <.05 for mesothelioma.[426] Mesothelioma was reported among carpenters in the Australian Mesothelioma Register.[452] Because of the high numbers of carpenters, they also account for the greatest number of a single occupational group exposed to asbestos in the Australian Mesothelioma Tumor Registry.[453] In an update of mortality among Texaco refinery workers, carpenters and other insulation-related trades were found to have an SMR of 411.[410] In a study of 27,362 members of the Carpenters' Union who died between 1987 and 1990, asbestosis had a PMR of 283 (95% CI = 158–457), and there were a total of 121 mesotheliomas.[454] A survey of 631 asbestos-exposed construction carpenters found excess pleural plaques and interstitial fibrosis.[455] In Northern Ireland between 1985 and 1994, carpenters and joiners were found to have a PMR of 397 for pleural cancers (mesothelioma) that was statistically significant at the 5% level (lower limit = 245 and upper limit = 607) as well as for asbestosis, which had a PMR of 628, also statistically significant (lower limit = 329 and upper limit = 1095).[456]

5.4.6 Custodial Workers, Laborers, and Maintenance Workers

Among the statistics from the Australian Mesothelioma Registry between 1980 and 1985, laborers represented the greatest percentage of jobs with mesothelioma (14.8%).[405] Among 11,685 members of the Laborers' International Union of North America who died between 1985 and 1988, there was a statistically significant elevated mortality risk for lung cancer (N = 1208, proportionate cancer mortality ratio [PCMR] = 1.06, 95% CI = 1.00–1.12) and 20 mesothelioma deaths.[457] Anderson et al.[458] x-rayed 457 school maintenance and custodial workers and found conditions consistent with asbestos-induced diseases, including pleural abnormalities, that could not be explained by work before that of their present occupation. Laborers at the schools with more than 20 years of employment had the highest prevalence of abnormalities. Churg and Warnock[459] found asbestos bodies in the lungs of 21 patients in the general population who had 300–9000 asbestos bodies/g, which the authors claim is a concentration frequently found in manual laborers among the general population who were not primary asbestos workers. Churg and Warnock concluded that laborers were at likely risk for occupational exposure to asbestos, thus confirming that laborers are at risk of developing an asbestos-related disease. Almost 660 custodians employed by the New York City Board of Education were examined between 1985 and 1987 for asbestos-related disease and 39% of those with 35 years of employment had abnormal films.[460] Eighty-four percent reported removing asbestos and 89% reported working in areas where asbestos was present and abated. In a study of male employees at one California school district, 13.3% of custodians were found to have asbestos-related disease, and because these were related to parenchymal and pleural fibrosis, it would indicate rather high exposures of asbestos to these custodial workers.[461] Oliver et al.[462] found pleural plaques above background and restrictive lung disease among 120 white male public school custodians in the Boston school district. Among the total group, the percentage of distribution of pleural plaques increased with latency for those having no other outside exposure to asbestos. In a multicentric (Paris, Caen, and Lyon) cross-sectional study of 227 custodian and maintenance workers in buildings containing friable asbestos-containing material and with generally low exposures (82% had fewer than 5 fibers/mL-years), the authors[463] found pleural thickening, particularly circumscribed pleural thickening, was significantly higher in the exposed group when compared with the nonexposed control group of 87 when it came to latency from first exposure but not with duration of exposure. No other significant differences were seen between the exposed and nonexposed groups. The authors[463] concluded there were no differences between profusion categories of the exposed versus nonexposed group because the cumulative asbestos exposures were probably insufficient, as was suggested by Doll and Peto,[304] who found such changes after 25 fibers/mL-years or higher.

5.4.7 Decorators

One case of pleural mesothelioma was reported in a female decorator where spray-on crocidolite asbestos was her only known exposure to asbestos.[464] When the new duty to manage asbestos regulation came out in England in May 2004, the notion that some occupational groups may be unwittingly exposed to asbestos identified decorators among them.[465]

5.4.8 Electricians

Selikoff and Hammond[466] included electricians as a trade with a high risk of asbestos-related disease, particularly in those employed in shipyards for more than 20 years. Electricians had a non-significant excess of mesothelioma with an RR of 1.29 on the basis of data from the Connecticut Tumor Registry.[426] In a study of more than 1000 welders and electricians of shipyard workers in England, nine cases of mesothelioma among electricians were recorded.[467] Coggon et al.[468] found from hospital registry data of 2942 cancer cases in four English counties between 1975 and 1980 that electricians were one group where mesotheliomas were found to cluster. Statistically significant lung cancer excess has also been reported among electricians by Menck and Henderson.[469]

In a survey of materials sprayed on the ceilings of 127 buildings throughout the United States, asbestos was found in approximately 50% of the buildings.[470] Chrysotile was the main fiber type identified. During renovation activities, the average fiber concentration in workers' breathing zones was less than 2 fibers/cm^3 but exceeded 0.1 fibers/cm^3, with some workers exposed to higher concentrations averaging 16.4 fibers/cm^3. Electricians were included among the workers studied. Electricians had a twofold excess of mesotheliomas in a study of national population-based registries linking cancer incidence from 1961 to 1979 with 1960 census data on industry and occupation for all employed individuals in Sweden.[471] A cross-sectional epidemiological study of a small group of nonshipyard electricians found asbestosis in 15 of them and in 25% for those with 20 years or more of service.[472] In a survey of unrecognized sources of asbestos exposure in British Columbia, the incidence of mesothelioma in electricians was elevated with an OR of 3.0 and a 95% CI of 0.08–12, although this was statistically insignificant.[433]

In a study which identified mesothelioma patients younger than 50 years exposed predominantly to amosite as determined by lung burden analysis, construction workers, predominantly electricians, and three other job titles were among those young patients with mesothelioma.[451] Swedish male electrical workers followed between 1961 and 1998 had an SIR for mesothelioma of 1.92 (95% CI = 1.49–2.44).[224] Cases of asbestosis were found to be elevated in several trades (between 20% and 30%), including electricians who experienced 24.4%.[473] In 1976, Harries et al.[474] reported ship-yard workers to have a 9.1% increase in mesothelioma. Singh et al.[475] studied a case of mesothelioma in an electrician who had been exposed to asbestos 35 years earlier. In a NIOSH Health Hazard Evaluation of a General Electric Plant in Evendale, Ohio,[476] two deceased electricians were found to have lung tissue samples containing 23 and 15.5 million asbestos fibers per gram, whereas lung tissue from those nonoccupationally exposed had only approximately 140,000 fibers/g. Both electricians had asbestosis and one had colon cancer. In two industrial areas in Northern Italy, Ciccone et al.[477] reported from a case–control study that electricians had an OR of 2.2 for lung cancer. An epidemiology study[478] of asbestos-related chest radiograph changes among a shipyard population on the U.S. West Coast found the prevalence ratio after age adjustment in high asbestos exposure shops to be 4.8 among electricians and mechanics in the shop. In the intermediate asbestos-exposed shop, electricians had a prevalence ratio of 2.47. In the two lowest asbestos-exposed shops, electricians had radiographic prevalence ratios of 2.17 and 1.50. Overall, the prevalence of pleural plaques was highest in workers who had ever smoked and who worked in shops that had the highest asbestos exposures. The prevalence ratio in this respect was 2.33 for smokers compared with 1.49 in non-smokers. The authors[478] concluded "the data presented in this article show that there is an exposure–response relationship between the asbestos exposure index and prevalence rates of pleural plaques in a shipyard workplace."

Huncharek and Muscat[479] reported mesothelioma in a 38-year-old nonshipyard electrician with a 15-year work history. In a series of case–control studies in New Zealand, the authors,[480] using the New Zealand Cancer Registry, identified electricians among one of the highest occupational groups for developing asbestos-related cancers. In a multicenter case–control study looking at lung cancers not attributed to tobacco smoke, electricians were found to have an adjusted OR of 1.7 (95%

CI = 1.1–2.9).[481] The authors[481] suggested that this higher risk for lung cancer may be due to exposure to asbestos experienced by their profession. Among Italian railroad workers, Maltoni et al.[482] found electricians to be second among the five highest job categories reporting the largest number of mesotheliomas.

NIOSH reported a PMR of 406, which was statistically significant at $p < .01$ for malignant neoplasms of the pleura.[483] A statistically significant excess of 10 mesotheliomas was reported to occur among 2300 Italian oil refinery workers, one of which was an electrician.[484] Peto et al.[485] reported that their analysis of occupations, as recorded on death certificates, included electricians among the largest high-risk group for mesotheliomas and that those in construction and building maintenance made up the largest group. In a survey of unrecognized sources of asbestos exposure in British Columbia,[433] the incidence of mesothelioma in electricians resulted in an OR of 3.0 with a 95% CI of .08–12 that, although statistically insignificant, was elevated. A NIOSH study[486] found a PMR of 2.4 for mesothelioma among electricians when evaluating mesothelioma trends of mortality and incidence in the United States. The Italian National Mesothelioma Registry found electricians to be one of the most common occupations for developing mesothelioma.[487]

Fiber drift is a significant exposure hazard as shown by measurements taken in the construction industry when they measured fiber counts from spraying asbestos onto buildings. The authors[281] found 70 fibers/mL at 10 ft. from the nozzle of the spray gun and 3 fibers/mL at 25 ft. from the nozzle. This shows that not only were the spray operators at risk of exposure but also the auxiliary workers such as carpenters, pipefitters, welders, electricians, plumbers, and so forth.

McElvenny et al. [488] described exposure to asbestos by many electricians as secondary exposure. Other reports have described electricians with pleural plaques mesothelioma or to be at potential risk of developing an asbestos-related disease.[489–492] Mesothelioma in electricians had the sixth highest PMR (264) among men aged 16–74 years in Great Britain between 1991 and 2000. In the construction industry in Great Britain, electricians with no other high risk jobs had a mesothelioma rate of 14.6 (95% CI = 7.5–28.4).[241] Coggon et al.[493] reported a PMR of 349 for electricians in the construction and engineering industries in the United Kingdom. Robinson et al.,[494] in a mortality study of the U.S. members of the International Brotherhood of Electrical Workers who worked primarily in the construction industry, reported PMRs for lung cancer of 117, for asbestosis of 247, and for mesothelioma of 356. McDonald et al.[451] reported an OR of 5.0 (5% CI = 3.4–7.1) among electricians in the construction industry in a case-referent study where most of the workers were employed before 1970.

5.4.9 Jewelers

Jewelers have been exposed to asbestos through the use of asbestos powder and have been found to develop pleural plaques alone and with asbestosis as well as mesothelioma.[471,495,496] Dossing and Langer[497] reported four cases among retired jewelers—two with pleural plaques and parenchymal changes, one with isolated pleural plaques, and one with only parenchymal infiltrates.

5.4.10 Mechanics

Pleural plaques were found in 41 car mechanics but in none of the referents; however, no apparent impairment was detected among 925 car mechanics and 109 referents as reported by Marcus et al.[498] Because pleural plaques are an indicator of asbestos exposure, the risk of asbestos disease among auto mechanics is possible. In the study by Dahlqvist et al.[499] of low-level exposure to asbestos among vehicle mechanics, the authors found slight small airway dysfunction and a dose–response relationship between asbestos exposure and closing volume, a finding not previously reported. The authors[499] suggested that such exposure initially might cause involvement of both terminal and respiratory bronchioles, which thereafter develops into diffuse interstitial fibrosis. Auto mechanics and plumbers had an increased rate of lung cancer in a case–control study of welders with exposure to asbestos.[500] In a survey of cancer by occupational groups, mechanics were among those with the highest incidence of pleural cancers over more than a 20-year period in Nordic Countries.[501] Mechanics had an increase in mesothelioma according to Australian mesothelioma registry data, indicating an increase within the asbestos user industries.[452] In a survey of Hungarian workers[197] with lung tumors who were exposed to asbestos, 72 of 297 patients (24%) had cumulative occupational asbestos exposures assessed below 25 fiber-years (between 0.01 and 23.9 fiber-years). Among this group, car and truck mechanics were identified.

5.4.11 Merchant Seamen

Studies have been conducted of merchant seamen involved in the building, maintenance, and repair of sea-going vessels, the majority of which have shown an excess of asbestos-related diseases, including asbestosis, lung cancer, and mesothelioma. Routine maintenance at sea can result in high exposures to asbestos when fibers are disturbed, become airborne, and are of respirable size, thus putting merchant seamen at an increased risk of developing asbestos-related diseases. In fact, the U.S. Maritime Commission studies found that long after the vessel had been at sea, it was not unusual to find flaking and cracking of asbestos-containing materials because of the vibration and motion of the vessel at sea. Therefore, the hazards of asbestos exposures were not confined to shipbuilders alone but also to the vessel's crew.[502] In some studies, asbestos-induced lung changes were detected in more than 40% of radiographs studied. One study of radiological abnormalities among 3324 U.S. merchant marine seamen found the highest prevalence of asbestotic changes among those who served in the engine department (391/920; 42.5%) when compared with other departments (deck: 301/820, 36.6%; steward: 278/981, 28.4%) or multiple departments (167/541, 30.9%).[503] Further, Selikoff et al.[503] estimated that all vessels delivered before 1975 contained extensive asbestos-insulating material aboard and that most vessels delivered between 1975 and 1978 might have some asbestos in the form of insulating cement on machinery casings, although most other uses of asbestos aboard ship had been reduced.

In 1918, the first report of radiological change among asbestos-exposed workers included those of a marine fireman.[51] Selikoff et al.[503] further referenced reports of subsequent incidences of parenchymal fibrosis, pleural plaques, pseudo-tumors, lung cancer, and mesothelioma. In their study of marine engineers, Jones et al.[504] reported knowledge of mesothelioma in addition to asbestotic pleural changes. Greenberg[505] reported that seamen experienced an excess mortality from cancer for the past 100 years and that in a preliminary mortality analysis of a small population of merchant seamen, two cases of malignant mesothelioma were identified, and that in the United Kingdom's National Mesothelioma Register, 28 cases were reported in seamen, which represents a "markedly excessive" number. Two mesotheliomas were reported among Greek merchant seamen—one in a marine engineer with 35 years service and the other in a deck department seaman with 25 years service.[506] A mortality study of Italian merchant seamen[507] reported one mesothelioma and an excess of respiratory cancer (36 observed vs. 19.8 expected), drawing the authors[507] to conclude that because of the observation of a mesothelioma, asbestos may have been responsible for the excess respiratory cancers. A 79-year-old man was found to have pleural plaques on x-ray 6 years before he developed lung cancer.[508] He had been a farmer the majority of his life, but at age 26 years he had served as a boiler man on a battle cruiser for 1 year during World War II, which was his only known exposure to asbestos. He was a 26-pack-year smoker and had 3348 asbestos bodies per gram dry lung tissue. In a case–control study of merchant seamen between 1960 and 1980,[509] lung cancer was shown to have increased with duration of employment and had an OR of 1.68 (95% CI = 1.17–2.41) for engine crews after 3 years whereas deck officers did not. Deck officers on icebreakers had an increased OR of 3.41 (95% CI = 1.23–9.49) after 20 or more years of employment. The same study found that mesothelioma among engine room workers was increased to 9.75 (95% CI = 1.88–50.6) after 20 years latency. Kidney cancer among deck officers increased after 3 years of employment (OR = 2.15, 95% CI = 1.14–4.08). Swedish seamen from the Gothenburg area had an SIR of 7.43 (95% CI = 3.54–13.72) in 1960 and when followed through 1970 had an SIR of 4.27 (95% CI = 0.80–12.63).[224] Overall, Swedish seamen had an SIR of 2.83 (95% CI = 1.41–5.09). Cancer incidence among marine engineers was elevated in those followed between 1955 and 1998 for both lung cancer (SIR = 1.2, 95% CI = 1.0–1.5) and for stomach cancer (SIR = 1.3, 95% CI = 1.0–1.5).[510] When controlled for smoking through questionnaires on a sample of the cohort (n = 1501), the lung cancer risk was elevated (SIR = 1.4, 95% CI = 1.2–1.8) as was the risk for mesothelioma (SIR = 4.8, 95% CI = 1.3–12.3) and urinary bladder cancer (SIR = 1.3, 95% CI = 1.0–1.8) after 40-years latency. A series of 50 seamen from the Trieste-Monfalcone area of Italy were diagnosed with pleural mesothelioma between 1973 and 2003.[511] They ranged in age between 53 and 91 years. Twenty-four were in the Italian Navy, 17 in the Italian Merchant Navy, and 9 in both. Asbestos bodies were found in 55% of 38 necropsy cases. Asbestos bodies were elevated in the lung (between 2100 and 7000 per gram of dried tissue). Latency ranged from 33 to 72 years (mean = 56.1). The authors[511] concluded that although the seamen showed signs of less intense exposure than shipyard workers, their latency was longer. Airborne asbestos has been generally low in seamen; however, this can vary depending upon the work being done on the ship both at sea or in port. Lemen[512] reported on two ships in port stating that PCM samples ranged from 0.001 to 0.152 fibers/cm^3 and greater than 5 μm in length, and in ships at sea the concentrations were somewhat lower. However, samples taken at the Long Beach Naval Shipyard during asbestos removal operations were much higher, with average counts of 40 fibers/mL and some as high as 150 fibers/mL, showing that ships maintained at sea could generate exposures in these higher ranges. A paper examining historical industrial hygiene data onboard maritime shipping vessels between 1978 and 1992 found PCM in crew quarters, common areas, and so forth, to be around 0.004 fibers/mL with samples in the engine room and machine shops somewhat higher at 0.010 fibers/mL.[513] In this reanalysis of historic samples, the authors[513] reported approximately 1.3% of the samples exceeded 0.1 fibers/mL, but none were above 1 fiber/mL. In 1978, 17.0% of 53 samples were above the 0.01 fibers/mL OSHA Standard, which was the highest percentage for any 1 year reported. Most other years were none except for the year 1980 in which 5.7% exceeded the OSHA Standard. Both reports show concentrations below many other occupational groups, but as I, Lemen,[512] pointed out, the activity is very influential to the amount of exposure, and it should not be concluded that the risk is negligible when certain operations onboard ship, whether at sea or in port, can expose seamen to very high concentrations of airborne asbestos fibers. The finding of asbestos-related disease and cancers including mesothelioma reported in this section on merchant seamen attest to the elevated risks among some seamen.

5.4.12 Painters

At the Devonport Dockyard, 53 deaths from mesothelioma were observed in workers employed since 1966. Painters were found to have been one of the most affected.[229] Painters were found to have a mesothelioma SIR of 199 using union records to search tumor registries.[514] In a case–control study of New York painters and members of the International Brotherhood of Painters and Allied Trades,[515] a 3.6-fold excess of lung cancer was identified. Painters using spackling compounds known to have contained asbestos had an estimated OR of 4.33 (95% CI = 1.40–13.96) when compared with cancer controls and an OR of 6.33 (95% CI = 2.04–19.68) compared with noncancer controls.

A study of occupational risks in Sweden between 1961 and 1979 found painters had an SIR for pleural mesothelioma of 2.31 ($p < .05$). In British Columbia, 51 incident cases of mesothelioma were compared with 154 population-based controls where painters were found to have an OR = 4.5 (95% CI = 1.0–24).[433]

5.4.13 Petrochemical Workers

The U.S. Bureau of Mines published an information circular in November 1936 outlining "Some Problems of Respiratory Protection in the Petroleum Industry, with suggestions for their Solution."[516] In this circular, they specifically mentioned asbestosis caused by breathing "fine particles" of asbestos. They further stated that the dust need not be visible to be dangerous and that no one seemed to be able to state with exactness the safe size and number of dust particles that might be in the air without causing harm. The circular provided detailed measures to protect workers from these "fine particles" and concluded by stating that the "forward-looking employer will take steps to become fully informed."

"Because it is the duty of industry to protect its employees and because no comprehensive survey of the hazards incident to occupational dust problems had yet been made, it was felt that here was an opportunity to render a service to the petroleum industry and its employees by making such a survey." These were the words of Willard J. Denno, MD, in the forward to the survey of Dust Producing Operations in the Production of Petroleum Products and Associated Activities sponsored by the Standard Oil Company (New Jersey) in July 1937.[517] This survey reported on the use of insulation within the petrochemical industry and discussed the hazards associated with the use of asbestos-containing insulation and outline measures for reducing the hazard. This survey reviewed the medical literature to date, which found that asbestos dust did not seem to be readily handled by the protective mechanism of the respiratory system. The author of the survey report, Roy Bonsib, used much of the knowledge he gained from the 1937 survey to author *Safeguarding Petroleum Refineries and Their Workers* for the ILO, which he published in 1943.[518] This report[518] discussed the many hazards found in petroleum refineries, one of which was asbestos, and recommended preventive methods to protect workers from asbestos-related diseases.

In 1949, the Standard Oil Company (New Jersey) commenced a "Summary of the Plant Industrial Hygiene Problems" authored by Berry et al.[519] The report was marked *Company Confidential—Not For Publication In Present Form*. The report discussed the extensive use of asbestos in the refinery and the problem with high concentrations of asbestos dust. The report also discussed asbestos and its relationship to fibrosis and cancer of the lungs and identified various trades at risk, including brick masons and helpers, insulators, laborers, and pipe benders.

Between 1949 and 1957, an industry-wide effort was sponsored by the Medical Advisory Committee of the American Petroleum Institute to assess the possible skin cancer hazard to petroleum workers; however, this study was terminated on July 1, 1956, primarily because of the lack of cooperation within the industry itself.[520] The terminated report found that the proportion of tumors of the digestive system and peritoneum was much larger than that found in the United States as a whole.

In 1960, two cases of primary malignant mesothelioma of the pleura were reported in a 57- and 58-year-old refinery foremen.[521] The first case had previously been reported in detail by the author in 1956.[522] Many additional studies since 1960 have discussed the hazards of asbestos in the petroleum refinery industry.[523–538] In follow-up to a 1992 study of a Canadian petroleum company,[539] with the exception of mesothelioma, no clear excesses in work-related mortality were observed. For mesothelioma, no cases were observed in women and the risk for men increased overall to an SMR of 3.51 (95% CI = 2.25–5.22). An SMR of 8.68 (95% CI = 5.51–13.03) was observed in the operating segments mainly among mechanical workers and pipefitters. Cancers of the large intestine, except the rectum, were also higher than expected with a significant SMR of 1.98 (95% CI = 1.24–3.00) in the marine section of employment.[540] Satin et al.,[541] in an update of two California petroleum refineries between 1950 and 1995, found no excess of mortality for any asbestos-related diseases. Although the study consisted of a very large number of person-years at risk, criticism has been levied that because of the strong healthy worker effect, the study suffered from dilution, which may indicate a comparison bias concealing association.[542] For those asbestos-related diseases of long latency, the inclusion of workers employed after December 31, 1980, could also dilute the cohort for risk of long latent diseases like mesothelioma, which generally has a much longer latency period and masks any causal associations. Five mesotheliomas were reported in the cohort by death certificate. In addition, the authors should have attempted to segregate those with potential exposure to asbestos from those with no potential exposure.[*]

An update of the mortality data from a refinery in Louisiana found three mesotheliomas but could not calculate an SMR for comparison with national data, as the authors[544] stated, because no mortality rates were available for mesothelioma. However, when the authors[544] compared this mortality to data from the SEER program, they calculated a nonstatistical excess SMR of 2.16 (95% CI = 0.44–6.30). As the expected mortality was calculated using SEER incidence rates, this may be misleading. This study had a total of 68,881 person-years among the 3579 men making up the cohort and, when compared with the most recent mesothelioma mortality data from Louisiana that reports 1.4 deaths occurring out of each 100,000 population, this study's expected mortality from mesothelioma may have been overestimated, thus underestimating the SMR and its 95% CI.[544,545]

5.4.14 Plasterers and Drywall Workers

Nicholson et al.,[546] in a survey of men applying and finishing tape and spackle at the joints of wallboard, found that 60% of the personal samples exceeded the recommended exposure limit by NIOSH of 2 fibers/cm^3 greater than 5 µm in length per milliliter, and two-thirds of the 69 workers with at least 10 years exposure had radiographic abnormalities (37 of 63; 59%). The authors[546] suggested that asbestos disease was an important hazard in this industry.

Rohl et al.,[287] in a study of consumer spackling and patching compounds, found asbestos in 5 of 15 spackling and patching compounds and in all 10 drywall taping compounds. Using both optical and electron microscopes, the asbestos fibers ranged in length from 0.25 to 8.0 µm, and those shorter than 5 µm in length would only be found using electron microscopy and not the PCM method. Both spackling and taping compounds consisted of most fibers <3 µm in diameter or length. Using PCM, it was found that airborne concentrations of 5 fibers/mL of air were common and that they lingered in the air at high concentrations even after 15 min. Furthermore, it was found that for every visible fiber seen using the PCM method, there were 200 to 1000 that could only be seen using the electron microscope. These findings have further implications to their use in home repair than just to the worker, but also to the family members because the fibers stay airborne for long periods of time. According to the authors,[287] none of the samples had warning labels.

Fischbein et al.[547] further confirmed the risk of asbestos-related disease among drywall construction workers. Residential and commercial drywall workers were found to have exposures to concentrations of asbestos dust as high as 12.4 fibers/cm^3 from dry joint compound, mixing of a paste premix produced 1.2–3.2 fibers/cm^3, and that when sanding the drywall, the highest concentrations were encountered at 2.1–24.2 fibers/cm^3. Dry sweeping of the waste resulted in concentrations of 4–25.5 fibers/cm^3.[548]

In a PMR study of unionized construction plasterers and cement masons,[549] statistically significant elevated mortality occurred among plasterers for asbestosis (PMR = 1657, $p < .01$) and lung cancer (PMR = 162, $p < .01$). Forty mesotheliomas were recorded out of 9449 death certificates examined individually. Of the 3745 cancer deaths included in the study cohort, only four mesotheliomas were found. The authors[549] stated that although the risk was elevated (PMR = 188), it was statistically insignificant, and although one-third of the cohort were plasterers, 50% died of mesothelioma. The author's[549] pointed out that the underreporting of mesothelioma ($n = 4$) in their cohort was because the ICD code for mesothelioma did not include all sites where mesothelioma can occur,

---

[*] A note concerning the HWE that Richard Monson states in his text *Occupational Epidemiology*, 2nd ed., "However, it might be argued that because of the HWE (or because of some other bias), SMRs greater than the all-causes SMR should be considered in excess. Intuitively, one assesses such excess by dividing each cause-specific SMR by the all-causes SMR to obtain a 'corrected' SMR (CSMR)."[543]

and thus most mesotheliomas were coded into other death categories. As a result, those mesotheliomas not coded as mesothelioma were not counted by the National U.S. Death Index, resulting in a large undercount of mesothelioma deaths. Of the 40 mesotheliomas, 24 were not specified as to site, 7 were categorized as pleural mesothelioma or pleural cancer (unspecified) and 9 were categorized as being of the lung (unspecified). The risk of lung cancer among plasterers continued to be elevated among those entering the union after 1970. In cement masons, stomach cancer was statistically significant (PCMR = 133, $p < .01$).[549]

In a study of asbestos exposure during drywall abatement work,[550] it was found that personal time-weighted average samples ranged from 0.12 to 3.16 fibers/cm³, which were above the current OSHA PEL of 0.1 fibers/cm³. Lange and Thomulka,[550] upon further study, concluded that when abatement workers were trained and followed OSHA requirements as well as the Pennsylvania Department of Labor and Industry requirements concerning friable asbestos-containing materials, exposures might be kept low and the likelihood of exceeding the OSHA standard was less than 5%.

NIOSH, in conjunction with the National Center for Health Statistics, reported between 1987 and 1996 that various work groups had extremely elevated PMRs for pleural malignancies, including plasterers, at 11.61 (95% CI = 3.76–27.13).[245]

5.4.15 Plumbers and Pipefitters

Among mesothelioma cases from the Connecticut Tumor Registry,[426] plumbers and pipefitters had an RR of 3.87 with a p value of <.05. In a preliminary case–control study of welders conducted by Jockel et al.,[551] auto mechanics and plumbers had an increased rate of lung cancer probably associated with asbestos. A cross-sectional study found plumbers and pipefitters, especially plumbers, exposed to asbestos had an excess of radiographic abnormalities.[552] In a survey of unrecognized sources of asbestos exposure in British Columbia, the incidence of mesothelioma in plumbers and pipefitters resulted in an OR of 8.3 (95% CI = 1.5–86).[433] In a study of radiologic and pulmonary function effects of asbestos-induced pleural thickening,[553] 19% had parenchymal fibrosis and 29% had pleural thickening. Those with pleural thickening had decrements in pulmonary function with pleural abnormalities increasing with length of exposure. Small airway disease was found among 701 Copenhagen plumbers in which 23 were never smokers and who had removed asbestos insulation and had intermittently been exposed to high levels of asbestos for about 25 years without being exposed to welding fumes.[554] Bilateral pleural thickening was found in 28 (18.3%) of 153 plumbers and pipefitters employed in building construction.[555] In a study of 7121 members and retirees of the United Association of Plumbers and Pipefitters in California who died between 1960 and 1979, PMRs were elevated for lung cancers (PMR = 1.41) and 16 mesotheliomas were identified.[556] The SIR for pleural mesothelioma was 4.56 (95% CI = 3.42–5.95) among Swedish male plumbers followed between 1961 and 1998.[224] Gaskets, which are used by plumbers and pipefitters, have been shown to release respirable fibers of asbestos exceeding both the previous 15 min and current 30 min OSHA excursion limits and, in some cases, the OSHA 8 h TWA.[557]

5.4.16 Power Plant Workers

Asbestos has been used in power-generating plants for thermal insulation of steam pipes and turbines. Asbestos can be found in many electric conductors such as electrodes wrapped with asbestos-containing yarn. Cable and wiring may also contain asbestos insulation, as does field-coil wrapping used on electrical machinery.[46] Laggers (pipefitters) stripping asbestos off steam pipes, generating clouds of asbestos-containing dust, were found to have pneumoconiosis.[558] As warned by Bonsib,[517] the use of asbestos outside of the manufacturing process could pose a problem. In 1963, another article[324] warned that controls for asbestos must be expanded beyond the mining and manufacturing industries to other industries, including power stations.

Fontaine and Trayer[559] noted that the Tennessee Valley Association had been engaged in asbestos control for about 30 years (i.e., 1945) and reported levels of asbestos, even when using control measures, reached 4.7 fibers/cm^3. The authors[559] noted that not only were control measures to be used, but training was a key factor in controlling asbestos. Other studies have validated the existence of asbestos use within the electric power-generating industry.[560–562] In general, asbestos fibers counts have been low except in areas where mixing of asbestos for insulation occurs and evidence of ferruginous bodies have been found in the sputum of workers in power plants.[563] In 1975, at the 18th International Conference on Occupational Health in Brighton England, which I attended, a paper by Dr. J. Bonnell was presented on insulation workers (laggers) from British power plants in which eight mesotheliomas were discussed. The authors[564] stated that in 1949, a case of asbestosis was reported in a lagger employed at a power plant for 13 years. Bonnell et al.[564] indicated that these cases of asbestos-related diseases presented in his paper were not indicative of the measure of the prevalence or the incidence of the diseases because many of the cases were only diagnosed after retirement. Cammarano et al.[565] found an excess mortality of cancer associated with asbestos in an Italian thermoelectric power plant where asbestos, mainly amosite, was used as an insulating material on turbines, boilers, and pipes and where workers were exposed during periodic removal for maintenance. These cancers included lung, laryngeal, stomach, and colon cancer. Forastiere et al.[566] also reported an excess of respiratory cancers in Italian thermoelectric power plant workers, especially among maintenance workers, suggesting past exposure to known respiratory carcinogens, including asbestos.

Two cases of mesothelioma have been described in detail in a clerk and an insulator at an electric power-generating plant in Israel.[567] Another paper from the International Agency for Research on Cancer (IARC) reiterates that asbestos was used in electricity-generating plants and that asbestos is carcinogenic.[568] A Russian study[569] found insulation workers in thermoelectric power plants had asbestos exposures in concentrations sufficient to cause disease and that these exposures were above maximum allowable concentrations in Russia. Four mesotheliomas were reported among workers at three Italian power plants and three additional mesotheliomas were reported by physician records from Tuscany.[570] The cases ranged in age from 46 to 60 years and exposures ranged from 21 to 40 years. Three cases were among maintenance workers, one case was an insulator, one case was a handler of asbestos-containing insulation products, one case was a cleaner, and the last case was a clerk.

In a study of active male workers of Electricite de France-Gaz de France in association with asbestos exposure,[534] asbestosis was stated to have an OR of 57.4 (95% CI = 17.0–194.0) in the highest exposure group. Pleural cancer had an OR of 4.8 (95% CI = 1.2–19.8) and lung cancer had significant ORs of 2.0 (95% CI = 1.3–3.2) and 1.9 (95% CI = 1.2–3.0) in the two highest exposure groups. The cell type most related to asbestos-exposed cases was squamous. Laryngeal cancers showed a tendency toward a nonsignificant increase in ORs in the highest exposure categories but disappeared when adjusted for confounders. The authors[534] concluded that their study showed that occupational exposure to asbestos could increase the risk of pleural cancers in areas of the plant where exposures were not considered high as compared with other industrial settings.

Asbestos exposure accounted for significant excesses of lung and pleural cancers in men employed in Danish utility companies.[571] Although a study of geothermal power plants at Larderello, Italy, reported no significant excess of mortality from asbestos-related cancers, two cases of mesothelioma were found among the less than 40% of the workforce with any exposure to asbestos.[572] Although one of the mesotheliomas occurred in a worker with prior asbestos exposure before working at the power plant, the other did not. The overall mortality indicated a significant healthy worker effect and, with the known use of asbestos-containing materials in the plant, may have had a more significant meaning than that concluded by the authors. Three cases of fatal extrapulmonary neoplasm were reported among power plant workers in Israel who were exposed to asbestos.[573] A low prevalence of 1.3% in asbestos-related lung abnormalities was reported among 3063 power plant maintenance workers.[574] The authors[574] stated this represented the success of prevention in the control of asbestos in this industry.

A Lebanese study group studied the cancer incidence among Australian nuclear industry workers and found pleural cancers to be in excess (SIR = 17.71, 95% CI = 7.96–39.43), although no association with radiation exposure was established; thus, a strong link to asbestos was indicated.[575] A mortality study of U.K. electrical generation and transmission workers between 1973 and 2002 reported significant excess deaths in male power plant workers from neoplasms of the pleura (observed 129 vs. 30.3 expected; SMR = 426, 95% CI = 356–506) and from peritoneal cancer (14 observed vs. 7.6 expected; SMR = 185, 95% CI = 101–310).[576]

5.4.17 Railroad Workers

The knowledge of the American Railway Association Medical and Surgical Section as it pertains to dust, asbestos exposures, and disease dates back to the 1930s.[292,577–585] Their first entry in 1932 discusses dust as an industrial hazard which demands attention and causes pneumoconiosis, pathologically described as fibrosis of the lungs.[577] A discussion of the prevention of pneumoconiosis stated: "Dust pathology of the lungs can be prevented in two ways, first, by the adequate and proper use of water to wet down the dust at the point of its origin; second, by forced ventilation to quickly remove the dust particles and replace this with clear air."

The next entry in 1933 also discussed ways to control dust, stating: "The subject of dust as an industrial hazard has been presented for consideration by the committee. The subject cannot be considered as inherently [as] a railroad problem; however, it may arise in connection with various lines of work [in the railroad industry], and when it does so, presents a problem which demands attention ... use of water to wet down the dust at the point of origin, or by forced ventilation to remove the dust particles. In the event that neither of these methods is practicable, respirators should be made available to employees [sic] who are required to work in the presence of the dust."

In 1935, at the 15th meeting of the Association of American Railroads Medical and Surgical Section,[292] the term *asbestosis*, the pneumoconiosis caused specifically from breathing asbestos fibers, was used: Pneumoconiosis (pneumon—lung; konis—dust) is a condition that may be caused by any kind of dust entering the lung; but we as railroad surgeons are undoubtedly more interested in silicosis and asbestosis than other types. "... asbestosis is caused by breathing fine fibres of asbestos which consists of magnesium calcium silicate. Asbestosis is not a common condition but it causes extensive pulmonary fibrosis and takes on a more rapid course than does silicosis."

The minutes of the Association of American Railroads Medical and Surgical Section continued to specifically recommend prevention methods, including education, eliminating dust, wetting down the dust, use of respirators, and analysis of the work air to ensure that the suppression of the dust was effective. These were specifically discussed for the years 1935, 1937, 1939, 1940, 1951, 1952, 1953, 1957, and 1958.[292,577–585]

Asbestos has been used in the railroad industry in a variety of ways, including insulation for railroad shops, wrapping around the boilers of locomotives, insulation in the driving cabins and carriages of locomotives, in asbestos cement ties, and for other heat-transfer protection.[482,586] Railroad workers at risk of exposure to asbestos include workers engaged in repair, demolition, technical control, maintenance (including machinists), handling waste materials, and railroad construction and maintenance. Other workers at risk of exposure to asbestos include locomotive engineers, electricians, joiners, painters, laborers, brake men, station maintenance workers, pipefitters, riggers, insulators, fitters, finishers, polishers, mechanics, and other ancillary workers who work in close proximity to others directly exposed to asbestos. There have been numerous reports of asbestos-related diseases in railroad workers.[482,586–589]

It was reported in 1997 by the announcement of the French railroad SNCF that 30 rail workers had died since 1988 from asbestos-related disease, whereas another 120 current or former employees had been diagnosed with health conditions related to on-the-job exposure to asbestos.[590] The main French rail workers' union estimated that asbestos-related health conditions kill 97 rail workers annually.[590]

Railroad carriage construction and repair workers experienced elevated risks of lung cancer (26 cases; SMR of 124, 90% CI = 87–172), pleural cancer (5 cases; SMR of 1327, 90% CI = 523–2790), laryngeal cancer (9 cases; SMR = 240, 90% CI = 126–420), and multiple myeloma (3 cases; SMR of 429, 90% CI = 117–1109). Liver cancer and pancreatic cancer were also in excess.[591]

5.4.18 Roofers

Pneumoconioses and other NMRDs were reported in a group of union roofers and waterproofers (PMR of 115, 95% CI = 103–128).[592] The authors[592] concluded that asbestos could have been a factor in their cause. In a radiographic study of 410 roofers compared with a control group, 14.4% of roofers had small, irregular opacities found more frequently than that in the controls.[593] Exposure to asbestos occurred as a result of machining asbestos-containing roofing cement. The study also identified three lung cancers.

Christiani and Greene,[594] in cooperation with the Roofers International Union Local No. 3, conducted a medical survey of union members. The survey included 271 workers with 10 or more years membership in the union. Sixty-nine of the 271 participating had a mean age of 52 and a mean number of years as a roofer of 29 years. Forty-six of the survey group had evidence of pleural disease; however, parenchymal abnormalities were uncommon with only two having radiologic fibrosis after having worked 20 or more years. No relationship was noted between the radiologic abnormalities and smoking.

Lange and Thomulka[550] were among the very few to evaluate asbestos exposure among roofers during controlled abatement activities. They[550] concluded that, in their small study, if outlier samples were removed, there was a probability that about 30% of the 5% of those exposed to asbestos would have experienced exposures that exceeded the OSHA PEL and that 95% would fall within two standard deviations of not exceeding the PEL. Overall, the study suggested that, during abatement, exposure was low, but because the airborne samples were not normally distributed and exhibited large variation, additional investigations were warranted to best assess such asbestos exposures during asbestos abatement activities.

Another study from Germany of some 40 building sites during normal roofing activities using corrugated asbestos cement sheets found light microscopy measurements of more than 100 fibers/mL greater than 5 µm in length when the sample was taken within the dust cloud caused by the grinding machine.[595] When measured near the head of the worker, the concentration was between 0.6 and 41 fibers/mL greater than 5 µm in length during the cutting process with a mean of the 9 samples of 20 fibers/mL. Because cutting appeared to amount to about 6% of the working time per day, the daily mean would be around 1.2 fibers/mL. The daily mean for roofers using corrugated sheet was calculated to be around 0.6 fibers/mL. The authors[595] estimated that peak concentrations of fine chrysotile dust might be more than 8 mg/m^3 as determined by using the Tyndallometer. The authors[595] commented that roofers who were not cutting were exposed as bystanders to a similar degree.

According to a NIOSH survey,[596] roofers as an occupation have the most number of workers potentially exposed to asbestos. In a study sponsored by the Bitumen Water Proofing Association of the United Kingdom evaluating carcinogenic agents of the Bitumen Waterproofing Industries of Finland and Denmark, the study[597] concluded that exposure to asbestos, which was previously high, was now much lower. Four cases of asbestos-related disease were identified from the Finnish Register of Occupational Disease from 1993 to 2002 showing past exposures to have been significant. In Finland and Denmark, exposures to bitumen roofers occurred during demolition work of old asbestos cement roofs.[597]

According to another study sponsored by The Monsey Products Company and The Henry Company, roof coating product companies, a simulation study of five asbestos-containing commercial roofing products sold from the 1950s through the 1970s found a low probability that asbestos will become airborne during manipulation of coating and cement-type roofing products such as those tested.[598] Calculated TWAs were above background (0.0002 fibers/mL) ranging from 0.0003 to 0.002 fibers/mL but well below the OSHA TWA of 0.1 fibers/mL. The results of this study are in contrast to that of Rodelsperger et al.[595] mentioned previously. Additionally, replacement, repair, or destruction (demolition) of asbestos cement roofs can be an exposure problem to the worker and the environment around the roof. Campopiano et al.[599] studied 40 cement roofs in various states of deterioration in Italy. They found that although a significant release of asbestos fibers may not be observed from cement roofs, evidence of prior release of a high quantity of asbestos fibers found in gutters was evidence that continued relapse of asbestos occurs and creates a big problem through uptake of the asbestos fibers into the environment. The authors[599] emphasized the importance of training workers or operators in evaluating the conditions of the roofs by using multiple methods to determine the friability of the asbestos within the roofs to allow sound decisions to be made to protect the workers and the environment.

5.4.19 Rubber Workers

The risk of lung cancer was found to be significant among rubber workers exposed in the early stages of production when exposure to asbestos-contaminated talc and carbon black can occur. The authors[600] concluded that either asbestos or carbon black could play an etiological role. For carbon black, weak associations were found for lung cancers according to the IARC,[601] who concluded there was inadequate evidence for the carcinogenicity of carbon black to humans, while there was sufficient evidence that carbon black was carcinogenic to experimental animals. The overall IARC evaluation of carcinogenic risk placed carbon black in Group 2B (possibly carcinogenic to humans). Thus, the combined role of asbestos and carbon black needs further investigation to evaluate the risk of lung cancers from asbestos in the rubber industry. Stomach cancer was also increased among rubber workers who worked in the early production stages of mixing and weighing, which the authors[600] concluded might point to the role of either asbestos-contaminated talc or carbon black, but their results did not support the causal role of nitrosamines. The role of carbon black in the etiology of stomach cancer is not supported. In looking further at a cohort of German rubber workers followed for mortality between January 1, 1981 and December 31, 1991, Straif et al.[602] observed reported lung cancer risk among those rubber workers exposed to asbestos and talc. Stomach cancers were also elevated and were associated with exposure to asbestos. The authors[602] concluded the risks were associated with asbestos and dust, although was statistically insignificant.

5.4.20 Shipyard Workers

It has been known that shipyards have contributed to the increase in asbestos-related diseases because of their vast use of large quantities of asbestos.[603,604] Data on asbestos-related diseases and asbestos exposure have been reported from around the world in jobs within the shipyard industry.[605–685,125] Exposures within shipyards have been measured dating back to 1946 when Fleischer et al.[323] found that pipecoverers doing band sawing experienced exposures to asbestos between 1 and 73 mppcf, during cement mixing from 31 to 84 mppcf, and during installation between 11 and 142 mppcf. Harries[34] measured asbestos fibers when applying amosite thermal insulation to pipes to range from 9 to 40 fibers/cm^3, removal of the thermal pipe amosite insulation between 29 and 1040 fibers/cm^3, and removal of spray-on asbestos between 112 and 1906 fibers/cm^3. In 1971, Harries[686] again sampled asbestos at shipyards and found that removal of lagging (insulation) in the boiler room ranged from 24.7 to 186.4 fibers/cm^3, during application of pipe lagging in the boiler room ranged from 0.13 to 5 fibers/cm^3, and during removal of pipe and machine lagging ranged from 0.16 to 3021 fibers/cm^3.

5.4.21 Smelter Workers

Smelter workers in New Caledonia had excesses of lung cancer and nasal sinus cancers that were thought to be the result of the carcinogenicity of nickel. Langer et al.[687] speculated the lung cancer cause may be, in part, due to the nickeliferous ores from at least one major smelter in New Caledonia, which came from serpentine host rocks containing large amounts of chrysotile asbestos. Analysis indicated the ores were contaminated with asbestos and that, when mined, the miners are exposed. In an exposure assessment of aluminum smelter workers, 40% of smelter workers were found to have been exposed to asbestos.[688]

5.4.22 School Teachers

Case reports of four mesotheliomas have been reported among two male and two female school teachers, aged 60, 52, 43, and 64 years, who worked in buildings containing asbestos.[689] Twelve cases of mesothelioma were reported among school teachers from Wisconsin, nine of whom had no other known exposure to asbestos than from asbestos-containing materials found within the buildings where they taught.[690] Bang et al.[486] reported at the American Public Health Association Meeting in 2003 that their analysis of mesothelioma in the United States resulted in a PMR of 2.1 for mesothelioma in elementary school teachers.

5.4.23 Steel Workers

Analyzing asbestos bodies in lung tissue from 252 patients older than 40 years, Churg and Warnock found that only 12% of white-collar men, 32% of blue-collar men not in construction or steel-mill work, 45% of steelworkers, and 65% of construction workers had more than 100 asbestos bodies per gram of lung tissue.[459] A study of steel workers in Belgium found an increased prevalence of asbestos bodies particularly among maintenance workers, production workers, and in workers reporting no asbestos exposure compared with controls.[691] Kronenberg et al.[692] reported that among 898 steel workers screened as of April 1990, 43% ($n = 67$) had restrictive pulmonary function; 22% ($n = 35$) had pleural disease; 22% ($n = 34$) had cancer of the lung, larynx, or gastrointestinal tract; 13% ($n = 20$) had fibrosis ≥ILO grade1/0; and one had mesothelioma. Overall, 17.5% ($n = 157$) had abnormalities.

Asbestos-containing materials used in some parts of the steel mills included protective gloves, protective clothing, refractory bricks on hot tops, liner boards, and asbestos blankets used for covering ladles, often being discarded on the pouring pit floor. Studies of steelworkers have found elevated risks of lung cancer in areas where asbestos was used; however, the role of asbestos has not been specifically assessed because of the difficulty of separating other carcinogenic exposures within the mills.[693–695] Asbestos bodies have been found among steelworkers, indicating the possible role of asbestos in the etiology of lung cancers.

5.4.24 Sulfate Mill Workers

Among 2480 men between 40 and 75 years of age at death and observed between 1960 and 1989 found that lung cancer (OR = 1.6, 90% CI = 1.1–2.3) and pleural mesotheliomas (OR = 9.5, 90% CI = 1.9–48) were significantly elevated, which the authors[696] suggested was probably due to asbestos exposure.

5.4.25 Welders

In 1936, Carl Hohan Jacobson of Copenhagen[697] described the first case of acute primary asbestosis in a welder using asbestos-covered electrodes while welding rails and boilers. On examination of one of the electrodes that the patient used, the asbestos found in the packing was actinolite, which is more resistant to acids.

Welders in shipyards had higher rates of parenchymal fibrosis and mesothelioma.[229] Thirteen of 306 shipyard welders had small irregular opacities of International Labour Organization/International Union Against Cancer (ILO/UICC) category 1/1 or more. When strict clinical criteria were followed, 3% were diagnosed with parenchymal fibrosis as compared with 0.5% from a random sample who did not have pleural or parenchymal lesions over the same timeframe. The authors[698] concluded that although welders were at risk of asbestos-related disease, pleural lesions may not only be merely markers of exposure but may be a source for identifying those at risk of developing parenchymal fibrosis.

Five deaths from pleural mesothelioma, unrelated to the type of welding, has drawn attention to the risk of exposure to asbestos during welding activities.[699] Lung cancer was increased among arc welders in Germany (SMR = 113) as was mesothelioma.[700] Asbestos bodies were found in 40.1% of welders during examination of their bronchoalveolar lavage fluid and 39.5% in lung tissue. The intensity of exposure to welding increased the retention of the asbestos bodies, which the authors[701] suggested could well increase the risk of fibrotic and malignant lung disease. Among Norwegian boiler welders, 50 cases of lung cancer were observed when 37.5 were expected (CRR = 1.3333, 95% CI = 0.99–1.76) and three cases of pleural mesothelioma versus 1.1 expected (CRR = 2.73, 95% CI = 0.56–7.97) were observed.[702] Welders in Sweden had an SIR of 1.86 (95% CI = 1.20–2.75) between 1961 and 1998.[224]

5.5 TAKE HOME AND COMMUNITY EXPOSURES TO ASBESTOS

"It inevitably tends to lower the social status and self-respect of work people if they have to go back to their homes in the same untidy condition" (J. S. Haldane[703]).

Take-home asbestos on worker's clothes, shoes, or hair can cause household exposure as can proximate residential exposure to asbestos sources. These types of exposures and their resultant disease manifestations are outlined very effectively in the NIOSH Report to Congress on Workers' Home Contamination Study,[286] which was conducted under The Workers' Family Protection Act (29 U.S.C. 671a). In this report, NIOSH concluded: "… families of asbestos-exposed workers have been at increased risk of pleural, pericardial, or peritoneal mesothelioma, lung cancer, cancer of the gastrointestinal tract, and nonmalignant pleural and parenchymal abnormalities as well as asbestosis."

It has been known for many years that the best method to control diseases associated with exposure to asbestos was to control the exposure to the dust containing the asbestos fibers.[130] As early as 1897, Netolitzky,[704] a physician reporting on lung disease among textile workers, also observed illness among their family members. In 1913, it was suggested that street clothes should not be worn in work areas and that work clothes should be removed before leaving the factory, thus preventing industrial poisons from being carried away from the workplace and exposing nonworkers to the industrial hazard.[705] Kober and Hayhurst[706] advised that street clothes should not be worn at work and that changing rooms and washing facilities be furnished by the employer at the workplace. The ILO, in their Standard Code of Industrial Hygiene published in 1934,[707] recommended that "In dusty trades, cloakrooms, washing accommodations, and eventually douche-baths, separate from the workrooms, should be provided for the workers." The Code also stated that "Such smoke, fumes and gas should be rendered harmless before being passed into the outside air."[707] In 1940, the Germans issued "Guidelines for the Prevention of Health Hazards from Dust in Asbestos Manufacturing Plants," which specifically mentions that street garments must not be left in the working area and that the retained dust on working clothes must be removed at regular intervals.[708]

In 1943, the U.S. Public Health Service published in their *Manual of Industrial Hygiene and Medical Service in War Industries*[709] the importance of cleanliness so that the worker did not carry workplace exposures out of the workplace. The Manual[709] stated that "[I]t is highly necessary that workers have adequate washing facilities. This implies enough washstands or showers and a sufficient quantity of hot water as well as cold. There should also be adequate time to enable thorough cleansing, change of clothes and dressing between the end of work and the time when transportation facilities are available. Many plants give too little time between the end of work and the bus home." The report further stated: "The work clothes should be provided and laundered by the employer" and that "[T]he employer should, without expense to the employees, furnish proper boots or shoes for the use of the employees while at work in such places." As can be seen from the above-cited references, concern for take-home exposure and the release of toxic materials from the factory were of major concern.

Specifically, by 1943, documentation of the effects of these take-home and environmental contamination concerns were appearing in the literature. Good and Pensky[710] reported a few cases in workers' wives of eruptions resembling their husbands' from halowax acne (cable rash). The authors[710] suspected the cases in the wives to have been the result of contact with work clothes and from laundering shirts and underwear. In 1965, two events documented asbestos take-home exposure and environmental exposure to asbestos with disease. The first was the publication by Newhouse and Thompson,[256] reporting mesothelioma among persons with a history of living with asbestos workers and of cases in persons living in the neighborhood of asbestos factories. At a meeting of the New York Academy of Sciences published in December 1965,[711] discussion of the Newhouse and Thompson[256] findings and the Wagner et al.[219] findings of community disease in South Africa, first published in 1960, was rereported at the New York Academy of Sciences meeting.[711] The Kiviluoto[712] finding of bilateral pleural calcification in a 50-year-old woman whose only known exposure to asbestos was living in the immediate vicinity of an asbestos mill and playing with asbestos as a child was also reported at the New York Academy of Sciences meeting in 1965.

Subsequent to the events of 1965, many studies have shown the effects of take-home asbestos exposure and of community environmental exposures. Navratil and Trippe[713] of Czechoslovakia found that 9 of 155 persons living in the neighborhood of an asbestos factory had radiographic evidence of pleural calcification, with or without other signs of asbestosis, when only 0.53 were expected. They also found that 4 of 114 persons older than 20 years who were relatives of factory workers had radiographic changes when only 0.39 were expected. Finally, they found 28 (0.34%) of 8127 persons older than 40 years who lived in the same district of the factory, but not in the immediate neighborhood of the factory, had pleural calcification. Lieben and Pistawka,[254] from the Pennsylvania Department of Health, reported several cases of mesothelioma from neighborhood and household exposure to asbestos. Anderson et al.[714–716] and Anderson[717] reported on familial exposure to asbestos and disease, showing both nonmalignant and malignant disease occurring in family members not otherwise exposed to asbestos. Among households with at least 20 years latency, Kilburn et al.[638] found radiographic evidence of asbestosis (profusion 1/0) in 11.3% of wives of shipyard workers when only a 0.6% prevalence was reported among California women and 0% was reported among Michigan women with prevalence increasing up to 32% in wives with the longest latency period. Of the shipyard workers, 1% were insulators; however, 25% of the wives with asbestosis were the wives of insulators.[639] In 1991, Joubert et al.[718] followed household contacts from one amosite factory in New Jersey and found 28% died of lung cancer, 23% died of gastrointestinal tract cancer, and 9% died from mesothelioma. The authors[718] stated this represented two times that was expected on the basis of national estimates. Magnani et al.[719] reported that among family members of Italian cement workers, four pleural tumors (one mesothelioma) were observed when only 0.5 were expected and that six lung cancers were observed when only four were expected. This represented a significantly elevated SMR of 792.3 for cancer of the pleura among domestically exposed women. The authors[719] reported that the plant had no laundering facilities, and therefore the work clothes were laundered at home.

Many other community studies,[638–640,718–719] case–control studies,[259,421,653,720–722] and according to NIOSH[286] some 17 case reports and 22 case series reports have also discussed take-home asbestos exposure and subsequent disease development as well as neighborhood exposure to asbestos and disease. A population-based case–control study was carried out in six areas from Italy, Spain, and

Switzerland.[233] Fifty-three cases without evidence of occupational exposure to asbestos compared with 232 controls found that domestic exposure was associated with an increased risk (OR = 4.81, 95% CI = 1.8–13.1). The authors[233] suggested that cleaning asbestos-contaminated clothes, handling asbestos material, and the presence of asbestos material susceptible to damage may have been the cause. The estimated OR for those living near sources of asbestos was 11.5 (95% CI = 3.5–38.2).

A meta-analysis by the IARC[723] found that the RR of pleural mesothelioma from household exposure ranged between 4.0 and 23.7 with a summary risk estimate of 8.1 (95% CI = 5.3–12). For neighborhood exposures, the RR ranged between 5.1 and 9.3 (a single RR of 0.2 was reported) and a summary estimate of 7.0 (95% CI = 4.7–11). The authors[723] concluded that although their analysis found a positive causal association between household and neighborhood exposures to asbestos and mesothelioma, at present, the data did not allow any estimate of the magnitude of risk from general environmental exposures.

Placenta transfer of asbestos fibers have been reported, which suggests that in the absence of a maternal history of an asbestos-related occupation, environmental exposures may have played a role.[724] Additionally, one study[288] observed 12 of 16 dogs with mesothelioma had a history of asbestos exposure. Nine dogs lived in a house with a family member who had an asbestos-related occupation or hobby, five lived in households where insulation or home remodeling had occurred, and five others lived in residential proximity to industrial sources of asbestos. It is interesting that, when using a method to equate dog to human age, the mesotheliomas were occurring at similar ages in dogs as in humans. In a study of individuals not exposed occupationally to asbestos, short fibers (<5 μm in length) were predominant in the omentum and mesentery, only one fiber greater than 5 μm in length was found, and there was a low fiber burden in the lung. The findings were in contrast to those found in occupationally exposed persons who died of mesothelioma and which were linked to the lung fiber burden, the number of asbestos bodies, the total amphibole burden, and the average fiber length and aspect ratio.[265] An evaluation of the residents of Da-yao, China, found lifetime environmental exposure to crocidolite asbestos to have significantly higher rates of pleural plaques, asbestosis, lung cancer, and mesothelioma.[165] The authors[165] reported an annual mortality rate of mesothelioma ranging from 85 to 365 per million when only two to three were expected in the general population. The lung cancer and mesothelioma ratio was very low (1.2–3.0), even when the prevalence of smoking was quite high (80%). Pleural plaques were prevalent in 11 % of the residents 20 years or older and in 20% of those older than 40 years.

The IHF, first called the Air Hygiene Foundation (1936–1941), was formed.[124] The IHF was founded by the Mellon Institute with membership consisting of a group of large industrial corporations. The IHF conducted medical and industrial hygiene surveys of various industries, including the asbestos industry. It also published proceedings of its meeting and also the IHD. The annual meetings were covered by various trade journals and news media like the *Wall Street Journal* and the *New York Times* as well as wire services like the Associated Press and the United Press International.

Beginning in April 1960, the IHD published an abstract showing asbestos contamination as far as 600 m from the factory,[725] as did one other report of exposure from a region near a mine and factory.[726] In July 1963, the IHD published an abstract of the results of some 500 consecutive autopsies in subjects 15 years or older.[727] The findings suggested environmental contamination to urban residents not occupationally exposed to asbestos and that this contamination in the community might be of etiological significance in mesothelioma development. Subsequently, the IHD continued to report the dangers of community exposures to asbestos.[711,727–733] Any company that was a member of the IHF would have received these reports.

In addition, on March 3, 1969, the law firm of Davies, Hardy, Loeb, Austin, and Ives of New York City sent the minutes of the Health and Safety Council/Asbestos Cement Products Association meeting held on February 18, 1969, to several asbestos companies, many of whom attended the council meeting.[734] In these minutes, it was reported "... that mesothelioma occurred among workers as well as among people who live near crocidolite workings" (so-called *neighborhood cases*).

Finally, on October 4, 1982, Dr. Homan of the Bushy Run Research Center sent a copy of Dr. Selikoff's paper on "Household Risks with Inorganic Fibers" to Mr. Sicard of the Union Carbide Corporation, in which Dr. Selikoff specifically discussed family contact and asbestos-related disease.[735] From these data and correspondence, it is clear that take-home exposure poses a real risk to the family and to those living in contaminated environmental areas.

5.6 HUMAN EVIDENCE OF DISEASE BY FIBER TYPE

When discussing the results of his landmark study on asbestos and its association with mesothelioma, Dr. Christopher Wagner concluded: "These experiments suggest that other dusts may be 'carcinogenic' if they reach the pleural cavity. It is probable from the cases of carcinomata of the lung in patients, with asbestosis reported from overseas, and in the four cases from amosite miners, and the one from a chrysotile miner in our series, that the other types of asbestos are associated with pulmonary malignancy" (Wagner JC. The Pathology of Asbestosis in South Africa. Thesis presented for the degree of Doctor of Medicine in the Department of Pathology of the University of the Witwatersrand; 1964).

This section will discuss evidence of the toxicity of the major commercial forms of asbestos. The studies discussed do not include all the studies on each fiber type but were selected as representative of the knowledge as it developed for the toxicity of a particular asbestos fiber type.

5.6.1 Anthophyllite

Anthophyllite is a member of the amphibole group with a chemical composition of $(Mg, Fe+^2)_7 \cdot (Si_8O_{22}(OH, F)_2)$ and was principally produced in Finland up until 1974 where it was widely used.[9,736] Asbestos-related diseases have been reported by Meurman et al.,[737–739] Tuomi et al.,[740] Karjalainen et al.,[741] and Rom et al.[742]

In a study of two mines with 1092 miners of which 248 were deceased and with less than 5% lost to follow-up, the authors[739] found a statistically excess of lung cancers in those with more than 10 years of exposure (8 observed vs. 2.4 expected; SMR = 3.33, 95% CI = 1.44–6.57)[*] and an overall excess of asbestosis (10 expected vs. 3 observed; SMR = 3.33, 95% CI = 1.60–6.13).[†] They[739] calculated the RR for nonsmoking asbestos workers to be 1.4, for smokers to be 12, and for smoking asbestos workers to be 17. The number of deaths (43) was small, especially for those with more than 10 years of exposure. There were no reports of mesothelioma or gastrointestinal cancers among this cohort, and the authors suggested more follow-up of the cohort as latency increased.

In a study of 793 anthophyllite miners and millers, PMRs were calculated for smokers and nonsmokers and compared with Finnish rates.[737] The PMR for lung cancer was significantly elevated for the heavily exposed asbestos miners and millers. Asbestosis was elevated in smokers and nonsmokers alike. The authors[737] reported the multiplicative nature between smoking and anthophyllite exposure, with an RR for nonsmoking asbestos workers of 1.6, smokers not exposed to asbestos of 12, and asbestos workers who were smokers of 19. In comparing the total deaths between 1936 and 1977, 44 lung cancers were observed when 22 were expected (SMR = 2.0, 95% CI = 1.45–2.68).[‡] Although the results were compatible with both multiplicative and promoter models, the study had only one nonsmoking asbestos worker with lung cancer for comparison.

---

[*] The 95% CI exact calculated by R. Lemen.
[†] The 95% CI exact calculated by R. Lemen.
[‡] The 95% CI exact calculated by R. Lemen.

Tuomi et al.[740] compared 19 mesotheliomas in Finland with 15 randomly selected controls and found 0.5 to 370 million fibers per gram of dry lung tissue in the mesothelioma group and from less than 0.01 to 3.2 million fibers per gram of dry lung tissue in the autopsy control group. In six mesotheliomas, anthophyllite fibers predominated whereas the rest of the cases were predominated by amphiboles with few chrysotile fibers identified.

Karjalainen et al.[743] reported four cases of mesothelioma among 999 anthophyllite miners and millers followed through 1991. Three were pleural mesotheliomas, and one was peritoneal meso-thelioma. There were 503 deaths within the cohort. Each case had long latencies between 39 and 58 years and worked within the anthophyllite mines and mills between 13 and 31 years. All had asbestosis and were smokers. Between 270 and 1100 million anthophyllite fibers per gram of dry lung tissue were found after TEM analysis and appeared thicker with smaller aspect ratios than had been reported among crocidolite fibers found in the lungs of mesothelioma patients.

Meurman et al.[738] reported four mesotheliomas when only 0.1 was expected (RR = 40, 95% CI = 10.90–102.42)[*] of 736 male miners and millers from two anthophyllite mines. Men had an excess of total cancers (SIR = 1.7, 95% CI = 1.4–1.9) and lung cancer (SIR = 2.8, 95% CI = 2.2–3.6), whereas there were no such excesses among 156 women in the cohort. The authors[738] reported that lung can-cer among the men increased with both extent of exposure and amount of smoking.

Karjalainen et al.[744] reported how anthophyllite had been mined and used in Finland between 1915 and 1975. When comparing the asbestos body formation, they[744] reported that in those exposed mainly to anthophyllite, the asbestos bodies were greater when compared with those exposed mainly to crocidolite/amosite and that the anthophyllite fibers were longer than those of crocidolite/amosite found in lung tissue.

Karjalainen et al.[741] reported that the increasing trend in mesothelioma had been slowing down in Finland during the 1990s in those younger than 55 years but was still increasing for those older than 65 years. It is thought that the number of cases will be less than 100 during the 2000s with about 40–50 cases in men and 10–20 in women with about 40–50 of the total cases occupationally connected. This is probably reflective of the strict regulations concerning the use and importation of asbestos into Finland for many years. It has been reported that about 90% of all pleural and 50% of all peritoneal mesotheliomas are work-related.

Rom et al.[742] reported a case of pleural mesothelioma in a 38-year-old man who lived near a plant that used anthophyllite asbestos exclusively between the ages of 8 and 17 years and who had no history of occupational exposure to asbestos. Anthophyllite fibers were >5 μm in length in lung tissue compared with 3 μm from a general population study.

In a study of 54 individuals with pathologically diagnosed mesothelioma, Dodson et al.[745] found that tremolite in the tissue most often was associated with the finding of anthophyllite. They also found that the majority of fibers were short fibers less than 8 μm in length; however, longer fibers were also found.

Mesothelioma had not been recognized from exposure to anthophyllite until much later than the three other major commercial fiber types—amosite, chrysotile, and crocidolite. It is now clear that mesotheliomas occur among anthophyllite asbestos-exposed workers.[740,743,746,747]

5.6.2 Amosite

Amosite is a member of the amphibole group with a chemical composition $(Mg, Fe+^2)_7 \cdot (Si_8O_{22}(OH)_2)$ [cummingtonite–grunerite]. It was mainly used in asbestos cement sheet, thermal insulation, and roofing products and commonly referred to as brown asbestos.[9,10,736] Various studies have shown the causal association between exposure to amosite and the development of asbestosis, lung cancer, and mesothelioma.[219,251,748–755] Studies continue to confirm such associations and not all are listed here.

[*] Calculated by RAL.

Dr. J. C. Wagner et al.[219] reported a 32-year-old white man who worked as a bookkeeper at an amosite mine in the Transvaal area of South Africa who developed mesothelioma (their case no. 24). As a child, he lived up to age 7 years in Kuruman, South Africa, in an area with crocidolite and amosite mines nearby. His only subsequent contact with asbestos was at the amosite mine. The authors[219] described the amosite mining area of Transvaal as, until recently, being on a small scale, with no settlements near the mines, and that due to the long latency for mesothelioma development, this was likely the reason for the scarcity of disease.

Wagner[756] found amosite produced earlier and more marked lesions than those produced in animals exposed to chrysotile. He also found that asbestosis was progressive in monkeys and rabbits. Asbestos bodies occurred in the lungs of animals exposed to amosite, chrysotile, and crocidolite.

Schepers[757] described a rabbit exposed to amosite for a year developed marked fibrosis as did a monkey exposed for 15 months. In addition, Schepers described the North Eastern Transvaal area of South Africa stating: "... young children, completely included within large shipping bags, trampling down fluffy amosite asbestos, which all day long came cascading down over their heads." Several children had radiologic asbestosis with cor pulmonale before the age of 12 years. Schepers saw many employees with "marked pleural sclerosis" in all black laborers and one white manager. In some, the pleura was more than an inch thick and very radiodense. Schepers described not being alerted to pleural mesothelioma, but after seeing his first case sometime later, "I 'knew' what had occurred." Dr. Schepers questioned the statistics presented by Sluis-Cremer,[758] comparing the finding of more disease in the workers in the crocidolite areas of Kuruman and Koegas as they were perennial workers with longer exposures than that of the Bantu personnel in the North Eastern Transvaal area who were mostly short-term transient laborers and more difficult to follow-up. Dr. Schepers questioned why Dr. Sluis-Cremer did not report on the fate of those miners he had seen with pleural thickening or the fate of the children who worked packing bags with asbestos.

Godwin and Jagatic[422] questioned an earlier letter to the *JAMA* stating the problem with mesothelioma relates only to crocidolite and pointed out evidence of mesothelioma had been reported from exposure to other fiber types, including chrysotile and amosite.

Wagner and Berry[759] reported mesothelioma occurring after exposing Wistar rats to amosite; however, the tumors occurred later than that in rats exposed to chrysotile and crocidolite. Another experiment with intrapleural inoculation of amosite asbestos produced mesotheliomas in specific pathogen resistance (SPR) rats and standard rats, with tumors occurring after a longer period for amosite than for chrysotile or crocidolite.[760]

Fibrotic reactions were found in rodents exposed to amosite, chrysotile, and crocidolite asbestos with amosite provoking the strongest response, especially in guinea pigs.[761] However, no tumors in any species exposed to amosite developed tumors, and although chrysotile and crocidolite induced mesothelioma, there were none in the amosite group.

Selikoff et al.[749] studied a group of 230 men formerly employed in an amosite manufacturing factory and found 14 deaths due to asbestosis, 43 cancers overall when 8.5 were expected (SMR = 5.10; 95% CI = 3.66–6.81), 25 deaths from lung cancer when approximately 2.4 or less were expected (SMR = 10.42, 95% CI = 6.74–15.38), 5 deaths from mesothelioma (the authors indicated that at that time the tumor was sufficiently rare in general populations that no U.S. data existed), and 5 gastrointestinal cancers when 1.6 were expected (SMR = 3.13, 95% CI = 1.01–7.29).*

Webster[762] reported two cases of mesothelioma in workers with amosite only exposure and nine cases of lung cancer out of 262 miners. The majority of miners in the Transvaal area where amosite was mined were Bantu and smoked less than the mixed race miners.

Reeves[763] observed a malignancy incidence of 5% in rats exposed to amosite dust in the atmosphere, including lung tumors and mesothelial tumors of the pleura.

---

* Calculated by RAL.

Seidman et al.[764] identified 933 men who worked in an amosite asbestos manufacturing plant. After eliminating those with prior asbestos exposure or working with asbestos after leaving the plant, or those lost to follow-up, the cohort was reduced to 820 men. Only 313 men worked in the plant for more than a year. The authors[764] observed that, using length of time as a surrogate for asbestos dosage, the shorter the duration of work, the longer the latency for an adverse effect and the smaller the magnitude of adverse mortality. In addition to length of exposure, the time elapsed since ceasing work was an important indicator of an adverse effect, indicating that continued follow-up is necessary to determine the magnitude of adverse effects on former workers. Direct heavy exposures for those described as already at "cancer ages" resulted in increased mortality in shorter periods after onset of work (5–14 years); however, this trend was not seen in younger workers at onset of employment (those in their twenties). These findings indicate the latency period depends not only on dosage but also on age at onset of exposure. Fourteen mesotheliomas, 93 lung cancers, and 30 asbestosis deaths were identified through best available evidence. Death certificate information only underreported the incidence significantly among factory workers. The authors[764] compared the mortality of the amosite factory workers with a cohort of 17,800 insulation workers. Asbestosis deaths and lung cancer deaths were similar, but mesothelioma deaths were higher in the insulation workers (3% vs. 88%, respectively). The latency was much longer for the factory workers than the insulation workers, which indicates that death trends of the insulation worker will be much higher over the same latency and that mixed exposures may carry a higher risk than exposures to principally one fiber type, or that intensity of exposure is higher among the insulation workers.

Seidman et al.[752] reported additional follow-up 7 years later on a cohort of 820 men from the amosite manufacturing plant making thermal pipe insulation. More than 50% of the workers ($n = 583$) had greater than 20 years since onset of work. Lung cancer mortality, using best evidence of death, reported an SMR of 287 ($n = 111$); mesothelioma of the pleura occurred in eight of the workers and in the peritoneum in nine of the workers. For laryngeal, buccal, and pharyngeal cancers, the SMR was 192 ($n = 7$); for colon–rectal cancers, the SMR was 190 ($n = 11$); and for noninfectious pulmonary diseases of which 31 were attributed to asbestosis, the SMR was 489 ($n = 46$). The authors[752] found that the lower the dose, the longer the latency for adverse mortality and the smaller the magnitude of the effect.

Finkelstein[753] reported on the mortality of workers in an Ontario factory manufacturing amosite pipe insulation and block insulation between 1956 and 1974. Seven deaths or 58% of those 10 years or greater from first employment were due to cancer. Four (25%) were due to lung cancer and two aged 47 and 49 years, were due to peritoneal mesothelioma. Two asbestosis deaths occurred in men aged 42 and 53 exposed more than 2 years and after 10 years of latency from first employment. There were no deaths from gastrointestinal cancers. The author[753] stated the study was very small and the statistical power to detect excess risk was limited.

Ribak et al.[754] reported on continued follow-up of the cohort first identified by Selikoff et al.[749] and then expanded by Seidman et al.[752] In this follow-up, they[754] identified 17 cases of mesothelioma (8 pleural and 9 peritoneal). Death certificates were less accurate in identifying the cases than clinical diagnosis at death. No exposure measurements were given, but exposure was estimated to be as high as 50 fibers/mL. The fiber type was mainly amosite, but some chrysotile had been used in the factory. Survival was shortest for peritoneal mesothelioma (5.4 months after diagnosis) compared with pleural mesothelioma (12.5 months after diagnosis).

Levin et al.[755] examined 222 death certificates out of 1130 former asbestos pipe-manufacturing workers from a plant in Tyler, Texas (earlier identified by Johnson et al. in 1982).[751] They found an excess of deaths from respiratory cancers (SMR = 277, 95% CI = 193–385), four pleural mesotheliomas and two peritoneal mesotheliomas. The analysis showed a dose–response trend for respiratory cancers with duration of exposure and that an excess occurred in those with less than 6 months of work at the plant (SMR = 268, 95% CI = 172–399). The plant used amosite exclusively for pipe manufacturing since its beginning in 1954 until the plant's closure in 1972.

5.6.3 Chrysotile

Chrysotile, the most commonly used asbestiform variety accounting for some 95%+ of the asbestos ever used, is found in the serpentine mineral group with a chemical formula of $Mg_6Si_4O_{10}(OH)_8$. The nonfibrous forms of this serpentine mineral are lizardite and antigorite. As compared with the amphiboles, the chrysotile fiber is generally finer with high flexibility and good heat resistance. Chrysotile is commonly referred to as *white asbestos*.[9,10,736] The issue of chrysotile-tremolite contamination has been a matter of debate. In fact, most deposits of chrysotile contain trace amounts of tremolite. Canadian chrysotile is said to be contaminated with fibrous tremolite[765] and considered to be less than 1%. The world's largest deposits of chrysotile asbestos are found in Russia at the Bazhenovsk deposit in the town of Asbest close to Ekaterinburg City and accounts for 20% of world production.[766] This mining area has been mined since 1889 and samples taken and analyzed by phase-contrast optical microscope and SEM found only chrysotile and no amphibole minerals; however, lung tissue analysis did find tremolite.[330]

In an analysis of lung tissue of six Chinese chrysotile miners,[767] all bulk samples contained amphibole asbestos (measuring about 0.002–0.310 wt.% lung tissue) with tremolite fibers found in every sample. Few studies have examined the impurities of Chinese chrysotile, with the exception of qualitative analyses of the Qilian mine, which showed a "little amount" of amphibole, and the Chaoyang mine in Liaoning Province, which also found a small amount of tremolite.[767]

Zimbabwe is also a major producer of chrysotile asbestos, and tremolite was not reported in samples taken for medical study.[768,769] In samples taken from a mine and mill in Balangero, Italy, another major deposit of chrysotile, no tremolite was detected in any of the samples of chrysotile.[770]

Before the OSHA of 1970, little information had been developed separating out the various fiber types; however, what was done showed that chrysotile was both fibrogenic and carcinogenic. To show some of these early results, I will run through some experimental and toxicologic studies on chrysotile and then follow through with human case reports, clinical reports, pathological tissue analysis, and epidemiologic studies implicating chrysotile in the etiology of asbestos-induced cancers.

5.6.3.1 Experimental and Toxicological Studies on Chrysotile Asbestos

Simson[65] reported fibrosis and golden yellow bodies in the lungs of guinea pigs similar to those found in humans. The animals were exposed 2 h/day for 50 days in 1925 to chrysotile. The results from animal bioassays presented a strong case for the toxicity of chrysotile. Wagner et al.,[771] then with the Medical Research Council, United Kingdom, had shown that commercial grade, predominantly short fiber Canadian chrysotile, which was used primarily for paint and plastic tile fillers, could induce mesotheliomas when injected intrapleurally into rats and induce primary lung neoplasms when the animals were exposed by inhalation. Not only does it appear that chrysotile is as potent as crocidolite and other amphiboles in inducing mesothelioma after intrapleural injections,[772] but also equally potent in inducing pulmonary neoplasms after inhalation exposure.[773] Wagner et al.[773] stated that in terms of degree of response related to the quality of dust deposited and retained in the lungs of rats, chrysotile appeared to be much more fibrogenic and carcinogenic than the amphiboles.

The experimental and epidemiological data are quite extensive on the toxicity of chrysotile, as seen by the following discussions.

The first real experimental study of chrysotile was conducted by the Saranac Laboratory of the Edward I. Trudeau Foundation and was published in 1951; however, the studies on asbestosis had begun some 20 years previous. Although some data were presented by the organizer of the studies (Dr. Leroy U. Gardner, 1942) before his death, the paper published by Arthur J. Vorwald, Thomas M. Durkan, and Philip C. Pratt was the first to give a complete result of the entire experimental investigations into asbestos. Controversy has surrounded the results and publication or lack thereof of the Saranac Laboratory studies; therefore, for a compelling discussion, I would refer the reader to papers by Phillip E. Enterline and Garrit W. H. Schepers published in the *American Journal of Industrial Medicine*.[774,775]

Vorwald et al.[776] described inhalation studies as ones "... on which great reliance is placed when estimating the degree to which a dust might constitute a respiratory hazard to industrial workers." Such inhalation studies can "... reveal whether the dust can be inhaled, pass the natural defense barriers of the body and reach the pulmonary tissue in quantities sufficient to cause damage." Thus far, the studies of the Saranac Laboratory have shown that inhalation of chrysotile can produce asbestos bodies only in the lungs of a few species such as man, guinea pigs, and white mice. Chrysotile produces fibrosis in man, guinea pigs, cats, rabbits, and rats, but not in mice or dogs. The first inhalation studies conducted on asbestos at Saranac Laboratory began in 1928. Petrographic analysis showed long chrysotile to be up to 50 μm in length and approximately 75% chrysotile, with 15% serpentine, 5% magnetite, 2% brucite, and the remaining 3% calcite, chloritic, and micaceous minerals. Only a trace of quartz was observed. Another preparation of the chrysotile fiber was called King's floats, which was composed and based on particles (except chrysotile) smaller than 10 μm and reported from particle counts to be composed of 14% chrysotile, 40% serpentine, 12% magnetite, 18% carbonates, 12% talc, and 4% other minerals. For chrysotile, fibers up to 200 μm long were included. Short fiber contained before ball milling contained a preponderance of fibrous chrysotile and platy (nonfibrous) serpentine. Percentage composition was 17% chrysotile, 55% serpentine, 10% magnetite, 2% quartz, 5% brucite, and 11% other minerals, including dolomite, actinolite, and tremolite. Results of the experiments with King's floats asbestos dust produced peribronchiolar fibrosis in guinea pigs but not in rabbits or rats. In animals infected with tuberculosis, guinea pigs, after termination of 2 years of exposure to asbestos dust, did not show progressive disease, which was opposite to disease progression after exposure to quartz.

When looking at inhalation exposure to short asbestos fibers, tissue reaction was slower than with King's floats dusts and, according to the authors, shows that factors not chemical in nature are more important in fibrosis. The guinea pig and the white rat were the only two to have peribronchiolar fibrosis, whereas the cat reacted with an atypical subpleural fibrosis and the rabbit only slight parenchymal fibrosis.

The results of long fiber inhalation found strong evidence that long fibers were chiefly responsible for asbestosis. Reactions in guinea pigs developed earlier and became more extensive in spite of smaller concentrations of atmospheric dust and a lower mineral content in the lungs. Typical peribronchiolar fibrosis was also produced in cats.

Vorwold et al.,[776] in their intratracheally injected studies, found that grinding unheated chrysotile (<3 μm) destroyed its ability to cause fibrosis when injected into guinea pigs. At 1 month, considerable inflammatory edema and cellular proliferation and localization of dust particles about the bronchioles occurred; at 2 months, only slight proliferative reaction occurred; and at 6–12 months, widely scattered small mononuclear phagocytes occurred. Also at 12 months, a few microscopic patches of thin alveolar wall thickening occurred with some adenomatoid changes in portions of air spaces abutting the thickened bronchi, but there was no asbestos body formation. With the larger size dust particles containing chrysotile (20–50 μm long), distinct fibrosis occurred and, after 12 months, well-developed peribronchial and intrabronchial adenomatoid areas of fibrosis produced considerable distortion. There were more peripheral patches of pneumonitis with eosinophilic infiltration, and some were being transformed into fibrous tissue, which seemed to be precursors of the localized, diffuse patches of thin alveolar wall fibrosis seen elsewhere. It appears that unheated, long fiber chrysotile produced typical peribronchiolar fibrosis and that the ball milled fibers less than 3 μm in length failed to cause fibrosis.

When looking at the source of long fiber chrysotile, the Thetford Quebec Canadian chrysotile injected intratracheally into guinea pigs produced distinct fibrosis and that chrysotile from Arizona with low iron content (0.2%) produced virtually identical fibrosis as well as asbestos bodies.

The fibrosis in the low iron chrysotile occurred before the asbestos bodies were seen and was in a well-formed cellular state at 1 month. At 2 months, minute foci of well-matured fibrosis about the bronchioles occurred; at 6 months, mature fibrosis with evidence of contraction and considerable chronic pneumonitis with infiltration of the lymphocytes and eosinophils occurred; and at 9 months, small intrabronchiolar fibrosis plugs with foci of more delicate fibrosis occurred at the periphery.

In summary, when long fiber chrysotile was heated and its structure changed, it lost its ability to cause fibrosis. When tested on various species of animals, including guinea pigs, rats, and rabbits, but not mice or dogs, the long fiber chrysotile asbestos produced peribronchial fibrosis of the lung similar to human asbestosis after being exposed by inhalation or intratracheal injection.[776]

Although continuing his animal studies, J. C. Wagner reported that these studies have shown that all types of asbestos have produced mesothelioma in rats. Because all fiber types cause mesothelioma in rats, although they have very different chemical structures, Wagner concluded it was unlikely that the chemistry of the fiber types explained the carcinogenicity of asbestos. Wagner further stated that the most interesting point obtained from these studies was that mesothelioma is associated with the presence of fine fibrous material within the pleural cavity and that physical characteristics are important factors in the carcinogenicity of the fibers. Wagner pointed to both Stanton[348] and Timbrell[778] as elaborating this position.[772,773,777]

Davis et al.,[779] in further animal experiments, found inhalation of chrysotile dust caused significantly more lung fibrosis than crocidolite or amosite, even when the number of fibers were similar. Also, chrysotile-containing dust was the only dust that induced cancers—both adenocarcinomas and squamous cell carcinomas. The chrysotile findings conformed to a dose–response effect as seen between the administration of 10 mg versus 2 mg, which produced lower numbers of bronchial carcinomas. Using an SEM, the authors[779] found that chrysotile dust had many more fibers more than 20 µm in length than did crocidolite or amosite; thus, the authors[779] concluded that chrysotile was much more fibrogenic than the two amphiboles tested and that the long fibers were the most dangerous. However, the authors[779] questioned the "long fiber theory" that just long fibers were responsible for the carcinogenicity and suggested that unbroken surface area appeared to be important and that continuous surface area was provided by long fibers and might account for their toxicity. The authors[779] suggested this on the basis of a study by Karp et al.,[780] where unbroken plastic implants with very small holes were effective carcinogens and those containing larger holes were much less dangerous.

Hiett,[781] experimenting with guinea pigs exposed by inhalation to chrysotile and amosite, found that the animals exposed at 8 months were most sensitive to functional changes when exposed to chrysotile than when they were exposed at 3 months of age. Duration of exposure was not related to functional disturbances as was the age at time of exposure. The functional and pathological changes in the lungs occurred after 40 weeks in animals exposed at 8 months but not until 70 weeks in those exposed at 3 months. No fibrotic reactions were seen during 70 weeks in animals exposed to amosite. Hiett thought the difference between chrysotile and amosite might be related to the greater inflammatory blocking of the small airways by the chrysotile fibers, thus obstructing the clearance of the fibers to a greater degree. Hiett felt this experiment was an indication that lung function tests sensitive to airways disease would be effective in early detection of asbestosis in humans.

Intratracheal instillation of chrysotile into 133 adult male Syrian golden hamsters resulted in histological and physiological changes, cytologic findings, and generation of inflammatory mediators by alveolar macrophages.[782] Within days after only one instillation, hamsters developed patchy bronchopneumonia with equal involvement of the terminal airways along with adjacent alveolar tissue and a gradual shift of the inflammatory process to the peripheral alveolar tissue after day 60. Airflow obstruction and air trapping occurred and accompanied the histological changes. Beginning at 24 h after instillation and persisting throughout 6 months, a striking increase was noted in the proportion of neutrophils recovered by bronchoalveolar lavage. The authors[782] concluded that the hamster was a good model in which to study asbestosis and pulmonary fibrosis.

Wagner et al.[783] compared Italian talc to chrysotile asbestos in animal inhalation studies using caesarian-derived Wistar rats. Three samples of chrysotile included UICC Canadian chrysotile, grade 7 Canadian chrysotile from the Belle Mine, and a super fine sample (SFA) from the Normandy Mine in Canada were used. The UICC cloud of dust had the highest fiber counts with fibers of all lengths. In the first experiment, 48 rats were injected intrapleurally with 20 mg of respirable dust and mesothelioma developed with all asbestos samples: 18 occurred with SAF, 13 with grade 7, and 5 with the UICC sample. None occurred in the talc-exposed or saline controls. In the second experiment, the rats were exposed to clouds of approximately 1 mg/m^3 for 35 h per week for 3, 6, and 12 months. Cancer occurred in all chrysotile types with the most (10 tumors) occurring in the UICC-exposed sample. One mesothelioma occurred among the SFA-exposed rats. Fibrosis occurred after 3 months and progressed after cessation of exposure with all samples, including the talc-exposed animals, with the greatest scores in the asbestos-exposed rats. No malignant tumors occurred in the rats exposed to Italian talc. The impurities of the UICC sample included brucite and pyroaurite, silicates of talc, and chlorite; the grade 7 contained brucite, chlorite, talc, and traces of tremolite; the SFA sample contained pyroaurite with some talc and chlorite; and the Italian talc contained impurities of chlorite and quartz. No tremolite was reported in the SFA sample given to the rats where mesothelioma occurred, and lung tumors occurred in both the UICC- and SFA-exposed animals where neither samples contained tremolite. In fact, the grade 7 chrysotile with traces of tremolite produced the smallest number of lung tumors.[771,783]

Platek and Groth[784] of NIOSH conducted an inhalation study of short chrysotile asbestos fibers exposing the animals to mean air concentrations of 1 mg/mL with a ratio of short to long >5 μm of 265:1. Rats autopsied after 1, 3, 6, 12, and 18 months since initiating exposure showed little or no pathologic reaction to the inhaled asbestos. Asbestos fibers were not seen in the lung by light microscopy but were seen in alveolar macrophages when examined by electron microscopy. Further analysis of this study after the lifetime of the rats is warranted as is examination of tissue external from the lung. Cynamolgus monkeys were also exposed, but no results were reported because the observation time was too short.

A model for studying asbestos-induced pulmonary disease used Balb/c-mice, which were exposed to 10.9 mg/m^3 chrysotile for 2 h daily, 5 days per week for up to 2.5 months. The first changes histologically were influxes of macrophages at 4–5 days. As this progressed, asbestos body formation occurred as did diffuse focal interstitial fibrosis by 1 year. After termination of exposure and 12 to 18 months later, 92% of the exposed mice developed lung tumors compared with 10% of the controls.[785]

In studying the production of mast cells following asbestos exposure, Wagner et al.[786] found that Wistar rats exposed to Rhodesian (Zimbabewian) and Canadian chrysotile asbestos dust for 7 h daily, 5 days a week, for up to 24 months produced the largest number of mast cells in the lung interior as did anthophyllite compared with other asbestos types. The mast cells increased at least 100 times between fibrosis grades 1 and 5 to 8. For these reasons, the authors[786] concluded that mast cells were associated with interstitial fibrosis induced by asbestos exposure in rats.

Brody[787] found that rats, after 1 h of exposure to chrysotile via nose only, accumulated macrophages in significant numbers. Overall, Brody's experiment to understand the initial cellular events which result in asbestosis found that asbestos fibers impacting on air space surfaces activated serum derived complement components of the alveolar lining layer to produce a chemotactic factor which could attract other cells influencing the development of emphysematous or fibrotic lung responses. The brief chrysotile exposure in rats was accompanied by local thickening of the epithelium and interstitium. Brody[787] concluded that these appeared to be the earliest measurable morphologic alterations from inhalation of asbestos.

Rats (8 weeks old, male, CD-1) were exposed to chrysotile asbestos via nose only inhalation to respirable mass concentrations of 15 mg/m^3 for 1 h. They were then sacrificed immediately after exposure, or at 24 h, 8 days, 2 weeks, or 1 month after exposure. The findings indicated that as time passed, there was a progressive decrease in fiber number and mass as well as significant changes in the fiber dimensions retained in the lungs. Twenty-three percent of the respirable fraction was deposited in the lungs and that after 1 month there was still 19% present.[788]

Rats were exposed via nose only to aerosols of 14.6 mg/m³ chrysotile asbestos for 1 or 5 h, then sacrificed at 0, 48, 72, or 192 h and the lungs removed. The lungs were examined by SEM and the macrophages were examined by x-ray energy spectrometry and SEM. Findings indicated that alveolar macrophages accumulated on alveolar duct bifurcations within 48 h and that phagocytic and chemotactic capacities of the macrophages were impaired, which could relate to the pathogenesis of asbestos-related lung disease.[789]

A study using chrysotile asbestos found it can induce clotting activation in vitro and that a subsequent decrease in activity of clotting factors occurs, which results in fibrin formation around asbestos particles.[790]

Craighead et al.[791] found that after injection into the abdominal cavity of rats at 6 to 23 months with both crocidolite and chrysotile, they both produced mesotheliomas that were similar to those found in humans in relationship to growth patterns and histological features.

Glickman et al.,[288] while studying 18 dogs with mesothelioma, found one dog with only chrysotile in its lungs and whose owner's only known exposure to asbestos was as a pipefitter in a shipyard. The number of fibers in the dog's lungs was 3.1×10^6 compared with the controls with a range of 0.323×10^6 to 2.9×10^6. This is a curious finding because a pipefitter would be expected to have had amphibole exposure.

5.6.3.2 Case Reports, Pathological Analysis, and Epidemiology of Predominantly Chrysotile Asbestos

The first evidence of lung cancer and mesothelioma among chrysotile workers was reported in 1952 when Cartier[792] reported two cases of pleural mesothelioma, five cases of bronchogenic carcinoma, and one case of mediastinal lymphosarcoma with pulmonary metastasis among 11,000 asbestos workers in the Canadian mines working between 1940 and 1950. Two of the lung cancer cases did not have preexisting asbestosis.

In 1958, Braun and Truan[793] reported lung cancer in a cohort of chrysotile asbestos miners from Quebec, Canada. However, less than 4% of the cohort had died by the end of the study; thus, any findings should be considered unreliable when making judgments concerning the risk of lung cancer or mesothelioma among this cohort. Nine confirmed and three additional lung cancer deaths were recorded when the authors[793] reported that six were expected compared with the general population of the Province of Quebec. The authors stated: "On the basis of what are believed to be complete and reliable data, it seems fair to conclude that the asbestos miners in the Province of Quebec do not have a significantly higher death rate for lung cancer than do comparable segments of the general population." To make such a statement when only 4% of the cohort was deceased was clearly premature. This study was funded by the Quebec Asbestos Mining Association and performed by the IHF.

In 1964, Elwood and Cochrane[794] studied 1165 men and 268 women who worked in a factory using chrysotile only asbestos for 6 months or more during the period 1936–1962. Only 885 of both the men and the women were traced and of those only 13% of the men and 5% of the women had died. One mesothelioma in a man exposed to asbestos before the study period and 11 lung cancers were reported. When the authors[794] looked at those lung cancers with 15 years or more latency, there were 7 reported when 3.02 were expected, which was a doubling of the number but not a statistically significant finding. Because of the short latencies and with 12% lost to follow-up, this study was limited in its power to determine any excesses in asbestos-related diseases, especially long latent diseases including lung cancers and mesothelioma.

In 1965, it was reported by Kogan et al.[795] that immunobiological reactivity was suppressed in asbestosis patients and more so in those exposed to chrysotile than to the anthophyllite form of asbestos. The complement titer was the most clearly suppressed and preceded both clinical and radiological signs of asbestosis. The degree of suppression increased with duration of exposure. The authors[795] reported that persons with both asbestosis and high exposure to asbestos developed lesions peculiar to autoimmunologic disease. These occurred in a rise to gamma-globulin and anti-complementary activity of the serum.

In 1966, Kogan et al.[796] reported that short fiber chrysotile asbestos and serpentine dust both exert a fibrogenic effect on pulmonary tissue, but that chrysotile asbestos exerted the greatest effect. In another paper from 1966, Kogan et al.[797] reported on the mortality of lung cancer as being three times higher among Russian chrysotile workers than that in the adjacent town and that the town's lung cancer mortality was twice that of the region. They also reported that 9% of those with asbestosis died of lung cancer and it was also higher among women workers.

In 1968, Godwin and Jagatic[422] sent a letter to the *JAMA* questioning the presumption that mesothelioma involved only those exposed to crocidolite asbestos. They[422] pointed out examples of mesothelioma in persons exposed to chrysotile asbestos, including a 43-year-old worker with a history of weaving chrysotile brake linings, a 50-year-old man who worked for 5 years in a Canadian asbestos mine and who showed x-ray diffraction evidence of only chrysotile in his body, and the induction of mesothelioma in the pleura of rats who inhaled chrysotile along with the development of mesothelioma in hamsters and mice following chrysotile administration.

With the passage of the OSHAct of 1970, more information continued to be published on the hazards of exposure to chrysotile asbestos. Champion[798] reported two cases of mesothelioma, one of which was attributed to exposure to chrysotile asbestos. It was also at this time that a series of epidemiologic studies began on Canadian chrysotile asbestos miners and millers, who continue to be followed to the present. The first of these epidemiologic studies was conducted by McDonald and coworkers from the McGill University in Montreal, Quebec, Canada, in the Province where the major Canadian chrysotile mines are located.

In 1971, McDonald et al.[799] reported on the mortality of chrysotile asbestos miners in the mines and mills of Québec. Their primary purpose was to "define as accurately as possible the quantitative relationship between exposure to chrysotile asbestos and the incidence of lung cancer." Of 11,788 persons identified as born between 1891 and 1920 and who worked in the mining industry, 88.4% were traced and, of these, 2457 (23.6%) had died. Overall, the mortality of the cohort was lower than expected, but in the highest exposure group it was 20% higher than that in other groups of workers. Three mesotheliomas were reported and 97 deaths were attributed to lung cancer. In the highest exposure category, respiratory cancers were five times higher compared with workers with the lowest exposure. Because about 12% overall were lost to follow-up, the results could likely underestimate the true rates of mortality. The highest lost to follow-up were in the older age category and in less than the 10-year employment category. Twenty-three cases of asbestosis were reported, and the greatest occurrence was in those workers with between 10 and 29 years of employment. The authors[799] do not give a latency analysis; therefore, it is impossible to determine what the power of the study is for the detection of long latent diseases associated with asbestos exposures, such as cancer. In a later paper authored by Liddell, McDonald and Thomas,[800] they criticized this first study as "not the best possible. It relied on cumulative mortality (ignoring era and age of death), allowed imperfectly for losses to view, and used a rather inflexible method of calculating expectations from an external standard, while the selection of sub-cohorts rendered particularly difficult the investigation of interactions."

Following this first report by McDonald et al., Navarátil and Trippé[801] reported on a plant processing asbestos products using both Soviet and Canadian chrysotile. In their x-ray survey of approximately 800 workers, they found a little more than 5% ($n = 42$) had pleural calcifications and more than half showed radiologic signs of asbestosis. When looking at 114 blood relatives of asbestos workers and 115 inhabitants in the neighborhood of the factory, 3.5% ($n = 4$) of the relatives and 5.8% ($n = 9$) from the neighborhood had pleural calcifications. The percentage of pleural calcifications in the general population ($n = 8133$) of the district was only 0.34% ($n = 28$). Thus, this study[801] shows direct exposures as well as proximity to those exposed (bystander) or by living in the neighborhood of the factory can be affected by the chrysotile asbestos, barring other exposures have not occurred to sources of asbestos.

In studying the area where the largest deposits of chrysotile are located, Kogan et al.[802] found the total cancer mortality rate among Russian Urals asbestos miners and millers was 1.6 times higher when compared with the general population. The period of investigation was between 1948 and 1967. Lung cancer in men was two times higher. For women, the total cancer rates were less than expected in the mines and somewhat higher in the mills (1.3); however, for lung cancer, the female rates were 2.1 times higher in the mines and 1.4 times higher in the mill workers than that of the general population. When looking at miners older than 50 years, the rates of lung cancer were much higher. For men, the rate was 4.9 in mining and 5.9 in milling, and for women, the rate was 9.5 in mining and 39.8 in milling. No mesotheliomas were reported nor were the total number of miners and millers in the total cohort reported.

In 1973, McDonald[803] reported that in the cohort of the Quebec chrysotile mining industry, the total deceased had increased to 2950 (30%) and that five pleural mesotheliomas had since been reported compared with three in the first study. There were 129 respiratory cancers when the number expected for the totality of Quebec was 139, but for the mining region it was only 93. This meant that asbestos workers had an occurrence of respiratory cancer 34% above that of the local population. The percentage of respiratory cancers increased as estimated dust exposures increased, with that in the highest dust category having about three times that of the lowest, but when comparing those with more than 30 years employment, the difference was about five times greater than those employed less than 1 year and in the lowest exposure category. When McDonald compared the Quebec cohort with a smaller cohort from Italy (about one-tenth of the size), the results were fairly similar; however, no mesotheliomas were reported in the Italian cohort, but one mesothelioma did occur in the neighborhood around the Italian mine, whereas four additional cases attributed to domestic exposure were reported in Quebec. When McDonald looked at several other chrysotile production areas, he found one additional mesothelioma in Cyprus where chrysotile production had begun in 1904. Therefore, McDonald reported 11 cases of mesothelioma associated with chrysotile production or in its vicinity among the three geographic areas he looked at. He also concluded that the eight cases in his cohort were at least four times that expected. It is of interest that McDonald mentioned this was a very small number of mesotheliomas considering that 30,000 persons have been employed in the Quebec industry and that many times this number have been exposed at home or in the general environment.

In a study by McDonald's wife Alison and two other researchers,[804] they reported 165 cases of primary malignant mesothelial tumors between 1960 and 1968 in a Canadian National Survey and an additional 71 cases reported between 1968 and 1970. Of these, a panel of pathologists reviewed 180 of the cases and certified 99 as being mesothelioma while being uncertain in 12 cases. The authors[804] stated that more in the certain category had exposure to asbestos, but this came from, as best I can see, the most available source but not from personal interviews with next of kin. Therefore, the question is how many of these were a result of exposure from the Canadian Chrysotile mine and mills versus environmental or occupational exposure to end products manufactured from chrysotile originating from the mines?

In the first reported look at the Ballangero chrysotile mine in Italy, Rossiter[805] reported in 1973 on cancers related to this fiber type. There were no reported mesotheliomas; however, there was a slight excess of lung cancer deaths. From the Czechoslovakia data where only Russian chrysotile was used, Rossiter reported 54 cases of asbestosis, 8 lung cancers, and 2 mesotheliomas. This shows an excess risk of lung cancer as well as asbestosis and mesothelioma from the Czechoslovakian data, but evidence from the larger group (25,000) of asbestos workers in the Russian chrysotile mining industry were lacking and needed to be compared with the Czechoslovakian data. Rossiter reported that in the Selikoff national survey of 1092 deaths among insulation workers before amphibole asbestos (amosite) was used pre-1935 in this industry, the lung cancer risks were a result of chrysotile exposure. Rossiter pointed out that Pooley, in a nonstatistical analysis of fiber type in mesothelioma cases, stated it was unlikely that chrysotile dissolved completely in the lung, although physical breakdown, relocation, and removal could occur. This is because examination of tissue from persons occupationally exposed to chrysotile has shown at least as many fibers as are found in tissue of those exposed to amphiboles.

Timbrell[778] pointed out that because UICC Canadian chrysotile has produced mesotheliomas, this suggests that present techniques are inadequate to detect and quantify asbestos fibers in tissue, especially very fine chrysotile fibers. (Note that this observation in 1973 should have brought into question the conclusions of many epidemiology studies that used or continued to use PCM and SEM to measure fiber burden when making statements on the causative fiber type in disease causation). Timbrell also pointed out that because short chrysotile fibers are virtually straight, they will behave aerodynamically like amphibole fibers and that aerodynamic properties seem to govern the biological response. These findings suggest that there may be major differences in exposures at different points of asbestos use in the industry and that this is supported by the high health risks found in the asbestos textile trade.

Morgan[806] reported that by 1973, the evidence suggested that both asbestosis and lung cancer appeared to be unrelated to fiber type but that a dose–response relationship as dose increased was the most important risk factor. He also concluded that animal studies confirmed that when the various fiber types were intrapleurally inoculated, chrysotile was just as effective as crocidolite in producing mesothelioma.

Wagoner et al.[299] studied 3367 asbestos textile, friction, and packing industry workers employed at least 1 year or more between January 1, 1940, and December 31, 1962, and followed through January 1, 1968. There were 655 (19%) deceased and 231 (7%) lost to follow-up. The plant used mainly chrysotile and less than 1% amphiboles. Malignant neoplasms were found in excess and statistically significant at the $p < .05$ level with an SMR of 122 (95% CI = 1.01–1.46). Cancers of the respiratory system and NMRDs were statistically significant at the $p < .01$ level with SMRs of 244 (95% CI = 1.79–3.26) and 206 (95% CI = 1.61–2.59), respectively. The respiratory cancers and the NMRDs followed a dose–response pattern, with those having more than 20 years latency having the highest significant excess. More than 50% of the lung cancer deaths occurred less than 6 months after termination of employment. A somewhat similar pattern occurred for the NMRDs, with 41.5% dying less than 6 months after termination of employment. No cases of mesothelioma were reported. Because of the small percentage of decedents and the high percent lost to follow-up, future evaluation might reveal a different pattern of mortality. Less than one-fourth of the cohort were deceased and the follow-up was only 93%; therefore, further follow-up might yield more information on the risks of mesothelioma in this cohort.

Enterline and Henderson[807] studied 1348 retirees from the asbestos industry and concluded that men exposed only to chrysotile after adjustment for cumulative dust exposure* had a respiratory cancer mortality rate 2.4 times that expected. However, for men exposed to both chrysotile and crocidolite, the mortality rate was 5.3 times that expected. Seven hundred fifty-four deaths occurred, of which 733 death certificates were located. Eighteen deaths were determined to be from asbestosis with no trend as to age. In this study, only men exposed to amosite or chrysotile alone were studied. Data on crocidolite did not allow it to be studied alone. Although the cohort did not have complete smoking histories, the data that were available on smoking suggested that the differences in respiratory risk were not due to differences in smoking habits. Although the number of retirees with amosite only exposure was small, the findings of those using amosite in combination with other

---

* The adjustment assumes that the cumulative dust exposures at time of retirement for each group had been the same as the equivalent average dust exposure for the total cohort.

types of asbestos did not differ from the risk seen for men exposed only to chrysotile asbestos. Of 1013 men exposed only to chrysotile asbestos, there was a clear dose–response relationship and little doubt that chrysotile had carcinogenic or co-carcinogenic properties. These authors[807] suggested there might be a threshold for chrysotile and respiratory cancer only; however, no conclusions could be made for its relationship to mesothelioma. The authors[807] pointed out that studies of retirees have been criticized as representing a survivor population and possibly a group less susceptible to the toxic effects of asbestos or other toxins.

In 1974, McDonald et al.[808] reported nine cases of mesothelioma associated with the Quebec chrysotile mining and milling industry. Seven (five in the cohort studied) had been employees and the other two were women whose fathers worked in the industry. On the basis of this study evaluating respiratory signs and symptoms, the authors suggested that a 1% risk of clinically significant disease was not reached until a worker had between 2 and 4 million particles per cubic foot exposure as calculated for a 50-year working life. This could not be applied to the two mesothelioma cases in women as exposure data were not reported for the household exposures. When Gibbs and LaChance[809] placed side-by-side midget impinger–membrane filter samples taken at five mines and mills in Quebec, they found that the correlation was poor and no single conversion factor could be justified. This is in contrast to the conversion factor used by many where 6 fiber/mL is equal to 1 mppcf.

A random sample of 1027 workers out of 6180 men working on October 31, 1966, in eight constituent companies of the Quebec Asbestos Mining Association was selected.[810] A second sample was selected to increase the number of older men to bring the random sample up to 1268 men. One thousand sixty-nine (83%) agreed to be tested during 1967–1968, and completed results were obtained for 1034 men. Five pulmonary function tests were used, and a normal profile was found in 44.3% of the workers. Restrictive and obstructive function profiles occurred with equal frequency in 12.8% and 12.2%, respectively, and both were associated with radiologic asbestosis. Because these occurred infrequently in nonsmokers, the authors[810] concluded that a synergistic association existed between smoking and the harmful effects of asbestos exposure on lung function. By implication, the authors[810] suggested this was true for lung fibrosis. The authors[810] suggested that the use of a polyvalent test such as the vital capacity should be most appropriate for early detection of abnormality in the Quebec chrysotile asbestos production industry. The authors[810] pointed to differences in the health effects of asbestos exposure in one industry compared with another and in one type of operation compared with another and may well be explained in terms of differences in the levels of dust exposure and/or particle size distribution. Furthermore, the authors[810] suggested this experience in the primary mining and milling of pure chrysotile asbestos might not be directly applicable to secondary industries concerned with the further processing of this fiber.

Weiss[811] studied a small number of men hired during 1935–1945 in a chrysotile asbestos products factory who had worked 1 year or more and who were alive on January 1, 1945. The follow-up traced 94% of the men. Unfortunately, Weiss did not do a latency analysis but did compare those with less than 5 years employment with those greater than 5 years and found that mortality was 50% higher in the latter group, which Weiss attributed to age. Two cases of asbestosis occurred among 25% of the cohort who were deceased by the end of the study period on December 31, 1974. Because Weiss did not analyze by latency, the man-year analysis in this paper showed that two-thirds of the population had less than 20 years latency, meaning that the power of the study was further limited to determine the true magnitude from the longer latent asbestos-related diseases like mesothelioma and other cancers. Closer examination of this study[811] suggested several possible explanations for the favorable mortality experience of these workers. First, the study population was small ($n = 264$), and only 66 (25%) workers had died at the time of analyses. Second, the analyses included larger observation periods, which were less than 25 or 30 years from the onset of initial exposure. Frequently, asbestos-associated disease does not manifest until after 25 years from initial exposure. Third, the age distribution of the study population was not listed, which may have played an important role in the mortality patterns of these workers and is interesting because the author[811] attributed the higher mortality in the greater than 5 years of employment to age. Fourth, more than 50% of the workers studied were employed for less than 4 years but with no idea as to their subsequent latency from termination. Given these uncertainties makes the author's[811] conclusion rather questionable, which was: "While the dearth of pertinent information makes for an unsatisfactory state of *affairs*, the favorable experience of the cohort reported in the current study suggests that the hazard of chrysotile in asbestos products manufacturing is minimal. The results are consistent with what is known of the relative dangers of chrysotile, amosite, and crocidolite."

In a cross-sectional clinical study of 485 active chrysotile miners from Baie Verte, Newfoundland, 50 (10%) had one or more radiographic abnormalities commonly associated with asbestos exposure.[812] Pleural changes, including fibrosis and calcification, were present in 3%, and the abnormalities increased with duration of employment. Fifteen percent of those with more than 10 years employment had abnormal x-rays, whereas 5% of those with less than 5 years employment had abnormal films. Abnormalities were also more prevalent in those with heaviest exposures (12%) compared with 7% among the least exposed. This study was not designed to detect asbestos-related disease of long latency such as mesothelioma or other cancers as it was a cross-sectional medical evaluation only.

In their first monograph on asbestos, the IARC[813] concluded that all forms of asbestos, including chrysotile asbestos, caused all asbestos-related diseases, including asbestosis, lung cancer, and mesothelioma. They also concluded: "At present, it is not possible to assess whether there is a level of exposure in humans below which an increased risk of cancer would not occur."

Studying radiological changes more than 20 years in relation to chrysotile exposure in Quebec, Liddell et al.[814] found abnormalities most related to time from first employment. The study consisted of 267 men who were Quebec chrysotile mine and mill workers, each with five chest radiographs spanning an average of 20 years. Of the 150 men with normal x-rays on their first film, 45 (30%) had some radiological change in subsequent films over more than a 20-year period. Changes were weakly related to age. The study was conducted in three phases: Phase 1 measured the degree of abnormality to age when first employed, years from first employment, average dust concentrations, and if a smoker. Phase 2 looked at 150 men whose earliest films were normal and followed until any change occurred or until the last film was taken. The stimulus variables for this phase included age at first film showing change, if a smoker, and dust concentrations over the period of employment up to 5 years before change occurred. Phase 3 looked at those whose first film was abnormal and then followed the possible progression in subsequent films, examining factors that may have contributed to the changes. This phase consisted of 111 men. Overall, dust levels were considerably lower at the town of Asbestos than at Thetford Mines, and Thetford had more abnormality from small opacities and considerably more pleural changes of all types except obliteration of the costophrenic angle.

McDonald's[815] continuing studies of the Quebec chrysotile miners and millers had found 11 mesotheliomas as of 1977—4 from the town/area of Asbestos and 7 from the Thetford Mines area. Two cases from Thetford had questionable diagnoses, but all were pleural and occurred in men employed between 19 and 53 years, but no latency periods were defined. McDonald stated that at the Thetford Mines "There is therefore no good reason to doubt chrysotile exposure as the cause." When compared with the chrysotile miners in Italy where one mesothelioma was reported, which accounted for 0.30% of all deaths, the Quebec miners and millers accounted for 0.24% of all deaths attributed to mesothelioma.

By 1977, Peto[816] concluded that the 2 fibers/cm³ was too high for chrysotile. In his reanalysis of the British Occupational Hygiene Society study of 679 men in an asbestos textile factory, up to 10% of the men exposed for 50 years to chrysotile asbestos at concentrations of 1 to 2 fibers/cm³ were likely to die of asbestos-induced disease.

Elena[817] looked at a small number of workers engaged in the manufacture of chrysotile asbestos cement and brake linings in Cuba. Out of the 123 workers, there were 17 cases of pleural changes. Most of those affected were workers with 5 years or more exposure.

Robinson et al.[300] followed up a study of the chrysotile textile, friction, and packing plant previously reported by Wagoner et al. in 1973, which now had 98% follow-up with one-third of the population deceased. The plant used more than 99% chrysotile per year except for 3 years during World War II when amosite was used due to U.S. naval specifications, which increased its use from <1% to approximately 5% of the total use during these 3 years. Crocidolite asbestos use was always less than 1% of the total asbestos used. Nine hundred twelve deaths among men occurred when 714.3 would have been expected ($p < .01$). Total malignant neoplasms, diseases of the heart, NMRD, and suicides were found in significant excess among men. Malignant diseases of the respiratory tract accounted for a large part of the total cancer deaths (49 observed vs. 36.1 expected; $p < .05$), although many of the heart disease death certificates indicated that occupationally induced respiratory disease was a direct contributing cause of death in 29 of the white male asbestos workers. The excesses of NMRDs did not include bronchitis, acute upper respiratory infection, influenza, or pneumonia, implying other diseases including pneumoconiosis as the cause (76 observed vs. 16.4 expected; $p < .01$). The NMRDs had a latency effect as the years since onset of employment increased, as did the ratios of disease being greatest after 30 years since employment. Suicide deaths were in excess in men only, and the excess followed an increasing trend through the second latency interval since onset of employment. The authors[300] could not rule out an association between the suicides and asbestos-related diseases. In the Robinson et al. study,[300] 17 mesotheliomas were observed compared with none in the earlier analysis by Wagoner et al. in 1973, which could have been due to the lower follow-up or the increased longer latency. There were five pleural mesotheliomas, six peritoneal mesotheliomas, and six with sites unspecified. In three of the five pleural mesotheliomas, the medical records indicated preexisting asbestosis, whereas five of the six peritoneal mesotheliomas had asbestosis, as did two of the unspecified cases. In case series studies of mesothelioma in the general population, a male-to-female ratio of 3:1 was seen, whereas in studies of asbestos workers, no difference in the ratio or a slightly elevated rate for women was seen as in this study where the population rate was 2.7/10,000 for women and 1.9/10,000 for men. In this study,[300] 4.8% of workers developed mesothelioma. With only one-third of the study cohort deceased, further follow-up would be necessary to determine the full extent of asbestos-related disease, especially those of longer latency like cancers.

Rubino et al.[818] examined 56 retired Italian chrysotile asbestos miners who had retired 3 years before the study. X-rays before retirement were compared with those taken after retirement. Thirty-two percent of the retired miners had irregular opacities, 19.6% had pleural changes, and 39% had both parenchymal and pleural changes. The authors[818] found disease progression in 7 of the 18 workers with radiological signs of disease.

Rubino et al.[819] also evaluated the mortality of more than 900 miners in the Balangero mine in Northern Italy from 1946 to 1975. The mine was a pure chrysotile mine started in 1916 in the foothills of the Alps about 30 km from Turin. This was the second study of the mine, the first being by Ghezzi et al.[820] in 1972, which found no indication of an increase of lung cancer in the miners, and a proportional mortality study showed a similarity with the Quebec miners as reported by McDonald in 1973. Rubino et al.[819] had followed the cohort to 1975 and found 9 deaths attributed to asbestosis and 11 deaths to lung cancer. A death attributed to mesothelioma was not supported upon further histologic examination. No excess was seen in the lung cancers compared with the national Italian rate except for the last 5 years of observations when the SMR rose to 206 where all but two of the lung cancers occurred. Ten of the lung cancers occurred in the higher exposure group of more than 101+ fiber/years for an RR of 2.89. All of the lung cancer cases were smokers. This group of miners and millers continued be followed into the future and the results will be discussed later in this chapter.

Weill et al.[821] looked at the influence of dose and fiber types on malignancy when comparing those exposed to chrysotile and/or crocidolite in two New Orleans cement building materials plants. The cohort consisted of anyone who was ever employed for at least one continuous month before

January 1, 1970. The report focused on 5615 employees with at least 20 years of follow-up. Only 601 (11%) were deceased as of December 31, 1974, and 91% of the death certificates were found and coded by the Eighth Revision of the ICD. Five dust categories were evaluated. No excess mortality occurred in any exposure group other than respiratory cancers and only in those within the two highest dust categories of 101–200 and >200 mppcf-years occurring in a dose–response pattern as years since initial exposure occurred. Two mesotheliomas were diagnosed but did not make the cohort because both died less than 20 years since first employment, being 18 and 19 years. One of the mesotheliomas occurred in a man whose only known exposure was to chrysotile, whereas the other had exposure to chrysotile and crocidolite. The authors[821] suggested that mesothelioma may be underdiagnosed in this cohort and that other studies suggested mesotheliomas do occur in those with less than 20 years since initial exposure to asbestos.

In a further analysis using the case–control method, cancer patients were found to have higher exposures than did the matched controls (164.1 and 77.8 mppcf-years, respectively) and were statistically significantly different in the two highest dust categories of 100–200 or >200 mppcf-years. Respiratory cancers occurred in those exposed to both fiber types with the highest rate occurring in the mixed exposure group (those exposed to chrysotile with intermittent exposures to crocidolite). The importance of this study was that those exposed solely to chrysotile developed malignancies; however, the magnitude of the potency of chrysotile or crocidolite could not be compared by this study because only 11% of the total cohort were deceased, meaning that 89% of the cohort was still alive and the mortality patterns were very preliminary.[821,822]

McDonald et al.[823] continued reporting on the birth cohort of Quebec asbestos miners and millers that they had started studying in 1966 and which were described earlier in this chapter. This follow-up was presented at the Second Wave conference of Dr. Selikoff sponsored by the New York Academy of Sciences in 1979 and published in the *Annals of the New York Academy of Sciences*. In 1966, they had traced 88.4% of the original 11,788 members of the cohort and reported 23.6% had died. In this latest follow-up, they had now traced 90.1% of the now 11,379 cohort members with 44.3% now deceased. The authors[823] explained the reduced number from the original cohort was "due to improvement in information, which permitted more stringent application of admission criteria and better recognition of situations in which the same employee had been registered separately with different companies or under different names." This left the reader to assume that the 164 difference was due to duplication. The follow-up was still less than suitable for adequate analysis with almost 10% having vital status unknown and less than half the cohort deceased. The authors[823] pointed out that less than 2% were lost to follow-up after 1935. This larger group lost to follow-up before 1935 might contain some with longer latency and thus at higher risk of the longer latent diseases such as cancer. However, the authors[823] did show patterns of increasing mortality, which was now slightly greater than expected in men (SMR = 1.06; 4350 observed vs. 4107 expected). As the authors[823] pointed out, the comparison between the 1966 findings and those as of 1975 was not entirely compatible. However, there are some indications of an increasing trend in deaths due to pneumoconiosis, respiratory cancers, and mesotheliomas. With the additional 11 years of latency, the total deaths in men were now about 47% higher, pneumoconiosis 39% higher, respiratory cancers 62% higher, and mesotheliomas 70% higher. These increasing trends for pneumoconiosis and respiratory cancers tended to follow the increase in the amount of dust exposure. As for mesotheliomas, the authors[823] identified another two cases through 1977 with all occurring after more than 20 years latency from first exposure and 9 having 20 or more years of employment and only 3 with less than 20 years of employment. Although the authors[823] expected that mesotheliomas would continue to increase because of the long latency for mesothelioma, they felt that their overall excess would be less than for crocidolite. The authors[823] reported that the major occupational concern for these chrysotile miners and millers was due to respiratory cancers and fibrosis. Although the authors[823] found a linear relationship for respiratory cancers and dust exposures, they stated that developing a threshold for regulatory purposes would be difficult due to the conversion limitations between impinger counts and fiber counts, something they intended to work on in future analysis of the cohort.

Sebastien et al.[824] found that when comparing parenchymal samples with pleural samples, almost all fibers in the pleura were chrysotile fibers, but no single fiber type predominated in parenchymal samples. The authors[824] concluded that lung parenchymal retention was not a good indicator of fiber type or dose and that autopsy measurements of fiber concentration could be unreliable because of fiber translocation from the lung due to penetration and clearance.

Churg and Warnock,[825] when looking at the lungs of 21 urban dwellers with fewer than 100 asbestos bodies per gram of lung, a level previously associated with environmental and not occupational exposures, found that 80% of the fibers were chrysotile with 90% less than 5 µm long. Twenty percent of the amosite, crocidolite, and anthophyllite were longer than 10 µm and in accord with the types of fibers seen in asbestos bodies of these patients. The short fiber chrysotile was preferentially deposited subpleurally. The authors[825] concluded that substantial amounts of asbestos, mainly chrysotile and noncommercial amphiboles, were present in the average lung of an urban dweller. The authors[825] also reported that most of these fibers were too small to form asbestos bodies or to be seen by PCM.

Nicholson et al.[826] established a cohort of 544 miners from Thetford Mines, Quebec, Canada, who were employed during 1961 and had at least 20 years of seniority in one of four companies mining or milling chrysotile asbestos. The lists were obtained from the union representing the workers. All were traced and their vital status determined. One hundred seventy-eight (33%) of the 544 miners were deceased for which 172 death certificates were found. Information on the six without death certificates was obtained from hospital records or autopsy protocols and an additional 130 of the deceased had clinical, surgical, or pathologic data to supplement the information on the death certificate. Overall, 25 lung cancers (19%), 24 asbestosis (18%), and 1 mesothelioma (0.7%) were identified among the additional 130 decedents. For the entire number of deaths, there were 28 lung cancers when 11.1 were expected (OR = 2.52, 95% CI = 1.68–3.65). None were expected for the 26 asbestosis deaths or the 1 mesothelioma death. The highest number of lung cancers, asbestosis, and mesothelioma deaths was greatest after 40 years latency. There were no lung cancers observed less than 30 years from onset of employment; however, there were 11 lung cancers between 30 and 39 years latency, 24 between 40 and 49 years, and 14 with greater than 50 years. For asbestosis, three deaths occurred between 20 and 29 years latency, eight deaths between 30 and 39 years, eight deaths between 40 and 49 years, and seven deaths after 50 years. The one mesothelioma occurred after 40 years latency. When comparing the miners and millers to similar cohorts of factory workers or insulation workers having similar times since onset of exposure, the authors[826] found that asbestosis was similar between the miners and millers and the factory workers and insulation workers. For lung cancer, this was true for miners and millers and the factory workers but higher in the insulation workers. Mesothelioma was much less in the miners and millers when compared with factory workers and insulation workers. It is unclear from the paper if total follow-up was similar between all three groups, which could have an influence on the validity of the comparison between the three groups.

Acheson and Gardner[827] reported in their analysis of previously published work that when amphiboles and chrysotile exposures occurred together, a synergistic effect occurred. Their analysis used findings of Pooley, which compared fiber types in the lung matched to controls and calculated the RR. Simply put, Acheson and Gardner[827] found that those with chrysotile only in their lungs had an RR of 6, those with amphiboles alone in their lungs had an RR of 12, and for a mixture of both the RR jumped to 61. The RR also reacted similarly when classifying fiber burdens by nil, low, and high. However, in 1980 Acheson and Gardner[828] reported using a new fiber analysis technique counting fibers per mg rather than fibers per electron microscopic grid. This change did not allow direct comparisons with previous findings, but when using the new technique, the synergistic effect was not evident and the risk for mesothelioma from high chrysotile exposure and low amphibole exposure turned out to be half the risk for persons with low chrysotile and low amphibole, which was a rather curious finding. When high concentrations of amphiboles and low concentrations of chrysotile were present in the lung samples, the risk was four and a half times greater than those with low concentrations of both chrysotile and amphiboles. When both chrysotile and amphiboles were found in high concentrations, the risk was three times higher. Low concentrations in the lungs were <1000 fibers/mg lung tissue and high concentrations were >1000 fibers/mg.

In 2009, Peto[241] reported that protracted exposure suggested that asbestos acted both early and late in mesothelioma induction; therefore, chrysotile exposure could increase the lifelong mesothelioma risk in those whose lungs contained persistent amosite or crocidolite.

Boutin et al.[829] reviewed radiographs of 166 chrysotile mine and mill workers from Canari, Corsica. The mine opened in 1948 and closed in 1965. The authors[829] had been following this cohort since 1975, and the workers, at the time of the report in 1980, were 14 years since the mine closure. According to the authors,[829] the exposures were to "relatively pure chrysotile ore," with concentrations of 85 to 267 mppcf for a limited exposure of 11.3 years. Forty-seven percent of the workers had abnormal radiographs. Parenchymal fibrosis occurred in 19.3%, 6.6% had bilateral pleural changes, and 21.2% had parenchymal fibrosis and bilateral pleural changes. The dust weighted-time exposure was significantly higher in those with severe fibrosis or bilateral pleural thickening. The authors[829] reported that age, smoking, and exposures were similar in all workers and thus indicated the importance of dust exposures in asbestos-related disorders.[*]

Acheson and Gardner,[831] using data from McDonald's latest data on chrysotile miners and millers, estimated that if they allowed about half of the mortality attributed to chrysotile was due to lung cancer and the other half due to other asbestos-related causes, notably asbestosis, then a 2% excess mortality would occur with a range of 1–5 fibers/mL. This, however, is dependent on the conversion factor used to convert mppcf to fibers per milliliter. Specifically, for chrysotile and pleural mesothelioma, the authors[831] concluded that the only data related to dose of dust and mortality came from the McDonald et al. 1980 data, which was based on only 10 cases. In these data, the risk of mesothelioma was almost 10 times greater in the most heavily exposed workers when compared with those with the least exposure.

Peto[832] studied the incidence of pleural mesothelioma among workers in a chrysotile asbestos textile plant in the United Kingdom. The cohort included 567 men first employed before 1951 and 143 employed before 1933. Follow-up was through 1978. The first mesothelioma occurred in 1936 and was called *endothelium of the pleura*. The second mesothelioma did not occur until 1968, indicating that the disease might have been missed clinically in the intervening years according to the author. Fourteen cases total were observed in this cohort. The cohort was broken into three cohorts. The first included 69 men with 20 or more years of exposure with more than 10 employed before 1933. The second included 74 men with 20 or more years of exposure with less than 10 employed before 1933. The third included 424 men with 10 or more years of exposure employed between 1933 and 1950. In the first cohort of 69 men, there were two mesotheliomas; in the second cohort of 74 men, there were five mesotheliomas; and in the third cohort of 424 men, there were seven mesotheliomas. The shortest latency was 23 years with the remainder greater than 23 years and up to 50+ years since first exposure. In the first cohort, there were 13 lung cancers when 1.57 were expected (RR = 8.28, 95% CI = 4.4–14.2),[†] in the second cohort, there were 7 lung cancers when 3.54 were expected (RR = 1.98, 95% CI = 0.8–4.1),[‡] and in the third cohort, there were 22 lung cancers when 13.85 were

---

[*] Later studies of goats grazing in the area of the tailings of the mines in Corsica found both chrysotile and tremolite in their lungs. However, chrysotile fibers shorter than 5 μm were predominant in the parietal pleura, indicating their ability to translocate from the parenchymal lung to the parietal pleura where mesothelioma occurs. Seventy-eight percent and 86% of the tremolite found in the lung and parietal pleural samples were longer than 5 μm.[830]

[†] RR calculated by RAL.

[‡] Ibid.

expected (RR = 1.59, 95% CI = 1.0–2.4).[*] Although dust levels were "dramatically reduced" from 1933 onwards, the incidence of pleural mesothelioma did not appear to be substantially lowered in men employed since this date and remained as high as the rates reported among workers in a factory that processed much larger quantities of crocidolite. Peto[832] stated one explanation for this was that the risk of developing mesothelioma, although affected by early exposure, was substantially lower in men whose exposure was either reduced or had ceased than that in those whose exposure was maintained. Citing Jones et al.,[833] Peto pointed out that short or brief exposure to crocidolite could cause mesothelioma years later, but this had not been demonstrated for chrysotile. Peto also suggested the high incidence of asbestosis in those employed before 1933 in cohort 1 might have played a role in the reduction of mesotheliomas when compared with the lower rate of asbestosis in cohort 3 or those who were employed after 1933, which had an incidence of only 13%. The mesotheliomas were unrelated to age, which might suggest, according to Peto's speculation, that many human cancers might be entirely due to passage of time since exposure to a carcinogenic agent rather than the progressive breakdown of immunological or other growth control mechanisms. Also, the extent of exposure to crocidolite in this cohort was not accurately known and appeared to be much lower than other cohorts; therefore, it appears unlikely that occasional exposure to crocidolite was the major cause of the mesotheliomas in this cohort of chrysotile textile workers.

A 1980 IARC publication by Jones et al.[833] looked at 93 cases of confirmed mesothelioma in 1976 of which 86 had sufficient tissue for mineralogy. Originally, Jones et al.[833] received postmortem material on 117 cases, which had been diagnosed by the referring pathologist as being mesotheliomas or needing a definite diagnosis. In 1976, 209 deaths were certified as due to malignant neoplasm of the pleura in the United Kingdom. Therefore, less than half were included in this survey. In this limited study, chrysotile fibers were not present in the lungs of mesothelioma patients any more frequently than that in the controls. Four cases had no amphibole fibers in their lungs, although two of these only had chrysotile and the other two had no fibers in their lungs. These findings supported further findings of the low biopersistence of chrysotile in the lung. The findings may have also been marginally affected by the method used by Pooley and Clark,[834] which recognized that extensive preparation of the material might lead to alterations in both physical and chemical properties of the fibers. This process had not shown major changes with the amphiboles, the only exception being with chrysotile where some dispersion of aggregates could lead to production of extrafine fibrils, but the authors[834] reported these had been shown to produce only very small statistical changes in the size distribution of the chrysotile extracted from the biological samples.

McDonald et al.[835] continued to follow-up the original chrysotile cohort of Canadian asbestos miners and millers that had begun in 1966 and reported on in 1971, 1973, 1974, and 1977. During the 12-year period since the studies began, four stages of analysis had been done, which have been closely consistent. These analyses have shown essentially a linear relationship between length of service, exposures based on dust concentrations (mppcf) and lung cancer, pneumoconiosis and the total number of deaths. As reported in the paper presented at the New York Academy of Sciences Conference in 1979, a little less than half of the cohort was diseased (44.3%). In trying to look at exposure comparisons, the authors[835] pointed out the difficulties of comparing mppcf measurements with fiber per milliliter measurements and pointed to the extreme challenges in doing so. Although some estimates have been suggested such as a ratio of 3 to 7 fibers per 1 mppcf of dust, the authors[835] felt it was closer to the range of 1 to 5 fibers per 1 mppcf of dust. Whatever the range, it is at best speculative as the authors pointed out. The authors[835] also pointed out that smoking was a confounding factor and, by their belief, suggested that smoking had an additive effect whereas others believe it is a multiplicative effect or that lung cancer will not increase in the absence of smoking. The authors[835] took this a step further and speculated that before the advanced dust suppression systems were in place in the early 1950s, the lung cancer risk was equivalent to heavy smoking, but with the

---

[*] Ibid.

lowering of the dust levels to 1 mppcf, this would be equivalent to smoking one cigarette per day.[*] The authors[835] pointed to the factors that related to the validity of their survey by stating it was only as good as the environmental and mortality records on which it was based. They stated that many environmental measurements were taken after 1950, but that pre-1950, they could only estimate. As to their 10% overall lost to follow-up, the authors[835] stated that almost all were employed for a short time before 1935 and that since 1935 less than 2% were lost to follow-up. The authors pointed to the bias of death certificate studies and suggested that because of "diagnostic bias" by physicians writing the death certificates, those dying from respiratory disease with a known history of dust exposure may more likely be diagnosed as having pneumoconiosis, whereas others without such history would not. They also pointed out that because of compensation concerns, it might account for the higher rate of necropsies in those with pneumoconiosis (52%) and that this might overflow into those causes of death such as cancer of the lung and other organs that are underdiagnosed without necropsy. They stated that this would not affect the overall validity of the exposure–response relationship for total deaths but could have an effect on pneumoconiosis or lung cancer. They pointed out the healthy worker effect as a problem in cohort studies but discounted it as a major obstacle in this study because of the similarity of SMRs for all causes in short- and long-term employees overall.

McDonald et al.[835] found an excess of gastrointestinal cancers of the upper gastrointestinal tract in those highly exposed to dust and with 20 or more years of total service (SMR = 289 for esophagus and stomach), but not the lower. Nevertheless, they reported some evidence of an exposure–response trend. For those with 20 years total service, they[835] found a dose–response effect with both lung cancer (SMR = 2.65 in the "very high" exposure category) and pneumoconiosis (SMR = 101.52 in the "very high" exposure category). Lung cancers occurred in both nonsmokers and smokers and with a greater incidence in nonsmokers as dose increased, which was not evident in smokers. The study could not distinguish between additive or multiplicative models for smoking and exposure. The authors[835] reported pleural mesotheliomas in ten men and one woman. The authors[835] concluded: "By their nature, epidemiological surveys, however large, cannot achieve greater precision than the one described here. Hence, the clear importance of deciding whether a linear exposure–response model should be adopted, if only for practical reasons." This conclusion is apparently drawn from their earlier statement that "only the greatly enhanced SMRs for those with high and very high exposure allow the conclusion that there was a response to exposure."[†]

Liddell and McDonald[836] studied two cohorts of chrysotile miners and millers to determine the predictability of signs and symptoms including earlier x-rays for future mortality. One cohort of 11,379 workers had 1543 (33.8%) deaths by the end of 1975 and had one x-ray read that was taken before 1967. The other cohort was composed of 988 male workers who were examined in 1967–1968 through questionnaires on respiratory symptoms and smoking, lung function tests, and for whom six B-readers had assessed their 1966 x-rays using the U/C classification. By the end of 1975, 130 (13.2%) of the men studied in 1966 had died. Although these cohorts studied could have selection bias because of the requirement of having been x-rayed, several trends did occur. Total mortality was greater in the men who smoked, had radiographic abnormalities, or who were exposed to heavy dust. The indirect evidence was strong in showing no sign of a threshold for the exposure–response relationship for either lung cancer or pneumoconiosis. From this, the authors[836] concluded that employees exposed long enough to exhibit dust-related changes in their x-rays must have inevitably and already been at an increased risk of death from their asbestos-related diseases, meaning that periodic medical examination might be limited for protection unless the readings were valid and had prognostic significance. The authors[836] commented that the association between pulmonary fibrosis and lung cancer in asbestos workers was more a matter of theoretical interest

---

[*] In reading the paper, this appears as pure speculation with no scientific foundation.
[†] This paper demonstrates why even very large retrospective-prospective cohort epidemiology studies alone are inadequate for determining a threshold concentration for asbestos when attempting to measure effect at low concentrations.

and medicolegal importance, which their study did not answer. Smoking confounded their findings. In cohort 1 where only one reader read the x-ray, the SMR for lung cancer of 1.77 implied an occupational excess of perhaps 52 deaths, many by virtue of the interaction between asbestos and smoking. The authors[836] concluded it was impossible to specifically identify the excess cases individually, but by making a series of assumptions, the authors[836] pushed their data beyond its findings. They assumed that of the 118 lung cancers in cohort 1, that if all 33 with small opacities occurred in the 52 excess deaths from lung cancer, then this would suggest that most but not all lung cancers attributable to chrysotile exposure in mining and milling probably had small parenchymal opacities before death. Their assumption was based on the finding that 49 of the 52 excess lung cancer deaths had "less than normal" x-rays where small opacities would occur.* No such analysis was made of cohort 2 where all x-rays were read by all six B-readers.

Viallat et al.[837] followed up further progression of radiologic abnormalities among 166 former male workers in a chrysotile mine in Corsica and compared them to 156 matched controls. Forty-seven (47%) percent of ex-workers 13 years after end of exposure found 19.3% with fibrosis of the lung of category 1.1 using the ILO U/C radiological classification, 7% with bilateral pleural changes only, and 21.1% with both pleural and parenchymal changes. These findings led the authors[837] to conclude that asbestos-induced lesions progressed at various rates and was dependent upon dust exposure (higher in those more heavily exposed), whereas in this study, age, tobacco consumption, and length of exposure were similar in all those exposed. See also the report by Viallat et al. in 1983.[837]

Dr. Gail McKeown Eyssen[838] picked 270 men out of 11,000 who had worked wholly or predominantly in chrysotile mining and milling in Quebec and whose most recent chest radiograph was taken in 1971 plus 4 earlier taken at 5-year intervals. Using the ILO U/C 1971 classification and designating 0/1 and below as normal, Dr. Eyssen used five B-readers to evaluate the series of films for each man. The B-readers differed greatly in the number of subjects as normal on the first (earliest) film compared with abnormal (53% vs. 97%, respectively). They also differed on those "attacked," being those normal on earliest film then abnormal on later films by 24% to 96%, respectively. The B-readers did agree that on those attacked, the radiographic pattern usually showed small opacities of chest wall thickening. In the ILO U/C scheme, asbestosis was usually characterized by the characteristic small irregular opacities appearing in the lower lung zones; however, as these came from nonepidemiological surveys, Eyssen's study did come from such a survey. Dr. Eyssen's study found that although there was a slight trend for irregular opacities to be recorded less often in the upper zones, only one of the B-readers found the preponderance of rounded opacities to be in the upper lung zones, and there was slightly more tendency for the right lung to be affected than the left. The main finding was that there was little consistency among B-readers, although they were all well trained using standard ILO U/C films. Liddell[814] also found considerable interobserver variability in the assessment of the shape and size of small opacities as well as affected lung zones. The overall message from this study is that when x-rays are used as a clinical tool, there is no reason to believe they are less variable than those read for epidemiologic studies. Thus, it is emphasized that the chest radiograph is only one tool to be used in diagnosing asbestosis and must be used in conjunction with clinical signs and symptoms and occupational history.

Dement et al.[839] studied a textile plant in South Carolina with 768 men employed 6 months or more and found statistically significant excess mortality for lung cancer and NMRDs. Lung cancer deaths increased with years of employment, and none occurred before 15 years from initial employment. One case of mesothelioma and 15 cases of asbestosis were reported. Using cumulative dose as the exposure variable and the SMR for disease risk, strong dose–response relationships were

---

* The author feels that in these studies, the authors have gone beyond the limits of the data in making these assumptions and notes that the study's authors (Liddell and McDonald) indicate the study was sponsored by a grant from the Institute of Occupational and Environmental Health of the Quebec Asbestos Mining Association.

observed for lung cancer and NMRDs with a linear fit being the best to describe the dose–response curve for both. Lung cancer was significantly in excess at the lowest cumulative fiber exposure category of less than 10,000 fiber/cm^3/days. The authors[839] identified potential confounders as age, race, sex, and calendar time period, which their methodology dealt with. Both comparison populations and smoking posed larger confounding problems. The death rates chosen for this population were those of white men for the entire United States because using local rates would have elevated the expected number due to asbestos exposures from the shipyard industry, which was the peak industry in the area where lung cancer rates were as much as 75% higher than that of the entire United States. As for smoking patterns, those in the asbestos workers were very similar to those found in the United States. When using conversion factors for converting mppcf to fibers/mL, there are always questions of accuracy, and although this study tried to take into account the differences from operation to operation as fiber morphology can change, the important finding was the consistency of a dose–response with the principle asbestos-related diseases—asbestosis and lung cancer. The finding of only one mesothelioma in the cohort or 0.5% of the deaths raises the question of underdiagnosis. However, other cohorts exposed to mainly chrysotile have shown similar findings, although as latency increases, such a finding might change as it did in the Robinson et al.[300] study where no mesotheliomas were reported in the first analysis of the cohort by Wagoner et al.[299] and the 17 recorded by the 1979 analysis.

Drs. McDonald and Fry[840] published a preliminary report of mesothelioma incidence from three American asbestos factories. In this study sponsored by the Quebec Asbestos Mining Association, no mesotheliomas were found in a friction manufacturing plant in Connecticut, one case of mesothelioma was found in a South Carolina textile manufacturing plant, and 18 mesotheliomas were found in a Pennsylvanian textile, friction, and packing manufacturing plant. Not a great deal can be derived from this report as to the real exposures to the various types of asbestos fibers except that the three plants used mainly chrysotile. The authors[840] described the Pennsylvanian plant as a mixed exposure plant; however, authors who studied this plant in detail reported that the asbestos type used in this plant was 99% chrysotile (see Robinson et al., 1979).[300] McDonald and Fry[840] concluded that a possibility of missed cases might have occurred in factories A and B and the inclusion of persons with short and low exposures in their three cohorts raised some problems.

In a study of workers in the Havelock chrysotile mines and mills in Swaziland, McDermott et al.[841] compared two groups of workers radiologically and by pulmonary function testing results. The mine had been in full operation since the 1930s with a workforce of about 2000 Africans and 100 Europeans. An attempt was made to trace all men who had been employed for 10 years or more before 1970, which produced a list of 748 men. Of the 748 men, 185 were still employed, 153 had left but still lived in Swaziland, 200 had moved, and 210 had died. Out of the group of 338 still living in Swaziland, there were 270 Swazis and 68 Europeans, of which 235 Swazis and 36 Europeans participated in chest radiographs and examination and completed occupational history questionnaires. Of those eligible for the study, 46% participated, 28% were deceased, and 26% had moved away from the area. Because of this distribution, the results of the study reflected less than half of the eligible population for study and the remainder represented the active workforce and those that chose to stay in Swaziland near the mining area. Thus, the representativeness of the study cohort was unclear because over half of those eligible were not included and possibly the sickest were included in those deceased workers not in the study. Twenty-nine percent of the men had category 1 or more pneumoconiosis, 4.5% had category 2, and 1.5% had category 3. Not surprisingly, almost twice those in the dustiest jobs had the most abnormal results in both pulmonary function and x-ray grade profusion not related to aging alone. When looking at a second group consisting of mill workers who were exposed to much higher concentrations of dust than those in the mine or in surface jobs included in group 1, there were 224 men eligible with a mean age of 33 years, and all worked in the mill for at least 1 year. Exposures within the dustiest categories more than doubled the estimated annual decline in pulmonary function and also doubled the rate of progression of dust-related lung disease. Smoking did not account for the differences in either lung function or lung disease as the authors found no significant difference between smokers and nonsmokers. The first study found considerable deterioration of lung function and an increase of small opacities profusion except in one area of the mill, that being the rock crushing plant. The second study of younger men exposed for shorter periods confirmed the results from the first study group. When compared with the Quebec miners, the difference between those with category 1 parenchymal change was quite different, with the Quebec miners experiencing about 5% whereas the Swaziland group experienced about 30%. The Italian chrysotile mining group experienced an incidence of 29.8% for parenchymal change category 1/1 or greater, whereas the Corsican chrysotile men experienced an incidence of 40.3%. It is important to note that this study and those in Italy, Corsica, and Quebec all show chrysotile miners and millers at risk of both radiologic changes and pulmonary decrements as a result of exposure to chrysotile. Although the radiological results from Swaziland, Italy, and Corsica were similar, those for Canadian miners and millers were much lower and seemed to be the outlier for which no explanation was rendered.

In a follow-up of the preliminary report by McDonald and Fry in 1982 and supported by the Quebec Asbestos Mining Association, McDonald et al.[842] published another paper in 1982 on the Pennsylvania plant. Several more specific conclusions were drawn about this plant. In this study, the authors[842] reported 14, not 18, mesotheliomas from the Pennsylvania plant as they did in the preliminary report. Second, the authors reported that the "Lines fitted to relative risks derived from SMRs in this [Pennsylvania plant] and the textile plant studied in South Carolina were almost identical in slope." Third, the authors[842] concluded that the findings from the Pennsylvania plant supported the conclusion reached by the South Carolina study that lung cancer risk was much greater in textile processing than in chrysotile mining and milling and speculated this might be true for the friction products industry. Finally, the authors[842] stated a much greater risk of mesothelioma from exposures to processes where even quite small quantities of amphiboles were used had been confirmed.

Mortality experience was evaluated in two factories where women manufactured gas masks.[843] One factory used crocidolite only while making gas masks for the military during World War II. The masks were made by hand. In the other factory that used chrysotile asbestos to make gas masks for civilians during World War II, the masks were mass produced by mechanical means. The two plants—one in Leyland and the other in Blackburn, England—included 757 and 576 women, respectively. The identities of the women were found by searching the National Health Service Central Register of every resident in September 1939 of Leyland, Preston, and Blackburn whose occupations at that time indicated they were manufacturing gas masks. The vital status as of June 30, 1980, was ascertained. About one-third of each group was deceased at the end of the study period, and the majority was in their 60s at the time of the study. The excess deaths in Leyland were mainly due to cancer, which was not true in Blackburn. In Leyland, there was a pronounced excess of deaths from lung and ovarian cancers.[*] There were five deaths from mesothelioma in Leyland and one from Blackburn. The authors[843] attributed the differences between the two plants as possibly because of the following: (1) Leyland used crocidolite while Blackburn used chrysotile, (2) the Leyland gas masks were made by hand and those in Blackburn were made by mechanical means, and (3) the Leyland factory had been operational longer than the Blackburn facility. These last two differences could have resulted in higher doses and longer duration of exposure to the women in Leyland than in Blackburn. The authors[843] also pointed out that prior occupational histories were unknown for the women from either plant. Also, the authors[843] reported three additional mesotheliomas from the Blackburn plant, and each had amphiboles in their lung tissue.[†] One of the three may have worked in another plant in Blackburn where crocidolite was used.

---

[*] IARC now recognizes ovarian cancers as asbestos related (IARC, 2009).

[†] Acheson et al. did not specify the type of amphibole found in the lung samples, but this is not an uncommon finding for persons exposed to chrysotile as tremolite can be a contaminate and also may be a good measure of the original, but no

In a preliminary report by Rowlands et al.[845] looking at lung samples from 47 Quebec miners and millers and using TEM, the authors found tremolite in the samples similar to chrysotile, suggesting that much of the chrysotile fibers were removed from the lung while the contaminate amphibole tremolite remained. Few people had more than one million fibers of crocidolite or amosite in their lung samples. The authors[845] cited two case–control studies of mesothelioma by Jones et al.[833] and McDonald et al.,[835] where both groups of authors pointed out that the critical level of amosite or crocidolite in the lung of apparent etiological significance was one million fibers per gram dried lung tissue and that smaller concentrations were found equally in both their cases and controls. Rowlands et al.[845] found lung content of amosite and crocidolite in the Quebec miners and millers mainly below one million fibers per gram of dry lung tissue. Rowlands et al.[845] suggested that although tremolite was found in similar quantities to chrysotile in their study of 47 Quebec miners and millers' lungs, it was unlikely that tremolite rather than chrysotile had a role in the miners' asbestosis. Rowlands et al.[845] suggested it was difficult to know what the fate of the chrysotile was as to penetration of the chrysotile into alveolar spaces and whether it was different than that of tremolite because they received and evaluated only paraffin blocks for which they did not know where, in the lung, they came from.

In an asbestos plant manufacturing textiles, friction, and packaging products using 99% chrysotile, an excess of non-Hodgkin's lymphoma was found (7 observed vs. 3.28 expected; SMR = 2.13, 95% CI = 0.86–4.40).[846] Although statistically insignificant, the authors[846] reported that an earlier study of the same plant identified five additional hematopoietic and lymphatic malignancies. Additionally, the authors[846] reported that animal experiments revealed reticulosarcomas in rats administered with chrysotile asbestos orally or by intratracheal injection along with benzopyrene. They further suggested that a possible etiology for non-Hodgkin's lymphoma was supported by findings that thoracic lymph nodes were important points in the clearance pathway of asbestos fibers in animals and humans.

In a chrysotile mine in Corsica, which closed, a comparison between radiographic changes of 133 ex-workers from 1965 to 1979 revealed the prevalence of grade 1/1 or more parenchymal fibrosis had risen from 14% to 40% and the change in bilateral pleural lesions had risen from 6% to 27%.[837] Progression of parenchymal changes occurred in 39% of workers who had normal findings in 1965 and in 63% of those with grade 1/1 parenchymal fibrosis since 1965. The authors[837] noted that these changes occurred in those who were older and those with longer exposures to the highest dust concentrations and who were heavier smokers.

Churg[844] found a significant difference of about twice as much fibers in pulmonary asbestos burden of the lungs between nine chrysotile asbestos miners with asbestos airways disease (early asbestosis) with no evidence of classic asbestosis on pathologic examination with matched miners without asbestos airways disease. Churg discounted this because of being sufficiently small enough to suggest other factors may have been involved in the genesis of the small airway lesions. Churg[844] also found contaminant amphiboles (tremolite, actinolite, and anthophyllite) probably from the chrysotile ore. He found a strong correlation between the amount of chrysotile and amphiboles, suggesting that amphiboles might be a good measure of the original chrysotile burden.

Liddell[847] reported from the large Canadian chrysotile mining population that in those workers with more than 20 years of employment, out of 3291 deaths between 1951 and 1975, there were 230 lung cancers, 276 abdominal cancers, and 10 mesotheliomas. This resulted in a PMR for mesothelioma of 3/1000 when compared with other chrysotile studies (worldwide) that found 2/1000. Liddell[847] observed that when working with amphiboles, this rate climbed to 40/1000. In a survey of Quebec, Liddell observed that the rates for mesothelioma were similar to the overall Quebec rates but were substantially higher in Montreal. He also estimated the rates in Canada of the annual

---

longer present chrysotile burden and substantial amounts of asbestos, mainly chrysotile and noncommercial amphiboles, are found in the average lung of the urban dweller (Churg and Warnock, 1979; Churg, 1983).[844]

incidence of mesothelioma in the mid-1980s to be $3/10^6$ in men and $1/10^6$ in women, with about two-thirds of the men exposed occupationally to asbestos. Liddell[847] suggested the ratio of lung and gastrointestinal cancers to mesothelioma to be 3.3:1 after a review of 33 cohort studies. Liddell[847] concluded the nonoccupational annual incidence of mesothelioma in Canada was about $1/10^6$ (about 24 cases per year) for both men and women. Finally, Liddell[847] believed that, in Canada, deaths in the general population due to tumors attributed to asbestos would be about 105 per year or a PMR of 0.6/1000 and even lower (0.25) if one assumed that all were asbestos-related and that the ratio between lung and digestive cancers and mesothelioma was indeed 3.3:1.

In a study of 16 owners of dogs with mesothelioma, Glickman et al.[288] matched 32 owners of dogs without mesothelioma to determine if the owner's occupational and medical history and their dog's medical history, lifestyle, diet, exposure to asbestos, or their owner's or a household member's asbestos-related hobbies or occupation as well as the use of flea repellants on the dogs, were significantly related to the increased risk of mesothelioma. Lung tissue of three of the dogs with mesothelioma and one dog with squamous cell carcinoma of the lung had higher concentrations of chrysotile fibers than did the lungs of the control dogs.

Dement et al.[848] conducted a retrospective mortality study of 1261 asbestos workers using chrysotile to produce textiles in a South Carolina plant. The cohort consisted of workers employed one or more months between January 1, 1940, and December 31, 1965, and followed through December 31, 1975. In addition to determining vital status, cumulative exposures and estimated fiber concentrations were calculated. The final cohort status was 927 alive (73.5%), 308 deceased (24.2%), and 26 unknown (2.1%). Of those deceased, 205.66 were expected, and no significant mortality occurred until 15 years after their initial employment. Of the 24 deaths in the nonmalignant respiratory category, 17 were attributed to asbestosis or pulmonary fibrosis and 6 of 105 cardiovascular deaths mentioned either asbestosis or pulmonary fibrosis as contributing causes. Thirty-five lung cancers were observed when 11.10 were expected (SMR = 315, 95% CI = 2.20–4.39). One peritoneal mesothelioma was identified.

Both lung cancer and asbestosis require long latencies before becoming clinically evident. Exposure response analysis for lung cancer showed a significant excess for all but the lowest exposure stratum where five lung cancers were observed when 3.58 were expected, but after that, all exposure stratum showed excesses cumulating with an SMR of 1818 in the highest exposure stratum where a linear function appeared the best fit. For asbestosis and pulmonary fibrosis, a strong increasing trend in incidence density with exposure was observed, with the highest exposure stratum 50 times greater than the lowest. The exposure–response pattern increased faster than predicted by a linear function. The highest exposure category had only two cases with a wide CI; therefore, this observation should be considered as only a tentative observation. The comparison population was the entire United States. Lung cancer rates for the United States and the State of South Carolina where the plant was located were approximately equal, but those in the county where the plant was situated were 75% higher for white men, which might reflect the presence of shipyard industries in addition to the plant being studied. Smoking was found to be nearly identical to that of the U.S. white male comparison population and that of the white male plant employees. These data predict that significantly elevated mortality risks for lung cancer and asbestosis are predicted at cumulative exposures of 100 fibers/mL-years in the asbestos textile industry, which equates to the current OSHA standard of the time of 2 fibers/mL. This study was supported by NIOSH.[848]

In 1984 at the Royal Commission on Matters of Health and Safety Arising from the Use of Asbestos in Ontario,[849] evidence was put forth by several scientists that tremolite, as reported by Mr. Ross Hunt,* "may be every bit as much a concern as crocidolite." Hunt's statement was based

---

* Mr. Ross Hunt was with the Research Unit of the BBA Group PLC formally known as British Belting and Asbestos and testified to the Royal Commission on June 16, 1982. Hunt's statement may be the first to introduce tremolite as the causative agent in the induction of mesothelioma among chrysotile-exposed workers.

on findings by Dr. Fred D. Pooley that in three cases of mesothelioma in Cyprus, tremolite was the only asbestos fiber found. Pooley had also reported finding large quantities of tremolite in 20 lung samples from the Canadian mining industry supplied by Dr. JC McDonald. Also, Rowlands et al.[845] reported finding similar quantities of tremolite and chrysotile in 47 lung samples from Quebec miners and millers, none of which had asbestosis or mesothelioma. JC McDonald then went on to "speculate" that mesothelioma among the Quebec miners "heretofore attributed to chrysotile may be due to tremolite exposure." A preliminary report by JMG Davis of pure tremolite inhalation exposure to rats suggested that tremolite was very harmful to rats and "may be more harmful than chrysotile." However, with these statements to the Commission, the final report of the Royal Commission stated: "Neither actinolite nor tremolite has been used in sufficient quantities commercially to engage detailed investigation of their health effects." The report stated that talc miners studied by Kleinfeld et al. found increased deaths due to lung cancer mortality and one death from peritoneal mesothelioma among 250 upper New York miners of talc contaminated by tremolite and, to a lesser extent, anthophyllite. With this additional evidence from the New York talc miners at hand, the Royal Commission stated: "While this evidence indicates a possible health risk from tremolite exposure, in our judgment there are not yet sufficient data to come to any firm conclusions. However, we do point out that to the extent that tremolite contaminates mines in Ontario, and to the extent that it is used commercially, its health effects warrant further scientific investigation." Thus, in the Royal Commission's eyes, data were lacking in 1984 to implement tremolite as a cause of mesothelioma over that known to be caused by chrysotile (see later section on tremolite for further discussion).

Liddell et al.[850] published a paper to define the relationship between chrysotile exposure in fiber terms and death. The cohort studied began in 1966 and contained 11,379 people born between 1891 and 1920 who had worked in the asbestos mines and mills of Quebec for a month or more before 1967. This cohort had previously been reported in 1980 by McDonald et al. and constituted the same subjects of this study. As of the end of 1975, there were a total of 634 deaths: 245 due to lung cancers, 46 due to pneumoconiosis, 21 due to laryngeal carcinoma, 154 due to esophageal and stomach cancers, 88 due to colon and rectal cancers, and 80 other abdominal sites. For each death, referents were randomly selected from among those male workers in the cohort born in the same year and known to have survived to a greater age. For each case and its referents, exposures accumulated up to 9 years before death had been obtained. Mesothelioma was not discussed in this report but were matched, and they and other subjects brought the total number of subjects to 2217. The authors[850] converted mppcf to fibers by multiplying mppcf by 3.5. When looking at exposure categories, the authors[850] found a clear dose–response trend with pneumoconiosis and lung cancer and cancer of the esophagus and stomach and none for laryngeal, colon, rectal, or abdominal cancers. When looking at lung cancer and smoking, a similar dose–response occurred both by pack years and by dose alone. The authors[850] concluded the asbestos-smoking interaction appeared intermediate between multiplicative and additive, but the evidence was less in favor of additive. Keep in mind that conversion from mppcf to fibers/mL has been troublesome. The authors[850] stated: "We cannot claim precision or certainty for our estimates only that the available data—more plentiful in this industry than most others—were used to the best of our ability." The decision by Liddell et al.[850] to eliminate exposures for a period of 9 years before death was not based on any scientific authority. In fact, recently it has been shown that protracted exposure suggests that asbestos acts both early and late in mesothelioma induction[241]; therefore, without further evidence, the elimination of exposure in the last 9-year period was not justified.

Churg et al.[851] looked at lung samples from 6 deceased men diagnosed with mesothelioma out of 90 autopsies performed on long-term Quebec chrysotile industry workers. Five had only chrysotile components in their lungs, including the contaminate tremolite, while the sixth had substantial amounts of amosite. In the five with chrysotile components, the number of chrysotile fibers was 64 million/gram and up to 540 million/gm tremolite fibers as compared with nonexposed subjects who, on average, had a range of 0.6 to 23 million/gm chrysotile and 0.3 to 58 million/gm tremolite/amphiboles. The sixth had 44 million/gm chrysotile, 54 million/gm tremolite/amphibole, and 70 million/gm amosite. Fiber sizes were similar between the exposed and nonexposed group. The ratios between the exposed chrysotile patients and the reference population ranged from 2.8:1 to 9.3:1.

In measuring chrysotile asbestos in the urine of exposed workers during production of roofing tars and asphalt sealers, six male workers and six comparisons with no occupational exposure to asbestos, Finn and Hallenbeck[852] found higher concentrations in the exposed worker group. One exposed worker and three comparisons had urinary values that were not significantly different than the field blanks. After adjustment for the field blank values, five exposed workers had fibers ranging from 9000 to 514,000 fibers/mL as compared with a range of 4600 to 6000 fibers/mL in three comparisons. Fiber mass was also higher in the exposed workers (0.04–8.68 ng/mL) and 0.02 to 0.03 ng/mL in the comparison group. The personal air samples ranged from 0 to 0.16 fibers/mL as 8-h TWAs, which led the authors to conclude that chrysotile asbestos can appear in the urine of workers exposed to airborne concentrations lower than the OSHA ceiling and that asbestos can appear in lower concentrations in the general population.

In a study of friction production workers from a Connecticut plant, no mesotheliomas were observed, although an increased SMR for respiratory cancers occurred in men working less than 1 year (SMR = 167.4) and more than 1 year (SMR = 136.7).[853] The plant used chrysotile from Canada until 1957 when some anthophyllite was added to make paper discs and bands and between 1964 and 1972 when approximately 400 lb. of crocidolite was handled experimentally on a few occasions in the laboratory. The study cohort included anyone employed for one calendar month or more before January 1, 1959, and who had a social security number and name that matched with data in the U.S. Social Security files. Vital status was established until December 31, 1977. Of the men, 3513 (96.5%) were traced and 1267 (36%) had died. Death certificates were obtained for 1228 (96.9%). Follow-up on the women was less successful, and no analysis was reported in the paper. Although dust measurements were reported using impinger counts pre-1970 and fiber counts thereafter, no comparisons were attempted. The authors[853] reported impinger levels around 1–5 mppcf in the 1930s but gave no idea of the numbers of samples taken for either impinger or fiber counts, and it appears that just estimates were given in the tables produced in the paper by the authors. Thus, it is difficult to understand the accuracy or validity of the levels. Twenty-two percent of the cohort had reached greater than 20 years employment. In this study, 803 (65%) deaths occurred in those with more than 20 years latency. The study results are hard to interpret because the authors[853] did not give expected numbers of deaths for each category, only SMRs. Thus, tests of significance are hard to calculate. Additionally, this cohort only had 36% of the workers traced as deceased, meaning 64% of the cohort were still alive and the magnitude of diseases of longer latency would not show up until their future mortality was know. Also, although small, the 39 with missing death certificates might also hold important information that would reflect on the final outcome of this cohort. Thus, studies such as this must be followed up to understand the true risk of disease from work in this cohort of friction plant employees, and these results must be viewed with caution. Any judgments as to risk at this time are limited and may be misleading. It should be noted this study was supported by the Quebec Asbestos Mining Association.

A study[854] of the prevalence of atypical cytology among male workers employed in three chrysotile mines in the Province of Quebec found workers aged 25 years, when first starting work, had increased abnormal cytology with both years of asbestos exposure and when the exposure index was measured by fibers per cubic centimeter.

A study[855] was conducted of temporal patterns of exposure and the development of nonmalignant pulmonary abnormalities among chrysotile workers in Canada. The strongest relationship for parenchymal fibrosis was cumulative exposure, whereas early exposure, residence time of dust in the lung, time since first exposure, and the number of years having greater than 5 mppcf exposures were important factors for pleural fibrosis. Airflow limitations related more to smoking, dust effects, and early exposure. For chronic bronchitis, significant factors were constant exposure, smoking, and early exposure. Airway reactivity related significantly to early and recent dust exposure, age, and smoking. All of these findings led the authors[855] to conclude that, after taking into account smoking and age, asbestos exposure was an important contributing factor in the development of pulmonary abnormalities.

In looking at the extent and nature of pathologic changes in small airways induced by asbestos, Wright and Churg[856] looked at 36 nonasbestotic, long-term chrysotile miners comparing them to 36 matched controls with no history of asbestos exposure. Their results found that the asbestos-containing mineral dust produced a generalized fibrosis of the small airways which was greater than that produced by cigarette smoking alone. The changes to the lungs appeared even when the lungs were no different from ordinary cigarette smoker's lungs. They[856] also found that the pathological changes in the small airways were not just confined to the respiratory bronchioles but also affected the membranous bronchioles. Finally, they found that pigmentation was a relatively poor marker of exposure to dust and of pathological changes. The pigmentation was not different than the controls, although the miners had more dust exposures and more severe fibrosis in their membranous bronchioles.

Gardner et al.[857] conducted a follow-up study of workers from a chrysotile manufacturing asbestos cement plant in England. The follow-up consisted of 2167 subjects employed between 1941 and 1983. No significant excesses of asbestos-related diseases were found, except for a nonstatistical excess of lung cancer among 87 workers exposed to ≥5 fibers/mL with 5 observed and 2.2 expected (observed/expected = 2.24, 95% CI = 073–5.23). These findings were not surprising to the authors[857] who attributed this to the relatively low airborne fiber levels (>90% were exposed to less than 0.1 fiber/mL) as well as their conclusion that the power of the study was limited.

Hughes et al.[858] reported mesothelioma risk from a cement manufacturing plant in New Orleans that used predominantly chrysotile, but crocidolite was used in pipe production. Eight mesotheliomas were reported and seven had mixed exposure to chrysotile and crocidolite, whereas one had only chrysotile exposure.

In a further analysis of chrysotile mining areas in Russia, Kogan and Berzin[859] reported that mesothelioma was almost six times higher in the area of the asbestos industry than the regional average. Four of seven mesotheliomas investigated in the asbestos industry area showed intense exposure to asbestos-containing dust. The conclusions by the authors[859] were that "it was demonstrated that the dust of chrysotile asbestos ores is capable of increasing the risk of mesothelioma formation, although final practical conclusions require more long-term observations."

In 1987, Hughes et al.[860] gave an expanded publication of their previously reported studies of asbestos cement manufacturing plants in New Orleans. They examined the mortality of 6931 employees of the two plants. In plant 1, 1592 (62%) were alive, 886 (34.5%) were deceased, and 87 (3.4%) were lost to follow-up. In plant 2, 2936 (67.2%) were alive, 1257 (28.8%) were deceased, and 173 (4%) were lost to follow-up. In this follow-up of their 1979 and 1980 reports, the cohort was larger by 1316 workers (20%). This difference was not discussed in this latest report, and it is not clear whether all cohort members were production workers or whether nonproduction workers with little or no exposure were included. The results indicated that the ratio of observed deaths to that expected were similar in the 20 or more years after initial exposure categories. In plant 1 where small amounts of amosite were used along with predominantly chrysotile, excess malignancies were primarily due to lung, colon-rectal, urinary, and residual cancers, although none were statistically significant. The 20 residual cancers were primarily cancers of unspecified sites and secondary respiratory/digestive cancers. Two were pneumoconiosis. In plant 2 where crocidolite was used continuously in the pipe operation, statistically significant excesses of lung cancer (107 observed vs. 74.3 expected; $p < .01$) and residual cancers (42 observed vs. 29.4 expected; $p < .01$) as well as a statistically insignificant excess of stomach cancers were reported. The unspecified cancers were primarily unspecified/ill-defined sites ($n = 26$) and secondary respiratory/digestive cancers ($n = 6$).

Five were due to pneumoconiosis. Since all operations in plant 1 occurred in one building, it was difficult to judge exposure variation. In plant 2, the authors were able to place workers into two groups—those exposed to both crocidolite and chrysotile and those exposed to chrysotile only. The risk of lung cancer in the two groups in plant 2 showed similar levels and trends and, if eliminating the shortest-term workers, an increasing trend with cumulative asbestos exposure in both groups. The authors[860] found no significant differences in risk of lung cancer between fiber types. Six mesotheliomas occurred (two in plant 1 and four in plant 2). Four additional mesotheliomas occurred outside the cohort definition in plant 2. The mesotheliomas in plant 1 were short-term workers, each with less than 1 year, with one citing previous employment as a longshoreman. Duration of the eight cases in plant 2 had employment ranging from 5 months to 42 years and all but one had exposure to both chrysotile and crocidolite. The authors[860] noted an inverse relationship between latency and age at initial employment, with those exposed at the earliest ages having the longest latency times before death. The crocidolite pipe workers in plant 2 were exposed approximately four times longer than the other workers, and plant 1 workers were, on average, 5 years older than those in plant 2 at age of hire. Sixty-three percent of the workers in plant 1 were black and 49% in plant 2 were black. When using a case–control analysis, the authors[860] found a statistically significant relationship between duration of employment, proportion of time in the pipe area, and work in the pipe area with increased risk of mesothelioma. When evaluating lung cancer risk with smoking, the authors[861] found similar smoking patterns in both plants. In plant 2 where exposure to chrysotile could be compared with chrysotile plus crocidolite exposure, the dose–response relationship was similar for workers exposed only to chrysotile and those exposed to both fiber types. On the basis of this study, no firm conclusions can be drawn. It is interesting that the authors concluded: "The existing evidence is so convincing that continued failure to differentiate between fiber types by governmental regulatory agencies such as the U.S. Occupational Safety and Health Administration is difficult to justify." Their conclusion is interesting because their own study shows no difference between lung cancer risk by fiber type and they had previously concluded in this paper that "We conclude that although the across study comparisons of Doll and Peto suggest greater risk of lung cancer from exposure to amphibole compared with chrysotile alone, firm conclusions on this issue cannot yet be drawn." This study was funded, in part, by the Quebec Asbestos Mining Association.

Huncharek,[419] as part of an epidemiological study of diffuse pleural mesothelioma by the Canadian Tumor Reference Center, looked at 37 cases of mesothelioma, and of these, 1 worked as a brake mechanic, 1 as an elevator mechanic, and 1 did railroad brake banding. Tissue samples from the pleura of the auto mechanic showed 99% of the fibers to be chrysotile and 1% amosite. The author felt this should lead to other investigations into the role of chrysotile in the etiology of mesothelioma.

Finkelstein[861] reported a cohort of 324 men exposed to chrysotile in a manufacturing plant making construction materials in Ontario, Canada, where one pleural mesothelioma was identified and there was an elevated risk of lung cancer among long-term employees. The 324 men had been employed at the plant during 1960 or later. The pleural mesothelioma occurred in 1959, which was outside the parameter of the cohort, and worked as a beater operator where the excess of lung cancer among the cohort occurred (RR = 0.2, 95% CI = 2.25–23.3). The plant also used coal tar pitch, but none of the beater operators were directly exposed to it. Two squamous cell carcinomas of the skin were reported in the cohort—one of the chest wall and one of the scrotum. Coal tar pitch has a known association with skin cancer. The cohort was small, no exposure data existed, and smoking histories were lacking, but the area where the lung cancer and respiratory diseases were different than the controls in the case–control study was in the beater area where the most exposure and use of chrysotile occurred. As for smoking, Siemiatycki et al.[862] had stated: "It is unlikely, however, that there would be substantial variation in smoking habits among the various occupational groups at the factory, and differences in smoking are unlikely to explain the associations with job found in the case–control analysis." Finkelstein[861] made two observations: (1) that the findings confirmed the hazards of uncontrolled exposure to chrysotile asbestos and (2) that it was disheartening that 200 years after the first description of scrotal cancers as an occupational disease,[*] workplace-associated cancer was still occurring.

In another study by Finkelstein[863] of the mortality of 1657 men and women employed in two automotive parts manufacturing factories using chrysotile, the author found an increase of laryngeal cancer and an elevated rate of lung cancer. However, when Finkelstein conducted a case–control analysis of both laryngeal cancer and lung cancer, no associations were supported. Finkelstein reported two suspected pleural mesotheliomas, although the cause of death had been recorded as lung cancer. The first man began work in 1952 and was diagnosed in 1966. The man had undergone biopsy of a pleural mass that the pathologist diagnosed as pleural mesothelioma. The second mesothelioma was in a man who began work in 1968 and died in 1981. A biopsy specimen had been obtained, but the pathologists were unable to make a firm diagnosis. A pathology consultant to the Workers' Compensation Board reported the morphologic features were fully consistent with mesothelioma. It should be noted that both men had short latency periods but not out of the range associated with occupational exposure and latency of greater than 10 years.[166]

Thus, up until 1990 epidemiologic evidence combined with animal and experimental data supported the role that all fiber types, including chrysotile, were responsible in the etiology of lung cancer and mesothelioma as well as other cancers. Reports continue to support these findings as found in the IARC 2009 reevaluation of asbestos.[301] However, it is important to note that with the report of Dr. Pooley[864] in 1976 that lung tissue from 20 cases of diagnosed asbestosis from Canadian miners and millers who had fibrous minerals other than chrysotile in their lungs, including tremolite, was when speculation by industry-supported scientists suggested that chrysotile may not be the cause of asbestos-related diseases in this population. The samples of lung tissue were supplied by Dr. Corbert McDonald to Dr. Pooley. This laid the foundation to introduce doubt into the notion that chrysotile was the cause of asbestos-related diseases among workers exposed to Canadian chrysotile. Then in 1982, Rowlands, Gibbs, and A. D. McDonald (wife of J. C. McDonald),[845] using a TEM, examined 47 autopsy lung samples from Quebec miners and found tremolite in approximately similar quantities to chrysotile along with crocidolite and amosite in smaller amounts. They[845] knew that the tremolite was found in very small quantities in the chrysotile ore. They[845] then summarized that the chrysotile must be leaving the lung through some mechanism. Using this information, Dr. Corbet McDonald testified to the Royal Commission on Matters of Health and Safety Arising from the Use of Asbestos in Ontario. Dr. J. C. McDonald, during his testimony, went so far as to speculate that the mesothelioma among the Quebec miners heretofore attributed to chrysotile may be due to tremolite exposure. Dr. McDonald based this speculation on the findings of Pooley[864] and Rowlands et al.[845] as well as citing Dr. John M. G. Davis who testified that "he had just completed an inhalation study with pure tremolite. While the study had been completed at the time of his testimony in January 1982, not all of the data had been analyzed. However, Dr. Davis suggested that his experiment appeared to indicate that tremolite is very harmful to rats and may be more harmful than chrysotile" (see Royal Commission footnote 210).[849] From this point on, the foundations were laid that implemented tremolite as the cause of mesothelioma among the Canadian mining population. This speculation has lead scientists to try to examine populations of persons exposed to as pure chrysotile as possible to determine chrysotile's role in lung cancer and mesothelioma etiology. The following discussion expands on the role of chrysotile alone as a cause of cancer, especially mesothelioma.

Simson[65] reported fibrosis and golden-yellow bodies in the lungs of guinea pigs similar to those found in humans. The animals were exposed 2 h/day for 50 days in 1925 to chrysotile. The results

---

[*] Sir Percivall Pott made this finding in a study of chimney sweeps in 1775 and was considered the first person to associate occupational exposures to cancer. See Pott P. Cancer scroti. In: *Chirurgical observations*. London, England: Hawes, Clark & Collins; 1775. p. 63–69.

from animal bioassays present a strong case for the toxicity of chrysotile. Wagner et al.,[771] then with the Medical Research Council, United Kingdom, have shown that commercial grade, predominantly short fiber Canadian chrysotile, which is used primarily for paint and plastic tile fillers, can induce mesotheliomas when injected intrapleurally into rats and can induce primary lung neoplasms when the animals are exposed by inhalation. Not only does it appear that chrysotile is as potent as crocidolite and the other amphiboles in inducing mesotheliomas after intrapleural injections but is also equally potent in inducing pulmonary neoplasms after inhalation exposure.[773] In terms of degree of response related to the quality of dust deposited and retained in the lungs of rats, chrysotile appears to be much more fibrogenic and carcinogenic than the amphiboles.[773]

Epidemiologic evidence combined with the animal data supports the role that all fiber types, including chrysotile, are responsible in the etiology of lung cancer and mesothelioma as well as other cancers. Although most of these studies are of cohorts of workers who were exposed to chrysotile contaminated with low levels of tremolite, an amphibole form of asbestos, several studies revealed a substantially increased risk of developing mesothelioma from exposure to chrysotile that did not contain any tremolite contamination. In the first study, Piolatto et al.[770] examined a cohort of 1094 chrysotile production workers employed at the mine and mill in Balangero, Italy, a site where no tremolite was detected in any of the samples of chrysotile. Among the 427 deaths, the authors[770] discovered two mesothelioma cases—one confirmed pathologically and one based on radiographic findings and on examination of pleural fluid.

In another similar study, Cullen and Baloyi[768,769] examined the records of Zimbabwean miners and millers who had been certified as having an occupational lung disease. Like the chrysotile ore mined in Balangero, Italy, no tremolite was detected in any of the samples. The authors estimated that 6647 Zimbabweans were engaged in the mining and milling operations at two mines: Shabani and Goths. Among the chosen cohort of 27 miners with sufficient documentation, the authors discovered one mesothelioma case proven by biopsy, one mesothelioma proven by postmortem, and one probable mesothelioma based on radiographic findings. They also reported one case of asbestosis with probable mesothelioma versus lung cancer based on chest radiograph and having a pleural mass develop 5 years later.

Rogers et al.[865] examined 221 cases of definite and probable mesothelioma obtained from the Australian Mesothelioma Surveillance Program.[866] Among these cases, Rogers et al.[865] recorded a substantial number of mesothelioma patients in whom the only detectable type of asbestos was chrysotile (see Table 9 in his paper), with evidence of a dose–response effect as reflected in a trend toward an increasing OR at relatively low fiber concentration of less than 10^6 fibers/g of dry lung tissue ($\log_{10} = 5.5–6$; OR = 8.67).

A 25-year longitudinal study of workers exposed to amphibole-free chrysotile found two confirmed cases of mesothelioma among the exposed workers.[868] The RR for all cancers, adjusted for smoking and age, was 4.29 (95% CI = 2.17–8.46). The authors[868] reported that analysis of four commercial samples of asbestos used in the Chongqin chrysotile asbestos plant under study were shown to contain less than 0.001% tremolite fiber, which is less than the detection limit for amphibole contamination using x-ray diffraction analysis and analytical TEM as used in this study. It has been reported that samples of Chinese chrysotile are contaminated with tremolite; however, like the findings of the Zimbabwe UICC samples contaminated with anthophyllite, the findings from the Chinese mines cannot be equated to those reported by the authors[868] from their own analysis of the samples representing those taken from their study. In 2009, Yano et al.[868] reported another mesothelioma from chrysotile only exposure in a man working in a plant where no amphiboles were used. The lungs of the man, however, did contain tremolite, which the authors[868] attributed to contamination of the chrysotile. This finding points to the difficulty of finding a pure chrysotile-exposed population without contamination, especially from tremolite.

In addition to the studies of uncontaminated "pure" chrysotile, there have been several studies of populations exposed to chrysotile ore and who processed chrysotile products containing trace amounts of tremolite. In the mining context, Camus et al.[392] compared mortality among women in two chrysotile asbestos mining areas in the Province of Quebec with mortality among women in 60 control areas. While focusing on lung cancer mortality, the authors[392] discovered a statistically significant increase in mesotheliomas as evidenced by an SMR of 7.63 (95% CI = 3.06–15.73).

With regard to processed products composed of principally chrysotile asbestos, Nokso-Koivisto and Pukkala[869] examined a cohort of 8391 members of the Finnish Locomotive Drivers' Association during 1953 and 1991. The authors[869] found a statistically significant fourfold risk of mesothelioma. In another study of railroad workers predominantly exposed to chrysotile asbestos, Mancuso[870] arrived at a similar conclusion. Out of a cohort of 181, there were 156 deaths, 14 of which were identified as mesotheliomas, constituting 34% of all cancer deaths in the study.

A study of workers employed in an asbestos textile, friction, and packing manufacturing facility using 99% chrysotile asbestos observed 17 deaths from mesothelioma, representing 4.3% of the deaths.[300] Amphiboles had only been used for a few years during World War II and accounted for a very small amount of the total asbestos used at this facility.

Dement and Brown,[356] in a cohort of chrysotile textile workers, found an overall excess of respiratory cancer with an SMR of 2.25 (95% CI = 1.85–2.71) and an SMR of 2.24 (95% CI = 1.83–2.72) for pleural mesothelioma. The chrysotile fibers came exclusively from Quebec, British Columbia, and Rhodesia. During the manufacturing process, the fibers mixed with cotton were sprayed with a light mineral oil, which saturated it to about 4%, and by the time it reached the spinning looms, the oil had diminished to less than 1%. Some have claimed this study's findings might be a result of the mineral oil treatment; however, the authors[356] found during a case–control analysis that only a slight exposure–response reduction occurred for lung cancer when adjusted for the mineral oil exposures, thus leading the authors[356] to conclude the mineral oil exposures were insignificant. An update of this cohort[871] where the majority of the cohort (64%) were now deceased found that all causes of death exceeded the expected standard mortality rate (SMR = 1.33, 95% CI = 1.28–1.39), and this was true for all cancers (SMR = 1.27, 95% CI = 1.16–1.39). Lung cancer had an SMR = 1.87 (95% CI = 1.09–2.99), and esophageal cancer had an SMR = 1.87 (95% CI = 1.09–2.99). Pneumoconiosis and other respiratory diseases were also in excess (SMR = 4.81, 95% CI = 3.84–5.94). There were three mesotheliomas among the cohort. There also was a clear dose–response relationship for lung cancer.

Loomis et al.[872] described the mortality of workers employed for at least 1 day between January 1, 1950, and December 31, 1973, among three plants in North Carolina, producing asbestos textile products. There were 2583 deaths out of the 5770 workers included in the cohort. Lung cancer accounted for 277 deaths (SMR = 1.95, 95% CI = 1.73–2.19), and all cancers had an SMR = 1.41 (95% CI = 1.31–1.53). SMR from pleural cancer, mesothelioma, and pneumoconiosis were also elevated. The authors[872] found the risk of lung cancer (RR = 1.102 per 100 fiber-year/mL, 95% CI = 1.044–1.164) and asbestosis (RR = 1.249, 95% CI = 1.186–1.316) increased with cumulative fiber exposure. Pneumoconiosis had 73 deaths (SMR = 3.48, 95% CI = 2.73–4.38), mesothelioma accounted for four deaths (SMR = 10.92, 95% CI = 2.98–27.96), and there were four pleural cancer deaths (SMR = 12.43, 95% CI = 3.39–31.83).

In a second paper by Loomis et al.,[873] the authors examined and estimated the exposure to asbestos fibers of specific sizes from workers at three asbestos textile plants in North Carolina using chrysotile asbestos. Their evaluation employed the use of TEM. All 3803 workers employed in the three plants had worked at least 1 day between January 1, 1950, and December 31, 1973. When comparing the TEM results for total cumulative exposures to PCM methods, the fiber exposures were far greater using the TEM (mean = 989.4 fiber-years/mL lagged 10 years vs. 59.2 fiber-years/mL lagged 10 years). The authors[873] found the risk of lung cancer increased with exposure to longer, thinner fibers and that some evidence showed the effects were most pronounced for long fibers between 0.25 and 1.0 μm in diameter. The authors[873] found that "Goodness of fit and strength of association with lung cancer tended to increase in models for fibers >10 μm in length, but similar results were obtained for very short fibers ≤1.5 μm long and for fibers >3 μm in diameter." This led the authors to conclude: "There is still uncertainty about the relative carcinogenicity of specific fiber-size fractions, however."

Sturm et al.[874] reviewed 843 cases of mesothelioma recorded in the German Federal State of Saxony-Anhalt between 1960 and 1990. Sixty-seven cases representing 14% of the total were directly attributable to sole exposure to chrysotile asbestos.

When comparing animal studies to human response on the basis of epidemiologic studies, Kuempel et al.[875] of NIOSH concluded that chrysotile toxic doses in rats compared with that in humans. Their analysis found that the rat-based risk estimates for lung cancer compared with humans were reasonably concordant to those for the Canadian miners and millers studies, whereas those compared with textile workers were much higher, indicating that humans may be more sensitive. However, fiber size studies were not done, but there was evidence that textile workers may have been exposed to longer fibers than those found in the Canadian cohorts.

The 1984 Report of the Royal Commission on Matters of Health and Safety Arising from the Use of Asbestos in Ontario concluded: "All fibre types can cause all asbestos-related diseases, …."[849] This supports the finding of reported cases of mesothelioma among brake mechanics exposed to chrysotile.[416] Furthermore, Mancuso[870,876] contends on the basis of his analysis of railroad machinists that commercial chrysotile asbestos causes mesothelioma and that the risk is greater than previously asserted. There is further concern that chrysotile is rarely found in its pure form and that most chrysotile deposits are contaminated with tremolite, which is agreed by experts to be a toxic form of asbestos.[877] In a review of the evidence, scientists from NIOSH concluded: "Given the evidence of a significant lung cancer risk, the lack of conclusive evidence for the amphibole hypothesis, and the fact that workers are generally exposed to a mixture of fibers, we conclude that it is prudent to treat chrysotile with virtually the same level of concern as the amphibole forms of asbestos."[333]

Three publications highlight the fact that the majority of the world's medical community considers chrysotile to be a cause of pleural and peritoneal mesothelioma. In 1997, a multidisciplinary gathering of 19 pathologists, radiologists, occupational and pulmonary physicians, epidemiologists, toxicologists, industrial hygienists, and clinical and laboratory scientists held a meeting in Helsinki, Finland, to agree on criteria for attribution of disorders of the lung and pleura in association with asbestos.[166] Collectively, the group had published more than 1000 articles on asbestos and asbestos-associated disorders. The consensus of the group was that *all types* of malignant mesothelioma can be induced by asbestos, with the amphiboles showing greater carcinogenic potency than chrysotile.

The second publication[335] was a monograph devoted specifically to chrysotile asbestos that was prepared by the International Programme on Chemical Safety in conjunction with the World Health Organization. After an extensive review of the world's literature, this group concluded that "commercial grades of chrysotile have been associated with an increased risk of pneumonoconiosis, lung cancer and mesothelioma in numerous epidemiological studies of exposed workers."

Chrysotile fibers are much more chemically and biologically reactive than amphibole fibers and because of this reactivity with the tissues, they lose their structural elements and divide into smaller fibrils, making their recognition difficult by the usual analytical methods. In fact, many of the fibers are removed from the lung and exhaled back through the bronchi or are removed by the lymphatic system to other organs of the body.[779,878–880] The concentration of dust in the lungs of rats exposed to Canadian chrysotile was only 1.8–2.2% of the dust concentration in the lungs of animals exposed to amphiboles after 24 months of inhalation exposure. Yet the lung tumor incidence and degree of pulmonary fibrosis was similar in all groups. These findings support the idea that chrysotile fibers cause more cellular injury, fibrosis, and lung cancer than the amphiboles while at the same time are less readily detected in the tissue after the damage is done. Churg et al.[881] concluded that the failure of chrysotile to accumulate in the lung was a result of preferential chrysotile clearance during the first few days to weeks after exposure and that dissolution played no role in the clearance, and that the preferential clearance might be a result of fragmentation and rapid removal of the chrysotile fibers. This is supported by Roggli et al.,[788] who concluded, as do others, that chrysotile does not accumulate in lung tissue because they are broken down into smaller fibrils that rapidly clear from the lung. Such chrysotile fibers have been missed by their technique, which counts only fibers longer than 5 µm in length. They also concluded that long, thin fibers would likewise be missed because chrysotile content is poorly detected by SEM and thus fiber burden is a poor indicator of total chrysotile exposure and that other information must be sought to address the question of total fiber burden of chrysotile. Suzuki et al.[882] in reviewing 92 consecutive cases of mesothelioma observed that the major asbestos type identified in mesothelial tissues was chrysotile when compared with the chrysotile fiber burden in the lungs of the same cases (79.0% vs. 28.3%). Dogs with mesothelioma had higher concentrations of chrysotile in their lungs than did the control dogs.[883] McDonald et al.[451] suggested that because of low biopersistence, autopsy tissue cannot be reliably used to evaluate the contribution of chrysotile in the etiology of mesothelioma; however, they contended that "… to the extent that tremolite is a valid marker, our results suggest that (chrysotile's role) is small." The question remains as to the validity of tremolite found in the lung tissue as a valid marker for past chrysotile exposures.

Malorni et al.[884] suggested that fiber penetration can rearrange the cytoskeletal apparatus of the cell and this could indicate an interaction between chrysotile fibers and the normal mitotic process as giant multinucleated cells are formed. Churg et al.[885] further believes that short fibers may be more fibrogenic than previous animal data suggested and deserved further study.

Biologic plausibility seeks to determine if the theory of causation fits known mechanisms of injury causation. Although it is impossible to have a complete understanding of the mechanisms of cancer causation, the biologic facts known about the various asbestos fibers and how they cause disease are consistent with the postulate that chrysotile asbestos fibers are capable of producing mesotheliomas. First, it has long been known that it is not the chemical composition of the various asbestos fibers that is important in their ability to produce disease but rather that the health effects of asbestos are related primarily to the asbestos fibers' morphology, shape, and size. Many researchers contend that the potency of crocidolite is related to its thin diameter. Similarly, chrysotile fibers have a tendency to cleave longitudinally, creating extremely thin fibrils.

Second, it is universally accepted that chrysotile asbestos is carcinogenic and capable of causing or contributing to the development of lung cancer.

Third, mesotheliomas develop in the pleura, peritoneum, and other serosal surfaces of the body. It is universally accepted that chrysotile is a cause of cancer in the lung and that it also migrates to the mesothelial linings of the body.[882,886] Sebastien et al.[824] found that all fibers in the pleura were chrysotile when there was no predominance in parenchymal samples, which led the authors to conclude that lung parenchymal retention was not a good indicator of total fiber body burden in tissue. Translocation of asbestos fibers to other organs is also well documented. In addition, a series of 168 cases of mesothelioma reviewed by Suzuki and Yuen[332] confirmed the following:

1. Asbestos fibers were present in almost all of the lung and mesothelial tissues from the mesothelioma cases.
2. The most common types of asbestos fibers in the lung were an admixture of chrysotile with amphiboles, amphibole alone, and occasionally chrysotile alone. In mesothelial tissues, most asbestos fibers were chrysotile.
3. In lung tissue, amosite fibers were greatest in number followed by chrysotile, crocidolite, tremolite/actinolite, and anthophyllite. In mesothelial tissues, chrysotile fibers were 30.3 times more common than amphiboles.
4. In some mesothelioma cases, the only asbestos fibers detected in either lung or mesothelial tissue were chrysotile fibers.
5. The average number of asbestos fibers in both lung and mesothelial tissues was two orders of magnitude greater than the number found in the general population.
6. The majority of asbestos fibers in lung and mesothelial tissues were shorter than 5 µm in length.

Because chrysotile is carcinogenic and is present in high concentrations in the mesothelial linings where mesothelioma develops, it is biologically plausible that it causes or contributes to the cause of mesothelioma. This has been shown by many mechanistic and molecular studies that indicate how chrysotile may cause mesothelioma. Fiber penetration can rearrange the cytoskeletal apparatus of the cell and this could indicate an interaction between the chrysotile fibers and the normal mitotic process as giant multinucleated cells are formed. These studies indicate that chrysotile penetrates the cell, enters the nucleus, and induces abnormal chromosome formations in dividing cells.[884] Some of these abnormalities include the deletion of the p53 gene growth.[887] Inhaled chrysotile asbestos induced at the fiber deposition site showed expression of p53 protein, which suggests that the p53 protein can accumulate in lung tissue after chrysotile exposure. Additionally, a study of the phosphorylation of the p53 protein in A549 human pulmonary epithelial cells exposed to asbestos found that chrysotile asbestos, on a per-weight basis, was more potent in inducing Serl5 phosphorylation and accumulation of the p53 protein than was crocidolite.[888] Another study[889] indicated particle stimulation chemiluminescence (CL) production by polymorphonuclear leukocytes has been used to evaluate the pathogenicity of mineral fibers, understanding that reactive oxygen metabolites as measured by CL are etiopathogenically related to fiber toxicity. These findings may indicate that neither the total number nor the specific range of fiber dimensions are solely determinate of the CL production, and thus other physiochemical factors like surface reactive characteristics of milled fibers may play a role in the etiology of disease. Pott[890] questioned fiber dimension as a reliable yardstick for carcinogenic dose and whether inhalation studies of rats as a surrogate for human inhalation effects were misleading in that rats are known obligatory nose breathers. These findings bring into question the Stanton et al.[891] hypothesis that fiber diameter and length are the only determinates of the carcinogenicity of fibers. Pott[890] also addressed the use of intrapleural and intraperitoneal injection when examining the carcinogenic potential of inorganic fibers, which has been criticized emphatically. Pott[890] concluded that the consistency of such an argument was not supported when, for example, the inhalation studies with crocidolite did not result in lung tumors or mesothelioma although the fiber concentrations in the lung were very high. These epidemiological findings, along with the results of experimental studies, leave no doubt that the scientific evidence supports the carcinogenicity of chrysotile asbestos alone in the induction of mesothelioma.[892]

5.6.4 Crocidolite

Crocidolite is the asbestiform (fibrous) of riebeckite minerals of the amphibole group with a chemical formula of $Na_2Fe_3^{2+}Fe_2^{3+}Si_8O_{22}(OH,F)$. It is often referred to as *blue asbestos* and is more brittle with harsher texture, which explains why it is not used in a lot of commercial products such as friction products due to its ability to score brake drums.[893,894] Within Precambrian banded ironstone terrains are found the majority of the world's crocidolite deposits in South Africa and Western Australia.[895] Studies and reports of workers exposed to crocidolite have well established its causal association with all asbestos-related diseases, including asbestosis, lung cancer, and mesothelioma.[762,896–899]

The first study to look at and bring much attention to fiber type was the series of 33 case reports of mesothelioma published by Wagner et al. in 1960, which was discussed in detail under the section on mesothelioma. However, it might be of interest to mention some of the findings and conclusions from Dr. J. C. Wagner's thesis presented for the degree of Doctor of Medicine in the Department of Pathology of the University of Witwatersrand. This thesis was published after Wagner et al.'s original paper in 1960, and the last reference date in the thesis was 1961. Dr. Wagner was first asked to investigate respiratory disease among asbestos-exposed workers by Dr. Ian Webster, then Deputy Director of the Pneumoconiosis Research Unit, in August 1954. The first case of mesothelioma in Wagner's series came to necropsy in February 1956 and was of a 36-year-old Bantu man thought to have tuberculous pleurisy with an empyema following repeated aspiration. The clinical features were described by Martiny in 1956.[900] The average latency in the series of 75 cases who gave a history of occupational or environmental exposure was 44.7 years. There were 78 total cases examined in this Thesis by the end of August 1961 (75 pleural and 3 peritoneal). The youngest case involved a 21-year-old whose mother cobbed asbestos and, as was the custom, probably brought him along to the cobbing site at an age as early as 3 weeks. The oldest case was that of a 99-year-old in which little was known except the age of the patient from the hospital record. Dr. Wagner's conclusions in his thesis were as follows: (1) asbestosis is a serious and widespread disease in South Africa, (2) the two types of asbestos mainly produced in South Africa can cause pulmonary fibrosis in man and experimental animals, (3) insufficient material from chrysotile miners is included in this series for comparisons to be made, (4) problem is not confined to people employed by the industry but to a certain extent to those living in the vicinity of the mines and mills, (5) only crocidolite dust was implicated in 75 of the mesotheliomas in this series but insufficient evidence to state if other types of asbestos are implicated, and (6) experimental intrapleural inoculation of crocidolite asbestos dusts, chrysotile dusts, and pure silica have produced mesothelioma in rats.

In 1961, Sleggs et al.[23] detailed the findings of 34 cases of mesothelioma the authors had investigated. Originally, the 33 cases reported by Wagner et al. in 1960 had been reported but only 30 had been clinically investigated by the authors. In the paper by Sleggs et al.,[23] eight new cases were reported of which four were under the care of the authors. They also had radiographic findings on the 34 cases. The authors gave some history of the mining in the North West Cape and described this area as the most extensive in the world, extending 20 miles south of the Orange River and north to the Bechuanaland border, covering some 8000 square miles. The type of asbestos throughout the area was crocidolite, also known as *Cape Blue*, and pointed out the crocidolite was the fibrous form of riebeckite. The mining in the Prieska district in 1893 was spreading northward and in 1908 production began in the Kuruman district. Hand cobbing occurred until the first crushing mill was built in 1915 in Koegas in the south. Following this, a large mill was built in Kuruman and operated between 1926 and 1931 and was located within 300 yards of the city's main street. Other mills then began opening in other areas around the mine. Until the report of Wagner et al. in 1960, the authors stated six cases of mesothelioma had been clinically described—one by Doll[168] in 1955, two by Cartier[214] in 1952, and three by Van der Schoot[216] in 1958.

In the 34 mesothelioma cases described in the Wagner et al. paper, the latency was between 20 and 60 years. Little investigation had been done in the Transvaal mining area, and no cases had been reported, which the authors thought was possibly due to the shorter period of time the Transvaal mines had been in operation or possibly because the type of asbestos was chrysotile and not Cape Blue. Some crocidolite and amosite asbestos, both amphiboles, were also mined around this area. Of the 34 cases, 24 were men and 10 were women. Six of the men were younger than 40 years and lived in the area all their lives, and four were miners. Only one, a nursing sister who died at age 60 years, had never lived in the area or had any known exposure to asbestos. Three women lived in the Transvaal area and had never or only occasionally visited the North West Cape after leaving school. Three other women had engaged in cobbing asbestos in their homes. Seven men worked in the mines and two were born and raised in the district but did not engage in mining. Four others worked in the asbestos industry—two were boilermakers who lagged locomotive boilers, one worked during the war manufacturing asbestos protective devices for fighting aircraft fires, and one worked as a boilermaker in a Cape factory, which got its asbestos from the Cape asbestos fields. In one family, both the father and the daughter died of mesothelioma, and in two other cases, a sibling had radiologic evidence of asbestosis. Pleural effusions always developed and often, unless the fluid was drained, could obliterate the pleural space. In about a third of the cases, radiologic signs of asbestosis were present. Pleural changes took the form of bilateral pleural thickening, pleural adhesions, and rather characteristic dense calcified plaques. In the majority of cases,[23] no evidence of preceding pleural or pulmonary asbestosis was found, but these cases, upon further investigation, invariably showed unilateral pleural involvement in the form of diffuse thickening or effusion. In the late stages, secondary spread may occur, and in eight cases this spread occurred to the peritoneal area. In this case series,[23] 27 of the 34 cases had right-sided lesions and in no case was the meso-thelioma initially bilateral; however, radiographs showed bilateral changes due to asbestosis in 10 cases. Asbestos bodies were found in 30% of the cases.

In 1939, 1500 miles north of Perth, Australia, deposits of crocidolite were discovered at Wittenoom and by 1943 production of the deposit had commenced. Three hundred to 400 work-ers were at the mine, but because of the heat and lack of amenities, most of the workers consisted of new migrants and led to a very high turnover in the labor force. By 1966 the mine had closed. Fewer than 20% of the men had worked there 3 years or longer. The mine was very dusty and health concerns began by 1948 by the Australian Health Department. Even with controls for dust, the situ-ation was never good. From the very beginning, the miners had initial clinical examinations and annual periodic chest x-rays until 1957 when annual clinical examinations were added. Pulmonary function testing was never routine but rather was done when indicated by examination or radiologic findings. The first migrant worker found to have developed pulmonary tuberculosis was a 33-year-old man who, in 1958, underwent a lobectomy and the specimen showed asbestosis. Two others suffered from pneumoconiosis but were classified as silicotics. Since 1958, a total of 103 men have developed pneumoconiosis. Thirty-three were excluded from further analysis because of previous dust exposures, mixed mine or mill history, and/or insufficient clinical data. As the mine increased production and with continued poor conditions, pulmonary disease began to appear even after short periods of time. The average length of time at the mill before disease developed was about 5.25 years, with a range between 1 and 14 years, and in the mine it was 6.6 years with a range of 3 to 12 years and an average age of 40 to 45 years. The rapidity of the disease was described as: "A man with 2 years' exposure in the mill might have a normal chest x-ray and no signs or symptoms in 1 year, but be found to have dyspnoea, finger clubbing, basal crepitations and an abnormal chest x-ray the following year." In this paper, two developed lung cancer and both were heavy smokers. One pleural mesothelioma occurred in a worker who was in the mill between 1947 and 1949 and whose tumor developed in 1960. The high labor turnover made further follow-up difficult. The dumping of the mine tailings for road surfacing exposed the townspeople and children of the area to the risk of asbestos-related diseases. The author[896] expected much more disease to develop in former miners, millers, town folks, and children.

In October 1956, the South African Institute for Medical Research was asked to investigate the noticeable number of cases of pleural carcinoma among people living in the North Western Cape area. This was instigated by the finding of mesothelioma in a white man after a pleural biopsy in Johannesburg. In a very confusing paper by Sleggs[901] in 1970, a description of this investigation was given, which I will try to describe. However, I suggest the researcher with in-depth interest obtain and read the paper themselves. At the time, Sleggs indicated they believed there was a marked asso-ciation between tuberculosis and mesothelioma among the family groups of all races. One medical officer x-raying families of nonwhite asbestos workers said they had not seen a case of mesothelioma since 1966. Sleggs[901] described the asbestos exposure as often minimal in the North Western Cape and that childhood exposure appeared important. Sleggs intimated that other dusts like laterite and the type of climate might be implemented in the number of cases. He stated casual exposure to asbestos and other dusts could occur later on in life among the people in the North Western Cape and that asbestos by itself could not be wholly blamed, although it must play a part in the etiology of the tumors. He indicated that mesotheliomas were reported with no asbestos in the lungs. In this paper,[901] Sleggs described the population in the Vryburg and Kuruman districts as having large Bantu homelands and described the climate as long, hot summers and brief, cold, rainless winters, which have many windless days, whereas spring has windy months and dust storms, sometimes quite heavy. As a result, lung resections and other specimens have shown dust deposition in the male patients who had no mining history. By 1966, a lobectomy specimen from a 12-year-old Bantu girl from southeast of Kimberely showed dust deposition. In the other age groups, asbestos bodies were found in lung smears on postmortem survey. Sleggs[901] stated that with mining excluded, the main occupations were outdoors in nature and contributed to the dust hazard, as did travel on dusty roads. Finally, the Bantu men were described as of low physical standard and generally did not have a full working life, having only worked when needed and having several occupations during their lifetime. Sleggs[901] placed the cases into two categories—those with fluid and showing some pleural thickening on x-ray after aspiration and those presenting as a solid peripheral opacity on x-ray with no fluid. For diagnosis, it was only through pleural biopsy with the exact decision left to the pathologist. Thinking these cases arose from tubular scar tissue in the lungs, their investigation turned to look for relatives with tuberculosis, which began in 1958, but by 1962, with the increasing mesothelioma cases in the nonwhites, this search intensified. The cases now consisted of 141 cases (32 white, 32 colored, and 77 Bantu). The early cases were mostly white. Of the white cases, 24 had pleural effusion, 16 of these occurring on the right, and 8 had solid tumors. Out of the 32 white cases, 12 were women and 11 presented with fluid. Of the colored patients or Euroafricans up to 1968, there were 32 cases of which 25 were mesothelioma. One man had abdominal mesothelioma. There were 24 men and 8 women, of which one was pregnant and another nursing a baby. Eighteen had fluid and 12 of the cases were right sided on initial presentation. There were 77 Bantu patients, one of which, a female patient, had abdominal mesothelioma. Fifty-one (35 men and 16 women) presented with fluid and 28 had initial right-sided presentation. Eight were diagnosed with peripheral carcinoma and, of the remaining 43, four had insufficient material to review and seven had mislaid slides from which a diagnosis could be confirmed. Twenty-six (15 men and 11 women) presented without fluid and another 8 were diagnosed with peripheral carcinoma. Two (one man and one woman) had tuberculosis beforehand. Sleggs[901] concluded that air pollution by asbestos or any dust had an effect on the *Mycobacterium tuberculosis* or, for that matter, other bacteria and believed that in some cases this might lead to mesothelioma or a peripheral carcinoma. Sleggs also, when speculating on cause, mentioned a possible genetic cause or a favorable but unidentified factor in the accompanying air pollution. Finally, Sleggs[901] went into a discussion of focal repetition dissemination to spread tuberculosis, describing repetition pleurisy, and concluding repetition might have an effect.

Studies continue to date describing the capabilities of crocidolite asbestos to cause asbestos-related diseases and its strong propensity to cause mesothelioma. I will briefly mention a few of significance that the reader may want to explore further. In comparing the use of crocidolite and chrysotile in two factories manufacturing gas masks during World War II, McDonald and McDonald[902] showed the differences of mesothelioma occurring in greater prevalence among those using crocidolite than chrysotile. In the chrysotile section, I discussed these differences in much detail and refer the reader to that section of the chapter. I have also discussed a similar situation among cement manufacturing facilities in New Orleans[821] where crocidolite was used more at one site than the other. It was also found that more mesotheliomas were reported at the site where crocidolite was more prevalent.[821]

Crocidolite has only been mined in South Africa and Western Australia. Western Australian mining began in the 1930s in Wittenoom Gorge and became full-scale operational by 1943 and ending in 1966. The first case of mesothelioma was diagnosed in 1960 and many more have subsequently occurred. In a study[903] of 138 patients, mesothelioma was the most likely diagnosis. One hundred twenty-five were men, 134 had pleural mesothelioma, and 4 had peritoneal mesothelioma. Their ages ranged from 22 to 82 years, and only two cases occurred under the age of 35 years in one man and one woman. Seventy-six had certain or probable exposure to Western Australian crocidolite, 56 in the mine or mill, 11 in state government railway shops, 1 who handled empty sacs that once contained crocidolite, and the remainder employed in transport or as laggers, plumbers, boilermakers, fitters, or carpenters, or in the manufacturing of asbestos cement, in building construction, in the manufacture of sealants for beer barrels, the manufacture of fire brick, the assembly of gas masks, or the loading and unloading of ships. Four had no known occupational exposure but had lived in the town of Wittenoom either as children or as adults. Three of the four with peritoneal mesothelioma had worked in the asbestos mine or mill and the exposure history of the fourth was unknown. The latency ranged from 11 to 50 years and for those with known exposures at Wittenoom, either occupational or environmental, it ranged from 2 months to 29 years (mean 3.8 years). Exposure measurements were made only near the end of operations and were heavy (as high as 80–100 fibers/mL).[903]

In an update published in 1988,[898] the follow-up continued to the end of 1980. The cohort consisted of 6506 men and 411 women whose names were searched in the death registry of all Australian states from January 1, 1943, to December 31, 1980. The authors[898] calculated the number of deaths using two different censoring dates: (1) December 31, 1980, for SMR1 and (2) the last date known to be alive for SMR2. All subjects were censored at age 85 years if they were not known to be dead before that time. Most of the workforce was of either Australian or British origin. For the men where their known worksite was known, 31% worked in the heaviest exposure area—the mill. The women (80%) on the other hand did not work in the mills, the mine or other on-site operations, but rather in the town. Despite the men working in the heavy exposure area, most did not accumulate more that 10 fibers/mL-years because of their short work histories. Only 5.5% accumulated more than 100 fibers/mL-years. The medium exposures for men were 6.0 fibers/mL-years and 0.5 fibers/mL-years for women. Follow-up was poor—73.2% for men and 58.0% for women. This was most apparent in the short-term workers (<1 month) and in the lowest exposure groups. The low number of deaths in women precluded much analysis or conclusions. One death out of the 10 neoplasms among the women was due to pleural mesothelioma. In the men, there were 32 pleural mesotheliomas. Statistically elevated observations for SMR2 only were observed for neoplasms of the stomach (17 observed for SMR2 = 1.90, 95% CI = 1.18–3.06) and for both SMR1 and SMR2 in neoplasms of the trachea, bronchus, and lung (91 observed for SMR1 = 1.60, 95% CI = 1.31–1.97; and SMR2 = 2.64, 95% CI = 2.15–3.24). There was only one death from peritoneal mesothelioma. Pneumoconiosis had elevated SMRs (34 observed for SMR1 = 15.1, 95% CI = 10.8–21.1; and SMR2 = 25.5, 95% CI = 18.2–35.7) under both schemes, as did cirrhosis of the liver (25 observed for SMR1 = 2.53, 95% CI = 1.71–3.74; and SMR2 = 3.94, 95% CI = 2.66–5.83) and peptic ulceration only on censor scheme SMR2 (12 observed for SMR2 = 2.48, 95% CI = 1.41–4.37). Mortality was associated with dose in mesothelioma only after 20 years or more since first exposure, which was longer than that for lung cancers. Latency for pneumoconiosis was even shorter after first exposure.

In 1989 de Klerk et al.[904] looked at the dose–response relationship between exposure to crocidolite alone and the incidence of lung cancer in the same cohort as studied by Armstrong et al. in 1988. de Klerk et al.[904] found an increase with increasing duration of employment to an OR of 2.2 (95% CI = 1.1–4.5) for five or more years. The OR for years of employment as a continuous variable was 1.11 a year (95% CI = 1.04–1.19). There was an observed small increase in the OR for the period between 11 and 20 years after first employment, but this was statistically insignificant. There was little evidence to support either year of first employment or worksite with any effect on lung cancer. The data clearly indicated a stronger effect for duration of employment than for exposure intensity. This was also true for pleural mesothelioma, with no deaths in those employed for 90 days or less. Three deaths occurred in those with up to 183 days of employment, and thereafter, the longer periods had a 10-fold or higher increase in mortality, with little indication of a gradient of increasing mortality with increasing duration of employment. For pleural mesothelioma, year of first employment was related to substantially lower mortality if employed in or after 1957 (OR = 0.2, 95% CI = 0.1–0.8). There was an eightfold increase in mortality after 16–20 years from first employment and a 20-fold increase after 20+ years from first employment. This study[904] revealed no evidence of mortality from cancer of the stomach or any index of exposure. In conclusion, the authors[904] found evidence of mortality from lung cancer related to duration of employment and intensity of exposure with the greatest between 10 and 20 years after initial employment. They confided this was expected if smoking and asbestos exposures occurred in this fairly heavy smoking cohort and that asbestos acted as an intermediate or late-stage carcinogen in lung cancer development. In addressing those lost to follow-up in the cohort (73.2% men and 58% women), the authors[904] felt their methods of tracing and sources used would unlikely miss any deaths from pleural mesothelioma or more than a few from lung cancer or stomach cancer, and that the effect of this large percentage lost to follow-up would be slight.

In 1986, Botha et al.,[905] while looking at the effects of exposure on mortality from crocidolite in South Africa between 1968 and 1980 and in individuals aged 35 to 74 years, found that high crocidolite districts comprised less than 1% of the population but accounted for 7% of the asbestosis/mesothelioma deaths in white men, 35% in black men, 20% in white women, and 49% in black women. SMRs were elevated almost 10-fold for all races in the high crocidolite districts. This study[905] found that although high in South African coloreds, stomach cancers more than doubled when exposed to crocidolite.

These studies, although not all inclusive, show the ability of crocidolite to cause all asbestos-related diseases during the early history of crocidolite usage and exposure as well as disease patterns. Although this fiber is no longer of major commercial use, its legacy will linger for many years as cleanup and disposal of old applications continue. This is particularly true in the abandoned crocidolite minefields around Kuruman, South Africa, where mesothelioma rates remain among the highest in the world. I recently visited the area and saw first hand the extent of devastation and risk placed on the remaining population after the asbestos mining companies left the area with only their deadly legacy left behind. Remediation has slowly begun in this area, but because of the lack of funds, is moving very slowly with no foreseeable end in sight, thus allowing the trail of death from the mining company's past to travel into the future.

5.6.5 Tremolite

Tremolite is one of the tremolite–actinolite minerals and is found in the amphibole group; although it is often referred to only as tremolite, it has a chemical formula of Ca_2 $(Mg, Fe^{2+})_5$... $(Si_8O_{22}$ $(OH, F)_2)$. Tremolite is often found as an contaminate of chrysotile asbestos or talc.[893] It has been suggested that milling will remove the tremolite from the chrysotile; however, this is not universally accepted.[437] Studies have established tremolite's ability to cause all asbestos-related diseases, including asbestosis, lung cancer, and mesothelioma.[906–908] Persons in New Caledonia using a pure form of tremolite to mix a whitewash called "po" have shown a risk of pleural mesothelioma, which is strongly associated with its use.[909] Other studies have shown similar associations with tremolite-containing whitewashes in Cyprus, Greece, Turkey, and Corsica where environmental exposures to tremolite deposits occur.[910,911] Associations with lung cancer have been much fewer and seem to be complicated with potential confounding factors, that is, alcohol, diet, occupational exposures, and smoking. Yazicioglu et al.[912] reported an excess of mesotheliomas in areas where tremolite-containing "po" was used.

5.6.6 Talc

Talc is a specific and naturally occurring mineral described as a hydrated magnesium silicate $(Mg_3Si_4O_{10}(OH)_2)$ but can occur in intergrowths where it is contaminated with the asbestos material actinolite, anthophyllite, chrysotile, tremolite, and silica.[736,913] The health effects of tremolite have been discussed earlier. Large doses of talc have resulted in adverse inflammatory pulmonary responses, cough, tachycardia, and cyanosis.[913] Talcosis, a disease caused by the inhalation of talc, has been described in detail in many of the occupational medicine textbooks.[914] When contaminated, talc can cause diseases associated with the type of contaminate, that is, asbestos can cause pleural thickening, asbestosis, lung cancer and mesothelioma, and silica can cause silicosis and lung cancer.[915]

Epidemiological studies of talc miners and millers have demonstrated such diseases in a manner similar to the radiological patterns of silicosis—discrete opacities in the mid-lung (3–5 mm);

asbestosis—diffuse, interstitial fibrosis in the lower lung zones; and mixed patterns of both diseases.[913]

WC Dreessen[916] of the U.S. Public Health Service published the ill effects of tremolite-containing talc among 57 workers exhibiting such effects after 10 years of exposure. Dreessen and Dalla Valle[917] further described such findings among 66 workers in two Georgia talc mines and concluded the changes were permanent. Further epidemiologic studies confirmed the presence of talc-related diseases among New York State talc miners and millers.[143,144,918–920]

Cancers have been reported among talc-exposed workers. Kleinfeld et al.[921] reported 12 respiratory cancer deaths when 3.7 were expected in workers exposed to talc contaminated with anthophyllite and tremolite (calculated: RR = 3.24, 95% CI = 1.67–5.67). Lamm et al.[922] reported an SMR for respiratory cancers of 246 among 705 male talc workers, but as the excess mortality occurred among those employed less than 1 year, the authors[922] were unable to associate it with their exposure to talc. Thomas and Stewart[923] of the National Cancer Institute (United States) reported that as latency increased among workers exposed to talc and quartz for 1 year between 1939 and 1966, the SMR for lung cancer rose from 250 to 364 among those exposed for 15 or more years. Other such studies have not shown such associations.[924,925] However, the IARC[926] concluded there was adequate evidence that talc contaminated with asbestos causes cancer in humans, although there was inadequate evidence that uncontaminated talc causes cancer.

Talc has had many uses in both industry and in consumer products and when it has been obtained from geographical deposits where it is contaminated with asbestos-containing materials, it poses a significant hazard to the downstream user and results in a risk to asbestos-related diseases.

5.6.7 Vermiculite

Vermiculite is a member of the phyllosilicate group of minerals with a typical formula of $(Mg,Ca,K,Fe^{II})_3(Si,AL,Fe^{II})_4O_{10}(OH)_2O4H_2O$ (http://www.schundler.com/techverm.htm). Like talc, vermiculite, a naturally occurring mineral, can occur in areas where other naturally occurring minerals are found and thus contaminated. One form of contamination is from the tremolite form of asbestos. In the United States in 1881, Robert Rannie and his partner dug a 40-ft. shaft hoping to get gold but instead discovered vermiculite, which was later commercialized by Edward Alley in 1919, who had observed its unique characteristic of expanding to a large, lightweight, puffy material that did not burn. The vermiculite product was then named *zonolite* and was found to expand up to 15 times its original size when heated to 2000°F. In 1963, an industrial hygiene study at the Zonolite Company by Ben Wake found 6.2%–22.5% tremolite in samples of vermiculite.[927]

Peipins et al.[928] reported radiographic abnormalities consistent with asbestos-related pulmonary diseases, as had Lockey et al.,[929] among workers in an Ohio fertilizer plant using vermiculite from the mining community of Libby, Montana. Lockey et al.[929] found workers with daily TWA exposures of 0.031–0.415 fibers/cm^3 similar to those encountered by community residents in the mining community to have significantly elevated radiographic pleural changes as well as chest pain. Very high exposures to tremolite–actinolite were reported in the Libby vermiculite dry mill by NIOSH before 1964 to be as high as 168 fibers/cm^3 in the working areas, 182 fibers/cm^3 encountered by sweepers, and 13 fibers/cm^3 in the quality control laboratory.[930] They also found that exposures in the mine before 1971 ranged between 9 and 23 fibers/cm^3 for drillers and less than 2 fibers/cm^3 for the nondrilling jobs.

Vermiculite contaminated with asbestos, such as found in Libby, Montana, have resulted in not only the miners and mill workers developing asbestos-related diseases at an alarming rate but also the residents in the community around the Libby mine. NIOSH looked at 575 men hired before 1970 for at least 1 year and found SMRs of 223.2 (95% CI = 136.3–344.7) for lung cancer and 243.0 (95% CI = 148.4–375.3) for NMRD.[930] Both lung cancer and NMRD SMRs increased with fiber-year exposures, thus showing a dose–response relationship.[930]

McDonald et al.,[931] in their most recent follow-up of a cohort from the Libby, Montana, vermiculite mine and community, recorded elevated SMRs for lung cancer (SMR = 2.40), NMRD (SMR = 3.09), and reported 12 deaths ascribed to mesothelioma among 406 vermiculite mine workers followed until 1999 and employed before 1963. The authors[931] concluded that using an all-cause linear model, a 14% increase in mortality would occur among the mine workers exposed occupationally to 100 fibers/mL-years and a 3.2% increase for the general population if exposed for 50 years at ambient concentrations at the current OSHA PEL of 0.1 fibers/mL.

When McDonald et al.[932] looked at another smaller cohort of vermiculite workers in South Carolina exposed to lower levels of tremolite in the ore, out of 194 men only 4 deaths from lung cancer were observed when 3.31 (SMR = 121) would have been expected. PCM and ATEM fiber counts found low concentrations up to 0.32 fibers >5 μm/cm^3 and tremolite–actinolite accounted for 47.6% of the settled dust. The mortality study included those workers working 6 months or more before January 1, 1971, and followed through January 1, 1986. The mean duration of employment was 9.2 years, and the average mean from beginning of employment to death was 19.7 years. Because only 51 deaths had thus far occurred (26% of the cohort) and the follow-up period rather short, the resultant incidence of mesothelioma would have been difficult to ascertain until further follow-up was obtained. At the time of the study,[932] no deaths from pneumoconiosis or mesothelioma were observed.

Hessel and Sluis-Cremer[933,934] found similar results in a cross-sectional study among black vermiculite workers exposed to "very little asbestos" at the Palabora Vermiculite Mine in South Africa. Two cases of small opacities were observed—one with 1/0 and t/t opacities in a worker with 22.5 years as an operator and the other with 1/1 and p/s opacities who worked in a duster job for 19.5 years. No dose–response trend was noted, lung function was comparable with the control groups as were respiratory symptoms, and the authors stated that because of the nature of their study (cross-sectional), the risk of mesothelioma could not be excluded.

Vermiculite contaminated with asbestos can provide significant hazards to its users and has been used in consumer products for more than 80 years. Its uses have included: generic applications such as loose fill, absorbents, industrial heat insulation, soil conditioners, asbestos substitutes, fire protection; construction applications such as acoustic finishes, fire protection, floor and roof screed, roof insulation, gypsum plaster, loft insulation, sound deadening; agricultural applications such as animal feed, fertilizer, pesticides, seed encapsulant, soil conditioner; and horticultural applications such as potting mixes, root cuttings, seed germination, and sowing composts.[935]

REFERENCES

1. Jones RH. *Asbestos and Asbestic: Their Properties, Occurrences and Use.* London: Crosbey Lockwood and Son; 1897.
2. Agricola G, De Re Metallica, Dover Publications, New York, 1556 [translated from Latin edition by Herbert Clark Hoover and Lou Henry Hoover, The Mining Magazine, 1912, London, 1950 edition].
3. Noro L. Occupational and "non-occupational" asbestosis in Finland. *Am Ind Hyg Assoc J* 1968;29:195.
4. Gilray CG. Asbestos. In: *The History of Silk, Cotton, Linen, Wool, and Other Fibrous Substances*, Gilroy CG, ed. New York: Harper & Brothers; 1845: 392–399; Chapter III.
5. Carroll-Porgzynski CZ. *Asbestos from Rock to Fabric.* Manchester, England: The Textile Institute; 1956.
6. Pliny The Elder. Natural History: A Selection. Translated with introduction and notes by John F. Healy, Penguin Books, 360, 2004; Pliny, Natural History, Books 36–37. Loeb Classical Library, Translated by D. E. Eichholz, 43–113, 2006.
7. Keyaler JG, *Keyaler's Travels.* Translated 1760, ii, 292, 1760.
8. Latham RE, Ed. *The Travels of Marco Polo.* London: Penguin Books; 1958; pp. 89–90.
9. Liddell D, Miller K. *Mineral Fibers and Health.* Boca Raton, FL: CRC Press; 1991.
10. Selikoff IJ, Lee DHK. *Asbestos and Disease.* New York: Academic Press; 1978; 559 pp.

11. Baxter J. *A Pound of Paper: Confessions of a Book Addict*. London, UK: Doubleday; 2003.

12. Brodeur P. The Magic Mineral. *The New Yorker Magazine*, October 12, 1968.

13. Brodeur P. *The Magic Mineral: Asbestos and Enzymes*. New York: Ballantine Books; 1972; p. 2.

14. Maines R. *Asbestos & Fire Technological Trade-Offs and The Body of Risk*. Rutgers University Press, 2005.

15. Anonymous. Asbestos mining in Vermont. *Asbestos* 1921;2(9):41.

16. Hendry NW. The geology, occurrences and major uses of asbestos. *Ann NY Acad Sci* 1965;132:12.

17. Hueper WC. *Occupational Tumors and Allied Diseases*. Springfield, IL: Charles C. Thomas; 1942; 896 pp.

18. Hueper WC. Occupational and nonoccupational exposures to asbestos. *Ann NY Acad Sci* 1965;132:184–195.

19. Morinaga K, Kishimoto T, Sakatani M, et al. Asbestos-related lung cancer and mesothelioma in Japan. *Ind Health* 2001;39:65.

20. Wagner JC. The pathology of asbestosis in South Aftica. Doctoral Thesis. Medicine in the Department of Pathology, University of the Witwatersrand; 1961.

21. Cilliers JJ, Le R, Genis, Genis JH. Crocidolite asbestos in the Cape Province. In: *Proceedings of the Fourth Annual Congress on Geol. South Africa*, 1961, p. 1.

22. Hall AL. *Asbestos in the Union of South Africa, 2nd ed*. Pretoria: Govt. Printer; 1930.

23. Sleggs, CA, Marchand P, Wagner JC. Diffuse pleural mesotheliomas in South Africa. *J S Afr Med Assoc* 1961;35:28.

24. Sluis-Cremer GK. Asbestosis in South African asbestos miners. *Environ Res* 1970;3:310.

25. Raybestos-Manhattan, Friction product facts, 1968.

26. Anonymous. Asbestos production, United States of America. *Asbestos* 1948;30:22.

27. Cirkel F. *Asbestos—Its Occurrence, Exploitation and Uses*. Ottawa, Canada: Govt. Printing Bureaul; 1910.

28. Bowles O. Asbestos, Vol. 403, U.S. Department of Interior, Bureau of Mines, Bull., U.S. Govt. Printing Office, Washington, DC, 1937, p. 9.

29. Anonymous. Asbestos product manual. C.W. Trainer Manufacturing Co., Boston, MA, 1903.

30. Anonymous. *The Asbestos Fact Book, 3rd ed.*, Asbestos, Vol. 54, August, 1953, p. 3 (later edition 1970).

31. Berger H. *Asbestos Fundamentals—Origin, Properties, Mining*. New York: Chemical Publishing Co.; 1963.

32. Anonymous. *Asbestos*, September, 1953, p. 8.

33. Anonymous. *Asbestos*, November, 1958, p. 10.

34. Harries PG. Asbestos hazards in naval dockyards. *Ann Occup Hyg* 1968;11:135–145.

35. Harries PG. Asbestos dust concentrations in ship repairing: a practical approach to improving asbestos hygiene in naval dockyards. *Ann Occup Hyg* 1971;14:241.

36. Scientific American. *Gradual Ascendency of the United States as an Asbestos Producer*. Munn & Co., Inc., Publishers, New York, N.Y., 155, August 12, 1916.

37. Hoffman FL. Mortality from respiratory diseases in dusty trades, Inorganic Dusts, Bulletin of Bureau of Labor Statistics, No. 231 (Industrial Accidents and Hygiene, Series 17), U.S. Bureau of Labor, Washington, D.C., 1918; p. 458.

38. Heisler C II. South African asbestos seeks market. Commerce Reports, Bureau of Foreigh and Domestic Commerce, E.E. Pratt, Chief, Nos. 1=76, Vol. 1, Nineteenth Year, January, February, and March, Washington, Government Printing Office, 1916.

39. Saborsky AD. Glass wool health insulation in Europe. *J Amer Ceram Soc* 1923;6:674.

40. Oliver T. Pulmonary asbestosis in its clinical aspects. *J Industr Hyg* 1929;9(11):483–485.

41. Anderson AM. Historical sketch of the development of legislation for injurious and dangerous industries in England. In: *Dangerous Trades*, Oliver T, ed. New York: Dutton; 1902.

42. Dean L. *Factories and Workshops: Annual Report for 1899*. Great Britain, London; 1899.

43. Murray HM. Statement before the committee in the minutes of evidence. In *Report of the Departmental Committee on Compensation for Industrial Disease*, London, H.M. Stationery Office, p. 127, 1907.

44. Auribault M. Note sur l'hygiene et la securite des ouvriers dans les filateurs et tissages d'amiante, *Bull. Insp. Trav.*, Paris, 14, 120, 1906; in Selikoff IJ and Lee DHK, *Asbestos and Disease*, Academic Press, New York, San Francisco, London, 1978, 559 pp.

45. Scarpa L. Industria dell'amianto e tuberculosi. In: *Proceedings of the 18th International Medical Congress*, 1908, p. 358, in Selikoff IJ and Lee DHK, Asbestos and Disease, Academic Press, New York, 1978, 559 pp.

46. Merewether ERA, Price CW. Report on the effects of asbestos dust on the lungs and dust suppression in the asbestos industry I. Occurrence of pulmonary fibrosis and other pulmonary affections in asbestos workers II. Processes giving rise to dust and methods for its suppression, H.M. Stationery Office, London, 1930.

47. Collis. Dusty processes. In: *Factories and Workshops: Annual Report for 1910*. London, 1911, H.M. Inspectorate of Factories, UK.

48. Anonymous. Industrial diseases, The American Association for Labor Legislation, American Legislation Review, Pub. 17, 1912.

49. Fahr T. Asbestosis-pneumoconiosis. *Munch Med Woch* 1914;61:625.

50. Pancoast HK, Miller TG, Landis HRM. A roentgenologic study of the effects of dust inhalation upon the lungs. *Trans Assoc Am Phys* Read 1917, 1918;31:97.

51. Pancoast HK, Pendergrass EP. A review of our present knowledge of pneumoconiosis, based upon roentgenologic studies, with notes on the pathology of the condition. *Am J Roentgenol Radium Ther* 1925;14(5):381.

52. Tweedale G. *Magic Mineral to Killer Dust Turner & Newall and the Asbestos Hazard*. Oxford: Oxford University Press; 2000.

53. Howker E. Asbestos: The lies that killed. *New Statesman*, August 28, 2008.

54. Cooke WE. Fibrosis of the lungs due to the inhalation of asbestos dust. *Brit Med J* 1924;2:147.

55. Cooke WE, Hill CF. Pneumoconiosis due to asbestos dust. *J Roy Micr Soc* 1937;47:232.

56. McDonald S. Histology of pulmonary asbestosis. *Brit Med J* 1927;2:1025.

57. Cooke WE. Asbestos dust and curious bodies found in pulmonary asbestosis. *Brit Med J* 1929;2:578.

58. Williams MG, Dodson RF, Dickson EW, Fraire AE. An assessment of asbestos body formation in extrapulmonary sites: liver and spleen. *Tox Indust Health* 2001;17:1.

59. Cooke WE. Pulmonary asbestosis. *Brit Med J* 1927;2:1024.

60. Roggli VL, Pratt PC. Asbestosis. In: *Pathology of Asbestos-Associated Diseases*, Roggli VL, Donald Greenberg S, Pratt PC, eds. Boston: Little, Brown and Company; 1992.

61. Craighead JE, Abraham JL, Chrug A, Green FHY, Kleinerman J, Pratt PC, Seemayer TA, Vallyathan V, Weill H. The pathology of asbestos-associated diseases of the lungs and pleural cavities: Diagnostic criteria and proposed grading schema. Report of the Pneumoconisosi Committee of the College of American Pathologists and the National Institute for Occupational Safety and Health. *Arch Pathol Lab Med* 106(11):October 8, 1982.

62. Crouch E, Churg A. Ferruginous bodies and the histologie evaluation of dust exposure. *Am J Surg Pathol* 1984;8(2):109–116.

63. McLarty JW, Greenberg SD, Hurst GA, Spivey CG, Seitzman LH, Hieger LR, Farley ML, Mabry LC. The clinical significance of ferruginous bodies in sputa. *J Occup Med* 1980;22(2):92–96.

64. Sporn TA, Roggli VL. Asbestosis. In *Pathology of Asbestos-Associated Diseases*, Roggli VL, Oury TD, Sporn TA, eds., 2nd ed. Springer; 2003.

65. Simson FW. Pulmonary asbestosis in South Africa [abstract]. *Brit Med J* 1928;July–December:258.

66. JAMA. Pulmonary asbestosis—Editorial. *J Am Med Assoc* 1928;90:119.

67. Seiler HE. A case of pneumoconiosis. *Brit Med J* 1928;11:982.

68. Gloyne SR. The presence of the asbestos fiber in the lesions of asbestos workers. *Tubercle* 1929;10:404.

69. Stewart MJ. A method of examining the sputum for asbestosis bodies. *Brit Med J* September 28, 1929;682.

70. Greenberg MG. Professor Matthew Stewart: asbestosis research 1929–1934. *AJIM* 1997;32:562–569.

71. Stewart MJ, Haddow AC. Demonstration of the peculiar bodies of pulmonary asbestosis ("asbestosis bodies") in material obtained by lung puncture and in the sputum. *J Pathol Bacterial* 1929;32:172.

72. Wood WB. Pulmonary asbestosis. Radiographic appearances in skiagrams of the chests of workers in asbestos. *Tubercle* 1929;10:353–363.

73. Bridge JC. Remarks on occupational dust. *Brit Med J* 1929;II:1143.

74. Klokov AL. Significance of investigation of function of cardiopulmonary system in early diagnosis of asbestosis. *Soviet Med* 1960;24:98.

75. Haslam JFC, Cowell SJ. *Recent Advances in Preventive Medicine*. Philadelphia: P. Blakiston's Son & Co. Inc.; 1930.

76. Anonymous. Asbestos, 1930.

77. Drinker P, Hatch T. *Industrial Dust Hygienic Significance, Measurement and Control*. New York and London: McGraw-Hill Book Company, Inc.; 1936.

78. Merewether ERA, Price CW. Report on effects of asbestos dust on the lungs and dust suppression in the asbestos industry. Printed and published by His Majesty's Stationary Office, London, 1930.

79. Notes and Memoranda. *The Engineer* April 4, 1930;149:379.

80. Pulmonary asbestosis. *Lancet* 1930;1:870.

81. Merewether ERA. The occurrence of pulmonary fibrosis and other pulmonary affections in asbestos workers. *J Indus Hyg* 12930;12(4):239.

82. Seiler HE. A case of pneumoconiosis. *Brit Med J* December 1, 1928:982.

83. Engineering, Mineral dust in factories, *Engineering*, May 2, 1930;129:577–578.

84. Mills RG. Pulmonary asbestosis: Report of a case. *Minn Med J* 1930;13:495.

85. Compensation act to be extended to asbestosis. *J Am Med Assoc* 1930;94:2078.

86. Fishbein M. *A History of the American Medical Association 1847 to 1947*. Philadelphia: W.B. Saunders Co.; 1947, p. 992.

87. Wood WB, Page DS. A case of pulmonary asbestosis: Death from tuberculosis two years after first exposure to the dust. *Tubercle* January 1930;157.

88. Wood WB, Gloyne SR. Pulmonary asbestosis. *Lancet* 1930;1:445.

89. Soper WB. Pulmonary asbestosis. A report of a case and a review. *Am Rev Tuberc* 1930;22:571.

90. ILO. Asbestos. *Occupation and Health Encyclopaedia of Hygiene, Pathology and Social Welfare*, Vol. 1, A-H. Geneva: International Labour Organization; 1930.

91. Pedley FG. Asbestosis. In *Industrial Hygiene*, Pedley FG, Cunningham JG, eds., 1930, pp. 576–577, in Pedley FG. Asbestosis. *J Can Med Assoc* 1930;2:253–254.

92. Greenberg M. The doctors and the dockers. *Am J Indust Med* 2004;45:573–581.

93. Fitzhugh GW. Memorandum of the Supervisor, Actuarial Division, Group Life and Health Section, to Dr. McDonnell, 1935. Cited by Castleman BI, 1996, in *Asbestos: Medical and Legal Aspects*, 4th ed., Aspen Law and Business.

94. Lynch KM, Smith WA. Pulmonary asbestos II. *Am Rev Tuberculosis* 1931;XXIII:643–660.

95. Ramazzini B. *Diseases of Workers*, 1713 [Translated from the Latin text *DeMorbis Artificum* of 1713, Wilmer Cave Wright, transi. Intr. George Rosen, The New York Academy of Medicine, Harper Publishing Company, Published in 1964].

96. Adams F. *The Genuine Works of Hippocrates*. Baltimore: The Williams & Wilkins Company; 1939.

97. Sparks JW. Pulmonary asbestosis. *Radiology* 1931;17:1249.

98. Schuster NH. Pulmonary asbestosis in a dog. *J Pathol Bact* 1931;34:75 (also as discussed in Ellman, 1933 and 1934).

99. Gye WE, Purdy WJ. The poisonous properties of colloidal silica. *Br J Exp Pathol* 1922;iii:75.

100. Mavrogordato A. Publication of the South African Institute for Medical Research, No. 15, 1922.

101. Lancet. German work on pulmonary asbestosis. *Lancet* July 9, 1932;2:92–93.

102. Buttner-Wobst W, Trillitzsch O. Die Bergflaschslunge (asbestosis) und was der Deutsche Artz von ilu wissen muss. *Die Tuberkulose* 1931;xi, 11:11–14.

103. Gerbis H. Ucko, Uber asbestosis der lungen. *Ver f Inn Med z Gerlin, Sitz*. 1931;V.7.

104. Timmermans FD. Asbestosis. *Zentralbl f. Gewerbehyg* 1931;8:280–288; 307–309.

105. U.K., Report on conferences between employers and inspectors concerning methods for suppressing dust in asbestos textile factories. Printed and published by His Majesty's Stationery Office, London, 1931.

106. Russell AE. Effects of dust upon the respiratory system, Conference Proceedings. Industrial Commission of Wisconsin. Democrat Printing, Madison, Wisconsin, 1932, p. 180.

107. Ellman P. Pulmonary asbestosis. *Lancet* 1933;252.

108. Dee P. Inhalational lung diseases. In *Imaging of Diseases of the Chest*, Armstrong P, Wilson AG, Dee P, Hansell DM, eds., 3rd ed. Mosby; 2000: 467–503.

109. Weinberger SE. *Principles of Pulmonary Medicine*, 4th ed. Philadelphia: Saunders; 2004.

110. Webster I. Asbestosis in non-experimental animals in South Africa. *Nature* February 2, 1963;506.

111. NRC. *Animals as Sentinels of Environmental Health Hazards*. National Research Council. 71, 1991.

112. Ellman P. Pulmonary asbestosis. *Proceedings of the Royal Society of Medicine* 1933;526.

113. Lynch KM, Smith WA. Asbestosis bodies in sputum and lung. *JAMA* August 30, 1930;95(9):659–661.

114. Gloyne SR. The morbid anatomy and histology of asbestosis. *Tubercle* 1933;14:550–558.

115. Merewether ERA. A memorandum on asbestosis. *Tubercle* 1933;XIV:109.

116. Donnelly J. Pulmonary asbestosis. *Am J Publ Health* 1934;23:1275.

117. Page RC. A study of the sputum in pulmonary asbestosis. *Am J Med Sci* 1933;189:41–55.

118. Stock GA. Pulmonary asbestosis. *Med Bull Vet Admin* 1933;10:126–129.

119. Wood WB, Gloyne SR. Pulmonary asbestosis. *Lancet* December 22, 1934;1383.

120. Gray RN. *Attorneys' Textbook of Medicine*. Albany, NY: Matthew Bender & Company; 1931.

121. Fulton WB, Dooley A, Mathews JL, Houtz RL. Asbestosis, Commonwealth of Pennsylvania, Department of Labor and Industry, *Special Bulletin* 42, 1935.

122. Lanza AJ, McConnell WJ, Fehnel JW. Effects of the inhalation of asbestos dust on the lungs of asbestos workers. *United States Public Health Reports* 1935;50:1.

123. Shull JR. Asbestosis: A roentgenologic review of 71 cases. *Radiology* 1936;27:279.

124. McMahon JF. Progress report—Air hygiene foundation, Mellon Institute of industrial Research, March 11, University of Pittsburgh & Castleman, B.I., 1990. *Asbestos: Medical and Legal Aspects*, 3rd ed., Prentice-Hall, Law and Business, Englewood Cliffs, NJ, 1939.

125. Castleman BI. *Asbestos: Medical and Legal Aspects*, 3rd ed. Englewood Cliffs, NJ: Prentice Hall Law & Bussiness; 1990.

126. Lanza AJ. Asbestosis. *J Am Med Assoc* 1936;106:368.

127. Donnelly J. Pulmonary asbestosis: Incidence and progress. *J Industr Hyg Tox* January–December 1936;18:222–228.

128. Egbert DS, Geiger AJ. Pulmonary asbestosis and carcinoma. Report of a case with necropsy findings. *Am Rev Tuberculosis* 1936;36:143–150.

129. McPheeters SB. A survey of a group of employees exposed to asbestos dust. *J Ind Hyg Toxicol* 1936;18(4):229.

130. Drinker P, Hatch T. *Industrial Dust—Hygienic Significance, Measurement and Control*. New York and London: McGraw-Hill Book Company Inc. 1936; p. 76.

131. Dreessen WD, Dallavalle JM, Edwards TL, Miller JW, Sayers RR. A study of asbestosis in the asbestos textile industry, *Public Health Bulletin* 241, U.S. Treasury Department, Public Health Service, 1938.

132. Gardner LU. Recent developments in relation to silicosis. *Industr Med* February 1940;9(2):45–49. The pathology and roentgenographic manifestations of pneumoconiosis, Annual Report of The Saranac Laboratory for the Study of Tuberculosis of the Edward L, Trudeau Foundation for the Year 1940. Saranac Lake, N.Y.: 1–33, 1940.

133. Johnstone RT. Asbestosis. In: *Occupational Diseases. Diagnosis, Medicolegal Aspects and Treatment*. Philadelphia and London: W.B. Saunders Company; 1941:318–354.

134. Brown EW. Industrial hygiene and the Navy in national defense. *War Med* 1941;1:2–14.

135. Drinker P. The health and safety program of the U.S. Maritime Commission and the U.S. Navy in contract shipyards. *JAMA* March 13, 1943;822–823.

136. Bettes JA, Jr. The story of the asbestos textile industry in the United States. *Asbestos* August 1972:1–12.

137. Lanza AJ. *Silicosis and Asbestosis*. London, New York, Toronto: Oxford Medical Publications; 1938.

138. Fleisher WE, Viles FJ, Gade RL, Drinker P. A health survey of pipe covering operations in constructing Naval vessels. *J Indusr Hyg Tox* 1946;28(1):9–16.

139. Wegelius C. Changes in the lungs in 126 cases of asbestosis observed in Finland. *Acta Radiologica* 1947;28:139–152.

140. Smith KW. Pulmonary disability in asbestos workers. *AMA Arch Indust Health* 1955;12:198.

141. Thomas DL. Pneumonokoniosis in Victorian industry—Asbestosis. *Med J Austral* 1957;1:75.

142. Sander OA. Silicosis and asbestosis—Diagnosis, prevention and treatment. *Am J Surg* 1955;90(7):115.

143. Porro FW, Patton JR, Hobbs AA. Pneumoconiosis in the talc industry. *Am J Radiol* 1942;47(4):507.

144. Siegal W, Smith AR, Greenburg L. The dust hazard in tremolite talc mining, including roentgenologic findings in talc workers. *Am J Roentgenol Radium Ther* 1943;49(1):11.

145. Smith AR. Pleural calcification resulting from exposure to certain dusts. *Am J Radiol* 1952;67(3):375.

146. Jacob G, Bohlig H. Die rontggenologischen komplikationen der lungenasbestose. *Fortschritte Auf dem Gebiete Der Rontgenstrahlen veeinigt mit Rontgenpraxis* 1955;83(4):515.

147. Fehre W. Ueber doppelseitige Pleuraverkalkungen infolge beruflicher Staubeinwirkungen. *Fortschr Rontegenstr* 1956;85(1):16.

148. Frost J, George J, Moller. Asbestosis with pleural calcification among insulation workers. *Dan Med Bull* 1956;3:202.
149. Cai SX, Zhang CH, Zhang X, Morinaga K. Epidemiology of occupational asbestos-related diseases in China. *Ind Health* 2001;39:75.
150. Kilviluoto R. Pleural calcification as a roentgenologic sign of non-occupational endemic anthophyllite asbestos. *Acta Radiol* suppl. 194, Stockholm, 1960, pp. 7–67.
151. McMillan G, Rossiter CE. Development of radiological and clinical evidence of parenchymal fibrosis in men with non-malignant asbestos-related pleural lesions. *Brit J Ind Med* 1982;39:54.
152. Sheers G. Asbestos—Associated disease in employees of Devonport Dockyard. *Ann NY Acad Sci* 1979;330:281.
153. Rosenstock L, Hudson LD. Nonmalignant asbestos-induced pleural disease. *Seminars Resp Med* 1986;7(3):197–202.
154. Rosenstock L, Barnhart S, Heyer NJ, et al. The relation among pulmonary function, chest roentgenographic abnormalities, and smoking status in an asbestos-exposed cohort. *Am Rev Resp Dis* 1988;138:272.
155. Becklake MR, Bagatin E, Neder JA. Asbestos-related diseases of the lungs and pleura: uses, trends and management over the last century. *Int J Tuberc Lung Dis* April 2007;11(4):356–369.
156. Hillerdal G. Pleural plaques—Occurrence, exposure to asbestos, and clinical importance, *Acta Universitatis Upsaliensis*, Uppsala, Sweden, 1980, p. 363.
157. Rosenstock L. Asbestosis and asbestos-related pleural disease. In *Textbook of Clinical Occupational and Environmental Medicine*, Rosenstock L, Cullen MB, eds. Philadelphia, London, Toronto, Montreal, Sydney, Tokyo: W.B. Saunders Company; 1994:260.
158. Dodson RF, Williams MG, Corn CJ, et al. A comparison of asbestos burden in lung parenchyma, lymph nodes, and plaques. *Ann NY Acad Sci* 1991;643:53.
159. Dodson RF, Williams MG, Corn CJ, et al. Non-asbestos fibre burden in individuals exposed to asbestos. In *Mechanisms in Fibre Carcinogenesis*, Brown RC, Hosking JA, Johnson NF, eds. New York: Plenum Press; 1991:29.
160. Karjalainen A. Epidemiologie and clinical aspects of asbestos-related diseases. *Proceedings of the Asbestos Symposium for the Asian Countries*, Vol. 3, Japan, September 2002;26–27.
161. Fletcher DE. A mortality study of shipyard workers with pleural plaques. *Brit J Ind Med* 1972;29:142–145.
162. Edge JR. Asbestos-related disease in Barrow-in-Furness. *Environ Res* 1976;11:244.
163. Edge JR. Incidence of bronchial carcinoma in shipyard workers with pleural plaques. *Ann NY Acad Sci* 1979;330:289.
164. Hillerdal G. Radiological changes as markers of environmental exposure and environmental risk of lung cancer and mesothelioma 2001, Asbestos Health Effects Conference, U.S. Environmental Protection Agency, Oakland, CA, May 24–25, 2001.
165. Luo S, Liu X, Mu S, Tsai SP, Wen CP. Asbestos-related disease from environmental exposure to crocidolite in Da-yao, China. I. Review of exposure and epidemiological data. *Occup Environ Med* 2003;60(1):35–42.
166. Tossavainen A, Henderson DW, Rantanen J, et al. Consensus Report, "Asbestos, asbestosis, and cancer: the Helsinki criteria for diagnosis and attribution." *Scand J Work Environ Health* 1997;23:311–316.
167. Merewether ERA. *Annual Report of the Chief Inspector of Factories for the Year 1947*. London: HMSO; 1949, p. 78.
168. Doll R. Mortality from lung cancer in asbestos workers. *Brit J Ind Med* 1955;12:81.
169. Buchanan WD. Asbestosis and primary intrathoracic neoplasms. *Ann NY Acad Sci* 1965;132:507.
170. Gloyne SR. Two cases of squamous carcinoma of the lung occurring in asbestosis. *Tubercle* 1935;17:5–10.
171. Lynch KM, Smith WA. Pulmonary asbestosis III: carcinoma of lung in asbestos-silicosis. *Am J Can* 1935; XXIV:56–64.
172. Hillerdal G. Pleural plaques and risk for bronchial carcinoma and mesothelioma: A prospective study. *Chest* 1994;105:144–150.
173. Karjalainen A. Occupational asbestos exposure, pulmonary fiber burden and lung cancer in the Finnish population. An academic dissertation, Finnish Institute of Occupational Health and University of Helsinki, 1994;pp. 1–66.
174. Cullen MR. Controversies in asbestos-related lung cancer. *Occup Med State Art Rev* 1987;2:259–272.

175. Broderick A, Fuortes LJ, Merchant JA, Galvin JR, Schwartz DA. Pleural determinants of restrictive lung function and respiratory symptoms in an asbestos-exposed population. *Chest* 1992;101(3):684.

176. Roggli VL, Hammar SP, Pratt PC, et al. Does asbestos or asbestosis cause carcinoma of the lung? *Am J Ind Med* 1994;26:835–838.

177. Abraham JL. Asbestos inhalation, not asbestosis, causes lung cancer. *Am J Ind Med* 1994;26:839–842.

178. Jones RN, Hughes JM, Weill H. Asbestos exposure, asbestosis, and asbestos-attributable lung cancer. *Thorax* 1996;51 (Supp. 2):59–515.

179. McDonald JC, Hansell D, Newman Taylor A, et al. Is lung cancer related to asbestos exposure in the absence of pulmonary fibrosis? A case-referent study. *Am J Resp Crit Care Med* 1994;149:A405.

180. Koskinen K, Pukkala E, Reijula K, Karjalainen A. Incidence of cancer among the participants of the Finnish Asbestos Screening Campaign. *Scand J Work Environ Health* 2003;29(1):64–70.

181. Balashazy I, Hofmann W, Heistracher T. Local particle deposition patterns may play a key role in the development of lung cancer. *J Appl Physiol* 2003;94(5):1719.

182. Hammond EC, Selikoff IJ, Seidman H. Asbestos exposure, cigarette smoking, and death rates. *Ann NY Acad Sci* 1979;330:473.

183. Segarra F, Monte MB, Ibanez PL, Gonzalez AG, Nicolas JP. Asbestosis in the industries of the Barcelona area. *Am J Insust Med* 1980;1:149–158.

184. Blennerhassett J, Farlow D, Glass W, et al. Asbestos exposure and disease: Notes for medical practitioners. *Occup Safety Health Serv* 1995:1–14.

185. Morinaga K, Yokoyama K, Sakatani M, Yamamoto S, Sera Y. Lung cancer mortality among the asbestosis by smoking habit. *Proceedings of the Seventh International Conference on Occupational Lung Diseases, 372.* Geneva: ILO; 1993.

186. Lee PN. Relation between exposure to asbestos and smoking jointly and the risk of lung cancer. *Occup Environ Med* 2001;58:145.

187. Berry G, Liddell FDK. The interaction of asbestos and smoking in lung cancer: A modified measure of effect. *Ann Occup Hyg* 2004;48(5):459–462.

188. McFadden D, Wright J, Wiggs B, Chrug A. Cigarette smoke increases the penetration of asbestos fibers into airway walls. *Am J Pathol* 1986;123(1):95–99; McFadden D, Wright JL, Wiggs B, Churg A. Smoking inhibits asbestos clearance. *Am Rev Respir Dis* March 1986;133(3):372–374.

189. Liddell FDK, Armstrong BG. The combination of effects on lung cancer of cigarette smoking and exposure in Quebec Chrysotile miners and millers. *Ann Occ Hyg* 2002;46(1):5–13.

190. Gustavsson P, Nyberg F, Pershagen G, Schéele P, Jakobsson R, Plato N. Low-dose exposure to asbestos and lung cancer: Dose–response relations and interaction with smoking in a population-based case-referent study in Stockholm, Sweden. *Am J Epidemiol* 2002;156(11):1016.

191. Reid A, de Klerk NH, Ambrosini GL, Berry G, Musk AW. The risk of lung cancer with increasing time since ceasing exposure to asbestos and quitting smoking. *Occup Environ Med* 2006;63(8):509–512.

192. Knox JF, Holmes S, Doll R, Hill ID. Mortality from lung cancer and other causes among workers in an asbestos textile factory. *Brit J Ind Med* 1968;25:298.

193. Elmes PC, Simpson MJC. Insulation workers in Belfast III. Mortality 1940–66. *Brit J Ind Med* 1971;28:226.

194. Churg A. Malignant mesothelioma in British Columbia in 1982. *Cancer* 1985;55(3):672–674.

195. Morinaga K, Kishimoto T, Sakatani M, Akira M, Yokoyama K, Sera Y. Epidemiology of occupational asbestos-related diseases in China. *Ind Health* 2001;39(2):75–83.

196. Muscat JE, Stellman SD, Richie JP, Wynder EK. Lung cancer risk and workplace exposures in black men and women. *Environ Res* 1998;76:78.

197. Mándi A, Posgay M, Vadász P, et al. Role of occupational asbestos exposure in Hungarian lung cancer patients. *Arch Environ Contam Toxicol* 2000;73(8):555.

198. Pohlabeln H, Wild P, Schill W, Ahrens W, Jahn I, Bolm-Audorff U, Jöckeel K-H. Asbestos fibre years and lung cancer: A two phase case-control study with expert exposure assessment. *Occup Environ Med* 2002;59:410.

199. Stayner L, Smith R, Bailer J, Gilbert S, Dement J, Brown D, Lernen RA. Exposure-response analysis of risk of respiratory disease associated with occupational exposure to chrysotile asbestos. *Occup Environ Med* 1997;54:646–652.

200. Dement JM, Brown DP. Cohort mortality and case-control studies of white male chrysotile asbestos textile workers. *J Occ Med Tox* 1993;2(4):1–18.

201. Selikoff IJ, Hammond EC. Health hazards of asbestos exposure. *Ann NY Acad Sci* 1979;330.

202. Mullan RJ, Murthy LM. Occupational sentinel health events: An up-dated list for physician recognition and public health surveillance. *Am J Ind Med* 1991;19:775–799.

203. Wagner E. Das tuberkelahnliche lymphadenom. *Arch Heilk* 1870;11:495–525.

204. Adami JG. *Principles of Pathology*. Philadelphia: Lea and Febiger; 1908.

205. Kemperer P, Rabin CB. Primary neoplasms of pleura: Report of five cases. *Arch Pathol* 1931;11:385–412.

206. Hill AB. Asbestos and mesothelioma of the pleura [Abridged]. *Proc Roy Soc Med* 1966;59:57.

207. Wedler HW. Lung cancer in asbestosis patients. *Deutsche Arch Klin Med* 1943;191:189–209; Wedler HW, Asbestosis and lung cancer. *Deutsche Medizinische Wochenschrig* 1943;69:575.

208. Bonser GM. Occupational cancer. *Am J Clin Path* 1955;25:126–134.

209. Wyers H. That legislative measures have proved generally effective in the control of asbestosis. M.D. Thesis. University of Glasgow, United Kingdom, 1946.

210. Mallory TB, Castleman B, Parris EE. Case records of the Massachusetts General Hospital #33111. *N Engl J Med* 1947;236:407.

211. Doig AT. Other lung diseases due to dust. *Postgraduate Med J* December 1949;XXV:639–648.

212. Wyers H. Asbestosis. *Postgraduate Med J* December 1949;25:631.

213. Smith WE. Survey of some current British and European studies of occupational tumor problems. *AMA Arch Indust Hyg Occup Med* March 1952;5(3):185 [see discussion of Dr. Paul Cartier, L'Annonciation, Oue., Canada p. 262 & Dr. Smith].

214. Cartier P. Abstract of discussion. *Arch Ind Hyg Occup Med* 1952;5:262.

215. Leicher F. Primary epithelial tumor of the peritoneum in asbestosis. *Archiv fur Gewerbepathologie und Gewerbehygiene* 1954;13:382–392.

216. Van der Schoot HCM. Asbestosis and pleural tumors. *Netherlands J Med* 1958;102(I):1125–1126.

217. Konig. Asbestosis. *Arch Gewerbvepath Gewerbehyg* 1960;18:159.

218. Keal EE. Asbestosis and abdominal neoplasms. *Lancet* 1960;II:1211.

219. Wagner JC, Sleggs CA, Marchand P. Diffuse pleural mesothelioma and asbestos exposure in the North Western Cape Province. *Brit J Ind Med* 1960;17:260.

220. Mancuso TF, Coutler EJ. Methodology in industrial health studies. The cohort approach, with special reference to an asbestos company. *Arch Environ Health* 1963;6:210.

221. Selikoff IJ, Churg J, Hammond EC. Asbestos exposure and neoplasia. *JAMA* 1964;188:22.

222. Selikoff IJ, Chrug JC, Hammond EC. Relation between exposure to asbestos and mesothelioma. *N Engl J Med* March 18, 1965;272(11):560–565.

223. McDonald AD, McDonald JC. Mesothelioma as an index of asbestos impact. In: *Banbury Report* 9, Schneiderman M, Peto R, eds. Cold Spring Harbor, NY: Cold Springs Harbor Laboratory; 1981:73.

224. Hemminki K, Li X. Time trends and occupational risk factors for pleural mesothelioma in Sweden. *JOEM* 2003;45(4):451–455.

225. Jarvholm B, Englund A, Albin M. Pleural mesothelioma in Sweden: An analysis of the incidence according to the use of asbestos. *Occup Environ Med* 1999;56:110–113.

226. Newhouse ML, Berry G. Predictions of mortality from mesothelial tumors in asbestos factory workers. *Brit J Ind Med* 1976;33:147.

227. Jones JSP, Pooley FD, Smith PG, Berry G, Sawle GW, Madeley RJ, Wignall BK, Aggarwal A. The consequences of exposure to asbestos dust in a wartime gas mask factory. *INSERM* 1980;92:637–653.

228. Hobbs MST, Woodward S, Murphy B, Musk AW, Elder JE. The incidence of pneumoconiosis, mesothelioma and other respiratory cancers in men engaged in mining and milling crocidolite in Western Australia. In: *Biological Effects of Mineral Fibers*, Vol. 2, Wagner JC, ed. Lyon, France: IARC; 1980: 615–626.

229. Sheers G, Coles RM. Mesothelioma risks in a naval dockyard. *Arch Environ Health* 1980;35(5):276–282.

230. Pinherio GA, Antao VCS, Bang KM, Atifield KM. Malignant mesothelioma surveillance: A comparison to ICD 10 mortality data with SEER incidence data in nine areas of the United States. *Int J Occup Environ Health* 2004;10(3):251–255.

231. Weill H, Hughes JM, Churg AM. Changing rends in US mesothelioma incidence. *Occup Environ Med* 2004;61:438–441.

232. Price B, Ware A. Mesothelioma trends in the United States: An update based on surveillance, epidemiology, and end results program data for 1973 through 2003. *Am J Epidemiol* 2004;159(2):107–112.

233. Magnani C, Agudo A, Gonzalez CA, et al. Multicentric study on malignant pleural mesothelioma and non-occupational exposure to asbestos. *Brit J Cancer* 2000;83(1):104.

234. Peto J, Decarli A, La Vecchia C, Levi F, Negri E. The European mesothelioma epidemic. *Brit J Cancer* 1999;79(3–4):666–672.

235. Kjellstrom T, Smartt P. Increased mesothelioma incidence in New Zealand: The asbestos cancer epidemic has started. *NZ Med J* 2000;113(1122):485–490.

236. Hemminki K, Li X. Time trends and occupational risk factors for pleural mesothelioma in Sweden. *J Occup Environ Med* 2003;45(4):456–461.

237. Hillerdal G. Mesothelioma: cases associated with non-occupational and low dose exposures. Review article on cases of mesothelioma associated with non-occupational and low levels of exposure to asbestos. *Occup Environ Med* 1999;56(8):505.

238. Leigh J, Driscoll. Malignant mesothelioma in Australia, 1945–2002. *Int J Occup Environ Health* 2003;9:206–217.

239. Steenland K, Burnet C, Lalich N, Ward E, Hurrell J. Dying for work: The magnitude of US mortality from selected causes of death associated with occupation. *Am J Ind Med* 2003;43:461.

240. Rake C, Gilham C, Hatch, J, Darnton A, Hodgson J, Peto J. Occupational, domestic and environmental mesothelioma risks in the British population: A case-control study. *Br J Cancer* March 3, 2009;100:1175–1183.

241. Peto, J, Rake C, Gilham C, Hatch J. Occupational, domestic and environmental mesothelioma risks in Britain. A case-control study. *Health and Safety Executive Research Report* 2009;696.

242. Neumann V, Gunthe S, Mulle KM, Fischer M. Malignant mesothelioma—German mesothelioma register 1987–1999. *Int Arch Occup Environ Health* 2001;74(6):383–395.

243. Suzuki Y. Pathology of human malignant mesothelioma—Preliminary analysis of 1,517 mesothelioma cases. *Ind Health* 2001;39:183–185.

244. Ariad S, Barchana M, Yukelson A, Geffen DB. A worrying increase in the incidence of mesothelioma in Israel. *Isr Med Assoc J* 2000;2(11):828–832.

245. NIOSH. Work-related lung disease surveillance report 1999, U.S. Department of Health and Human Services, Public Health Service, Centers for Disease Control and Prevention, National Institute for Occupational Safety and Health, 1999; pp. 138–139.

246. NIOSH. Work-related lung disease (WoRLD) surveillance report, CDC/NIOSH, National Institute for Occupational Safety and Health, DHHS (NIOSH) Publication No. 2008-143, September 2008.

247. Tagnon I, Blot WJ, Stroube RB, et al. Mesothelioma associated with the shipbuilding industry in coastal Virginia. *Cancer Res* 1980;40(11):3875–3879.

248. Newhouse ML, Berry G, Wagner JC, Purok ME. A study of the mortality of the female asbestos worker. *Brit J Ind Med* 1972;29:134.

249. Hammond EC, Selikoff IJ. Relation of cigarette smoking to risk of death of asbestos-associated disease among insulation workers in the United States. In: *Proceedings of the Conference on the Biological Effects of Asbestos*, Bogovuski PI, Gilson JC, Pinurell V, Wagner JC, eds. International Agency for Research on Cancer, Lyon, France, 1973: 312.

250. Selikoff IJ. Asbestos disease in the United States, 1918–1975. *Rev Franc Mal Resp* 1976;4(1):7.

251. Selikoff IJ, Seidman H. Evaluation of selection bias in a cross-sectional survey. *Am J Ind Med* 1991;20(5):615–627.

252. Talcott JA, Thurber WA, Kantor AF, Gaensler EA, Danahy JF, Antman KH, Li FP. Asbestos-associated diseases in a cohort of cigarette-filter workers. *N Engl J Med* 1989;321:1220–1223.

253. Gilson JC. Asbestos cancer: past and future hazards [Abridged]. *Proc Roy Soc Med* 1973;66:395.

254. Lieben J, Pistawka H. Mesothelioma and asbestos exposure. *Arch Environ Health* 1967;14:559.

255. Elmes PC, McCaughey WTE, Wade OL. Diffuse mesothelioma of the pleura and asbestos. *Brit Med J* 1965;I:350.

256. Newhouse ML, Thompson H. Mesothelioma of pleura and peritoneum following exposure to asbestos in the London area. *Brit J Ind Med* 1965;22:261.

257. McEwen J, Fiunlayson A, Mair A, Gibson AAM. Mesothelioma in Scotland. *Brit Med J* 1970;4:575.

258. McDonald AD, Harper A, El Attar OA, McDonald JC. Epidemiology of primary malignant mesothelial tumours in Canada. *Cancer* 1970;26:914.

259. Rubino GF, Scanetti G, Conna A, Palestro G. Epidemiology of pleural mesothelioma in northwestern Italy (Piedmont). *Brit J Ind Med* 1972;29:436.

260. Ashcroft T. Epidemiological and quantitative relationships between mesothelioma and asbestos on Tyneside. *J Clin Pathol* 1973;26:436.

261. Hain E, Dalquen P, Bohlig H, et al. Retrospective study of 150 cases of mesothelioma in Hamburg. *Int Arch Arbeitsmed* 1974;33:15.

262. Zielhuis RL, Versteeg JPJ, Planteydt HT. Pleural mesothelioma and exposure to asbestos: A retrospective case-control study in The Netherlands. *Int Arch Occup Environ Health* 1975;36:1.

263. McDonald JC, McDonald AD. The epidemiology of mesothelioma in historical context. *Fur Resp J* 1996;9(9):1932–1942.

264. Pinto C, Soffritti C, Maltoni C. Ignored occupational risks of asbestos mesothelioma. *La Medicina del Lavoro* 1995;86(5):484.

265. Dodson RF, O'Sullivan MF, Brooks DR, Bruce JR. Asbestos content of omentum and mesentery in non-occupationally exposed individuals. *Toxicol Ind Health* 2001;17(4):138–143.

266. Bonser GM, Faulds JS, Stewart MJ. Occupational cancer. *Am J Clin Pathol* 1955;25:126.

267. Enticknap JB, Smither WJ. Peritoneal tumours in asbestosis. *Brit J Ind Med* 1964;21:20.

268. Heard BE, Rogers W. The pathology of asbestosis with reference to lung function. *Thorax* 1961;16:264.

269. Frenkel M, Jager H. Mesothelioma peritonei in asbestosis pulmonuim. *Jaarb Kankeronderz Kankrtbestrijd Ned* 1961;11:99 (Translated by the Department of Health, Education, and Welfare, Division of Occupational Health in January 1964).

270. Thomson JG. Mesothelioma of pleura or peritoneum and limited basal asbestosis. *SA Med J* 1962;36:759.

271. Hourihane DB. The pathology of mesotheliomata and an analysis of their association with asbestos exposure. *Thorax* 1964;19:268.

272. Owen WG. Diffuse mesothelioma and exposure to asbestos dust in the Merseyside area. *Brit Med J* 1964;5403:214.

273. Mann RH, Grosh JL, O'Donnell WM. Mesothelioma associated with asbestosis. *Cancer* 1966;19:521.

274. O'Donnell WM, Mann RH, Grosch JL. Asbestos, an extrinsic factor in the pathogenesis of bronchogenic carcinoma and mesothelioma. *Cancer* 1966;19(4):1143 (Abstracted in the Industrial Hygiene Bulletin of May 1966).

275. Kobayashi Y, Murakami R, Ogura J, Yamamoto K, Ichikawa T, Nagasawa K, Hosone M, Kumazaki T. Primary pericardial mesothelioma: A case report. *Eur Radiol* 2001;11(11):2258–2261.

276. Churg A, Warnock ML, Bensch KG. Malignant mesothelioma arising after direct application of asbestos and fiber glass to the pericardium. *Am Rev Resp Dis* 1978;118(2):419.

277. Paterson, A., Grundy R, de Goyet J, Raafat F, Beath S, McCarthy A. Congenital malignant peritoneal mesothelioma. *Pediat Radiol* 2002;33(1):73–74.

278. NIOSH. Exposure to asbestiform compounds. Unpublished provisional data as of 7/1/90. National Occupational Exposure survey (1981–1983), National Institute for Occupational Safety and Health. Cincinnati, OH: U.S. Department of Health and Human Services, Public Health Service, Centers for Disease Control. February 27, 1991.

279. Lloyd JW. Asbestos: Asbestos exposure during servicing of motor vehicle brake and clutch assemblies. *Curr Intell Bull* August 8, 1975:5.

280. Nicholson WJ, Pirkel G, Selikoff IJ. Occupational exposure to asbestos: Population at risk and projected mortality—1980–2030. *Am J Ind Med* 1982;3:259–311.

281. Reitze WB, Nicholson WJ, Holaday DA, Selikoff IJ. Application of sprayed inorganic fiber containing asbestos: occupational health hazards. *Am Ind Hyg Assoc J* 1972;33:179–191.

282. Cook PM, Olson GF. Ingested mineral fibers: Elimination in human urine. *Science* 1979;204:195.

283. Bohlig H, Hain E. Cancer in relation to environmental exposure, *Biological Effects of Asbestos*, IARC Scientific Publication; 1973;8:217–221.

284. Nicholson WJ. The comparative mortality experience of three cohorts of asbestos workers. *Proceedings of the 18th International Congress Occupational Health*, Abstract; 55, 1975.

285. Anderson HA, Lilis R, Daum SM, Selikoff IJ. Household-contact asbestos neoplastic risk. *Ann NY Acad Sci* 1876;271:311.

286. NIOSH. Report to Congress on Workers' Home Contamination Study conducted under the Workers' Family Protection Act (29 U.S.C. 671a). National Institute for Occupational Safety and Health. Cincinnati, Ohio: U.S. Department of Health and Human Services, Public Health Service, Centers for Disease Control and Prevention; September, 1995.

287. Rohl AN, Langer AM, Selikoff IJ. Exposure to asbestos in the use of consumer spackling, patching and taping compounds. *Science* 1975;189(4202):551.

288. Glickman LT, Domanski LM, Maguire TG, Dubielzig RR, Churg A. Mesothelioma in pet dogs associated with exposure of their owners to asbestos. *Environ Res* 1983;32:305–313.

289. Pancoast HK, Miller TG, Laudin HRM. A roentgenologic study of the effects of dust inhalation upon the lunge. *Am J Roentgenol* 1918;5:129.

290. HMSO. Memorandum on the industrial disease of silicosis and asbestosis, His Majesty's Stationary Office, July, 1932.

291. American Railway Association. *Proceedings of the 13th Annual Meeting of the Medical and Surgical Section*. Stevens Hotel, Chicago, IL, June 26–27, 1933; 72.

292. Association of American Railroads. *Proceedings of the 15th Annual Meeting of the Medical and Surgical Section*. Chalfonte-Haddon Hall, Atlantic City, NJ, June 10–11, 1935; 89.

293. Ellman P. Pulmonary asbestosis: Its clinical, radiological, and pathological features, and associated risk of tuberculosis infection. *J Ind Hyg* 1933;XV(4):165.

294. Mayer E, Kaltreider NL, Pendergrass EP, Princi F, Sander OA, Vorwald AJ, Wright GW, Hames LN. The pneumoconioses. *Arch Environ Health* 1963;7:130.

295. Holleb HB, Angrist A. Bronchogenic carcinoma in association with pulmonary asbestosis. *Am J Pathol* 1942;18:123.

296. Selikoff IJ, Chrug J. Biological effects of asbestos. *NY Acad Sci* 1965;132:1–766.

297. Selikoff IJ, Hammond EC, Churg J. Mortality experience of asbestos-related workers, 1943–1968. In: *Pneumoconiosis*, Shapiro HA, ed. Johannesburg: Oxford University Press; 1970.

298. Dohner VA, Beegle RG, Miller WT. Asbestos exposure and multiple primary tumors. *Am Rev Resp Dis* 1975;112:181.

299. Wagoner JK, Johnson WM, Lernen RA. Malignant and nonmalignant respiratory disease mortality patterns among asbestos production workers. In: *Congressional Record-Senate Proceedings and Debates of the 93rd Congress*, First Session, 199, part 6, U.S. Government Printing Office, Washington, DC, S-4660, 1973.

300. Robinson CF, Lemen RA, Wagoner JK. Mortality patterns, 1940–1975 among workers employed in an asbestos textile friction and packing products manufacturing facilities. In: *Dust and Disease*, Lernen RA, Dement JM, eds. Park Forest, IL: Pathotox Publishers; 1979: 131.

301. Straif K, Benbrahim-Tallaa L, Baan R, et al. Special Report: Policy. A review of human carcinogens-Part C: metals, arsenic, dusts, and fibres. International Agency for Research on Cancer, WHO, www.thelancet.com/oncology; 10, May, 2009.

302. Parkes WR. Asbestos-related disorders. *Brit J Dis Chest* 1973;67:261.

303. Acheson ED, Gardner MJ. *Asbestos: The Control Limit for Asbestos*. Prepared for the U.K. Health and Safety Commission, HMSO, London, 1983.

304. Doll R, Peto J. *Asbestos—Effects on Health of Exposure to Asbestos*. London: HMSO; 1985.

305. MacLure M. Asbestos and renal adenocarcinoma: A case-control study. *Environ Res* 1987;42:353.

306. Selikoff IJ, Lilis R, Nicholson WJ. Asbestos disease in United States shipyards. *Ann NY Acad Sci* 1979;330:295–311.

307. Raffn E, Korsgaard B. Asbestos exposure and carcinoma of the penis. *Lancet* 1987;11:1394.

308. Bravo MP, Rey-Calero JD, Conde M. Bladder cancer and asbestos in Spain. *Rev Epidemiol* 1988;36:10.

309. Doniach I, Swettenhau KV, Hathorn MKS. Prevalence of asbestos bodies in a necropsy series in East London: association with disease, occupation and domiciliary address. *Brit J Ind Med* 1975;32:16.

310. Kagen E, Solomon A, Cochrame JC, et al. Immunological studies of patients with asbestosis. I. Studies of the cell-mediated immunity. *Clin Exp Immunol* 1977;18:261.

311. Gerber MA. Asbestosis and neoplastic disorders of the hematopoietic systems. *Am J Clin Pathol* 1970;53:204.

312. Kishimoto T, Okada K, Sato T, et al. Evaluation of double cancers of the lung and stomach. *Gan No Rinsho* 1988;34(11):1565.

313. Meiklejohn A. Silicosis and other fibrotic pneumoconiosis. In: *Industrial Medicine and Hygiene*, Vol 3, Merewether ERA, ed. London: Butterworth & Co. Publishers Ltd.; 1956: Chapter 1.

314. Holmes H. *The Secret Life of Dust—From the Cosmos to the Kitchen Counter, the Big Consequence of Little Things*. Hoboken, NJ: John Wiley & Sons Inc.; 2001.

315. Merewether ERA. Dusts and the lungs with particular reference to silicosis and asbestosis. *The Medical Press & Circular Supplement*, 1938: xi–xvii.

316. Cook WA. The occupational disease hazard. *Ind Med* 1942;11(4):193.
317. Hemeon WCL. Sight-perception dust scale—Tables 1–8, *Plant and Process Ventilation*. New York: The Industrial Press; 1955: 15.
318. Oliver T. *Dangerous Trades*. EP Dutton and Co., New York and John Murray, London; 1902.
319. The Chief Inspector of Factories, 1910. *Annual Report for the Year 1910*. London, England: HM Stationery Office; 1911.
320. Willson F. The very least an employer should know about dust and fume diseases. *Safety Eng* 1931; LXII(5):317–318.
321. Bloomfield JJ, Dallavalle JM. The determination and control of industrial dust. *Pub Health Bull* 1935;217.
322. Selikoff IJ, Greenberg M. A landmark case in asbestosis. *JAMA* 1991;265(7):898.
323. Fleischer WE, Viles FJ, Gade RL, Drinker P. A health survey of pipe covering operations in constructing Navy vessels. *J Ind Hyg Tox* 1946;28(1):9–16.
324. Leathart GI, Sanderson JT. Some observations on asbestosis. *Ann Occup Hyg* 1963;6:63.
325. Marr W. Survey of William Marr, Chief industrial hygienist at the Long Beach Naval Shipyards, T/P Exhib 146, Glover v. Johns-Manville Corp. v. United States of America, 1964.
326. Selikoff IJ, Churg J, Hammond EC. The occurrence of asbestosis among asbestos insulation workers. *Ann NY Acad Sci* 1965;132:139.
327. Balzer JL, Cooper WC. The work environment of insulating workers. *Am J Ind Hyg* 1968;29(3):222–227.
328. Dodson RF, Mark AL, Atkinson AL, O'Sullivan M. Stability of ferruginous bodies in human lung tissue following death, embalmment, and burial. *Inh Tox* 2005;17L:789–795.
329. Dement JM. Carcinogenicity of asbestos—Differences by fiber type? *Proceedings of the 2001 Asbestos Health Effects Conference*. Oakland, CA: U.S. Environmental Protection Agency, May 24–25, 2001.
330. Tossavainen A, Riala R, Kamppl R, et al. Dust Measurements in the Chrysotile Mining and Milling Operations of Uralasbest Company, Asbest, Russia, Finnish Institute of Occupational Health, Finland, National Institute for Occupational Safety and Health, Morgantown, USA, Russian Academy of Medical Sciences, Institute of Occupational Health, Moscow, Russia and Medical Research Center for Prophylactic and Health Protection of Industrial Workers, Ekaterinburg, Russia, Helsinki, 1996.
331. Suzuki Y, Kolynema N. Translocation of inhaled asbestos fibers from the lung to other tissues. *Am J Ind Med* 1991;19:701–704.
332. Suzuki Y, Yuen SR, Asbestos fibers contributing to the induction of human malignant mesothelioma. *Ann N Y Acad Sci* 2002;982:160–176.
333. Stayner LT, Dankovic DA, Lernen RA. Occupational exposure to chrysotile asbestos and cancer risk: A review of the amphibole hypothesis. *Am J Publ Health* 1996;86(2):179.
334. Rodelsperger K, Jockei K-H, Pohlabeln H, Romer, Woitowitz H-J. Asbestos and man-made vitreous fibers as risk factors for diffuse malignant mesothelioma: Results from a German hospital-based case-control study. *Am J Ind Med* 2001;39:262.
335. IPCS. Environmental Health Criteria 203: Chrysotile asbestos, International Program on Chemical Safety. World Health Organization; 1998: 107.
336. NIOSH. Workplace exposure to asbestos: Review and recommendations, DHHS (NIOSH) Publication 81-103. NIOSH-OSHA Asbestos Work Group, April. U.S. Department of Health and Human Services, Public Health Service, Centers for Disease Control, National Institute for Occupational Safety and Health, U.S. Department of Labor, Occupational Safety and Health Administration; 1980.
337. NIOSH. Revised recommended asbestos standard. DHEW (NIOSH) Publication 77-169, U.S. Department of Health, Education, and Welfare, Public Health Service, Centers for Disease Control, National Institute for Occupational Safety and Health; December, 1976.
338. Iwatsubo Y, Pairon JC, Boutin C, et al. Pleural mesothelioma: Dose-response relation at low levels of asbestos exposure in a French population-based case-control study. *Am J Epidemiol* 1998;1948(2):133.
339. Valic F. The asbestos dilemma: I. Assessment of risk. *Arh Hig Tada Toksikol* 2002;53:153.
340. Roach SA. Measurement of airborne asbestos dust by instruments measuring different parameters: Discussion. *Ann N Y Acad Sci* 1965;132(1):336.
341. DOL. Title 29, Labor. *Federal Register*, 25, No. 36; 1543, Saturday, February 20, Washington, Part II, 1960.
342. Cooper WC. Asbestos as a hazard to health—Fact and speculation. *Am Acad Occup Med Arch Environ Health* 1967;15:285.

343. Lane RE. Hygiene standards for chrysotile asbestos dust. *Ann Occup Hyg* 1968;2(2):47.

344. Ayer HE, Lynch JR, Fanney JH. A Comparison of impinger and membrane filter techniques for evaluating air samples in asbestos plants. *Ann N Y Acad Sci* 1965;132(Article 1):274–287.

345. Peck AS, Serocki JJ. Airborne asbestos measurement: Preliminary findings, identify a new source of variability in the membrane filter method. *Am Ind Hyg Assoc J* 1985;46(3):B14–B16.

346. Loomis D, Dement JM, Wolf SH, Richardson DB. Lung cancer mortality and fiber exposures among north carolina asbestos textile workers. *Occup Environ Med* doi:10.1136/oem.2008.044362 published online March 11, 2009.

347. Dodson RF, Atkinson MAL. Measurements of asbestos burden in tissues. *Ann N Y Acad Sci* 2006;1076:281–291.

348. Stanton MF, Wrench C. Mechanisms of mesothelioma induction with asbestos and fibrous glass. *J Natl Cancer Inst* 1972;48:797.

349. Stanton MF, Laynard M, Tegeris A, et al. Relation of particle dimension to carcinogenicity in amphibole asbestoses and other fibrous minerals. *JNCI* 1981;67(5):965.

350. Greenberg M, Fibers S. *Am J Indust Med* 1984;5:421–422 [personal correspondence from Dr. Morris Greenberg, 23 May 2003].

351. Wagner JC, ed. *Biological Effects of Mineral Fibres, International Agency for Research on Cancer*, World Health Organization, IARC Scientific Publications 30 and INSERM Symposia Series Volume 92, Lyon, France, Vols. 1 and 2, 1980.

352. Wylie AG, Virta RL, Segreti JM. Characterization of mineral population by index particle: Implication for the Stanton hypothesis. *Environ Res* 1987;43:427–439.

353. Dement JM, Wallingford KM. Comparison of phase contrast and electron microscopic methods for evaluation of occupational asbestos exposures. *Appl Occup Environ Hyg* 1990;5:242.

354. Sebastien P, Janson K, Gaudichet A, Hirsch A, Bignon J. Asbestos retention in human respiratory tissues comparative measurements in lung parenchyma and in parietal pleura. In: *Biological Effects of Mineral Fibres*, Vol. 1, Wagner JC, ed. World Health Organization, International Agency for Research on Cancer, IARC Scientific Publications No. 30; 1980: 237–246.

355. Oberdorster G. Fiber characteristics, environmental and host factors as determinants of asbestos toxicity. *Proceedings of the 2001 Asbestos Health Effects Conference*, U.S. Environmental Protection Agency, May 24–25, Oakland, CA; 2001.

356. Dement JM, Brown DP. Cohort mortality and case control studies of white male chrysotile asbestos textile workers. *J Occup Med Toxic* 1993;2(4):355.

357. Fubini B. The physical and chemical properties of asbestos fibers which contribute to biological activity. *Proceedings of the 2001 Asbestos Health Effects Conference*, U.S. Environmental Protection Agency, May 24–25, Oakland, CA; 2001.

358. Boffetta P. Health effects of asbestos exposure in humans: A quantitative assessment. *Med Lav* 1998;89(6):4714.

359. Bignon J, Monchaux G, Sebastien P, Hirsch A, Lafuma J. Human and experimental data on translocation of asbestos fibers through the respiratory system. *Ann N Y Acad Sci* 1979;330:745–750.

360. Richmond CR. Plutonium-health implications for man. The importance of non-uniform dose-distribution in an organ. *Health Phys* 1975;29(4):525–537.

361. Yeager H, Jr., Russo DA, Yanez M, Gerardi D, Nolan RP, Kagan E, Langer AM. Cytotoxicity of a short-fiber chrysotile asbestos for human alveolar macrophages: Preliminary observations. *Environ Res* 1983;30(1):224–232.

362. Dodson RF, Atkinson MAL, Levin JL. Asbestos fiber length as related to potential pathogenicity: A critical review. *Am J Ind Med* 2003;44:291.

363. ERG. Report on the peer consultation workshop to discuss a proposed protocol to assess asbestos-related risk, Eastern Research Group Inc., Prepared for: USEPA, Contract 68-C-98-148, work assignment 2003-05. Final Report, May 30, 2003.

364. Sappington CO. Preface, *Essentials of Industrial Health*. Philadelphia, J.B. Lippincott Company; 1943.

365. ACGIH. Proceedings of the Eighth Annual Meeting of the American Conference of Governmental Industrial Hygienists (ACGIH), Cincinnati, OH; April 7–13, 1946.

366. DOL. Safety and health standards for contractor performing federal contracts under the Walsh-Healey public contract, US Department of Labor; 1952.

367. DOL. *Federal Register*: 4025, March 27, 1964.

368. DOL. *Federal Register.* 14041, October 10, 1967.
369. ACGIH. Asbestos—All Forms, Supplemental documentation of threshold limit values—Appendix D. *Transactions of the 30th Annual Meeting of the American Conference of Governmental Industrial Hygienists*, St. Louis, Missouri, May 12–14, 1968: 188–191.
370. DOL. Title 41—Public contracts and property management, chap. 50—public contracts, Department of Labor, *Federal Register*, 34(96), Tuesday, May 20, 1969.
371. ACGIH. Documentation of the threshold limit values for substances in workroom air, Third Edition. *American Conference of Governmental Industrial Hygienists*; 1971: 17–19.
372. OSHA. *Occupational Safety and Health Act of 1970*, Public Law 91-596, 91st Congress, S-2193, December 29, 1970.
373. OSHA. Title 29—Labor, Ch. XVII—Occupational Safety and Health Administration, Department of Labor. Part 1910—Occupational Safety and Health Standards. *Federal Register*, 36(105), Saturday, May 29, 1971.
374. NIOSH. Criteria for a recommended standard ... Occupational Exposure to Asbestos. National Institute for Occupational Safety and Health. HSM 7 10267, second printing. U.S. Department of Health, Education, and Welfare, Public Health Service, Center for Disease Control, 1972.
375. OSHA. Standard for exposure to asbestos dust. *Federal Register* 1972:37(110):11318–11322.
376. OSHA. Occupational exposure to asbestos. Notice of proposed rulemaking, Occupational Safety and Health Administration, Part II. Department of Labor, October 9, 1975.
377. NIOSH. Revised Recommended Asbestos Standard DHEW (NIOSH) Publication 77169. U.S. Department of Health, Education, and Welfare, Public Health Service. Centers for Disease Control. National Institute for Occupational Safety and Health, 1976.
378. NIOSH/OSHA. Workplace exposure to asbestos: review and recommendations, DHHS (NIOSH) Publication 81-103, NIOSH-OSHA Asbestos Work Group, U.S. Department of Health and Human Services, Public Health Service, Centers for Disease Control, National Institute for Occupational Safety and Health, U.S. Department of Labor, Occupational Safety and Health Administration, 1980.
379. OSHA. Asbestos: emergency temporary standard (ETS) 48 FR 51085, U.S. Department of Labor, Occupational Safety and Health Administration, Washington, DC, November 4, 1983.
380. OSHA. Occupational exposure to asbestos. Regulatory history, 29 CFR Parts 1910, 1915, and 1926. RIN: 1218-AB25, Department of Labor. 59:40964-41162, 2009.
381. OSHA. Final rule: asbestos. 51 FR 22612. U.S. Department of Labor, Occupational Safety and Health Administration, Washington, DC, June 20, 1986.
382. OSHA. Occupational exposure to asbestos, tremolite, anthophyllite, and actinolite—Final rules; amendment. *Federal Register* 1988;53(178):35610–35629.
383. OSHA. Occupational exposure to asbestos, tremolite, anthophyllite and actinolite, Department of Labor Occupational Safety and Health Administration, 29 CFR Parts 1910 and 1926 [Docket Number H-033-d], 1992.
384. NIOSH. Comments to the docket number H-033-d, occupational exposure to asbestos, tremolite, anthophyllite and actinolite, Department of Labor Occupational Safety and Health Administration, 29 CFR Parts 1910 and 1926, National Institute for Occupational Safety and Health, CDC, USPHS, Department of Health and Human Services, 1992.
385. OSHA. Occupational exposure to asbestos—Final rule. *Federal Register* 1994;59(153):40964–41158.
386. OSHA. 2004. www.OSHA.gov.
387. Peto J. Fibre carcinogenesis and environmental hazards, in *Non-occupational Exposure to Mineral Fibres*, Bignon J, Peto J, and Saracci R, Eds., Lyon, France, International Agency for Research on Cancer, IARC Scientific Publications 90, 457–470, 1989.
388. Brownson RC, Alavanja MC, Chang JC. Occupational risk factors for lung cancer among nonsmoking women: A case-control study in Missouri (United States). *Cancer Causes Control* September 1993;4(5):449–454.
389. Jarvholm B, Larsson S, Hagberg S, Olling S, Ryd W, Toren K. Quantitative importance of asbestos as a cause of lung cancer in a Swedish industrial city: A case-referent study. *Eur Respir J* 1993;6(9):1271–1275.
390. van Loon AJM, Kant IJ, Swaen GMH, Goldbohm RA, Kremer AM, van den Brandt PA. Occupational exposure to carcinogens and risk of lung cancer: Results from the Netherlands cohort study. *Occup Environ Med* November 1997;54(11):817–824.

391. Jockel KH, Ahrens W, Jahn I, Pohlabeln H, Bolm-Audorff U. Occupational risk factors for lung cancer: A case-control study in West Germany. *Int J Epidemiol* August 1998;27(4):549–560.

392. Camus M, Siemiatycki J, Meek B. Nonoccupational exposure to chrysotile asbestos and the risk of lung cancer. *N Engl J Med* 1998;333(22):1585–1571.

393. WHO. Occupational exposure limit for asbestos, WHO/OCH/89.1, Office of Occupational Health, Word Health Organization, Geneva, 1989.

394. Addingley CG. Discussion. *Ann N Y Acad Sci* 1965;132:335.

395. Wells J. Discussion. *Ann N Y Acad Sci* 1965;132:335.

396. Selikoff IJ, Hammond EC, Churg J. Asbestos exposure, smoking and neoplasia. *JAMA* 1968;204:706.

397. Berry G, Newhouse ML, Turok M. Combined effect of asbestos exposure and smoking on mortality from lung cancer in factory workers. *Lancet* 1972;ii:476.

398. Weiss W. Cigarette smoking, asbestos and pulmonary fibrosis. *Am Rev Resp Dis* 1971;104:223.

399. Terry LL. Smoking and health: Report of the advisory committee to the Surgeon General of the Public Health Service. U.S. Department of Health, Education, and Welfare, Public Health Service Publication No. 1103, 1964.

400. Breslow L, Honglin L, Rasmussen G, Abrams HK. Occupations and cigarette smoking as factors in lung cancer. *Am J Publ Health* 1954;44:171–181.

401. Owen WG. Mesothelial tumors and exposure to asbestos dust. *Ann N Y Acad Sci* 1965;132:674.

402. Oels HC, Harrison Jr, EG, Carr DT, Bernatz PE. Diffuse malignant mesothelioma of the pleura: A review of 37 cases. *Chest* 1971;60(6):564–570.

403. Hasan FM, Nash G, Kazemi H. The significance of asbestos exposure in the diagnosis of mesothelioma: A 28-year experience from a major urban hospital. *Am Rev Resp Dis* 1977;115:761–768.

404. Sheers G, Coles RM. Mesothelioma risks in a Naval dockyard. *Arch Environ Health* September/October 1980;35(5):276–282.

405. Yeung P, Rogers A. An occupation-industry matrix analysis of mesothelioma cases in Australia 1980–1985. *Appl Occup Environ Hyg* 2001;16(1):40.

406. Anton-Culver H, Culver BD. An epidemiologic study of asbestos-related chest x-ray changes to identify work areas of high risk in a shipyard population. *Appl Ind Hyg* 1989;4(5):110.

407. Hessel PA, Melenka LS, Michaelchuk D, Herbert FA, Cowie RL. Lung health among plumbers and pipefitters in Edmonton, Alberta. *Occup Environ Med* 1998;55(10):678.

408. Vineis P, Ciccone G, Magnino A. Asbestos exposure, physical activity and colon cancer: A case-control study. *Tumori* 1993;79(5):301.

409. Demers RY, Neale AV, Robins T, Herman SC. Asbestos-related pulmonary disease in boilermakers. *Am J Ind Med* 1990;17(3):327.

410. Divine BJ, Hartman CM, Wendt JK. Update of the Texaco mortality study 1947–93: Part II, Analyses of specific causes of death for white men employed in refining, research, and petrochemicals. *Occup Environ Med* 2000;57(2):143.

411. Syamlal G, Bang KM, Wood JM. National trends in asbestosis mortality, 1990–1999. APHA 131st Annual Meeting and Exposition. San Francisco, CA: American Public Health Association, November 1, 2003.

412. Bang KM, Pinheiro GA, Wood JM. Mortality trends in malignant neoplasm of the pleura—United States, 1979–1998. *Am J Epidemiol* 2004 June;159(11)(Suppl):S78.

413. Ascoli V, Calisti R, Carnovale-Scalzo C, Nardi F. Malignant pleural mesothelioma in bakers and pastry cooks. *Am J Ind Med* 2001;40(4):371.

414. Greenburg M, Lloyd Davies TA. Mesothelioma register 1967–68. *Brit J Ind Med* 1974;31:91–104.

415. Bianchi C, Brollo A, Ramani L, Bianchi T, Giarelli L. Asbestos exposure in malignant mesothelioma of the pleura: a survey of 557 cases. *Ind Health* 2001;39(2):161–167.

416. Langer AM, McCaughey WTE. Mesothelioma in a brake repair worker. *Lancet* 1982;2:1101.

417. Ziem G. Three case reports of mesothelioma in brake mechanics. In: *Asbestos: Medical and Legal Aspects*, Castleman B, ed. New York, NY: Harcourt Brace Jovanovich; 1984.

418. EPA, Yorkshire Television. "Alice: A Fight for Life." July 14, 1982. Mesothelioma in a 10-year-old son of brake mechanic described and filmed, in guidance for preventing asbestos disease among auto mechanics, U.S. Environmental Protection Agency, EPA-560-OPTS-86-002, June, 1986.

419. Huncharek M, Muscat J, Capotorto JV. Pleural mesothelioma in a brake mechanic. *Brit J Ind Med* 1989;46:69–71.

420. Rohl AN, Langer AM, Wolff MS, Weisman I. Asbestos exposure during brake lining maintenance and repair. *Environ Res* 1976;12:110–126.

421. Vianna NJ, Polan AK. Non-occupational exposure to asbestos and malignant mesothelioma in females. *Lancet* 1978;1(8073):1061–1063.

422. Godwin MC, Jagatic G. Asbestos and mesothelioma. *JAMA* 1968;204(11):151.

423. Faigout DA. Environmental release of asbestos from commercial product shaping. Project summary, EPA/600/S2-85/044, Environmental Protection Agency, August 1985.

424. Paustenbach DJ, Richter RO, Finley BL, Sheehan P. An evaluation of the historical exposures of mechanics to asbestos in brake dust. *App Occup Environ Hyg* 2003;18:786–804.

425. Rushton L, Alderson MR, Nagarajah CR. Epidemiological survey of maintenance workers in London transport executive bus garages and Chiswick works. *Brit J Ind Med* 1983;40:340–345.

426. Teta MJ, Lewinsohn HC, Meigs JW, Vidone RA, Mowad LZ, Flannery JT. Mesothelioma in Connecticut, 1955–1977. Occupational and geographic associations. *J Occup Med* 1983;25(10):749.

427. Rodelsperger K, Jahn H, Bruckel B, Manke J, Paur R, Woitowitz HJ. Asbestos dust exposure during brake repair. *Am J Ind Med* 1986;10(1):63.

428. Wong O. Chrysotile asbestos, mesothelioma and garage mechanics—Letter to the editor. *Am J Ind Med* 1992;21:449.

429. Jarvholm B, Brisman J. Asbestos associated tumours in car mechanics. *Brit J Ind Med* 1988;45:645.

430. Hansen ES. Mortality of auto mechanics. *Scand J Work Environ Health* 1989;15:43–46.

431. Spirtas R, Heineman EF, Bernstein L, et al. Malignant mesothelioma: Attributable risk of asbestos exposure. *Occup Environ Med* 1994;51:804.

432. Woitowitz HJ, Rodelsperger K. Mesothelioma among car mechanics. *Ann Occup Hyg* 1994;38(4):635.

433. Teschke K, Morgan MS, Checkoway H, Franklin G, Spinelli JJ, van Belle G, Weiss NS. Mesothelioma surveillance to locate sources of exposure to asbestos. *Can J Publ Health* 1997;88(3):163.

434. Henderson DW. Friction products (e.g., brake linings), World Trade Organization—WT/DS135/R, 300, 2001.

435. Lemen RA. Asbestos in brakes: exposure and risk of disease. *Am J Ind Med* 2004;45:229–237.

436. Butnor KJ, Sporn TA, Roggli VL. Exposure to brake dust and malignant mesothelioma: A study of 10 cases with mineral fiber analyses. *Ann Occup Hyg* June 2003;47(4):325–330.

437. Roggli VL, Sharma A, Butnor KJ, Sporn T, Vollmer RT. Malignant mesothelioma and occupational exposure to asbestos: a clinicopathological correlation of 1445 cases. *Ultrastruct Pathol* 2002;26:55–65.

438. Finkelstein MM. Asbestos fibre concentrations in the lungs of brake workers: Another look. *Ann Occup Hyg* 2008;52:455–461; doi:10.1093/annhyg/men036: 1-7.

439. Finkelstein MM, Dufresne A. Inferences on the kinetics of asbestos deposition and clearance among chrysotile miners and millers. *AJIM* April 1999;35(4):401–412.

440. Hessel PA, Teta MJ, Goodman M, Lau E. Mesothelioma among brake mechanics: An expanded analysis of a case-control study. *Risk Anal* 2004;24(3):547–552.

441. Finley BL, Richter RO, Mowat FS, Mlynarek S, Paustenbach DJ, Warmerdam JM, Sheehan PJ. Cumulative asbestos exposure for US automobile mechanics involved in brake repair (circa 1950s–2000). *J Exp Sci Environ Epi* 2007;17:644–655; doi:l0.l038/sj.jes.7500553: 1–12.

442. Cohen HJ, Van Orden DR. Asbestos exposures of mechanics performing clutch service on motor vehicles. *J Occup Environ Hyg* March 2008;5(3):148–156.

443. Jiang GC, Madl AK, Ingmundson KJ, Murbach DM, Fehling KA, Paustenbach DJ, Finley BL. A study of airborne chrysotile concentrations associated with handling, unpacking, and repacking boxes of automobile clutch discs. *Regul Toxicol Pharmacol* June 2008;51(1):87–97. Epub March 18, 2008.

444. Madl AK, Scott LL, Murbach DM, Fehling KA, Finley BL, Paustenbach DJ. Exposure to chrysotile asbestos associated with unpacking and repacking boxes of automobile brake pads and shoes. *Ann Occup Hyg* August 2008;52(6):463–479. Epub May 31, 2008.

445. Blake CL, Van Orden DR, Banasik M, Harbison RD. Airborne asbestos concentration from brake changing does not exceed permissible exposure limit. *Regul Toxicol Pharmacol* August 2003;38(1):58–70.

446. Lorimer WV, Rohl AN, Miller A, Nicholson WJ, Selikoff IJ. Asbestos exposure of brake repair workers in the United States. *Mt Sinai J Med* 1976;43:207–218.

447. Atkinson MAL, Dodson RF. Response to letter from Paustenbach et al. *AJIM* 2006;49:62–64.

448. Nicholson WJ. Estimates of occupational mortality from past and projected exposure to asbestos. *Proceedings of the World Symposium on Asbestos*. Canadian Asbestos Information Centre, Montreal, Quebec, Canada: 136–149, May 25, 26, 27, 1982.

449. Wang E, Dement JM, Lipscomb H. Mortality among North Carolina construction workers, 1988–1994. *Appl Occup Environ Hyg* 1999;14(1):45.

450. Salg J, Alterman T. A proportionate mortality of bricklayers and allied craftsmen (IUBAC) 1986–1991. *Am J Ind Med* January 2005;47(1):10–19.

451. McDonald JC, Edwards CW, Gibbs AR, Lloyd HM, Pooley FD, Ross DJ, Rudd RM. Case-referent survey of young adults with mesothelioma: II. Occupational analyses. *Ann Occup Hyg* 2001;45(7):519.

452. Yeung P, Rogers A, Johnson A. Distribution of mesothelioma cases in different occupational groups and industries in Australia, 1979–1995. *Appl Occup Environ Hyg* 1999;14(11):759.

453. Leigh J, Driscoll T. Malignant mesothelioma in Australia, 1945-2002. *Int J Occup Environ Health* 2003;9:206–217.

454. Robinson CF, Petersen M, Sieber WK, Palu S, Halperin WE. Mortality of Carpenters' Union members employed in the U.S. construction or wood products industries, 1987–1990. *Am J Ind Med* 1996;30(6):674.

455. Garcia-Closas M, Christiani DC. Asbestos-related diseases in construction carpenters. *Am J Ind Med* 1995;27(1):115.

456. O'Reilly D, Reid J, Middleton R, Gavin AT. Asbestos-related mortality in Northern Ireland: 1985–1994. *J Public Health Med* 1999;21(1):95.

457. Stern F, Schulte P, Sweeney MH, Fingerhut M, Vossenas P, Burkhardt G, Kornak MF. Proportionate mortality among construction laborers. *Am J Ind Med* 1995;27(4):485.

458. Anderson HA, Hanrahan LP, Higgins DN, Sarow PG. A radiographie survey of public school building maintenance and custodial employees. *Environ Res* 1992;59(1):159.

459. Churg A, Warnock ML. Analysis of the cores of asbestos bodies from members of the general population: patients with probable low-degree exposure to asbestos. *Am Rev Resp Dis* 1979;120(4):781.

460. Levin SM, Selikoff IJ. Radiological abnormalities and asbestos exposure among custodians of the New York City Board of Education. *Ann N Y Acad Sci* 1991;643:530.

461. Balmes JR, Daponte A, Cone JE. Asbestos-related disease in custodial and building maintenance workers from a large municipal school district. *Ann N Y Acad Sci* 1991;643:540.

462. Oliver LC, Sprince NL, Greene R. Asbestos-related disease in public school custodians. *Am J Ind Med* 1991;19(3):303–316.

463. Matrat M, Pairon JC, Paolillo AG, Joly N, Iwatsubo Y, Orlowski E, Letourneux M, Ameille J. Asbestos exposure and radiological abnormalities among maintenance and custodian workers in buildings with friable asbestos-containing materials. *Int Arch Occup Environ Health* 2004;77(5):307–312.

464. Schneider J, Rodelsperger K, Bruckel B, Kleineberg J, Woitowitz H-J. Pleural mesothelioma associated with indoor pollution of asbestos. *J Cancer Res Clin Oncol* 2001;127:123.

465. Bunn R. Duty deadline. *Health and Safety at Work* July 2003;25(7):21.

466. Selikoff IJ, Hammond EC. Asbestos-associated disease in United States shipyards. *CA Cancer J Clin* March/April 1978;28(2):87–99.

467. Newhouse ML, Oakes D, Woolley AJ. Mortality of welders and other craftsmen at a shipyard in NE England. *Br J Ind Med* June 1985;42(6):406–410.

468. Coggon D, Pannett B, Osmond C, Acheson ED. A survey of cancer and occupation in young and middle aged men. I Cancers of the respiratory tract. *Br J Industr Med* 1986;43:332–338.

469. Menck HR, Henderson BE. Occupational differences in rates of lung cancer. *J Occup Med* December 1976;18(12):797–801.

470. Paik NW, Walcott RJ, Brogan PA. Worker exposure to asbestos during removal of sprayed material and renovation activity in buildings containing sprayed material. *Am Ind Hyg Assoc J* 1983;44(6):428.

471. Malker HSR, McLaughlin JK, Malker BK, Stone BJ, Weiner JL, Ericsson LE, Blot WJ. Occupational risks for pleural mesothelioma in Sweden 1961–1979. *J Natl Cancer Inst* 1985;74:61.

472. Hodgson MJ, Parkinson DK, Sabo S, Owens GR, Feist JH. Asbestosis among electricians. *J Occup Med* 1988;30(8):638.

473. Kilburn KH, Warshaw RH. Asbestos disease in construction, refinery, and shipyard workers. *Ann N Y Acad Sci* December 31, 1991;643:301–312.

474. Harries PG. Experience with asbestos disease and its control in Great Britain's naval dockyards. *Env Res* 1976;11:261–267.

475. Singh G, Whiteside TL, Dekker A. Immunodiagnosis of mesothelioma. use of antimesothelial cell serum in an indirect immunofluorescence assay. *Cancer* 1979;43:2288–2296.

476. Parrish RG, Hartle R, Groth D. HHE Report No. HETA-83-044-1596, General Electric plant, Evendale, Ohio. National Institute for Occupational Safety and Health; 1985.

477. Ciccone G, Mirabelli D, Ronco G, Troia B, Vineis P. Occupation and lung cancer in two industrialized areas of northern Italy. *Int J Cancer* 1988;41(3):354–358.

478. Anton-Culver H, Culver BD, Kurosaki T. An epidemiologic study of asbestos-related chest x-ray changes to identify work areas of high risk in a shipyard population. *Appl Ind Hyg* 1989;4(5):110–118.

479. Huncharek M, Muscat J. Pleural mesothelioma in a non-shipyard electrician. *Br J Ind Med* 1990;47(1):68.

480. Kawachi I, Glass W. Lung cancer, smoking and exposure to asbestos in New Zealand. *J Occup Health Safety Aust N Z* February 1991;7(1):43–47.

481. Morabia A, Markowitz K, Garibaldi K, Wynder EL. Lung cancer and occupation: Results of a multi-centre case-control study. *Br J Ind Med* 1992;49:721–727.

482. Maltoni C, Pinto C, Mobiglia A. Mesotheliomas due to asbestos used in railroads in Italy, in the third wave of asbestos disease: exposure to asbestos in place. *Ann N Y Acad Sci* 1991;643:347.

483. Robinson CF, Halperin WE, Alterman T, et al. Mortality patterns among construction workers in the United States. *Occ Med* 1995;10(2):269–283.

484. Gennaro V, Ceppi M, Boffetta P, Fontana V, Perrotta A. Pleural mesothelioma and asbestos exposure among Italian oil refinery workers. *Scand J Work Environ Health* 1994;20(3):213–215.

485. Peto J, Hodgson JT, Matthews FE, Jones JR. Continuing increase in mesothelioma mortality in Britain. *Lancet* March 4, 1995;545:535–539.

486. Bang KM, Wood JM, Syamlal G, Castellan RM. Recent malignant mesothelioma mortality and incidence in the United States. Presented at the 131st Annual Meeting (November 15–19) of the American Public Health Association, Thursday, November 18, Abstract #55389, 2003.

487. Nesti M, Marinaccio A, Gennaro V, et al. Epidemiologic surveillance for primary prevention of malignant mesothelioma: The Italian experience. *Med Lav* July–August 2005;96(4):338–346.

488. McElvenny DM, Darton AJ, Price MJ, Hodgson JT. Mesothelioma mortality in Great Britain from 1968 to 2001. *Occ Med* 2005;55:79–87.

489. Ohyagi S, Kagamimori S, Hillerdal G, Saitoh N, Hosoda Y, Shishido S, Iwai K. Study on prevalence of pleural plaques in miniature x-ray films in Japan and Sweden. *Ind Health* 1985;23(2):127–134.

490. Enterline PE, McKiever MF. Differential mortality from lung cancer by occupation. *J Occup Med* 1963;5(6):283–290.

491. Montomoli L, Spisso M, Romeo R, Spina D, Ghiribelli C, Sartorelli P. Work related mesothelioma: analysis of cases discovered at the Section for Occupational Medicine and Toxicology of Siena University during the years 2000–2007. *G Ital Med Lav Ergon* July–September 2007;29(3 Suppl):332–333.

492. Sullivan PA. Vermiculite, respiratory disease, and asbestos exposure in Libby, Montana: Update of a cohort mortality study. *Environ Health Perspect* April 2007;115(4):579–585.

493. Coggon D, Innkip H, Winter P, Pannett B. Differences in occupational mortality from pleural cancer, peritoneal cancer, ans asbestosis. *Occup Env Med* 1995;52:775–777.

494. Robinson CF, Petersen M, Palu S. Mortality patterns among electrical workers employed in the U.S. construction industry, 1982–1987. *AJIM* December 1999;36(6):630–637.

495. Kern DG, Frumkin H. Asbestos-related disease in the jewelry industry: report of two cases. *Am J Ind Med* 1988;13:407.

496. Kern DG, Hanley KT, Roggli VL. Malignant mesothelioma in the jewelry industry. *Am J Ind Med* 1992;21:409.

497. Dossing M, Langer SW. Asbestos-induced lung injury among Danish jewelry workers. *Am J Ind Med* 1994;26(6):755.

498. Marcus K, Jarvholm BG, Larsson S. Asbestos-associated lung effects in car mechanics. *Scand J Work Environ Health* 1987;13(3):252.

499. Dahlqvist M, Alexandersson R, Hedenstierna G. Lung function and exposure to asbestos among vehicle mechanics. *Am J Ind Med* 1992;22(1):59.

500. Jockei KH, Ahrens W, Bolm-Audorff U. Lung cancer risk and welding—Preliminary results from an ongoing case-control study. *Am J Ind Med* 1994;25(6):805.

501. Andersen A, Barlow L. Work related cancer in Nordic countries. *Scand J Work Environ Health* 1999;25(2):1–116.

502. Polland LD. The American Merchant Marine and the asbestos environment. A report by the Maritime Administration, Division of Naval Architecture, Office of Ship Construction, US Department of Commerce, 40 pp, 1979.

503. Selikoff IJ, Lilis R, Levin G. Asbestotic radiological abnormalities among United States merchant marine seamen. *Brit J Ind Med* 1990;47:292.

504. Jones RN, Diem JE, Ziskand MM, Rodregues M, Weill H. Radiographic evidence of asbestos effects in American marine engineers. *J Occup Med* 1984;26(4):281–284.

505. Greenberg. Cancer mortality in merchant seamen. *Ann N Y Acad Sci* 1991;643:321–332.

506. Varouchakis G, Velonakis EG, Amfiochiou S, Trichopoulos D. Asbestos in strange places: Two case reports of mesothelioma among merchant seamen. *Am J Ind Med* 1991;19(5):673.

507. Rapiti E, Turi E, Forastiere F, Borgia P, Comba P, Perucci CA, Axelson O. A mortality cohort study of seamen in Italy. *Am J Ind Med* 1992;21:863.

508. Hiraoka T, Watanabe A, Usuma Y, Mori T, Kohyama N, Takata A. An operated case of lung cancer with pleural plaques: its asbestos bodies, fiber analysis and asbestos exposure. *Ind Health* 2001;29:194.

509. Saarni H, Pentti J, Pukkala E. Cancer at sea: a case-control study among male Finnish seafarers. *Occup Environ Med* 2002;59:6133.

510. Rafnsson V, Sulem P. Cancer incidence among marine engineers, a population-based study (Iceland). *Cancer Causes Contr* 2003;14(1):29.

511. Bianchi C, Bianchi T, Grand G. Malignant mesothelioma of the pleura among seafarers. *Med Lav* 2005;96(6):490–495.

512. Lemen RA. Statement of Richard A. Lemen before the Subcommittee on Coast Guard and Navigation and the Committee on Merchant Marine and Fisheries of the United States House of Representatives. Shipboard Asbestos Exposure, Serial No. 96-41, 1980.

513. Murbach DM, Madl AK, Unice KM, Knutsen JS, Chapman PS, Brown JL, Paustenbach DJ. Airborne concentrations of asbestos onboard maritime shipping vessels (1978–1992). *Ann Occup Hyg* 2008;52(4):267–279.

514. Whorton MD, Schulman J, Larson SR, Stubbs HA, Austin D. Feasibility of identifying high-risk occupations through tumor registries. *J Occup Med* 1983;25(9):657–660.

515. Stockwell H. Lung cancer among painters. The School of Public Health of the Johns Hopkins University in conformity with the requirements for the degree of Doctor of Science, Baltimore, MD, 1983.

516. Kintz GM, Fowler HC. Some problems of respiratory protection in the petroleum industry, with suggestions for their solution, Information Circular, Department of the Interior—Bureau of Mines, 1936.

517. Bonsib RS. *Dust Producing Operations in the Production of Petroleum Products and Associated Activities*, Standard Oil Company, New York, NY, 1937.

518. Bonsib RS. *Safeguarding Petroleum Refineries and Their Workers*, International Labour Office, Montreal, Reprinted from the Industrial Safety Survey, Vol. XIX, No. 2, 1943.

519. Berry C, Hammond JW, Bonsib RS, Hendricks NV. Report on summary of the plant industrial hygiene problems, April 12, Medical Department, Research Section, Standard Oil Company (New Jersey), New York, 1949.

520. Kettering Laboratory. An epidemiological study of cancer among employees in the american petroleum industry, Department of Preventive Medicine and Industrial Health, College of Medicine, University of Cincinnati, Cincinnati, OH, March 1958.

521. Eisenstadt HB, Wilson FW. Primary malignant mesothelioma of the pleura. *Lancet* 1960;80:511.

522. Eisenstadt HB. Malignant mesothelioma of the pleura. *Dis Chest* November 1956;30:549–556.

523. Meyer WH, Church FW. Industrial hygiene aspects of mechanical operations in a petroleum refinery. *Med Bull* 1961;21(2):256–265 (Abstract).

524. Lilis R, Daum S, Anderson H, Andrews G, Selikoff IJ. Asbestos among maintenance workers in the chemical industry and in oil refinery workers. In: *Biological Effects of Mineral Fibres*, Wagner JC, ed. International Agency for Research on Cancer, Scientific Publication 30, INSERM symposia Series, Vol. 92, Lyon, 1980: 795–810.

525. HHE. Exxon Corporation, Bayway Refinery and Chemical Plant, Linden, NJ, HETA 81-372-1727, National Institute for Occupational Safety and Health, CDC, USPHS, Department of Health and Human Services, 1981.

526. Wong O, Raabe GK. Critical review of cancer epidemiology in petroleum industry employees, with a quantitative meta-analysis by cancer site. *Am J Ind Med* 1989;15:283–310.

527. Rosenman KD. Asbestos-related x-ray changes in refinery workers. *Ann N Y Acad Sci* 1991;643:390–396.

528. Mehlman MA. Dangerous and cancer-causing properties of products and chemicals in the oil-refining and petrochemical industries. Part IX: Asbestos exposure and analysis of exposures. *Ann N Y Acad Sci* 1991;643:368–389.

529. Mehlman MA. Diseases in workers exposed to asbestos in the oil refining and petrochemical industries. In: *The Identification and Control of Environmental and Occupational Diseases: Asbestos and Cancers*, Mehlman MA, Upton A, eds. Princeton, NJ: Princeton Scientific Publishers Co. Inc.; 1994: 189–211.

530. Honda Y, Delzell E, Cole P. An updated study of mortality among workers at a petroleum manufacturing plant. *J Occup Environ Med* 1995;37(2):194–200.

531. Collingwood KW, Raabe GK, Wong O. An updated cohort mortality study of workers at a northeastern United States petroleum refinery. *Int Arch Occup Environ Health* 1996;68(5):277–288.

532. Finkelstein MM. Asbestos-associated cancers in the Ontario refinery and petrochemical sector. *Am J Ind Med* 1996;30(5):610–615.

533. Finkelstein M. Mesothelioma in oil refinery workers. *Scand J Work Environ Health* 1996;22(1):67.

534. Imbernon E, Goldberg M, Bonenfant S, Chevalier A, Guenel P, Vatre R, Dehaye J. Occupational respiratory cancer and exposure to asbestos: a case-control study in a cohort of workers in the electricity and gas industry. *Am J Ind Med* 1995;28(3):33.

535. Tsai SP, Waddell LC, Gilstrap EL, Ransdell JD, Ross CE. Mortality among maintenance employees potentially exposed to asbestos in a refinery and petrochemical plant. *Am J Ind Med* 1996;29(1):89–98.

536. Tsai SP, Gilstrap EL, Cowles SR, Snyder PJ, Ross CE. Long-term follow-up mortality study of petroleum refinery and chemical plant employees. *Am J Ind Med* 1996;29(1):75–87.

537. Dement JM, Hensley L, Kieding S, Lipscomb H. Proportionate mortality among union members employed at three Texas refineries. *Am J Ind Med* 1998;33:327–340.

538. Gennaro V, Finkelstein MM, Ceppi M, et al. Mesothelioma and lung tumors attributable to asbestos among petroleum workers. *Am J Ind Med* 2000;37:275–282.

539. Schnatter AR, Theriault G, Katz AM, et al. a retrospective mortality study within operating segments of a petroleum company. *Am J Ind Med* 1992;22:209.

540. Lewis R, Schnatter AR, Katz AM, et al. Updated mortality among diverse operating segments of a petroleum company. *Occup Environ Med* 2000;57:595.

541. Satin KP, Bailey WJ, Newton KL, Ross AY, Wong O. Updated epidemiological study of workers at two California petroleum refineries, 1950–1995. *Occup Environ Med* 2002;59:248.

542. Parodi S, Montanaro F, Ceppi M, Gennaro V. Mortality of petroleum refinery workers. *Occup Environ Med* 2003;60:304–305.

543. Monson RR. *Occupational Epidemiology*, 2nd ed. Baco Raton, FL: CRC Press; 1990.

544. Tsai SP, Wendt JK, Cardarelli KM, Fraser AE. A mortality and morbidity study of refinery and petrochemical employees in Louisiana. *Occup Environ Med* 2003;60:627.

545. NIOSH. Work-related lung disease surveillance report 2002, U.S. Department of Health and Human Services, Public Health Service, Centers for Disease Control and Prevention, National Institute for Occupational Safety and Health, 2003: 159–168.

546. Nicholson WJ, Rohl A, Fischbein SA, Selikoff IJ. Occupational and community asbestos exposure from wallboard finishing compounds. *Bull N Y Acad Med* 1975;51(10):1180.

547. Fischbein A, Langer AM, Rohl AN, Selikoff IJ. Drywall construction and asbestos exposure. *Am Ind Hyg Assoc J* 1979;40(5):402–407.

548. Verma DK, Middleton CG. Occupational exposure to asbestos in the drywall taping process. *Am Ind Hyg Assoc J* 1980;41(4): 264–269.

549. Stern F, Lehman E, Ruder A. Mortality among unionized construction plasterers and cement masons. *Am J Ind Med* 2001;39(4):373.

550. Lange JH, Thomulka KW. An evaluation of personal airborne asbestos exposure measurements during abatement of dry wall and floor tile/mastic. *Int J Environ Health Res* 2000;10:5.

551. Jockel K-H, Almerns W, Bohm-Audortt U. Lung cancer risk and welding-preliminary results from an ongoing case-control study. *AJIM* 1994;33(4):313–320.

552. Hessel PA, Melenka LS, Michaelchuk D, Herbert FA, Cowie RL. Lung health among boilermakers in Edmonton, Alberta. *Am J Ind Med* 1998;34(4):38.

553. Rosenstock L. Roentgenographic manifestations and pulmonary function effects of asbestos-induced pleural thickening. *Toxicol Ind Health* 1991;7(1–2):81.

554. Dossing M, Groth S, Vestbo J, Lyngenbo O. Small-airways dysfunction in never smoking asbestos-exposed Danish plumbers. *Int Arch Occup Environ Health* 1990;62(3):209–212.

555. Sprince NL, Oliver LC, McLoud TC. Asbestos-related disease in plumbers and pipefitters employed in building construction. *J Occup Med* 1985;27(10):771.

556. Cantor KP, Sontag JM, Heid MF. Patterns of mortality among plumbers and pipefitters. *Am J Ind Med* 1986;10(1):73.

557. Longo WE, Egeland WB, Hatfield RL, Newton LR. Riber release during the removal of asbestos-containing gaskets: A work practice simulation. *App Occ Env Hyg* 2002;17(1):55–62.

558. Davis I. A pilot investigation into the occurrence of pneumoconiosis in large power stations in South Wales. *Brit J Ind Med* 1953;10:111–113.

559. Fontaine JH, Trayer DM. Asbestos control in steam-electric generating plants. *Am Ind Hyg Assoc J* 1974;36(2):126–130.

560. Mosley CL. Health hazard evaluation determination report HE-79-136-668, Shoreham Nuclear Power Plant, Shoreham, Long Island, New York, NIOSH, CDC, USPHS, Department of Health and Human Services, Cincinnati, OH, 1980.

561. Millette JR, Mount MD. A study determining asbestos fiber release during the removal of valve packing. *Appl Occup Environ Hyg* 1993;8(9):790–793.

562. Boelter FW, Crawford GN, Podraza DM. Airborne fiber exposure assessment of dry asbestos-containing gaskets and packings found in intact industrial and maritime fittings. *Am Ind Hyg Assoc J* 2002;63(6):732–740.

563. Hirsch A, Di Menza L, Carre A, Harf A, Perdrizet S, Cooreman J, Bignon J. Asbestos risk among full-time workers in an electricity-generating power station. *Ann N Y Acad Sci* 1979;330:137.

564. Bonnell JA, Bowker JR, Browne RC, Erskine JF, Fernandez RHP, Massey PMO. A review of the control of asbestos processes in the Central Electricity Generating Board, Proceedings of the XVIII International Congress on Occupational Health, Brighton, England, 1975.

565. Cammarano G, Crosignani P, Berrino F, Berra G. Cancer mortality among workers in a thermoelectric power plant. *Scand J Work Environ Health* 1984;10(4):259.

566. Forastiere F, Pupp N, Maglioola E, Valesini S, Tidel F, Perucci CA. Respiratory cancer mortality among workers employed in thermoelectric power plants. *Scand J Work Environ Health* 1989;15:383–386.

567. Lerman Y, Finkelstein A, Levo Y, Tupilsky M, Baratz M, Solomon A, Sackstein G. Asbestos-related health hazards among power plant workers. *Brit J Ind Med* 1990;47(4):281.

568. Boffetta P, Cardis H, Vainio H, et al. Cancer risks related to electricity production. *Eur J Cancer* 1991;27(11):1504–1519.

569. Kovalevskii EV. Hygienic evaluation of contact with asbestos-containing dusts at thermoelectric power plants. *Med Tr Prom Ekol* 1993;9–10:17.

570. Crosignani P, Forastiere F, Petrelli G, et al. Malignant mesothelioma in thermoelectric power plant workers in Italy. *Am J Ind Med* 1995;27(4):573.

571. Johansen C, Olsen JH. Risk of cancer among Danish utility workers—A nationwide cohort study. *Am J Epidemiol* 1998;147(6):548.

572. Pira E, Turbiglio M, Maroni M, Carrer P, La Vecchia C, Negri E, Iachetta R. Mortality among workers in the geothermal power plants at Larderello, Italy. *Am J Ind Med* 1999;35:536–539.

573. Ron IG, Ron H. Extrapulmonary neoplasms among asbestos-exposed power plant workers. *Int J Occup Environ Health* 1999;5(4):304–306.

574. Iachetta R, Pira E, Maroni M, Bosio D, Di Prisco ML. Epidemiologic research on asbestos related disease in ENEL SpA electricity production plant maintenance. *G Ital Med Lav Ergon* July–September 2003;25(3):396–397.

575. Habib RR, Abdallah SM, Law M, Kaldor J. Cancer incidence among Australian nuclear industry workers. *J Occup Health* 2006;48:358–365.

576. Nichols L, Sorahan T. Mortality of UK electricity generation and transmission workers, 1973–2002. *Occup Med* 2005;55:541–548.

577. American Railway Association. *Proceedings of the 12th Annual Meeting of the Medical and Surgical Section*, Pennsylvania Hotel, New York City, June 13–14, 1932, pp. 60–62.

578. Association of American Railroads. *Proceedings of the 17th Annual Meeting of the Medical and Surgical Section*, Hotel Traymore, Atlantic City, NJ, June 7–8, 1937, pp. 19–20.

579. Association of American Railroads. *Proceedings of the 19th Annual Meeting of the Medical and Surgical Section*, Stevens Hotel, Chicago, IL, June 15–16, 1939, p. 37.

580. Association of American Railroads. *Proceedings of the 20th Annual Meeting of the Medical and Surgical Section*, Pennsylvania Hotel, New York, N.Y., June 10–11, 1940, pp. 28–29.

581. Association of American Railroads. *Proceedings of the 31st Annual Meeting of the Medical and Surgical Section*, Chicago, IL, April 2, 1951, p. 38.

582. Association of American Railroads. *Proceedings of the 32nd Annual Meeting of the Medical and Surgical Section*, Chicago, IL, March 31, 1952, p. 35.

583. Association of American Railroads. *Proceedings of the 32nd Annual Meeting of the Medical and Surgical Section*, Chicago, IL, April 6, 1953, pp. 34–35.

584. Association of American Railroads. *Proceedings of the 37th Annual Meeting of the Medical and Surgical Section*, White Sulphur Springs, WV, March 28–30, 1957, p. 24.

585. Association of American Railroads. *Proceedings of the 38th Annual Meeting of the Medical and Surgical Section*, Edgewater Park, MS, March 24–26, 1958, p. 81.

586. Mancuso TF. Mesotheliomas among railroad workers in the United States. In the Third Wave of Asbestos Disease: Exposure to Asbestos in Place. *Ann N Y Acad Sci* 1991;643:333.

587. Mancuso TF. Mesothelioma among machinists in railroad and other industries. *Am J Ind Med* 1983;4:501.

588. Schenker MB, Garshick E, Munoz SR, Woskie SR, Speizer FE. A population-based case-control study of mesothelioma deaths among U.S. railroad workers. *Am Rev Resp Dis* 1986;134:461.

589. Malker HSR, Weiner JA, McLaughlin JK. Mesothelioma among Swedish railroad workers. *Acta Oncol* 1990;11:203.

590. Anonymous. Workers, management arguing over risk at French railroad: First dispute since ban. *Occup Safety Health Rep* 1997;26(38):1299.

591. Battista G, Belli S, Comba P, et al. Mortality due to asbestos-related causes among railway carriage construction and repair workers. *Occup Med (Lond)* 1999;49(8):536.

592. Stern FB, Ruder AM, Chen G. Proportionate mortality among unionized roofers and waterproofers. *Am J Ind Med* 2000;37(5):478–492.

593. Breuer G, Stander B. X-ray findings in roofers after long-term exposure to machining dust from asbestos cement. *Arbeitsmedizin Sozialmedizin Praeventivmedizin* November 1982;17(11):275–278.

594. Christiani DC, Green R. Asbestos disease in commercial roofers: radiologic signs. In: *VIIth International Pneumoconioses Conference*, NIOSH/ILO; Poster Session III; 1990:1414–1417.

595. Rodelsperger K, Woitowitz HJ, Krieger HG. Estimation of exposure to asbestos-cement dust on building sites. Biological Effects of Mineral Fibres, IARC Scientific Publication No. 30, International Agency for Research on Cancer, 1980: 845–853.

596. NIOSH. http://www.cdc.gov/noes. National Institute for Occupational Safety and Health, Centers for Disease Control and Prevention, 2011.

597. Anttila P, Heikkilä, P, Mäkelä, Schlünssen V, Priha E. Retrospective exposure assessment for carcinogenic agents in bitumen waterproofing industry in Finland and Denmark. *Ann Occ Hyg* 2009;51(2):139–151.

598. Mowat F, Weidling R, Sheehan P. Simulation tests to assess occupational exposure to airborne asbestos from asphalt-based roofing products. *Ann Occ Hyg* 2007;51(5):451–462.

599. Campopiano A, Ramires D, Zakrzewska AM, Ferri R, D'Annibale A, Pizzutelli G. Risk assessment of the decay of asbestos cement roofs. *Ann Occ Hyg* 2009;53(6):627–638.

600. Straif K, Chambless L, Weiland SK, et al. Occupational risk factors for mortality from stomach and lung cancer among rubber workers: An analysis using internal controls and refined exposure assessment. *Int J Epidemiol* 1999;28:1037.

601. IARC. *Printing Processes and Printing Inks, Carbon Black and Some Nitro Compounds*, IARC Monographs on the evaluation of carcinogenic risks to humans, Vol. 65, International Agency for Research on Cancer, Lyon, France, 1996.

602. Strait K, Kell U, Taeger D, Holthenrich D, Sun Y, Bungers M, Welland SK. Exposure to nitrosamines, carbon black, asbestos, and talc and mortality from stomach, lung, and laryngeal cancer in a cohort of rubber workers. *Am J Epidemiol* 2000;152(4):297–306.

603. Corn JK, Starr J. Historical perspective on asbestos: Policies and protective measures in World War II shipbuilding. *Am J Ind Med* 1987;11:359.

604. Hammond EC, Selikoff IJ. Asbestos-associated disease in United States shipyards. *Cancer J Clin* 1978;28(2):87.

605. Anton-Culver H, Culver BD, Kurosaki T. Immune response in shipyard workers with x-ray abnormalities consistent with asbestos exposure. *Brit J Ind Med* 1988;45:464–468.

606. Baba K. Indications of an increase of occupational pleural mesothelioma in Japan. *Sangyo Ika Daigaku Zasshi* 1983;5(1):3–15.

607. Begin R, Gauthier JJ, Desmeules M, Ostiguy G. Work-related mesothelioma in Quebec, 1967–1990. *Am J Ind Med* 1992;22(4):531–542.

608. Bell A. Industrial hygiene and occupational health studies in Australian (New South Wales) shipyards, Division of Occupational Health and Pollution Control, Health Commission of New South Wales Preprint (Paper 9), Paper presented at the International Shipyard Health Conference, Los Angeles, December 13–15, 1973, p. 28.

609. Bell A. Industrial hygiene and occupational health studies in Australian (New South Wales) shipyards. *Environ Res* 1976;11(2):198–212.

610. Bianchi C, Grandi G, DiBonito L. Diffuse pleural mesothelioma in Trieste. A survey based on autopsy cases. *Tumori* 1978;64(6):565–570.

611. Bianchi C. Asbestos-related mesothelioma in the Monfalcone area. *Pathologica* 1981;73:649–655.

612. Bianchi C, Brollo A, Ramani L, Zuch C. Asbestos-related mesothelioma in Monfalcone, Italy. *Am J Ind Med* 1993;24(2):149–160.

613. Blot WJ, Harrington JM, Toledo A, Hoover R, Health CW Jr, Rraumeni JF Jr. Lung cancer after employment in shipyards during World War II. *NEJM* 1978;299(12):620–624.

614. Blot WJ, Stone BJ, Fraumeni JF Jr, Morris LE. Cancer mortality in U.S. counties with shipyard industries during World War II. *Environ Res* 1979;18:281–290.

615. Blot WJ, Fraumeni JF Jr. Lung cancer mortality in the United States: Shipyard correlations. *Ann N Y Acad Sci* 1979;330:313–315.

616. Blot WJ, Morris LE, Stroube R, Tagnon E, Fraument JF. Lung and laryngeal cancers in relation to shipyard employment in coastal Virginia. *J Natl Can Inst* 1980;65(3):571–575.

617. Blot WJ, Fraumeni JF Jr. Cancer among shipyard workers. In: *Quantification of Occupational Cancer*, Banbury Report 9, Peto R, Schneiderman M, eds., Cold Spring Harbor Laboratory, 1981: 37–46.

618. Bohlig H, Hain E. Cancer in relation to environmental exposure. *Biological Effects of Asbestos*, IARC Scientific Publication 8, 1973: 217–221.

619. Bovenzi M, Stanta G, Antiga G, Peruzzo P, Cavallieti F. Occupational exposure and ling cancer risk in a coastal area of northeastern Italy. *Int Arch Occup Environ Health* 1993;65(1):35–41.

620. Churg A. Malignant mesothelioma in British Columbia in 1982. *Cancer* 1985;55(3):672–674.

621. Connelly RR, Spirtas R, Myers MH, Percy CL, Fraumeni JF Jr. Demographic patterns for mesothelioma in the United States. *JNCI* 1987;78(6):1053–1060.

622. Danielsen TE, Langard S, Anderson A. Incidence of lung cancer among shipyard welders investigated for side-rosis. *Int J Occup Environ Health* 1998;4(2):85–88.

623. Dodson RF, Williams MG Jr, Corn CJ, Brollo A, Bianchi C. Asbestos content of lung tissue, lymph nodes, and pleural plaques from former shipyard workers. *Am Rev Resp Dis* 1990;142(4):843–847.

624. Eisenstadt HB, Levine BW. Pleural effusion in asbestosis. *NEJM* 1974;290(18):1025.

625. Ferris BG Jr, Ranadive MV, Peters JM, Murphy RL, Burgess WA, Pendergrass HP. Prevalence of chronic respiratory disease. Asbestosis in ship repair workers. *Arch Environ Health* 1971;23:220–225.

626. Fletcher DE. A mortality study of shipyard workers with pleural plaques. *Brit J Ind Med* 1972;29:142–145.

627. Forman SA. US Navy shipyard occupational medicine through World War II. *J Occup Med* 1988;30(1):28–32.

628. Fournier-Massey G, Wong G, Hall TC. Retired and former asbestos workers in Hawaii. *Am J Ind Med* 1984;6(2):139–153.

629. Ghezzi L, Maranzana P, Zannini D. Considerations on asbestosis in the Piedmont, Liguria and Lombardy regions. *Med Del Lav* 1971;62(2–3):111–119.

630. Hain E, Bohlig H, Klosterkotter W, Schutz A, Woitowitz HJ. Asbestos: Health hazards, limiting values, prevention. *Staub Reinhaltung der Luft* 1973;33(2):51–57.

631. Harries PG. Experience with asbestos disease and control in Great Britain's naval dockyards, Medical Research Unit, H.M. Dockyard (Reprint Paper 19). Paper presented at the International Shipyard Health Conference, Los Angles, December 13–15, 1973.

632. Hinds MW. Mesothelioma in shipyard workers. *West J Med* 1978;128(2):169–170.

633. Holaday DA, Reitze WB. Shipyard procedures guide helps all insulation men. *Insulation Hygiene Progress Reports* 1971;3(4):1–4.

634. Holaday DA, Reitze WB. Control of exposure to asbestos-containing dust in shipyards. *Occup Saf Health Ser* 1972;40:53–58.

635. Hull CJ, Doyle E, Peters JM, Garabrant DH, Bernstein L, Preston-Martin S. Case-controi study of lung cancer in Los Angeles county welders. *Am J Ind Med* 1989;16(1):103–112.

636. Jarvholm B, Sanden A. Estimating asbestos exposure: A comparison of methods. *J Occup Med* 1987;29(4):361–363.

637. Jones RN, Diem JE, Ziskand MM, Rodregues M, Weill H. Radiographic evidence of asbestos effects in American marine engineers. *J Occup Med* 1984;26(4):281–284.

638. Kilburn KH, Warshaw R, Thornton JC. Asbestosis, pulmonary symptoms and functional impairment in shipyard workers. *Chest* 1985;88(2):254–259.

639. Kilburn KH, Lilis R, Anderson HA, Boylen CT, Einstein HE, Johnson SJS, Warshaw R. Asbestos disease in family contacts of shipyard workers. *Am J Publ Health* 1985;75(6):615–617.

640. Kilburn KH, Warshaw R, Thornton JC. Asbestos disease and pulmonary symptoms and signs in shipyard workers and their families in Los Angeles. *Arch Int Med* 1986;146(11):2213–2220.

641. Kilburn KH, Warshaw R, Thornton JC. Signs of asbestosis and impaired pulmonary function in woman who worked in shipyards. *Am J Ind Med* 1985;8(6):545–552.

642. Kilburn KH, Warshaw RH, Boylen CT, Thornton JC. Respiratory symptoms and functional impairment from acute (cross-shift) exposure to welding gases and fumes. *Am J Med Sci* 1989;298(5):314–319.

643. Kilburn KH, Warshaw RH. Airway obstruction in asbestos-exposed shipyard workers: With and without irregular opacities. *Resp Med* 1990;84(6):449–455.

644. Kilburn KH, Warshaw R. Airway obstruction in asbestosis studied in shipyard workers. *Proceedings of the VIIth International Pneumoconiosis Conference*, Part I, Pittsburgh, Pennsylvania, August 23–26, 1988. NIOSH US Department of Health and Human Services, DHHS (NIOSH) Publication 90-108 Part I, 408–412, 1990.

645. Kilburn KH, Warshaw RH. Asbestos disease in construction, refinery and shipyard workers. *Ann N Y Acta Sci* 1991;643:301–312.

646. Kishimoto T, Okada K. The relationship between lung cancer and asbestos exposure. *Chest* 1988;94(3):486–490.

647. Kishimoto T. Evaluation of the distribution of ferruginous bodies and the kind of asbestos fibers in the lungs in lung cancer cases with definite occupational history of asbestos exposure. *Nihon Kyobu Shikkan Gakkai Zasshi* 1992;30(10):1796–1800.

648. Kishimoto T. Relationship between asbestos exposure and malignant pleural mesothelioma: occurrence near the old Japanese naval shipyard. *Nihon Kyobu Shikkan Gakkai Zasshi* 1994;32(Suppl.): 250–256.

649. Kolonel LN, Yoshizawa CN, Hirohata T, Myers BC. Cancer occurrence in shipyard workers exposed to asbestos in Hawaii. *Cancer Res* 1985;45(8):3924–3928.

650. Koskinen K, Rinne JP, Zitting A, Tossavamnen A, Kivekas J, Reijula K, Roto P, Husskonen MS. Screening for asbestos-induced diseases in Finland. *Am J Ind Med* 1996;30(3):241–251.

651. Koskinen K, Zitting A, Tossavainen A, Rinne JP, Roto P, Kivekas J, Reijula K, Husskonen MS. Radiographic abnormalities among Finnish construction, shipyard and asbestos industry workers. *Scand J Work Environ Heath* 1998;24(2):109–117.

652. Lemercier JP. Seine-maritime pleural mesothelioma register. *Revue Francaise des Maladies Respiratorer* 1978;6(2):209–211.

653. McDonald AD, McDonald JC. Malignant mesothelioma in North America. *Cancer* 1980;46(7):1650–1656.

654. McDonald JC, McDonald AD. Epidemiology of mesothelioma from estimated incidence. *Prev Med* 1977;6(3):426–466.

655. McDonald AD, McDonald JC. Epidemiology of malignant mesothelioma. In: *Asbestos-Related Malignancy*, Antman K, Aisner J, eds. Orlando, FL: Grane and Stratton Inc.; 1987: 31–55.

656. McDonald JC, McDonald AD. The epidemiology of mesothelioma in historical context. *Eur Resp J* 1996;9(9):1932–1942.

657. McMillan GHG. The health of welders in naval dockyards. *J Occup Med* 1983;25(10):727–730.

658. Marr WT. Asbestos exposure during naval vessel overhaul. *Ind Hyg J* 1964;25(10):264–268.

659. Meijers JMM, Planteydt HT, Slangen JJM, Swaen GMH, van Vliett C, Sturmans F. Trends and geograpnical patterns of pleural mesotheliomas in the Netherlands 1970–1987. *Brit J Ind Med* 1990;47:775–781.

660. Meijers JM, Planteydt HT, Slangen JJ, Swaen GM, van Vliet C, Sturmans F. Course and distribution of mortality of pleural mesothelioma in the Netherlands 1970–1987. *Ned Tijdschr Geneeskd* 1991;135(3):93–98.

661. Morinaga K, Kishimoto T, Sakatani M, Akira M, Yokoyama K, Sera Y. Epidemiology of occupational asbestos-related diseases in China. *Ind Health* 2001;39(2):75–83.

662. Murphy RLH Jr, Ferris BG Jr, Burgess WA, Worcester J, Gaensler EA. Effects of low concentration of asbestos, clinical, environmental, radiologie and epidemiologic observation in shipyard pipe coverers and controls. *NEJM* 1971;285(23):1271–1278.

663. Newhouse ML, Berry G. Predictions of mortality from mesothelial tumours in asbestos factory workers. *Brit J Ind Med* 1976;33(3):147–151.

664. Nicholson WJ, Lilis R, Frank AL, Selikoff IJ. Lung cancer prevalence among shipyard workers. *Am J Ind Med* 1980;1(2):191–203.

665. Ono T, Okada K, Kishimoto T, Ito H. Relationship between number of asbestos bodies in autopsy lung and pleural plaques on chest x-ray film. *Chest* 1989;95(3):549–552.

666. Pancoast HK, Miller TG, Landis HRM. A roentgenologic study of the effects of dust inhalation upon the lungs. *Am J Roentgenol (N S)* 1918;5:129.

667. Polakoff PL, Horn BR, Scherer OR. Prevalence of radiographie abnormalities among northern California shipyard workers. *Ann N Y Acta Sci* 1979;330:333–339.

668. Renke W, Chmielewski J, Felczak-Korzybska I, Winnicka A. Estimation of the noxious effects of asbestos dust of the workers of sea shipyards. *Bull Inst Marit Trop Med Gdynia* 1979;30(2):153–159.

669. Renke W, Rosik E. Distant health effects of using asbestos in shipyards and in cooperating plants. *Bull Inst Marit Trop Med Gdynia* 1993;44–45(1–4):5–11.

670. Rosenstock LR, Hudson LS. The pleural manifestations of asbestos exposure. *Occup Med* 1987;2(2):383.

671. Ross DJ, Sallie BA, McDonald JC. SWORD '94: Surveillance of work-related and occupational respiratory disease in the UK. *Occup Med (Lond)* 1995;45(4):175–178.

672. Rossiter CE, Harries PG. UK naval dockyards asbestosis study: Survey of the sample population aged 50–59 years. *Brit J Ind Med* 1979;36(4):281–291.

673. Sanden A, Jarvholm B. Cancer morbidity in Swedish shipyard workers 1978–1983. *Int Arch Occup Environ Health* 1987;59(5):455–462. (Published erratum appears in *Int Arch Occup Environ Health* 1987;59(6):623.)

674. Selikoff IJ, Hammond EC, Seidman H. Mortality experience of insulation workers in the United States and Canada, 1943–1976. *Ann N Y Acad Sci* 1979;330:91.

675. Selikoff IJ, Lilis R, Nicholson WJ. Asbestos disease in United States shipyards. *Ann N Y Acad Sci* 1979;330:295–311.

676. Spirtas R. Time trends and risk factors for mesothelioma. *Proceedings of the Fourth NCI/EPA/NIOSH Collaborative Workshop: Progress on Joint Environmental and Occupational Cancer Studies*, April 22–23, 1986, Rockville, Maryland, NIH Publication 88-2960, 1988: 391–400.

677. Stack BHR, Dorward AJ. Diffuse malignant pleural mesothelioma in Glasgow. *Brit J Dis Chest* 1981;75(4):397–402.

678. Stanbury M, Rosenman KD. A methodology for identifying workers exposed to asbestos since 1940. *Am J Publ Health* 1987;77(7):854–855. (Published erratum appears in *Am J Public Health* November 1987;77(11):1403.)

679. Tagnon I, Blot WJ, Stroube RB, Day NE, Morris LE, Peace BB, Fraumeni JF. Mesothelioma associated with the shipbuilding industry in coastal Virginia. *Cancer Res.* 1980;40(11):3875–3879.

680. Tola S, Killiomake PL, Pukkala E, Asp S, Korkala ML. Incidence of cancer among welders, platers, machinists and pipe fitters in shipyards and machine shops. *Brit J Ind Med* 1988;45(4):209–218.

681. Wallace JM, Oishi JS, Barbers RG, Batra P, Aberle DR. Bronchoalveolar lavage cell and lymphocyte phenotype profiles in healthy asbestos-exposed shipyard workers. *Am Rev Resp Dis* 1989;139(1):33–38.

682. Wollaston JF. Shipbuilding and ship repair. *Occup Med* 1992;42:203–212.

683. Wozniak H, Wiecek E. Asbestos and asbestos-related diseases. *Ann Agri Environ Med* 1996;3(1):1–8.

684. Wright WE, Sherwin RP. Histological types of malignant mesothelioma and asbestos exposure. *Brit J Ind Med* 1984;41(4):514–517.

685. Zielhuis RL, Versteeg JPJ, Planteijdt HT. Pleural mesothelioma and exposure to asbestos. *Int. Archiv, fuer Arbeits- und Umweltmedizin* 1975;36(1):1–18.

686. Harries PG. A comparison of mass and fibre concentrations of asbestos dust in shipyard insulation processes. *Ann Occup Hyg* 1971;14(3):235–240.

687. Langer AM, Rohl AN, Selikoff IJ, Harlow GE, Prinz M. Asbestos as a cofactor in carcinogenesis among nickel-processing workers. *Science* 1980;209(4454):420.

688. Ronneberg A. Mortality and cancer morbidity in workers from an aluminium smelter with prebaked carbon anodes—Part I: Exposure assessment. *Occup Environ Med* 1995;52(4):242.

689. Lilienfeld DE. Asbestos-associated pleural mesothelioma in school teachers: A discussion of four cases. *Ann N Y Acad Sci* 1991;643:454.

690. Anderson HA, Hanrahan LP, Schirmer J, Higgins D, Sarow P. Mesothelioma among employees with likely contact with in-place asbestos-containing building materials. *Ann N Y Acad Sci* 1991;643:550.

691. Corhay J-L, Delavignette J-P, Bury T, Saint-Remy P, Radermechker M-F. Occult exposure to asbestos in steel workers revealed by bronchoalveolar lavage. *Arch Environ Health* 1990;45(5):278.

692. Kronenberg RS, Levin JL, Dodson RF, Garcia JGN, Griffith D. Asbestos-related disease in employees of a steel mill and a glass bottle-manufacturing plant. *Ann N Y Acad Sci* 1991;643:397–403.

693. Redmond CK, Wieand HS, Rockette HE, Sass R, Weinberg G. NIOSH research report, long-term mortality experience of steelworkers. Division of Surveillance, Hazard Evaluations, and Field Studies, NIOSH, Cincinnati, Ohio, 118 pages, NIOSH-00115875, 1981.

694. Blot WJ, Brown LM, Pottern LM, Stone BJ, Fraumeni JF Jr. Lung cancer among long-term steel workers. *Am J Epidemiol* 1983;117(6):706–716.

695. Finkelstein MM. Lung cancer among steelworkers in Ontario. *Am J Ind Med* 1994;26(4):549–557.

696. Anderson E, Hagberg S, Neisson T, Persson B, Wingren G, Torén K. A case-referent study of cancer mortality among sulfate mill workers in Sweden. *Occup Environ Med* 2001;58(5):321–324.

697. Jacobson CJ. A case of acute pulmonary asbestosis. *Acta Med Scand* 1936;78(LXXVIII):482–488.

698. McMillan GH. The health of welders in naval dockyards. The risk of asbestos-related diseases occurring in welders. *J Occup Med* 1983;25(10):727.

699. Simonato L, Fletcher AC, Andersen A, et al. A historical prospective study of European stainless steel, mild steel, and shipyard welders. *Brit J Ind Med* 1991;48(3):145.

700. Becker N, Chang-Claude J, Frentzel-Beyme R. Risk of cancer for arc welders in the Federal Republic of Germany: results of a second follow up (1983–1988). *Brit J Ind Med* 1991;48(10):675.

701. Pairon JC, Martinon L, Iwatsubo Y, Vallentin F, Billon-Galland MA, Bignon J, Brochard P. Retention of asbestos bodies in the lungs of welders. *Am J Ind Med* 1994;25(6):793.

702. Danielsen TE, Langard S, Andersen A. Incidence of cancer among Norwegian boiler welders. *Occup Environ Med* 1996;53(4):231.

703. Haldane JS. Dust removal in factories. Delivered in a lecture at Oxford, 1908. In: *The Occupational Diseases—Their Causation, Symptoms Treatment and Prevention*, 1914, Gilman Thompson W, ed. D. New York and London: Appleton and Company; 1908: 383.

704. Netolitzky A. Gewerbehygiene. In: *Handb. Hyg.* (Th. Weyl. ed.), Vol. 2 (5), 1897, 102 pp.

705. Tolman WH, Kendall LB. *MCMXIII, Safety Methods for Preventing Occupational and Other Accidents and Disease*. New York: Harper & Brothers Publishers; 1913.

706. Kober GM, Hayhurst ER. *Industrial Health*. Philadelphia, PA: P. Blackiston's Sons; 1924: 24.

707. ILO. *Standard Code of Industrial Hygiene*, International Labour Office, Geneva. London: R. S. King & Son, Ltd.; 1934.

708. Reich. Guidelines for the prevention of health hazards from dust in asbestos manufacturing plants, Effective as of 1 August (see *Bulletin for Labor Practices in the Reich* No. 29/1940, III 263), 1940.

709. Gafafer WM. *Manual of Industrial Hygiene and Medical Service in War Industries*, Division of Industrial Hygiene, National Institute of Health, United States Public Health Service, W.B. Saunders Company, Philadelphia, 1943, pp. 168, 350–351.

710. Good CK, Pensky N. Halowax Acne ("Cable Rash") Cutaneous eruption in marine electricians due to certain chlorinated naphthalenes and diphenys. *Arch Derm Syph* 1943;48(3):254.

711. Thompson JG. Asbestos and the urban dweller. *Ann N Y Acad Sci* 1965;132:196.

712. Kiviluoto R. Pleural plaques and asbestos: Further observations on endemic and other nonoccupational asbestosis. *Ann N Y Acad Sci* 1965;132:235.

713. Navratil M, Trippe F. Prevalence of pleural calcification in persons exposed to asbestos dust, and in the general population in the same district. *Environ Res* 1972;5:210–216.

714. Anderson HA, Lilis R, Daum SM, et al. Household exposure to asbestos and risk of subsequent disease. In: *Occupational Carcinogenesis* (*Ann N Y Acad Sci* Vol. 271), Saffiotti U, Wagoner JK, eds. New York, NY: New York Academy of Sciences; 1976: 311.

715. Anderson HA, Lilis R, Daum S, et al. Household exposure to asbestos and risk of subsequent disease. In: *Dusts and Disease*, Lemen R, Dement J, eds. Chicago: Pathotox Publishers Inc.; 1979: 145–156.

716. Anderson HA, Lilis R, Daum SM, Selikoff IJ. Asbestosis among household contacts of asbestos factory workers. *Ann N Y Acad Sci* 1979;330:387–399.

717. Anderson HA. Family contact exposure. In *Proceedings of World Symposium on Asbestos*, Montreal, Canada;1983.

718. Joubert L, Seidman H, Selikoff IJ. Mortality experience of family contacts of asbestos factory workers. *Ann N Y Acad Sci* 1991;643:416–418.

719. Magnani C, Terracini B, Ivaldi C, et al. A cohort study on mortality among wives of workers in the asbestos cement industry in Casale Monferrato, Italy. *Brit J Ind Med* 1993;50:779–784.

720. Ashcroft T, Heppleston AG. Mesothelioma and asbestos on Tyneside—A pathological and social study. In *Proceedings of the International Conference on Pneumoconios*, Shapiro HA, ed. Johannesburg, South Africa: Oxford University Press; 1970: 177.

721. McEwen J, Finlayson A, Mair A, Gibson AAM. Asbestos and mesothelioma in Scotland. An epidemiological study. *Int Arch Arbeitsmed* 1971;28:301–311.

722. Whitwell F, Scott J, Grinshaw M. Relationship between occupations and asbestos fibre content of the lungs in patients with pleural mesothelioma, lung cancer and other diseases. *Thorax* 1977;32:377–386.

723. Bourdes V, Boffetta P, Pisani P. Environmental exposure to asbestos and risk of pleural mesothelioma: review and meta-analysis. *Eur J Epidemiol* 2000;16(5):4.

724. Haque AK, Vrazel DM, Uchida T. Assessment of asbestos burden in the placenta and tissue digests of stillborn infants in South Texas. *Arch Environ Contam Toxicol* 1998;35:532.

725. IHD. *Industrial Health News* 1960;24(4):365.

726. Tomic A. Public health and hygienic factors in the region of an asbestos mine and factory. *Higijena (Belgrade)* 1958;10:273–286.

727. IHD. *Industrial Health News* 1963;27(7).

728. Cuthbert J. Danger of asbestos for general population. *Munch Med Wochschr* 1967;109:1369–1372.

729. IHF. Abstracts, Volume II, 1965–1976, Pneumoconiosis Abstracts, IHD, 1976.

730. Thompson JG, Graves WM Jr. Asbestos as an urban air contaminant. *Arch Pathol* 1966;81:458–464.

731. Tabershaw IR. Asbestos as an environmental hazard. *JOM* 1968;10:32–37.

732. Gold C, Cuthbert J. Asbestos—A hazard to the community. *Publ Health (London)* 1966;80:261–270.

733. Langer AM, Selikoff IJ, Sastre A. Chrysotile asbestos in the lungs of persons in New York City. *Arch Environ Health* 1971;22:348.

734. Davies, Hardy, Loeb, Austin and Ives, Memorandum and Walls, Minutes of the Meeting of the Health and Safety Council/Asbestos Cement Products Association, February 18, 1969.

735. Homan, Letter to Mr. Sicard, Union Carbide Corporation. October 4, Bushy Run Research Center, Pennsylvania, 1982.

736. Campbell WJ, Blake RL, Brown LL, Cather EE, Sjokerg JJ. Selected silicate minerals and their ashes to form varieties—Mineralogical definitions and identification characterization, *Bureau of Mines Information Circular* 8751, United States Department of the Interior, Vol. 56, Washington, DC, 1977.

737. Meurman LO, Kiviluoto R, Hakama M. Combined effect of asbestos exposure and tobacco smoking of Finnish anthophyllite miners and millers. *Ann N Y Acad Sci* 1979;330:491.

738. Meurman LO, Pukkala E, Hakama M. Incidence of cancer among anthophyllite asbestos miners in Finland. *Occup Environ Med* 1994;51(6):421–425.

739. Meurman LO, Kiviluoto R, Hakama M. Mortality and morbidity among the working population of anthophyllite asbestos miners in Finland. *Br J Industr Med* 1974;31:105–112.

740. Tuomi T, Segerberg-Konttinen M, Tammilehto L, Towwavainen A, Vanhala E. Mineral fiber concentration in lung tissue of mesothelioma patients in Finland. *Am J Ind Med* 1989;16(3):247.

741. Karjalainen A, Mattson K, Pukkala E, Tammilehto L, Vainio H. Trends in mesothelioma incidence and occupational mesotheliomas in Finland in 1960–1995. *Scand Work Environ Health* 1997;23(4):266–270.

742. Rom WN, Hammar SP, Rusch V, Dodson R, Hoffman S. Malignant mesothelioma from neighborhood exposure to anthophyllite asbestos. *Am J Ind Med* 2001;40(2):211–214.

743. Karjalainen A, Meurman LO, Pukkala E. Four cases of mesothelioma among Finnish anthophyllite miners. *Occup Environ Med* 1994;51(3):212.

744. Karjalainen A, Nurminen M, Vanhata E, Vainio H. Pulmonary asbestos bodies and asbestos fibers as indicators of exposure. *Scand J Work Environ Health* 1996;11(1):34–38.

745. Dodson RE, Graef R, Shepherd S, O'Sullivan M, Levin J. Asbestos burden in cases of mesothelioma from individuals from various regions of the United States. *Ultrastruct Pathol* September–October 2005;29(5):415–433.

746. Tuomi T. Fibrous minerals in the lungs of mesothelioma patients: Comparison between data on SEM, TEM, and personal interview information. *Am J Ind Med* 1992;21(2):155.

747. Tammilehto L, Tuomi T, Tiainen M, Rautonen J, Knuutila S, Pyrhonen S, Mattson K. Malignant mesothelioma: clinical characteristics, asbestos mineralogy and chromosomal abnormalities of 41 patients. *Eur J Can* 1992;28A(8–9):1373.

748. Schepers GWH. Discussion. *Ann N Y Acad Sci* 1965;132:246.

749. Selikoff IJ, Hammond EC, Churg J. Carcinogenicity of amosite asbestos. *Arch Environ Health* 1972;25:183–186.

750. Seidman H, Lilis R, Selikoff I. Short-term asbestos exposure and delayed cancer risk. *Proceedings of the Third International Symposium on the Detection and Prevention of Cancer*, New York, April 26–May 1, 1976; in *Prevention and Detection of Cancer*, Nieburgs HE, Ed., Part 1. Prevention, Vol. 1. Etiology, Marcel Dekker, New York and Basel, 1977: 994.

751. Johnson WM, Lernen RA, Hurst GA, Spiegel RM, Liu FHY. Respiratory morbidity among workers in an amosite asbestos insulation plant. *J Occup Med* 1983;24(12):994.

752. Seidman H, Selikoff IJ, Gelb SK. Mortality experience of amosite asbestos factory workers: Dose-response relationships 5 to 40 years after onset of short-term work exposure. *Am J Ind Med* 1986;10:479.

753. Finkelstein MM. Mortality among employees of an Ontario factory manufacturing insulation materials from amosite asbestos. *Am J Ind Med* 1989;14:477.

754. Ribak J, Seidman H, Selikoff IJ. Amosite mesothelioma in a cohort of asbestos workers. *Scand J Work Environ Health* 1989;15:106.

755. Levin JI, McLarthy JW, Hurst GW, Smith AN, Frank AL. Tyler asbestos workers: Mortality experience in a cohort exposed to amosite. *Occup Envrion Med* 1998;55:155–160.

756. Wagner JC. Asbestosis in experimental animals. *Brit J Industr Med* 1963;29:1–12.

757. Schepers GWH. Discussion. *Ann N Y Acad Sci* 1965;132(1):246–247.

758. Sluis-Cremer GK. Asbestosis in South Africa: Certain geographical and environmental considerations. *Ann N Y Acad Sci* 1965;132(1):215–234.

759. Wagner JC, Berry G. Mesotheliomas in rats following inoculation with asbestos. *Br J Cancer* September 1969;23(3):567–581.

760. Wagner JC, Berry G, Timbrell V. Mesotheliomas in rats following the intra-pleural inoculation of asbestos. pneumoconiosis. In: *Proceedings of the International Conference*, Johannesburg, 1969, Shapiro HA, ed. Cape Town: Oxford University Press; 1970: 216–219.

761. Reeves AL, Puro HE, Smith RG, Vorwald AJ. Experimental asbestos carcinogenesis. *Environ Res* 1971;4:496–511.

762. Webster I. Asbestos and malignancy. *S Afr Med J* 1973;47:165–171.

763. Reeves AL. The carcinogenic effect of inhaled asbestos fibers. *Ann Clin Lab Sci* September–October 1976;6(5):459–466.

764. Seidman H, Selikoff IJ, Hammond E. C. (1\17\1): Short-term asbestos work exposure and long-term observation. *Ann N Y Acad Sci* 1979;330:61–90.

765. Liddell FDK, McDonald AD, McDonald JC. Dust exposure and lung cancer in Quebec chrysotile miners and millers. *Ann Occup Hyg* 1998;42(1):7.

766. Tossavainen A, Kovalevsky E, Vanhala, E, Tuomi T. Pulmonary mineral fibers after occupational and environmental exposure to asbestos in the Russian chrysotile industry. *Am J Ind Med* 2000;37:327.

767. Tossavainen A, Kotilainen M, Takahashi K, Pan G, Vanhala E. Amphibole fibres in Chinese chrysotile asbestos. *Ann Occup Hyg* 2001;45(2):145–152.

768. Cullen M, Baloyi R. Chrysotile asbestos and health in Zimbabwe: I. Analysis of miners and millers compensated for asbestos-related diseases since independence (1980). *Am J Ind Med* 1991;19:161–169.

769. Baloyi R. Exposure to asbestos among chrysotile miners, millers, and mine residents and asbestosis in Zimbabwe, Academic dissertation, University of Kuopic, Helsinki, Finland, 1989.

770. Piolatto G, Negri E, La Vecchia C, Pira E, Decarli A, Peto J. An update of cancer mortality among chrysotile asbestos miners in Balangero, northern Italy. *Brit J Ind Med* 1990;47:810–814.

771. Wagner JC, Berry G, Skidmore JW, Poole FD. The comparative effects of three chrysotiles by injection and inhalation in rats. In *Biological Effects of Mineral Fibres*, Vol. 1, International Agency for Research on Cancer, Lyon, IARC Scientific Publication 30, World Health Organization; 1979: 363.

772. Wagner JC, Berry G, Timbrell V. Mesotheliomas in rats following inoculation with asbestos and other materials. *Brit J Cancer* 1973;28:175.

773. Wagner JC, Berry G, Skidmore JW, Timbrel V. The effects of the inhalation of asbestos in rats. *Brit J Cancer* 1974;29(3):252.

774. Enterline PE. Early animal research on asbestos cancer. *Am J Ind Med* December 1993;24(6):783–785; author reply 787–791.

775. Schepers GW. Chronology of asbestos cancer discoveries: Experimental studies of the Saranac Laboratory. *Am J Ind Med* April 1995;27(4):593–606.

776. Vorwald AJ, Durkan TM, Pratt PC. Experimental studies of asbestosis. *Arch Industr Hyg Occup Med* January 1951;3(1):1–43.

777. Wagner JC, Berry G. Information obtained from animal experiments. In: *Biological Effects of Asbestos*. IARC Scientific Publication No. 8; 1973:265–288.

778. Timbrell V. Physical factors as etiological mechanisms. In: *Biological Effects of Asbestos*. IARC Scientific Publication No. 8; 1973: 295–303.

779. Davis JMG. Current concepts in asbestos fiber pathogenicity. In: *Dust and Disease*, Lemen RA, Dement JM, eds. Park Forest South, IL: Pathotox Publishers, Inc.; 1979: 45–49.

780. Karp RD, Johnson KH, Buoen LC, Ghobrial HKG, Brand I, Brand KG. Tumorigenesis by millipore filters in mice. *J Nat Cancer Inst* 1973;51:1275–1285.

781. Hiett DM. Experimental asbestosis: An investigation of functional and pathological disturbances. I. Methods, control animals and exposure conditions. *Br J Ind Med* 1978;35:129–134.

782. Glassroth JL, Bernardo J, Lucey EC, Center DM, Jung-Legg Y, Snider GL. Interstitial pulmonary fibrosis induced in hamsters by intratracheally administered chrysotile asbestos. *Am Rev Respir Dis* 1984;130:242–248.

783. Wagner JC. The complexities in the evaluation of epidemiologic data of fiber-exposed populations. In: *Dust and Disease*, Lemen R, Dement JM, eds. Park Forest, IL: Pathox Publishers; 1979: 37–40.

784. Platek SF, Groth DH. Chronic animal inhalation study of short (5 micrometers) asbestos fibers. NIOSH Contract-210-77-0151, May 1980: 447–469.

785. Bozelka BE, Sestini P, Gaumer HR, Hammad Y, Heather CJ, Salvaggio JE. A murine model of asbestosis. *Am J Pathol* 1983;112(3):326–337.

786. Wagner MMF, Edwards RE, Moncrieff CB, Wagner JC. Mast cells and inhalation of asbestos in rats. *Thorax* 1984;39(7):539–544.

787. Brody AR. The early pathogenesis of asbestos-induced lung disease. *Scan Electron Microsc* 1984;1:167–171.

788. Roggli VL, Brody AR. Changes in numbers and dimensions of chrysotile asbestos fibers in lungs of rats following short-term exposure. *Exp Lung Res* 1984;7:133–147.

789. Warheit DB, Chang LY, Hill LH, Hook GER, Crapo JD, Brody AR. Pulmonary macrophage accumulation and asbestos-induced lesions at sites of fiber deposition. *Am Rev Respir Dis* 1984;129:301–310.

790. Losito R, Dufresne M, Masse S, Caro J, Bilodeau G. Asbestos-related fibrin formation in human plasma. *Thromb Res* 1984;34(4):311–319.

791. Craighead JE, Akley NJ, Gould LB, Libbus BL. Characteristics of tumors and tumor cells cultured from experimental asbestos-induced mesotheliomas in rats. *Am J Pathol* December 1987;129(3):448–462.

792. Cartier P. Abstract of discussion. *Arch Industr Hyg Occ Med* March 1952;5(3):262–263.

793. Braun DC, Truan TD. Epidemiology study of lung cancer in asbestos miners. *AMA Arch Ind Health* June 1958;17(6):634–653.

794. Elwood PC, Cochrane AL, Benjamin LT, Seys-Prosser D. A follow-up study of workers from an asbestos factory. *Brit J Ind Med.* 1964;21:304–307.

795. Kogan FM, Gerasimenko AA, Bunimovich GI. The occurrence of certain immunobiological changes in asbestosis. *Gigiena i Sanitariya* 1965;30(5):184–191.

796. Kogan FM, Yu Troitskie S, Udilova NN. Date [sic] on the mechanism of fibrogenic action of asbestos dust. *Gigiena i Sanitariya* 1966;31(1):10–14.

797. Kogan FM, Yu Troitskii S, Gulevskaya MR. Carcinogenic effect of asbestos dust. *Hygiene and Sanitation*, Vol. 31, Environmental Protection Agency and National Science Foundation (Gigiena i Sanitariya), Washington, D.C.; 1966: 218–225.

798. Champion P. Two cases of malignant mesothelioma after exposure to asbestos. *Am Rev Resp Dis* 1971;103:821–826.

799. McDonald JC, McDonald AD, Gibbs GW, Siemletycki J, Rossiter CE. Mortality in the chrysotile asbestos mines and mills of Quebec. *Arch Environ Health* June 1971;22:677–686.

800. Liddell FDK, McDonald JC, Thomas DC. Methods of cohort analysis: Appraisal by application to asbestos mining. *J R Statist Soc A* 1977;140(4):469–491.

801. Navrátil M, Trippé F. Prevalence of pleural calification in persons exposed to asbestos dust, and in the general population of the same district. *Environ Res* 1972;5:210–216.

802. Kogan FM, Guselnikova NA, Gulevskaya MR. The cancer mortality rate among workers in the asbestos industry in the Urals. *Gig Sanit* 1972;37:29.

803. McDonald JC. Cancer in chrysotile mines and mills. In: *Biological Effects of Asbestos,* Bogovski P, Gilson JC, Timbrell V, Wagner JC, eds. International Agency for Research on Cancer, IARC Scientific Publications No. 8; 1973:189–194.

804. McDonald AD, Magner D, Eyssen G. Primary malignant mesothelial tumors in Canada, 1960-1968. A pathologic review by the mesothelioma panel of the Canadian Tumor Reference Centre. *Cancer* 1973;31(4):869–876.

805. Rossiter CE. Discussion summary. Cancer in relation to type of fibre, dose, occupation and duration of exposure. *Biological Effects of Asbestos*. International Agency for Research on Cancer. IARC Scientific Publication No. 8; 1973: 226–227.

806. Morgan A. Discussion summary. In: *Biological Effects of Asbestos*, Bogovski P, Gilson JC, Timbrell V, Wagner JC, eds. Lyon FR: International Agency for Research on Cancer; 1973:318–319.

807. Enterline PE, Henderson V. Type of asbestos and respiratory cancer in the asbestos industry. *Arch Environ Health* November 1973;27:312–317.

808. McDonald JC, Becklake MR, Gibbs GW, McDonald AD, Rossiter CE. The health of chrysotile asbestos mine and mill workers of Quebec. *Arch Environ Health* February 1974;28:61–68.

809. Gibbs GW, LaChance M. Dust-fiber relationships in the Quebec chrysotile industry. *Arch Environ Health* February 1974;28:69–71.

810. Fournier-Massey G, Becklake MR. Pulmonary function profiles in Quebec asbestos workers. *Bull Physiopath Resp* 1975;11:429–225.

811. Weiss W. Mortality of a cohort exposed to chrysotile asbestos. *JOM* November 1977;19(11):737–740.

812. Selikoff IJ. Clinical survey of chrysotile asbestos miners and millers in Baire Verte, Newfoundland 1976, Report to the National Institute of Environmental Health Sciences, December 22, USPHS, Department of Health and Human Services, Research Triangle, NC, 1977.

813. IARC. *Monographs on the Evaluation of Carcinogenic Risk of Chemicals to Man—Asbestos*, Volume 14. International Agency for Research on Cancer, Lyon, 1977.

814. Liddell D, Eyssen G, Thomas D, McDonald C. Radiological changes over 20 years in relation to chrysotile exposure in Quebec. *Inhaled Particles IV*, Part 2. Oxford: Pergamon Press; 1977: 799–813.

815. McDonald JC. Exposure relationships and malignant mesothelioma. *Proceedings of Asbestos Symposium*, Johannesburg, SA, October 3rd–7th, 1977, Glen HW, ed. National Institute for Metallurgy; 1978.

816. Peto J, Doll R, Howard SV, Kinlen LJ, Lewinsohn HC. A mortality study among workers in an English asbestos factory. *Brit J Ind Med* 1977;34:169–173.

817. Elena R. Lesiones pleurales en trabajadores del asbesto [Pleural lesions in asbestos workers]. Revista cubana de higiene y epidemiología. *La Habana, Cuba* September—December 1978;16(3):217–231.

818. Rubino GF, Newhouse M, Murray R, Scansetti G, Piolatto G, Aresini G. Radiologic changes after cessation of exposure among chrysotile asbestos miners in Italy. In: *Health Hazards of Asbestos Exposure (Ann N Y Acad Sci* vol. 330), Selikoff IJ, Hammond EC, eds. New York NY: New York Academy of Sciences;1979:157–161.

819. Rubino GF, Piolatto G, Newhouse ML, Scansetti G, Aresini GA, Murrary R. Mortality of chrysotile asbestos workers at the Balangero Mine, Northern Italy. *Brit J Ind Med* 1979;36:187–194.

820. Ghezzi I, Aresini G, Vigliani EC. II rischio di asbestosi in una miniera di amianto crisotilo. *La Medicina del Lavoro* 1972;5–6:33–56.

821. Weill H, Hughes J, Waggenspack C. Influence of dose and fiber type on respiratory malignancy risk in asbestos cement manufacturing. *Am Rev of Resp Dis* 1979;129:345–354.

822. Hughes J, Weill H. Lung cancer risk associated with manufacture of asbestos-cement products. In: *Biological Effects of Mineral Fibres*, Volume 2: IARC Scientific Publication No. 30; 1980: 627–635.

823. McDonald JC, Liddell FDK. Mortality in Canadian miners and millers exposed to chrysotile. In: Part 1. Asbestos Disease in Employed Groups. *Ann N Y Acad Sci* 1979;330:1–10, 1979.

824. Sebastien P, Janson X, Bonnaud G, et al. Translocation of asbestos fibers through respiratory tract and gastrointestinal track according to fiber type and size. In: *Dust and Disease*, Lernen RA, John M, eds. Forest Park South, IL: Dement, Pathox Publishers, Inc.; 1979: 65–86.

825. Churg A, Warnock MI. Asbestos fibers in the general population. *Am Rev Respir Dis* 1980;122:669–678.

826. Nicholson WJ, Selikoff IJ, Seidman H, Lilis R, Formby P. Long-term mortality experience of chrysotile miners and millers in Thetford Mines, Quebec. In: Part 1. Asbestos Disease in Employed Groups. *Ann N Y Acad Sci* 1979;330:11–22.

827. Acheson ED, Gardner MJ. Mesothelioma and exposure to mixtures of chrysotile and amphibole asbestos. *Arch Environ Health* 1979; July/August: 240–241.

828. Acheson ED, Gardner MJ. Possible synergism between chrysotile and amphibole asbestos. *Lancet* March 29, 1980;1(8170).

829. Boutin C, Viallat JR, Bellenfant M. Radiological features in chrysotile asbestos mine and mill workers in Corsica. In: *Biological Effects of Mineral Fibres*, IARC Scientific Publication No. 30, International Agency for Research on Cancer; 1980: 507–511.

830. Rey F, Dumortier P, Viallat JR, Broucke I, Boutin C, De Vuyst P. Chrysotile and tremolite asbestos fibres in the lungs and parietal pleura of Corsican goats. *Occ Envir Med* September 2002;59(9):643–646.

831. Acheson ED, Gardner MJ. Asbestos: scientific basis for environmental control of fibres. In *Biological Effects of Mineral Fibres*, IARC Scientific Publication No. 30, International Agency for Research on Cancer; 1980: 737–754.

832. Peto J. The incidence of pleural mesothelioma in chrysotile asbestos textile workers. In: *Biological Effects of Mineral Fibres*, IARC Scientific Publication No. 30, International Agency for Research on Cancer; 1980: 703–712.

833. Jones JSP, Pooley FD, Clark JJ, Owen WG, Roberts GH, Smith PG, Wagner JC, Berry G, Pollock DJ. The pathology and mineral content of lungs in cases of mesothelioma in the United Kingdom in 1976. In *Biological Effects of Mineral Fibres*, IARC Scientific Publication No. 30, International Agency for Research on Cancer; 1980: 187–200.

834. Pooley FD, Clark NJ. A comparison of fibre dimensions in chrysotile, crocidolite and amosite particles from samples of airborne dust and from post-mortem lung tissue speciments. In: *Biological Effects of Mineral Fibres*, IARC Scientific Publication No. 30, International Agency for Research on Cancer; 1980: 79–86.

835. McDonald JC, Liddell FDK, Gibbs GW, Eyssen GE, McDonald AD. Dust exposure and mortality in chrysotile mining, 1910-75. *Brit J Ind Med* 1980;37:11–24.

836. Liddell FDK, McDonald JC. Radiological findings as predictors of mortality in Quebec asbestos workers. *Brit J Ind Med* 1980;37:257–267.

837. Viallat JR, Boutin C, Pietri JF, Fondarai J. Late progression of radiographic changes in Canari chrysotile mine and mill ex-workers. *Arch Environ Health* January–February 1983;38(1):54–58.

838. Eyssen GM. Development of radiographic abnormality in chrysotile miners and millers. *Chest* August 1980;78(2 Suppl):411–414.

839. Dement JM, Harris Jr RL, Symons MJ, Shy C. Estimates of dose-response for respiratory cancer among chrysotile asbestos textile workers. *Am Occup Hyg* 1982;26(1–4):869–887.

840. McDonald AD, Fry JS. Mesothelioma and fiber type in three American asbestos factories—Preliminary report. *Scand J Work Environ Health* 1982;8(suppl 1):53–58.

841. McDermott M, Bevan MM, Elmes PC, Allardice JT, Bradley AC. Lung function and radiographic change in chrysotile workers in Swaziland. *Brit J Ind Med* 1982;39(4):338–343.

842. McDonald AD, Fry JS, Woolley AJ, McDonald JC. Dust exposure and mortality in an American factory using chrysotile, amosite, and crodidolite in mainly textile manufacture. *Brit J Ind Med* 1982;39:368–374.

843. Acheson AD, Gardner MJ, Pippard BC, Grime LP. Mortality of two groups of women who manufactured gas masks from chrysotile and crocidolite asbestos: A 40-year follow-up. *Brit J Ind Med* 1982;39:344–348.

844. Churg A. Asbestos fiber content of the lungs in patients with and without asbestos airways disease. *Am Rev Resp Dis* April 1983;127(4):470–473.

845. Rowlands N, Gibbs GW, McDonald AD. Asbestos fibres in the lungs of chrysotile miners and millers: A preliminary report. *Am Occup Hyg* 1982;26(1–4):411–415.

846. Waxweiller RJ, Robinson C. Asbestos and non-Hodgkin's lymphoma. January 1983;22:189–190.

847. Liddell FDK. Tumour incidence after asbestos exposure in the general population of Canada. *VDI-Berichte/Verein Deutscher Ingenieure* 1983;475:179–183.

848. Dement JM, Harris Jr RL, Symons MJ, Shy CM. Exposures and mortality among chrysotile asbestos workers. Part I: exposure estimates. *AJIM* 1983;4:399–419; Part II: mortality. *AJIM* 1983;4:421–433.

849. Dupre' JS, Mustard JF, Uffen RJ. Report of the Royal Commission on Matters of Health and Safety Arising from the Use of Asbestos in Ontario, Ontario Ministry of the Attorney General, Queen's Printer for Ontario, Toronto, 1984.

850. Liddell FD, Thomas DC, Gibbs GW, McDonald JC. Fibre exposure and mortality from pneumoconiosis, respiratory and abdominal malignancies in chrysotile production in Quebec, 1926–75. *Ann Acad Med Singapore* April 1984;13(2 Suppl):340–344.

851. Churg A, Wiggs B, Depaoli L, Kampe B, Stevens B. Lung asbestos content in chrysotile workers with mesothelioma. *Am Rev Respir Dis* 1984;130(6):1042–1045.

852. Finn MB, Hallenbeck WH. Detection of chrysotile asbestos in workers' urine. *Am Ind Hyg Assoc J* 1984;45(11):752–759.

853. McDonald AD, Fry JS, Woolley AJ, McDonald JC. Dust exposure and mortality in an American chrysotile asbestos friction products plant. *Brit J Ind Med* 1984;41:151–157.

854. Kobusch AB, Simard A, Feldstein M, Vauclair R, Gibbs GW, Bergeron F, Morissette N, Davis R. Pulmonary cytology in chrysotile asbestos workers. *J Chronic Dis* 1984;37(8):599–607.

855. Copes R, Thomas D, Becklake MR. Temporal patterns of exposure and nonmalignant pulmonary abnormality in Quebec chrysotile workers. *Arch Environ Health* March/April 1985;40(20):80–87.

856. Wright JL, Churg A. Severe diffuse small airways abnormalities in long term chrysotile asbestos miners. *Brit J Ind Med* 1985;42:556–559.

857. Gardner MJ, Winter PD, Pannett B, Powell CA. Follow up study of workers manufacturing chrysotile asbestos cement products. *Brit J Ind Med* November 1986;43(11):726–732.

858. Hughes JM, Hammad YY, Erill H. Mesothelioma risk in relation to duration and type of asbestos fiber exposure. *Am Rev Resp Dis* April 1986;133(4; Part 2):A33.

859. Kogan FM, Berzin SA. The frequency of mesothelioma of the pleura with exposure to chrysotile asbestos dust. *Gigivena truda i professional 'yye zaboleyaniya* 1986;9:9–12.

860. Hughes JM, Weill H, Hammad YY. Mortality of workers employed in two asbestos cement manufacturing plants. *Brit J Ind Med* 1987;44:161–174.

861. Finkelstein MM. Mortality among employees of an Ontario factory that manufactured construction materials using chrysotile asbestos and coal tar pitch. *AJIM* 1989;16:281–287.

862. Siemiatycki J, Warholder S, Dewar R, Wald I, Bėgin, Richardson D, Rosenman K, Görin M. Smoking and degree of occupational exposure: Are internal analyses in cohort studies likely to be confounded by smoking status? *Am J Ind Med* 1988;13:59–70.

863. Finkelstein MM. Mortality rates among employees potentially exposed to chrysotile asbestos at two automotive parts factories. *CMAJ* July 15, 1989;141:125–130.

864. Pooley FD. An examination of the fibrous mineral content of asbestos lung tissue from the Canadian chrysotile mining industry. *Environ Res* 1976;12:281–296.

865. Rogers AJ, Leigh J, Berry G, Ferguson DA, Mulder HB, Ackad M. Relationship between lung asbestos fiber type and concentration and relative risk of mesothelioma, a case-control study. *Cancer* 1991;67(7):1912–1920.

866. Henderson DW. Discussion of Dr. D.W. Henderson in European Communities—Measures Affecting Asbestos and Asbestos-Containing Products—Report of the Panel, World Trade Organization (WTO), September 18, 2000: 273.

867. Yano E, Wang Z-M, Wang M-Z, Lan Y-J. Cancer mortality among workers exposed to amphibole-free chrysotile asbestos. *Am J Epidemiol* 2001;154:538.

868. Yano E, Wang, Z-M, Wang X-R, Wang M-Z, Takata A, Kohyama N, Suzuki Y. Mesothelioma in a worker who spun chrysotile asbestos at home during childhood. *AJIM* April 2009;52(4):282–287.

869. Nokso-Koivisto, Pukkala E. Past exposure to asbestos and combustion products and incidence of cancer among Finnish locomotive drivers. *Occup Environ Med* 1994;51:330.

870. Mancuso TF. Relative risk of mesotheliomas among railroad workers exposed to chrysotile. *Am J Ind Med* 1988;13:639.

871. Hein MJ, Stayner L, Lehman E, Dement JM. Follow-up study of chrysotile textile workers: Cohort mortality and exposure-response. *Occup Environ Med.* 2007;64:616–625. Published online April 20, doi:10.1136/OEM.2006.031005, 2007.

872. Loomis D, Dement JM, Wolf SH, Richardson DB. Lung cancer mortality and fiber exposures among North Carolina asbestos textile workers. *Occup Environ Med.* 2009;66:535–542. Published online March 11, doi:10.1136/oem.2008.044362, 2009.

873. Loomis D, Dement J, Richardson D, Wolf S. Asbestos fiber dimensions and lung cancer mortality among workers exposed to chrysotile. *Occup Environ Med.* 2009;67:580–584. Published online November 5, doi:10.1136/oem.2009.050120, 2009.

874. Sturm W, Menze B, Krause J, Thriene B. Use of asbestos, health risks and induced occupational diseases in the former East Germany. *Toxicol Lett* 1994;72:317–324.

875. Kuempel ED, Dankovic DA, Smith RJ, Stayner LT. Concordance of rat and human data-based risk estimates for lung cancer from chrysotile asbestos. In *Proceedings of the 2001 Asbestos Health Effects Conference*, U.S. Environmental Protection Agency, May 24–25, 2001, Oakland, CA.

876. Mancuso TR. Responses to Drs. Churg and Green. Letter to the Editor. *Am J Ind Med* 1990;17:525.

877. Sebastien P, McDonald JC, McDonald AD, Case B, Harley R. Respiratory cancer in chrysotile textile and mining industries: exposure inferences from lung analysis. *Brit J Ind Med* 1979;46:180.

878. Marten M, Dirksen M, Puschel K, Lieske K. Distribution of asbestos bodies in the human organism. *Der Pathologe* 1989;10:114–117.

879. Davis JMG, Addison J, Bolton RE, Donaldson K, Jones AD. Inhalation and injection studies in rats using dust samples from chrysotile asbestos prepared by a wet dispersion process. *Brit J Exp Path* 1986;67:113–129.

880. Davis JMG, Adison J, Bolton RE, Donaldson K, Jones AD, Smith T. The pathogenicity of long versus short fibre samples of amosite asbestos administered to rats by inhalation and intraperitoneal injection. *Brit J Exp Path* 1986;67:415–430.

881. Churg A, Wright JL, Depaoli L, Wiggs B. Mineralogie correlates of fibrosis in chrysotile miners and millers. *Am Rev Respir Dis* 1989;139:891.

882. Suzuki Y, Kolynema N. Translocation of inhaled asbestos fibers from the lung to other tissues. *Am J Ind Med* 1991;19:701–704.

883. NRC. Animals as Sentinels of Environmental Health Hazards. National Research Council, National Academy Press, Committee on Animals as Monitors of Environmental Hazards; 1991: 160.

884. Malorni W, Losi F, Falchi M, Donelli G. On the mechanism of cell internalization of chrysotile fibers: An immunocytochemical and ultrastructural study 1990. *Environ Res* 1990;52:164–177.

885. Churg A, Wright JL, Gilks B, Depaoli L. Rapid short-term clearance of chrysotile compared with asmoite asbestos in the Guinea Pig. *Am Rev Resp Dis* 1989;139:885.

886. Sebastien P, Janson X, Gausichet A, Hirsch A, Bignon J. Asbestos retention in human respiratory tissues: Comparative measurements in lung parenchyma and in perietal pleura. *IARC Sei Pub* 1980;30:237–246.

887. Mishra A, Liu JY, Brody AR, Morris GF. Inhaled asbestos fibers induce p53 expression in the rat lung. *Am J Resp Cell Mol Biol* 1997;16(4):479–485.

888. Matsuoka M, Igisu H, Morimoto Y. Phosphorylation of p53 protein in A549 human pulmonary epithelial cells exposed to asbestos fibers. *Environ Health Perspect* 2003;111(4):509–512.

889. Iwata T, Yano E. Reactive oxygen metabolite production induced by asbestos and glass fibers: Effect of fiber milling. *Indust Health* 2003;41:32–38.

890. Pott F. Testing the carcinogenicity of fibers in laboratory animals: result and conclusions. In: *Contemporary Issues in Fiber Toxicology*, Warheit D, (Hrsg.), ed. Fiber Toxicity, San Diego: Academic Press; 1993: 395–424.

891. Stanton MF, Laynard M, Tegeris A, et al. Carcinogenicity of fibrous glass: pleural response in the rat in relation to dimension. *J Natl Cancer Inst* 1977;58:587–603.

892. Lemen RA. Chrysotile asbestos as a cause of mesothelioma: Application of the hill causation model. *Int J Occup Environ Health* 2004;10:233–239.

893. Miller K, Liddell D. *Mineral Fibers and Health*. Boca Raton, FL: CRC Press; 1991: 381 pp.

894. Sheehy JW, Cooper TC. Control of asbestos exposure during brake drum service. United States. National Institute for Occupational Safety and Health Cincinnati, Ohio, (DHHS (NIOSH) publication No. 89–121; 1989: 70 pp.

895. Gibbons W. Amphibole asbestos in Africa and Australia: Geology, health hazard and mining legacy. *J Geol Soc London* 2000;157:851–858.

896. McNulty JC. Asbestos exposure in Australia pneumoconiosis. In: *Proceedings of the International Conference*, Shapiro HA, ed., Johannesburg, Oxford University Press, Cape Town, 1969: 201–203.

897. Jones JS, Pooley FD, Smith PG. Factory populations exposed to crocidolite asbestos—A continuing survey. *IARC Sci. Publ.* 1976;13:117–120.

898. Armstrong BK, De Klerk NH, Musk AW, Hobbs MST. Mortality in miners and millers of crocidolite in Western Australia. *Brit J Ind Med* 1988;45:5.

899. Cappelletto F, Merler E. Perceptions of health hazards in the narratives of Italian migrant workers at an Australian asbestos mine (1943–1966). *Soc Sci Med* 2003;56(5):1047.

900. Martiny O. Primary mesothelioma of the pleura. *Proc Transvaal Mine Med Officers' Assoc* 1956;35:63–64.

901. Sleggs CA. Mesothelioma, including peripheral lung malignancy and tuberculosis in the North West Cape. In: *Pneumoconiosis, Proceedings of the International Conference*, Johannesburg 1969, Shapiro HA, ed. Cape Town: Oxford University Press; 1970: 225–236.

902. McDonald AD, McDonald JC. Mesothelioma after crocidolite exposure during gas mask manufacture. *Environ Res* 1978;17:340–346.

903. Armstrong BK, Musk AW, Gaker JE, et al. Epidemiology of malignant mesothelioma in Western Australia. *Med J Aust* July 21, 1984;141:86–88.

904. de Klerk NH, Armstrong BK, Musk AW, Hobbs MST. Cancer mortality in relation to measures of occupational exposure to crocidolite at Wittenoom Gorge in Western Australia. *Brit J Ind Med* 1989;46:529.

905. Botha JL, Irwig LM, Strebel PM. Excess mortality from stomach cancer, lung cancer, and asbestosis and/or mesothelioma in crocidolite mining districts in South Africa. *Am J Epid* 1986;123(1):30–40.

906. McDonald JC, McDonald AD, Armstrong B, Sebastien P. Cohort study of morality of vermiculite miners exposed to tremolite. *Brit J Ind Med* 1986;43(7):436–444.

907. Amandus HE, Wheeler R. The morbidity and morality of vermiculite miners and millers exposed to tremolite-actinolite: Part II. Mortality. *Am J Ind Med* 1987;11(1):15–26.

908. Wright RS, Abraham JL, Harber P, Burnett BR, Morris P, West P. Fatal asbestosis 50 years after brief high intensity exposure in a vermiculite expansion plant. *Am J Resp Crit Care Med* 2002;165(8):1145–1149.

909. Luce D, Bugel I, Goldberg P, et al. Environmental exposure to tremolite and respiratory cancer in New Caledonia: a case-control study. *Am J Epidemiol* 2000;151(3):259–265.

910. Baris YI, Bilir N, Artvinli M, Sahin AA, Kalyoncu F, Sebastien P. An epidemiological study in an Anatolian village environmentally exposed to tremolite asbestos. *Brit J Ind Med* 1998;45(12):838–840.

911. Rey F, Boutin C, Steinbauer J, et al. Environmental pleural plaques in an asbestos-exposed population of northeast Corsica. *Ew Resp J* 1993;6(7):978–982.

912. Yazicioglu S, Ilcayto R, Balci K, Sayli BS, Yorulmaz B. Pleural calcification, pleural mesotheliomas, and bronchial cancers caused by tremolite dust. *Thorax* 1980;35(8):564–569.

913. NIOSH. Occupational exposure to talc containing asbestos morbidity, mortality, and environmental studies of miners and millers. National Institute for Occupational Safety and Health, CDC, USPHS, Department of Health and Human Services, February 1980.

914. Rosenstock L, Cullen MB. *Textbook of Clinical Occupational and Environmental Medicine*. Philadelphia, PA: WB. Saunders Company; 1996.

915. IARC. Silica. In *Silica, Some Silicates, Coal Dust and Para-aramid Fibrils*. IARC Monographs on the Evaluation of Carcinogenic Risks to Humans, Vol. 68, International Agency for Research on Cancer, Lyon, FR; 1997: 41–242.

916. Dreessen WC. Effects of certain silicate dusts on the lungs. *J Ind Hyg* 1933;15(2):66–78.

917. Dreessen WC, Dalla Valle JM. The effects of exposure to dust in two Georgia talc mills and mines. *Publ Health Rep* 1935;50:131.

918. Siegal W, Smith AR, Greenburg L. The dust hazard in tremolite mining, including roentgenological findings in talc workers. *J Roentgenol Rad Ther* 1942;XLIX:11–29.

919. Siegal W, Smith A, Greenburg L. Study of talc miners and millers. *Ind Bull* 1943;22:3–12.

920. Kleinfeld M, Messite J, Tabershaw I. Talc pneumoconiosis. *AMA Arch. Ind. Health* 1955;12:66–72.

921. Kleinfeld M, Messite J, Zaki MH. Mortality experiences among talc workers: A follow-up study. *J Occup Med* 1974;16(5):345–349.

922. Lamm SH, Levine MS, Starr JA, Tirey S. Analysis of excess lung cancer risk in short-term employees. *Am J Epidemiol* 1988;127(6):1202–1209.

923. Thomas TL, Stewart PA. Mortality from lung cancer and respiratory disease among pottery workers exposed to silica and talc. *Am J Epidemiol* 1987;125(1):35–43.

924. Rubino GF, Scansetti G, Piolatto G, Romano CA. Mortality study of talc miners and millers. *J Occup Med* 1976;18(3):187–193.

925. Wergeland E, Andersen A, Baerheim A. Morbidity and mortality in talc-exposed workers. *Am J Ind Med* 1990;17(4):505–513.

926. IARC. IARC Monographs on the Evaluation of Carcinogenic Risks to Humans Overall Evaluations of Carcinogenicity: An Updating of IARC Monographs, Vois. 1–42, Supplement 7, International Agency for Research on Cancer, Lyon, France, 1987.

927. Montana Department of Environmental Quality. W.R. Grace File Review Summary. Chronological order of Events (CVID # 3726)—Montana State Governments (Mt.gov), updated October 26, 2009, Helena, MT; 2000.

928. Peipins LA, Lewin M, Campolucci S, et al. Radiographic abnormalities and exposure to asbestos-contaminated vermiculite in the community of Libby, Montana, USA. *Environ Health Perspect* 2003;111(14):1753–1759.

929. Lockey JE, Brooks SM, Jarabek AM, Khoury PR, McKay RT, Carson A, Morrison JA, Wiot JF, Spitz HB. Pulmonary changes after exposure to vermiculite contaminated with fibrous tremolite. *Am Rev Resp Dis* 1984;129(6):952–958.

930. Amandus HE, Wheeler R. The morbidity and mortality of vermiculite miners and millers exposed to tremolite-actinolite: Part 1, Exposure estimates. *Am J Ind Med* 1987;11(1):1–14.

931. McDonald JC, Harris J, Armstrong B. Mortality in a cohort of vermiculite miners exposed to fibrous amphibole in Libby, Montana. *Occup Environ Med* 2004;61(4):363–366.

932. McDonald JC, McDonald AD, Sebastien P, Moy K. Health of vermiculite miners exposed to trace amounts of fibrous tremolite. *Brit J Ind Med* 1988;45(9):630–634.

933. Hessel PA, Sluis-Cremer GK. Prediction equations for lung function in black industrial workers at Palabora Mining Company. *S Afr Med J* 1989;76(10):548–549.

934. Hessel PA, Sluis-Cremer GK. X-ray findings, lung function, and respiratory symptoms in black South African vermiculite workers. *Am J Ind Med* 1989;15(1):1–29.

935. Asbestos: Vermiculite. www.epa.gov/asbestos/verm.html, last accessed June 7, 2010. U.S. Environmental Protection Agency.

CHAPTER **6**

Asbestos and Carcinoma of the Lung

Douglas W. Henderson and James Leigh

CONTENTS

6.1 INTRODUCTORY COMMENTS ON ASBESTOS-RELATED LUNG CANCER

There is no doubt that asbestos—for example, amphibole asbestos such as crocidolite and amosite, and Canadian chrysotile—can cause lung cancer, most often in combination with cigarette smoke (causal coaction), and the International Agency for Research on Cancer has classified asbestos as a Group 1 carcinogen (i.e., a proven human carcinogen). It is also widely accepted that tobacco smoke and asbestos in combination play a more than additive causal role for lung cancer induction—that is, a synergistic effect by way of a multiplicative or submultiplicative interaction (see later discussion). Yet the criteria for causal attribution of lung cancer to asbestos have been beset with controversy for decades: disagreement has focused on the issue of whether asbestosis is an obligate precursor for assignment of causation or whether lung cancer can be attributed on the basis of cumulative asbestos exposure, with no requirement for asbestosis.[1] Recent reviews[2–5] have revisited this issue and at least two[2,4] concluded that asbestosis is the only "consistently reliable marker"[2] for asbestos-attributable lung cancer. This chapter concentrates on classic studies and recent literature on this subject.[*]

Further and more extensive discussion can be found in reviews by the present authors,[1,8–12] especially the extensive review in the journal *Pathology* in 2004[1]. This chapter is based in part on the more detailed discussion in Henderson et al.,[1] and it represents an update of the literature between 2004 and 2010. It also addresses the criticisms set forth by Cagle,[2] Gibbs et al.,[4] and Attanoos[5] on the cumulative exposure model and, specifically, the *Helsinki Criteria*.[13]

Deaths from lung cancer remain dominant among cancer deaths worldwide. In the United States alone, there were an estimated 160,390 deaths from lung cancer in 2007, and the incidence was estimated at 213,380 cases in 2006–2007.[14] Although lung cancer represents a multifactorial group of cancers in terms of causation, active cigarette smoking is the strongest causal factor by far in the general population: about 10%–15% of continuing smokers will develop lung cancer, but about 10% of lung cancers occur in lifelong nonsmokers.[14] Cigarette smoke is implicated in the causation of all four main histological types of lung cancer, with the strongest association for small cell carcinoma, followed by squamous cell carcinoma, with a lower but still elevated risk for adenocarcinoma.[15–17] Adenocarcinoma now represents the most common histological type of lung cancer in general, and among never smokers, the proportion of adenocarcinoma is as high as about 50%–70%.[14] In this context, epidermal growth factor receptor mutations are common in nonsmokers, whereas k-*ras* mutations (see later discussion), p53 transversion mutations and p16 promoter hypermethylation are more common in the cancers that occur among smokers.[14]

"Lung cancer" represents a multiphenotypic and multifactorial group of cancers. Other known or postulated causal factors include passive smoking,[16] air pollution, cooking fumes, inhalation of radon daughters and other radioactive substances, inhalation of asbestos fibers, exposure to heavy metals such as arsenic,[18] nutritional status, immune dysfunction, tuberculous infection, asthma and other chronic obstructive pulmonary diseases (COPDs), and finally, innate susceptibility to lung cancer (see Henderson et al.[1] and Chapter 4). Although cigarette smoking dominates the risk, the occurrence of lung cancer in any one individual in the general population involves potential or actual interactivity of multiple causal factors (e.g., tobacco smoke [direct and/or "second hand"], radon daughters, air pollution, and individual innate susceptibility to carcinogenesis by known lung carcinogens).

About 2%–12% or more of lung cancers can be related to occupational exposure to asbestos.[19–24] Alberg and Samet[25] estimated that approximately 90% of lung cancers are related to smoking, 9%–15% to occupational exposures, 10% to radon, and perhaps 1%–2% to air pollution. Axelson[26] has estimated that more than a quarter of all lung cancer cases in Sweden are related to occupational exposures. Similar proportions have been reported for Finland,[27] Norway,[28] and Denmark.[29]

---

[*] In this chapter, we have excluded meta-analyses of the asbestos-associated risk of lung cancer. As noted by Lemen,[6] meta-analysis was first envisioned as a technique to combine the findings in clinical trials, with comparability of study design and results. When data used for meta-analysis are beset with flaws such as major confounders and with heterogeneity between studies (as for lung cancer), the conclusions from the meta-analysis can be flawed. Blettner et al.[7] have commented along similar lines:

> ... Meta-analyses from published data are in general insufficient to calculate a pooled estimate since published estimates are based on heterogeneous populations, different study designs and mainly different statistical models [abstract] ... Meta-analyses using published data are, therefore, restricted and seldom useful to produce a valid quantitative estimate or to investigate exposure relations such as dose-response ... (p. 8).

For most occupational lung cancers, two or more carcinogens are implicated in the causation of the cancer, and for asbestos-related lung cancer, the two most frequent and important carcinogens are asbestos fibers and tobacco smoke—apart from innate susceptibility to either or both.[1] The synergistic interactivity between tobacco smoke and asbestos for the causation of lung cancer among asbestos workers stands in contrast to the singularity of asbestos in the causation of malignant mesothelioma worldwide.*

Asbestos-related lung cancer is substantially underrecognized in most industrialized nations. A ratio of about two "excess" lung cancers (observed minus expected) for each mesothelioma across cohorts of asbestos workers is widely cited (2:1).[21,32–35] In their study of East London asbestos factory workers for the years 1933–1980, Berry et al.[36] found a lung cancer–mesothelioma ratio of 1.55:1 on the basis of 232 lung cancer deaths versus 77 expected and 100 mesothelioma deaths. In 1995, Hutchings et al.[37] reported that asbestos exposure caused about equal numbers of "excess" deaths from lung cancer in the United Kingdom (~200; 749 observed, 549 expected) and mesothelioma (183) for the period 1968–1991—a ratio of 1.09:1 (see later discussion).

In its report on *Health and Safety Statistics*[38] for 2001, the Health and Safety Commission (HSC) in the United Kingdom commented that:

> ... In heavily exposed populations there have typically been at least as many, sometimes up to five times as many, excess lung cancers as there have been mesotheliomas. The ratio depends on a range of factors ... so one cannot be too precise about the overall ratio. A reasonable rule of thumb would be to allow for one or two extra lung cancers for each mesothelioma ... (HSC,[38] p. 101; see also the preceding HSC[39] report)

As an outcome of a general diminution of asbestos exposures over the years and changing smoking habits, the ratio is likely to decline to about 1:1 or less, taking into account the difference in the gradient of the dose–response line for asbestos-related lung cancer and mesothelioma.[37,38,40]

Nonetheless, the number of officially registered deaths from asbestos-induced diseases in the United Kingdom for the years 1929–1996 included 17,999 mesotheliomas ($M = 15,298$; $F = 2701$) and 1878 lung cancers—a lung cancer to mesothelioma ratio of about 0.1:1,[32] and this ratio was maintained with minor variation over the years 1988–2000 in figures published by the HSC, which acknowledged in its 2001 *Health and Safety Statistics* report that "... these figures [UK disablement awards for asbestos-related lung cancer] substantially underestimate the true extent of the disease."[38] Likewise, asbestos-related lung cancers were underrecognized in France before introduction of a compensation standard based on 10 or more years of occupational exposure.[41,42] Similar underrecognition occurs in Italy[43] and Japan.[44] There appears to be analogous underrecognition of asbestos-related lung cancers in New South Wales in Australia: as one example, the lung cancer–mesothelioma ratio in the 1998 Report of the New South Wales Dust Diseases Board was 0.09:1, on the basis of 96 mesotheliomas in comparison to nine "asbestos induced carcinomas of the lung."[1] Teschke and Barroetavena[45] also reported that lung cancer across British Columbia, Saskatchewan, and Ontario in Canada was undercompensated, mainly because of underrecognition and underreporting to compensation boards.

6.2 GENERAL CHARACTERISTICS OF ASBESTOS-ASSOCIATED LUNG CANCER

Apart from frequent but by no means invariable coexistence of benign tissue markers of asbestos exposure such as pleural plaques or diffuse pleural fibrosis, asbestos-related lung cancers show

---

* In the Cappadocian region of Turkey, fibrous erionite is a proven cause of mesothelioma,[30] and there is increasing evidence that radiation is implicated in the causation of a minority of mesotheliomas,[31] but each of these causes is dwarfed by the overwhelming importance of asbestos fibers, especially amphibole asbestos, for the causation of mesothelioma worldwide.

no clinical or pathologic differences from lung cancers in the general (and predominantly male) population. As stated by the HSC report on *Health and Safety Statistics 1998/99* for the United Kingdom:[39]

> ... There is no clinical feature by which lung cancers caused by asbestos can be definitively distinguished from cases in which asbestos has not been involved, and therefore many of these cases may not be recognized as asbestos related by the sufferers or by their doctors. (HSC,[39] p. 86)

- There appears to be no major difference in the proportion of peripheral versus central lung cancers in asbestos-exposed patients in comparison to those unexposed.[1,5] Paris et al.[46] found a trend toward a peripheral location for lung cancers in long-term ex-smokers (cessation for 10 years or more) with asbestos exposure (59%) versus those with no documented asbestos exposure (20%), but there were no significant differences in short-term ex-smokers (25% vs. 24%) or continuing smokers (33% vs. 26%).
- In the general population, upper lobe lung cancers predominate in a ratio of up to 2:1 or more. Although a predominance of lower lobe carcinomas among asbestos-exposed workers has been recorded,[47] no difference in the lobar distribution of lung cancer in asbestos workers was found in other studies. Lee et al.[48] found that lung cancers in asbestos-exposed individuals were located most often in the upper lobe; and in all three groups of asbestos-exposed patients studied by Roggli and Sanders[49] (asbestosis; plaques without asbestosis; neither plaques nor asbestosis), upper lobe cancers outnumbered lower lobe tumors in a ratio of almost 3:1.
- Asbestos-associated lung cancer incidence rates vary greatly from one occupational group to another. This heterogeneity is exemplified by the much greater lung cancer rate among the South Carolina (Charleston) asbestos textile workers than for the Quebec chrysotile miners and millers—although the Charleston textile workers used Canadian chrysotile almost exclusively.[50–52] The almost 30- to 50-fold difference in lung cancer risk[52,53] remains unexplained. The use of potentially carcinogenic oils in the Charleston textile industry, the coexistent exposure to amphibole asbestos fibers, and differences in fiber dimensions have all been mooted as potential explanations, but none has been proven responsible. For example, nested case-referent analysis of the Charleston cohort found no difference in risk for the use or nonuse of oils;[51,54] for those cases where lung tissue was available for analysis, the Quebec miners/millers actually had higher geometric mean counts for total amphibole fibers (tremolite + amosite/crocidolite) than the Charleston workers;[55] and fiber analysis did not find any significant differences in the dimensions of the amphibole fibers.[1,55–57]
- For asbestos-exposed patients with pleural plaques as the only tissue marker of past exposure or whose estimated cumulative exposure is small, the increase in the relative risk for lung cancer (RR_{LCA}) may be small (less than 1.5) after allowance for other factors such as tobacco smoke.[58–60] Cullen et al.[61] reported an RR_{LCA} of 1.91 for radiographic pleural abnormalities in the form of bilateral pleural thickening or plaques with or without calcification (95% confidence interval [CI] = 1.25–1.92), but this finding clearly did not separate out the risk for radiographically detected plaques alone as opposed to diffuse pleural thickening.
- The RR_{LCA} in asbestos-exposed populations is greater when cases of asbestosis are present than for analogous worker groups without identifiable cases of asbestosis,[62] and higher RRs for lung cancer are recorded for patients with progressive asbestosis than for those with clinically static asbestosis.[63] According to the cumulative exposure model for lung cancer induction by asbestos,[1] asbestosis is primarily a marker for substantial to heavy asbestos exposure, and the severity of asbestosis generally correlates with the fiber load in lung tissue,[64] accounting for the greater RR_{LCA} (see later discussion).

Roggli and Sanders[49] reported a study on the asbestos body (AB) and asbestos fiber content of lung tissue in 234 cases of lung cancer with "some history of asbestos exposure." The median AB and the total asbestos fiber content for fibers 5 μm or longer—mainly commercial amphiboles and primarily amosite—were >35 and 20 times higher, respectively, for 70 patients with histological asbestosis than for 44 patients with pleural plaques in the absence of asbestosis and 300 and 50 times higher, respectively, than the AB/fiber content for 120 patients without plaques or asbestosis (for whom the median AB/fiber content was about 28 and 8 times greater, respectively, than the control group). The median AB and the uncoated fiber counts for the plaque-only group were about 245 and >23 times greater, respectively, than the control group. There was overlap in the counts for ABs and fibers between all three noncontrol groups.

- Most lung cancers in asbestos workers—but by no means not all—develop in continuing smokers or ex-smokers, and there is a well-known synergy between cigarette smoke and asbestos for the causation of lung cancer, so that the combined effect is greater than the sum of the individual effects of tobacco smoke and asbestos (causal coaction; see following discussion). In epidemiologic studies, cigarette smoke is thus an important confounder and effect-modifying factor that needs to be considered in the evaluation of the causal role of asbestos for the development of lung cancer.[*] Likewise, it has been shown repeatedly that the cigarette smoke-related risk of lung cancer declines after cessation of smoking, and this too requires adjustment.[15,65,66] In the 1991 study on New Orleans asbestos cement workers reported by Hughes and Weill,[67] 25% were ex-smokers and 52% were current smokers. In a 2002 study of 214 asbestos workers in the United States, Osinubi et al.[68] found that 61 were never smokers (28.5%), 118 were ex-smokers (55%), and 35 were continuing smokers (approximately 16.5%): presumably, the high proportion of never smokers and ex-smokers (83.5%) reflects the success of smoking awareness and cessation campaigns over recent years in the general population.

6.3 SYNERGY BETWEEN CIGARETTE SMOKE AND ASBESTOS FOR THE CAUSATION OF LUNG CANCER: HUMAN AND EXPERIMENTAL EVIDENCE

Cigarette smoke and asbestos are thought to be complex carcinogens that can affect multiple steps in the multistage process of carcinogenesis[69] and to interact synergistically for the induction of lung cancer.[70] The composite effect among insulation workers and as derived from case-referent studies approximates a multiplicative model—which has been accepted by many authorities[16,69,71] for about the last 30 years.

The multiplicative model is exemplified in the following passage of text from a chapter by Gong and Christiani[71] on lung cancer, in a textbook on occupational lung diseases:

Both smoking and asbestos are highly relevant to the risk of developing lung cancer, and in an interactive (multiplicative) fashion. For the average individual in this population, smoking increased the risk of lung cancer by about 10-fold, and asbestos increased the risk by about 5-fold; the two together increased the risk by about 50-fold not 15-fold, compared with that of the nonsmokers who were unexposed to asbestos. If the figure of 53 is used to quantify the actual average risk in a smoker with asbestos exposure, its components are 1 for the base risk, 10 (10.85−1) for the smoking risk, 4 (5.17−1) for the asbestos risk, and 38 (53−1−10−4) for the risk that depends on the interaction between smoking and asbestos. It is readily evident that the interaction is of major importance.

Even so, there has been discussion in the literature concerning the relationship between cigarette smoking and asbestos for the induction of lung cancer, and the multiplicative model has been called into question. For example, Liddell[72] and Liddell and Armstrong[73] argue that a multiplicative model does not fit most data sets, whereas Lee[74] argues in support of the multiplicative model. As mentioned, the model that emerges from most case-referent studies and for insulation workers is a multiplicative interaction, whereas (according to Liddell and Armstrong[73]) the effect for the Quebec chrysotile miners/millers appears to approximate an additive effect (in an additive model, there is no interactive effect). According to Liddell,[72] one consequence of departure from a multiplicative model is that the RR_{LCA} from asbestos exposure is "about twice as high in nonsmokers [than] in smokers," and in a later analysis Berry and Liddell[75] concluded that the "... excess relative risk of lung cancer from asbestos exposure is about three times higher in nonsmokers than in smokers."

---

[*] A factor can be both a confounder and an effect modifier: it is treated as a confounder when one does not want to consider it as part of the cause–effect inference, and as an effect modifier when one does. This is the key medicolegal problem of asbestos/smoking in lung cancer.

However, data for the Quebec cohort are not relevant to, or appropriate for, assessment of amphibole or mixed amphibole–chrysotile exposures—such as mixed-fiber end-use exposures, for example, in the building construction industry—or for chrysotile textile workers.

In subsequent correspondence, it appears that Lee[76] and Liddell[77] are not as far apart from each other as might seem at first: there appears to be agreement that even if the joint effect is less than multiplicative (i.e., submultiplicative), an additive model does not fit most data sets, so that most authorities acknowledge that there is an interactive supra-additive effect between cigarette smoke and asbestos for lung cancer induction. Erren et al.[78] estimated that the excess lung cancer risk from simultaneous exposures to asbestos and tobacco smoke was greater than the sum of the two separate risks by a factor of 1.64. By definition and in biological terms, the interactive effect cannot be separated out or fractionated into the individual effects, although this is sometimes done mathematically (and artificially) for apportionment modeling.[9]

The exact mechanisms that underpin the synergy between tobacco smoke and asbestos for lung cancer induction are not fully understood. At least four mechanisms have been proposed as potential explanations, of which the two most likely appear to be the following[1,5,10]:

- Carcinogens in cigarette smoke such as benzo[a]pyrene may be adsorbed onto asbestos fibers (e.g., crocidolite or chrysotile), with subsequent delivery of the carcinogens into cells at high concentration.[79]
- Tobacco smoke may interfere with the clearance of asbestos from the lungs. Churg and Stevens[80] found elevated concentrations of asbestos fibers in the airway tissues of smokers in comparison to nonsmokers, for both amosite (~6-fold) and chrysotile (~50-fold), especially for short fibers (in comparison, parenchymal amosite fiber concentrations were comparable in the smoker and non-smoker groups).

In this chapter, we have omitted systematic discussion of data from in vivo experiments on animals such as rats for several reasons[10]: (i) there is known to be marked variation between species in their susceptibility to carcinogenesis mediated by asbestos, with humans about 100 times more susceptible than rats.[81,82] Apart from obvious genetic differences, the greater susceptibility of humans than rats may be explicable by anatomical differences of the upper respiratory passages; for example, rats are obligate nose breathers whereas humans when exerted are often mouth breathers. (ii) The airborne asbestos fiber concentrations used in animal experiments were many, many times greater than those for most if not all workplace circumstances for humans—so that fibrosis was an inevitable accompaniment of experimental exposures,[83–85] although Pott[86] considered that neoplasia and fibrosis seemed to be the end points of two independent pathways. (iii) The histological spectrum of lung tumors in rats, for example, is different from humans. Finally, to the best of our knowledge, (iv) many of the experimental studies carried out in the past did not investigate the combined effect of asbestos fiber and cigarette smoke inhalation[81] (see also Chapter 4).

However, recent in vivo and in vitro experiments have supported the epidemiologic evidence concerning the synergy in humans between asbestos and carcinogens known to be present in tobacco smoke:

- In 1993, Kimizuka et al.[87] investigated the co-carcinogenic effects of chrysotile and amosite asbestos with the tobacco smoke carcinogen benzo[a]pyrene (B[a]P) in hamster lungs. Between 18 and 24 months after the last instillation, the number of tumors was examined: in the chrysotile + B[a]P group, there were 37 tumors that included 16 carcinomas in 12 animals; and 30 tumors, including 11 carcinomas, in 12 animals were found in the amosite + B[a]P group. In the chrysotile + B[a]P group, all animals developed tumors, as did 92% in the amosite + B[a]P group: carcinomas were found in 83% and 67%, respectively. The numbers of tumors and carcinomas and the frequency of the tumor-bearing or carcinoma-bearing hamsters in the chrysotile + B[a]P and the amosite + B[a]P groups were significantly higher than those of the groups injected independently. Although the number of tumors or the frequency of tumor-bearing animals was higher in the chrysotile + B[a]P than the amosite + B[a]P group, the differences were not significant. The results were considered to indicate that both chrysotile and amosite can play an important role in the genesis of bronchogenic carcinoma.

- Harrison et al.[88] investigated the combined effect in the lungs of rats of simultaneous exposure to chrysotile asbestos and N-nitrosoheptamethyleneimine (NHMI) for the development of metaplastic, hyperplastic, and neoplastic lesions. The effects were more pronounced in males than in females and NHMI administration increased the frequency of hyperplastic lesions with augmentation by chrysotile (although this was not statistically significant), but a "promoting" effect of chrysotile was observed for the induction of lung tumors (all but two out of 11 primary tumors were in rats treated with both NHMI and chrysotile)—although this finding was not confirmable statistically because of the small number of tumors observed.

- Kamp et al.[89] found evidence that cigarette smoke extracts (CSEs) augmented amosite asbestos-induced alveolar epithelial cell injury by generating iron-induced free radicals that damage DNA. In this study,[89] amosite or CSE each resulted in dose–dependent toxicity to alveolar epithelial cells (WI-26 and rat alveolar type I-like cells), and the effects of CSE + amosite in combination were synergistic in A549 cells and additive in WI-26 cells. The authors[89] concluded that the data provided further support to the effect that asbestos and cigarette smoke are genotoxic to relevant target cells in the lung and that iron-induced free radicals may in part cause these effects.

- Loli et al.[90] investigated the mutagenic effects of amosite asbestos and B[a]P in the lungs of λ-lacI rats. In the first experiment, intratracheal instillation of both amosite and B[a]P in combination resulted in a supra-additive increase in mutation frequency in comparison to rats treated only with amosite or B[a]P. In the second experiment, intraperitoneal administration of B[a]P did not alter significantly the mutation frequency induced by amosite after either four or 16 weeks of treatment, and B[a]P-DNA adduct levels were unaffected by amosite co-treatment in both experiments. The authors concluded that the "… striking enhancement effect of B[a]P may provide a basis for understanding the suspected [sic] synergism of smoking on asbestos carcinogenesis." This group[91] also reported that DNA adducts induced by simultaneous B[a]P and man-made mineral fibers (MMMF) indicated a strong increase in the mutation frequency.

In addition, molecular studies in humans have suggested that "… asbestos enhances the mutagenicity of tobacco carcinogens and that it acts, at least in part, independent[ly] of the tissue damage responsible for fibrosis."[79] Nelson et al.[92] investigated k-ras codon 12 mutations among 84 male patients with adenocarcinoma of the lung for whom a work history was available, as well as a chest radiograph for all those who had a history of occupational exposure to asbestos. k-ras mutations were more prevalent in the patients with a history of occupational asbestos exposure (crude odds ratio [OR] = 4.8, 95% CI = 1.5–15.4) in comparison to those without asbestos exposure. The association remained after adjustment for age and pack-years smoked (adjusted OR = 6.9, 95% CI = 1.7–28.6). An index score that weighted for both the dates of exposure and its estimated intensity indicated that subjects with k-ras mutations had significantly greater asbestos exposures than those without such mutations ($p < .01$). A supra-additive effect of smoking and asbestos exposure on the percentage of k-ras mutations was shown (Fig. 2 in the original). The duration of exposure was not associated with k-ras mutations, but the time after initial exposure was significantly associated with mutation status. "The association between k-ras mutation and reported asbestos exposure was not dependent on the presence of radiographic evidence of asbestos-related disease."[92] The findings were considered to suggest "… that asbestos exposure increases the likelihood of mutation at k-ras codon 12 and that this process occurs independently of the induction of interstitial fibrosis."[92] In an earlier study, the same group of researchers[93] also found that asbestos exposure ($p < .01$) and a duration of more than 50 years of smoking ($p < .01$) were significantly associated with exon deletion from the fragile histidine triad (FHIT) gene.

6.4 LATENCY INTERVALS BETWEEN ASBESTOS EXPOSURE AND LUNG CANCER

Asbestos-related lung cancers are neoplasms of long latency, like mesothelioma. Menegozzo et al.[94] found that excess lung cancer mortality was "especially pronounced" at latency times longer than 10 years in a study of insulation workers in Italy. For workers producing asbestos-containing insulation materials, of whom 77% were employed for less than 2 years, Nicholson et al.[95] reported an elevated lung cancer relative risk that occurred within 10 years and then remained constant over the period of observation. On the basis of additional data for 17,800 U.S. insulation workers, they[95] stated the lung cancer risk develops independently of age and preexisting risk, and an increased lung cancer rate was detectable earlier for those workers first exposed in older age than those whose exposures commenced when young. Using pooled data from two German case-referent studies, Hauptmann et al.[96] calculated the effect of an increment of asbestos exposure on the OR for lung cancer (OR_{LCA}) was greatest at 10–15 years after that exposure and then declined if such exposure had ceased.

6.5 ASBESTOSIS AND LUNG CANCER: THE FIBROSIS–CANCER HYPOTHESIS

Lung cancer in asbestos workers was first recorded in anecdotal individual case reports as an autopsy finding in those with asbestosis (see Chapter 1). Lung cancer in association with any degree of asbestosis was subsequently declared a compensable disease in Germany in 1943[97] (see Chapter 1). This association was later reestablished by Doll[98] in 1955. Subsequently, a longstanding controversy arose as to whether it is the asbestosis itself that confers the increased risk/occurrence of lung cancer (designated as *the fibrosis–cancer model* in following discussion in this chapter; the *obligate precursor model*), as opposed to the bronchopulmonary burden of asbestos fibers with no requirement for asbestosis (*the cumulative exposure model*). Proponents of the fibrosis–cancer model seem divided among themselves on this issue: Hughes and Weill,[67] Churg,[99,100] and Gibbs et al.[4] argue that it is the process and occurrence of inflammation and interstitial fibrosis induced by asbestos fibers that are responsible, whereas Cagle[2] expresses agnosticism on this issue but argues that asbestosis is the only "consistent and reliable" marker for asbestos exposure of sufficient magnitude to increase significantly the risk of lung cancer. The fibrosis–cancer approach appears to be based on the following observations, at least four epidemiologic studies, as well as reviews on this issue by Weiss:[62,101]

- Nonasbestosis interstitial pulmonary fibrosis itself is accompanied by an increased risk/frequency of lung cancer (see later discussion).
- There is universal (or at least near-universal) scientific/medical agreement that clinical–radiographic asbestosis delineates at least a two- to five-fold or greater increase in the risk of lung cancer.[102]
- The radiographic–histologic study on deaths from lung cancer among insulation workers reported by Kipen et al.[103] Among 450 deaths from lung cancer, a chest radiograph suitable for assessment of pneumoconiosis was available for 219 cases; among those, 138 had sufficient nonneoplastic lung tissue for the assessment of fibrosis and all had evidence of parenchymal fibrosis, although there was no radiographic indication of fibrosis in 18% (cf. Hughes and Weill[67]).
- The autopsy study on amphibole miners in South Africa reported by Sluis-Cremer and Bezuidenhout[104]: Blacks were excluded from this study, which dealt with 399 autopsies (among 1165 deaths). Of 35 cases of lung cancer, 24 were associated with asbestosis, and there were 11 cases in men without asbestosis (all smokers). Standardized proportional mortality rates (SPMRs) were elevated in men with "slight" asbestosis (15 cases observed [O] vs. 3.6 expected [E]: SPMR = 416.7), and the SPMR was 562.5 for those with moderate to pronounced asbestosis (O/E = 9/1.6). The SPMR was 88.7 for 302 men without asbestosis (O/E = 11/12.4).
- The prospective chest x-ray–based study of 839 New Orleans asbestos cement factory workers reported by Hughes and Weill[67] in 1991. Of those who had died, the cause of death was coded from death certificates (153 cases). Radiographic lung opacities were used as the marker for asbestosis according to the International Labor Organization (ILO) classification for the pneumoconioses. For lung cancer, those with small opacities had a standardized mortality ratio (SMR) of 177.5 (O/E = 4/2.3), and the SMR was 432.5 for those with a chest x-ray ILO score of ≥1/0 (O/E = 9/2.1). There was no elevation of the SMR for those with no radiographic evidence of asbestosis (12 cases in all, including two with pleural abnormalities only). These authors[67] concluded that an "... excess risk of lung cancer was restricted to workers with x-ray film evidence of asbestosis, a finding consistent

with the view that asbestos is a lung carcinogen because of its fibrogenicity." The Hughes–Weill[67] study found no excess of lung cancer among asbestos cement workers "... without radiologically detectable asbestosis, even among long-term workers ... ." Gibbs et al.[4] commented that a subsequent review of the literature published in 1996[105] suggested that the "... weight of the scientific evidence ..." supported the conclusion that the "... excess risk of lung cancer was limited to those workers who had radiographic [i.e., chest x-ray] evidence of asbestosis." Weill was an author for all three publications[4,67,105]—so that this conclusion seems unsurprising. In contrast, we consider that the current "weight of scientific evidence" militates *against* the requirement of radiographic asbestosis, or asbestosis per se no matter how diagnosed (see later discussion).

- The study reported by Camus et al.[106] on lung cancer deaths (SMRs) among women 30 years or older with nonoccupational (environmental) asbestos exposure in two chrysotile mining areas of Quebec: The estimated mean exposure was 25 fibers/mL-years (fiber-years)* within a range of 5–125. The lung cancer SMR was 0.99 (95% CI = 0.78–1.25).
- In his most recent review, Weiss[62] supported the fibrosis–cancer model and concluded that "asbestosis is a much better predictor of excess lung cancer risk than measures of exposure and serves as a marker for attributable cases."
- Essentially, rejection of those epidemiologic studies that have shown an increased risk of lung cancer for asbestos-exposed workers without evidence of asbestosis.

The limitations of the three epidemiologic studies summarized above are discussed below, and Hessel et al.[3] have addressed the strengths and weakness of both the Sluis-Cremer and Bezuidenhout[104] and the Hughes–Weill[67] studies.

- The Kipen et al.[103] study: The asbestosis status by radiology and histology was unknown for 69% of the deaths in this study, and the histological diagnosis was made in the absence of detectable asbestos bodies in 6% of the cases.
- Sluis-Cremer and Bezuidenhout[104]: Hessel et al.[3] consider the strengths of this study to include histological confirmation of the diagnosis of lung cancer and asbestosis and well-documented occupational, medical, and smoking histories. The weaknesses include the selectivity of the cases that came to autopsy (399 cases [34%] out of 1165 deaths, blacks excluded). Henderson et al.[8] have also pointed out that the criteria used for the grading of asbestosis in this study are strange and do not correspond to existing systems of grading, or to standard terminology for the description of asbestosis (e.g., Sluis-Cremer and Bezuidenhout[104] referred to "organization of alveolar spaces" as one of the histological findings, but this is not generally acknowledged as one of the characteristic features of asbestosis; instead, it raises the issue of the organizing pneumonia that is common in patients with lung cancer, either distal to the cancer as a consequence of bronchial obstruction or as a more generalized terminal event). In addition, Sluis-Cremer and Bezuidenhout[107] later acknowledged that—when a multivariate logistic regression was carried out to allow for the grade of asbestosis—duration of exposure (the most accurately measurable parameter of cumulative exposure) accounted for most of the variation, although the grade of asbestosis remained a significant risk factor.
- The Hughes–Weill[67] study: Although extraordinary significance has been assigned to this study (in part because it was prospective), it has major limitations, as discussed by Henderson et al.[1,8,10] and Hessel et al.[3] There were only 25 lung cancer deaths in all: 10 in those with no lung abnormalities, 2 in those with pleural abnormalities only, and 13 in those with small opacities (4 in those with an ILO score of 0/1 and nine with a score of ≥1/0). Therefore, the Hughes–Weill study had "... very low power ..."[3] to answer the question that it sought to answer; only a few changes in the small numbers of lung cancers in each of the exposure groups (e.g., between 0/1 and ≥1/0) would have changed the result.[3] In addition, there were more smokers among those with small opacities than those without[3] (the presence of small opacities ≥1/0 was related not only to cumulative asbestos exposure but also to smoking, age, and the plant where the workers worked).

---

* Calculated by multiplying the average airborne asbestos fiber concentration as measured or estimated as fibers/mL, by the duration in years over which the exposure occurred, usually on the basis of a standard working year of 1920 h: 25 fiber-years would correspond to 5 fibers/mL over 5 years or 1 fiber/mL over 25 years.

- The Camus et al.[106] study: Taking into account the low lung cancer risk for the Quebec miners and millers in comparison to other industries, it seems unsurprising that this study yielded a null result. The authors[106] also pointed out that this study had low statistical power to detect small risks.
- The 1999 Weiss[62] review: This selective review of the literature—which excluded case-referent studies, autopsy-based investigations, and fiber burden analysis— "… supported the view that excess lung cancer risk occurs only among those cohorts where asbestosis also occurs," with the conclusion that asbestosis "… serves as a marker for attributable cases." This review[62] was the subject of critical editorial comment[108] in the journal where it appeared and, later, by Henderson et al.[1] The criticisms included the following:

   a) Weiss[62] referred to a lung cancer SMR of 3.11 for Quebec miners/millers with small opacities in chest radiographs. Banks et al.[108] pointed out that the SMR was also elevated at 3.30 in workers with radiographic abnormalities other than small opacities, and 11 of the 37 cases this in group had a large opacity, which is not a feature of asbestosis.

   b) Henderson et al.[1] also emphasized the following: "Weiss[62] cited one study[109] with data on the association between cumulative asbestosis and excess lung cancer mortality rates, which recorded an excess lung cancer death rate of 8.48 per 1000 among 884 workers with light/moderate exposure lasting ≤2 years—an exposure unlikely to be sufficient to induce clinical asbestosis, so that the asbestosis death rate was zero. The figure of 8.48/thousand was based on 24 lung cancer deaths observed minus 16.5 expected, which equates to 7.5/884 workers (SMR = 1.45, 95% CI = 0.93–2.16). Weiss[62] claimed that this "… small excess lung cancer death rate … is not statistically significantly different from no excess … ." However, if one theorizes that the asbestos-attributable *excess* lung cancer death rate is zero when there is no asbestos exposure—a zero exposure, zero effect model—and notes that the excess lung cancer death rate in the same study[109] was 19.49/1000 among those with light/moderate exposure lasting >2 years, when the asbestosis death rate was 3.61, then a trend to an increase in lung cancer SMR is evident even at light/moderate exposures of ≤2 years (no asbestosis): X_1^2 (trend) = 163.9, $p \ll .005$.[110]"

   c) Like Banks et al.,[108] Henderson et al.[1] also commented that the finding of increased rates of lung cancer in cohorts where asbestosis also occurs does not equate to *seriatim* occurrence of asbestosis and lung cancer in the *same* individual (i.e., the asbestosis and the lung cancers may affect different workers). In other words, this observation is equally explicable by a dose–response effect for each of asbestosis and lung cancer in worker groups with substantial asbestos exposure, without an obligate fibrosis–cancer sequence.

6.6 THE OCCURRENCE OF LUNG CANCER IN THE SETTING OF NONASBESTOS INTERSTITIAL LUNG DISEASE AND COPD

One of the seemingly stronger pieces of evidence in favor of the requirement for asbestosis to assign causation of lung cancer to asbestos is the occurrence of lung cancer in patients with diffuse interstitial lung disease (DILD) unrelated to asbestos exposure, such as idiopathic usual interstitial pneumonia (UIP)—also known as idiopathic pulmonary fibrosis (IPF) or cryptogenic fibrosing alveolitis (CFA).[5,100] In this context, Harris et al.[111] set forth a tabular summary of 14 clinical and autopsy case series where the prevalence of lung cancer in the setting of CFA varied from zero (0/42 cases of IPF at autopsy[112]) to 48%.[113] The corresponding figure for asbestosis is about 25%–50%.[5,114]

The high figure of 48% (40 of 83 UIP cases) was reported by Matsushita et al.[113] in a series of 3712 autopsies over a period of 20 years (1972–1992). In 15% of the UIP-associated lung cancers, there were multiple carcinomas. However, in this series, the UIP cancers were strongly associated with smoking, and only one of the UIP-related cancers was found in a nonsmoker. The rates for heavy smoking (>40 pack-years) were 74% for the UIP cases with lung cancer, 51% for lung cancers without UIP, 38.5% for UIP cases without cancer, and 27% for the control group. The authors[113] concluded that: "… smoking habit, especially heavy smoking, is one of the most important risk factors in developing lung cancer in UIP … smoking may also have an important role in the pathogenesis of UIP itself" (see below).

In another study from Japan, Nagai et al.[115] reported lung cancer in 38% of subjects with diffuse interstitial fibrosis who were smokers and in 11% of those who were nonsmokers (again indicating that smoking is an important confounding factor for assessment of the association between chronic DILD and lung cancer). In the study reported by Nagai et al.,[115] 88% of the tumors were peripheral in location, and the diagnosis in 27 of the 31 cases (87%) was established by transbronchial biopsy. However, in small transbronchial biopsies, the distinction between genuine lung cancer and reactive bronchioloalveolar epithelial proliferation as part of the interstitial disease is often problematic.

In a later study from Japan on multiple lung cancers associated with IPF,[116] 23 synchronous multiple lung cancers were observed among 154 lung cancer patients with associated IPF and 131 had a single lung cancer. However, in both the IPF-associated single and the multiple lung cancer groups, most tumors were observed in male patients (91% and 96%, respectively), and 94% and 100%, respectively, were smokers. Most of the tumors were found in the peripheral regions of the lung (91% and 98%, respectively). It was noted that the frequency of small cell carcinoma was significantly higher in the IPF-multiple lung cancer group (33%) in comparison with the IPF-associated single lung cancer group (14%) and the entire lung cancer group (12%). As mentioned above, it is known that the causal relationship between tobacco smoking and lung cancer is strongest for small cell carcinoma followed by squamous cell carcinoma.[17]

Other authors have commented on the inconsistency of the reported frequencies for the development of lung cancer in the setting of interstitial lung disease.[117]

In one of the first reports on the association between CFA and lung cancer, Turner-Warwick et al.[118] found lung cancer in 20 of 205 patients with CFA (9.8%) or 12.9% of the 155 patients who were followed to death. These authors reported a lung cancer RR of 14.1 for the patients with CFA in comparison to the general population of comparable age and gender, taking into account the lengths of follow-up of the CFA patients. The RR_{LCA} for male smokers with CFA (15 observed in comparison to 1.06 expected) was 14.2, and for nonsmokers there was only one case of lung cancer observed in comparison to 0.1 expected. For female smokers, two cases were found in comparison to 0.3 expected, giving an RR_{LCA} of 6.7. However, only one male and one female nonsmoker developed lung cancer. These authors[118] suggested there was an excess risk of lung cancer that was not entirely accounted for by age, sex, or smoking habit.

In a further series of cases reported from France,[119] 7 (25%) of 28 cases with diffuse interstitial fibrosis died from lung caner. The authors[119] found that the cancers were more often peripheral in distribution and lower lobe in location than for cases of lung cancer without pulmonary fibrosis.

In 2004, Abrahams et al.[120] recorded the frequency of primary pulmonary neoplasms among 214 lung transplant patients in the United States. Lung transplantation was most often carried out for emphysema, followed by cystic fibrosis and primary pulmonary hypertension; and there were 26 cases with UIP. Four neoplasms were found in explanted lungs among the entire group, representing a prevalence of 2%; and three out of the four cancers were found in the setting of emphysema. Adenocarcinoma was the most common cell type.

In 2010, Harris et al.[111] reported on the British Thoracic Society study on 588 cases of CFA, 11 years after entry into the cohort (the largest study on this issue of which we are aware). Four hundred eighty-eight patients had died (83%) and 46 (9%) were certified as having lung cancer. The SMR was 7.4 (95% CI = 5.4–9.9). Stratified analysis demonstrated increased lung cancer mortality among younger subjects, men, and ever smokers. From review by an independent expert panel, 25 patients (4%) were considered to have had at least moderate exposure to asbestos, with a lung cancer SMR of 13.1 (95% CI = 3.6–33.6) in comparison with 7.2 (95% CI = 5.2–9.7) for those with less or no asbestos exposure. Ever smoking was reported for 448 cases (73%). Most patients who died from lung cancer were men (87%), and all but two (96%) were ever smokers. The authors[111] concluded the findings confirmed an association between CFA and lung cancer "… although this relationship may not be causal … [the] … high rate of smoking and evidence that smokers present for medical attention earlier than nonsmokers suggests that smoking could be confounding this association."

It is also worth emphasizing that tobacco smoke is increasingly recognized as a causal factor for interstitial fibrosis,[121–124] yet few authorities would require tobacco smoke-related interstitial fibrosis (or COPD) as a requirement for causal attribution of lung cancer to tobacco smoke. In this context, numerous reports now link COPD with an increased risk of lung cancer after adjustment for other known causal factors, most notably tobacco smoking.[125–130] For example, Gao et al.[131] found that a family history of chronic bronchitis or pneumonia was associated with (i) an increased OR_{LCA} of 1.49 (95% CI = 1.23–1.80) for the chronic bronchitis group and (ii) a decreased OR_{LCA} of 0.73 (95% CI = 0.61–0.87) for the pneumonia group. In this context, a background of COPD as an independent variable for RR_{LCA} does not negate a causal relationship between asbestos and lung cancer. If this association is causal, it means only that an additional causal factor for lung cancer may be identifiable in some asbestos-exposed individuals who also smoked.

As reviewed by Henderson et al.,[1] there is increasing evidence for innate susceptibility to the induction of lung cancer by carcinogens such as tobacco smoke and asbestos, and a family history of lung cancer is an established risk factor. [131] After adjustment for smoking, Gao et al.[131] reported that the OR_{LCA} for a family history of lung cancer in a father, mother, or sibling was 1.41, 2.14, and 1.53, respectively. Ishikawa and Kohno,[132] on the basis of experimental studies on a mouse model, concluded that genetic factors seem to be involved in the pathogenesis of lung cancer in the setting of ILD (see Chapter 4).

Accordingly, the occurrence of lung cancer in the setting of diffuse ILD is less clear and is more problematic than has been claimed; and tobacco smoking appears to be an important confounding factor concerning this relationship.

6.7 THE ANATOMIC DISTRIBUTION OF ASBESTOSIS AND ASBESTOS-RELATED LUNG CANCERS

A major problem concerning the fibrosis–cancer hypothesis is the simple pathologic observation that the interstitial fibrosis of asbestosis affects distal lung tissues, beginning in the subpleural and bronchiolar zones, whereas the lung cancers among asbestos workers, including those with asbestosis, are frequently bronchus centered—so that there is an anatomic disjunction between asbestosis and lung cancer.[1,5,10,133] This disjunction is difficult to explain in terms of reactive oxygen species (ROS) and other free radicals and cytokines implicated in lung cancer induction as a consequence of the interaction between asbestos fibers and lung macrophages as part of asbestosis (i.e., the fibrosis–cancer model would invoke an inverse spatial relationship whereby ROS and other factors implicated in lung carcinogenesis would have a greater carcinogenic effect at presumably lower concentrations than at the sites where they are generated).

In contrast, the anatomic distribution of lung cancers among asbestos workers who were smokers appears to correlate with the differential concentrations of asbestos fibers. As mentioned previously, Churg and Stevens[80] found elevated concentrations of asbestos fibers in the airway tissues of smokers in comparison to nonsmokers, for both amosite and chrysotile, especially for short fibers; whereas parenchymal amosite fiber concentrations were comparable in the smoker and nonsmoker groups.

6.8 IS ASBESTOSIS A "CONSISTENT AND RELIABLE" MARKER FOR ATTRIBUTION OF LUNG CANCER TO ASBESTOS?

Our response to this rhetorical question is in the negative for early-stage asbestosis as encountered in the 21st century, which may be asymptomatic and not associated with significant impairment of lung function.[64]

As noted by Craighead[64] in 2008, "… the classical description of the overt, severe disease [asbestosis] … is largely of historical interest. Now the pathologist and clinician are challenged to diagnose a disease of only microscopical proportions that ... results in minimal symptomatology and little if any disability.... Rarely are these lesions ... evident radiologically, and symptoms attributable to asbestos disease are either not present or are obscured by underlying chronic obstructive pulmonary disease consequent to smoking."

Most cases of asbestosis are established on clinical and radiological grounds—as opposed to histological examination of lung tissue—as assessed by the following[134]:

1. A background of past asbestos exposure, usually moderate to heavy and typically but not invariably occupational in character, and often protracted over many years.
2. Clinical signs of interstitial fibrosis in the form of end-inspiratory crackles on auscultation of the lung fields, especially over the lower zones.
3. Detection of reticular-linear diffuse opacities in the lower zones of the lung fields on radiological examination.
4. Classically, restrictive impairment of lung function.
5. Usually, but not always, associated parietal pleural fibrous plaques and/or diffuse pleural fibrosis.

In an update for the diagnostic criteria for asbestosis published in 2010, Roggli et al.[134] commented that the first and third of these criteria are essential for the clinical diagnosis, especially when supported by the fifth. However, if one or more of criteria 5, 2, or 4 (in declining order of importance) are unfulfilled, the confidence index for the diagnosis declines correspondingly.

In relation to chest radiographs for the diagnosis of asbestosis, Peric et al.[135] reported a study of 210 workers with asbestos-related disorders whereby the radiographs were interpreted by two radiologists independently, according to the ILO classification. There was a 27% variation in agreement for the size of the changes and a 42% variation for their profusion. These authors commented that their study had "... revealed a significant disagreement in the estimated degree of pleural and parenchymal asbestos pulmonary disease."[*]

Adams and Crane[137] commented that: "In a study ... of histopathologically proven cases of asbestosis, plain chest radiographic findings were suggestive of asbestosis in only 11 of 25 cases. ... In addition to underdetection of asbestosis, plain chest radiographs may also result in overdiagnosis of asbestosis due to obscuration of the pulmonary parenchyma by overlying pleural plaques, diffuse pleural thickening and even extrapleural fat deposits."

The same authors[137] commented further that even high-resolution CT (HRCT) "... is not infallible. None of the HRCT signs of asbestosis are diagnostic," and they can occur as either isolated or combined abnormalities in disorders other than asbestosis.

Roggli et al.[134] commented:

Asbestosis typically presents with small irregular opacities at the lung bases. As the disease progresses these opacities coalesce and become more coarse leading to a honeycomb pattern of small cysts. Association with pleural plaques increases the specificity of the diagnosis. However, there are significant problems associated with the chest radiograph and the diagnosis of asbestos associated complications. The chest radiograph is normal in 10–18% of patients with biopsy proven asbestosis and at least 10% of pleural disease is not identified. It is estimated that the positive predictive value for an abnormal chest radiograph alone is approximately 40%. The positive predictive value may be lower if the prevalence of asbestosis in the study population is less that 5%.

Conventional CT and HRCT are more sensitive and specific than plain chest radiography in the diagnosis of both parenchymal and pleural disease related to asbestos. ... HRCT is most useful when the chest radiograph is normal or minimally abnormal. It should be noted that there is overlap between the HRCT appearances of asbestosis and usual interstitial pneumonia (UIP).

---

[*] Interobserver disagreement is also recorded for other interstitial diseases. In a European multicenter multidisciplinary study on idiopathic pulmonary fibrosis—in which 179 HRCT scans and 82 lung biopsies were evaluated by expert panels—Thomeer et al.[136] reported an interobserver agreement (kappa coefficient) of .40 for the HRCT scans and .30 for the "histology readers." The level of agreement was assessed as "... only fair to moderate," but the diagnosis of IPF "... in expert centres ..." assessed as good (87.2%), although the diagnosis of IPF initially proposed by a respiratory specialist was rejected in 12.8%.

Case and Dufresne[138] also observed that the clinical diagnosis of asbestosis can be arbitrary and not consistently reproducible, and they refer to "an excess of idiopathic diffuse pulmonary fibrosis" among cases of lung cancer without asbestosis. Piekarski et al.[139] observed that medical criteria appear to be applied "arbitrarily and inconsistently" for compensation, including claims for asbestosis, and the likelihood of claim acceptance was unrelated to the severity of the radiographic abnormalities for one series of patients who filed claims for nonmalignant asbestos diseases during the 1980s in Washington. In the Delphi study carried out by Banks et al.[140] (see later discussion), there was a consensus that "... chest radiographic changes of a profusion level 1/0 small irregular opacities are a good screening tool but lack specificity for an accurate diagnosis of asbestosis. HRCT should be performed to increase the specificity of these chest radiographic findings."

It is the present authors' experience that in adversarial medicolegal proceedings, there is frequent dispute over a clinical–radiological diagnosis of early-stage asbestosis, related to the following areas of disagreement among expert radiologists and respiratory physicians:

- Dispute over whether or not there is acceptable radiological evidence of genuine lower-zone interstitial fibrosis as opposed to transpulmonary bands as a consequence of asbestos-related pleural fibrosis without asbestosis—and hence the specificity of the radiological findings. As discussed earlier, small irregular opacities are not themselves specific for asbestosis and can occur as a consequence of cigarette smoking.
- Disagreement concerning the diagnosis of asbestosis in the absence of radiologically demonstrable asbestos-related pleural disease.
- Allied to these observations, dispute as to whether the occupational history delineates cumulative asbestos exposure of a character and magnitude appropriate for a diagnosis of asbestosis. In other words, the history of cumulative exposure is an important factor for a probabilistic clinical–radiological diagnosis of asbestosis, as it is for the cumulative model of lung cancer induction by asbestos with no requirement for an intermediary step of asbestosis.
- Allied to all of the above, the issue of whether any demonstrable interstitial disease represents idiopathic UIP or some other DILD, as opposed to asbestosis.

Even when biopsy or autopsy lung tissue is available, we have encountered cases where expert pulmonary pathologists disagreed over a diagnosis of asbestosis, as related to the following factors:

- Dispute as to whether there is a genuine increase in interstitial fibrous tissue in cases of early-stage disease.
- Dispute as to whether early-stage fibrosis represents bona fide asbestosis or whether it represents tobacco smoke-related airways disease. Roggli et al.[134] commented: "These early stages of the disease [asbestosis] are diagnostically problematical as similar centriacinar fibrosis is often seen in cigarette smokers and is characteristic of mixed dust pneumoconiosis. Fibrosis limited to the walls of the bronchioles does not represent asbestosis."
- Dispute as to whether there are sufficient numbers of asbestos bodies for a diagnosis. Churg[141] has stated in the past that the finding of a single AB is sufficient, whereas others require more, and a recent update on the diagnostic criteria[134] states that "... two or more asbestos bodies per square centimeter of a 5-μm-thick lung section in combination with interstitial fibrosis of appropriate pattern are indicative of asbestosis. Fewer asbestos bodies do not necessarily exclude a diagnosis of asbestosis but evidence of excess asbestos would then require quantitative studies performed on lung digests."
- When only a few asbestos bodies are present, and there is prominent (seemingly disproportionate) interstitial fibrosis—so that there is dispute as to whether the disease represents asbestosis or idiopathic UIP in someone coincidentally exposed to asbestos[142] (see also detailed discussion of this issue in the judgment in the *Sabin v. BRB* case in the United Kingdom[143]).
- Finally, rare cases of asbestosis are recorded where asbestos bodies cannot be found, presumably related to an incapacity of alveolar macrophages to coat asbestos fibers with an iron–protein complex to form asbestos bodies.[8,13] Such cases are diagnosable only by analysis of the asbestos fiber burden in lung parenchyma, preferably by electron microscopy, either transmission or scanning.

6.9 ESTIMATES OF CUMULATIVE ASBESTOS EXPOSURE AND ASBESTOSIS

As mentioned in the preceding discussion, asbestosis is characteristically an outcome of substantial asbestos exposures, usually occupational and protracted over years (although in their 1934 paper on 100 cases of asbestosis, Wood and Gloyne[144] recorded the development of asbestosis in an 18-year-old van boy who had mixed asbestos in an open yard for a period of about 2.5 years). The 1984 Ontario Royal Commission[145] found that the occurrence of asbestosis was unlikely with a cumulative exposure of less than 25 fiber-years; others[141,146] set the range for the development of asbestosis at 25–100 fiber-years, and a Chinese chest x-ray study on workers involved in asbestos products manufacture reported a 1% prevalence of early-stage asbestosis at a cumulative exposure level of 22 fiber-years.[54] However, histological examination is known to be more sensitive and specific for a diagnosis of asbestosis than chest radiographs or conventional computerized tomography scans. Green et al.[147] reported that histological asbestosis was usually present in autopsy lung tissue from South Carolina textile workers with exposures above 20 fiber-years, and a few cases were encountered at estimated cumulative exposures of 10–20 fiber-years. In an analysis of cases in the German Mesothelioma Register, Fischer et al.[148] reported that a boundary requirement for 25 fiber-years of asbestos exposure for a diagnosis of asbestosis—including minimal histological asbestosis—would lead to underdiagnosis of 42% of cases and false-positive diagnosis in 24%.

However, although the frequency of asbestosis and its severity increase as exposures increase, depending on the industry concerned, not all heavily exposed workers are so diagnosed during their lifetimes (about 80%–95%). For the asbestos textile industry in the United Kingdom and on the basis of data from 1930, Craighead[64] gives a frequency rate for asbestosis of 26% at 5–9 years of employment, rising to 81% at 20+ years (17/21 subjects). In 1965, Selikoff et al.[149] reported on the frequency of presumed asbestosis among insulation workers in the United States wherein the percentage with an abnormal chest x-ray rose from 10% at 0–9 years latency to 94% for 40+ years; and in the 40+ group, Grade 1 asbestos was found in 29%, Grade 2 in 42%, and Grade 3 in 23%.[53]

The present authors' files include cases of lung cancer associated with proven heavy occupational asbestos exposure but without histological asbestosis. These include, for example, a worker involved in asbestos cement manufacture for whom an autopsy lung tissue asbestos body count varied from approximately 17,000 to 94,000 per gram of wet lung, and there was an uncoated crocidolite + amosite fiber count of about $40–108 \times 10^6$ fibers of any length with an aspect ratio of 3:1 or more per gram of dry lung (well within the "asbestosis" range for the same laboratory).[8] In addition, lung cancer in another worker involved in insulation work that included the spraying of asbestos—with an undisputed estimated cumulative exposure of about 800 fiber-years—was accompanied by innumerable asbestos bodies in histological sections of his lung tissue at autopsy, but there was no interstitial fibrosis.

6.10 THE CUMULATIVE EXPOSURE MODEL FOR LUNG CANCER CAUSATION BY ASBESTOS

According to the cumulative exposure model, asbestos-attributable lung cancer is related to the burden of asbestos fibers resident in bronchopulmonary tissues, with no requirement for preexisting or coincident asbestosis. The model derived from epidemiologic studies approximates a linear dose–response effect with no clearly delineated threshold[1,54] (e.g., see Hodgson and Darnton[150]), but the gradient of the dose–response line is much flatter than the analogous line for pleural mesothelioma. However, there is some evidence that the gradient is steeper at lower exposures than at higher exposures where there is some evidence of a less steep gradient[151,152] (as suggested by Hodgson and Darnton[150] for pleural mesothelioma). In their review of 17 cohort studies for which measures of cumulative exposure were available, Hodgson and Darnton[150] found the increase in risk per fiber-year of exposure for amphibole fibers (crocidolite and amosite were about equipotent, with an increment in risk of about 5% per fiber-year) was greater than for chrysotile exposures (approximately 0.1%–0.5% per fiber-year)—although the South Carolina chrysotile textile workers had a much greater risk at equivalent exposures (approximately 6.5% for men and 4.5% for women; approximately 2%–3% for the entire cohort[50]), which Hodgson and Darnton[150] considered to be "untypically high."

From epidemiologic analysis, a direct linear relationship has been demonstrated between lung cancer relative risk and cumulative exposure to asbestos (see Henderson et al.[1]), including chrysotile and the amphiboles, expressed as

$$RR_{LCA} = 1 + K_L \times E,$$

where RR_{LCA} is the relative risk for lung cancer, E represents cumulative asbestos exposure (fiber-years), and K_L is the industry-specific slope of the relationship expressed as the increase in the excess lung cancer risk ($RR_{LCA}-1.0$) per fiber-year of exposure. The value of K_L varies across cohorts, that is, from 0.0001 to 0.002 (0.01%–0.2% per fiber-year) in chrysotile miners (0.03% for Quebec miners, in Hodgson and Darnton,[150] Table 2) and for friction products manufacture, to 0.003 to 0.09 (0.3%–9% per fiber-year) in cohorts of asbestos cement, asbestos textile, and insulation workers;[1,150,153] whereas, in a case-referent study from Stockholm, Gustavsson et al.[151] recorded a 14% increase in risk per fiber-year at low exposures (see later discussion).

The cumulative exposure model with no requirement for asbestosis is based mainly on the following observations:

- The presence of asbestosis delineates at least a two- to fivefold or greater increased risk of lung cancer, depending on the severity of the asbestosis and, if it is present, whether it is progressive or not. In this context, asbestosis is usually a marker for substantial asbestos exposure, with higher mean lung tissue asbestos fiber burdens than for other asbestos-related disorders. In this circumstance, asbestosis and lung cancer represent different outcomes of increased concentrations of asbestos fibers in bronchopulmonary tissue.
- Asbestos (all types) has been declared by the International Agency for Research on Cancer as a Group 1 carcinogen (a proven human carcinogen).
- Asbestos (especially the amphibole forms such as crocidolite and amosite) appears to be a complete carcinogen for the mesothelium. It seems unlikely that the same fibers are entirely noncarcinogenic for the lung.
- Studies on bronchopulmonary epithelial cells in culture (where fibrosis cannot be invoked as a mechanism). For example, Panduri et al.[154] reported that amosite asbestos stimulates A549 cell p53 promoter activity and messenger RNA and protein expression, and the asbestos-induced p53 promoter activity occurred as early as 1 h after exposure and which persisted over 24 h. Hei and Piao[155] produced in vitro evidence of malignant transformation of a human papillomavirus–immortalized bronchial epithelial cell line by a single 7-day "treatment" with chrysotile (see also Chapter 4).
- Epidemiologic studies have demonstrated an increased risk of lung cancer among asbestos workers without clinical, radiological or histological evidence of asbestosis, after adjustment for smoking (past or continuing), and with evidence of a dose–response effect.
- Epidemiologic studies have also demonstrated an increase in the relative risk or OR_{LCA}, after adjustment for smoking (and other possible causal factors), with exposures insufficient to induce asbestosis (see following discussion). Collectively, such studies amount to strong evidence against the fibrosis–cancer model (falsification[156,157]).
- The cumulative exposure model is not beset with the problem of anatomic disjunction between the sites where interstitial fibrosis develops and those sites where many of the lung cancers are located.

Some epidemiologic studies on asbestos-associated lung cancer do not include data on the presence or absence of asbestosis and will not be considered further in this chapter. Both Henderson et al.[1]

and Hessel et al.[3] reviewed studies on asbestos-associated lung cancer where there was no evidence of asbestosis. In this context, Hessel et al.[3] reviewed the strengths and weaknesses of nine studies, two of which concluded that asbestosis is a requirement for assignment of a causal-contributory effect to asbestos,[67,104] and seven where there was no radiographic evidence of asbestosis.[47,58,158–162]

Therefore, in this chapter we concentrate on the two studies[61,163] considered and criticized by Gibbs et al.[4] in their 2007 editorial review (both were published in the same year as Hessel et al.[3]), and on those studies that have demonstrated an increased lung cancer risk in the setting of quantified exposures too low to have induced asbestosis.

1. The Cullen et al.[61] β-Carotene and Retinol Efficacy Trial (CARET) for the possible chemoprevention of lung cancer study: This was a prospective randomized trial of 3897 men in the United States who were "heavily exposed" to asbestos for 9–17 years. Men with less than 5 years of work in a "heavily exposed occupation," never smokers, and those who had ceased smoking for more than 15 years were excluded (i.e., the study focused on those with a high risk of lung cancer). Duration of exposure was used as a surrogate for "dose." The study adjusted for smoking and time since quitting. Some 241 lung cancers were observed. The subgroup of men with a normal chest radiograph at baseline and more than 40 years of exposure in high-risk trades had a lung cancer rate about fivefold higher than men with 5–10 years of exposure. This study also showed clear evidence of a significant dose–response trend for an increasing RR of lung cancer with increasing duration of exposure (Table 6.1).

The criticisms leveled by Gibbs et al.[4] at this study include: (i) "… serious flaws in regard to … changed purpose"; (ii) no quantitative estimates of exposure were possible, so that "… years of exposure in asbestos-exposure jobs, 80% of them in shipyards and construction, were a crude surrogate of exposure," with further comment that jobs in shipyards "… have extremely variable and nonquantifiable asbestos exposures"; (iii) there was an "inexplicable synergy" between "… treatment and asbestosis in the associated lung cancer risk"; and (iv) the radiographs were read by only a single B reader at each of the CARET centers.

As a response to these criticisms, we would comment that one of the strengths of a prospective cohort study of this type is that the data collected can be applied to the assessment of one or more issues different from the question for which the study was originally designed: by itself, this does *not* represent a serious flaw as claimed by Gibbs et al.[4] Another strength is the fact that the study was a stratified internal analysis (see Henderson et al.[1]) and, in fact, the reference group for the effect of

Table 6.1 Lung Cancers Among Work-History–Eligible Asbestos-Exposed Participants with an ILO Rating of Less Than 1/0,[a] in the CARET Trial, 1989–2002

	Overall			
	Total Number	Number of Lung Cancer Cases	Relative Risk	95% CI
Years in a high-risk trade				
<10	272	6	1.00 (reference)	
11–20	570	23	2.07	0.82–5.19
21–30	720	30	2.50	0.97–6.42
31–40	441	26	3.15	1.12–8.85
>40	86	12	5.17	1.61–16.6
p for trend			.007	

Note: [a] On the preceding page of the paper, the ILO score is given as <0/1.
Source: Modified from Table 5 of Cullen, M.R., Barnett, M.J., Balmes, J.R., et al. *Am. J. Epidemiol.* 161, 260–270, 2005.

increasing duration of exposure was not an unexposed population, but those with less than 10 years work in high-risk trade (tending to underestimation of risk). It is known that asbestos exposures in shipyards were highly variable (this issue was discussed at some length by Henderson et al.[1]); however, inclusion of workers with "low-dose" exposures among those with heavy exposures results in underestimation of causal effects (i.e., a bias toward a null result).

The data did not allow Cullen et al.[61] to derive precise quantitative estimates of exposure, but duration of exposure in a high-risk occupation can be substituted for assessments of "dose" expressed as fiber-years and is the most accurately measurable parameter of cumulative exposure:[10] it is widely used (e.g., by the Industrial Injuries Advisory Council [IIAC][102] in the United Kingdom). In addition, Roggli et al.[164] found a positive correlation between duration of asbestos exposure and the lung tissue content of asbestos bodies and uncoated commercial amphibole fibers. On average, those with direct exposures had higher concentrations of asbestos bodies and fibers than those whose exposures were indirect, and shipyard workers on average had higher asbestos concentrations than nonshipyard workers.

Again, one of the strengths of the Cullen et al.[61] study is that it demonstrated a highly significant trend with increasing duration of exposure (p for trend .007). Another strength is that it contained about 9.5-fold more lung cancers than the Hughes–Weill study (241 vs. 25).

In relation to the B-reader issue, Cullen et al.[61] investigated this by way of a nested analysis, whereby the Seattle panel reread a sample of 48 radiographs from each CARET site, with exact agreement in 44%–50% and agreement within one minor category in 77%–91%.

Cullen et al.[61] did not set forth any explanation for the unanticipated synergy between the intervention arm and the chest radiographic abnormalities, but by itself this observation does not vitiate the duration–response effect between asbestos exposure and lung cancer risk in the absence of radiographic asbestosis. One might speculate that this observation could reflect pulmonary toxicity related to the β-carotene/retinol administered as part of the intervention arm, but at the doses administered, these antioxidants appear to be free of significant side effects (see the *Cochrane Database of Systematic Reviews*).[*]

Cullen et al.[61] considered the issue of whether the increased risk might have been explicable by subclinical, radiologically undetected asbestosis or—when there was a significant time delay between the chest radiographs and the recognition of the lung cancer—that asbestosis may have developed during that time interval. Therefore, they[61] commented that the "... finding of increased lung cancer risk in men without radiographic evidence of fibrosis is noteworthy, but we can neither confirm nor refute the contention that asbestosis obligatorily mediates the relation between exposure and cancer."

2. The Reid et al.[163] study: This study investigated 1196 former workers in the Wittenoom blue asbestos industry in Western Australia and 792 residents enrolled in a Cancer Prevention Programme who were assigned randomly to take either β-carotene or retinyl palmitate. This study included numerical estimates of cumulative exposure (fiber-years) and it adjusted for smoking. During the period 1990–2002, there were 58 cases of lung cancer. Of the lung cancer cases, 36% had asbestosis in comparison to 12% of the study participants. Continued tobacco smoking was the strongest predictor for lung cancer (OR = 26.5, 95% CI = 3.5–198), but radiographic asbestosis (OR = 1.94, 95% CI = 1.09–3.46) and asbestos exposure (OR = 1.21 per fiber/mL-year, 95% CI = 1.02–1.42, p = .026) were also associated with an increased rate. Cumulative asbestos exposure (hazard ratio [HR] = 1.31 per log fiber/mL-year), ex-smoking (HR = 7.07), and current smoking (HR = 21.8) were all significantly associated with lung cancer risk in those without radiographic asbestosis at the start of the study. Reid et al.[163] also addressed the issue of any statistical interaction between asbestos exposure and asbestosis in their association with lung cancer and found no significant interaction (HR = 0.82, 95% CI = 0.59–1.13, p = .23). They[163] concluded the "... findings support the hypothesis that it is the asbestos fibres per se that cause lung cancer, which can develop with or without the presence of asbestosis."

---

[*] Accessible at http://www2.cochrane.org/reviews/.

Table 6.2   Relative Risk of Lung Cancer by Quartiles of Cumulative Asbestos Exposure for Stockholm County, Sweden

Asbestos Exposure (fiber-years)	Mean Cumulative Exposure in Class (fiber-years)	Number of Cases	Number of Referents	RR Crude (95% CI)	RR Adjusted 1 (95% CI)[a]	RR Adjusted 2 (95% CI)[b]
None	0	833	2024	1.0	1.0	1.0
>0–0.50	0.29	42	84	1.20 (0.82–1.76)	1.25 (0.81–1.92)	1.23 (0.80–1.89)
0.51–0.88	0.70	34	81	1.01 (0.67–1.53)	0.96 (0.61–1.51)	0.89 (0.56–1.41)
0.89–1.49	1.16	62	90	1.65 (1.18–2.30)	1.59 (1.09–2.32)	1.48 (1.01–2.17)
≥1.5	4.03	71	85	2.05 (1.48–2.84)	1.83 (1.27–2.65)	1.68 (1.15–2.46)

Sources: Modified from Table 4 in Gustavsson, P., Jakobsson, R., Nyberg, F., et al. *Am. J. Epidemiol.* 152, 32–40, 2000. And reproduced from Henderson, D.W., Rodelsperger, K., Woitowitz, H.J., Leigh, J. *Pathology* 36, 517–550, 2004, with permission.
[a] Adjusted for age, selection year, smoking, residential radon levels, and environmental exposure to nitrogen dioxide.
[b] RRs were in addition adjusted for occupational exposure to diesel exhausts and combustion products.

Again, Gibbs et al.[4] have criticized the Reid et al.[163] study on grounds similar to those they advanced against the Cullen study,[61] together with some others. Although Reid et al.[163] did set forth numerical estimates of cumulative exposure (fiber-years), Gibbs et al.[4] argued that for the Wittenoom residents included in the study, "… general environmental fiber sampling must be considered inadequate for construction of individual cumulative exposures." In this context, the data for Wittenoom are in principle no different from the approach in other equivalent epidemiologic studies such as Camus et al.[106] Gibbs et al.[4] also commented that because the Wittenoom industry and environment involved exposure to pure crocidolite and "… the universe of asbestos-exposed workers contains almost none exposed *only* to crocidolite, any results from this are clearly not generalizable." We agree: the Wittenoom data are not *directly* extrapolable to other asbestos exposures. But in a sense this is beside the point: the issue is whether crocidolite fibers (cumulative exposure per se) can result in an increased risk of lung cancer in the absence of detectable asbestosis—which the Reid et al.[163] study supports—whereas adherents of the fibrosis–cancer model argue that they cannot, and many past mixed-fiber exposures in Australia and the United Kingdom included crocidolite fiber exposure.

A number of epidemiologic studies have detected an increased lung cancer rate at exposures considered insufficient for the induction of asbestosis, and these are considered below:

• The South Carolina asbestos (chrysotile) textile cohort[50,51]: In their studies on those textile workers, Dement et al.[50] found an SMR of 2.59 and a standardized risk ratio (SRR) of 2.63 for white males (95% CI = 1.20–5.75) at exposures as little as 2.7–6.8 fiber-years (for white males, the SMR and the SRR were 1.96 and 2.03, respectively, for exposures in the range 6.8–27.4 fiber-years; for the same group, the SMR and the SRR were 3.08 and 2.95 at 27.4–109.5 fiber-years and 8.33 and 6.60, respectively, when the exposure was >109.5 fiber-years). An estimated cumulative exposure of 2.7–6.8 fiber-years fell below the level at which Green et al.[147] identified histological asbestosis on autopsy lung tissue among workers comprising this cohort. Furthermore, the predicted fibrosis score at 2.7–6.8 fiber-years would also have been in the range for the reference group.[147]

• The Gustavsson et al.[151,152] studies: In a population-based case-referent study on 1042 lung cancer cases and 2364 referents in Sweden, Gustavsson et al.[151] found an unexpectedly high asbestos-related lung cancer risk at low exposures (Table 6.2), with a 14% increase in lung cancer risk per fiber-year of exposure.

- Gustavsson et al.[152] later reported a follow-up study on 1038 cases and 2359 referents for lung cancer risk among men in Stockholm for the period 1985–1990 related to low-dose occupational exposure to asbestos (mainly chrysotile and end-use exposures). This study adjusted for other occupational exposures and environmental pollutants, including radon (as for the earlier paper[151]). It also took smoking into account, including ex-smokers and lifelong nonsmokers, the amount smoked, and potential misclassification of smoking habits. Asbestos exposure was assessed from the airborne fiber measurements, taking into account changes in asbestos levels over "calendar periods." Cumulative exposures were estimated with blinding for the case/referent status of the individuals, as in the preceding publication.[151] The exposure estimates were based on a survey of asbestos exposures in Swedish workplaces between 1969 and 1973 involving 2400 samples at 35 workplaces, which was considered to have been representative of 70%–75% of the asbestos imported into Sweden at that time.[152] Twenty percent of the cases and 14.4% of the referents had been exposed to asbestos for at least 1 year and the cumulative exposures were low, ranging from background only to a maximum of 20.4 fiber-years. These authors found the risk of lung cancer increased as cumulative exposure increased according to an almost linear relationship, with a joint effect with smoking that was submultiplicative. The calculated risk at a cumulative dose of 4.0 fiber-years was 1.90 (95% CI = 1.32–2.74) and was 5.38 among never smokers and 1.55 for current smokers (the approximately 3.5-fold greater effect in nonsmokers appears to correlate reasonably well with the difference reported by Berry and Liddell[75]). Gustavsson et al.[152] claimed their study appeared to have reasonable precision up to about 5.0 fiber-years but gave no information on higher cumulative exposures.
- The Carel et al.[165] study: This case-referent study on paper and pulp industry workers across 13 nations did not detect any increment in lung cancer risk in comparison to age-specific and period-specific national mortality rates. However, on stratified internal analysis, there was a trend in mortality for both lung cancer and pleural cancer, weighted for the individual probability of asbestos exposure and its duration. The lung cancer SMR was 1.44 for exposures amounting to ≥0.78 fiber-years in comparison to 0.01 fiber-years or less (95% CI = 0.85–2.45); and for pleural cancer at the same compared levels of exposure, the SMR was 2.43 (95% CI = 0.43–13.63).
- The Meguellati-Hakkas et al.[166] study: This study addressed lung cancer mortality among telephone linesmen in France who were exposed to asbestos at low levels during installation of telephone cables. Three hundred and eight (308) lung cancer deaths were identified, and exposure to asbestos and to other occupational carcinogens was assessed according to a job-exposure matrix. The RR for lung cancer death was 2.1 (95% CI = 1.1–4.0) associated with an estimated exposure of approximately 2.0 fiber-years in comparison to workers with less than 0.5 fiber-year of exposure. The mean annual exposure or exposure duration was not clearly related to lung cancer, and adjustment for other occupational lung carcinogens did not change this finding. The authors concluded that the observed mortality from lung cancer associated with asbestos exposure at low levels was higher than the prediction on the basis of linear downward extrapolation from highly exposed occupational cohorts.

Henderson et al.[1] have discussed several studies in Germany on lung cancer relative to estimated cumulative asbestos exposure.[167–170] In a pooled analysis of two studies,[167,168] ever exposure to asbestos (after adjustment for smoking) was associated with an OR of 1.41 (95% CI = 1.24–1.60); and there was a clear dose–response relationship with an OR of 1.79 (95% CI 1.39–2.30) for >2500 days of exposure. For a subsample of 301 cases and 313 controls, the OR_{LCA} in relation to an estimated 25 fiber-years of exposure was found to be 1.99 (95% CI = 1.20–3.30) in a logistic regression model, adjusted for smoking and stratified for the age and origin of the patients.[1] In a two-phase case-referent study, Pohlabeln et al.[171] derived results "consistent with a doubling of the lung cancer risk with 25 fiber-years asbestos exposure." In an analysis of two German case-referent studies, Hauptmann et al.[96] found that the OR_{LCA} was 1.8 (95% CI = 1.2–2.7) for subjects who had worked for 3–7 years in a job with potential exposure to asbestos, and it was 2.4 (95% CI = 1.7–3.4) for work in similar jobs for ≥8 years in comparison to never-exposed subjects. Estimates of fiber-years of exposure in Germany are based on the 90th percentile concentration of airborne fiber concentrations measured in multiple workplaces in Germany (9974 membrane filter counts, 1600 konimeter counts and 15,316 gravimetric measurements). The use of the 90th percentile has been criticized,[4] but Rödelsperger and Woitowitz have defended this approach in Henderson et al.[1] Among other reasons, they point out that:

> … the database for the BK-Report [in Germany] does not deal with a random sample of workplace situations but a selection, where there is routine supervision and airborne fibre concentrations may be lower than in unsupervised workplaces elsewhere, although the airborne fibre concentrations were measured in the absence of protective measures such as dust extraction equipment. In such supervised workplaces, fibre concentrations in excess of the limit values are normally followed by measures to reduce exposures—the efficacy of those measures being evaluated by further measurements—so that action is taken to maintain exposures at levels lower than those expected for workplaces without such scrutiny.

So far as we are aware, there is only one study that has evaluated lung cancer risk in relation to the concentration of amphibole fibers in lung tissue—namely, that reported by Karjalainen et al.[172] in 1994. This study was based on 113 lung cancer patients treated surgically in comparison to 297 autopsy referents from the Finnish population. Lung tissue fiber analysis was carried out for amphibole fibers longer than 1 μm by scanning electron microscopy at a magnification of 5000×. In comparison to a reference group with a tissue concentration of less than 1,000,000 fibers per gram of dry lung, the lung cancer OR increased to 1.7 for concentrations in the range 1.0–4.99 million fibers per gram of dry lung and to 5.3 for concentrations of 5.0 million or more. When two cases of asbestosis and seven cases of minor "histological fibrosis compatible with asbestosis" were excluded, the age-adjusted OR_{LCA} was still elevated at 2.8 (95% CI = 0.9–8.7, p = .07) in association with asbestos fiber concentrations of 5.0 million or more fibers per gram of dry lung; and for asbestos fiber counts in the range 1.0–4.99 million, the OR_{LCA} was 1.5 (95% CI = 0.8–2.9, p = .19). Churg[100] has criticized this study on the basis that these results failed to reach significance in terms of p values—thereby proving that "significance" lies only with the cases of fibrosis.[100] However, what is important in this study is the trend from a low to a higher OR_{LCA} with transition from an intermediate fiber count (1.0–4.99 million) to the higher value of ≥5.0 million. If one excludes the nine cases of fibrosis and assumes that two were in the high fiber group (≥5.0 million fibers per gram of dry lung) and seven were in the intermediate fiber group of 1.0–4.99 million (and assuming that the clinical asbestosis cases were in the heaviest exposure group and that the mild histological fibrosis cases were in the intermediate exposure group), the crude lung cancer ORs can be recalculated as 2.85 and 1.8, respectively, as consistent as possible with the age-adjusted ORs of 2.8 and 1.5 in the original paper; trend testing then yields χ^2_1 (trend) = 7.2 (p < .01). It is also possible from the data in the Karjalainen et al.[172] paper to recalculate the OR for adenocarcinoma only, after exclusion of all cases with any fibrosis. Assuming that all were in the high fiber group, the OR remains significantly elevated at 2.65 (95% CI = 1.11–6.26, p < .001) for a count >1.0 million compared with <1.0 million.

On the basis of these considerations, we consider the case for the cumulative exposure model to be compelling, with no threshold identified for the asbestos-related lung cancer risk. However, and as noted earlier in this chapter, causation of lung cancer is multifactorial, cigarette smoking being the strongest single causal factor for lung cancer in the general population and among the asbestos-exposed. The problem is to delineate indices of cumulative exposure at which the asbestos exposure has made a significant causal contribution to the development of a particular lung cancer as a matter of probability, usually but not always by causal coaction with cigarette smoke. If one considers a construction worker with exposure to asbestos (mixed-fiber type) amounting to, say, 0.1 fiber-year and who is also a continuing heavy smoker, the likely causal contribution by asbestos would be trivial, even taking synergy into account. For an equivalent worker with mixed-fiber asbestos exposure amounting to, say, 50 fiber-years, the asbestos-imposed rate ratio would be 2.0 or more, depending on the fiber types in the airborne dust. Therefore, between the causal effect in the first of these scenarios and the causal contribution in the second, there has been a switch from nonsignificance to significance. The exercise then becomes a matter of assessing on a probability basis the point (or, rather, cumulative "dose") at which this transition occurs. That is what the Helsinki Criteria[13] attempted to do.

6.11 THE CUMULATIVE EXPOSURE MODEL AND THE HELSINKI CRITERIA

For an individual case of lung cancer, the Helsinki Criteria[13] promulgated in 1997 set exposure estimates or indices at which the lung cancer RR is estimated to be 2.0 or more which, it is argued, confers an attributable fraction of 0.5, calculated from $(RR - 1/RR) = (2-1)/2$—often considered to equate to a probability of causation (POC) of 50%[102,173] (see later discussion and footnotes in p. 295).

Asbestosis is not a *sine qua non* of the Helsinki Criteria for attribution of lung cancer to asbestos, but instead the criteria also focus upon cumulative exposure to asbestos as assessed clinically (exposure history; estimates of cumulative exposure) or pathologically (asbestos bodies or uncoated fiber concentrations within lung tissue)[13]:

> Because of the high incidence of lung cancer in the general population, it is not possible to prove in precise deterministic terms that asbestos is the causative factor for an *individual* patient, even when asbestosis is present. However, attribution of causation requires *reasonable* medical certainty on a probability basis that the agent (asbestos) has caused or contributed materially to the disease. The likelihood that asbestos exposure has made a substantial contribution increases when the exposure increases. Cumulative exposure, on a probability basis, should thus be considered the main criterion for the attribution of a substantial contribution by asbestos to lung cancer risk. For example, relative risk is roughly doubled for cohorts exposed to asbestos fibers at a cumulative exposure of 25 fiber-years or with an equivalent occupational history, at which level asbestosis may or may not be present or detectable.

The Helsinki Criteria include the following indices of exposure for attribution of lung cancer to asbestos:

- Asbestosis diagnosed clinically, radiologically, or histologically. In this setting, asbestosis is significant mainly as a surrogate for cumulative exposures comparable to the exposure indices that follow; or
- A concentration of 5,000–15,000 ABs or more per gram dry lung tissue, or an equivalent uncoated fiber burden of ≥2.0 million amphibole fibers (>5 μm in length) per gram of dry lung tissue or ≥5.0 million amphibole fibers >1 μm in length. The criteria also recommend that when the AB concentration is <10,000 per gram of dry lung tissue, the count should be supplemented by an uncoated fiber burden analysis using electron microscopy.

These uncoated fiber counts refer only to the amphibole types of asbestos. Because of faster clearance rates, chrysotile does not accumulate within lung tissue to the same extent as the amphiboles. Although it might be assumed that a substantially elevated concentration of chrysotile fibers in lung parenchyma is indicative of substantial exposure because of shorter half-lives within lung tissue than the amphiboles, longitudinal splitting of the fibers as part of the clearance process may increase the number of fibers counted.[23] Therefore, occupational histories are considered to be a better indicator of lung cancer risk from chrysotile than fiber burden analysis.[13] A lung amphibole fiber burden within the range recorded for asbestosis in the same laboratory should be assigned a significance similar to that of asbestosis[13] (but see reference 143).

- Or an estimated cumulative exposure to asbestos of 25 fiber-years or more (see following discussion); or
- An occupational history (the only means for assessment of latency) of 1 year of heavy exposure to asbestos (such as the manufacture of asbestos products, asbestos spraying, insulation work with asbestos materials, and demolition of old buildings) or 5–10 years of moderate exposure (such as construction or shipbuilding). The criteria go on to state that a twofold risk of lung cancer can be

reached with exposures less than 1 year in duration if the exposure is of extremely high intensity (e.g., the spraying of asbestos insulation materials); and
*   A minimum latency interval of 10 years.

According to the criteria, pleural plaques are insufficient by themselves for the probabilistic attribution of lung cancer to asbestos:[13]

> Because pleural plaques may be associated with low levels of asbestos exposure, the attribution of lung cancer to asbestos exposure must be supported by [other parameters of exposure such as] an occupational history of substantial exposure or measures of asbestos fiber burden.

In 2005, the IIAC[102] in the United Kingdom revisited the criteria for attribution of lung cancer to asbestosis (the existing criteria were asbestosis, or at least unilateral diffuse pleural fibrosis). The IIAC rejected the Helsinki Criterion of 25 fiber-years, in part because this quantum of exposure was unlikely to be valid for all occupational groups (and asbestos fiber types). Equally, the IIAC did not address AB or fiber counts for the purpose of attribution. From a requirement for an asbestos-related lung cancer RR of 2.0 or more, the IIAC[102] determined that:

> … lung cancer can be attributed to occupation where workers have been exposed to substantial asbestos exposure. Workers with substantial asbestos exposure are those where asbestosis is present, or [in the absence of asbestosis] workers in the following categories: asbestos textile workers, asbestos sprayers, asbestos insulation workers including those applying and removing asbestos-containing materials in shipbuilding. The Council recommends that workers in the jobs listed require at least 5 years asbestos exposure before 1975 or at least 10 years asbestos exposure after 1975 to fulfill the terms of prescription. Recent evidence indicates that diffuse pleural thickening is an unreliable marker of asbestos exposure and the Council recommends removing the requirement for the presence of diffuse pleural thickening from the terms of prescription ….

The Helsinki Criteria[13] commented that bilateral diffuse pleural thickening is frequently an outcome of moderate to heavy exposures sufficient to induce asbestosis in some individuals, so that it was assigned significance equivalent to that of asbestosis for the purposes of attribution. The IIAC decision to remove pleural thickening from the attributional criteria in the United Kingdom seems to have been based in part on the paper by Smith et al.,[174] who suggested that diffuse pleural fibrosis is an unreliable marker of heavy exposure. In contrast, Miles et al.[175] commented:

> The prevalence of both DPT [diffuse pleural thickening] and pleural plaques increases significantly with past occupational exposure to asbestos, duration and intensity of exposure. Thus, workers who have worked in occupations with heavy exposure (e.g., laggers, insulators) are more likely to have pleural disease than those with moderate or minimal exposures.

However, for lung cancer patients with substantial asbestos exposure and DPT, attribution can be based on the exposure history or other indices of substantial exposure, apart from the DPT itself.

6.12 CRITICISMS OF THE HELSINKI CRITERIA

Some of the more serious criticisms set forth by Gibbs et al.[4] concerning the Helsinki Criteria include: (i) the increase in lung risk per fiber-year of asbestos exposure set forth in those criteria; (ii) the retrospective estimates of asbestos exposure, for example, as expressed as fiber-years; and (iii) the assessment of the AB and uncoated asbestos fiber concentrations in lung tissue as set forth in those criteria.

Hereunder, we address those criticisms:

*   The Helsinki Criteria state that the risk of lung cancer increases by 0.5%–4% per fiber-year of asbestos exposure. Gibbs et al.[4] are (rightly) critical of the use of the upper end of this range for derivation of the 25 fiber-year criterion—pointing out that although use of the upper boundary for

this risk would correspond to 25 fiber-years for a twofold increase in risk, the lower boundary would require 200 fiber-years for the same increase. Yet they themselves indicate the estimated increase in risk per fiber-year varies across different industries (from 0.01% to 9%) so that the Helsinki estimate is near the mid-point of this range (especially if one takes Gustavsson et al.[151] into account, so that the percentage increase per fiber-year ranges from 0.01% to 14%). We agree that a "broad brush" approach as embodied in *Helsinki* can no longer be applied across all industries and exposure circumstances. The Helsinki Criteria are arguably overconservative for amphibole-only exposures (a figure of 20 fiber-years of exposure would be appropriate as an epidemiologic average estimate for crocidolite-only and amosite-only exposures); they are arguably overgenerous for chrysotile-only exposures (except for textile exposures, for which a boundary figure of 25 fiber-years is arguably reasonable). Importantly, the risk estimates for exposures in "special" industries do not seem applicable for the risks assessed with end-use exposures. On the basis of case-referent studies on end-use mixed-fiber exposures (now the most frequent type of exposure across industrialized nations; see preceding discussion), the Helsinki figure of 25 fiber-years seems appropriate.

- In their editorial, Gibbs et al.[4] commented, "What really matters in terms of causing an asbestos-related lung cancer is the amount of fibers deposited in the lungs and their retention. Cumulative exposure estimates are a surrogate for this." (Which essentially represents a restatement of the cumulative exposure model, but most proponents of the fibrosis–cancer model go a step further and invoke the fibrosis induced by asbestos as an obligatory step in the pathway from asbestos fiber inhalation and deposition to cancer.)

Allen Gibbs et al.[4] are then skeptical about the precision of estimates of cumulative exposure ("... false precision ..."). Graham Gibbs and Berry[176] have commented that "... evaluation of exposure is complex but a key consideration in risk assessment." They go on to state that "... all too often it is the weak link inasmuch as reliable quantitative information is not available." Yet estimates of cumulative exposure expressed as fiber-years are standard in epidemiologic cohort studies, and some estimates of cumulative exposure (e.g., durations of exposure within a single cohort) are essential for evaluation of dose–response effects for at least two reasons: (i) to establish criteria for the protection of workers; and (ii) for the prediction of future numbers of the diseases in question.[176] In their criticisms, Allen Gibbs et al.[4] appear to critique and challenge not only the Helsinki Criteria but also the standard approaches in general for exposure–response assessment as part of cohort and case-referent studies on asbestos.

Exposure estimates are most precise and have greatest predictive value when they involve serial measurements of airborne fiber concentrations over time for various work activities within a single population of workers and allow for changes in methodology—especially if the exposures were individualized or stratified for different patterns of work and exposure within the single study group. The proportional imprecision is least significant in terms of causal assessment for heavy exposures as assessed from work histories. For example, if an exposure of 800 fiber-years is too high by a factor of two, the "true" result of 400 fiber-years still constitutes "heavy" exposure. It is when the estimates are much lower (e.g., estimates around 25 fiber-years and below) that large proportional imprecision occurs.

For many mixed chrysotile–amphibole asbestos exposures at sites of end use of asbestos-containing materials (notably in the building construction industry), there were no measured estimates of asbestos exposures, so that interpolated estimates of exposure on the basis of estimated equivalent exposures in other similar industries are fraught with substantial imprecision. The Helsinki Criterion of 25 fiber-years was promulgated primarily from a European perspective whereby there were cogent estimates of asbestos exposures as assessed from serial measurements of airborne asbestos fiber concentrations for various workplaces as discussed above, for example, in Sweden and in Germany, and those estimates had been correlated with lung tissue asbestos fiber concentrations.

In adversarial medicolegal cases in Australia, the present authors have encountered cases where different industrial/occupational hygienists have advanced wildly disparate estimates of cumulative asbestos exposures (with exceedingly low and reciprocally high estimates of cumulative asbestos exposure estimates for a particular case—sometimes with incompatibility between a low fiber-year estimate and the presence of tissue markers of substantial exposure, such as the presence of asbestos bodies in lung tissue and even histological asbestosis).

In these circumstances and when there are widely different estimates of cumulative asbestos exposure, we abandon fiber-year estimates and base attribution upon the work history (as reflected in Helsinki, and now in the United Kingdom).[*]

- Gibbs et al.[4] are also critical of semiquantitative terms such as "light," "moderate," and "heavy" exposure. Yet those expressions do not pretend any numerical "precision" for cumulative estimates, and analogous terms are widely used in relation to a diagnosis of asbestosis (work history). In general, the boundaries between these three levels of cumulative exposure are poorly delineated and subjective, but one can state that an insulation worker actively involved in the spraying of "limpet" asbestos[177] for 10 years or more has sustained "heavy" exposure, as would an insulation worker in a shipyard for 20 years. As discussed by Henderson et al.,[1] the same assessment would not apply to shipyard office personnel far removed from the places where the insulation work was carried out, and it would not apply to someone who carried out home renovation work for a few months using asbestos cement building materials ("light" only). For a carpenter in the building construction industry for 5–10 years and who cut asbestos cement materials with a power saw, one can assess the exposure as probably "moderate."
- Gibbs et al.[4] are also critical of the counts of asbestos bodies and uncoated amphibole fibers specified by the Helsinki Criteria (see above). They[4] point out that the median count of amphibole fibers vary from one cohort to another: 16 million fibers per gram dry lung for a cohort of naval dockyard workers and 106 million for workers in an asbestos products factory. It is acknowledged that the arithmetic or geometric mean and the median counts vary from one exposure group to another and from one laboratory to another for the same sample—which is why the Helsinki Criteria also refer to a lung fiber burden with the range of asbestosis for the same laboratory. Rather than the mean or median fiber counts, we would advocate an amphibole fiber count at or in excess of the lower 95% CI for the fifth percentile count in cases of asbestosis for that laboratory.
- Although the paper by Fischer et al.[148] found a poor correlation between exposures estimated as fiber-years versus the lung tissue asbestos fiber concentration, this seems explicable by their use of "total asbestos fiber concentration" instead of the amphibole fiber count only as specified in the Helsinki Criteria and as discussed by Henderson et al.[1,178] In his study on mesothelioma patients, Rödelsperger[179] found that: "A relationship is demonstrated between asbestos fibre dose estimated from the interview and concentration of amphibole fibres from lung tissue analysis. From this, a dose of 25 fibre-years corresponds to an amphibole fibre concentration of 2 fibres/mg" (i.e., 2 million amphibole fibers per gram of dry lung for fibers longer than 5 mg; abstract and p. 307).

Tuomi et al.[180] had earlier found a correlation between definite exposure to asbestos for mesothelioma patients versus smaller fiber counts for those with probable, possible and unlikely/unknown exposure. For nine reference male office workers, the counts were all less than one million. In Belgian studies on resected lung tissue from patients with lung cancer, it was found that a count ≥5000 asbestos bodies corresponded to "significant occupational exposure" amounting to about 10 fiber-years and about equivalent to five million fibers per gram of dry lung.[181,182] Mollo et al.[183] also found a correlation between the RR for adenocarcinoma of lung and the count of asbestos bodies. Finally, as mentioned earlier, Roggli[164] found that the concentration of asbestos bodies and uncoated amphibole fibers in lung tissue correlated with the duration of exposure as assessed from work histories.

Even so, it should be recognized that lung fiber analyses are subject to substantial variation and uncertainty. For example, there can be up to about a two- to threefold variation in fiber counts

---

[*] In the Sabin case in the United Kingdom concerning a disputed diagnosis of asbestosis versus UIP,[143] there was remarkably good agreement between estimates of exposure carried out by expert "consulting engineers" commissioned by both the plaintiff's and the defendant's lawyers: 42 and 47.2 fiber-years, respectively.

between tissue sampled from different sites in the same lung, rarely up to 10-fold, and up to about threefold variation between aliquots of the same tissue digest[184] (Roggli and Sharma[185] refer to a coefficient of variation of about 10% for counting of the same sample on different occasions). There is also scope for subjectivity in fiber counting in the decision on how many fields to count, counting of fibers crossing grid bars, and counting of aggregated fibers. Analysis of paraffin blocks, as often used in compensation cases, is not optimal because solvent extraction can result in fiber loss and a low count.[184] In addition to these and other factors, the fiber analysis is usually carried out many years after an individual's asbestos exposure ceased, and the counts do not take into account fiber clearance so that they do not correspond to the tissue concentration of fibers when the disease in question was evolving[185] (e.g., Wittenoom crocidolite fibers have a tissue half-life of several years, with an estimated clearance rate of 10%–15% per year[186,187]). Nonetheless, it is widely acknowledged that the tissue concentration of biopersistent fibers is a major determinant of asbestos-related diseases.[185]

The reality is that both retrospective estimates of cumulative exposure expressed as fiber-years and lung mineral content analyses are subject to error: neither is truly "objective."

6.13 GENERAL ACCEPTANCE OF THE CUMULATIVE EXPOSURE MODEL AND THE DELPHI STUDY REPORTED BY BANKS ET AL.[140]

With some variation from the Helsinki Criteria, the cumulative exposure approach—with no requirement for antecedent or coexistent asbestosis—is accepted for the purposes of compensation by authorities in the United Kingdom, France, Belgium, Germany, Denmark, Norway, Sweden, and Finland.[1,10]

The cumulative exposure approach is also supported by the results of an international computer-based Delphi study on asbestos-related diseases[140] (an approach originally devised by the RAND Corporation to gain consensus on contentious issues). The database PubMed was searched for all people in the world with three or more first-author publications on asbestos-related diseases for the period 1991–2002. Multiple questions were posed to the participants, who responded on a graded scale from 0 (strongly disagree) to 10 (strongly agree).

- Proposition 17 was: "Workers who have significant asbestos exposure (but who do not have asbestosis) are at increased risk of bronchogenic carcinoma." The median score was 9 and the p value was .0001. In round 2, the consensus on this proposition was ranked as "very good" and accepted (the majority ratio for agreement was about 13:1).
- Proposition 15 was: "In an asbestos exposed worker without asbestosis and with lung cancer, the recognition of asbestosis among co-workers with similar exposures is sufficient to attribute the worker's lung cancer to asbestos exposure." The median score was 8 and the p value was .0001, and it was considered that a consensus had been reached.
- Proposition 8 was: "Nonsmoking workers with significant asbestos exposure (without asbestosis) have at least double the risk of bronchogenic carcinoma compared with nonsmoking workers with low level exposure." The median score was 7.5 and the p value was .0609, and it was considered that no consensus had been reached.
- Proposition 13 was: "Workers who smoke cigarettes and have significant asbestos exposure (without asbestosis) have at least double the risk of bronchogenic carcinoma to nonexposed smokers." The median score was 9 and the p value was .003, but it was considered that no consensus had been reached.

No consensus was obtained for some other questions, in part because the wording (according to our perception) was ambiguous. For example, Proposition 1 was: "A heavy asbestos exposure (sufficient to cause asbestosis) with sufficient latency is necessary to establish asbestos exposure as causative for lung cancer (clarified from round 1)." To us, it is unclear whether this proposition implies that exposure insufficient to cause asbestosis is sufficient (more likely) or whether asbestosis is necessary (which would introduce an incompatibility with Proposition 17).

6.14 IS A RELATIVE RISK OF 2.0 OR MORE NECESSARY TO ATTRIBUTE LUNG CANCER TO ASBESTOS?

The Helsinki Criteria are arguably conservative for attribution of lung cancer to asbestos except for nontextile chrysotile-only exposures in that they require indices of exposure that would confer an RR of 2.0 or more related to asbestos exposure for the probabilistic attribution of lung cancer to asbestos (i.e., a 100% increase in risk in comparison to a reference group). However, it can be argued that this RR is overly restrictive (see also Greenland[188]). For example, the requirement for an RR = 2.0 or more is based on the concept of the attributable fraction, which in turn is derived from RRs or ORs assessed as an average across a population or occupational group[189,190]—but it does not follow that the RR for each and every member of that group has an RR = 2.0.*

Absolute associative or causal effects involve assessment of the actual numbers of cases or incidences, whereas relative effects involve assessment of ratios; hence, RR represents the ratio of the incidence for cases seen in the *exposed* group divided by the incidence for the same disease in the *controls* (obviously, for diseases such as lung cancer, allowance must be made for confounding factors/effect modifiers such as tobacco smoke, among others). Therefore, RR = (I_e/I_c), where I = incidence, e = exposed, and c = controls. By definition, RR = 1.0 for the control group. RR = 1.1 represents a 10% increase in risk, RR = 1.2 is a 20% increase in risk, and so on, so that RR = 2.0 represents a 100% increase in risk.†

To assign the mean properties of an entire class to each and every individual comprising that class has been called the *fallacy of complex division* and, as emphasized by Pirie,[191] this exercise ultimately descends into absurdity:

> An entertaining version of the fallacy is called the fallacy of complex division, and assumes that sub-classes of the whole share the same properties as the entire class. In this version, we meet the average British couple with their 2.2 children, out walking their 0.7 of a cat with a quarter of a dog. They have 1.15 cars, which they somehow manage to fit into only a third of a garage.

The point is that there is nothing magical about an RR = 2.0 as opposed to say 1.1, it is simply that the stronger the association (and the higher the RR/OR) when calculated as a mean across a class/population, the less likely it is to be affected by known and unknown confounding factors than when the RR/OR is only slightly greater than 1.0. The RRs for lung cancer related to passive (secondhand) smoking are generally in the range of 1.15–1.2 to about 2.0 at most,[16,192] but few authorities would dismiss a causal-contributory role for passive smoking in an otherwise never smoker with no other identifiable causal factor for lung cancer.

Henderson et al.[1] have emphasized that although epidemiologic investigations have been very effective for the detection and estimates of the net or average causal effects of various carcinogens across populations or groups as reflected in cohort or case-referent studies—and for public health estimates, planning and policy—they are less appropriate for assessment of the probability of causation for an *individual* person with the disease in question because of the following factors, among many others:

- Differential exposures to the carcinogen within the cohort or the cases group for case-referent studies—unless the exposure estimates are individualized or stratified for different patterns of work and exposure.

---

* Rockhill et al.[189] comment that the population-based AF does not address probability of causation for a specific case of disease nor does its estimation enable epidemiologists to discriminate between those cases caused by, and those not caused by, the risk factors under consideration. See also Greenland.[190]

† It should also be emphasized that "risk" in this context is no theoretical construct. Rather, it represents the ratio of the actual number of observed cases in the study group relative to the control/reference group. "Rate ratio" would be preferable but "relative risk" is well entrenched. Because RR is derived as an average across a population/group, it is unlikely to correspond to the individual risk for each and every individual making up the population under study because individual risks will vary from one individual to another. Therefore, although the mean RR/OR value is suitable for public health policy planning and for assessment of causal effects on a population-wide basis, it is inappropriate simply to extrapolate the mean RR/OR to each and every individual comprising the population.

- Changes over time in exposures and smoking habits across the cohort/group unless the parameters of exposure/smoking are evaluated longitudinally over time.
- Differential clearance of asbestos fibers from bronchopulmonary tissues, related to differences in the proportions of asbestos fiber types for mixed asbestos exposures and fiber dimensions as well as the efficacy of host clearance mechanisms as influenced by a variety of factors that include innate and acquired differences in the capacity for fiber clearance.
- Finally, differential innate/genetic susceptibility or resistance to the carcinogen(s).[193–195] Such susceptibility factors are now implicated to explain why, apart from chance alone, some smokers develop lung cancer whereas others with equivalent smoking habits (or heavier smokers) do not. Detailed discussion of this topic lies beyond the scope of this chapter (see Henderson et al.[1] and Chapter 4), but the factors implicated include a family history of cancer,[131] the fragile histidine triad (FHIT) gene,[93,196] and polymorphisms for the xeroderma pigmentosum,[197] myeloperoxidase (MPO),[198,199] and glutathione-S-transferase[198] genes, and the capacity for DNA repair,[194] among others.

In the context of biological variability in relation to carcinogenesis, even in the hypothetical situation where each individual comprising a worker population sustained exactly the same inhaled "dose" of asbestos, some will develop asbestos-related cancer and some (most) will not. Accordingly, for a cancer/no-cancer result, genetic susceptibility/resistance (G_S/G_R) will influence the outcome so that some individuals (G_S) are at greater risk of cancer than others (G_R) at the same level of exposure. It follows that those with cancer (e.g., lung cancer) are more likely to come from the G_S pool than the G_R. On this issue, Henderson et al.[1] commented:

> Given the emerging evidence on G_S/G_R for lung cancer, for both cigarette smoke and (to a far lesser extent) asbestos, and taking into account the complexity of the multiple genes and polymorphisms implicated so far, it seems that individuals comprising any population will vary in their susceptibility to (and risk from) these carcinogens. Therefore, one can deduce that the risk derived as an average or mean across entire cohorts/populations will tend to underestimate the risk for those with a G_S profile (RR_{GS}) and to overestimate risk for those with G_R (RR_{GR}). It also follows that those with the disease in question are more likely to have G_S for that disease and therefore be at greater risk than either: (i) those who are resistant (G_R); or (ii) the average/mean risk [i.e., $RR_{GS} > (RR_{GS} + RR_{GR})/2$], even if the variation in risk from the mean is only very small.

6.15 A MODIFIED SET OF CRITERIA FOR ATTRIBUTION

We consider that the criteria for probabilistic attribution of lung cancer to asbestos should conform as closely as possible to the prevailing scientific evidence, despite imperfections in exposure assessments. In this context, we consider that the evidence supports the cumulative exposure model for lung carcinogenesis by asbestos, as opposed to a tissue marker of convenience for substantial exposure (asbestosis)—on the basis that a clinical–radiological diagnosis of early-stage asbestosis is often problematic and is disputed in medicolegal proceedings in our experience, and not all asbestos-exposed workers develop asbestosis, even when heavily exposed.

Suggested modified criteria include the following:

- A nondisputed or majority clinical–radiological or histological diagnosis of asbestosis as a marker for substantial cumulative asbestos exposure; or
- The occurrence of asbestosis among other workers in the same workforce carrying out similar work for similar durations of time and at similar times; or
- A nondisputed or majority estimate of cumulative exposure to asbestos of 25 fiber-years or more for mixed-fiber end-use exposures to asbestos, for example, in the building construction industry and for insulation work. For amphibole-only (amosite or crocidolite) exposures, a nondisputed estimated cumulative exposure of 20 fiber-years, and 25 fiber-years for asbestos textile workers. For chrysotile-only exposures, most notably the Canadian chrysotile miners and millers and friction products exposures, 200 fiber-years; or

- A history of at least 5 years of asbestos exposure before 1975 or 5–10 years after 1975 for asbestos textile workers, asbestos insulation workers including those applying and removing asbestos-containing materials in shipbuilding, power stations, railways, workshops, and others in close proximity to such work—especially when it was carried out in confined and poorly ventilated workplaces—or a duration of one year for work that involved consistent or frequent spraying of asbestos insulation. We have excluded Canadian chrysotile miners/millers and friction products workers from this assessment; or
- For never smokers or those who had ceased smoking 30 years or more before the diagnosis of lung cancer, cumulative exposure amounting to 5 fiber-years or exposure amounting to one-third of the durations for work set forth in the preceding paragraph; or
- A concentration of asbestos bodies or uncoated amphibole fibers at or in excess of the lower 95% CI for the fifth percentile count in cases of asbestosis, for the same laboratory (for fibers of the same length), for mixed-fiber end-use exposures. For pure amphibole fiber exposures, greater concentrations are required to correspond to 25 fiber-years (see Henderson et al.[1]). The uncoated fiber counts are applicable only to the amphibole types of asbestos. Because of faster clearance rates, chrysotile does not accumulate within lung tissue to the same extent as the amphiboles; therefore, for chrysotile-only exposures, fiber counts should not be used and the occupational history should be substituted.
- And a minimum latency interval of 10 years.

These modified criteria are proposed primarily for statutory compensation where smoking is generally not taken into consideration. In a litigation situation where tobacco exposure can be considered, either as caused by a joint tortfeasor or as an example of contributory negligence, different approaches may be needed and apportionment methods applied, although apportionment modeling is artificial. In the individual case, when both asbestos and tobacco smoking are implicated, both would have acted to some extent in the process of carcinogenesis on the basis of the biological evidence of interaction (synergy) as discussed earlier in this chapter—so that asbestos will have made some contribution to causation of the lung cancer, even at cumulative exposures substantially less than 25 fiber-years.

6.16 CONCLUSION

Debate on the fibrosis–cancer versus the cumulative exposure model for asbestos causation of lung cancer is related mainly to the issue of the criteria for compensation and (in some jurisdictions) adversarial medicolegal proceedings. However, the overall implications and significance are wider and concern assessment of the overall burden of asbestos-related cancer across society and its prevention are therefore necessary for public health planning and policy. If causation of lung cancer were considered to be restricted only to those with clinical–radiological asbestosis, estimates of asbestos-induced cancer would be reduced by a stroke almost to the numbers of mesotheliomas, and this approach would be inconsistent with the lung cancer to mesothelioma ratios found across epidemiologic studies.

On the other hand, after introduction of the 25 fiber-year approach in Germany (where compensation is essentially an automated bureaucratic excise for those on the asbestos register), the lung cancer–mesothelioma ratio rose to 1.24:1 for the period 1995–2000, so that the ratio corresponds closely to the epidemiologic evidence as opposed to the underrecognition of asbestos-related lung cancers elsewhere (Table 6.3).

Conflict-of-Interest Statement: The authors have prepared reports on asbestos exposure and lung cancer for the courts in Australia, for example, the Dust Diseases Tribunal in New South Wales and in other courts in Australia and the United Kingdom, and have given courtroom testimony on this issue. Neither author has any affiliation with the asbestos industry or any nonprofessional group that lobbies for or against the industry.

Table 6.3   Cases of Asbestos-Related Cancers (LCAs) in the United Kingdom, 1988–2000, as
Assessed by Special Medical Boards, in Comparison with Compensated Cases in
Germany, 1986–2000, and to Excess Lung Cancer to Mesothelioma Ratios from Two
Other Reports

	United Kingdom			Germany		
Year	Asbestos-Related LCAs	Meso	Ratio of Lung Cancer to Meso	Asbestos-Related LCAs (Including Laryngeal Carcinoma Since 1997) (BK4104)	Meso (BK4105)	Ratio of Respiratory Tract Cancer to Meso (BK4104/ BK4105)
1986				38	172	0.22:1
1987				53	198	0.27:1
1988	59	479	0.12:1	100	228	0.44:1
1989	54	441	0.12:1	125	273	0.46:1
1990	58	462	0.13:1	129	296	0.44:1
1991	55	519	0.11:1	171	315	0.54:1
1992	54	551	0.10:1	223	350	0.64:1
1993	72	608	0.12:1	388	416	0.93:1
1994	77	583	0.13:1	545	495	1.10:1
1995	55	685	0.08:1	648	503	1.29:1
1996	51	642	0.08:1	726	535	1.36:1
1997	26	553	0.05:1	672	534	1.26:1
1998	42	590	0.07:1	723	575	1.26:1
1999	38	620	0.06:1	776	617	1.26:1
2000	42	652	0.06:1	697[a]	670[a]	1.04:1
1995–2000	254	3742	0.07:1	4242	3434	1.24:1
Excess lung cancer to mesothelioma ratio in Hutchings et al.[37]						1.09:1
Excess lung cancer to mesothelioma ratio: Berry et al.[36]: about 5100 asbestos factory workers in east London—232 lung cancer deaths observed; 77 expected; SMR (O/E) = 3.01 (95% CI = 2.6–3.4); 100 mesothelioma deaths (52 pleural; 48 peritoneal).						1.55:1

Notes: Meso = mesothelioma. For the United Kingdom, asbestos-related lung cancers comprise only cases of
primary carcinoma of lung with either asbestosis or pleural thickening; until April 1997, only cases of bilateral pleural thickening were accepted; thereafter, unilateral pleural thickening was also allowed (now
disallowed[102]).

Asbestos-related lung cancers for Germany include those fulfilling the criterion of 25 fiber-years of exposure, introduced in 1992. See also Baur and Czuppon,[200] where the 1995 asbestos-associated lung cancer
to mesothelioma ratios are 2.16:1 for reported cases, 1.29:1 for "recognized" cases, and 1.29:1 for cases
compensated for the first time. From 1997, the numbers of lung cancer cases include laryngeal carcinomas
related to 25 fiber-years or more exposure to asbestos by an extension to the existing German lung cancer
category BK4104.[200] On this basis, the number of laryngeal carcinomas attributed to asbestos is
small—15 cases of laryngeal carcinoma were "recognized" in 1995[200]—and would have only a slight effect
on the lung cancer to mesothelioma ratio; for example, if there were 25 cases of laryngeal cancer attributed
to asbestos for 1999, the excess lung cancer to mesothelioma ratio would be 1.22:1. See also pre-1997
lung cancer to mesothelioma ratios.

[a]   German data for 2000 represent a personal communication to Prof. Hans-Joachim Woitowitz.

Sources: The United Kingdom figures are from the Health and Safety Commission Reports, Health and Safety
Statistics 1998/99, HSE Books, London, 1999 and Health and Safety Statistics 2000/01, HSE Books,
London, 2001. Table reproduced from Henderson, D.W., Rodelsperger, K., Woitowitz, H.J., Leigh, J.
Pathology 36, 517–550, 2004 with permission; see that paper (Table 1) for sources of data.

REFERENCES

1. Henderson DW, Rodelsperger K, Woitowitz HJ, Leigh J. Schleuchenpflug T, Friedenreich C. After Helsinki: A multidisciplinary review of the relationship between asbestos exposure and lung cancer, with emphasis on studies published during 1997–2004. *Pathology* 2004;36:517–550.
2. Cagle PT. Criteria for attributing lung cancer to asbestos exposure [editorial]. *Am J Clin Pathol* 2002;117:9–15.
3. Hessel PA, Gamble JF, McDonald JC. Asbestos, asbestosis and lung cancer: A critical assessment of the epidemiological evidence. *Thorax* 2005;60:433–436. http://www.thoraxjnl.com.
4. Gibbs A, Attanoos RL, Churg A, Weill H. The "Helsinki Criteria" for attribution of lung cancer to asbestos exposure: How robust are the Criteria? *Arch Pathol Lab Med* 2007;131:181–184.
5. Attanoos R. Lung cancer associated with asbestos exposure. In: *Asbestos and Its Diseases*, Craighead JE, Gibbs AR, eds. Oxford: Oxford University Press; 2008: 172–189.
6. Lemen RA. Epidemiology of asbestos-related diseases and the knowledge that led to what is known today. In: *Asbestos: Risk Assessment, Epidemiology, and Health Effects*, Dodson RF, Hammar SP, eds. Boca Raton, FL: CRC Press; 2006: 201–308.
7. Blettner M, Sauerbrei W, Schlehofer B, Schleuchenpflug T, Friedenreich C. Traditional reviews, meta-analyses and pooled analyses in epidemiology. *Int J Epidemiol* 1999;28:1–9.
8. Henderson DW, Roggli VL, Shilkin KB, Hammar SP, Leigh J. Is asbestosis an obligate precursor for asbestos-induced lung cancer? In: *Sourcebook on Asbestos Diseases*, Vol 11, Peters GA, Peters BJ, eds. Charlottesville: Michie; 1995: 97–168.
9. Leigh J, Berry G, de Klerk NH, Henderson DW. Asbestos-related lung cancer: Apportionment of causation and damages to asbestos and tobacco smoke. In: *Sourcebook on Asbestos Diseases*, Vol 13, Peters GA, Peters BJ, eds. Charlottesville: Michie; 1996: 141–166.
10. Henderson DW, de Klerk NH, Hammar SP, Hillerdal G, Huuskonen M, Leigh J, et al. Asbestos and lung cancer: Is it attributable to asbestosis, or to asbestos fiber burden? In: *Pathology of Lung Tumors*, Corrin B, ed. New York: Churchill Livingstone; 1997: 83–118.
11. Henderson DW, Leigh J. An Australian perspective on the Helsinki Criteria for the attribution of lung cancer to asbestos. *Pathol Int* 2004;54(Suppl. 1): S442–S451.
12. Leigh J, Henderson D. Lung cancer related to asbestos exposure: Causation and compensation. *J Occup Health Safety–Aust NZ* 2006;22:449–462.
13. Helsinki Workshop 1997 Participants' Consensus Report. Asbestos, asbestosis, and cancer: The Helsinki criteria for diagnosis and attribution. *Scand J Work Environ Health* 1997;23:311–316.
14. Dubey S, Powell CA. Update in lung cancer 2007. *Am J Respir Crit Care Med* 2008;177:941–946.
15. Simonato L, Agudo A, Ahrens W, Benhamou E, Benhamou S, Boffetta P, et al. Lung cancer and cigarette smoking in Europe: An update of risk estimates and an assessment of inter-country heterogeneity. *Int J Cancer* 2001;91:876–887.
16. International Agency for Research on Cancer (IARC). Lung cancer. In: *World Cancer Report*, Stuart BW, Kleihues P, eds. Lyon: IARC; 2003: 182–187.
17. De Stefani E, Boffetta P, Ronco AL, Brennan P, Correa P, Deneo-Pellegrini H, et al. Squamous and small cell carcinomas of the lung: Similarities and differences concerning the role of tobacco smoking. *Lung Cancer* 2005;47:1–8.
18. Qiao YL, Taylor PR, Yao SX, Erozan YS, Luo XC, Barrett MJ, et al. Risk factors and early detection of lung cancer in a cohort of Chinese tin miners. *Ann Epidemiol* 1997;7:533–541.
19. Tossavainen A. Asbestos, asbestosis and cancer: Exposure criteria for clinical diagnosis. Asbestos, asbestosis and cancer. *People and Work Research Reports* 14. Helsinki: Finnish Institute of Occupational Health; 1997: 8–27.
20. Van Loon AJ, Kant IJ, Swaen GM, Goldbohm RA, Kremer AM, van den Brandt PA. Occupational exposure to carcinogens and risk of lung cancer: results from The Netherlands cohort study. *Occup Environ Med* 1997;54:817–824.
21. Mándi A, Posgay M, Vadász P, Major K, Rödelsperger K, Tossavainen A, et al. Role of occupational asbestos exposure in Hungarian lung cancer patients. *Int Arch Occup Environ Health* 2000;73:555–560.
22. World Health Organization (WHO). *Environmental Health Criteria 211: Health Effects of Interactions Between Tobacco Use and Exposure to Other Agents*. Geneva: WHO; 1999.
23. Rödelsperger K, Mándi A, Tossavainen A, Brückel B, Barbison P, Woitowitz H-J. Inorganic fibres in the lung tissue of Hungarian and German lung cancer patients. *Int Arch Occup Environ Health* 2000;74:133–138.

24. Case BW. Asbestos, smoking, and lung cancer: Interaction and attribution [commentary]. *J Occup Environ Med* 2006;63:507–508. doi:10.1136/oem.2006.027631.

25. Alberg AJ, Samet JM. Epidemiology of lung cancer. *Chest* 2003;123(Suppl.):21S–49S.

26. Axelson O. Alternative for estimating the burden of lung cancer from occupational exposures: Some calculations based on data from Swedish men. *Scand J Work Environ Health* 2002;28:58–63.

27. Nurminen M, Karjalainen A. Epidemiologic estimate of the proportion of fatalities related to occupational factors in Finland. *Scand J Work Environ Health* 2001;27:161–213 [erratum *in Scand J Work Environ Health* 2001;27:295].

28. Kjuus H, Langard S, Skjaerven R. A case-referent study of lung cancer, occupational exposures and smoking. III. Etiologic fraction of occupational exposures. *Scand J Work Environ Health* 1986;12:210–215.

29. Kvale G, Bjelke E, Heuch I. Occupational exposure and lung cancer risk. *Int J Cancer* 1986;37:185–193.

30. Emri S, Demir AU. Malignant pleural mesothelioma in Turkey, 2000–2002. *Lung Cancer* 2004;45 (Suppl. 1):S17–S20.

31. Travis LB, Fossa SD, Schonfeld SJ, McMaster ML, Lynch CF, Storm H, et al. Second cancers among 40,576 testicular cancer patients: Focus on long-term survivors. *J Natl Cancer Inst* 2005; 97:1354–1365.

32. Howie R. Asbestos-induced deaths in the United Kingdom. In: *Sourcebook on Asbestos Diseases*, Vol. 19, Peters GA, Peters BJ, eds. Charlottesville: Lexis; 1999:219–238.

33. Barroetavena MC, Teschke K, Bates DV. Unrecognized asbestos-induced disease. *Am J Ind Med* 1996;29:183–185.

34. Tulchinsky TH, Ginsberg GM, Iscovich J, Shihab S, Fischbein A, Richter ED. Cancer in ex-asbestos cement workers in Israel, 1953–1992. *Am J Ind Med* 1999;35:1–8.

35. Ulvestad B, Kjaerheim K, Martinsen JI, Damberg G, Wannag A, Mowe G, et al. Cancer incidence among workers in the asbestos-cement producing industry in Norway. *Scand J Work Environ Health* 2002;28:411–417.

36. Berry G, Newhouse ML, Wagner JC. Mortality from all cancers of asbestos factory workers in east London 1933–80. *Occup Environ Med* 2000;57:782–785.

37. Hutchings S, Jones J, Hodgson J. Asbestos-related diseases. In: *Occupational Health Decennial Supplement No. 10*, Drever F, ed. London: Office of Population Censuses (OPCS), Health & Safety Executive (HSE); 1995: 136–152.

38. Health and Safety Commission. *Health and Safety Statistics 2000/01*. London: HSE Books; 2001.

39. Health and Safety Commission. *Health and Safety Statistics 1998/99*. London: HSE Books; 1999.

40. Peto J, Decarli A, La Vecchia C, Levi F, Negri E. The European mesothelioma epidemic. *Br J Cancer* 1999;79:666–672.

41. Hindry M. Asbestos-related disease compensation in France. In: *Sourcebook on Asbestos Diseases*, Vol. 16, Peters GA, Peters BJ, eds. Charlottesville: Lexis; 1997: 423–448.

42. De Lamberterie G, Maitre A, Goux S, Brambilla C, Perdrix A. How do we reduce the under-reporting of occupational primary lung cancer [in French]. *Rev Mal Respir* 2002;19:190–195.

43. Mollo F, Magnani C, Bo P, Burlo P, Cravello M. The attribution of lung cancers to asbestos exposure: A pathologic study of 924 unselected cases. *Am J Clin Pathol* 2002;117:90–95.

44. Kishimoto T, Ohnishi K, Saito Y. Clinical study of asbestos-related lung cancer. *Ind Health* 2003;41:94–100.

45. Teschke K, Barroetavena MC. Occupational cancer in Canada: What do we know? *Can Med Assoc J* 1992;147:1501–1507.

46. Paris C, Benichou J, Saunier F, Metayer J, Brochard P, Thiberville L, et al. Smoking status, occupational asbestos exposure and bronchial location of lung cancer. *Lung Cancer* 2003;40:17–24.

47. Karjalainen A, Anttila S, Heikkilä L, Kyyrönen P, Vainio H. Lobe of origin of lung cancer among asbestos-exposed patients with or without diffuse interstitial fibrosis. *Scand J Work Environ Health* 1993;19:102–107.

48. Lee BW, Wain JC, Kelsey KT, Wiencke JK, Christiani DC. Association of cigarette smoking and asbestos exposure with location and histology of lung cancer. *Am J Respir Crit Care Med* 1998;157:748–755.

49. Roggli VL, Sanders LL. Asbestos content of lung tissue and carcinoma of the lung: A clinicopathologic correlation and mineral fiber analysis of 234 cases. *Ann Occup Hyg* 2000;44:109–117.

50. Dement JM, Brown DP, Okun A. Follow-up study of chrysotile asbestos textile workers: Cohort mortality and case–control analyses. *Am J Ind Med* 1994;26:431–447.

51. Dement JM, Brown DP. Lung cancer mortality among asbestos textile workers: A review and update. *Ann Occup Hyg* 1994;38:525–532, 412.

52. McDonald JC. Unfinished business: The asbestos textiles mystery [editorial]. *Ann Occup Hyg* 1998;42:3–5.

53. Craighead JE. Diseases associated with asbestos industrial producers and environmental exposure. In: *Asbestos and Its Diseases*, Craighead JE, Gibbs AR, eds. Oxford: Oxford University Press; 2008: 39–93.

54. World Health Organization. *Environmental Health Criteria 203: Chrysotile Asbestos*. Geneva: WHO; 1998.

55. Sebastien P, McDonald JC, McDonald AD, Case B, Harley R. Respiratory cancer in chrysotile textile and mining industries: Exposure inferences from lung analysis. *Br J Ind Med* 1989;46:180–187.

56. World Trade Organization Dispute Settlement Report WT/DS135. European communities—Measures concerning asbestos and asbestos-containing products. Geneva: World Trade Organization; 2000. See also WTO Dispute Settlement Reports 2001. Vol. VIII (DSR 2001: VIII). Cambridge: Cambridge University Press; 2004: 3303–4047.

57. Case BW, Dufresne A, McDonald AD, McDonald JC. Asbestos fiber type and length in lungs of chrysotile textile and production workers: fibers longer than 18 μm. *Inhal Toxicol* 2000;12(Suppl. 3):411–418.

58. Hillerdal G. Pleural plaques and risk for bronchial carcinoma and mesothelioma: A prospective study. *Chest* 1994;105:144–150.

59. Hillerdal G, Henderson DW. Asbestos, asbestosis, pleural plaques and lung cancer. *Scand J Work Environ Health* 1997;23:93–103.

60. Koskinen K, Pukkala E, Martikainen R, Reijula K, Karjalainen A. Different measures of asbestos exposure in estimating risk of lung cancer and mesothelioma among construction workers. *J Occup Environ Med* 2002;44:1190–1196.

61. Cullen MR, Barnett MJ, Balmes JR, Cartmel B, Redlich CA, Brodkin CA, et al. Predictors of lung cancer among asbestos-exposed men in the β-Carotene and Retinol Efficacy Trial. *Am J Epidemiol* 2005;161:260–270.

62. Weiss W. Asbestosis: a marker for the increased risk of lung cancer among workers exposed to asbestos. *Chest* 1999;115:536–549. [published erratum appears in *Chest* 1999;115:1485].

63. Oksa P, Klockars M, Karjalainen A, Huuskonen MS, Vattulainen K, Pukkala E, et al. Progression of asbestosis predicts lung cancer. *Chest* 1998; 113:1517–1521.

64. Craighead JE. Benign pleural and parenchymal diseases associated with asbestos exposure. In: *Asbestos and Its Diseases*, Craighead JE, Gibbs AR, eds. Oxford: Oxford University Press; 2008: 139–171.

65. Doll R, Peto R, Wheatley K, Gray R, Sutherland I. Mortality in relation to smoking: 40 years' observations on male British doctors. *Br Med J* 1994;309:901–911.

66. International Agency for Research on Cancer. *Reversal of Risk after Quitting Smoking. IARC Handbooks of Cancer Prevention: Tobacco Control*, Vol 11. Lyon: IARC; 2007.

67. Hughes JM, Weill H. Asbestosis as a precursor of asbestos related lung cancer: Results of a prospective mortality study. *Br J Ind Med* 1991;48:229–233.

68. Osinubi OY, Afilaka AA, Doucette J, Golden A, Soriano T, Rovner E, et al. Study of smoking behavior in asbestos workers. *Am J Ind Med* 2002;41:62–69.

69. Vainio H, Boffetta P. Mechanisms of the combined effect of asbestos and smoking in the etiology of lung cancer. *Scand J Work Environ Health* 1994;20:235–242.

70. Boffetta P. Health effects of asbestos exposure in humans: A quantitative assessment. *Med Lav* 1998;89:471–480.

71. Gong MN, Christiani DC. Lung cancer. In: *Occupational Disorders of the Lung: Recognition, Management, and Prevention*, Hendrick DJ, Burge PS, Beckett WS, Churg A, eds. London: Saunders; 2002: 305–326.

72. Liddell FD. The interaction of asbestos and smoking in lung cancer. *Ann Occup Hyg* 2001;45:341–356.

73. Liddell FD, Armstrong BG. The combination of effects on lung cancer of cigarette smoking and exposure in Quebec chrysotile miners and millers. *Ann Occup Hyg* 2002;46:5–13.

74. Lee PN. Relation between exposure to asbestos and smoking jointly and the risk of lung cancer. *Occup Environ Med* 2001;58:145–153.

75. Berry G, Liddell FD. The interaction of asbestos and smoking in lung cancer: A modified measure of effect. *Ann Occup Hyg* 2004;48:459–462.

76. Lee PN. Joint action of smoking and asbestos exposure on lung cancer: Author's reply. *Occup Environ Med* 2002;59:495–496.

77. Liddell FD. Joint action of smoking and asbestos exposure on lung cancer. *Occup Environ Med* 2002;59:494–495;discussion 5–6.

78. Erren TC, Jacobsen M, Piekarski C. Synergy between asbestos and smoking on lung cancer risks. *Epidemiology* 1999;10:405–411.

79. Nelson HH, Kelsey KT. The molecular epidemiology of asbestos and tobacco in lung cancer. *Oncogene* 2002;21:7284–7288.

80. Churg A, Stevens B. Enhanced retention of asbestos fibers in the airways of human smokers. *Am J Respir Crit Care Med* 1995;151:1409–1413.

81. Fattman CL, Chu CT, Oury TD. Experimental models of asbestos-related diseases. In: *Pathology of Asbestos-Associated Diseases*, 2nd ed., Roggli VL, Oury TD, Sporn TA, eds. New York: Springer-Verlag; 2004: 256–308.

82. Pott F. Asbestos use and carcinogenicity in Germany and a comparison with animal studies. *Ann Occup Hyg* 1994;38:589–600.

83. Wagner JC, Berry G, Skidmore JW, Timbrell V. The effects of the inhalation of asbestos in rats. *Br J Cancer* 1974;29:252–269.

84. Davis JMG, Beckett ST, Bolton RE, Donaldson K. The effects of intermittent high asbestos exposure (peak dose levels) on the lungs of rats. *Br J Exp Pathol* 1980;61:272–280.

85. Davis JMG, Cowie HA. The relationship between fibrosis and cancer in experimental animals exposed to asbestos and other fibers. *Environ Health Perspect* 1990;88:305–309.

86. Pott F, Dungworth DL, Heinrich U, Muhle H, Kamino K, Germann P-G, et al. Lung tumours in rats after intratracheal instillation of dusts. *Ann Occup Hyg* 1994;38(Suppl. 1):357–363.

87. Kimizuka G, Azuma M, Ishibashi M, Shinozaki K, Hayashi Y. Co-carcinogenic effect of chrysotile and amosite asbestos with benzo(a)pyrene in the lung of hamsters. *Acta Pathol Jpn* 1993;43:149–153.

88. Harrison PTC, Hoskins JA, Brown RC, Pigott GH, Hext PM, Mugglestone MA. Hyperplastic and neoplastic changes in the lungs of rats treated concurrently with chrysotile asbestos and *N*-nitrosoheptamethyleneimine. *Inhal Toxicol* 2000;12(Suppl. 3):167–172.

89. Kamp DW, Greenberger MJ, Sbalchierro JS,Preusen SE, Weitzman SA. Cigarette smoke augments asbestos-induced alveolar epithelial cell injury: Role of free radicals. *Free Radic Biol Med* 1998;25:728–739.

90. Loli P, Topinka J, Georgiadis P, Dusinska M, Hurbankova M, Kovacikova Z, et al. Benzo[a]pyrene-enhanced mutagenesis by asbestos in the lung of λ-lacI transgenic rats. *Mutat Res* 2004;553:79–90.

91. Topinka J, Loli P, Hurbakova M, Kovacikova Z, Volkovova K, Wolff T, et al. Benzo[a]pyrene-enhanced mutagenesis by man-made mineral fibres in the lung of λ-lacI transgenic rats. *Mutat Res* 2006;595:167–173.

92. Nelson HH, Christiani DC, Wiencke JK, Mark EJ, Wain JC, Kelsey KT. K-ras mutation and occupational asbestos exposure in lung adenocarcinoma: asbestos-related cancer without asbestosis. *Cancer Res* 1999;59:4570–4573.

93. Nelson HH, Wiencke JK, Gunn L, Wain JC, Christiani DC, Kelsey KT. Chromosome 3p14 alterations in lung cancer: Evidence that FHIT exon deletion is a target of tobacco carcinogens and asbestos. *Cancer Res* 1998;58: 1804–1807.

94. Menegozzo M, Belli S, Borriero S, Bruno C, Carboni M, Grignoli M, et al. Mortality study of a cohort of insulation workers [in Italian]. *Epidemiol Prev* 2002;26:71–75.

95. Nicholson WJ, Perkel G, Selikoff IJ, Seidman H. Cancer from occupational asbestos exposure projections 1980–2000. In: *Quantification of Occupational Cancer*, Peto R, Schneiderman M, eds. New York: Cold Spring Harbor Laboratory; 1981: 87–111.

96. Hauptmann M, Pohlabeln H, Lubin JH, Jockel KH, Ahrens W, Bruske-Hohlfeld I, et al. The exposure–time–response relationship between occupational asbestos exposure and lung cancer in two German case–control studies. *Am J Ind Med* 2002;41:89–97.

97. Proctor RN. *The Nazi War on Cancer*. Princeton: Princeton University Press; 1999.

98. Doll R. Mortality from lung cancer in asbestos workers. *Br J Ind Med* 1955;12:81–86.

99. Churg A. Asbestos, asbestosis, and lung cancer. *Mod Pathol* 1993;6:509–510.

100. Churg A. Neoplastic asbestos-induced disease. In: *Pathology of Occupational Lung Disease*, 2nd ed., Churg A, Green FHY, eds. Baltimore: Williams & Wilkins 1998: 339–391.

101. Weiss W. Asbestos-related pleural plaques and lung cancer. *Chest* 1993;103:1854–1859.

102. Industrial Injuries Advisory Council (UK). Asbestos-related diseases: report by the Industrial Injuries Advisory Council in Accordance with Section 171 of the Social Security Administration Act 1992 Reviewing the Prescription of the Asbestos-Related Diseases. London: HMSO; 2005. http:// www.iiac.org.uk.

103. Kipen HM, Lilis R, Suzuki Y, Valciukas JA, Selikoff IJ. Pulmonary fibrosis in asbestos insulation workers with lung cancer: a radiological and histopathological evaluation. *Br J Ind Med* 1987;44:96–100.

104. Sluis-Cremer GK, Bezuidenhout BN. Relation between asbestosis and bronchial cancer in amphibole asbestos miners. *Br J Ind Med* 1989;46:537–540.

105. Jones RN, Hughes JM, Weill H. Asbestos exposure, asbestosis, and asbestos-attributable lung cancer. *Thorax* 1996;51(Suppl. 2):S9–S15.

106. Camus M, Siemiatycki J, Meek B. Nonoccupational exposure to chrysotile asbestos and the risk of lung cancer. *N Engl J Med* 1998;338:1565–1571.

107. Sluis-Cremer GK, Bezuidenhout BN. Relation between asbestosis and bronchial cancer in amphibole asbestos miners [reply to letter]. *Br J Ind Med* 1990;47:215–216.

108. Banks DE, Wang ML, Parker JE. Asbestos exposure, asbestosis, and lung cancer [editorial; comment]. *Chest* 1999;115:320–322.

109. Newhouse ML, Berry G, Wagner JC. Mortality of factory workers in east London 1933–80. *Br J Ind Med* 1985;42:4–11.

110. Henderson DW, Leigh J. Asbestos and lung cancer: a selective up-date to The Helsinki Criteria for individual attribution. *People and Work Research Reports* 36. Helsinki: Finnish Institute for Occupational Health; 2000: 3–18.

111. Harris JM, Johnston ID, Rudd R, Taylor AJ, Cullinan P. Cryptogenic fibrosing alveolitis and lung cancer: The BTS study. *Thorax* 2010;65:70–76.

112. Daniels CE, Yi ES, Ryu JH. Autopsy findings in 42 consecutive patients with idiopathic pulmonary fibrosis. *Eur Respir J* 2008;32:170–174.

113. Matsushita H, Tanaka S, Saiki Y, Hara M, Nakata K, Tanimura S, et al. Lung cancer associated with usual interstitial pneumonia. *Pathol Int* 1995;45:925–932.

114. Wells C, Mannino DM. Pulmonary fibrosis and lung cancer in the United States: analysis of the multiple cause of death mortality data, 1979 through 1991. *South Med J* 1996;89:505–510.

115. Nagai A, Chiyotani A, Nakadate T, Konno K. Lung cancer in patients with idiopathic pulmonary fibrosis. *Tohoku J Exp Med* 1992;167:231–237.

116. Mizushima Y, Kobayashi M. Clinical characteristics of synchronous multiple lung cancer associated with idiopathic pulmonary fibrosis: a review of Japanese cases. *Chest* 1995;108:1272–1277.

117. Daniels CE, Jett JR. Does interstitial lung disease predispose to lung cancer? *Curr Opin Pulm Med* 2005;11:431–437.

118. Turner-Warwick M, Lebowitz M, Burrows B, Johnson A. Cryptogenic fibrosing alveolitis and lung cancer. *Thorax* 1980;35:496–499.

119. Rouetbi N, Battikh M, el Kamel A. Diffuse interstitial pulmonary fibrosis and bronchial cancer. *Rev Pneumol Clin* 1999;55:370–372.

120. Abrahams NA, Meziane M, Ramalingam P, Mehta A, DeCamp M, Farver CF. et al. Incidence of primary neoplasms in explanted lungs: Long-term follow-up from 214 lung transplant patients. *Transplant Proc* 2004;36:2808–2811.

121. Baumgartner KB, Samet JM, Stidley CA, Colby TV, Waldron JA. Cigarette smoking: A risk factor for idiopathic pulmonary fibrosis. *Am J Respir Crit Care Med* 1997;155:242–248.

122. Kawabata Y, Hoshi E, Murai K, Ikeya T, Takahashi N, Saitou Y, et al. Smoking-related changes in the background lung of specimens resected for lung cancer: A semiquantitative study with correlation to postoperative course. *Histopathology* 2008;53:707–714.

123. Mizuno S, Takiguchi Y, Fujikawa A, Motoori K, Tada Y, Kurosu K, et al. Chronic obstructive pulmonary disease and interstitial lung disease in patients with lung cancer. *Respirology* 2009;14:377–383.

124. Katzenstein AL, Mukhopadhyay S, Zanardi C, Dexter E. Clinically occult interstitial fibrosis in smokers: classification and significance of a surprisingly common finding in lobectomy specimens. *Hum Pathol* 2010;41:316–325.

125. Turner MC, Chen Y, Krewski D, Calle EE, Thun MJ. Chronic obstructive pulmonary disease is associated with lung cancer mortality in a prospective study of never smokers. *Am J Respir Crit Care Med* 2007;176:285–290.

126. Wilson DO, Weissfeld JL, Balkan A, Schragin JG, Fuhrman CR, Fisher SN, et al. Association of radiographic emphysema and airflow obstruction with lung cancer. *Am J Respir Crit Care Med* 2008;178:738–744.

127. De Torres JP, Zulueta JJ, Wisnivesky JP. Emphysema and airway obstruction as risk factors for lung cancer. *Am J Respir Crit Care Med* 2008;178:1187.

128. Koshiol J, Rotunno M, Consonni D, Pesatori AC, De Matteis S, Goldstein AM, et al. Chronic obstructive pulmonary disease and altered risk of lung cancer in a population-based case–control study. *PLoS One* 2009;4:e7380.

129. Lee G, Walser TC, Dubinett SM. Chronic inflammation, chronic obstructive pulmonary disease, and lung cancer. *Curr Opin Pulm Med* 2009;15:303–307.

130. Schwartz AG, Cote ML, Wenzlaff AS, Van Dyke A, Chen W, Ruckdeschel JC, et al. Chronic obstructive lung diseases and risk of non-small cell lung cancer in women. *J Thorac Oncol* 2009;4:291–299.

131. Gao Y, Goldstein AM, Consonni D, Pesatori AC, Wacholder S, Tucker MA, et al. Family history of cancer and nonmalignant lung diseases as risk factors for lung cancer. *Int J Cancer* 2009;125:146–152.

132. Ishikawa N, Kohno N. Interstitial lung disease and lung cancer [in Japanese]. *Gan To Kagaku Ryoho* 2010;37:6–9.

133. Roggli VL, Hammar SP, Pratt PC, Maddox JC, Legier J, Mark EJ, et al. Does asbestos or asbestosis cause carcinoma of the lung? *Am J Ind Med* 1994;26:835–838.

134. Roggli VL, Gibbs AR, Attanoos R, Churg A, Popper H, Cagle P, et al. Pathology of asbestosis—An update of the diagnostic criteria: Report of the Asbestosis Committee of the College of American Pathologists and Pulmonary Pathology Society. *Arch Pathol Lab Med* 2010;134:462–480.

135. Peric I, Novak K, Barisic I, Mise K, Vuckovic M, Jankovic S, et al. Interobserver variations in diagnosing asbestosis according to the ILO classification. *Arh Hig Rada Toksikol* 2009;60:191–195.

136. Thomeer M, Demedts M, Behr J, Buhl R, Costabel U, Flower CD, et al. Multidisciplinary interobserver agreement in the diagnosis of idiopathic pulmonary fibrosis. *Eur Respir J* 2008;31:585–591.

137. Adams H, Crane MD. Radiological features of the asbestos-associated diseases. In: *Asbestos and Its Diseases*, Craighead JE, Gibbs AR, eds. Oxford: Oxford University Press; 2008: 269–298.

138. Case BW, Dufresne A. Asbestos, asbestosis, and lung cancer: observations in Quebec chrysotile workers. *Environ Health Perspect* 1997;105(Suppl. 5):1113–1119.

139. Piekarski C, Jennison EA, Parker JE. Workers' compensation for occupational lung disease: German–US parallels. In: *Occupational Lung Disease: An International Perspective*, Banks DE, Parker JE, eds. London: Chapman & Hall Medical; 1998: 83–93.

140. Banks DE, Shi R, McLarty J, Cowl CT, Smith D, Tarlo SM, et al. American College of Chest Physicians consensus statement on the respiratory health effects of asbestos: Results of a Delphi study. *Chest* 2009;135:1619–1627.

141. Churg A. Nonneoplastic disease caused by asbestos. In: *Pathology of Occupational Lung Disease*, 2nd ed., Churg A, Green FHY, eds. Baltimore: Williams & Wilkins; 1998: 277–338.

142. Gaensler EA, Jederlinic PJ, Churg A. Idiopathic pulmonary fibrosis in asbestos-exposed workers. *Am Rev Respir Dis* 1991;144:689–696.

143. White HHJ. Judgement in the Sabin v. BRB (Subsidiary) Case. Queens Bench High Court in the UK ncnEQ, Case No. HQ07XO3352. February 19, 2010.

144. Wood WB, Gloyne SR. Pulmonary asbestosis: A review of 100 cases. *Lancet* 1934;2:1383–1385.

145. Dupres JS, Mustard JF, Uffen RJ. *Report of the Royal Commission on Matters of Health and Safety Arising from the Use of Asbestos in Ontario* (3 vols). Toronto: Ontario Ministry of Government Services: Queen's Printer for Ontario; 1984.

146. Browne K. A threshold for asbestos-related lung cancer. *Br J Ind Med* 1986;43:556–558.

147. Green FH, Harley R, Vallyathan V, Althouse R, Fick G, Dement J, et al. Exposure and mineralogical correlates of pulmonary fibrosis in chrysotile asbestos workers. *Occup Environ Med* 1997;54:549–559.

148. Fischer M, Gunther S, Muller KM. Fibre-years, pulmonary asbestos burden and asbestosis. *Int J Hyg Environ Health* 2002;205:245–248.

149. Selikoff IJ, Churg J, Hammond EC. The occurrence of asbestosis among insulation workers in the United States. *Ann N Y Acad Sci* 1965;132:139–155.

150. Hodgson JT, Darnton A. The quantitative risks of mesothelioma and lung cancer in relation to asbestos exposure. *Ann Occup Hyg* 2000;44:565–601.

151. Gustavsson P, Jakobsson R, Nyberg F, Pershagen G, Järup L, Schéele P. Occupational exposure and lung cancer risk: a population-based case-referent study in Sweden. *Am J Epidemiol* 2000;152:32–40.

152. Gustavsson P, Nyberg F, Pershagen G, Scheele P, Jakobsson R, Plato N. Low-dose exposure to asbestos and lung cancer: Dose–response relations and interaction with smoking in a population-based case-referent study in Stockholm, Sweden. *Am J Epidemiol* 2002;155:1016–1022.

153. HEI-AR. *Asbestos in Public and Commercial Buildings: A Literature Review and Synthesis of Current Knowledge*. Cambridge, MA: Health Effects Institute–Asbestos Research; 1991.

154. Panduri V, Surapureddi S, Soberanes S, Weitzman SA, Chandel N, Kamp DW. P53 mediates amosite asbestos-induced alveolar epithelial cell mitochondria-regulated apoptosis. *Am J Respir Cell Mol Biol* 2006;34:443–452.

155. Hei TK, Wu LJ, Piao CQ. Malignant transformation of immortalized human bronchial epithelial cells by asbestos fibers. *Environ Health Perspect* 1997;105(Suppl. 5):1085–1088.

156. Popper K. *The Logic of Scientific Discovery*. London: Routledge Classics (originally published as *Logic der Forschung* in Vienna: Verlag von Julius Springer; 1935); 1959/2002.

157. Popper K. *Conjectures and Refutations: The Growth of Scientific Knowledge*. London: Routledge Classics; 1963/2002.

158. Martischnig KM, Newell DJ, Barnsley WC, Cowan WK, Feinmann EL, Oliver E. Unsuspected exposure to asbestos and bronchogenic carcinoma. *Br Med J* 1977;1:746–749.

159. Liddell FD, McDonald JC. Radiological findings as predictors of mortality in Quebec asbestos workers. *Br J Ind Med* 1980;37:257–267.

160. Wilkinson P, Hansell DM, Janssens J, Rubens M, Rudd RM, Newman Taylor A, et al. Is lung cancer associated with asbestos exposure without small opacities on the chest radiograph? *Lancet* 1995;345:1074–1078.

161. Finkelstein MM. Radiographic asbestosis is not a prerequisite for asbestos-associated lung cancer in Ontario asbestos-cement workers. *Am J Ind Med* 1997;32:341–348.

162. De Klerk NH, Musk AW, Glancy JJ, Pang SC, Lund HG, Olsen N, et al. Crocidolite, radiographic asbestosis and subsequent lung cancer. *Ann Occup Hyg* 1997;41(Suppl. 1):134–136.

163. Reid A, de Klerk N, Ambrosini GL, Olsen N, Pang SC, Berry G, et al. The effect of asbestosis on lung cancer risk beyond the dose related effect of asbestos alone. *Occup Environ Med* 2005;62:885–889.

164. Roggli VL. Malignant mesothelioma and duration of asbestos exposure: Correlation with tissue mineral fibre content. *Ann Occup Hyg* 1995;39:363–374.

165. Carel R, Boffetta P, Kauppinen T, Teschke K, Andersen A, Jappinen P, et al. Exposure to asbestos and lung and pleural cancer mortality among pulp and paper industry workers. *J Occup Environ Med* 2002;44:579–584.

166. Meguellati-Hakkas D, Cyr D, Stucker I, Fevotte J, Pilorget C, Luce D, et al. Lung cancer mortality and occupational exposure to asbestos among telephone linemen: A historical cohort study in France. *J Occup Environ Med* 2006;48:1166–1172.

167. Wichmann HE, Jöckel K-H, Molik B. *Luftverunreinigung und Lungenkrensrisiko—Ergebnisse einer Pilotstudie*. Bericht des Umweltbundesamtes 7/91. Berlin: Erich-Schmidt-Verlag; 1991.

168. Jöckel K-H, Ahrens W, Wichmann HE, Becher H, Bolm-Audorff U, Jahn I, et al. Occupational and environmental hazards associated with lung cancer. *Int J Epidemiol* 1992;21:202–213.

169. Jöckel KH, Ahrens W, Jahn I, Pohlabeln H, Bolm-Audorff U. et al. Occupational risk factors for lung cancer: a case–control study in West Germany. *Int J Epidemiol* 1998;27:549–560.

170. Jöckel K-H, Brüske-Hohlfeld I, Wichmann HEH. Lungenkrebsrisiko durch berufliche Exposition. In: *Forschritte in der Epidemiologie*, Wichmann HE, Jöckel K-H, Robta BPH, eds. Landsberg: Ecomed; 1998.

171. Pohlabeln H, Wild P, Schill W, Ahrens W, Jahn I, Bolm-Audorff U, et al. Asbestos fibreyears and lung cancer: A two phase case–control study with expert exposure assessment. *Occup Environ Med* 2002;59:410–414.

172. Karjalainen A, Anttila S, Vanhala E, Vainio H. Asbestos exposure and the risk of lung cancer in a general urban population. *Scand J Work Environ Health* 1994;20:243–250.

173. Working Party on Occupational Cancer of the Australasian Faculty of Occupational Medicine (AFOM) of the Royal Australasian College of Physicians. Occupational cancer: a guide to prevention, assessment and investigation. Sydney: AFOM; 2003.

174. Smith KA, Sykes LJ, McGavin CR. Diffuse pleural fibrosis: An unreliable indicator of heavy asbestos exposure? *Scand J Work Environ Health* 2003;29:60–63.

175. Miles SE, Sandrini A, Johnson AR, Yates DH. Clinical consequences of asbestos-related diffuse pleural thickening: A review. *J Occup Med Toxicol* 2008;3:20.

176. Gibbs GW, Berry G. Epidemiology and risk assessment. In: *Asbestos and Its Diseases*, Craighead JE, Gibbs AR, eds. Oxford: Oxford University Press; 2008: 94–119.

177. Tweedale G. Sprayed "limpet" asbestos: technical, commercial, and regulatory aspects. In: *Sourcebook on Asbestos Diseases*, Vol 20, Peters GA, Peters BJ, eds. Charlottesville: Lexis; 1999: 79–109.

178. Henderson DW. Commentary regarding the article by Fischer et al: fibre years, pulmonary asbestos burden and asbestosis. *Int J Hyg Environ Health* 2002;205:245–248; *Int J Hyg Environ Health* 2003;206:249–250.

179. Rödelsperger K. *Anorganische Fasern im menschlichen Lungengewebe. Lungenstaubfaseranalytik zur Epidemiologie der Risikofaktoren des diffusen malignen Mesothelioms (DMM).* [*Inorganic Fibres in Human Lung Tissue. Epidemiology of the Risk Factors for Diffuse Malignant Mesothelioma (DMM) Based on Lung Dust Fibre Analysis*]. Berlin: Bundesanstalt für Arbeitsmedizin; 1996.

180. Tuomi T, Huuskonen MS, Tammilehto L, Vanhala E, Virtamo M. Occupational exposure to asbestos as evaluated from work histories and analysis of lung tissues from patients with mesothelioma. *Br J Ind Med* 1991;48:48–52.

181. De Vuyst P, Missouni A, Van Muylen A, Rocmans P, Dumortier P. Systematic asbestos bodies counting in lung specimens resected for lung cancer. *Eur Respir J* 1997;10(Suppl. 25):19s.

182. Thimpont J, De Vuyst P. Occupational asbestos-related diseases in Belgium (epidemiological data and compensation criteria). In: *Sourcebook on Asbestos Diseases*, Vol. 17, Peters GA, Peters BJ, eds. Charlottesville: Lexis; 1998: 311–328.

183. Mollo F, Pira E, Piolatto G, Bellis D, Burlo P, Andreozzi A, et al. Lung adenocarcinoma and indicators of asbestos exposure. *Int J Cancer* 1995;60:289–293.

184. Rogers AJ. Determination of mineral fibre in human lung tissue by light microscopy and transmission electron microscopy. *Ann Occup Hyg* 1984;28:1–12.

185. Roggli VL, Sharma A. Analysis of tissue mineral fiber content. In: *Pathology of Asbestos-Associated Diseases*, 2nd ed., Roggli VL, Oury TD, Sporn TA, eds. New York: Springer; 2004: 309–354.

186. Berry G. Models for mesothelioma incidence following exposure to fibers in terms of timing and duration of exposure and the biopersistence of the fibers. *Inhal Toxicol* 1999;11:111–130.

187. Berry G, de Klerk NH, Reid A, Ambrosini GL, Fritschi L, Olsen NJ, et al. Malignant pleural and peritoneal mesotheliomas in former miners and millers of crocidolite at Wittenoom, Western Australia. *Occup Environ Med* 2004;61:e14.

188. Greenland S. Relation of probability of causation to relative risk and doubling dose: A methodologic error that has become a social problem. *Am J Public Health* 1999;89:1166–1169.

189. Rockhill B, Newman B, Weinberg C. Use and misuse of population attributable fractions. *Am J Public Health* 1998;88:15–19.

190. Greenland S. Attributable fractions: bias from broad definition of exposure. *Epidemiology* 2001;12:518–520.

191. Pirie M. *How to Win Every Argument: The Use and Abuse of Logic.* New York: Continuum; 2006.

192. Gorlova OY, Zhang Y, Schabath MB, Lei L, Zhang Q, Amos CI, et al. Never smokers and lung cancer risk: a case–control study of epidemiological factors. *Int J Cancer* 2006;118:1798–1804.

193. Spitz MR, Wei Q, Li G, Wu X. Genetic susceptibility to tobacco carcinogenesis. *Cancer Invest* 1999;17:645–659.

194. Spitz MR, Wei Q, Dong Q, Amos CI, Wu X. Genetic susceptibility to lung cancer: The role of DNA damage and repair. *Cancer Epidemiol Biomarkers Prev* 2003;12:689–698.

195. Spitz MR, Hong WK, Amos CI, Wu X, Schabath MB, Dong Q, et al. A risk model for prediction of lung cancer. *J Natl Cancer Inst* 2007;99:715–726.

196. Pylkkänen L, Wolff H, Stjernvall T, Tuominen P, Sioris T, Karjalainen A, et al. Reduced Fhit protein expression and loss of heterozygosity at FHIT gene in tumours from smoking and asbestos-exposed lung cancer patients. *Int J Oncol* 2002;20:285–290.

197. Hou SM, Falt S, Angelini S, Yang K, Nyberg F, Lambert B, et al. The XPD variant alleles are associated with increased aromatic DNA adduct level and lung cancer risk. *Carcinogenesis* 2002;23:599–603.

198. Brockmoller J, Cascorbi I, Henning S, Meisel C, Roots I. et al. Molecular genetics of cancer susceptibility. *Pharmacology* 2000;61:212–227.

199. Schabath MB, Spitz MR, Delclos GL, Gunn GB, Whitehead LW, Wu X. Association between asbestos exposure, cigarette smoking, myeloperoxidase (MPO) genotypes, and lung cancer risk. *Am J Ind Med* 2002;42:29–37.

200. Baur X, Czuppon AB. Regulation and compensation of asbestos diseases in Germany. In: *Sourcebook on Asbestos Diseases*, Vol 15, Peters GA, Peters BJ, eds. Charlottesville: Lexis; 1997: 405–419.

CHAPTER 7

Asbestos and Mesothelioma

Samuel P. Hammar

CONTENTS

7.1 INTRODUCTION

For extensive additional discussions concerning asbestos and mesothelioma, I (S.P.H.) refer the reader to Chapter 1 written by Douglas W. Henderson and James Leigh titled "The History of Asbestos Utilization and Recognition of Asbestos-Induced Diseases"; Chapter 5 written by Richard A. Lemen, specifically, Section 5.1.1 titled "History and Usage of Asbestors" and Section 5.1.7 titled "Mesothelioma"; and Chapter 4 written by Sonja Klebe and Douglas W. Henderson titled "The Molecular Pathogenesis of Asbestos-Related Disorders."

This chapter discusses the macroscopic, histological, histochemical, immunohistochemical, and ultrastructural features of malignant mesothelioma. Included in this chapter are the pathological differential diagnoses of mesothelioma, the clinical features of mesothelioma, the approach to the diagnosis, the staging of mesothelioma, and the prognosis.

Mesotheliomas are neoplasms that arise from the serosal lining of the body cavities, namely, the pleura (lung), the peritoneum (abdomen), and the pericardium (heart). These body cavities have a visceral layer, which covers the organs, and a parietal layer, which covers the body spaces. These body cavities are derived from the celomic cavity (Figure 7.1) that develops very early in embryogenesis and forms these cavities by partitioning membranes and other structures.

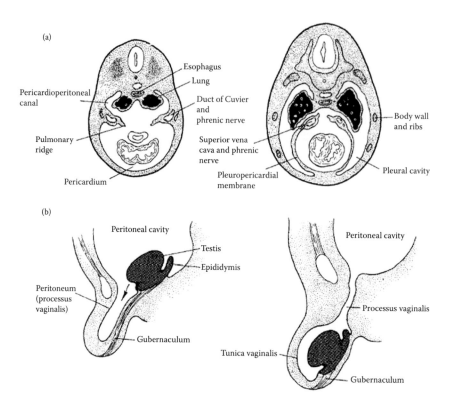

Figure 7.1 (a) Celomic cavity develops early in embryogenesis and is lined by a thin serosal membrane that gives rise to the pleura, peritoneum, and pericardium. (b) Tunica vaginalis is an invagination of the peritoneum.

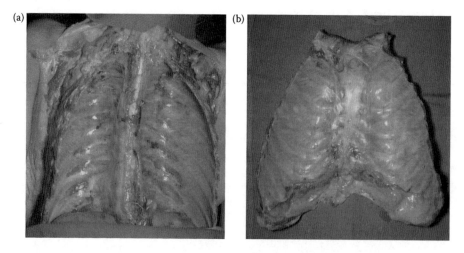

Figure 7.2 (a, b) This portion of the chest plate is covered by the shiny parietal pleura.

The serosal membranes have the thickness of a piece of ordinary cellophane (approximately 0.2 mm) and has the same clarity. The macroscopic appearance of the parietal and visceral pleura are shown in Figures 7.2 and 7.3.

The visceral and parietal pleural membranes are composed of an outer layer of meso-thelial cells with underlying elastic tissue, collagen, and spindle cells that we have termed

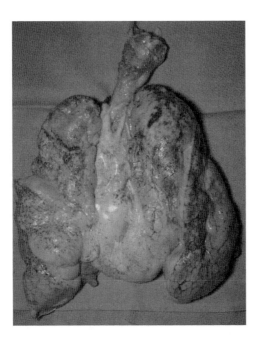

Figure 7.3   The lung is covered by the visceral pleura that frequently contains anthracotic material.

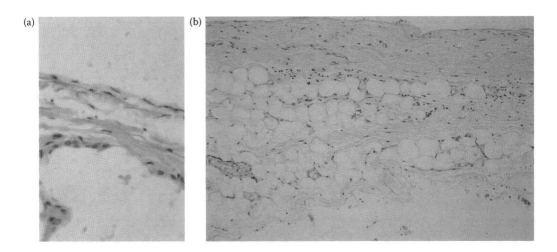

Figure 7.4   (a, b) The visceral and parietal pleura are composed of an outer layer of mesothelial cells that may be flattened or cuboidal and are separated by a basement membrane from a connective tissue layer composed of cells we termed *multipotential subserosal cells* that produce elastin and collagen (VVG stain).

multipotential subserosal cells. The same anatomy is seen in the peritoneal and pericardial cavities (see Figures 7.4–7.7).

Ultrastructurally, the mesothelial cells vary somewhat depending on how activated they are. When they are injured or activated by inflammation, the mesothelial cells frequently become cuboidal to columnar (Figures 7.8 and 7.9) and have long, thin, smooth microvilli that are not covered by a glycocalyx. With injury, the multipotential subserosal cells proliferate, producing reactive spindle cells (Figures 7.10 and 7.11).

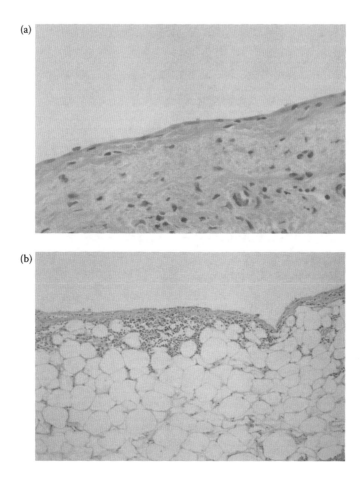

Figure 7.5 The (a) visceral peritoneum and the (b) parietal peritoneum are similar to the pleura.

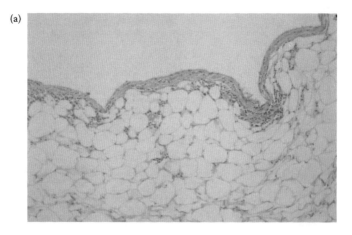

Figure 7.6 The (a) visceral pericardium and the (b) parietal pericardium are composed of the same cellular elements as in the pleura and peritoneum.

(b)

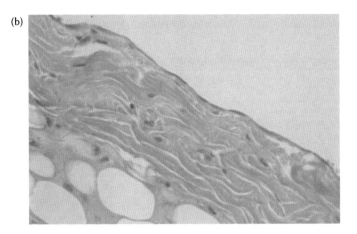

Figure 7.6 Continued.

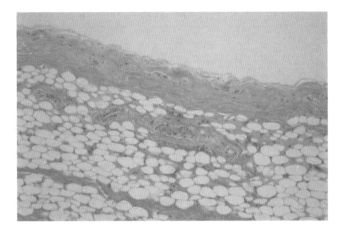

Figure 7.7 There is a layer of adipose tissue underlying the connective tissue of the pleura, peritoneum, and pericardium.

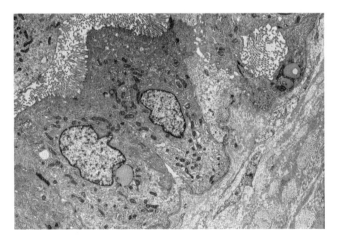

Figure 7.8 Ultrastructurally, the mesothelial cells are connected to each other by junctional complexes.

(a) 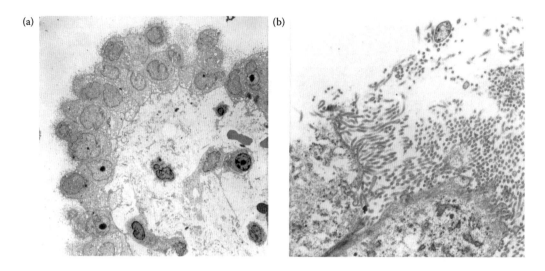 (b)

Figure 7.9   (a, b) Reactive and neoplastic mesothelial cells have long, thin, sinuous microvilli that are not covered by a glycocalyx.

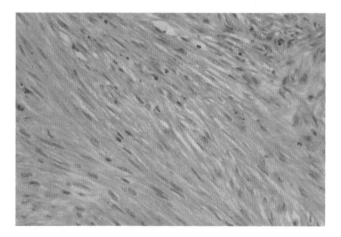

Figure 7.10   The multipotential subserosal cells are spindle-shaped cells.

Immunohistochemically, the normal and reactive epithelioid mesothelial cells express keratins 5 through 8 and 14 through 18 (Figure 7.12) and calretinin (Figure 7.13). The reactive mesothelial cells typically express desmin (Figure 7.14). The multipotential subserosal cells typically express keratin (Figure 7.15), vimentin (Figure 7.16), and alpha actin (Figure 7.17).

7.2 LOCATION OF MESOTHELIOMAS

The majority of mesotheliomas (90%–95%) occur in the chest cavity and are referred to as *pleural mesothelioma*. Approximately 5%–10% of all mesotheliomas occur in the peritoneal cavity and are referred to as *peritoneal mesothelioma*.

With respect to pericardial mesotheliomas, one must be aware that approximately 25% of pleural mesotheliomas directly invade the visceral and parietal pericardium and not infrequently directly invade the myocardium. Primary pericardial mesotheliomas are rare.

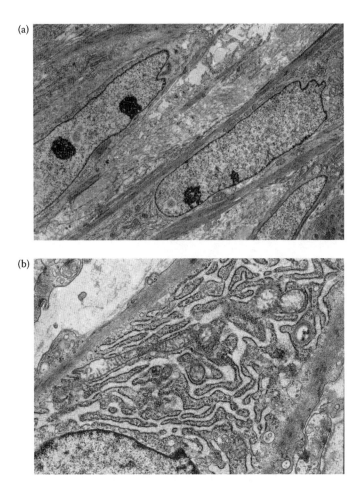

Figure 7.11 (a, b) The spindle cells have a prominent rough endoplasmic reticulum and intracytoplasmic filaments.

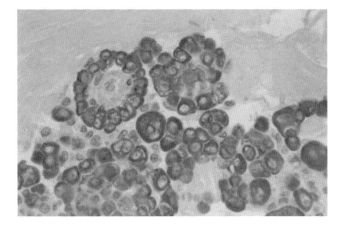

Figure 7.12 The pleural, peritoneal, and pericardial cells express low and high molecular weight keratin.

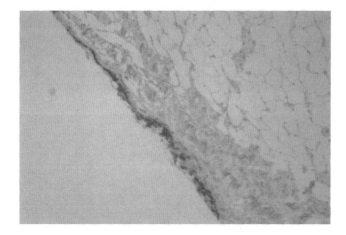

Figure 7.13 The mesothelial cells show cytoplasmic and nuclear staining for calretinin.

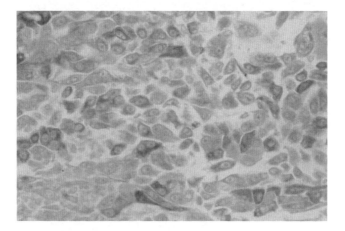

Figure 7.14 Benign reactive mesothelial cells typically express desmin.

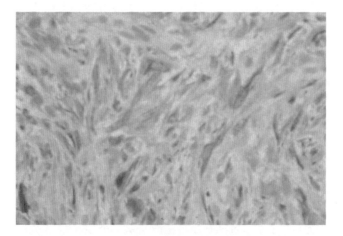

Figure 7.15 The multipotential subserosal cells show intense cytoplasmic immunostaining for cytokeratin.

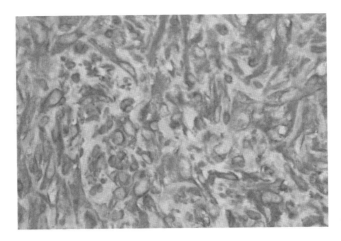

Figure 7.16 Vimentin is expressed in multipotential subserosal cells just as they would be in sarcomatoid mesotheliomas.

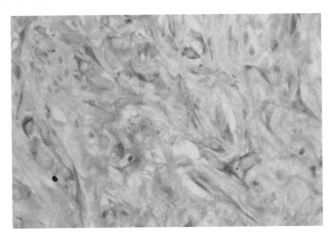

Figure 7.17 Alpha actin is expressed in reactive multipotential subserosal cells and in sarcomatoid mesotheliomas.

Mesotheliomas of the tunica vaginalis usually present as a hydrocele with or without an associated mass. Mesotheliomas of the tunica vaginalis must be distinguished from secondary spread from a peritoneal mesothelioma.

Primary mesotheliomas of the ovary are rare. The criteria for the diagnosis of ovarian mesothelioma include the presence of unilateral or bilateral ovarian enlargement, parenchymal replacement in the absence of significant peritoneal disease, or both. Most ovarian mesotheliomas are due to secondary involvement.

7.3 MACROSCOPIC FEATURES OF MESOTHELIOMA

The macroscopic appearance of mesothelioma is dependent on when the mesothelioma's progression is first observed. In patients with pleural mesothelioma, the earliest changes are of nodules on the visceral and parietal pleura (Figure 7.18). As the disease progresses, the nodules coalesce to form a rind of tumor that encases the lung (Figure 7.19). There may be total fusion between the visceral and the parietal pleura, although in some cases there is a cystic space between the

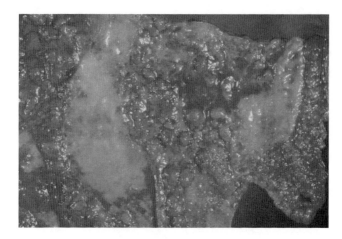

Figure 7.18   The earliest macroscopic feature of mesothelioma is small, white-yellow-gray nodules on the visceral and parietal layers. There is usually no significant difference in the number of tumor nodules on the visceral and parietal layers.

(a)

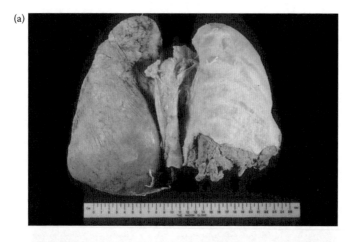

(b)

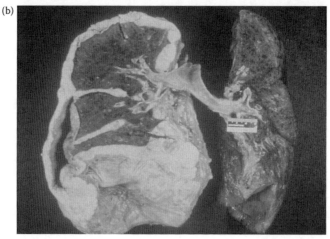

Figure 7.19   (a, b) The mesothelial tumor nodules coalesce to form a rind that encases the lungs.

mesothelioma's involvement of the visceral and parietal pleura (Figure 7.20). In general, pleural mesotheliomas are thicker at the base of the lung than they are at the apex (Figure 7.21).

It is common for mesotheliomas to directly invade the lung fissures (Figure 7.22). The thickness of the tumor invading the fissure can vary—sometimes being thinner than the rind encasing the lung and sometimes being about the same thickness (Figure 7.23).

It is not uncommon for mesotheliomas to invade the lung and chest wall. Mesotheliomas that invade the chest wall frequently have a nodular morphology (Figure 7.24). Sometimes the degree of invasion is so extensive that it almost obliterates the pulmonary parenchyma (Figure 7.25). Not

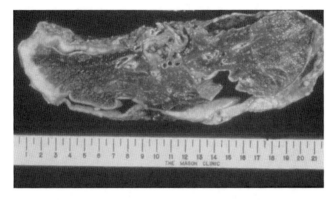

Figure 7.20 In pleural mesotheliomas, there may be a cystic space between the tumor involving the visceral and parietal pleura.

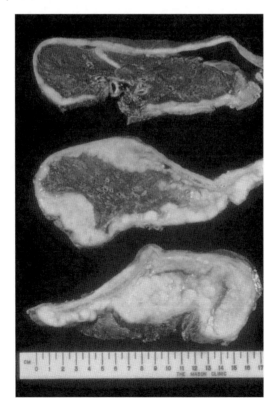

Figure 7.21 Pleural mesotheliomas are typically thicker at the base of the lung (chest cavity) than at the apex.

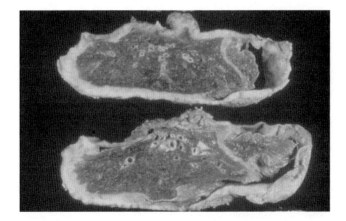

Figure 7.22   Pleural mesotheliomas frequently invade the fissures that separate the lobes of the lungs.

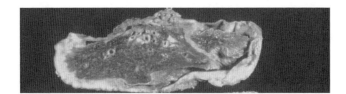

Figure 7.23   The mesothelioma invading the fissure is often thinner than the tumor forming the rind.

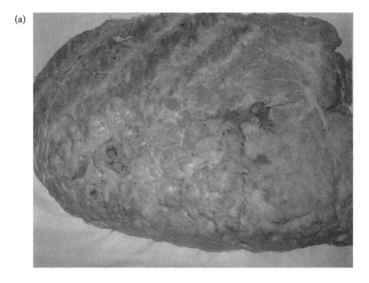

Figure 7.24   (a, b, c) Mesotheliomas frequently invade the chest wall or lung tissue, producing a nodular morphology.

(b)

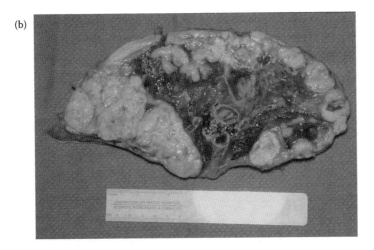

(c)

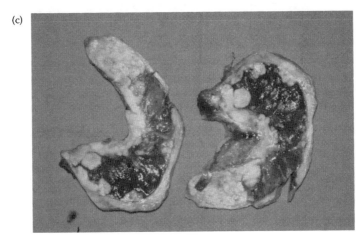

Figure 7.24 Continued.

infrequently, one may see a combination of tumor invading the chest wall, fibrofatty tissue, and muscular tissue frequently in association with plaques involving the pleura (Figure 7.26).

Pleural mesotheliomas not infrequently directly invade mediastinal tissue (Figure 7.27) and sometimes encase the trachea, esophagus, and aorta (Figures 7.28–7.30). They frequently metastasize to regional lymph nodes and sometimes present as hilar masses (Figures 7.31 and 7.32).

With respect to metastases, pleural mesotheliomas and peritoneal mesotheliomas can metastasize. Sarcomatoid mesotheliomas frequently metastasize to bone and, as will be discussed later, some sarcomatoid mesotheliomas may produce bone as part of their makeup. Mesotheliomas can metastasize to adrenal glands (Figure 7.33) and, not infrequently, to the opposite pleura as small nodules (Figure 7.34). They can metastasize extensively to the surface of the visceral pleura (Figure 7.35).

The morphology of peritoneal mesothelioma is also dependent upon at what point in time the tumor is identified. In the earliest phase, there are multiple nodules that involve the visceral and parietal peritoneum (Figure 7.36). As time passes, the tumor compresses/invades the peritoneal/pelvic tissue and surrounds the organs in the abdominal cavity, especially the intestine (Figures 7.37 and 7.38). In the end stage, the tumor almost completely obliterates the abdominal organs (Figure 7.39).

(a)

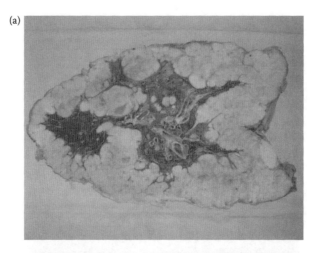

(b)

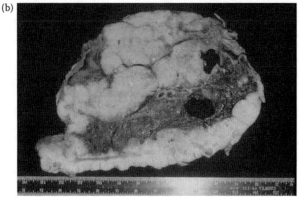

Figure 7.25   (a, b) Some pleural mesotheliomas invade and obliterate lung tissue.

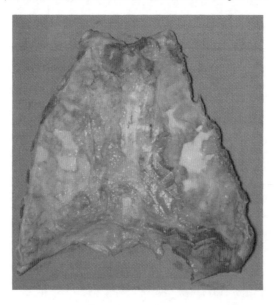

Figure 7.26   Pleural mesotheliomas invade chest wall, often in association with pleural plaque typical of plaque caused by asbestos.

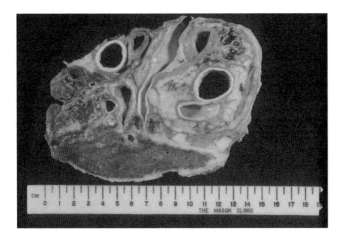

Figure 7.27 Mesotheliomas invade mediastinal tissue.

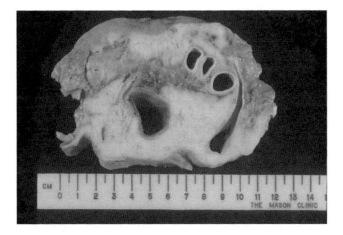

Figure 7.28 Pleural mesotheliomas may encase the trachea.

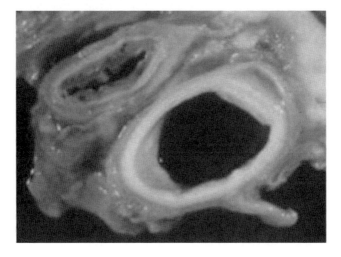

Figure 7.29 Pleural mesotheliomas may encase the esophagus and the aorta.

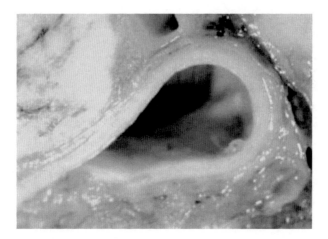

Figure 7.30   Pleural mesotheliomas may encase the aorta.

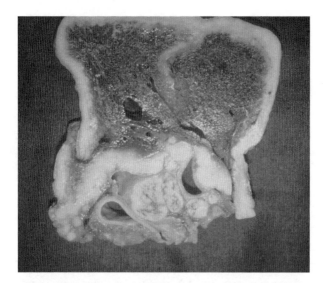

Figure 7.31   Mesotheliomas not infrequently metastasize to lymph nodes, producing hilar or umbilical masses.

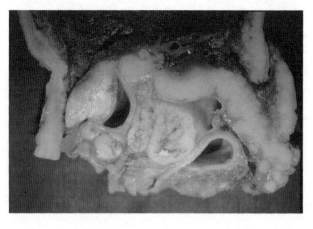

Figure 7.32   In this pleural mesothelioma, the tumor metastasized to a hilar lymph node, producing a mass.

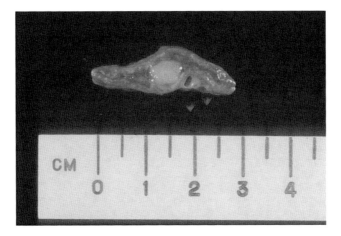

Figure 7.33   Mesotheliomas rarely metastasize to adrenal glands.

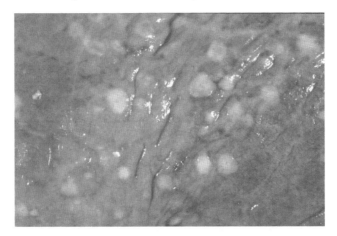

Figure 7.34   Metastases of pleural mesotheliomas to the opposite pleural surface is common.

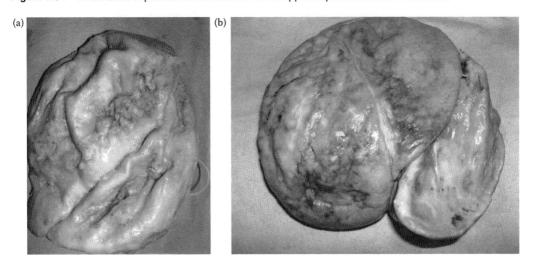

Figure 7.35   (a, b) This peritoneal mesothelioma metastasized to the pleural surface of both lungs.

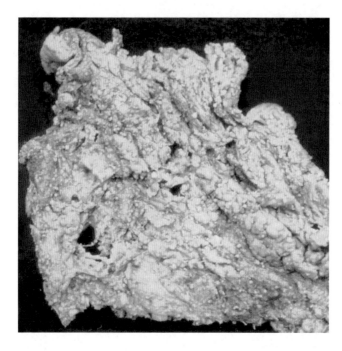

Figure 7.36 Like pleural mesotheliomas, peritoneal mesotheliomas begin as small nodules on the visceral and parietal peritoneum.

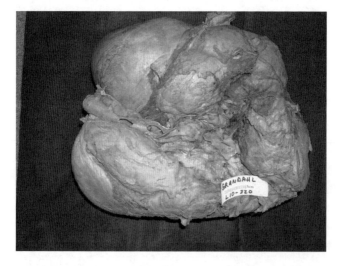

Figure 7.37 This peritoneal mesothelioma extensively involves the peritoneal cavity.

As stated earlier, it is not uncommon for pleural mesotheliomas to directly invade the visceral and parietal pericardium (Figure 7.40); therefore, it can be difficult to determine whether a mesothelioma involving the pericardium is primary or a metastases. In some instances, involvement of the myocardium is so extensive (Figure 7.41) that it is difficult to believe how a patient could survive with that degree of involvement.

Primary pericardial mesotheliomas are rare. Like other mesotheliomas, pericardial mesotheliomas grow in a diffuse distribution (Figure 7.42). As stated previously, one has to be aware that

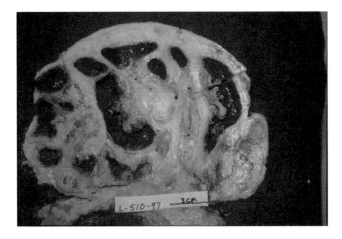

Figure 7.38 The bowel is extensively surrounded by this peritoneal mesothelioma.

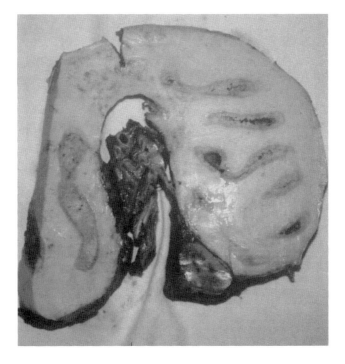

Figure 7.39 The "end-stage" macroscopic appearance of peritoneal mesothelioma.

pericardial involvement by mesothelioma can be a result of a pleural mesothelioma that is directly invading the pericardium.

There is a primary mesothelioma of the tunica vaginalis, which is a variant of peritoneal mesothelioma because the tunica vaginalis is an invagination of the peritoneum. Primary mesothelioma of the tunica vaginalis can present as isolated spherical masses in the scrotum or can present primarily in the spermatic cord or directly invade the peritoneal cavity (Figure 7.43).

There are rare mesotheliomas such as multicystic mesotheliomas, which usually occur in younger women and have a tendency to recur (Figures 7.44 and 7.45).

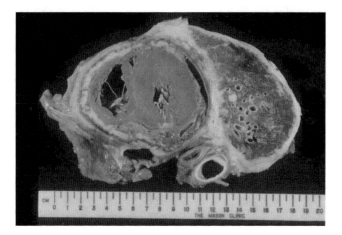

Figure 7.40 This pleural mesothelioma extensively involves the visceral and the parietal pericardium.

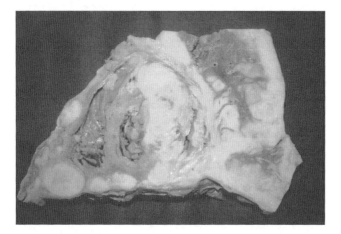

Figure 7.41 This pleural mesothelioma extensively invades the pericardium and the myocardium.

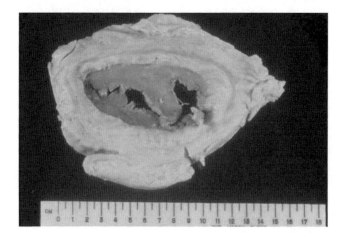

Figure 7.42 The heart is surrounded by tumor, the morphology being characteristic of a pericardial mesothelioma.

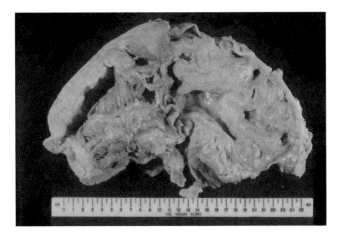

Figure 7.43 This mesothelioma originated in the tunica vaginalis, which is an invagination of the peritoneum.

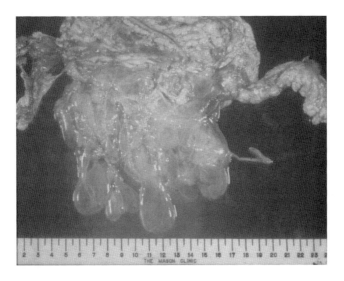

Figure 7.44 Rare mesotheliomas that typically occur in younger women exhibit a cystic morphology.

7.4 HISTOLOGICAL FEATURES AND CLASSIFICATIONS OF MESOTHELIOMA

Mesotheliomas are neoplasms that show a variety of histological patterns and can resemble many other malignant neoplasms. Therefore, histochemistry, immunohistochemistry, and electron microscopy are necessary to accurately diagnose suspected mesotheliomas. The simplest histological classification includes three general categories as listed in Table 7.1.

Desmoplastic mesotheliomas are a fairly common subtype of sarcomatoid mesothelioma. Sarcomatoid mesotheliomas show homologous differentiation producing spindle neoplasms producing collagen (fibrous tissue) or heterologous differentiation where they may form cartilage and bone. There is controversy as to whether mesotheliomas can exhibit vascular differentiation.

There are approximately 25 subtypes of epithelial mesothelioma, which are listed in Table 7.2.

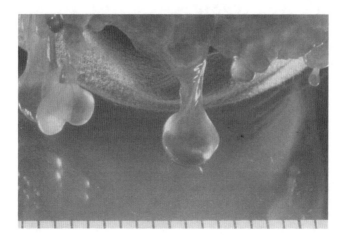

Figure 7.45   Cystic mesotheliomas are histologically benign and frequently recur.

Table 7.1   Histological Classification

Epithelial (epithelioid)
Sarcomatoid (sarcomatous, fibrous)
Biphasic (mixed, epithelioid-sarcomatoid)

Table 7.2   Epithelial Mesothelioma Subtypes

Adenoid Cystic	Microcystic
Adenomatoid	Mucin positive
Bakery (pastry) roll	Placentoid
Clear cell	Pleomorphic
Deciduoid	Poorly differentiated
Diffuse—not otherwise specified	Rhabdoid
Gaucher-like	Round cell
Glandular/acinar	Signet ring
Glomeruloid	Single file
Histiocytoid/epithelioid	Small cell
In association with excess amounts of hyaluronic acid or proteoglycan	Squamous
In situ	Tubulopapillary
Macrocystic	Well-differentiated papillary

7.4.1 Epithelioid Mesotheliomas Subtypes

7.4.1.1 Adenoid Cystic/Cystic

Mesotheliomas occasionally form glandular structures that resemble adenoid cystic carcinomas, such as those seen in salivary glands (Figures 7.46 and 7.47). In addition, there are mesotheliomas that are composed of small cysts made up of cells that frequently have attenuated cytoplasm and that often look benign. These cysts can be small (Figure 7.48) and sometimes are composed of larger cysts (Figure 7.49).

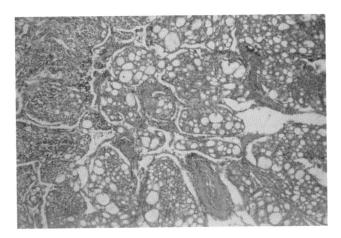

Figure 7.46   Adenoid cystic mesotheliomas are composed of multiple small cysts and resemble adenoid cystic carcinomas of salivary glands (low power magnification).

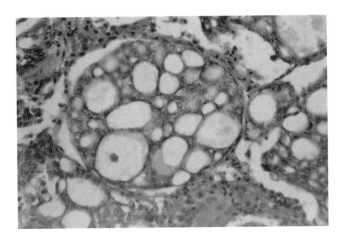

Figure 7.47   Adenoid cystic mesotheliomas are composed of multiple small cysts and resemble adenoid cystic carcinomas of salivary glands (high power magnification).

7.4.1.2 Clear Cell

Another rare form of mesothelioma that can cause confusion is that of a clear cell mesothelioma. In most cases, the clear cell morphology is due to the accumulation of glycogen and fat in the cells (Figure 7.50), although may be due to certain organelles in the clear cell mesotheliomas (Figure 7.51).[1]

7.4.1.3 Deciduoid

The largest round cell mesothelioma is referred to as a deciduoid mesothelioma. The term *deciduoid* is based on the morphologic similarity of these cells to progestationally stimulated endometrial stromal cells and placental cells. Deciduoid cells are typically large; usually round; have large nuclei and often prominent nucleoli; and have abundant glassy, eosinophilic cytoplasm (Figures 7.52 and 7.53). Often, the peripheral cytoplasm has a fibrillar appearance (Figure 7.54).

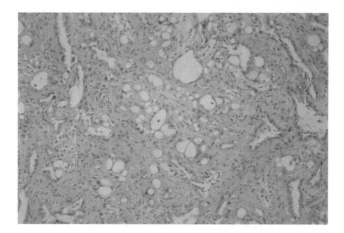

Figure 7.48   Some epithelial mesotheliomas are composed of small cysts.

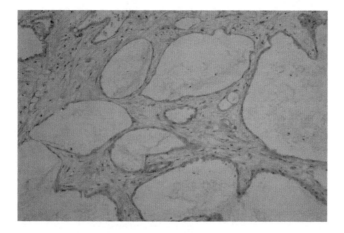

Figure 7.49   As expected, there are mesotheliomas composed of larger cysts.

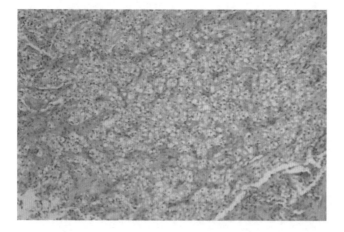

Figure 7.50   Clear cell mesothelioma resembles clear cell carcinoma of the kidney.

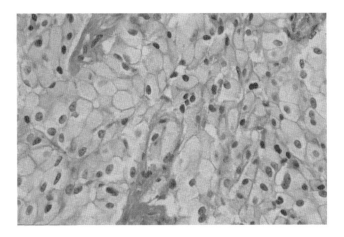

Figure 7.51 Some clear cell mesotheliomas contain numerous organelles.

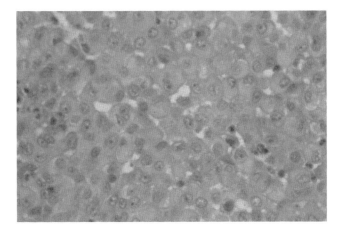

Figure 7.52 Deciduoid mesotheliomas are in the round cell category.

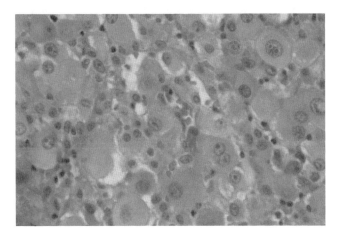

Figure 7.53 Deciduoid mesotheliomas are made up of large cells with abundant glassy eosinophilic cytoplasm with large, round nuclei and prominent nucleoli.

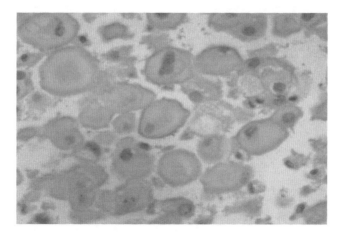

Figure 7.54 The cytoplasm of some deciduoid mesothelioma tumor cells has a fibrillar appearance.

Deciduoid mesothelioma was first described in 1985 in a 13-year-old girl[2] and was only confirmed as a mesothelioma after additional immunohistochemical studies were performed (see later discussion concerning deciduoid mesothelioma in this chapter).

7.4.1.4 Glandular/Acinar

Glandular mesotheliomas are composed of cells that form glandular structures similar to a primary pulmonary acinar adenocarcinoma (Figures 7.55 and 7.56). Sometimes mesotheliomas are made up of large columnar epithelial cells that contain eosinophilic cytoplasm that resemble mucin-producing adenocarcinomas (Figure 7.57).

7.4.1.5 Hyaluronic Acid- and Proteoglycan-Producing Mesotheliomas

Mesotheliomas can produce excess amounts of hyaluronic acid and proteoglycan. Nests of cells are suspended in this material that in hematoxylin and eosin–stained sections is pinkish-gray (Figures 7.58 and 7.59). This material stains positive with Alcian blue and is usually eradicated with pre-treatment with hyaluronic acid. The proteoglycan material is frequently formed by a granular bluish material (Figures 7.60 and 7.61) and can be somewhat eradicated by pre-treatment with hyaluronidase.

7.4.1.6 Pastry Roll

There are a few very rare patterns of epithelioid differentiation. These include a pattern I refer to as a *pastry roll* (Figures 7.62 and 7.63).

7.4.1.7 Placentoid

Some mesotheliomas have a histological appearance resembling chorionic villi (Figures 7.64 and 7.65).

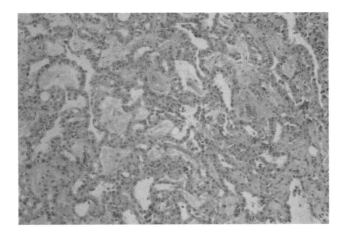

Figure 7.55 Glandular/acinar mesotheliomas are similar to glandular/acinar carcinomas, usually made up of cuboidal and/or columnar cells.

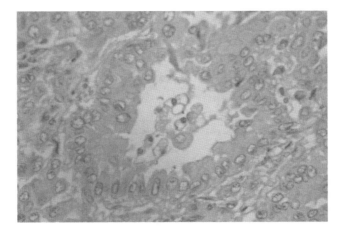

Figure 7.56 This glandular/acinar mesotheliomas is composed of tall columnar cells that resemble a primary pulmonary adenocarcinoma.

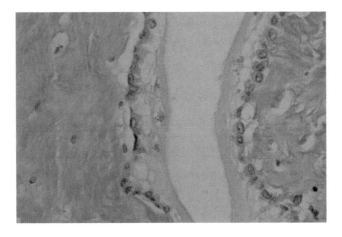

Figure 7.57 Rarely, acinar mesotheliomas appear as mucus-producing adenocarcinomas.

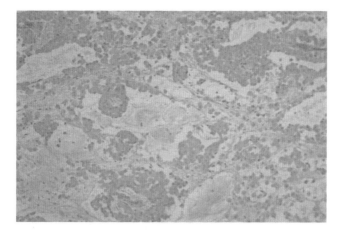

Figure 7.58   Normal mesothelial cells secrete hyaluronic acid and proteoglycan. Some epithelial mesotheliomas secrete excess amounts of hyaluronic acid.

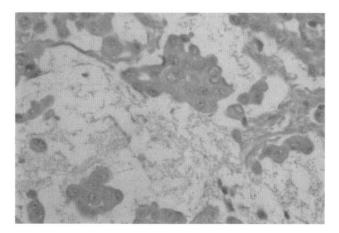

Figure 7.59   The neoplastic mesothelial cells are surrounded by this material that stains pinkish-gray in hematoxylin and eosin–stained sections.

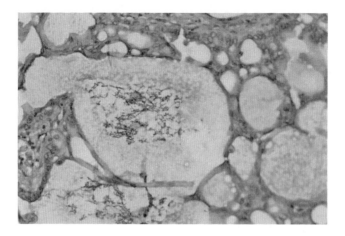

Figure 7.60   Proteoglycan-producing mesotheliomas are surrounded by bluish granular material.

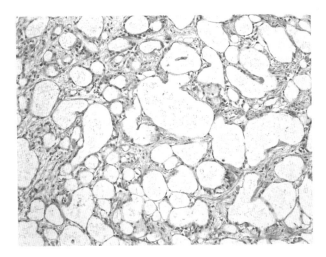

Figure 7.61 The proteoglycan material can be somewhat eradicated by pretreatment with hyaluronidase.

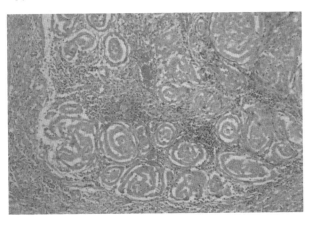

Figure 7.62 Some mesotheliomas are composed of uniform epithelial cells in a repeating circular configuration resembling a pastry roll (low power magnification).

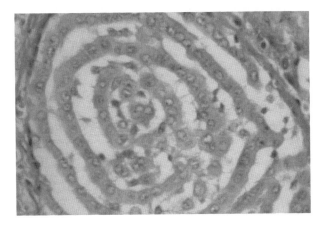

Figure 7.63 Some mesotheliomas are composed of uniform epithelial cells in a repeating circular configuration resembling a pastry roll (high power magnification).

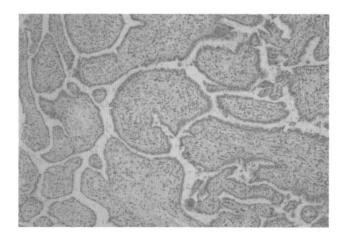

Figure 7.64 Placentoid mesotheliomas are occasionally formed by an outer layer of epithelioid cells that sur-
round spindle cell stromal cells and produce a pattern that looks like chorionic villi (low power
magnification).

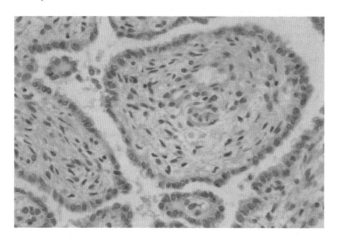

Figure 7.65 Placentoid mesotheliomas are occasionally formed by an outer layer of epithelioid cells that sur-
round spindle cell stromal cells and produce a pattern that looks like chorionic villi (high power
magnification).

7.4.1.8 Round Cell

Mesotheliomas can be composed of round cells and there is significant variability in the size of
these round cells (Figures 7.66 through 7.68).

7.4.1.9 Signet Ring

Rarely, mesotheliomas show signet ring differentiation very similar to that seen in a signet ring
carcinoma (Figure 7.69).

7.4.1.10 Single File

Some mesotheliomas grow in a single file arrangement similar to that seen in a lobular carcinoma
of breast (Figures 7.70 and 7.71). This is a nonspecific pattern but one that mesothelioma can assume.

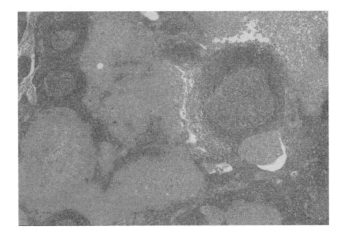

Figure 7.66 Round cell mesotheliomas can be composed of a uniform population of round cells that vary in size.

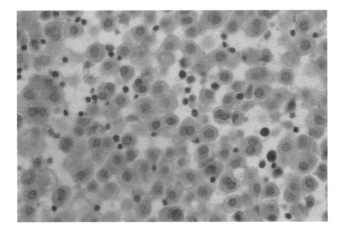

Figure 7.67 Some resemble alveolar macrophages.

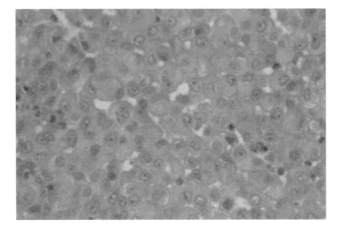

Figure 7.68 Others are composed of smaller round cells and larger round cells, the largest member of the group being deciduoid cells.

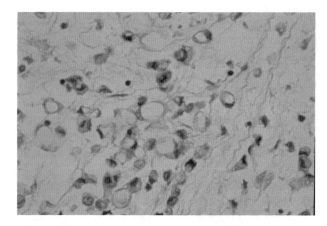

Figure 7.69 Neoplasms composed of signet ring cells are usually carcinomas. However, some mesothe-liomas are composed of signet ring cells and are confused with signet ring carcinoma.

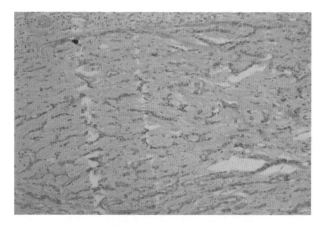

Figure 7.70 Many carcinomas, such as breast carcinomas, are composed of neoplastic cells that are arranged in a single file pattern. Epithelioid mesotheliomas can have this morphology (low power magnification).

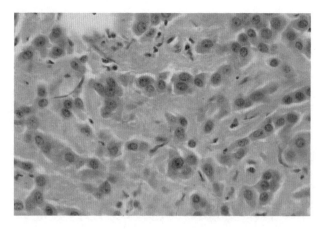

Figure 7.71 Many carcinomas, such as breast carcinomas, are composed of neoplastic cells that are arranged in a single file pattern. Epithelioid mesotheliomas can have this morphology (high power magnification).

7.4.1.11 Small Cell

Mesotheliomas can resemble small cell lung cancer and occasionally have a glomeruloid pattern (Figures 7.72 and 7.73). These mesotheliomas do not show neuroendocrine differentiation as is seen in typical small cell lung cancers. They do not express synaptophysin, chromogranin-A, neuron-specific enolase, and thyroid transcription factor-1 (TTF-1).

7.4.1.12 Squamous

Some mesotheliomas show areas of squamous differentiation (Figures 7.74 and 7.75). Perhaps this is not surprising in that there are reports of normal pleural mesothelial cells undergoing squamous metaplasia.

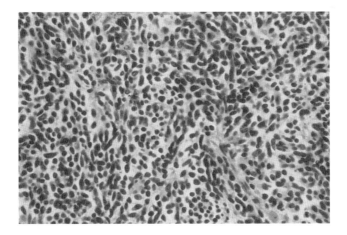

Figure 7.72 Rarely, mesotheliomas have a morphology almost identical to small cell lung cancer.

(a)

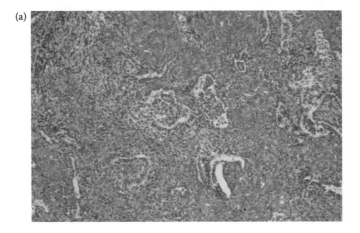

Figure 7.73 (a, b) Small cell mesotheliomas may have a glomeruloid morphology.

(b)

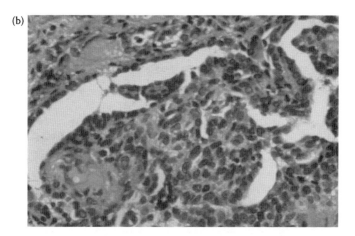

Figure 7.73   Continued.

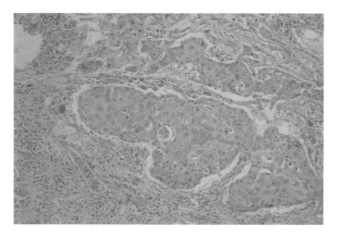

Figure 7.74   Rare epithelioid mesotheliomas show regions of squamous differentiation and by themselves resemble squamous cell carcinomas that occur in other parts of the body (low power magnification).

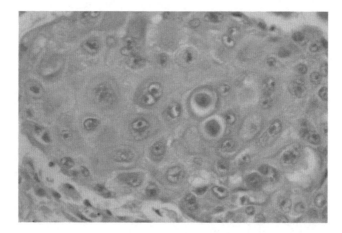

Figure 7.75   Rare epithelioid mesotheliomas show regions of squamous differentiation and by themselves resemble squamous cell carcinomas that occur in other parts of the body (high power magnification).

7.4.1.13 Tubulopapillary

Tubulopapillary mesothelioma is the most common epithelial subtype and is composed of relatively uniform cuboidal to occasionally columnar cells with centrally located nuclei that have fibrovascular cores or form small tubular structures (Figures 7.76 and 7.77). These may be associated with psammoma bodies (Figure 7.78), which is a nonspecific finding; although, in general, psammoma bodies are much more commonly seen in nonmesotheliomatous epithelial neoplasms than they are in papillary mesotheliomas. Occasionally, papillary mesotheliomas are composed of more pleomorphic cells (Figure 7.79).

7.4.2 Sarcomatoid Mesothelioma

Sarcomatoid mesotheliomas are neoplasms in which there is an absence of epithelioid differentiation. Some reports have stated a mesothelioma can be referred to as sarcomatoid if it has no more than 10% epithelial cell differentiation.[3] Pleural sarcomatoid mesotheliomas represent

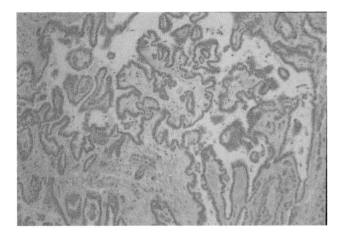

Figure 7.76 Tubulopapillary mesothelioma is the most common epithelial subtype and is composed of relatively uniform cuboidal or columnar cells with centrally located nuclei that have fibrovascular cores and form tubular structures (low power magnification).

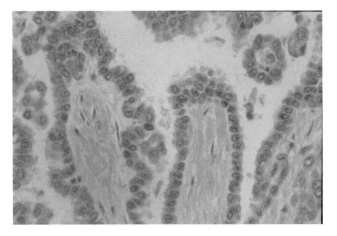

Figure 7.77 Tubulopapillary mesothelioma is the most common epithelial subtype and is composed of relatively uniform cuboidal or columnar cells with centrally located nuclei that have fibrovascular cores and form tubular structures (high power magnification).

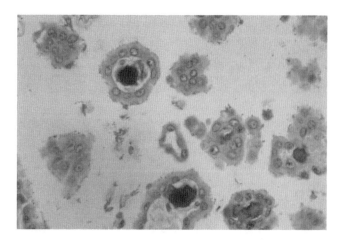

Figure 7.78   Tubulopapillary mesotheliomas may be associated with psammoma bodies, which are concentric layers of calcium often in close association with the tumor cells. Psammoma bodies can be seen in any tubulopapillary neoplasm and are much more common in carcinomas.

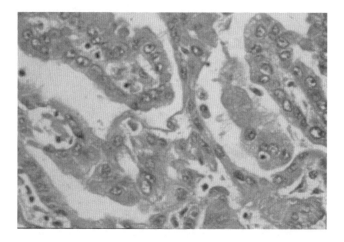

Figure 7.79   Occasionally, tubulopapillary mesotheliomas are composed of larger, more pleomorphic cells.

approximately 7%–22% of all pleural mesotheliomas. The usual histological pattern of sarcomatoid malignant mesothelioma resembles the pattern seen in soft tissue sarcomas such as a fibrosarcoma, a malignant fibrous histiocytoma, or a pleomorphic sarcomatoid neoplasm (Figures 7.80 through 7.83).

Sarcomatoid mesotheliomas can show heterologous differentiation, including leiomyoid differentiation resembling a leiomyosarcoma (Figure 7.84); chondroid differentiation resembling a chondrosarcoma (Figure 7.85); and osteoid differentiation resembling an osteosarcoma (Figure 7.86).[4-6] Patterns resembling neurogenic sarcoma and rhabdomyosarcoma have been described,[5] as well as a hemangioparacystic architecture, which requires differentiation from localized fibrous tumors of the pleura.

In my (S.P.H.) experience, the following criteria are useful for the diagnosis of sarcomatoid pleural mesothelioma:

• A confluent growth pattern of the tumor along the pleura. In limited biopsy specimens, the anatomical distribution and localization of the lesion may not be readily apparent. In this circumstance,

Figure 7.80 This sarcomatoid mesothelioma is composed of uniform spindle cells that resemble a soft tissue fibrosarcoma.

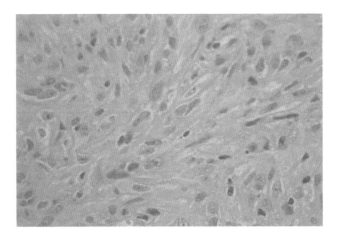

Figure 7.81 Sarcomatoid mesotheliomas can have the morphology of a malignant fibrohistiocytoma.

(a)

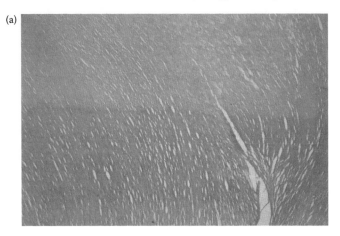

Figure 7.82 (a, b) Some sarcomatoid mesotheliomas are composed of hypocellular tissue with slit-like spaces, the findings characteristic of desmoplastic mesothelioma.

(b)

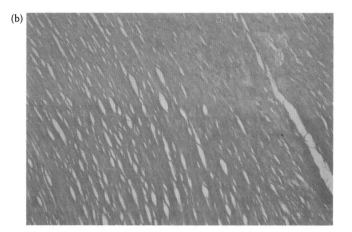

Figure 7.82 Continued.

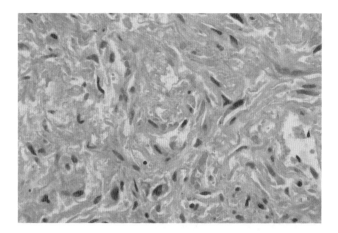

Figure 7.83 Sarcomatoid mesotheliomas may show a somewhat haphazard proliferation of neoplastic spindle cells.

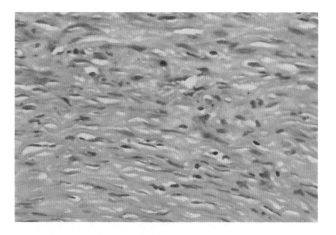

Figure 7.84 Sarcomatoid mesotheliomas may resemble leiomyosarcomas, being composed of spindle cells with cigar-shaped nuclei.

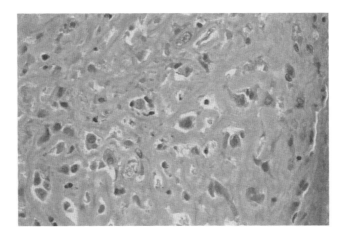

Figure 7.85 Sarcomatoid mesotheliomas may resemble chondrosarcomas.

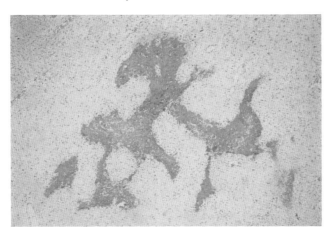

Figure 7.86 Bone formation may be extensive in sarcomatoid mesotheliomas.

the findings on radiographic investigation, including CT scans, can substitute as a useful surrogate for gross distribution.

- Sarcomas of extraserosal soft tissue or bone, sarcomatoid renal cell carcinoma (RCC), and amelanotic spindle cell melanoma should be excluded on clinical grounds, including organ imaging studies such as ultrasound or CT scans, or (importantly) from consideration of the past medical history of the patient in question.
- Cellularity, cytologic atypia, pleomorphism, and a mitotic index that are excessive for a benign fibrous lesion of the pleura. In other words, tissue that is overtly sarcomatoid in the context of lesions of the pleura with exclusion of reactive serosal fibrosis (benign fibrous pleuritis) from the histological appearance of the lesion in question, including the zonal pattern.
- Focal tumor necrosis.
- The presence of invasion. Note that most sarcomatoid mesotheliomas show a pattern of invasion into subpleural adipose tissue and, occasionally, deeper structures such as skeletal muscle.
- In the case of localized tumors in particular, a malignant localized fibrous tumor requires exclusion from the lesion by immunohistochemical studies, which is discussed later in this chapter.

Peritoneal mesotheliomas can exhibit a sarcomatoid morphology, although most peritoneal mesotheliomas have an epithelioid morphology.

7.4.3 Biphasic Mesothelioma

A mixed (biphasic) epithelial and sarcomatoid mesothelioma (Figures 7.87 through 7.91) is the most encountered histological pattern of malignant mesothelioma if enough sections are taken.[7] Approximately 30% of malignant mesotheliomas within a reported range of 24%–35% are biphasic.[3,5,6] Mixed histological patterns can be encountered in nonmesothelial tumors affecting the pleural and peritoneal cavities, most notably primary synovial sarcoma and a metastatic sarcomatoid carcinoma from the lung or other site such as the kidney or pancreas. The most accurate diagnosis of a biphasic mesothelioma requires a combination of immunohistochemistry, electron microscopy, and/or genetic studies.

Synovial sarcomas are characterized by the t(X:18) translocation,[8] whereas biphasic mesotheliomas are not.

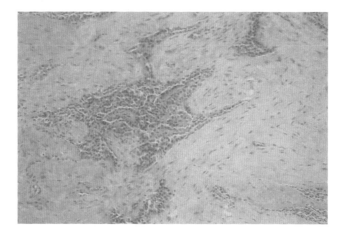

Figure 7.87 Typical biphasic mesothelioma composed of neoplastic epithelioid cells and neoplastic spindle cells.

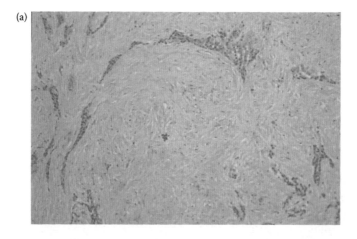

Figure 7.88 (a, b) The variability in biphasic mesotheliomas can be extensive, such as a desmoplastic sarcomatoid mesothelioma in association with a sparse epithelial component.

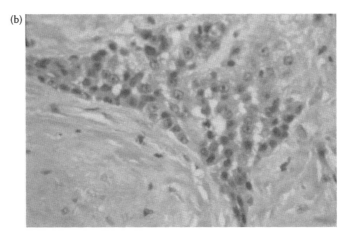

Figure 7.88 Continued.

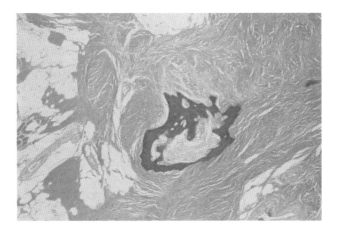

Figure 7.89 A heterologous sarcomatoid component (bone) is seen in this biphasic, predominantly desmo-plastic, mesothelioma.

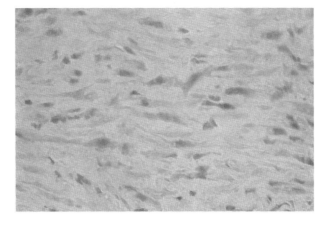

Figure 7.90 Differentiation of a sarcomatoid mesothelioma component from a reactive spindle cell prolifera-tion can be difficult.

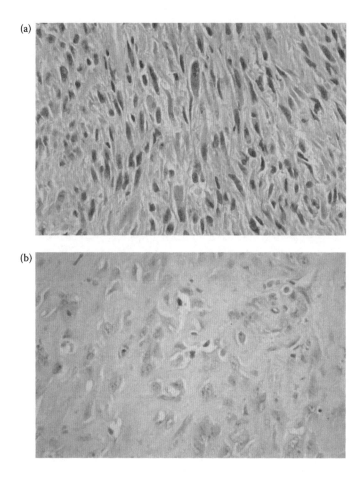

Figure 7.91   (a, b) Some biphasic mesotheliomas are composed of plump spindle cells and large neoplastic epithelioid cells.

7.4.4 Transitional Mesothelioma

Transitional mesothelioma is a type of mesothelioma we[9] described in 1986 after evaluating immunohistochemical differentiation of injured pleural tissue and mesotheliomas. Some mesotheliomas described by Dardick et al.[10] as poorly differentiated mesotheliomas would fit into this category. These mesotheliomas are composed of large, polygonal, plump, and occasionally spindle-shaped cells that usually show no specific differentiation, although they have features of both epithelioid and sarcomatoid mesotheliomas (Figures 7.92 through 7.95).

7.4.5 Pleomorphic Mesothelioma

Pleomorphic mesotheliomas are composed of generally large undifferentiated cells that have an epithelioid and/or sarcomatoid morphology (Figures 7.96 to 7.99). They can be confused with other pleomorphic cancers.[3]

7.4.6 Mesotheliomas Showing Variable Differentiation

In my (S.P.H.) experience, a significant number of mesotheliomas show various histological patterns. This can be extreme with as many as 10 different histological patterns (Figures 7.100 through 7.103).

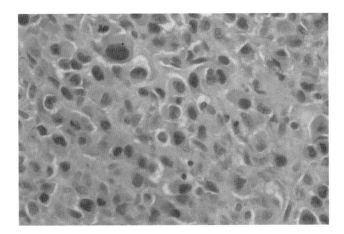

Figure 7.92 Mesotheliomas composed of large epithelioid cells and plump spindle cells. These are mesotheliomas that are "in between" epithelioid and sarcomatoid mesotheliomas and are referred to as *transitional*.

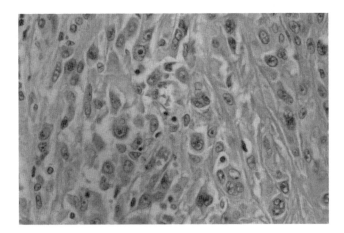

Figure 7.93 This transitional mesothelioma is composed of uniform plump cells.

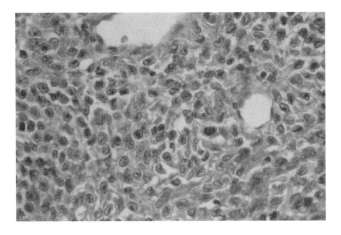

Figure 7.94 Transitional mesotheliomas may be misdiagnosed as an undifferentiated carcinoma or sarcoma.

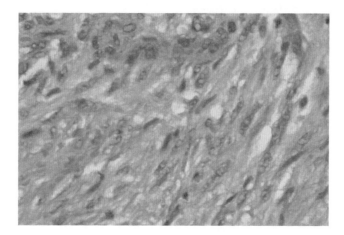

Figure 7.95   This transitional mesothelioma shows variation in the morphology of the neoplastic cells and could be confused with reactive multipotential subserosal cells.

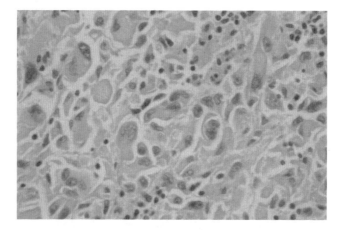

Figure 7.96   This pleomorphic mesothelioma is similar to pleomorphic carcinomas and is composed of large undifferentiated tumor cells.

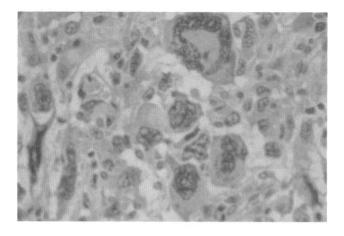

Figure 7.97   Pleomorphic mesotheliomas can be localized, as reported by Galateau-Sallé et al.[80]

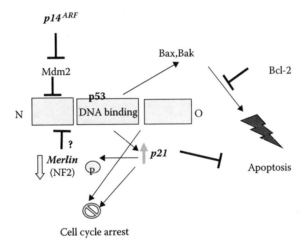

Figure 4.2 Alternative pathways of regulation of apoptosis. Apoptosis is a normal process that allows deletion of damaged and potentially dangerous cells, such as cells that contain irreparable DNA damage. There are several potential pathways that may lead to apoptosis, and the tumor suppressor p53 plays a central role. Mesotheliomas often express normal p53, but the p53 pathway is still commonly affected in mesotheliomas. Activated p53 may arrest the cell cycle via up-regulation of p21, a cyclin-dependent kinase, which has been found to be altered in some mesotheliomas. Depending on the cell type, p21 may not only induce cell cycle arrest but also initiate apoptosis directly. In addition, p21 phosphorylates merlin. Merlin is the gene product of the NF2 gene at chromosome 22 and has been found to be mutated in many mesotheliomas. Phosphorylation decreases function of merlin, which is thought to act as a tumor suppressor gene. Alternative pathways to apoptosis lead via the mitochondrial-bound proteins Bax and Bak, which are opposed by the antiapoptotic protein Bcl-2. This pathway is commonly affected in malignant tumors and also mediates apoptosis in alveolar epithelial cells exposed to asbestos. (With kind permission of Springer Science + Business Media: From Hammar SP, Henderson DW, Klebe S, Dodson RF. Neoplasms of the pleura, in J.F. Tomashefski, Jr. et al. (eds.), *Dail and Hammar's Pulmonary Pathology*, 3rd ed., vol. 2, p. 591, 2008.)

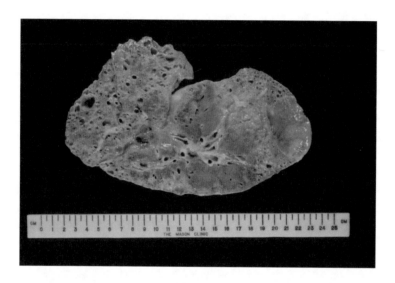

Figure 9.2 "End-stage" pulmonary fibrosis with honeycombing caused by asbestos. Macroscopic features are identical to those seen in idiopathic pulmonary fibrosis.

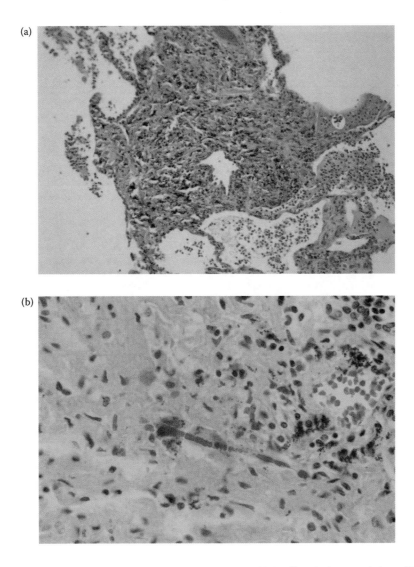

Figure 9.3 (a) Grade 1 asbestosis characterized by peribronchiolar fibrosis in association with asbestos bodies and other dusts. (b) Ferruginous body consistent with an asbestos body.

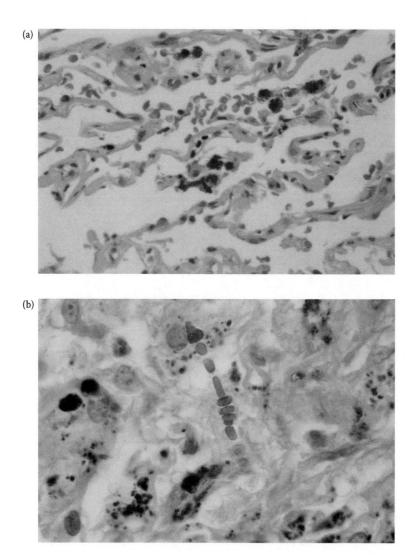

Figure 9.4 (a) Grade 2 asbestosis characterized by mild septal fibrosis of two layers of alveoli. (b) Asbestos body is associated with other dusts.

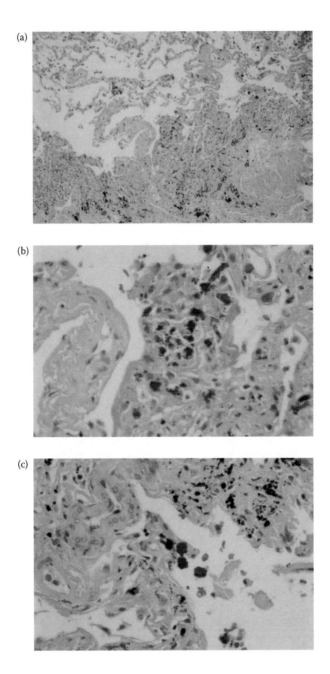

Figure 9.5 (a) Grade 3 asbestosis characterized by coalescence of fibrosis with involvement of two adjacent acinar units. (b and c) Several ferruginous bodies consistent with asbestos bodies in fibrotic lung tissue.

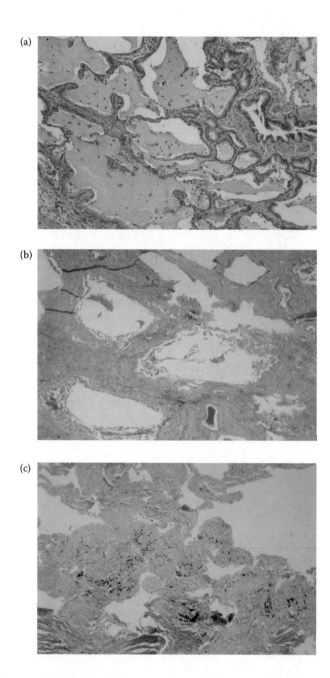

Figure 9.6 (a and b) Grade 4 asbestosis characterized by diffuse interstitial fibrosis with honeycombing. (c and d) Fibrosis in subpleural location, the region of most severe fibrosis in grade 4 asbestosis. (e) Asbestos body in dense connective tissue. (f) Asbestos bodies seen in filter preparation made from case of grade 4 asbestosis.

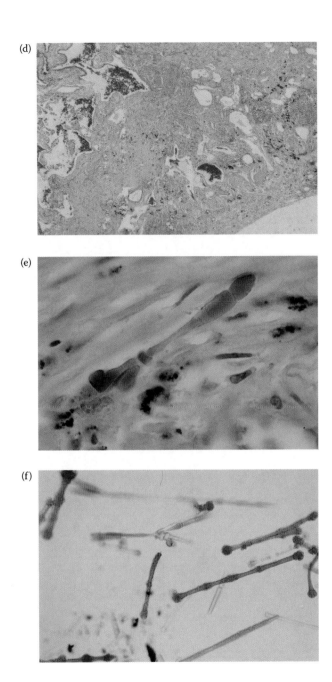

Figure 9.6 Continued.

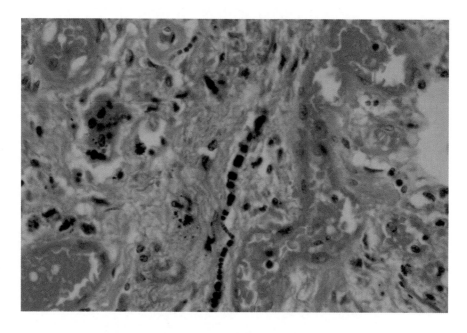

Figure 9.7 In this case of grade 4 asbestosis, it was difficult to identify asbestos bodies (arrow); however, high concentrations of asbestos fibers were found in lung tissue.

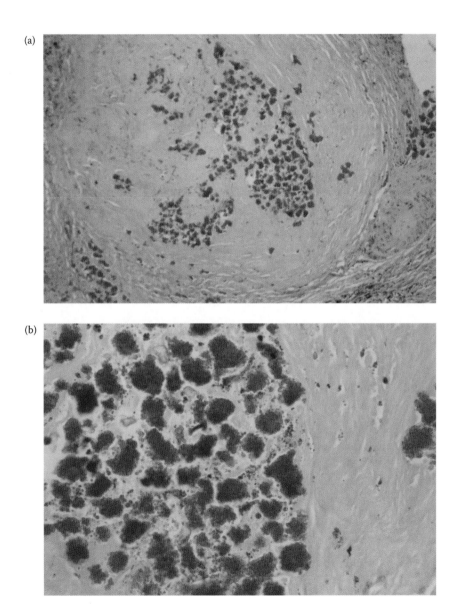

Figure 9.8 In this case, the patient's lung tissue contained numerous aggregates of asbestos bodies formed on anthophyllite cores.

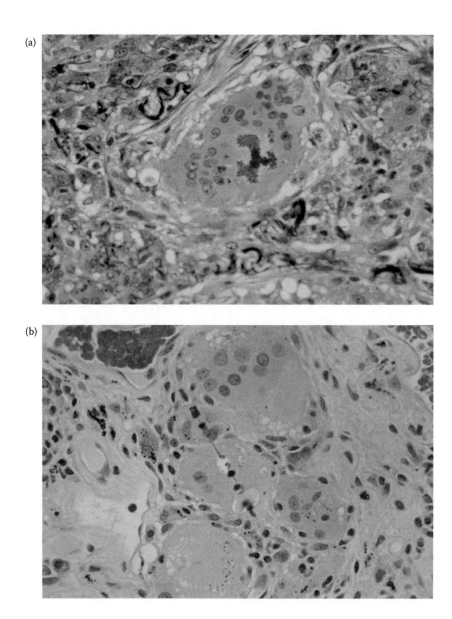

(a)

(b)

Figure 9.9 (a and b) Asbestos bodies are occasionally found in cytoplasm of multinucleated histiocytic giant cells; they are often fragmented.

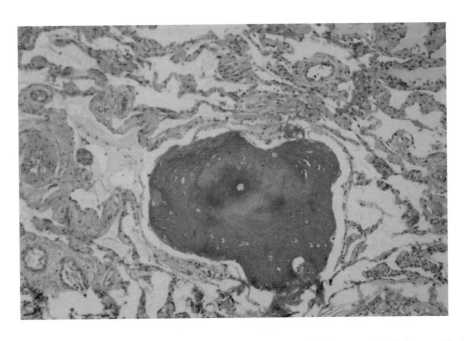

Figure 9.10 This area of grade 4 asbestosis shows a region of ossification, a relatively frequent finding in grade 4 asbestosis.

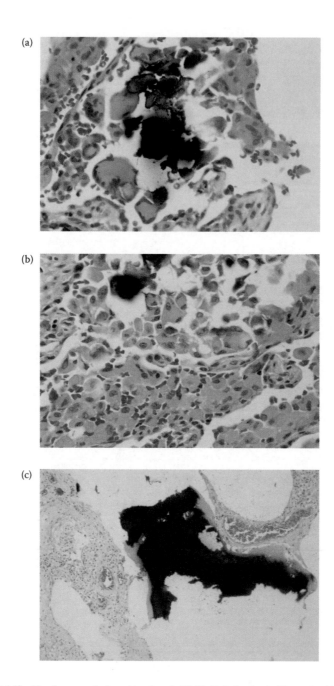

Figure 9.11 (a) Calcified bodies are clustered in alveoli. (b) Multiple laminated irregular blue bodies are seen. (c) Multiple blue bodies present with alveolar macrophages.

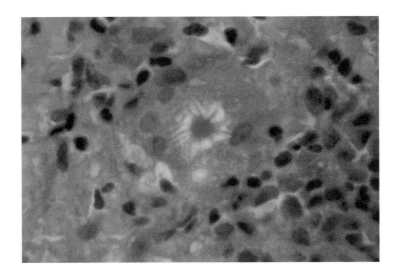

Figure 9.12 Asteroid body. Stellate inclusion, measuring 10 to 15 micrometers, in the upper right corner of a multinucleated giant cell.

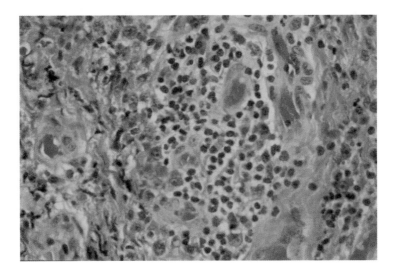

Figure 9.13 Cytoplasmic hyaline in alveolar cells. Dense ropelike glassy inclusion is surrounded by clear space in enlarged alveolar cells in center and upper right.

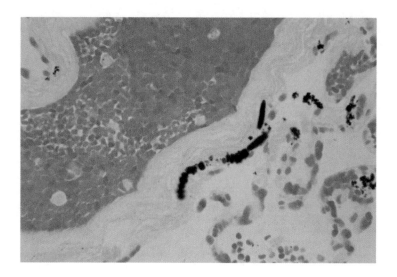

Figure 9.14　In many persons exposed to asbestos, asbestos bodies are frequently seen in the wall of blood vessels (iron stain).

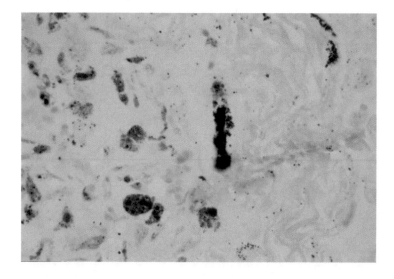

Figure 9.15　Not infrequently, abundant hemosiderin is present in lung tissue. In iron-stained sections, asbestos bodies are typically more intensely blue than the surrounding hemosiderin (iron stain).

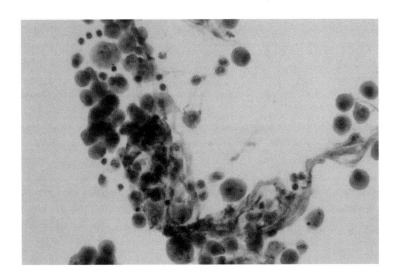

Figure 9.18 Representative region of cytocentrifuge preparation of bronchoalveolar lavage fluid from a patient with clinical features of asbestosis. Note the increased number of neutrophils.

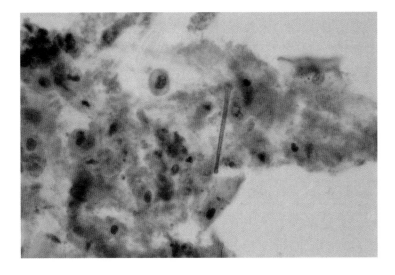

Figure 9.20 Amosite-cored ferruginous body obtained from digested lavage sample from individual occupationally exposed to this form of asbestos (transmission electron microscopy).

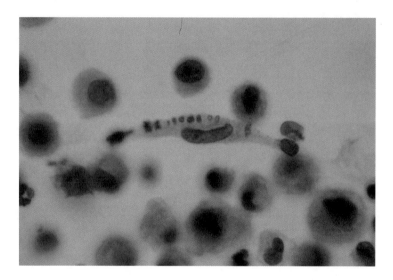

Figure 9.22 Thin section of embedded sputum shows ferruginous body (arrow) with associated macrophages and mucous material (transmission electron microscopy).

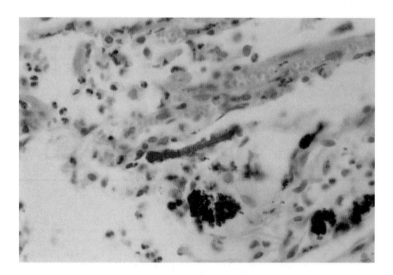

Figure 9.23 Transbronchial biopsy specimen from patient with clinical features of asbestosis shows a ferruginous body (arrow) consistent with an asbestos body.

(a)

(b)

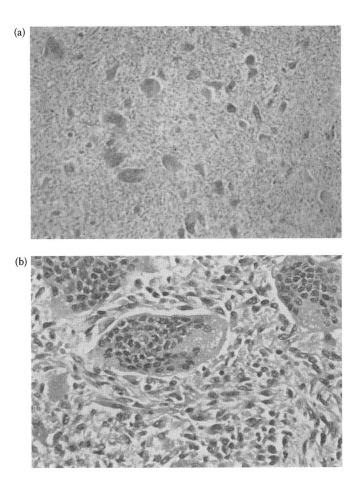

Figure 7.98 (a, b) Pleomorphic mesotheliomas can be associated with multinucleated macrophage giant cells.

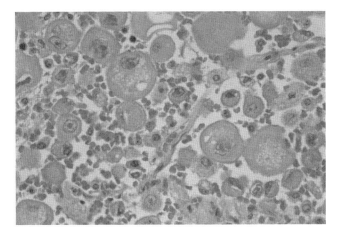

Figure 7.99 This pleomorphic mesothelioma is composed of large undifferentiated deciduoid-appearing cells admixed with plump spindle cells.

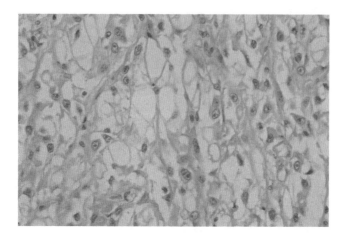

Figure 7.100 An example of mesothelioma showing variable differentiation. Figures 7.100–7.103 are from the same mesothelioma. This photo shows mesothelioma having a microcystic pattern.

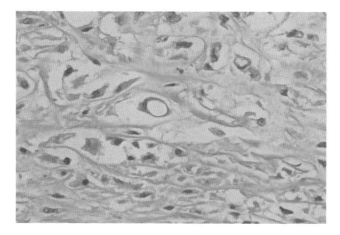

Figure 7.101 An example of mesothelioma showing variable differentiation. Figures 7.100–7.103 are from the same mesothelioma. This photo shows signet ring cells.

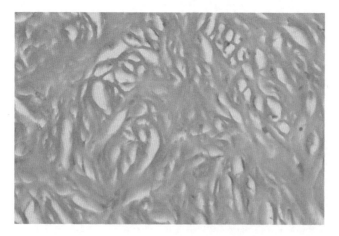

Figure 7.102 An example of mesothelioma showing variable differentiation. Figures 7.100–7.103 are from the same mesothelioma. This photo shows features of desmoplastic mesothelioma.

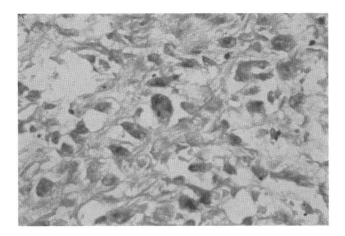

Figure 7.103 An example of mesothelioma showing variable differentiation. Figures 7.100–7.103 are from the same mesothelioma. This mesothelioma shows pleomorphic cells.

7.5 HISTOCHEMICAL FEATURES OF PLEURAL EPITHELIAL MESOTHELIOMA

The presence of carbohydrate/mucopolysaccharide substances in epithelioid tumor cells can be useful in differentiating epithelial mesotheliomas from primary pulmonary adenocarcinomas and other mucin-producing adenocarcinomas. The two main substances to be considered are mucin and glycogen. Mucin is a somewhat vague term and is frequently used synonymously with mucopolysaccharide, glycoprotein, proteoglycan, glycosaminoglycan, mucosubstance, and glycoconjugate. The protein portion of a glycoprotein is synthesized in the rough endoplasmic reticulum and the carbohydrate portion is added in the Golgi apparatus. Mucosubstances can be divided into highly acidic, weakly acidic, or neutral acidic substances. Glycogen is observed in the cytoplasm of epithelial mesotheliomas in up to 50% of cases and typically stain with a periodic acid Schiff (PAS) reagent. Glycogen can cause mesotheliomas to have a clear cell morphology and, if pretreated with diastase, there is a lack of staining (Figure 7.104). Many clear cell carcinomas of the lung represent neoplasms that contain significant amounts of glycogen. Approximately 20% of epithelial mesotheliomas produce highly acidic mucosubstances referred to as *hyaluronic acid* and *proteoglycan* (Figures 7.105 and 7.106), which can be identified with an Alcian blue or colloidal iron stain. A note of caution is that stromal connective tissue surrounding nests of epithelial mesothelial cells can be rich in hyaluronic acid and be misinterpreted as a positive reaction.

Approximately 65%–70% of pulmonary adenocarcinomas show intracytoplasmic staining for neutral or weakly acidic mucosubstances that can be identified with a PAS–diastase or a Mayer's mucicarmine stain. As I (S.P.H.) have reported, most pulmonary adenocarcinomas that show intracytoplasmic staining with PAS–diastase or Mayer's mucicarmine also show Alcian blue/colloidal iron staining.

I (S.P.H.) compared the histochemical and immunohistochemical stains of 10 epithelial mesotheliomas (diagnosis documented by ultrastructural examination) that were mucicarmine-positive and compared them with 10 pulmonary adenocarcinomas.[11] The adenocarcinomas were all primary lung adenocarcinomas that were mucicarmine-positive. The mucicarmine and PAS–diastase staining reaction in epithelial mesotheliomas resulted from the hyaluronidase acid production by these neoplasms. When tissue sections were pretreated with hyaluronidase, the intensity of the staining reaction with mucicarmine and PAS–diastase decreased or disappeared. However, in some cases—specifically those that showed intracellular droplet-like staining—the reaction was not eradicated by hyaluronidase. All mucin-positive epithelial mesotheliomas that we have examined have contained

(a)

(b)

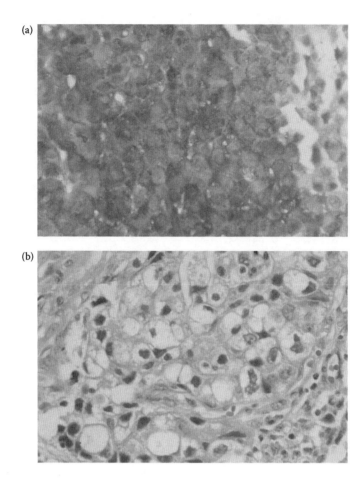

Figure 7.104   (a, b) This epithelioid mesothelioma contains glycogen in the cytoplasm that is identified by a positive PAS stain.

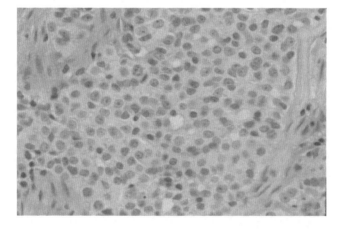

Figure 7.105   This epithelioid mesothelioma shows intracytoplasmic Alcian blue staining likely due to hyaluronic acid.

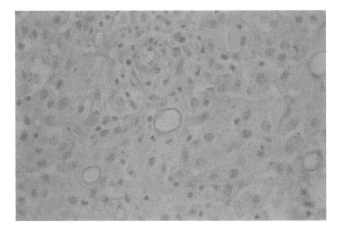

Figure 7.106   Colloidal iron staining of this epithelioid mesothelioma is due to intracytoplasmic proteoglycan or hyaluronic acid.

crystalloid material, which is described in the section on rare mesotheliomas (mucin-positive epithelial mesotheliomas).

Many adenocarcinomas commonly spread to the pleura such as those originating in the lung and breast and may not produce significant amounts of mucin. Therefore, some authorities consider mucin stains to be of limited or little value in the diagnosis of epithelioid mesothelioma.

7.6 IMMUNOHISTOCHEMICAL FEATURES OF MESOTHELIOMA

Immunohistochemistry is the primary diagnostic technique in differentiating epithelial mesothelioma from other types of epithelioid cancers and occasionally for differentiating sarcomatoid mesotheliomas from other types of sarcomatoid neoplasms.

7.6.1 Antibodies

Multiple antibodies have been used to diagnose mesothelioma. They have been most useful in differentiating epithelial mesotheliomas from pulmonary adenocarcinomas or from other adenocarcinomas/carcinomas. Immunohistochemistry is less useful in diagnosing sarcomatoid mesotheliomas and differentiating them from sarcomas and other spindle cell neoplasms.

Antibodies used to diagnose epithelioid mesotheliomas have been divided into three categories:

1. Antibodies that are relatively specific for mesothelial cells and epithelial mesothelioma cancer cells that, when positive, serve as a positive marker for epithelioid mesothelioma;
2. Antibodies that show no reaction with mesothelial cells or mesotheliomas and, when positive, serve as a negative marker for mesothelioma; and
3. Other antibodies that may react with mesothelial cells/epithelial mesotheliomas but which are relatively nonspecific.

Positive markers, negative markers, and other markers useful in diagnosing epithelial or biphasic mesotheliomas are shown in Tables 7.3, 7.4, and 7.5, respectively.

Table 7.3 Markers Usually Positive in Epithelial or Biphasic Mesotheliomas

Positive Mesothelial Markers	Comments
Calretinin	Currently regarded as the most sensitive and specific marker for epithelial mesothelial differentiation. The calretinin staining shows cytoplasmic and nuclear staining in epithelial mesothelioma.
CK5/6	Sensitive and specific for differential diagnosis of epithelial malignant mesothelioma versus adenocarcinoma but not suitable to distinguish ovarian serous and squamous cell carcinomas.
WT-1	Good sensitivity and specificity for epithelial mesotheliomas but possible difficulties with autopsy material. Cross-reactivity with renal cell carcinoma (RCC) is not a problem. The stain is nuclear.
D2-40 (podoplanin)	Similar sensitivities and specificities to calretinin, but less extensively studied. Cell membrane staining pattern.
Thrombomodulin	Variable in literature but considered useful in the distinction of malignant mesothelioma from metastatic adenocarcinoma. Avoids misdiagnosis of epithelioid hemangioendothelioma. Cell membrane staining pattern.
HBME-1	Variably regarded, but found useful if only membrane labeling is considered positive and if dilution is high (1:5000 to 1:15,000).
CD44S	High sensitivity but low specificity.
Mesothelin	Some consider it useful (if negative, epithelial malignant mesothelioma is less likely). However, there is no advantage over calretinin and other positive markers. The staining pattern is cell membrane.

Table 7.4 Markers Usually Negative in Epithelial Mesotheliomas or the Epithelial Component of Biphasic Mesotheliomas

Markers Positive in Carcinoma but Negative in Mesothelioma	Comments
CEA	Very useful for differential diagnosis of MM and adenocarcinoma; usually negative in RCC and ovarian/peritoneal serous carcinoma. Up to 10% of epithelial mesotheliomas may show staining.
CD15 (Leu-M1)	Well characterized and considered a good discriminator; useful in the distinction from RCC (most are positive) but does not reliably identify squamous cell carcinomas. Less frequent than initially reported in pulmonary adenocarcinomas.
B72.3	Variable reports. Sensitivity and specificity of 93% and 80%, respectively (meta-analysis).
Ber-EP4 and MOC31	Both antibodies recognize the same antigen. Less reliable than CEA or BG-8. There has been some labeling of mesotheliomas but may be useful in certain situations, for example, with metastatic breast carcinoma and pleural synovial sarcoma. Up to 20% of epithelial mesotheliomas show focal or diffuse cell membrane staining. Approximately 5% of epithelioid mesotheliomas show cell membrane staining for MOC31 in a cell membrane distribution.
BG-8	Reliable in distinguishing malignant mesothelioma from adenocarcinoma; labels 80% of squamous cell carcinomas, but does not label RCCs.
TTF-1	Useful for differential diagnosis of malignant mesothelioma and lung adenocarcinoma. Highly specific, but lack of labeling does not exclude lung adenocarcinoma. Squamous cell carcinomas of lung do not stain.

Immunohistochemistry has been used to differentiate benign from malignant mesothelial cell proliferations and was discussed in 2009 in a Consensus Statement issued by the International Mesothelioma Interest Group,[12] of which I (S.P.H.) am is a member. Immunohistochemical stains used to separate reactive mesothelial proliferations from mesothelioma are shown in Table 7.6.

Table 7.5   Other Useful Markers in the Diagnosis of Malignant Pleural Mesothelioma

Antibody	Utility/Comments
CK7 and CK20	Limited value to ascertain origin of secondary adenocarcinoma. Not useful for discriminating between mesothelioma and adenocarcinoma. Malignant mesothelioma may be CK7+ and CK20– or CK7+ and CK20+.
p63	Useful marker in distinguishing malignant mesothelioma from squamous cell carcinoma. Must remember that some epithelial mesotheliomas show squamous differentiation.
Gross cystic disease fluid protein	Limited usefulness in distinguishing malignant mesothelioma from metastatic breast carcinoma. Low sensitivity but high specificity.
CD10	Not specific enough to distinguish malignant mesothelioma from RCC because up to 54% of malignant mesotheliomas are positive for CD10.
Estrogen receptor protein (ER)	Useful in distinguishing malignant mesothelioma from serous carcinoma of ovary or peritoneum. Rarely (<.1%) of peritoneal mesotheliomas show ER protein staining. Significance uncertain.
Progesterone receptor protein (PR)	In conjunction with ER, useful in distinguishing malignant mesothelioma from serous carcinoma of ovary or peritoneum.
p53	Possibly some limited use in distinguishing reactive mesothelial hyperplasia from malignant mesothelioma.
Napsin A	Stains most pulmonary adenocarcinomas and RCCs, but not malignant mesotheliomas.

Table 7.6   Immunohistochemical Stains Used to Separate Reactive Mesothelial Proliferations from Malignant Mesothelioma

Antibody	Reactive Mesothelium	Malignant Mesothelioma
GLUT-1	0% positive	89% positive
EMA	20% positive	80% positive
p53	0% positive	45% positive
Desmin	85% positive	10% positive

7.7   ULTRASTRUCTURAL FEATURES OF MESOTHELIOMA

A variety of publications in the literature have illustrated the use of ultrastructural evaluation in identifying epithelioid mesotheliomas.[13–15] Ultrastructural evaluation is also helpful in ruling out mesothelioma by finding ultrastructural features that are not characteristic of an epithelial mesothelioma such as a pulmonary adenocarcinoma or a GI tract adenocarcinoma.

In general, the most specific feature of a well to moderately well-differentiated epithelial mesothelioma is the long, thin, sinuous microvilli that are not covered by a glycocalyx (Figure 7.107). There have been reports of measurements of the microvilli in epithelial mesotheliomas compared with the microvilli in adenocarcinomas, but in my (S.P.H.) opinion, this is not worthwhile in that these microvilli usually never arise from the cell in a straight line and therefore length–width dimensions are not useful. The lack of a glycocalyx is much more important than the length–width ratio of microvilli (Figure 7.108).

Well and moderately well-differentiated epithelial mesotheliomas typically show large desmosomes and junctional complexes connecting the neoplastic mesothelial cells to one another (Figures 7.109 through 7.110); this is characteristically seen in epithelial mesotheliomas but is not 100% specific. Likewise, most neoplastic epithelial mesothelial cells show large bundles of tonofilaments in their cytoplasm (Figure 7.111), which is not a specific feature.

In some cases where there is abundant hyaluronic acid or proteoglycan production by tumor cells, the microvilli are covered by grayish material that represents hyaluronic acid (Figure 7.112).

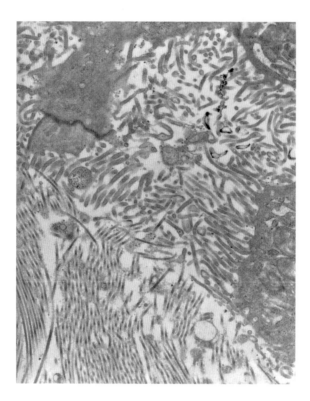

Figure 7.107 The most specific ultrastructural feature of an epithelial mesothelioma is the long, thin, sinuous microvilli.

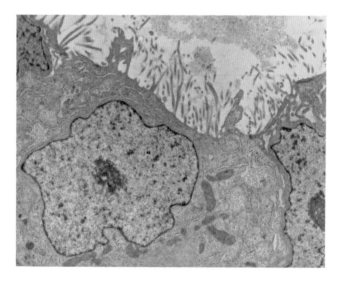

Figure 7.108 These mesothelial cancer cells were retrieved from paraffin and processed for electron microscopic evaluation. The neoplastic cells show long, thin microvilli.

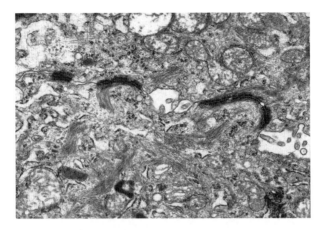

Figure 7.109 Most epithelial mesotheliomas are composed of cells that are connected by large desmosomes.

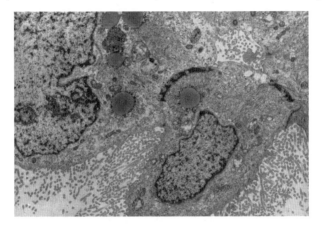

Figure 7.110 Epithelial mesothelioma cells are often connected to each other by junctional complexes.

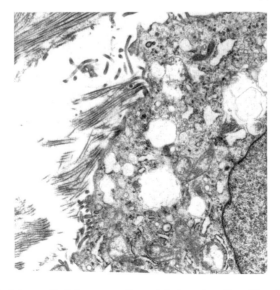

Figure 7.111 Most epithelial mesothelial cancer cells contain large bundles of tonofilaments.

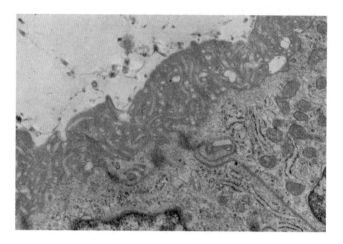

Figure 7.112 Some mesothelial cancer cells have microvilli that are covered by hyaluronic acid.

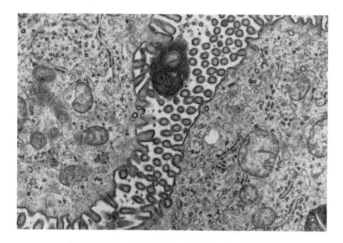

Figure 7.113 This primary pulmonary adenocarcinoma shows short microvilli and glycocalyceal bodies.

In addition, if one compares epithelial mesotheliomas to a well to moderately differentiated adenocarcinoma of the lung, the adenocarcinomas typically have short microvilli often associated with glycocalyceal bodies and a glycocalyx (Figure 7.113). In addition, most pulmonary adenocarcinomas and GI tract adenocarcinomas have rootlets (Figures 7.114 and 7.115), which are not seen in epithelial mesotheliomas.

In my (S.P.H.) experience, electron microscopy can be used when uncertainties remain concerning the diagnosis of mucin-producing epithelial mesotheliomas versus pulmonary adenocarcinomas. Electron microscopy can be regarded as the "gold standard" for diagnosing the epithelial component of a biphasic mesothelioma or an epithelioid mesothelioma. However, in everyday practice, immunohistochemistry has largely replaced electron microscopy at most institutions. Nonetheless, I (S.P.H.) believe electron microscopy still plays an important role in the independent validation of a diagnosis of an epithelioid mesothelioma. In addition, we continue to find electron microscopy useful, and often decisively so, including the use of deparaffinized and reprocessed biopsy tissue when the sample is small or where the histological appearance is somewhat variable, or when there is discordant immunohistochemical findings (Figures 7.116 and 7.117).

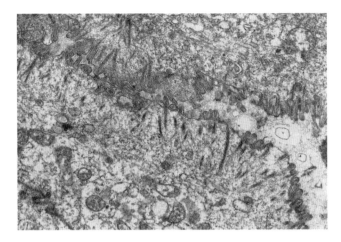

Figure 7.114 This primary pulmonary adenocarcinoma contains numerous rootlets.

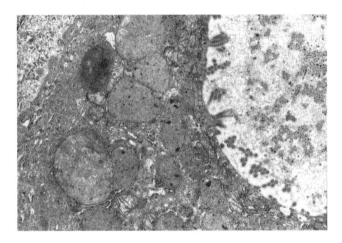

Figure 7.115 Most mucin-producing pulmonary adenocarcinomas and other adenocarcinomas contain rootlets that anchor the microvilli to the cytoplasm.

7.8 DNA ANALYSIS AND PROLIFERATIVE INDEX IN MALIGNANT MESOTHELIOMA

With the passage of time, DNA proliferative indexes have been used to evaluate a variety of neoplasms.[16–23] Ki-67 evaluation by immunohistochemistry is probably the most common evaluation of proliferative indices at this point in time. Ki-67 immunohistochemistry has been reported to have a sensitivity of 74%, a specificity of 86%, and a positive predictive value of 94% in detecting malignant mesothelioma.

Human telomerase reverse transcriptase was detected by immunohistochemistry with a sensitivity and specificity of 68% of cases. Cakir et al.[24] suggested that immunohistochemistry profiling for Ki-67 and human telomerase reverse transcriptase were useful in differentiating malignant and benign mesothelial lesions in routine formalin-fixed and paraffin-embedded material.

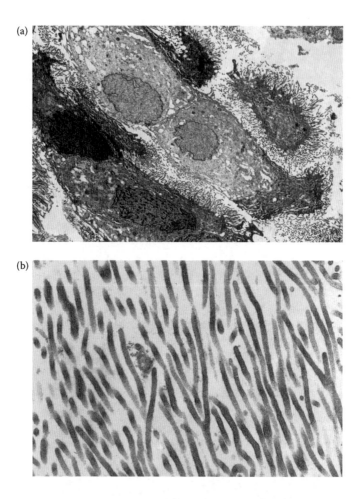

Figure 7.116   (a, b) In some instances where there is an uncertainty as to whether an epithelioid neoplasm is an adenocarcinoma or an epithelial mesothelioma, removal of tissue from the paraffin block can be useful. In this case, the microvilli had the features of an epithelial mesothelioma.

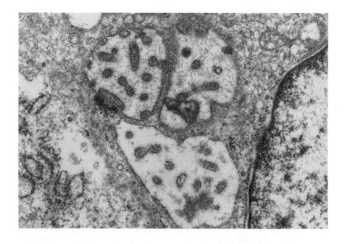

Figure 7.117   In this case, the microvilli had the features of an adenocarcinoma.

7.9 RARE/UNUSUAL MESOTHELIOMAS OR MESOTHELIAL PROLIFERATIONS

7.9.1 Benign Mesothelial Inclusions in Lymph Nodes/ Metastatic Mesotheliomas to Lymph Nodes

Mesotheliomas not infrequently metastasize to regional (hilar, bronchopulmonary, and mediastinal) lymph nodes.[5] Cases of metastatic mesothelioma to lymph nodes as a presenting finding of mesothelioma have been reported (Figure 7.118).[25–28] Sometimes, metastatic deposits require distinction from benign mesothelial inclusions within subpleural, bronchial, or mediastinal lymph nodes related to chronic inflammatory processes affecting the pleura and, occasionally, other serosal membranes (Figure 7.119).[29–31] This can create a problem. The International Mesothelioma Panel,[3] of which I (S.P.H.) am a member, recommends the diagnosis of metastatic mesothelioma within lymph nodes should be supported by either a diagnostic biopsy of a corresponding serosal membrane or radiologic evidence supportive of an underlying pleural mesothelioma, such as diffuse pleural thickening with encasement of the lung.

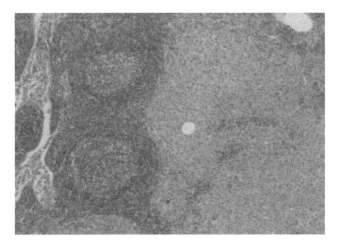

Figure 7.118 This lymph node was almost completely replaced by mesothelioma. The neoplastic mesothelial cells had the immunohistochemical features of an epithelial mesothelioma.

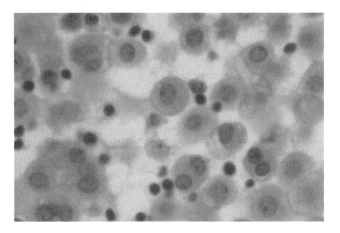

Figure 7.119 This lymph node contains benign mesothelial cells in the cortical sinuses. These can be mistaken for metastatic carcinoma or epithelial mesothelioma.

7.9.2 Adenomatoid Tumors

Adenomatoid tumors represent benign mesothelial proliferations characteristically occurring in the testis/epididymis of males and the cornu of the uterus of females.[32,33] Rarely, they have been identified in other locations such as the adrenal gland, heart, liver, mesentery of small intestine, peritoneum, omentum, pleura, mediastinal lymph nodes, and appendix.[34] Macroscopically, adenomatoid tumors are nonencapsulated and usually consist of a poorly delineated, firm, pale yellow mass (Figure 7.120). Histological examination shows unencapsulated mesothelial cells with microcystic spaces and complex tubules (Figure 7.121). The individual cells are cuboidal to flattened. The differential diagnosis includes lymphangioma. It is important to emphasize that antibody D2-40 identifies lymphatic endothelium and mesothelial cells.[35,36] Ultrastructurally, the tumor cells have the features of mesothelial cells (Figure 7.122). Pleural adenomatoid tumors[3,37,38] are exceedingly rare and typically represent small and clinically silent lesions. The differential diagnosis is that of a conventional malignant mesothelioma with a microcystic pattern.

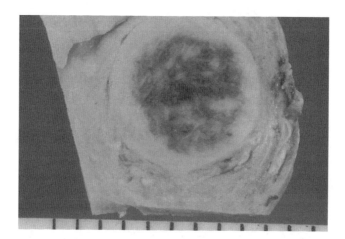

Figure 7.120 Uterine adenomatoid tumor can be confused with a carcinoma.

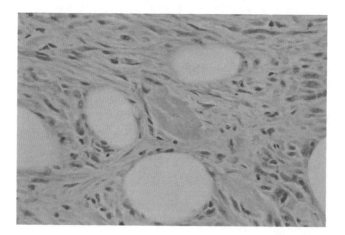

Figure 7.121 Adenomatoid tumor composed of cuboidal and squamoid mesothelial cells.

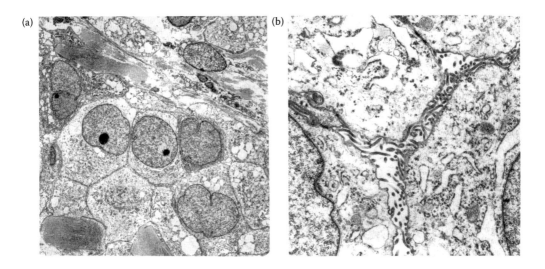

Figure 7.122   (a, b) Ultrastructural morphology of tumor cells in an adenomatoid tumor.

7.9.3 Well-Differentiated Papillary Mesothelioma

This entity has been reported predominantly in the peritoneum of young women but has also been reported in the pleura.[39–51] Rare examples of well-differentiated papillary mesothelioma (WDPM) have been encountered in the pericardium[52] and tunica vaginalis testis.[50,53] In (S.P.H.) was a coauthor of a report by Butnor et al.[50] concerning 14 cases of well-differentiated papillary epithelial mesothelioma, seven of which affected the pleura, six in the peritoneum, and one in the tunica vaginalis. Eleven patients were men and three were women. Six patients had a history of asbestos exposure. Nine cases had complete follow-up and six had clinical indolent disease, but one pursued an aggressive course. Histologically, WDPMs show an exophytic papillary proliferation of well-differentiated cuboidal cells with uniform nuclei and without invasion (Figures 7.123 and 7.124).

Galateau-Sallé et al.[51] reported a series of 24 cases (11 men and 13 women) of well-differentiated papillary epithelial mesothelioma affecting the pleura. The patients had a mean age of 60 years and an age range of 31 to 79 years. In 10 cases, invasion was present at the time of diagnosis but was strictly limited to the submesothelial layers with no extension into lung parenchyma or subpleural adipose tissue. The histological appearance of the tumors in two cases at the time of progression was similar to that of a conventional epithelioid mesothelioma. Occasional cases were almost indistinguishable from a well-differentiated epithelioid mesothelioma as shown in the fascicle concerning *Tumors of the Serosal Membranes* (third series), where Figure 4.16 was stated to represent a diffuse, predominantly papillary, epithelial mesothelioma and Figure 4.55, which was exactly the same photograph as 4.16, was stated to represent a well-differentiated papillary mesothelioma with an area of increased fibrosis.[54]

7.9.4 Noninvasive Atypical Mesothelial Cell Proliferation

The concept of mesothelioma in situ and discrimination between early-stage mesothelioma and reactive mesothelial hyperplasia is a complex issue. For a detailed discussion, see pages 642–648 of *Dail and Hammar's Pulmonary Pathology*, Third Edition, Volume 2.[55] It is my (S.P.H.) opinion that mesothelioma in situ is a real entity and is the precursor of invasive epithelial mesothelioma. Likewise, it is my (S.P.H.) opinion that most cases of what are referred to as atypical mesothelial proliferation are precursors of epithelial mesothelioma.

(a)
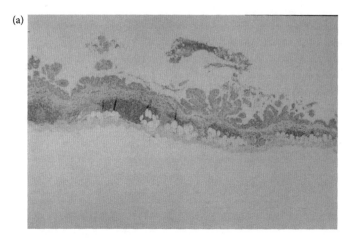

(b)
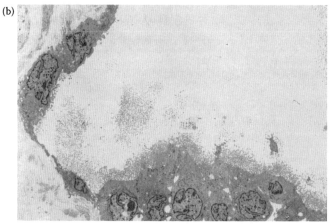

Figure 7.123   (a, b) This well-differentiated epithelial mesothelioma originated in the peritoneum. It is composed of a papillary proliferation of uniform cuboidal-columnar cells.

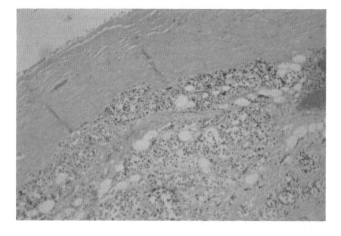

Figure 7.124   Some well-differentiated papillary epithelial mesotheliomas are caused by asbestos and are associated with hyaline plaques characteristic of plaque caused by asbestos.

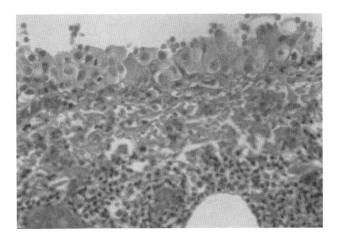

Figure 7.125   This mesothelial proliferation shows extensive in situ mesothelioma.

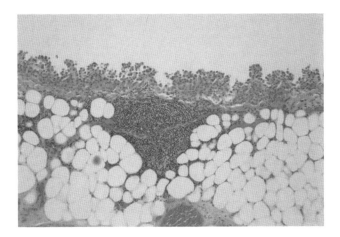

Figure 7.126   In this in situ mesothelial proliferation, there are focal papillary changes.

In situ epithelial mesothelioma is no different than any other in situ epithelioid neoplastic process. The cells are cytologically atypical, often with large nuclei and prominent nucleoli, but without invasion (Figures 7.125 and 7.126). In most cases, there is invasion (Figures 7.127 and 7.128).

7.9.5 Small Cell Mesothelioma

Some cases of mesothelioma are composed of cells that resemble small cell lung cancer (Figures 7.129 and 7.130). Pathologically, they can be difficult to differentiate from small cell lung cancer.[56–58] In general, small cell mesotheliomas do not show immunostaining for neuron-specific enolase, synaptophysin, chromogranin-A, and TTF-1. They usually show immunostaining for keratin and vimentin. Not infrequently, small cell mesotheliomas show other areas of differentiation that is more typical of mesothelioma, which makes it easier to diagnose (Figures 7.131 and 7.132).

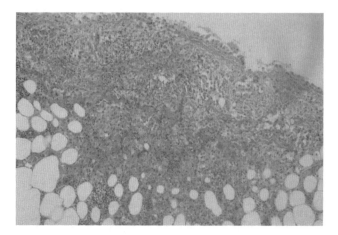

Figure 7.127   In this invasive epithelial mesothelioma, there are areas of in situ mesothelioma.

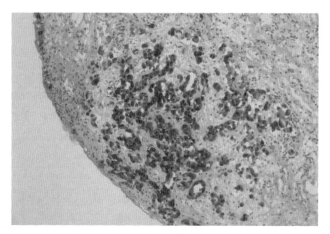

Figure 7.128   Invasive mesothelioma is seen in association with in situ mesothelioma (calretinin-stained section).

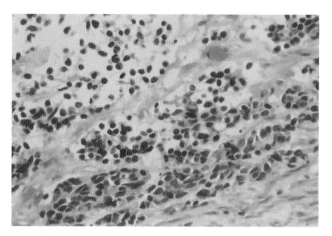

Figure 7.129   This small cell mesothelioma is composed of neoplastic cells that resemble small cell lung cancer.

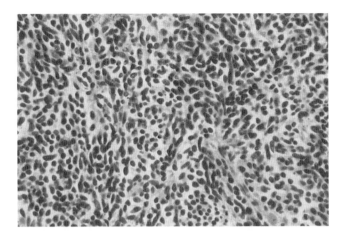

Figure 7.130   Small cell mesothelioma composed of cells resembling small cell lung cancer.

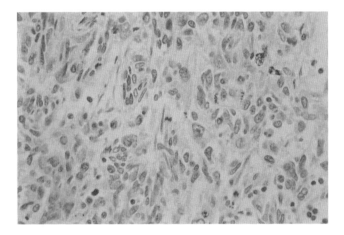

Figure 7.131   The majority of this neoplasm has the features of a small cell mesothelioma but in areas shows the features of an epithelial mesothelioma.

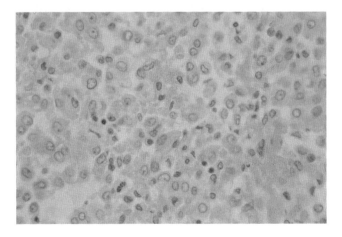

Figure 7.132   Areas of epithelial morphology are observed in this small cell mesothelioma.

7.9.6 Deciduoid Mesothelioma

In 1985, Talerman et al.[2] reported a case of deciduoid mesothelioma in a 13-year-old girl with no history of asbestos exposure. In 1994, Nascimento et al.[59] reported two cases of deciduoid peritoneal mesothelioma in young females, aged 23 and 24 years. In 2000, Ordòñez[60] reported four cases (three men and one woman) of mesothelioma with deciduoid features originating in the pleura. Two patients had a history of asbestos exposure. Shanks et al.[61] reported six cases (three men and three women) of deciduoid mesothelioma. Five of the six cases originated in the peritoneum and one in the pleura. In 2002, Serio et al.[62] reported two cases of malignant mesothelioma with deciduoid features arising in the pleura—one in a 73-year-old man with a history of occupational exposure to asbestos and the other in a 23-year-old female with a history of familial mesothelioma. Shia et al.[63] reported five new cases of deciduoid mesothelioma and 21 cases of deciduoid mesothelioma previously reported in the literature. Shia et al.[63] stated that the age range was 13–78 years (median = 53 years), with a slight female predominance (female-to-male ratio of 1.4:1). Fourteen (54%) of 26 cases occurred in the peritoneum. Seven (35%) of 20 patients had a documented history of asbestos exposure. I (S.P.H.) have seen more than 200 cases of deciduoid mesothelioma. They may be "pure" deciduoid mesotheliomas or may show focal differentiation with other patterns. Most occur in persons exposed to asbestos. Histologically, they are part of what I (S.P.H.) refer to as *the round cell group of mesotheliomas*, being large and having large nuclei, prominent nucleoli, and abundant eosinophilic cytoplasm (Figures 7.133 and 7.134). They usually show the typical immunohistochemical features of a well to moderately well-differentiated epithelial mesothelioma. Ultrastructurally, they have shorter microvilli and filaments in the outer part of the tumor cell (Figures 7.135 and 7.136).

7.9.7 Mucin-Positive Epithelial Mesothelioma

Approximately 5% of epithelial mesotheliomas show focal staining with Mayer's mucicarmine, PAS–diastase, and Alcian blue/colloidal iron with hyaluronidase. These are referred to as mucin-positive mesotheliomas.[64–67] These were first reported in an abstract, indicating the mucin-positive staining was due to the hyaluronic acid.[67] The readers are referred to the review article by Hammar et al.,[11] which cites all the critical references. In many instances, there can be several different mucin-positive staining patterns. The one that causes the most concern is the intracellular droplet-like

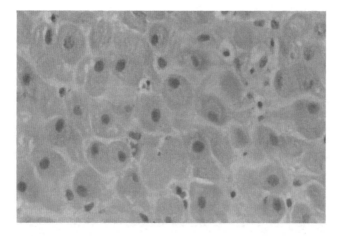

Figure 7.133 Deciduoid epithelial mesotheliomas are composed of large round cells with abundant eosinophilic cytoplasm. They resemble normal deciduoid cells as shown in this photograph.

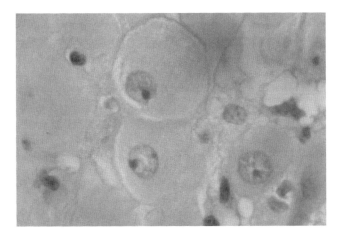

Figure 7.134 At higher magnification, most nuclei of deciduoid epithelial mesotheliomas have large nuclei and nucleoli.

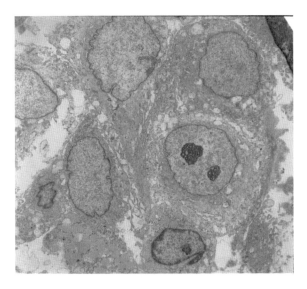

Figure 7.135 Ultrastructurally, the neoplastic deciduoid cells have relatively short microvilli, but they are not covered by a glycocalyx.

staining (Figures 7.137 and 7.138). Ultrastructurally, the cells of mucin-positive epithelial mesotheliomas show crystalloid inclusions (Figures 7.139 and 7.140), which in my (S.P.H.) opinion are only seen in this entity and not in any other neoplasm.

7.9.8 Gaucher Cell-Like Mesothelioma

A very rare type of mesothelioma exists that is composed of cells that resemble Gaucher cells (Figures 7.141 and 7.142). They usually are associated with more typical malignant mesothelial cells, but not always. Ultrastructurally, they show unique intracellular crystalloid material within the cisternae of the rough endoplasmic reticulum (Figures 7.143 and 7.144). Their ultrastructural morphology was first published by Henderson et al.[5]

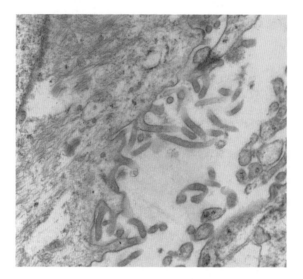

Figure 7.136 The neoplastic deciduoid cells contain cytoplasmic filaments.

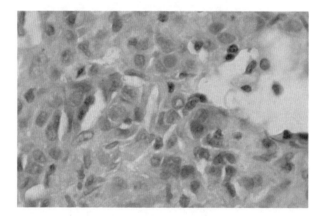

Figure 7.137 This epithelioid neoplasm contains intracellular mucicarmine-positive staining suggesting the diagnosis of a mucin-positive adenocarcinoma.

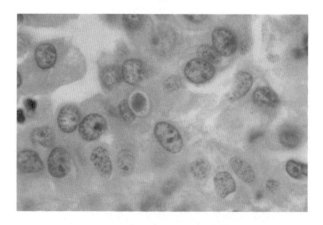

Figure 7.138 Intracellular PAS–diastase is observed in this epithelial neoplasm.

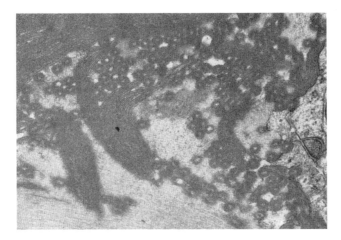

Figure 7.139 Ultrastructurally, mucin-positive epithelial mesotheliomas contain crystalloid structures which appear to be unique.

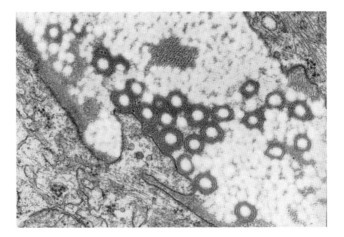

Figure 7.140 When seen in cross section, the crystalloid structures resemble the cross-sectional appearance of chrysotile asbestos.

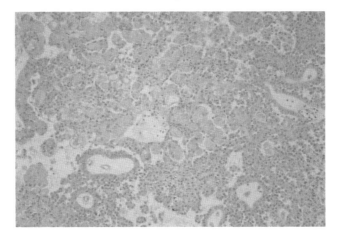

Figure 7.141 The neoplastic cells in this neoplasm resemble Gaucher cells.

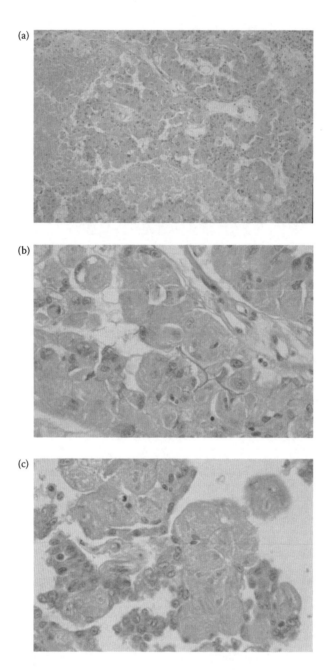

Figure 7.142   (a–c) At greater magnification, the tumor cells contain intracellular inclusions.

7.9.9 Desmoplastic/Sarcomatoid Mesothelioma of the Pleura and Its Distinction from Benign Fibrous Pleuritis

With the progression of time, pathologists have become more aware of the entity of desmo-plastic mesothelioma.[65,68–74] Desmoplastic mesothelioma is a variant of sarcomatoid mesothelioma and can be confused with hyaline pleural plaque and more cellular sarcomatoid mesotheliomas. Desmoplastic mesotheliomas form nodules in the pleura and have slit-like spaces (Figures 7.145 and 7.146). They usually show necrosis (Figure 7.147) and their cellularity is significantly less than a

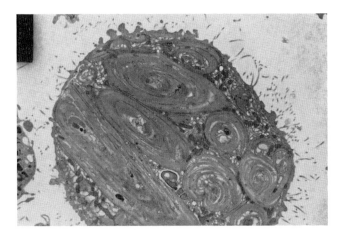

Figure 7.143   Ultrastructurally, the neoplastic cells contain parallel arrays with the cisterna of the rough endo-plasmic reticulum.

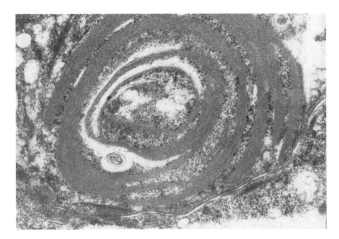

Figure 7.144   The inclusions are seen at a greater magnification.

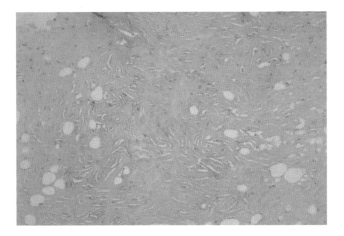

Figure 7.145   Desmoplastic mesotheliomas are composed of relatively hypocellular fibrous tissue with slit-like spaces between the tumor cells.

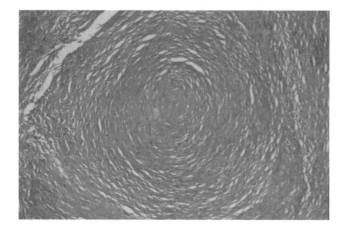

Figure 7.146   Desmoplastic mesotheliomas frequently show nodule formation.

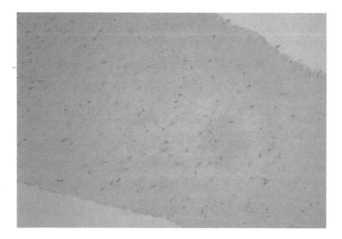

Figure 7.147   Desmoplastic mesotheliomas frequently show necrosis.

typical sarcomatoid mesothelioma (Figure 7.148). They do not show reactive changes that one sees in fibrosing pleuritis (Figures 7.149 and 7.150).

Desmoplastic mesotheliomas not infrequently directly invade lung tissue, metastasize to bone, and produce an organizing pneumonia in the lung (Figure 7.151). By immunohistochemistry, the tumor cells in desmoplastic mesothelioma express low molecular weight keratin, broad spectrum keratin, vimentin, and alpha actin. They typically do not exhibit immunostaining for CK5/6 and calretinin but may immunostain for CK7.

7.9.10 Lymphohistiocytoid Mesothelioma

In 1988, Henderson et al.[75] described three cases of malignant pleural mesothelioma that were initially thought to represent lymphoma. The authors[75] concluded that this type of mesothelioma was a variant of a predominantly sarcomatoid mesothelioma where the neoplastic cells had a histiocytoid morphology and were obscured by the intense inflammatory infiltrate of lymphocytes and plasma cells and, in one case, eosinophils, imparting a histological resemblance to either Hodgkin's disease or non-Hodgkin's lymphoma. The three cases represented only 0.8% of all cases pathologically

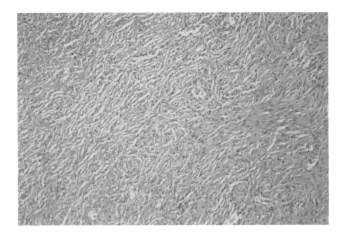

Figure 7.148 The cellularity of a "typical" sarcomatoid mesothelioma is compared with a desmoplastic mesothelioma.

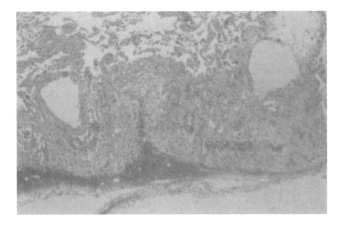

Figure 7.149 Fibrosing pleuritis is the primary differential diagnosis for desmoplastic mesothelioma. In fibrosing pleuritis, there is inflammation, vascular proliferation, and reactive cellularity with necrosis.

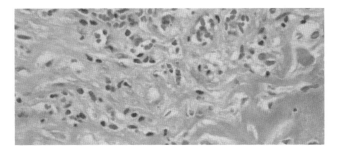

Figure 7.150 Another example of fibrosing pleuritis.

identified in the Australian Mesothelioma Register. Subsequently, cases were reported by Khalidi et al.[76] and by Yao et al.[77] In the report by Galateau-Sallé,[3] the Mesothelioma Pathology Group in France found cases of lymphohistiocytoid mesothelioma to represent less than 2% of their total cases. Of the 12 cases of lymphohistiocytoid mesothelioma described in the literature,[75–79] 11 were

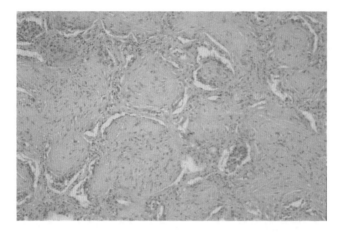

Figure 7.151 When desmoplastic mesothelioma invades the lung, the tumor cells fill up the alveoli that resembles organizing pneumonia.

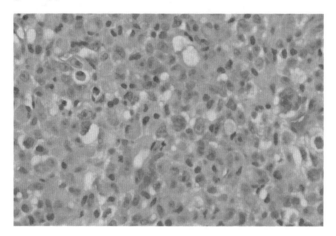

Figure 7.152 Lymphohistiocytoid mesothelioma resembles a lymphoma.

in a pleural location and one was in a peritoneal location. The age range was 31 to 74 years with a mean of 59 years.

I (S.P.H.) recently saw a peritoneal mesothelioma composed of large lymphoid cells that resembled Reed–Sternberg cells, the findings being characteristic with a lymphohistiocytoid mesothelioma (Figures 7.152 and 7.153).

The criteria for diagnosing lymphohistiocytoid mesothelioma are as follows:

1. A confluent pleura-based or, rarely, a peritoneal lesion with anatomic features indistinguishable from mesothelioma on imaging studies or at surgery;
2. A lymphoma-like appearance by light microscopy with scattered, dispersed, or indistinctly clustered atypical large histiocytoid cells;
3. Areas of transition to conventional spindle-cell sarcomatoid tissue or even small foci of epithelioid mesothelioma;
4. Cytokeratin and vimentin expression by large histiocytoid cells (Figures 7.154 and 7.155) and, occasionally, expression of mesothelial markers such as calretinin (Figure 7.156) or CK5/6, whereas the same large cells are devoid of lymphoid markers such as CD45, CD3, or CD20;
5. Evidence in some instances of mesothelial differentiation by electron microscopy, such as elongated serpentine microvilli devoid of a glycocalyx.

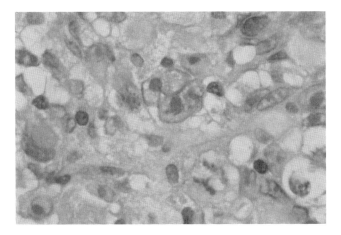

Figure 7.153 In some cases of lymphohistiocytoid mesothelioma, the neoplastic cells resemble Reed–Sternberg cells.

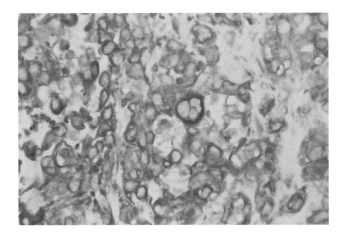

Figure 7.154 Lymphohistiocytoid mesothelioma showing cytokeratin expression of the neoplastic cells.

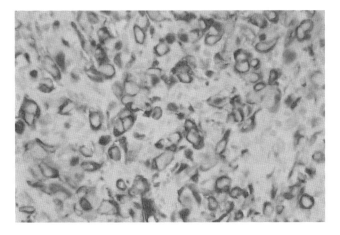

Figure 7.155 Vimentin expression of the neoplastic cells is seen in this lymphohistiocytoid mesothelioma.

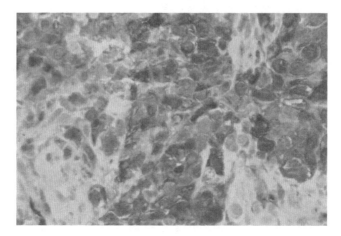

Figure 7.156   In this lymphohistiocytoid mesothelioma, the neoplastic cells express calretinin.

Henderson et al.[75] pointed out that this variant does not simply represent a prominent lymphocytic infiltration of an epithelioid mesothelioma but is a variant of a predominantly sarcomatoid mesothelioma where there is an intimate admixture with an intermingling of background histiocytoid tumor cells with tumor infiltrating lymphocytes, plasma cells, and, in some instances, eosinophils. Henderson et al.[75] also pointed out that focal areas of lymphohistiocytoid features can occur in sarcomatoid mesothelioma. Henderson et al.[75] suggested that the lymphohistiocytoid appearance presumably reflects an immunological response on the part of the host to the mesothelioma.

7.9.11 Pleomorphic Mesothelioma

Like other cancers, mesotheliomas can be composed of pleomorphic cells that can cause problems in diagnosing this type of mesothelioma unless the features are clearly known and pathologists are aware of these features. Pleomorphic mesotheliomas show extreme cellularity, nuclear atypia, hyperchromasia, and pleomorphism, thus producing a histological resemblance to an undifferentiated pleomorphic neoplasm (Figures 7.157 and 7.158). The neoplastic cells typically express pan keratin (Figure 7.159), vimentin (Figure 7.160), and, occasionally, mesothelial-specific markers such as calretinin (Figure 7.161). Some pleomorphic mesotheliomas have a rhabdoid morphology (Figures 7.162 through 7.164).

The diagnosis of pleomorphic mesothelioma, whether epithelial or sarcomatoid, can be based on the following findings:

1. A pleural-based tumor with an anatomic distribution that conforms to a diagnosis of mesothelioma, as revealed by imaging studies;
2. Transition from pleomorphic areas to other regions where the appearance is more characteristic of either an epithelial or sarcomatoid mesothelioma;
3. An immunohistochemical profile that conforms to a diagnosis of mesothelioma, either epithelial or sarcomatoid type, as opposed to a secondary carcinoma or a secondary sarcoma; and
4. Occasional ultrastructural evidence of mesothelial differentiation.

Galateau-Sallé et al.[80] recently reported on a series of 44 cases of malignant mesothelioma of the pleura with pleomorphic features in which 66% had a history of asbestos exposure. A localized pleural-based mass was observed in 16% of cases. Hyaline fibrous plaques were present in 4% of cases. The authors stated the findings suggested that malignant mesothelioma with pleomorphic

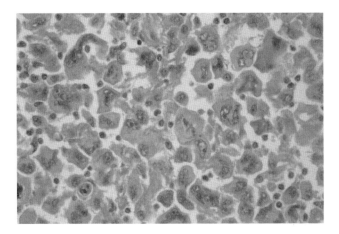

Figure 7.157   This pleomorphic mesothelioma is composed of large cells showing no specific differentiation.

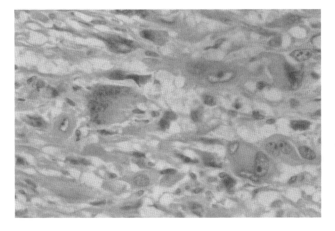

Figure 7.158   This pleomorphic mesothelioma is composed of large undifferentiated epithelioid and sarcoma-toid cells.

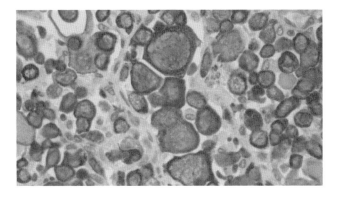

Figure 7.159   The pleomorphic cells usually express keratin.

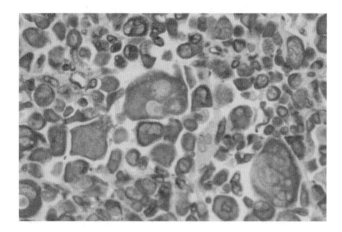

Figure 7.160 Vimentin is typically expressed in most pleomorphic mesotheliomas.

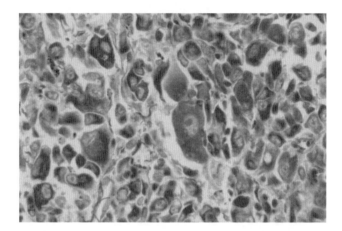

Figure 7.161 Calretinin expression is seen in many pleomorphic cells in this case.

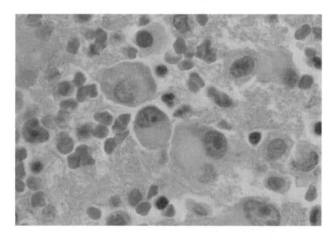

Figure 7.162 This pleomorphic mesothelioma is composed of cells that have a rhabdoid morphology.

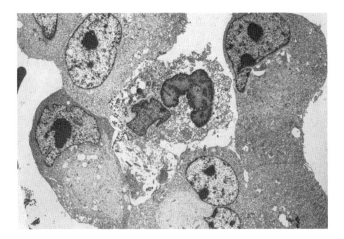

Figure 7.163   Ultrastructurally, the neoplastic cells have large nuclei with prominent, often multiple nucleoli.

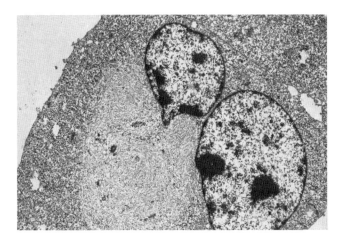

Figure 7.164   The neoplastic mesothelial rhabdoid tumor cells contain aggregates of cytoplasmic filaments that compress the nucleoli of the cells.

features was a distinct morphological variant of epithelioid ($p = .001$) and sarcomatoid ($p = .097$) malignant mesothelioma.

7.9.12 Localized Malignant Mesothelioma

In 1992, Henderson et al.[5] briefly referred to two cases of localized malignant pleural mesothelioma and additional cases were subsequently described by Crotty et al.[81] in 1996. In 2005, Allen et al.[82] described 23 cases of localized malignant mesothelioma (21 pleural and 2 peritoneal) and stated that 16 tumors showed histological features of diffuse epithelial mesothelioma, 6 had mixed epithelial and sarcomatous differentiation, and 1 was purely sarcomatous. Additional cases of localized malignant mesothelioma were published by Myers et al.,[83] Ojeda et al.,[84] Churg et al.,[85] and Okamura et al.[86] Galateau-Sallé et al.[80] pointed out that pleomorphic mesotheliomas can also be localized.

Localized pleural mesotheliomas occur in men and women in about equal frequency with an age range between 40 and 70 years.

The characteristic feature of localized malignant mesothelioma is a circumscribed or well-demarcated tumor that has the histological, immunohistochemical, and ultrastructural features essentially identical to diffuse epithelial, biphasic, and sarcomatoid mesotheliomas.

In the cases reported by Crotty et al.,[81] three of six cases treated with surgical excision had a disease-free survival for an extended period of time following resection, while the other three died within 2 years of the initial resection.

One should be aware that localized mesotheliomas exist and have the histological features of diffuse malignant mesothelioma.

I (S.P.H.) have encountered several cases of localized malignant mesothelioma that have not been published that have a clear history of exposure to asbestos. Therefore, there is no reason to think that asbestos does not have the potential to cause localized malignant mesothelioma just as asbestos causes diffuse malignant pleural mesothelioma.

7.10 CLINICAL FEATURES OF MESOTHELIOMA

7.10.1 Pleural Mesothelioma

The majority of patients diagnosed with pleural mesothelioma present in the exact same manner.[88–96] The most common presentation is shortness of breath (dyspnea) on exertion, which is almost always caused by a pleural effusion on the side where the tumor is eventually identified. Another common presentation is chest pain. The pain can radiate to a shoulder, the scapula, or sometimes to the spine. Rarely, the pain is referred to the neck, jaw, or flank. Another common symptom is weight loss. Patients with pleural mesotheliomas are sometimes thought to have an infectious process, and they frequently receive antibiotics with little or no improvement in their symptoms.

When the patient's symptoms fail to resolve, they are usually referred to a pulmonologist or surgeon and radiographs are obtained that identify the pleural effusion. The pleural effusion is usually treated by thoracentesis, with removal of the fluid, thus alleviating the patient's symptoms. Unfortunately, in most cases the pleural effusion rapidly recurs and produces the same/similar symptoms as seen during the initial presentation.

Some patients who are diagnosed with pleural mesothelioma exhibit malaise, night sweats, chills, weakness, fatigue, fever, and anorexia. They may have anemia, usually suggestive of iron deficiency anemia, but upon investigation the iron deficiency anemia is usually not identified by a GI bleed, and so forth. Another common finding in all types of mesothelioma is thrombocytosis. Approximately 25%–30% of all patients diagnosed with mesothelioma have an elevated platelet count ranging from slightly over normal (415,000–425,000 per microliter) to sometimes exceeding 1 million platelets per microliter. This is thought to be mediated by interleukin-6 and is a potential clinical problem. Of interest, when some patients respond to chemotherapy, their platelet count goes down, which is thought to not be due to chemotherapy but rather because the tumor has responded to chemotherapy, but may also be an effect caused by chemotherapy.

With the passage of time, many patients with mesothelioma will eventually develop pneumonia and some will develop cachexia of malignancy.

Some pleural mesotheliomas invade inferiorly and obstruct the inferior vena cava as it passes through the diaphragm. The obstruction of the inferior vena cava can result in marked lower extremity edema, producing what looks like elephantiasis.

7.10.2 Peritoneal Mesothelioma

Peritoneal mesothelioma is usually associated with abdominal pain, a distended abdomen, and bowel symptoms.[97,98] Peritoneal mesothelioma is not always considered in the differential diagnosis.

Not infrequently, patients will think they have gained weight. As described by me (S.P.H.)[99] some patients will present as having an infectious disease process with fever, elevated sedimentation rates, and increased white blood cell and platelet counts. Clinically, some patients will be extensively evaluated for a GI tract condition, which is usually negative. With the passage of time, changes in bowel habits, such as constipation, become a significant problem.

7.10.3 Pericardial Mesothelioma

Pericardial mesotheliomas are so rare that there is not enough information to describe how such patients present. Some patients develop pericardial effusions,[100] just like one would see with a pleural effusion or peritoneal effusion, with thickening of the pericardium. Pericardial mesothelioma must be distinguished from secondary involvement by pleural mesothelioma into the pericardium. Patients may have dyspnea, cardiac tamponade,[101] constrictive pericarditis,[102,103] cardiac failure, arrhythmias,[101] or tumor invading the atrium.[104] Pericardial mesothelioma may also present as a left atrial thrombus in patients with mitral stenosis.[105] The prognosis for pericardial mesothelioma is poor.[106]

7.10.4 Ovarian Mesothelioma

Patients with ovarian mesothelioma usually present with abdominal or pelvic pain, abdominal swelling, and/or with an adnexal mass found on pelvic examination or at laparotomy; tumors present as localized masses. The criteria for the diagnosis of ovarian mesothelioma include the presence of unilateral or bilateral ovarian enlargement, parenchymal replacement in the absence of significant peritoneal disease, or both. Most ovarian mesotheliomas are due to secondary involvement.[107]

7.10.5 Mesothelioma of the Tunica Vaginalis

Patients with malignant mesothelioma of the tunica vaginalis typically present with a hydrocele, with or without an associated mass.[108,109] The primary symptom is enlargement of the scrotum.[110] The preoperative diagnosis is usually that of a hydrocele, a suspected testicular tumor, epididymitis, a scrotal hernia, a spermatocele, or a post-traumatic testicular lesion.[110] They often present as localized masses.[111] This tumor must also be distinguished from secondary spread from a "typical" peritoneal mesothelioma.

7.11 APPROACH TO THE DIAGNOSIS

Because the development of pleural effusions or ascites is commonly seen in patients diagnosed with mesothelioma, it is not surprising that the fluid from the chest or abdominal cavity is analyzed to further evaluate the possibility of the development of mesothelioma. Generally, fluid is sent to the chemistry and cytology laboratory for analysis. In the chemistry laboratory, the typical tests that are performed are protein, glucose, cellularity, and lactic dehydrogenase—both of the fluid and of the serum. The fluid sent to the cytology laboratory is usually evaluated with a ThinPrep, a cytocentrifuged preparation, and/or a cell block preparation. Depending on the findings, one can determine whether the fluid is an exudate or transudate and whether the fluid contains atypical cells.

I (S.P.H.) have come to the conclusion that it is not possible to differentiate neoplastic mesothelial cells from reactive mesothelial cells and the cells of an adenocarcinoma—be it a lung adenocarcinoma or an adenocarcinoma from a site outside of the chest—on the basis of cytology alone. Nevertheless, there is information that is helpful in differentiating reactive mesothelial hyperplasia from mesothelioma or metastatic adenocarcinoma. This is shown in Table 7.7.

Table 7.7 Summary of Cytologic Discriminants between Reactive Mesothelial Hyperplasia, Epithelial Malignant Mesothelioma, and Secondary Adenocarcinoma

Feature	Reactive Mesothelial Hyperplasia/Mesotheliosis	Mesothelioma (Epithelial, Biphasic)	Metastatic Adenocarcinoma
Low power	Moderate to high cellularity	Cellular	Cellular
Cell population	Single epithelioid cell population ± inflammatory cells	Single epithelioid cell population	Classically dual epithelioid cell population but may be single malignant population
Cell disposition	Single cells; small 2-D clusters/sheets and clumps (<20 cells)	Single cells; large 3-D morules, (>50 cells); scalloped and complex outline of clusters; papillary structures; pseudoacini with collagen core	Large clusters (>12 cells) smooth "cannonball" outline; acini with peripheral nuclei; cells in single-file row
Cytologic features	Enlarged cells; enlarged central nucleus	Enlarged cells, nuclear-cytoplasmic (N/C) ratio same or less; range of cell sizes; many multinucleated cells, "cell-in-cell"; giant mesothelial cells; squamous-like cells	Enlarged cells; atypical and bizarre cells
Differentiating features	Fenestrations between the cells in clusters/sheets; central nuclei; bitonal staining cytoplasm (dense orange around nucleus to green-blue at periphery in PAP, denser centrally in DQ); peripheral fringe; cytoplasmic vacuoles may be present (no or only minimal diastase–PAS staining); atypia usually only moderate		Mucin vacuoles indenting nucleus, diastase–PAS-positive; nuclei peripheral; nuclei may be very atypical, often with coarse chromatin
Immuno-histochemistry (IHC)	Calretinin (nuclear); CK5/6; WT-1 (nuclear); HBME-1 (linear membrane); thrombomodulin (linear membrane); EMA: strong circumferential linear labeling more common in MM than reactive (clone E29), cytoplasmic labeling in adenocarcinoma		CEA; B72.3; CD15; BG8; site-specific markers, e.g., TTF-1, gross cystic disease fluid protein
Electron microscopy (EM)	Long slender serpentine microvilli; no glycocalyx		Short stubby microvilli; antennular glycocalyx

7.11.1 Reactive Mesothelial Cells versus Neoplastic Mesothelial Cells

Reactive mesothelial cells and neoplastic mesothelial cells can be very similar.[12] Immunohisto-chemical studies that are sometimes helpful in differentiating between the two include a combination of epithelial membrane antigen (EMA) and desmin. In a neoplastic process, the epithelial mesothelial cells typically show cell membrane staining for EMA, whereas the desmin stain is typically negative. In a reactive process, the opposite is true—the EMA stain is negative or shows minimal cell membrane staining while the desmin stain shows cytoplasmic staining.[112]

7.11.2 Immunohistochemistry

Immunohistochemistry can be easily applied to cell block preparations, just as one would do for any other type of histological specimen. The primary differential diagnosis with respect to a pleural epithelial mesothelioma and a peritoneal epithelial mesothelioma is between mesothelioma versus adenocarcinoma. There has been extensive discussion concerning immunohistochemistry with respect to how many antibodies should be used for evaluating positive markers and negative markers.[12,35,36,112–123] The most difficult differential diagnosis is between a pseudomesotheliomatous adenocarcinoma of the lung and a metastatic pseudomesotheliomatous adenocarcinoma and an epithelial mesothelioma.

Klebe et al.[114] performed a study to identify the minimal panel of antibodies necessary to distinguish between malignant mesothelioma and metastatic adenocarcinoma. The authors[114] used a standard of 12 antibodies (CAM5.2, CK5/6, HBME-1, calretinin, EMA, carcinoembryonic antigen [CEA], CD15, B72.3, TTF-1, WT-1, thrombomodulin, and BG8) and stated that positive staining for calretinin and lack of staining (negative immunostaining) for BG8 were sufficient for definite correlation with a diagnosis of mesothelioma, and that CD15 (LeuM1) provided further differentiating information in some cases. The authors[114] stated a panel of three antibodies was sufficient in most cases to diagnose or to exclude epithelial mesothelioma and that calretinin exhibited the strongest correlative power of these antibodies.

7.11.2.1 Markers for Differentiating between Epithelioid Pleural Mesothelioma and Lung Adenocarcinoma

Positive mesothelioma markers include calretinin, CK5/6, WT-1, and podoplanin (D2-40).

- Calretinin staining (cytoplasmic and nuclear) is shown in virtually all epithelioid mesotheliomas. The staining is often strong and diffuse. Note that 5%–10% of lung adenocarcinomas are positive for calretinin, but the staining is usually focal and cytoplasmic.
- D2-40 (podoplanin) is expressed in 86%–100% of mesotheliomas (cell membrane staining) and up to 7% of lung adenocarcinomas (focal staining).
- Cytokeratin 5/6 is expressed in 75%–100% of mesothelioma and 2%–19% of lung adenocarcinomas (focal staining).
- WT-1 is expressed in 43%–93% of mesotheliomas (nuclear staining) and is not expressed in lung adenocarcinomas (negative).

Positive lung adenocarcinoma markers include MOC-31, BG8 (Lewis^y), CEA, B72.3, BerEP4, and TTF-1.

- MOC-31 is expressed in 95%–100% of lung adenocarcinomas and 2%–10% of mesotheliomas (focal).
- BerEP4 is expressed in 95%–100% of lung adenocarcinomas (strongly positive) and up to 20% of mesotheliomas (focally positive), usually in a cell membrane distribution.
- BG8 (Lewis^y) is expressed in 85%–100% of lung adenocarcinomas and 3%–7% of mesotheliomas (focal reactivity).
- TTF-1 is expressed in 75%–85% of lung adenocarcinomas (nuclear staining) and is not expressed in mesotheliomas (negative staining).
- B72.3 is expressed in 75%–85% of lung adenocarcinomas and very few mesotheliomas.
- CEA is expressed in 50%–90% of lung adenocarcinomas and less than 5% of mesotheliomas (focal staining).
- CD15 (LeuM1) is expressed in 50%–70% of lung adenocarcinomas and is rarely expressed in mesotheliomas (focal staining).

7.11.2.2 Markers for Differentiating between Epithelioid Pleural Mesothelioma and Squamous Cell Carcinoma of the Lung

Positive mesothelioma markers include CK5/6, calretinin, WT-1, and D2-40 (podoplanin).

- WT-1 is expressed in up to 93% of mesotheliomas (nuclear staining) and is negative in squamous cell carcinomas of lung.
- Calretinin is expressed in virtually all mesotheliomas (nuclear and cytoplasmic staining) and in 40% of squamous cell carcinomas of lung (focal staining).

- D2-40 (podoplanin) is expressed in 86%–100% of mesotheliomas and in 50% of squamous cell carcinomas of lung; therefore, this stain is not considered useful.
- CK5/6 is expressed in 75%–100% of mesotheliomas and in 100% of squamous cell carcinomas of lung; therefore, this stain is not considered useful.

Positive squamous cell carcinoma of lung markers include CK5/6, MOC-31, BerEP4, BG8 (Lewis^Y), and p63.

- p63 is expressed in 100% of squamous cell carcinomas of lung (strong, diffuse nuclear staining) and 7% of mesotheliomas (often focally).
- MOC-31 is expressed in 97%–100% of squamous cell carcinomas of lung and in 2%–10% of mesotheliomas (focal staining).
- BG8 (Lewis^Y) is expressed in 80% of squamous cell carcinomas of lung and in 3%–7% of mesotheliomas (focal staining).
- BerEP4 is expressed in 87%–100% of squamous cell carcinomas of lung and in up to 20% of mesotheliomas (focal staining).
- CK5/6 is expressed in 100% of squamous cell carcinomas of lung and in 75%–100% of mesotheliomas; therefore, this stain is not considered useful.

7.11.2.3 Markers for Differentiating between Epithelioid Pleural Mesothelioma and Renal Cell Carcinoma

Positive epithelioid mesothelioma markers include CK5/6, calretinin, WT-1, mesothelin, and D2-40.

- Mesothelin is expressed in 100% of mesotheliomas and is negative in RCCs.
- D2-40 (podoplanin) is expressed in 86%–100% of mesotheliomas (cell membrane distribution) and is negative in RCCs.
- CK5/6 is expressed in 75%–100% of mesotheliomas and is negative is RCCs.
- Calretinin is expressed in virtually all mesotheliomas (strong, diffuse nuclear, and cytoplasmic staining) and is focally positive in 4%–10% of RCCs.
- WT-1 is expressed in 43%–93% of mesotheliomas (nuclear staining) and in 4% of RCCs.

Positive RCC markers include CD15 (LeuM1), MOC-31, BerEP4, BG8, RCC Ma, PAX2, and Napsin.

- CD15 (LeuM1) is expressed in 63% of RCCs and can show focal positive staining in mesotheliomas. Note that it can stain any necrotic tissue.
- RCC Ma is expressed in 50%–70% of RCCs and 8% of mesotheliomas (focal staining).
- MOC-31 is expressed in 50% of RCCs and in 2%–10% of mesotheliomas (focal staining).
- BerEP4 is expressed in 42% of RCCs and in up to 20% of mesotheliomas (focal staining); therefore, this stain is not considered useful.
- BG8 (Lewis^Y) is expressed in 4% of RCCs and in 3%–7% of mesotheliomas; therefore, this stain is not considered useful.
- PAX2 has been detected in 88% of clear cell RCCs, in 18% of papillary RCCs, and in 13% of chromophobe RCCs.
- Napsin A is expressed in 28% of papillary RCCs.

7.11.2.4 Markers for Differentiating between Malignant Peritoneal Mesothelioma and Papillary Serous Carcinoma

Positive peritoneal malignant mesothelioma markers include CK5/6, calretinin, WT-1, and D2-40.

- Calretinin is expressed in 85%–100% of malignant peritoneal mesotheliomas and in up to 38% of papillary serous carcinomas (usually cytoplasmic and not nuclear); therefore, this limits its use as a single marker.
- D2-40 is expressed in 93%–96% of malignant peritoneal mesotheliomas and in 13%–65% of papillary serous carcinomas; therefore, more data are required.
- CK5/6 is expressed in 53%–100% of malignant peritoneal mesotheliomas and in 22%–35% of papillary serous carcinomas; therefore, this stain is not considered useful.
- WT-1 is expressed in 43%–93% of malignant peritoneal mesotheliomas and in 89%–93% of papillary serous carcinomas; therefore, this stain is not considered useful.

Positive papillary serous carcinoma markers include CEA, B72.3, BerEP4, MOC-31, BG8, estrogen receptor (ER), and progesterone receptor (PR).

- MOC-31 is expressed in 98% of papillary serous carcinomas and in 5% of malignant peritoneal mesotheliomas.
- BerEP4 is expressed in 83%–100% of papillary serous carcinomas and in 9%–13% of malignant peritoneal mesotheliomas.
- BG8 is expressed in 73% of papillary serous carcinomas and in 3%–9% of malignant peritoneal mesotheliomas.
- B72.3 is expressed in 65%–100% of papillary serous carcinomas and in up to 3% of malignant peritoneal mesotheliomas; however, many show focal/trace staining.
- CEA is expressed in up to 45% of papillary serous carcinomas (mean = 20%); however, sensitivity is too low compared with other choices. CEA is negative in malignant peritoneal mesotheliomas.
- ER is expressed in 60%–93% of papillary serous carcinomas and is low to negative in up to 8% of malignant peritoneal mesotheliomas.
- PR has a lower sensitivity than ER but is uniformly negative in malignant peritoneal mesotheliomas. This stain may be of limited value if positive.

7.11.3 Pseudomesotheliomatous Lung Cancer

Pseudomesotheliomatous lung cancers are essentially identical to mesotheliomas, except that in most cases they have the typical immunohistochemical features of an adenocarcinoma versus an epithelial mesothelioma.

7.11.4 Other Neoplasms Arising in the Pleura

7.11.4.1 Synovial Sarcoma of the Pleura

Both biphasic and monophasic synovial sarcomas have been extensively documented in the literature[124–130] and can cause confusion between sarcomatoid mesotheliomas and biphasic mesotheliomas.[131–133] The most effective way to differentiate those entities is by determining fusion gene changes.[134–136]

7.11.4.2 Solitary Fibrous Tumors

Solitary fibrous pseudotumor are lesions that can be seen in many parts of the body, including the chest cavity.[137,138] They are typically composed of spindle cells and can be benign or malignant. They typically express vimentin, CD34, and may express CD117.[139,140] The malignant forms of localized fibrous tumors may fail to stain for CD34,[140] and a small portion of sarcomatoid mesotheliomas are negative for cytokeratin.[141] Evidence of malignancy is determined by necrosis,[142] hemorrhage, and more than four mitotic figures per 10 high power field.[137] In the parietal pleura, they can be sessile or have the appearance of a large tumor mass. They can be attached to the parietal pleura by a pedicle and can directly invade the lung.

7.11.4.3 Desmoid Tumors of the Pleura

Desmoid tumors of the pleura typically occur in the shoulder girdle region of the chest wall (shoulder region and chest wall). Primary desmoid tumors of the pleura and lung are extremely rare, although have been reported. Wilson et al.[143] reported four cases of pleural desmoids tumors (two men and two women; aged 16–66 years; mean of 44 years). Three patients presented with chest pain and one with dyspnea. Three tumors affected the parietal pleura and one affected the visceral pleura.

7.11.4.4 Calcifying Fibrous Pseudotumor of the Pleura

Calcifying fibrous tumor typically affects the subcutaneous and deeper soft tissues of the limbs, trunk, and neck of children, adolescents, and young adults,[6] but cases have been reported in relation to the chest wall,[144] mediastinum,[145,146] pleura,[147–150] peritoneum,[151] and mesentery.[152] Pinkard et al.[148] described three cases of pleural calcifying fibrous pseudotumors in young to middle-aged adults, aged 23, 28, and 34 years. Typically, pleural calcifying fibrous pseudotumors of the pleura are located in the inferior chest region and may represent either solitary mass lesions or multifocal tumor-like lesions measuring approximately 30 to 120 mm in greatest diameter.[6,147] One case with multiple pleural lesions was reported in a 29-year-old woman who had no symptoms referable to the tumor.[150]

On histological examination, calcifying fibrous pseudotumors comprise paucicellular fibrocollagenous tissue without a laminar (plaque-like) architecture accompanied by a sparse lymphoplasmacytic infiltrate and with variable numbers of rounded, calcified bodies of variable size resembling psammoma bodies. Points of distinction of calcifying fibrous pseudotumor from either desmoplastic malignant mesothelioma or solitary fibrous tumor include negative reactions for cytokeratins and CD34, whereas the fibroblastoid cells show positive staining for vimentin.[6] Pleural plaques are distinguishable by their paucicellular, laminated, and frequently hyalinized appearance. In addition, the pattern of psammoma-like calcification in calcifying fibrous pseudotumors differs from the finely punctate to sheet-like calcification seen in plaques.

A relationship to inflammatory myofibroblastic tumor has been noted,[153–155] but the pathogenesis of calcifying fibrous pseudotumor remains obscure. These lesions are entirely benign in character and are usually treated successfully by surgical extirpation; however, local recurrence has been recorded.[156]

7.11.4.5 Benign and Malignant Nerve Sheath Tumors

Rare nerve sheath tumors occur in the pleura, and can be benign or malignant.[157,158] The benign neoplasms typically show morphologic features of Verocay bodies with Antoni A and B areas and hyaline vascular changes. The malignant variants do not show the typical benign features of nerve sheath tumors. Immunohistochemical studies show S100 protein as being helpful in confirming the neurogenic origin of these neoplasms.

7.11.4.6 Inflammatory Myofibroblastic Tumors

These neoplasms are also referred to as *plasma cell granulomas* and *inflammatory pseudotumors.*[159] These tumors typically have the same morphology as in the lung, and are made up of proliferating spindle cells with predominantly plasma cells in the inflammatory cell infiltrate. There is a debate as to whether these are true neoplasms.[160]

7.11.4.7 *Epithelioid Hemangioendothelioma and Angiosarcoma of the Pleura*

Epithelioid hemangioendothelioma is a distinctive malignant angioformative neoplasm where the neoplastic endothelial cells are epithelioid and sometimes bland in appearance,[161] often arranged as solid sheets or in a linear fashion, and embedded in a hyaline or myxohyaline stroma.[3] These epithelioid endothelial neoplasms have been described in soft tissue,[161] bone, liver, and lung. In the lung, they were designated as intravascular bronchioloalveolar tumors before their endothelial character was recognized.[162] The epithelioid appearance of the neoplastic cells stands in contrast to the angioformative and papillary patterns of conventional angiosarcomas. Epithelioid hemangioendotheliomas in soft tissues are often considered to represent neoplasms intermediate in malignancy between conventional aggressive angiosarcomas and benign hemangiomas; however, they have the potential for local recurrence and metastatic spread.

In 1993, Battifora[163] reported pleural epithelioid hemangioendotheliomas mimicking mesothelioma. In 1996, Lin et al.[164] reported 14 cases of malignant vascular tumors of serous membranes mimicking mesothelioma. These epithelioid hemangioendotheliomas (epithelioid angiosarcomas) diffusely involving pleural, peritoneal, or pericardial cavities produced a clinical picture that closely simulated mesothelioma. The patients ranged in age from 34 to 85 years at the time of diagnosis, with a mean age of 52 years. The patients included two women and one man with peritoneal epithelioid hemangioendothelioma, eight men with pleural epithelioid hemangioendotheliomas, and three men with pericardial tumors. The histological appearance took the form of a diffuse sheetlike, clustered pattern of tumor cells with variable degrees of vascular differentiation. A tubulopapillary growth pattern was encountered in four cases. Nine cases showed varying numbers of spindle-shaped cells producing a focal biphasic architecture, heightening the resemblance to mesothelioma. The initial diagnoses made on those cases included mesothelioma, secondary adenocarcinoma, and leiomyosarcoma. On immunohistochemical analysis, they were characterized by extensive strong vimentin staining (14/14 cases) in the face of weak (4/14) to moderate (2/14) immunostaining for cytokeratins. The tumor cells expressed at least two of the four epithelial markers employed in the study (CD31, CD34, von Willebrand factor [factor VIII-related antigen; factor VIII-RAG], and *Ulex europaeus* agglutinin-1). Markers for mesothelial, epithelial, myoid, and neuronal differentiation were negative.

Additional cases of epithelioid hemangioendothelioma have been reported.[165–169] Not only do pleural epithelioid hemangioendotheliomas essentially mimic mesothelioma in their presentation and anatomical distribution, but the epithelioid appearance of the neoplastic cells can produce a pattern in hematoxylin and eosin–stained sections that is virtually indistinguishable from mesothelioma. The neoplastic cells can closely resemble epithelioid cells in malignant mesothelioma, being composed of sheets or as irregular clusters. In some areas, abortive vascular differentiation may be found. In many cases, the neoplastic cells possess empty-appearing intracytoplasmic vacuoles that appear on electron microscopic examination as rudimentary vascular lumina. The stroma of these tumors can vary from myxoid to hyaline, and there may be a spindle-cell sarcomatoid pattern mimicking a biphasic mesothelioma.

Clues to the correct diagnosis of an epithelioid hemangioendothelioma include the following:

- Negative to weak or only moderate immunostaining for cytokeratins in comparison with disproportionately prominent reactivity for vimentin.
- Absence of staining for mesothelial cell markers such as calretinin or HBME-1, or for carcinoma-related markers.
- Positive immunostaining for endothelial markers such as CD31, CD34, or factor VIII-RAG.

By electron microscopy, these tumors show features of endothelial differentiation, including the formation of rudimentary vascular structures, a surrounding basal lamina, and in some instances the presence of tubulated Weibel–Palade bodies in their cytoplasm.

7.11.4.8 Desmoplastic Round Cell Tumors

Desmoplastic round cell tumors that characteristically occur in young adults in the pelvic cavity have been reported in the pleura. These neoplasms have the same morphology as they do in the abdominal cavity, typically occurring as nests of small round cell tumors with dense fibrous cellular stroma.[170–172]

7.11.4.9 Pleuropulmonary Blastomas

Pleuropulmonary blastomas are rare neoplasms that occur predominantly in infants and in early childhood.[54,173] Pleuropulmonary blastoma is different from the pulmonary blastoma that typically occurs in adults. Pleuropulmonary blastomas are composed of primitive cells underneath an epithelium with a cambium layer-like appearance such as seen in sarcoma botryoides. Rhabdomyoblasts have been reported among the small cells.

7.11.4.10 Primitive Neuroectodermal Tumors

Primitive neuroectodermal tumors are part of the spectrum of small round cell tumors that include Ewing's sarcoma. These tumors have also been referred to as *Askin tumors* and are composed of sheets of small round cells with hyperchromatic nuclei that show areas of necrosis. Glycogen is frequently seen in the cytoplasm of these cells. By immunohistochemistry, they typically express CD99 and usually are negative for keratin, although may show some positive staining for chromogranin and synaptophysin.[174–176]

7.11.4.11 Pleural Lymphomas

There are two pleural lymphomas that are mentioned as part of the spectrum of lymphomas in the pleura. The first is a primary effusion lymphoma (PEL) and the second is a pyothorax-associated lymphoma.[177,178] The PELs are composed of large B lymphoid cells and are typically present in effusions without detectable tumor masses elsewhere in the body. PELs have been associated with herpes virus 8 and Kaposi's sarcoma and typically occur in individuals with AIDS.[179–181]

Pyothorax-associated lymphomas typically occur in persons with a chronic pyothorax, often decades after the initial injury. These were first reported in Japan. The pathogenesis is thought to be due to chronic anogenic stimulation analogous to mucosal-associated lymphomas.[182–184]

Diffuse large B-cell lymphomas have been reported to show pleuropulmonary involvement and typically have features that have immunoblastic and plasmacytoid differentiation.

Primary sclerosing mediastinal B-cell lymphomas occur most frequently in young females but can show pleuropulmonary involvement. These are thought to arise from perithymic B-lymphocytes and typically show immunostaining for CD45, CD20, and CD30. They do not express immunostaining for CD15.

Multiple myeloma has also been identified, primarily in the pleura, although is rare. The most recent report on lymphomas involving the pleura is by Vega et al.,[185] who showed clinicopathologic features of 34 patients with lymphoma. Other B-cell lymphomas have rarely been reported in the pleura.[186–188]

7.12 DIAGNOSTIC TECHNIQUES

There are a variety of techniques to obtain a specimen for evaluation to diagnose mesothelioma.

7.12.1 Cytologic Diagnosis

7.12.1.1 Fine-Needle Aspiration Biopsy

Fine-needle aspiration biopsies are frequently performed on patients who are eventually diagnosed with mesothelioma. These are usually cases where the pleura or peritoneum is identified to have nodularity or if the PET scan shows areas of diffuse increased standardized uptake values (SUV) activity in the pleura or peritoneal cavity.

7.12.1.2 Tru-Cut Biopsy

Tru-Cut biopsies can be done on pleural and peritoneal tissue, again with the idea that if one can localize the area(s) of activity or the mass(es), one has a chance to obtain a sample of tumor tissue that can be evaluated. The fine-needle aspiration biopsy specimens and the Tru-Cut biopsy specimens can be treated just like any other tissue specimen with the understanding that often the size of the specimen is significantly smaller than one would obtain with a video-assisted thoracoscopic biopsy.

7.12.1.3 Cytologic Diagnosis Controversy

There is significant controversy with respect to whether or not the diagnosis of mesothelioma can be made cytologically. The report from the International Mesothelioma Interest Group[12] suggested that cytologic evaluation was not consistently reliable in making a diagnosis of mesothelioma.

In my (S.P.H.) opinion, we have had very good correlation between cytological findings and VATS biopsy findings when diagnosing malignant mesothelioma. In most instances, the diagnosis is the same. The most important concern with respect to the cytologic diagnosis is that there has to be no question that the cells are neoplastic, just like any other cytology specimen. One other finding that is important is that the greater the number of atypical cells in the cytologic fluid specimen, the more likely this is to be a neoplastic process.

Sometimes, there are cases where there is significant inflammatory cells in the specimen such as neutrophils that can release CEA, which can coat the atypical cells and be interpreted as neoplastic cells that are CEA-positive. The same thing can occur with calretinin. This can lead to a misdiagnosis. In this situation, one has to be very certain about the diagnosis and use a wide spectrum of antibodies.

7.12.1.4 Electron Microscopy

Electron microscopy can be used in evaluating atypical cells in fluid specimens such as pleural or peritoneal fluid. It is usually fairly easy to determine if there are cells that have the morphology of mesothelial cells. What is more difficult, however, is differentiating reactive epithelial mesothelial cells from neoplastic mesothelial cells. It is my (S.P.H.) opinion that differentiating reactive epithelial mesothelial cells from neoplastic mesothelial cells cannot be done by ultrastructural evaluation (EM).

7.13 PATHOLOGICAL DIFFERENTIAL DIAGNOSIS

The primary differential diagnosis between an epithelioid mesothelioma is distinguishing it from another type of neoplasm that can look like an epithelioid mesothelioma. As shown in this chapter, epithelial mesotheliomas have a wide variety of histological appearances; therefore, one has to be aware of the variation in mesotheliomas with respect to ruling out another type of cancer. In cases where there seems to be difficulty in determining whether a tumor is or is not an epithelial mesothelioma, electron microscopy is usually helpful. The typical ultrastructural findings of a well to moderately well-differentiated epithelial mesothelioma include long, thin, sinuous microvilli; well-defined desmosomes; junctional complexes; and large numbers of intracellular tonofilaments.

7.13.1 Epithelioid Mesothelioma versus Adenocarcinoma of Lung

The most common type of cancer that epithelial mesotheliomas are mistaken for are adenocarcinomas—primarily, pulmonary adenocarcinomas, and, occasionally, metastatic adenocarcinomas from a site outside of the chest.

The immunohistochemical profile we perform in our laboratory to differentiate an epithelioid mesothelioma from a pulmonary adenocarcinoma includes pan cytokeratin, CK5/6, CK7, CK20, vimentin, HBME-1, calretinin, EMA, WT-1, D2-40, and mesothelin (Table 7.8). Occasionally, CA125, thrombomodulin, and CD10 are used. With respect to the negative immunohistochemical tests, our lab (PAKC/DSL) usually uses CEA and TTF-1, although other negative markers used to exclude a diagnosis of malignant mesothelioma include CD15 (LeuM1), BerEP4, B72.3, MOC-31, and BG8, which are positive in primary lung adenocarcinomas. One also has to recognize that a small percentage of epithelioid mesotheliomas will express markers that are seen in adenocarcinomas of the lung such as MOC-31, BG8, BerEP4, B72.3, CD15 (LeuM1), and CEA. Rarely, BerEP4 will show diffuse cell membrane staining of an epithelioid mesothelioma.

7.13.2 Epithelial Mesothelioma versus Primary Kidney Cancer

Some primary kidney cancers can cause difficulty in differentiating an epithelial mesothelioma from a primary kidney cancer. Kidney cancers, like mesothelioma, can show a great deal of variation in morphology.

Table 7.8   Panel of Antibodies Used in Our Laboratory (PAKC/DSL, Inc., P.S., Bremerton, WA)

	Cytokeratins (AE1/AE3, CK8/18)	CK5/6	CK7	CK20	Vimentin	HBME-1	Calretinin	EMA
Malignant mesothelioma	+	+	+	−	+/−	+*	+	+*
Lung adenocarcinoma	+	−/+	+	−/+	−/+	−/+**	−	+**
	WT1	D2-40	Mesothelin	CEA	CD15 (LeuM1)	B72.3	BerEP4 MOC31	TTF-1
Malignant mesothelioma	+	+	+	−	−	−	−/+	−
Lung adenocarcinoma	−	−	±	+	+	+/−	+	+

+, positive; −, negative; +/−, mostly positive; −/+, mostly negative; ±, may be positive or negative; *, linear, membrane related; **, cytoplasmic.

7.13.2.1 Papillary Renal Cell Carcinoma

The typical positive markers for a papillary RCC are AE1/AE3 keratin, vimentin, RCC, and alpha-methylacyl coenzyme A racemase (AMACR).[189]

7.13.2.2 Clear Cell Carcinoma of the Kidney

With respect to clear cell carcinoma of the kidney, the neoplastic cells are usually positive for low molecular weight keratin such as CAM5.2 keratin and CK18, AE1/AE3 keratin, EMA, vimentin, CAIX, CD10, PAX2, and PAX8. They usually show no immunostaining for high molecular weight keratin, CK5/6, CK7, CK20, and CEA.[189]

7.13.3 Squamous Cell Carcinoma of Lung versus Epithelioid Mesothelioma

With respect to squamous cell carcinomas of the lung, there can be overlap between immunohistochemical features. Squamous cell carcinomas typically express CK5/6 and high molecular weight keratin (34βE12), as do epithelioid mesotheliomas. Squamous cell carcinomas typically show immunostaining for p63, which is usually not expressed in epithelial mesotheliomas.[189]

7.13.4 Peritoneal Epithelioid Mesothelioma versus Peritoneal Carcinoma

With respect to peritoneal carcinomas, the primary differential diagnosis includes a serous ovarian carcinoma or a primary carcinoma of the peritoneum. These neoplasms can show some similar immunohistochemical findings such as with WT-1 and CA-125. They also express CEA, LeuM1, and B72.3. In contrast, peritoneal epithelioid mesotheliomas usually have the same pattern of reactivity as one would see in the pleural cavity. One potentially positive difference would be that primary peritoneal carcinomas and ovarian serous adenocarcinomas usually express ER protein, whereas peritoneal mesotheliomas are usually ER negative. There have been reports of a few cases of peritoneal mesotheliomas that express estrogen and progesterone receptor proteins.

7.13.5 Reactive Mesothelial Hyperplasia versus Infiltrating Epithelial Mesothelioma

It can be extremely difficult to differentiate reactive mesothelial hyperplasia from a superficially infiltrating epithelial mesothelioma. This has been described previously. Reactive mesothelial cells usually express cytoplasmic staining for desmin and do not show cell membrane staining for EMA. Likewise, GLUT-1 is typically positive in epithelial mesotheliomas but negative in reactive mesothelial cells. What I (S.P.H.) have found in most instances is that cases that are diagnosed as reactive atypical mesothelial hyperplasia turn out to be epithelial mesothelioma. I (S.P.H.) have evaluated one case in which I initially thought the process was an invasive epithelioid mesothelioma, whereas other well-respected pathologists did not. In that case, the patient was relatively stable for approximately 2 years and then developed recurrent pleural effusions and chest pain. The patient was subsequently rebiopsied and found to have an invasive epithelial mesothelioma.

7.13.6 Desmoplastic Mesothelioma versus Fibrosing Pleuritis

With respect to sarcomatoid lesions, one difficulty is differentiating between desmoplastic mesothelioma and fibrosing pleuritis. In general and as described previously, desmoplastic mesotheliomas frequently form nodules and have slit-like spaces between the tumor cells; they not infrequently show areas of necrosis. In contrast, benign fibrous pleuritis shows vascular proliferation that is usually perpendicular to the surface of the pleura. Also, there is a proliferation of multipotential subserosal cells with varying degrees of inflammation. One has to be aware, however, that fibrosing pleuritis can be infiltrative, just like a desmoplastic mesothelioma, and involve subparietal pleural fat. Immunohistochemistry is not helpful in resolving this differential diagnosis.

7.13.7 Synovial Sarcoma versus Sarcomatoid/Biphasic Mesothelioma

Synovial sarcomas are neoplasms that show biphasic features with an epithelial component or a monophasic morphology composed of spindle cells.[127,130,131] It is thought by some that biphasic synovial sarcomas might represent a carcinosarcoma. With respect to the epithelial component, the neoplastic cells typically show immunoreactivity for low molecular weight keratin (35βH11), chromosome-associated or desmoplakin, CEA, and, occasionally, S100 protein. They may also express immunoreactivity that is typically associated with Ewing's sarcoma/PNET.

The monophasic sarcomatoid tumor typically expresses vimentin but can express keratin. Synovial sarcomas have been reported in the chest cavity and have been reported to simulate mesotheliomas.

Synovial sarcomas have been associated in approximately 90% of cases with chromosomal translocation t(X;18) (p11.2;q11.2). This aberration is present in both the biphasic and the monophasic types. The break points have been cloned and have been shown to involve two novel genes: SSX (in chromosome X) and SYT (in chromosome 18). This results in a chimeric XYT-SSX.[190,191]

7.13.8 Localized Fibrous Tumors (Solitary Fibrous Tumors) versus Sarcomatoid Mesothelioma

Localized fibrous tumors (solitary fibrous tumors) can occur in all parts of the body, including the chest cavity, and can cause difficulty in differentiating them from sarcomatoid mesothelioma. Frequently, the solitary fibrous tumors are pedunculated, and a pedicle can be seen attached to the pleura. Sometimes, the pedicle is not seen. Solitary fibrous tumors typically are composed of spindle cells and can be difficult to differentiate from a sarcomatoid mesothelioma. The criteria for differentiating sarcomatoid mesothelioma from a localized (solitary) fibrous tumor of the pleura includes CD34-positive staining of the solitary fibrous tumor and, occasionally, CD117 and bcl2 staining of the solitary fibrous tumor. In contrast, the spindle cells of sarcomatoid mesotheliomas typically show immunostaining for broad spectrum keratin, low molecular weight keratin, vimentin, and, occasionally, alpha actin.

7.13.9 Calcifying Fibrous Pseudotumor versus Sarcomatoid Mesothelioma

Other spindle cell tumors that can occasionally cause difficulty in differentiating from a sarcomatoid mesothelioma include a calcifying fibrous pseudotumor. These are composed of dense hyalinized or laminated collagen with a few spindle cells and calcification and either dystrophic or psammomatous features. I (S.P.H.) have seen one calicifying fibrous pseudotumor that entirely encased the lung and was diagnosed by two pathologists as a desmoplastic mesothelioma. The patient underwent a radical extrapleural pneumonectomy and was free of disease several years later.

7.13.10 Desmoid Tumors of the Pleura/Desmoplastic Round Cell Neoplasms versus Sarcomatoid Mesothelioma

Some desmoid tumors of the pleura can resemble sarcomatoid mesothelioma, just as inflammatory myofibroblastic tumors. Also, desmoplastic round cell neoplasms can resemble mesotheliomas.

7.13.11 Pseudomesotheliomatous Epithelioid Hemangioendothelioma versus Epithelial Mesothelioma

There are occasional tumors that have an epithelioid morphology that can grow in a diffuse pleural distribution and resemble mesothelioma. These are composed of endothelial cells that have an epithelioid morphology and are referred to as *pseudomesotheliomatous epithelioid hemangio-endotheliomas*. The neoplastic cells are round or polygonal and can express keratin. They typically do not show markers for mesothelioma, such as calretinin. They express endothelial markers such as CD31 and Factor VIII. Ultrastructurally, the tumor cells may contain Weibel–Palade bodies in their cytoplasm.

7.13.12 Thymoma/Thymic Carcinoma, Melanoma, and Lymphoma versus Mesothelioma

Finally, there are other tumors that can occasionally cause problems with respect to diagnosis such as thymoma/thymic carcinomas, melanomas, and lymphomas. Most of these are fairly easy to differentiate from a mesothelioma, but one has to be aware of these other entities. Thymomas occasionally affect the pleura as a result of spread into the pleura from an anterior mediastinal thymoma[192] or as primary pleural thymomas.[193–197]

The main histological feature distinguishing lymphocyte-rich thymoma from lymphohistiocytoid mesothelioma is a subdivision of the thymoma by bands of fibrocollagenous tissue producing a lobulated architecture.

Rare cases of thymic carcinoma also exist. As reported by Attanoos et al.,[193,198] thymic epithelial cancers can show variable expression of CK5/6 and thrombomodulin. They generally do not show nuclear immunostaining for calretinin.

7.14 PATHOLOGICAL STAGING OF MESOTHELIOMA, TREATMENT, AND PROGNOSIS

In 2010, the American Joint Committee on Cancer published the seventh edition of the *Cancer Staging Manual*.[199] The TNM staging system for pleural mesothelioma is shown in Tables 7.9 and 7.10.

Historically, patients with malignant pleural mesothelioma who have potentially resectable disease have been treated with surgery, chemotherapy, and radiation.[200] With improvements in systemic and intrapleural treatment options, multimodality therapy has become more common. Systemic treatments largely consist of neoadjuvant chemotherapy with platinum doublets and, more recently, novel targeted agents such as dasatinib. Intrapleural strategies have included injection chemotherapy, chemotherapy with hyperthermic perfusion, gene therapy, and immunotherapy. Surgical treatment options include pleurectomy/decortication or extrapleural pneumonectomy. Adjuvant radiation therapy has been the only proven treatment modality that assists in preventing local–regional recurrence of mesothelioma after surgical resection. Investigation into the use of intraoperative radiation therapy and intensity-modulated radiation therapy in mesothelioma after extrapleural pneumonectomy (EPP) has been done, although high-dose intraoperative radiation therapy appears to be too toxic to administer after EPP and is largely no longer studied in this disease. However, the preliminary studies with intensity-modulated radiation therapy appear to be more promising with reports of an 87% local–regional disease control rate. The authors[200] stated additional clinical trials to define the optimal radiation therapy technique were needed. The use of neoadjuvant chemotherapy before surgery has become more common; however, it has not been shown to offer a survival

Table 7.9   TNM Staging/Clinical and Pathological Staging for Pleural Mesothelioma

	Primary Tumor (T)
TX	Primary tumor cannot be assessed
T0	No evidence of primary tumor
T1	Tumor limited to the ipsilateral parietal pleura with/without mediastinal pleura and with/without diaphragmatic pleural involvement
T1a	No involvement of the visceral pleura
T1b	Tumor involves the visceral pleura
T2	Tumor involving each of the ipsilateral pleural surfaces (parietal, mediastinal, diaphragmatic, and visceral pleura) with at least one of the following: • Involvement of diaphragmatic muscle • Extension of tumor from visceral pleura into the underlying pulmonary parenchyma
T3	Locally advanced but potentially resectable tumor Tumor involves all of the ipsilateral pleural surfaces (parietal, mediastinal, diaphragmatic, and visceral pleura) with at least one of the following: • Involvement of the endothoracic fascia • Extension into mediastinal fat • Solitary, completely resectable focus of tumor extending into/invading soft tissues of the chest wall • Nontransmural involvement of the pericardium
T4	Locally advanced, technically unresectable tumor Tumor involves all of the ipsilateral pleural surfaces with at least one of the following: • Diffuse extension/invasion or multifocal masses of tumor in the chest wall with or without associated rib destruction • Direct transdiaphragmatic extension/invasion of tumor to the peritoneum • Direct extension/invasion of tumor to the contralateral pleura • Direct extension/invasion of tumor to mediastinal organs • Direct extension/invasion of tumor into the spine • Tumor extending through the internal surface of the pericardium with or without a pericardial effusion; or tumor involving the myocardium
	Regional Lymph Nodes (N)
NX	Regional lymph nodes cannot be assessed
N0	No regional lymph node metastases
N1	Metastases in the ipsilateral bronchopulmonary or hilar lymph nodes
N2	Metastases in the subcarinal or ipsilateral mediastinal lymph nodes, including the ipsilateral internal mammary and peridiaphragmatic nodes
N3	Metastases in the contralateral mediastinal, contralateral internal mammary, and ipsilateral or contralateral supraclavicular lymph nodes
	Distant Metastasis (M)
M0 (clinical only)	No distant metastasis (no pathological M0; use clinical M to complete stage group)
M1	Distant metastasis

benefit. Chemotherapy agents typically used consist of cisplatin with pemetrexed (Alimta) and cisplatin with gemcitabine. Intrapleural chemotherapy has also been undertaken. Additional therapies include intrapleural gene therapy, intrapleural immunotherapy, adjuvant photodynamic therapy, and intrapleural chemotherapy plus intrapleural radiation therapy.[200]

Yan et al.[201] performed a systemic review on the efficacy of cytoreductive surgery combined with perioperative intraperitoneal chemotherapy for diffuse malignant peritoneal mesothelioma. The length of survival was dependent upon the aggressive versus indolent biologic behavior of the neoplasm. The authors[201] found that the median survival ranged from 34 to 92 months; 60%–88% survived 1 year, 43%–65% had a 3-year survival, and 29%–59% had a 5-year survival. The perioperative morbidity varied from 25% to 40% and mortality ranged from 0% to 8%. This study[201]

Table 7.10 Anatomic Stage—Prognostic Grouping for Pleural Mesothelioma

Group	T	N	M .
Stage I	T1	N0	M0
Stage IA	T1a	N0	M0
Stage IB	T1b	N0	M0
Stage II	T2	N0	M0
Stage III	T1, T2	N1	M0
	T1, T2	N2	M0
	T3	N0, N1, N2	M0
Stage IV	T4	Any N	M0
	Any T	N3	M0
	Any T	Any N	M1

was stated to demonstrate an improved overall survival as compared with historical controls using systemic chemotherapy and palliative surgery for malignant peritoneal mesothelioma.

Christensen et al.[202] stated they studied the relationship between asbestos exposure and survival outcome in malignant pleural mesothelioma in an effort to advance the understanding of the contribution of asbestos exposure to prognosis in those diagnosed with malignant pleural mesothelioma. The authors[202] studied cases of MPM patients enrolled through the International Mesothelioma Program at Brigham and Women's Hospital in Boston, Massachusetts. They used survival follow-up, self-reported asbestos exposure ($n = 128$), and a subset of cases ($n = 80$) with quantitative asbestos fiber burden measures. They found independent, significant associations between male sex and reduced survival ($p < .04$) and between nonepithelioid tumor histology and reduced survival ($p < .02$). After adjusting for covariates in a Cox model, the authors found that patients with low asbestos burden (0–99 asbestos bodies per gram wet weight) had a threefold elevated risk of death compared with patients with a moderate fiber burden (100–1099 asbestos bodies per gram wet weight). Patients with a high fiber burden (>1099 asbestos bodies per gram wet weight) had a 4.8-fold elevated risk of death versus those with moderate exposure. The authors[202] concluded that patient survival was associated with asbestos fiber burden and was perhaps modified by susceptibility.

Expected survival for those diagnosed with malignant mesothelioma is 1.4 to 13.9 months. Independent predictors of reduced survival include three or more of the following:

- Age 75 years or older
- Performance status of 1 or 2
- Nonepithelial histology or sarcomatoid subtype
- Pleural involvement
- Chest pain
- Platelet count greater than 400,000 per microliter
- WBC greater than 15,600 per microliter
- Lactate dehydrogenase greater than 500 IU/L

Independent predictors of increased survival include the following:

- Age 49 years or younger
- Performance status of 0
- Hemoglobin of 14.6 g/dL

7.15 RELATIONSHIP BETWEEN ASBESTOS AND THE DEVELOPMENT OF MESOTHELIOMA

7.15.1 Target Organs

The target organs in mesothelioma are the serosal membranes of the body cavities, specifically the pleura, the peritoneum, and the pericardium. The tunica vaginalis is an invagination of the peritoneum and therefore is classified as a peritoneal epithelioid mesothelioma.

It is generally thought that in the case of carcinogens causing cancer, what is important is the concentration of that carcinogen (i.e., asbestos) at the site where the tumor develops (e.g., pleura for pleural mesotheliomas, peritoneum for peritoneal mesotheliomas, and pericardium for pericardial mesotheliomas).

The exact amount of asbestos it takes to cause a mesothelioma in a certain location is unknown. The sequence of the molecular changes that eventually cause the formation of a single cancer cell is not totally understood, but there is overwhelming evidence that mutations in genes such as proto-oncogenes, tumor suppressor genes, DNA repair genes, and changes in the cell cycle and cell membrane receptors are part of the changes that occur in the development of a cancer such as mesothelioma.[203]

7.15.2 Dose–Response Relationship

There is abundant information in this book concerning the development of mesothelioma. In general, mesothelioma is a disease that has a dose–response relationship, which means that, with respect to asbestos, the greater the exposure to asbestos and the greater the inhalation of asbestos is into the lungs and body cavities, the greater the risk of an individual developing mesothelioma, although most persons exposed to asbestos will not develop an asbestos-related disease, perhaps with the exception of asbestosis and the occupation of insulators. The published information indicates it takes significantly less asbestos to cause mesothelioma than it does to cause lung cancer and asbestosis.

7.15.3 Concentration

The concentration of asbestos that is associated with asbestos-induced diseases such as mesothelioma, lung cancer, and asbestosis is variable, and there is no absolute concentration anyone can cite with respect to how much it takes for an individual person to develop an asbestos-related disease such as mesothelioma. The idea that there is individual susceptibility or genetic susceptibility seems reasonable on the basis of the evidence available.

With respect to what asbestos exposure causes mesothelioma, it is safe to say it is the injuries that occur as a result of exposure to asbestos that causes the development of a neoplasm. Obviously, with the information available that even people exposed to large amounts of asbestos such as insulators, only a relatively small percentage of them will develop mesothelioma, although at autopsy one can find very high concentrations of amphiboles and chrysotile asbestos in all insulators. In most instances, asbestos-related mesotheliomas develop in conditions in which there is a mixed exposure to amphiboles and chrysotile asbestos.

The factors involved as to whether one develops a mesothelioma include the dose a person is exposed to and an individual's susceptibility to the tumorigenic effect of asbestos. The study by Dodson et al.[204] concerning asbestos fiber types and concentrations in 55 cases of mesothelioma strongly indicates there is a wide range of concentrations of asbestos that one finds in the lungs of individuals who are exposed to asbestos and who develop mesothelioma. The range in our study was from 22,096 to 68,950,000, with the mean being approximately 4,500,000 and the median being approximately 694,444.

I (S.P.H.) do not believe every asbestos fiber an individual breathes into their lungs contributes to the development of mesothelioma. It is my opinion that when a person is exposed to asbestos fibers that are released into the air they breathe in an occupational or bystander setting, a certain number of fibers are deposited in the lungs, usually in the region of the respiratory bronchial and the alveolar duct. These asbestos fibers may stay in the lung or may translocate to other parts of the body. The mechanism by which they are translocated probably includes lymphatic transport, vascular transport, and possibly other methods of transport. With respect to what happens in pleural and peritoneal mesotheliomas, it is my opinion that a certain number of asbestos fibers translocate to the pleura and peritoneum where they have the ability to cause inflammatory/genetoxic injury that, over a significant amount of time (usually many years), damage many cells that form the serosal membrane and eventually form a cancer cell(s) that undergo clonal proliferation to produce a tumor mass that, when it becomes extensive enough, will cause symptoms in a patient due to physiological changes in the body.

The number fibers that are involved in causing the cellular changes that lead to the development of mesothelioma is unknown. Scientists have discovered that there are a number of mutations in mesothelial cancer cells in persons who died from mesothelioma.[205] It is not possible to retrospectively tell exactly at what point in time the cellular changes occurred that resulted in the development of a single cancer cell that underwent a clonal proliferation.

With respect to exposures that cause mesothelioma, it is my opinion the exposures are those that resulted from occupational exposure and/or bystander exposure, which are usually thousands to millions/billions times greater than what one would see in an exposure to asbestos in the ambient air in which there had not been any release of fibers from an asbestos-containing product.

It is not possible to specifically identify an individual fiber from the individual's occupational or bystander exposure that caused the cellular events that led to the development of mesothelioma. However, on the other hand, it is not possible for anyone to exclude the possibility these fibers did not contribute to cause the injury that led to the development of the mesothelioma.

If it was scientifically possible to determine exactly which fibers caused the injury, which exposure they came from, and how they contributed to the development of a mesothelioma over what period of time, then it might be possible to specifically state whether a certain asbestos-containing product a person was exposed to in an occupational or bystander setting was or was not a contributing factor in causing the mesothelioma. At this point in time, it is not possible to do that.

7.15.4 Genetic Susceptibility

In the article published in 2008 by Neri et al.,[206] the authors stated that many studies in the last decade have shown that polymorphism in the genes involved in xenobiotic and oxidative metabolism or in DNA repair processes might play an important role in the etiology and pathogenesis of malignant pleural mesothelioma, lung cancer, and other nonneoplastic conditions, including asbestosis and pleural plaques. The authors[206] stated the most commonly studied *GSTM1* polymorphism showed for all asbestos-related diseases, there was an increased risk in association with the null genotype, possibly linked to its role in the conjugation of reactive oxygen species. The authors[206] stated that the studies focused on *GSTT1* null and *SOD2 Ala16Val* polymorphisms gave conflicting results, whereas promising results came from studies on alpha-1 antitrypsin in asbestosis and *MPO* in lung cancer. Among genetic polymorphisms associated to the risk of malignant pleural mesothelioma, the *GSTM1* null genotype and two variant alleles of *XRCC1* and *XRCC3* showed increased risks in a subset of studies. Results for the *NAT2* acetylator status, *SOD2* polymorphism, and *EPHX* activity were conflicting. The authors stated the major limitations in the study design, including the small size of the study groups, affected the reliability of these studies. Technical improvements such as the use of high-throughput techniques would help to identify molecular pathways regulated by candidate genes.

7.15.5 Attribution

With respect to attribution of causation in mesothelioma, it is worthwhile to remember the points made in the Helsinki Consensus Report,[207] which were as follows:

- Malignant mesothelioma can be induced by all asbestos types (chrysotile, amphiboles) with amphiboles showing greater carcinogenic potency than chrysotile;
- A lung fiber count exceeding the background range for the laboratory in question, or the presence of radiographic or pathological evidence of asbestos-related tissue injury (e.g., asbestosis or pleural plaques), or histopathologic evidence of abnormal asbestos content (e.g., asbestos bodies in histological sections of lung) should be sufficient to relate a case of pleural or peritoneal mesothelioma to asbestos exposure on a probability basis; and
- In the absence of such markers, a history of significant occupational, domestic, or environmental exposure to asbestos will suffice for attribution.

There is evidence that peritoneal mesotheliomas are associated with higher levels of asbestos exposure than pleural mesotheliomas, but even this is not absolute.[208] For example, the concentration of asbestos in lung tissue in patients with peritoneal mesothelioma reported by Oury et al.[209] showed a significant difference in concentrations from one case to another. Likewise, in the publication by Dodson et al.,[205] which included five peritoneal mesotheliomas, there was significant variation in the concentration of asbestos in lung tissue from such persons. The publication by Welch et al.,[210] which was a case–control epidemiology study, showed cases of peritoneal mesothelioma associated with low-level exposure to asbestos.

From another perspective, specifically the study Dodson and I performed on omentum and mesenteric tissue in patients with mesothelioma,[211] we found that the type of asbestos found in the omentum and mesentery was the same as that found in the lung, but, in contrast, the concentration found in the omentum and mesentery was very low compared with that found in the lung. If the amount of asbestos found in the omentum and mesentery is what it takes to cause peritoneal mesothelioma, then one could say it takes very little asbestos to cause mesothelioma.

In some circumstances, exposures such as those occurring among household members may approach occupational levels.[212–214]

The question is unresolved as to whether or not a case of mesothelioma in which the lung fiber count falls within the range recorded for unexposed urban dwellers is caused by asbestos. More information is needed regarding the interpretation of fiber burdens in the pleura or samples of tumor tissue before these measures can be used for the purpose of attribution.

The Helsinki Consensus Report[207] suggested that the following points needed to be considered in the assessment of occupational etiology:

- A great majority of mesotheliomas are due to asbestos exposure.
- Mesothelioma can occur in cases with low asbestos exposure. However, very low background environmental exposure carries an extremely low risk.
- Approximately 80% of mesothelioma patients had some occupational exposure to asbestos, and therefore a careful occupational and environmental history should be obtained.
- An occupational history of brief or low-level exposure should be considered sufficient for mesothelioma to be designated as occupationally related.
- A minimum of 10 years from the first exposure is required to attribute mesothelioma to asbestos exposure, although in most cases the latency interval is longer (e.g., on the order of 30–40 years).

7.15.6 Environmental

There is published evidence that a background/ambient level of asbestos exposure exists in the environment that is sufficient to cause mesothelioma.[215–221]

For example, in a study[215] carried out in the city of Shuba El-Kheima in greater Cairo concerning asbestos and the exposure–response relationship with mesothelioma, the study evaluated the prevalence of malignant pleural mesothelioma due to occupational and environmental (nonoccupational) exposure to asbestos among persons who worked in a chrysotile concrete-producing plant and in persons living in an area nearby the plant. Eighty-eight cases of mesothelioma were diagnosed, 87 in the exposed group. The risk of mesothelioma was stated to be higher in the environmentally exposed group than in other groups and was higher in females than males. The prevalence of mesothelioma increased with increased cumulative exposure to asbestos.

Pan et al.[216] conducted a case–control study of residential proximity to naturally occurring asbestos with malignant mesothelioma in California. The study included 2354 men and 554 women diagnosed with malignant mesothelioma who were reported to the California Cancer Registry between 1988 and 1997. These were matched to control subjects with pancreatic cancer. Age-adjusted logistic regression analysis showed that occupations with a high probability of occupational exposure to asbestos in men such as boilermaker, insulator, plumber, pipefitter, steamfitter, sheet metal worker, electrician, and painter were strongly associated with mesothelioma risk, whereas few female cases and control subjects had occupations with a high probability of occupational asbestos exposure. Among all subjects, the odds ratio (OR) for mesothelioma for a 10-km increase in nearest distance was 0.943 (95% confidence interval [CI] = 0.895–0.922). The authors[216] found that residential proximity to naturally occurring asbestos showed an independent and dose–response association with mesothelioma risk. The authors[216] stated that their findings were biologically plausible in view of the known strong association between occupational asbestos exposure and mesothelioma and the observation of an association between naturally occurring asbestos and mesothelioma in other areas of the world.

In a report published by the Health and Safety Executive in March 2009, Peto et al.[218] stated that asbestos exposure was common in the workplace, with 65% of male and 23% of female controls having worked in occupations that were classified as medium or high risk. The increase in female cases in the United Kingdom, many with no identifiable exposure to asbestos, suggested widespread environmental contamination from industrial and construction activities.

Rake et al.,[219] in another case–control study of occupational, domestic, and environmental mesothelioma risk in the British population, stated that the cumulative female mesothelioma death rate by age 70 was more than three times higher in the United Kingdom (0.037%) than that in the United States (0.012%). The authors[219] stated that if this was due to differences in asbestos exposure, more than two-thirds of mesotheliomas in British women born since the 1930s were caused by asbestos, far more than the 38% that were attributed to identifiable exposures to asbestos in their study. A similar conclusion was suggested by the threefold increase in the death rate in British women between 1975–1979 and 2000–2004. The authors[219] stated this implied that at least 30% of female cases (around 100 per year) were caused by environmental asbestos exposure or by occasional or ambient exposure in occupational settings classified as low risk. If so, there would presumably be a similar number in men. The authors[219] stated that many apparently spontaneous mesotheliomas were therefore likely to be due to an increase in ambient asbestos exposure that coincided with the widespread occupational exposures of the 1960s and 1970s.

A report by Maule et al.[220] of environmental asbestos exposure and mesothelioma risk in association with high levels of asbestos pollution from an asbestos cement factory around Casale Monferrato, Italy, stated their study provided strong evidence that asbestos pollution from an industrial source greatly increased mesothelioma risk. Furthermore, the authors[220] stated that the relative risk from occupational exposure was underestimated and was markedly increased when adjusted for residential distance.

Kurumatani and Kumagai[221] investigated the magnitude of the risk among residents with no occupational exposure to asbestos and who lived within a 300-m radius of a former large asbestos cement pipe plant in Amagasaki, Japan, where crocidolite and chrysotile asbestos were used. The authors[221] stated there were 73 mesothelioma deaths (35 men and 38 women) identified with no occupational exposure to asbestos. The standardized mortality ratio (SMR) of mesothelioma was 13.9 (95% CI = 5.6–28.7) for men and 41.1 (95% CI = 15.2–90.1) for women. When the study area was divided into five regions by relative asbestos concentration, the SMR of mesothelioma declined for both sexes in a linear dose-dependent manner with concentration. The regions with a significant elevated SMR reached 2200 m from the plant in the same direction in which the wind predominantly blew. The authors[221] concluded neighborhood exposure to asbestos can pose a serious risk to residents across a wide area.

7.15.7 Background

Because of the extensive and longstanding use of asbestos, the ambient air in the United States contains minute amounts of asbestos. These ambient air concentrations are generally known as the "background level" and have been reported in United States cities to range from 0.00005 to 0.00023 fibers/cc, which is tens of thousands of times less than the current permissible exposure limit of 0.1 fibers/cc established in 1994.[222]

It is my opinion that *background* is a vague term that has not been well defined. Asbestos concentrations in the air that have been evaluated show a significant degree of variation. How one defines background is going to be arbitrary as it pertains to determining whether a certain background concentration is capable of causing mesothelioma. For example, if one assumes the air that was breathed in the Northwest Cape Provence of South Africa in the 1950s and 1960s was a background concentration, then there were definite cases of mesothelioma that occurred from that exposure. Likewise, if one concludes the background exposure to asbestos in Libby, Montana, from tremolite/Libby amphibole containing vermiculite material was background, then there were definite cases of mesothelioma occurring in that background situation. Likewise, if one agrees that the concentration of air in the Wittenoom Mine area in the 1940s–1950s was background, then there were a significant number of cases of mesothelioma that resulted from that exposure.

7.15.8 Low-Level Exposure

In 1999, Hillerdal[223] acknowledged that amphiboles were more tumorigenic in causing mesothelioma than chrysotile. Hillerdal[223] reported several cases of low-level exposure to asbestos and the development of mesothelioma and stated: "There is no proof of a threshold value—that is, a minimal lower limit below which asbestos fibers cannot cause the tumour—and thus it is plausible that even such low exposure can cause mesothelioma (even if the risk is extremely low)."

In a case–control study by Iwatsubo et al.[224] in 1998, the authors found an excess of pleural mesothelioma in the lowest exposure group with an estimated total exposure between 0.001 and 0.49 fibers/mL-years. The study included 405 cases and 387 controls. Twenty-three percent (23%) of the cases and 35% of the controls had been exposed to less than 0.5 fibers/mL-years. A gradient was observed with the cumulative exposure index (CEI). The OR rose from 1.2 (95% CI = 0.8 to 1.8) for the lowest exposure category (<0.5 fibers/mL-years) to 8.7 (95% CI = 4.1–18.5) for the highest category (more than 10 fibers/mL-years). Among women, the OR for possible or definite exposure was 18.8 (95% CI = 4.1–86.2). The results concerning the time-related pattern of exposure revealed a significantly elevated OR among workers whose exposure to asbestos was intermittent (OR = 1.8, 95% CI = 1.3–2.6). The OR was much greater, however, for continuous exposure (OR = 5.7, 95%

CI = 3.4–9.7). The median CEI within each category (<0.5, 0.5–0.99, 1–9.99, and ≥10 fibers/mL-years) was similar among intermittent and continuous exposure cases, except in the highest class of CEI (≥10 fibers/mL-years) where it was 0.1, 0.65, 3.5, and 38.7 fibers/mL-years for the intermittent exposure groups and 0.075, 0.65, 3.1, and 71.3 fibers/mL-years for the continuous groups, respectively. Iwatsubo et al.[224] stated their results indicated that mesothelioma cases occurred below a cumulative exposure of 5 fibers/mL-years and perhaps less than 0.5 fibers/mL-years. They could not examine mesothelioma risk according to fiber type because their study design (i.e., case–control study in a general population) did not allow them to identify those subjects whose exposure was only to chrysotile fibers. The authors[224] concluded they found a clear dose–response relationship between cumulative exposure to asbestos and pleural mesothelioma in a population-based case–control study with retrospective assessment of exposure. A significant excess of mesothelioma was observed for levels of cumulative exposure that were probably far below the limits adopted in many industrial countries during the 1980s.

Rödelsperger et al.[225] concluded there was a distinct dose–response relationship, even at extremely low levels of asbestos exposure, with exposures from >0 to <0.15 fibers/cc-yrs showing a significantly increased risk of mesothelioma. Rödelsperger et al.[225] stated: "In addition to asbestos exposure at the workplace, contact in the household and environmental exposure to asbestos are established causes of diffuse malignant mesothelioma. ... It has been demonstrated that the time since initial exposure and the type of asbestos are important for the quantification of the risk .... Nevertheless, it has recently been demonstrated that an increase of risk may occur even below a cumulative exposure of a few fiber years (fibers/ml × years) .... This is true although the amphibole fibers in the lung tissue do not seem to be a good indicator of the fiber content of the pleura, where chrysotile fibers are predominantly observed .... The original aim of this study was to investigate not only asbestos, but also man-made vitreous fibers and other inorganic fibers as causal factors of the diffuse malignant mesothelioma."

In an abstract presented at the International Mesothelioma Interest Group Meeting, Rolland et al.[226] evaluated the risk of pleural mesothelioma in a French population-based case–control study between 1998 and 2002. The authors[226] studied 19 French districts within the National Mesothelioma Surveillance Program covering 25% of the French population. The report was based on 467 confirmed cases (80% men, 41–93 years old) and 868 controls matched for sex, age, and district. The authors[226] found that among men, the highest risk was observed for the occupations of plumbers, pipefitters, and sheet metal workers and for the industries of ship repair, asbestos products, metal products, and construction. The authors[226] stated that a significant dose–response relationship was found between cumulative occupational asbestos exposure and pleural mesothelioma, even for the lowest category (greater than 0–0.07 fibers/mL-years; OR = 2.8, 95% CI = 1.7–4.7).

The Environmental Health Criteria 203 report concerning chrysotile asbestos stated: "exposure to chrysotile asbestos poses increased risk for asbestosis, lung cancer, and mesothelioma in a dose-dependent manner. No threshold has been identified for carcinogenic risk."[227]

In the article by Hodgson and Darnton,[228] there is extrapolation information with regard to crocidolite that at 0.01 fibers/mL-years, there are 20 deaths per 100,000 exposed with the highest arguable estimate 100 and the lowest two cases. Even at the lowest estimate of two cases per 100,000 exposed, this would be in excess of 20 times that which is considered to be the background level for mesothelioma development, which is approximately one to two cases per million people per year.

With respect to amosite, at a level of cumulative exposure of 0.01 fibers/mL-years, the estimate is 3 deaths per 100,000 exposed, with the highest arguable estimate 20 and the lowest insignificant.[228]

For chrysotile, the risk for development of mesothelioma at 0.01 fibers/mL-years was stated to be probably insignificant, although the highest arguable estimate was 1 death per 100,000 exposed, which would still be 10 times that of background.[228]

Hodgson and Darnton[228] stated: "Taking this evidence together, we do not believe there is a good case for assuming any threshold for mesothelioma risk."

In an update by Hodgson and Darnton[229] in 2009 concerning mesothelioma risk from chrysotile asbestos, the authors[229] stated that the risk of mesothelioma caused by chrysotile derived from these data was higher by a factor of 10 than that which emerged from their meta-analysis. The authors[229] stated these new results strengthened the case for the proposition that the per-fiber risk of mesothelioma from chrysotile textile plants was greater than it was in the mines. Whether this applied to other settings was stated to be unclear.

With respect to mixed exposures, Dr. Andrew Darnton was contacted via e-mail by Mr. Jim Watson on February 15, 2006. Dr. Darnton replied: "To use our model to predict risk for a single exposure episode you need a cumulative exposure (i.e. exposure concentration × time), the type of asbestos and the age." Dr. Darnton stated: "We have not at this point developed a method to extend the model to estimate risks for multiple exposures to different mixes of asbestos type across extended periods." Since most occupational exposures to asbestos are mixed exposures, it would appear to be difficult to apportion a certain contribution of mesothelioma to a certain exposure in a person who had mixed exposure unless there was very precise information available.

The current permissible exposure limit (PEL) is 0.1 fibers/cc-years (effective in 1994). It should be recognized that these data are based on the National Institute for Occupational Safety and Health (NIOSH) 7400 method. The findings are recognized as very conservative regarding the actual numbers of aerosol/potentially respirable asbestos fibers in many environments in that the fibers are too short (<5 µm) to be included in the count scheme or too thin to be detected by light microscopy. The studies referred to above provide evidence that there can be an increased incidence of mesothelioma at concentrations lower than 0.1 fibers/cc-years. As stated in the *Federal Register* in 1986,[230] even at that concentration there was an excess of seven cases per 100,000 people exposed. The 1986 *Federal Register* also pointed out that at that level there would be cases of mesothelioma. Therefore, the lowest concentration of asbestos that can produce mesothelioma is currently unknown.

Several agencies have commented that there is no safe level of exposure to asbestos:

- NIOSH, 1976: "excessive cancer risks have been demonstrated at all fiber concentrations studied to date. Evaluation of all available human data provides no evidence for a threshold or a 'safe' level of asbestos exposure."
- NIOSH, 1980: "All levels of asbestos exposure studied to date have demonstrated asbestos related disease ... there is no level of exposure below which clinical effects do not occur."
- USPHS, 1980: "It is important to point out that when a permissible level for exposure (PEL) to a certain carcinogen is set by OSHA, there is no implication that such a level is safe. To the contrary, it is the agency's policy that any occupational exposure to a carcinogen carries with it some risk of disease, even if it cannot be easily or precisely measured."
- NIOSH, 1986: "a linear, no threshold, dose–response relationship. ... Any asbestos exposure carries with it some increased risk of asbestos related disease."
- OSHA, 1994: "reducing exposure to 0.1 fibers/cc would further reduce, but not eliminate, significant risk. The 0.1-fiber/cc level leaves a remaining significant risk."
- WHO, 1998: "Exposure to chrysotile asbestos poses increased risks for asbestosis, lung cancer and mesothelioma in a dose-dependent manner. No threshold has been identified for carcinogenic risks."
- WTO, 2000: "... the experts confirm the position of the European Communities according to which it has not been possible to identify any threshold below which exposure to chrysotile would have no effect. The experts also agree that the linear relationship model, which does not identify any minimum exposure threshold, is appropriate for assessing the existence of a risk. We find therefore that

no minimum threshold level of exposure or duration of exposure has been identified with regard to the risk of pathologies associated with chrysotile, except for asbestosis."

7.16 SUMMARY

There is a dose–response relationship between the amount of asbestos to which an individual is exposed and the risk of developing mesothelioma. I believe this concept is accepted in the medical and scientific communities. The greater the exposure to asbestos or inhalation of asbestos, the greater the risk is of developing mesothelioma.

There is evidence that there is genetic susceptibility to malignant pleural mesothelioma and other asbestos-associated diseases.

There is published evidence that a background/ambient level of asbestos exists in the environment that is sufficient to cause mesothelioma. With respect to background concentrations, it is my opinion that "background" is a vague term that has not been well defined.

In my opinion, an exposure of 0.1 fibers/cc-years within the latency period is a sufficient exposure to cause mesothelioma. Latency in this context means that one would ordinarily not expect to see a mesothelioma until at least 15 years after exposure. There is a steep gradient of increased risk for mesothelioma above the cumulative exposure level of 0.1 fibers/cc-years. In other words, once an individual has had that level of exposure to a particular asbestos-containing product or class of products, the incidence of mesothelioma rises significantly with additional exposures, even if the exposure was less than 0.1 fibers/cc-years.

I and many other scientists in the field of asbestos disease agree with the following statement by Dr. Douglas Henderson, a well-known expert in asbestos-related disease:

> When one is faced with multiple exposures to asbestos, the following points emerge, specifically for mesothelioma induction, provided that the characteristics and time for each exposure are appropriate for a biological effect: (i) it is not valid to point to one exposure among the others and incriminate it as the sole cause of a mesothelioma, with exoneration of the other exposures; (ii) it is not valid to point to one exposure among the others and exonerate it from a causative role in the development of a mesothelioma, and to incriminate all the others; (iii) when there are multiple episodes of exposure as a background to mesothelioma, it is often the case that each exposure in isolation would be sufficient for attribution of the mesothelioma to asbestos. … In such circumstances, it is not the presence or absence of an effect that is in question, but the magnitude of each effect in proportion to the others.

REFERENCES

1. Ordóñez NG, Myhre M, Mackay B. Clear cell mesothelioma. *Ultrastruct Pathol* 1996;20:331–336.
2. Talerman A, Chilcote RR, Montero JR, et al. Diffuse malignant peritoneal mesothelioma in a 13-year-old girl. *Am J Surg Pathol* 1985;9:73–80.
3. Galateau-Sallé F, ed. International mesothelioma panel: Brambilla E, Cagle PT, Churg AM, et al. *Pathology of Malignant Mesothelioma*. London: Springer; 2006.
4. Henderson DW, Rodelsperger K, Woitowitz H-J, et al. After Helsinki: A multidisciplinary review of the relationship between asbestos exposure and lung cancer, with emphasis on studies published during 1997–2004. *Pathology* 2004;36:517–550.
5. Henderson DW, Shilkin KB, Whitaker D, et al. The pathology of mesothelioma, including immunohistology and ultrastructure. In: *Malignant Mesothelioma*, Henderson DW, Shilkin KB, Langlois SL, Whitaker D, eds. New York: Hemisphere; 1992: 69–139.
6. Churg A, Cagle PT, Roggli VL. *Tumors of the Serosal Membranes*. Washington DC: American Registry of Pathology/Armed Forces Institute of Pathology; 2006.

7. Roggli VL, Kolbeck J, Sanfilippo F, et al. Pathology of human mesothelioma: Etiologic and diagnostic considerations. *Pathol Annu* 1987;22:91–131.

8. Bégueret H, Galateau-Sallé F, Guillou L, et al. Primary intrathoracic synovial sarcoma: A clinicopathologic study of 40 t(X:18)-positive cases from the French Sarcoma Group and the Mesopath Group. *Am J Surg Pathol* 2005;29:339–346.

9. Bolen JW, Hammar SP, McNutt MA. Reactive and neoplastic serosal tissue: A light-microscpic, ultrastructural and immunocytochemical study. *Am J Surg Pathol* 1986;10:34–47.

10. Dardick I, Al-Jabi M, McCaughey WTE, et al. Ultrastructure of poorly differentiated diffuse epithelial mesotheliomas. *Ultrastruct Pathol* 1984;7:151–160.

11. Hammar SP, Bockus DE, Remington FL, Rohrbach KA. Mucin-positive epithelial mesotheliomas: A histochemical, immunohistochemical and ultrastructural comparison with mucin-producing pulmonary adenocarcinomas. *Ultrastruct Pathol* 1996;20:293–325.

12. Husain AN, Colby TV, Ordóñez NG, et al. Guidelines for pathologic diagnosis of malignant mesothelioma: a consensus statement from the International Mesothelioma Interest Group. *Arch Pathol Lab Med* 2009;133:1317–1331.

13. Hammar SP. Mesothelioma. In: *Practical Pulmonary Pathology*, Sheppard MN, ed. Boston: Little, Brown and Edward Arnold; 1995: 264–288.

14. Suzuki Y, Churg J, Kannerstein M. Ultrastructure of human malignant diffuse mesothelioma. *Am J Pathol* 1976;85:241–262.

15. Klima M, Bossart MI. Sarcomatous type of malignant mesothelioma. *Ultrastruct Pathol* 1983;4:349–358.

16. Croonen AM, van der Valk P, Herman CJ, Lindeman J. Cytology, immunopathology and flow cytometry in the diagnosis of pleural and peritoneal effusions. *Lab Invest* 1988;10:725–732.

17. Hafiz MA, Becker RL Jr, Mikel UV, Bahr GF. Cytophotometric determination of DNA in mesotheliomas and reactive mesothelial cells. *Anal Quant Cytol Histol* 1988;58:120–126.

18. Frierson HF, Mills SE, Legier JF. Flow cytometric analysis of ploidy in immunohistochemically confirmed examples of malignant mesothelioma. *Am J Clin Pathol* 1988;90:240–243.

19. Burmer GC, Rabinovitch PS, Kulander BG, Rusch V, McNutt MA. Flow cytometric analysis of malignant pleural mesothelioma: Relationship to histology and survival. *Hum Pathol* 1989;20:777–783.

20. Dazzi H, Thatcher N, Hasleton PS, Chatterjee AK, Lawson AM. DNA analysis by flow cytometry in malignant pleural mesothelioma: Relationship to histology and survival. *J Pathol* 1990;162:51–55.

21. Tierney G, Wilkinson MJ, Jones JSP. The malignancy grading method is not a reliable assessment of malignancy in mesothelioma. *J Pathol* 1990;160:209–211.

22. El-Nagar AK, Ordonez NG, Garnsey L, Batsakis JG. Epithelioid pleural mesotheliomas and pulmonary adenocarcinomas: A comparative DNA flow cytometric study. *Hum Pathol* 1991;22:972–978.

23. Esteban JM, Sheibani K. DNA ploidy analysis of pleural mesotheliomas: Its usefulness for their distinction from lung adenocarcinomas. *Mod Pathol* 1992;6:626–630.

24. Cakir C, Gulluoglu MG, Yilmazbayhan D. Cell proliferation rate and telomerase activity in the differential diagnosis between benign and malignant mesothelial proliferations. *Pathology* 2006;38:10–15.

25. Kim BS, Varkey B, Choi H. Diagnosis of malignant pleural mesothelioma by axillary lymph node biopsy. *Chest* 1987;91:278–281.

26. Sussman J, Rosai J. Lymph node metastasis as the initial manifestation of malignant mesothelioma: Report of six cases. *Am J Surg Pathol* 1990;14:819–828.

27. Lloreta J, Serrano S. Pleural mesothelioma presenting as an axillary lymph node metastasis with anemone cell appearance. *Ultrastruct Pathol* 1994;18:293–298.

28. Wills EJ. Pleural mesothelioma with initial presentation as cervical lymphadenopathy. *Ultrastruct Pathol* 1995;19:389–394.

29. Henderson DW, Comin CE, Hammar SP, et al. Malignant mesothelioma of the pleura: Current surgical pathology. In: *Pathology of Lung Tumors*, Corrin B, ed. New York: Churchill Livingstone; 1997: 241–280.

30. Colby TV. Benign mesothelial cells in lymph node. *Adv Anat Pathol* 1999;6:41–48.

31. Sion-Vardy N, Diomin V, Benharroch D. Hyperplastic mesothelial cells in subpleural lymph nodes mimicking metastatic carcinoma. *Ann Diagn Pathol* 2004;8:373–374.

32. Walker AN, Mills SE. Surgical pathology of the tunica vaginalis testis and embryologically related mesothelium. *Pathol Annu* 1988;23;2:125–152.

33. Nogales FF, Isaac MA, Hardisson D, et al. Adenomatoid tumors of the uterus: An analysis of 60 cases. *Int J Gynecol Pathol* 2002;21:34–40.

34. Yeh CJ, Chuang WY, Chou HH, Jung SM, Hsueh S. Multiple extragenital adenomatoid tumors in the mesocolon and omentum: Case report. *APMIS* 2008;116:1016–1019.

35. Ordóñez NG. The diagnostic utility of immunohistochemistry in distinguishing between epithelioid mesotheliomas and squamous carcinomas of the lung: A comparative study. *Mod Pathol* 2006;19:417–428.

36. Ordóñez NG. Podoplanin: A novel diagnostic immunohistochemical marker. *Adv Anat Pathol* 2006;13:83–88.

37. Kaplan MA, Tazelaar HD, Hayashi T, et al. Adenomatoid tumors of the pleura. *Am J Surg Pathol* 1996;20:1219–1223.

38. Handra-Luca A, Couvelard A, Abd Alsamad I, et al. Adenomatoid tumor of the pleura. *Ann Pathol* 2000;20:369–372.

39. Kannerstein M, Churg J, McCaughey WTE, Hill DP. Papillary tumors of the peritoneum in women: Mesothelioma or papillary carcinoma. *Am J Obstet Gynecol* 1977;127:306–314.

40. Goepel JR. Benign papillary mesothelioma of peritoneum: A histological, histochemical and ultrastructural study of six cases. *Histopathology* 1981;5:21–30.

41. Burrig KF, Pfitzer P, Hort W. Well-differentiated papillary mesothelioma of the peritoneum: A borderline mesothelioma. Report of two cases and review of literature. *Virchows Arch A Pathol Anat Histopathol* 1990;417:443–447.

42. Daya D, McCaughey WT. Well-differentiated papillary mesothelioma of the peritoneum: A clinicopathologic study of 22 cases. *Cancer* 1990;65:292–296.

43. Lovell FA, Cranston PE. Well-differentiated papillary mesothelioma of the peritoneum. *AJR Am J Roentgenol* 1990;155:1245–1246.

44. Daya D, McCaughey WT. Pathology of the peritoneum: A review of selected topics. *Semin Diagn Pathol* 1991;8:277–289.

45. Lammer F, Scherrer C, Hacki WH. Well-differentiated papillary mesothelioma of the peritoneum: Rare, but prognostically important differential diagnosis. *Schweiz Med Wochenschr* 1991;121:954–956.

46. Bouvier S, Baron O, Nomballais F, et al. Well-differentiated papillary mesothelioma of the peritoneum: An attenuated malignant tumor—Review of the literature apropos of a case. *Bull Cancer* 1994;81:104–107.

47. Mangal R, Taskin O, Franklin R. An incidental diagnosis of well-differentiated papillary mesothelioma in a woman operated on for recurrent endometriosis. *Fertil Steril* 1995;63:196–197.

48. Hoekman K, Tognon G, Risse EK, et al. Well-differentiated papillary mesothelioma of the peritoneum: A separate entity. *Eur J Cancer* 1996;32A:255–258.

49. Shukunami K, Hirabuki S, Kaneshima M, et al. Well-differentiated papillary mesothelioma involving the peritoneal and pleural cavities: Successful treatment by local and systemic administration of carboplatin. *Tumori* 2000;86:419–421.

50. Butnor KJ, Sporn TA, Hammar SP, Roggli VL. Well-differentiated papillary mesothelioma. *Am J Surg Pathol* 2001;25:1304–1309.

51. Galateau-Sallé F, Vignaud JM, Burke L, et al. Well-differentiated papillary mesothelioma of the pleura: A series of 24 cases. *Am J Surg Pathol* 2004;28:534–540.

52. Sane AC, Roggli VL. Curative resection of a well-differentiated papillary mesothelioma of the pericardium. *Arch Pathol Lab Med* 1995;119:266–267.

53. Chetty R. Well differentiated (benign) papillary mesothelioma of the tunica vaginalis. *J Clin Pathol* 1992;45:1029–1030.

54. Battifora H, McCaughey WTE. Tumors of the serosal membranes. *Atlas of Tumor Pathology*. 3rd Series, Fascicle 15. Washington, DC: Armed Forces Institute of Pathology; 1995: 33, 50.

55. Hammar SP, Henderson DW, Klebe S. Dodson RF. Neoplasms of the pleura. In: *Dail and Hammar's Pulmonary Pathology*, 3rd ed., Tomashefski JF Jr, ed. New York: Springer; 2008: 642–648.

56. Mayall FG, Gibbs AR. The histology and immunohistochemistry of small cell mesothelioma. *Histopathology* 1992;20:47–51.

57. Falconieri G, Zanconati F, Bussani R, Di Bonito L. Small cell carcinoma of lung simulating pleural mesothelioma: Report of 4 cases with autopsy confirmation. *Pathol Res Pract* 1995;191:1147–1152.

58. Krismann M, Müller K-M, Jaworska M, Johnen G. Pathological anatomy and molecular pathology [of mesothelioma]. *Lung Cancer* 2004;45S:S29–S33.

59. Nascimento AG, Keeney GL, Fletcher CD. Deciduoid peritoneal mesothelioma. An unusual phenotype affecting young females. *Am J Surg Pathol* 1994;18:439–445.

60. Ordóñez NG. Epithelial mesothelioma with deciduoid features: Report of four cases. *Am J Surg Pathol* 2000;24:816–823.

61. Shanks JH, Harris M, Banerjee SS, et al. Mesotheliomas with deciduoid morphology: A morphologic spectrum and variant not confined to young females. *Am J Surg Pathol* 2000;24:285–294.

62. Serio G, Scattone A, Pennella A, et al. Malignant deciduoid mesothelioma of the pleura: Report of two cases with long survival. *Histopathology* 2002;40:348–352.

63. Shia J, Erlandson RA, Klimstra DS. Deciduoid mesothelioma: A report of 5 cases and literature review. *Ultrastruct Pathol* 2002;26:355–363.

64. Ernst CS, Atkinson BF. Mucicarmine positivity in malignant mesothelioma. *Lab Invest* 1980;42:113–114.

65. McCaughey WTE, Colby TV, Battifora H, et al. Diagnosis of diffuse malignant mesothelioma: Experience of a US/Canadian mesothelioma panel. *Mod Pathol* 1991;4:342–353.

66. Benjamin CJ, Ritchie AC. Histological staining for the diagnosis of mesothelioma. *Am J Med Technol* 1982;48:905–908.

67. MacDougall DB, Wang SE, Zibar BL. Mucin-positive epithelial mesothelioma. *Arch Pathol Lab Med* 1992;116:874–880.

68. Kannerstein M, Churg J. Desmoplastic diffuse malignant mesothelioma. In: *Progress in Surgical Pathology*, Fenoglio CM, Wolff M, eds. New York: Masson; 1980: 19–29.

69. Cantin R, Al-Jabi M, McCaughey WT. Desmoplastic diffuse mesothelioma. *Am J Surg Pathol* 1982;6:215–222.

70. Du Bray ES, Rosson FB. Primary mesothelioma of the pleura: A clinical and pathologic contribution to pleural malignancy, with report of a case. *Arch Intern Med* 1920;26:715–737.

71. Mangano WE, Cagle PT, Churg A, et al. The diagnosis of desmoplastic malignant mesothelioma and its distinction from fibrous pleurisy: A histologic and immunohistochemical analysis of 31 cases including p53 immunostaining. *Am J Clin Pathol* 1998;110:191–199.

72. Wilson GE, Hasleton PS, Chatterjee AK. Desmoplastic malignant mesothelioma: A review of 17 cases. *J Clin Pathol* 1992;45:295–298.

73. Battifora H, McCaughey WTE. Tumors of the serosal membranes. *Atlas of Tumor Pathology*, 3rd series, fascicle 15. Washington, DC: Armed Forces Institute of Pathology; 1995.

74. Machin T, Mashiyama ET, Henderson JAM, McCaughey WTE. Bony metastases in desmoplastic pleural mesothelioma. *Thorax* 1988;43:155–156.

75. Henderson DW, Attwood HD, Constance TJ, et al. Lymphohistiocytoid mesothelioma: a rare lymphomatoid variant of predominantly sarcomatoid mesothelioma. *Ultrastruct Pathol* 1988;12:367–384.

76. Khalidi HS, Medeiros LJ, Battifora H. Lymphohistiocytoid mesothelioma: An often misdiagnosed variant of sarcomatoid mesothelioma. *Am J Clin Pathol* 2000;113:649–654.

77. Yao DX, Shia J, Erlandson RA, Klimstra DS. Lymphohistiocytoid mesothelioma: A clinical, immunohistochemical and ultrastructural study of four cases and literature review. *Ultrastruct Pathol* 2004;28:213–228.

78. Dorfmüller P, Krismann M, Müller K-M. Mesotheliomas with leukocytic infiltration: Aspects of differential diagnosis. *Pathologe* 2004;25:349–355.

79. Robinson BW, Robinson C, Lake RA. Localised spontaneous regression in mesothelioma—Possible immunological mechanism. *Lung Cancer* 2001;32:197–201.

80. Galateau-Sallé F, Le Stang N, Astoul P, et al. Malignant mesothelioma of the pleura with pleomorphic features: A series of 44 cases. *Mod Pathol* 2010;402A.

81. Crotty TB, Myers JL, Katzenstein AL, et al. Localized malignant mesothelioma: A clinicopathologic and flow cytometric study. *Am J Surg Pathol* 1994;18:357–363.

82. Allen TC, Cagle PT, Churg AM, et al. Localized malignant mesothelioma. *Am J Surg Pathol* 2005;29:866–873.

83. Myers J, Tazelaar H, Katzenstein AL, et al. Localized malignant epithelioid and biphasic mesothelioma of the pleura: Clinicopathologic, immunohistochemical, and flow cytometric analysis of 3 cases. *Lab Invest* 1992;66:115A.

84. Ojeda HF, Mech K, Jr, Hicken WJ. Localized malignant mesothelioma: A case report. *Am Surg* 1998;64:881–885.

85. Churg AM. Localized pleural tumors. In: *Diagnostic Pulmonary Pathology*, Cagle PT, ed. New York: Marcel Dekker; 2000: 719–735.

86. Okamura H, Kamei T, Mitsuno A, et al. Localized malignant mesothelioma of the pleura. *Pathol Int* 2001;51:654–660.

87. Umezu H, Kuwata K, Ebe Y, et al. Microcystic variant of localized malignant mesothelioma accompanying an adenomatoid tumor-like lesion. *Pathol Int* 2002;52:416–422.

88. Hasleton PS. Pleural disease. In: *Spencer's Pathology of the Lung*, 5th ed. New York: McGraw Hill; 1996.

89. Adams VI, Unni KK, Muhm JR, et al. Diffuse malignant mesothelioma of pleura: Diagnosis and survival in 92 cases. *Cancer* 1986;58:1540–1551.

90. Law M, Hodson M, Turner-Warnick M. Malignant mesothelioma of the pleura: Clinical aspects and symptomatic treatment. *Eur J Respir Dis* 1984;65:162–168.

91. Boutin C, Rey F, Gouvernet J, et al. Thoracoscopy in pleural malignant mesothelioma: A prospective study of 188 consecutive patients. *Cancer* 1993;72:394–404.

92. Jordan K, Kwong J, Flint J, et al. Surgically treated pneumothorax. *Chest* 1991;111:280–285.

93. Mannes G, Gouw A, Berendsen H, et al. Mesothelioma presenting with pneumothorax and interlobar tumour. *Eur Respir J* 1991;4:120–121.

94. Ruffie P, Feld R, Minkin S, et al. Diffuse malignant mesothelioma of the pleura in Ontario and Quebec: A retrospective study of 332 patients. *J Clin Oncol* 1989;7:1157–1168.

95. Sheard J, Taylor W, Soorae A, et al. Pneumothorax and malignant mesothelioma in patients over the age of 40. *Thorax* 1991;46:584–585.

96. Walz R, Koch H. Malignant pleural mesothelioma: Some aspects of epidemiology, differential diagnosis and prognosis. *Pathol Res Pract* 1990;186:124–134.

97. Attanoos RL, Gibbs AR. Peritoneal mesothelioma: Clinicopathological analysis of 227 cases from the U.K. Mesothelioma Register. *Arch Anat Cytol Pathol* 1998:376.

98. Van Gelder T, Hoogsteden HC, Versnel MA, et al. Malignant peritoneal mesothelioma: A series of 19 cases. *Digestion* 1989;43:222–227.

99. Hammar SP. Malignant peritoneal mesothelioma mimicking mesenteric inflammatory disease: Critical commentary. *Pathol Res Pract* 1994;190:623–626.

100. Patel J, Sheppard MN. Primary malignant mesothelioma of the pericardium. *Cardiovasc Pathol* 2011;20:107–109.

101. Turk J, Kenda M, Kranjeck I. Cardiac tamponade caused by primary pericardial mesothelioma. *N Engl J Med* 1991;325:814.

102. Watanabe A, Sakata J, Kawamura H, et al. Primary pericardial mesothelioma presenting as constrictive pericarditis: A case report. *Jpn Circ J* 2000;64:385–388.

103. Kainuma S, Masai T, Yamauchi T, et al. Primary malignant pericardial mesothelioma presenting as pericardial constriction. *Ann Thorac Cardiovasc Surg* 2008;14:396–398.

104. Lin TS, Chen MF, Lee YT. Pericardial mesothelioma with intracardiac invasion into the right atrium. *Cardiology* 1994;85:357–360.

105. Miyamoto Y, Nakano S, Shimazaki Y, et al. Pericardial mesothelioma presenting as left atrial thrombus in a patient with mitral stenosis. *Cardiovasc Surg* 1996;4:51–52.

106. Nilsson A, Rasmuson T. Primary pericardial mesothelioma: Report of a patient and literature review. *Case Rep Oncol* 2009;2:125–132.

107. Clement P, Young R, Scully R. Malignant mesotheliomas presenting as ovarian masses: A report of nine cases, including two primary ovarian mesotheliomas. *Am J Surg Pathol* 1996;20:1067–1080.

108. Jones MA, Young RH, Scully RE. Malignant mesothelioma of the tunica vaginalis: A clinicopathologic analysis of 11 cases with review of the literature. *Am J Surg Pathol* 1995;19:815–825.

109. Tolhurst SR, Lotan T, Rapp DE, et al. Well-differentiated papillary mesothelioma occurring in the tunica vaginalis of the testis with contralateral atypical mesothelial hyperplasia. *Urol Oncol* 2006;24:36–39.

110. Plas E, Riedl CR, Pflüger H. Malignant mcsothclioma of the tunica vaginalis testis: Review of the literature and assessment of prognostic parameters. *Cancer* 1998;15:2437–2446.

111. Attanoos RL, Gibbs AR. Primary malignant gonadal mesotheliomas and asbestos. *Histopathology* 2000;37:150–159.

112. Attanoos RL, Griffin A, Gibbs AR. The use of immunohistochemistry in distinguishing reactive from neoplastic mesothelium. A novel use for desmin and comparative evaluation with epithelial membrane antigen, p53, platelet-derived growth factor-receptor, P-glycoprotein and Bcl-2. *Histopathology* 2003;43:231–238.

113. Hammar SP, Dacic S. Immunohistology of lung and pleural neoplasms. In: *Diagnostic Immunohistochemistry: Theranostic and Genomic Applications*, 3rd ed., Dabbs DJ, ed. Philadelphia, PA: Saunders; 2010: 369–463.

114. Klebe S, Nurminen M, Leigh J, Henderson DW. Diagnosis of epithelial mesothelioma using tree-based regression analysis and a minimal panel of antibodies. *Pathology* 2009;41:140–148.

115. Fowler LJ, Lachar WA. Application of immunohistochemistry to cytology. *Arch Pathol Lab Med* 2008;132:373–383.

116. Kushitani K, Takeshima Y, Amatya VJ, et al. Immunohistochemical marker panels for distinguishing between epithelioid mesothelioma and lung adenocarcinoma. *Pathol Int* 2007;57:190–199.

117. Yaziji H, Battifora H, Barry TS, et al. Evaluation of 12 antibodies for distinguishing epithelioid mesothelioma from adenocarcinoma: Identification of a three-antibody immunohistochemical panel with maximal sensitivity and specificity. *Mod Pathol* 2006;19:514–523.

118. Ordóñez NG. D2-40 and podoplanin are highly specific and sensitive immunohistochemical markers of epithelioid malignant mesothelioma. *Hum Pathol* 2005;36:372–380.

119. Ordóñez NG. The immunohistochemical diagnosis of mesothelioma: A comparative study of epithelioid mesothelioma and lung adenocarcinoma. *Am J Surg Pathol* 2003;27:1031–1051.

120. Ordóñez NG. Immunohistochemical diagnosis of epithelioid mesotheliomas: A critical review of old markers, new markers. *Hum Pathol* 2002;33:953–967.

121. Ordóñez NG. Role of immunohistochemistry in differentiating epithelial mesothelioma from adenocarcinoma: review and update. *Am J Clin Pathol* 1999;112:75–89.

122. Marchevsky AM, Wick MR. Evidence-based guidelines for the utilization of immunostains in diagnostic pathology: pulmonary adenocarcinoma versus mesothelioma. *Appl Immunohistochem Mol Morphol* 2007;15:140–144.

123. Dabbs DJ, ed. *Diagnostic Immunohistochemistry: Theranostic and Genomic Applications*, 3rd ed. Philadelphia, PA: Saunders; 2010.

124. Corson JM, Weiss LM, Banks-Schlegel SP, Pinkus G. Keratin proteins and carcinoembryonic antigen in synovial sarcomas: An immunohistochemical study of 24 cases. *Hum Pathol* 1984;15:615–621.

125. Nakamura T, Nakata K, Hata S, et al. Histochemical characterization of mucosubstances in synovial sarcoma. *Am J Surg Pathol* 1984;8:429–434.

126. Abenoza P, Manivel JC, Swanson PE, Wick MR. Synovial sarcoma: Ultrastructural study and immunohistochemical analysis by a combined peroxidase–antiperoxidase/avidin–biotin–peroxidase complex procedure. *Hum Pathol* 1986;17:1107–1115.

127. Fisher C. Synovial sarcoma: Ultrastructural and immunohistochemical features of epithelial differentiation in monophasic and biphasic tumors. *Hum Pathol* 1986;17:996–1008.

128. Ordóñez NG, Mahfouz SM, Mackay B. Synovial sarcoma: An immunohistochemical and ultrastructural study. *Hum Pathol* 1990;21:733–749.

129. Dickersin GR. Synovial sarcoma: A review and update, with emphasis on the ultrastructural characterization of the nonglandular component. *Ultrastruct Pathol* 1991;15:379–402.

130. Fisher C. Synovial sarcoma. *Ann Diagn Pathol* 1998;2:401–421.

131. Gaertner E, Zeren H, Fleming MV, et al. Biphasic synovial sarcomas arising in the pleural cavity: A clinicopathologic study of five cases. *Am J Surg Pathol* 1996;20:36–45.

132. Nicholson AG, Goldstraw P, Fisher C. Synovial sarcoma of the pleura and its differentiation from other primary pleural tumors: A clinicopathological and immunohistochemical review of three cases. *Histopathology* 1998;33:508–513.

133. Jawahar DA, Vuletin JC, Gorecki P, et al. Primary biphasic synovial sarcoma of the pleura. *Respir Med* 1997;91:568–570.

134. Dos Santos NR, de Bruijn DR, Balemans M, et al. Nuclear localization of SYT, SSX and the synovial sarcoma-associated SYT-SSX fusion proteins. *Hum Mol Genet* 1997;6:1549–1558.

135. De Leeuw B, Balemans M, Olde Weghuis D, Geurts van Kessel A. Identification of two alternative fusion genes, SYT-SSX1 and SYT-SSX2, in t(X;18)(p11.2;q11.2)-positive synovial sarcomas. *Hum Mol Genet* 1995;4:1097–1099.

136. Brett D, Whitehouse S, Antonson P, et al. The SYT protein involved in the t(X;18) synovial sarcoma translocation is a transcriptional activator localised in nuclear bodies. *Hum Mol Genet* 1997;6:1559–1564.

137. England DM, Hochholzer L, McCarthy MJ. Localised benign and malignant fibrous tumour of the pleura. *Am J Surg Pathol* 1989;13:640–658.

138. Briselli M, Mark EJ, Dickersin GR. Solitary fibrous tumour of the pleura: Eight new cases and review of 360 cases in the literature. *Cancer* 1981;47:2678–2689.

139. Flint A, Weiss SW. CD-34 and keratin expression distinguishes solitary fibrous tumour (fibrous mesothelioma) of pleura from desmoplastic mesothelioma. *Hum Pathol* 1995;26:428–431.

140. Yokoi T, Tsuzuki M, Yatabe Y, et al. Solitary fibrous tumor: Significance of p53 and CD34 immunoreactivity in its malignant transformation. *Histopathology* 1998;32:423–432.

141. Cavazza A, Rossi G, Agostini L, et al. Cytokeratin-positive malignant solitary fibrous tumour of the pleura: An unusual pitfall in the diagnosis of pleural spindle cell neoplasms. *Histopathology* 2003;43:606–608.

142. Moran CA, Suster S, Koss MN. The spectrum of histologic growth patterns in benign and malignant fibrous tumour of the pleura. *Semin Diagn Pathol* 1992;9:169–180.

143. Wilson RW, Galateau-Sallé F, Moran CA. Desmoid tumors of the pleura: A clinicopathologic mimic of localized fibrous tumor. *Mod Pathol* 1999;12:9–14.

144. Reed MK, Margraf LR, Nikaidoh H, Cleveland DC. Calcifying fibrous pseudotumor of the chest wall. *Ann Thorac Surg* 1996;62:873–874.

145. Dumont P, de Muret A, Skrobala D, et al. Calcifying fibrous pseduotumor of the mediastinum. *Ann Thorac Surg* 1997;63:543–544.

146. Jeong HS, Lee GK, Sung R, et al. Calcifying fibrous pseudotumor of mediastinum: A case report. *J Korean Med Sci* 1997;12:58–62.

147. Erasmus JJ, McAdams HP, Patz EFJ, et al. Calcifying fibrous pseudotumor of the pleura: Radiologic features in three cases. *J Comput Assist Tomogr* 1996;20:63–65.

148. Pinkard NB, Wilson RW, Lawless N, et al. Calcifying fibrous pseudotumor of pleura: A report of three cases of a newly described entity involving the pleura. *Am J Clin Pathol* 1996;105:189–194.

149. Nascimento AE, Ruiz R, Hornick JL, Fletcher CD. Calcifying fibrous 'pseudotumor': Clinicopathologic study of 15 cases and analysis of its relationship to inflammatory myofibroblastic tumor. *Int J Surg Pathol* 2002;10:189–196.

150. Hainaut P, Lesage V, Weynand B, et al. Calcifying fibrous pseudotumor (CFPT): A patient presenting with multiple pleural lesions. *Acta Clin Belg* 1999;54:162–164.

151. Kocova L, Michal M, Sulc M, et al. Calcifying fibrous pseudotumor of visceral peritoneum. *Histopathology* 1997;31:182–184.

152. Ben-Izhak O, Czernobilsky B. Calcifying fibrous pseudotumor of the mesentery presenting with acute peritonitis: case report with immunohistochemical study and review of the literature. *Int J Surg Pathol* 2001;9:249–253.

153. Van Dorpe J, Ectors N, Geboes K, et al. Is calcifying fibrous pseudotumor a late sclerosing stage of inflammatory myofibroblastic tumor? *Am J Surg Pathol* 1999;23:329–335.

154. Hill KA, Gonzalez-Crussi F, Chou PM. Calcifying fibrous pseudotumor versus inflammatory myofibroblastic tumor: A histological and immunohistochemical comparison. *Mod Pathol* 2001;14:784–790.

155. Sigel JF, Smith TA, Reith JD, Goldblum JR. Immunohistochemical analysis of anaplastic lymphoma kinase expression in deep soft tissue calcifying fibrous pseudotumor: Evidence of a late sclerotic phase of inflammatory myofibroblaastic tumor? *Ann Diagn Pathol* 2001;5:10–14.

156. Maeda A, Kawabata K, Kusuzaki K. Rapid recurrence of calcifying fibrous pseudotumor (a case report). *Anticancer Res* 2002;22:1795–1797.

157. Fletcher C, Krishman A, Mertens F. *Tumor of Soft Tissue and Bone*. Lyon: WHO/IARC Press; 2002.

158. Ordóñez NG, Tornos C. Malignant peripheral nerve sheath tumor of the pleura with epithelial and rhabdomyoblastic differentiation: Report of a case clinically simulating mesothelioma. *Am J Surg Pathol* 1997;21:1515–1521.

159. Galateau-Sallé F, ed. International Mesothelioma Panel: Brambilla E, Cagle PT, Churg AM, et al. Differential diagnosis: non-mesothelial tumors of serosal cavity: sarcomas. In: *Pathology of Malignant Mesothelioma*. London: Springer; 2006: 169.

160. Snyder CS, Dell-Aquila N, Munson P, et al. Clonal changes in inflammatory pseudotumor of lung. *Cancer* 1995;76:1545–1549.

161. Weiss SW, Enzinger FM. Epithelioid hemangioendothelioma: A vascular tumor often mistaken for carcinoma. *Cancer* 1982;50:970–981.

162. Colby TV, Koss MN, Travis WD. *Tumors of the Lower Respiratory Tract*. Washington DC: Armed Forces Institute of Pathology; 1995.

163. Battifora H. Epithelioid hemangioendothelioma imitating mesothelioma. *Appl Immunohistochem* 1993;1:220–221.
164. Lin BT-Y, Colby T, Gown AM, et al. Malignant vascular tumors of the serous membranes mimicking mesothelioma. *Am J Surg Pathol* 1996;20:1431–1439.
165. Attanoos RL, Dallimore NS, Gibbs AR. Primary epithelioid haemangioendothelioma of the peritoneum: An unusual mimic of diffuse malignant mesothelioma. *Histopathology* 1997;30:375–377.
166. Crotty EJ, McAdams HP, Erasmus JJ, et al. Epithelioid hemangioendothelioma of the pleura: clinical and radiologic features. *AJR Am J Roentgenol* 2000;175:1545–1549.
167. Zhang PJ, Livolsi VA, Brooks JJ. Malignant epithelioid vascular tumors of the pleura: Report of a series and literature review. *Hum Pathol* 2000;31:29–34.
168. Sporn TA, Butnor KJ, Roggli VL. Epithelioid haemangioendothelioma of the pleura: An aggressive vascular malignancy and clinical mimic of malignant mesothelioma. *Histopathology* 2002;41(Suppl. 2):173–177.
169. Al-Shraim M, Mahboub B, Neligan PC, et al. Primary pleural epithelioid haemangioendothelioma with metastases to the skin: A case report and literature review. *J Clin Pathol* 2005;58:107–109.
170. Sapi Z, Szentirmay Z, Orosz Z. Desmoplastic small round cell tumor of the pleura: A case report with further cytogenetic and ultrastructural evidence of mesothelial "blastemic" origin. *Eur J Surg Oncol* 1999;25:633–634.
171. Venkateswaran L, Jenkins JJ, Kaste SC, et al. Disseminated intrathoracic desmoplastic small round-cell tumor: A case report. *J Pediatr Hematol Oncol* 1997;19:172–175.
172. Liu J, Nau MM, Yeh JC, et al. Molecular heterogeneity and function of EWS-WT1 fusion transcripts in desmoplastic small round cell tumors. *Clin Cancer Res* 2000;6:3522–3529.
173. Manivel JC, Priest JR, Watterson J, et al. Pleuropulmonary blastoma: The so-called pulmonary blastoma of childhood. *Cancer* 1988;62:1516–1526.
174. Dehner LP. Primitive neuroectodermal tumor and Ewing's sarcoma. *Am J Surg Pathol* 1993;17:1–13.
175. Perlman EJ, Dickman PS, Askin FB, et al. Ewing's sarcoma—Routine diagnostic utilization of MIC2 analysis: A Pediatric Oncology Group/Children Cancer Group Intergroup Study. *Hum Pathol* 1994;25:304–307.
176. Weidner N, Tjoe J. Immunohistochemical profile of monoclonal antibody O13: Antibody that recognizes glycoprotein p30/32MIC2 and is useful in diagnosing Ewing's sarcoma and peripheral neuroepithelioma. *Am J Surg Pathol* 1994;18:486–494.
177. Yiakoumis X, Pangalis GA, Kyrtsonis MC, et al. Primary effusion lymphoma in two HIV-negative patients successfully treated with pleurodesis as first-line therapy. *Anticancer Res* 2010;310:271–276.
178. Sekine A, Hagiwara E, Hashiba Y, Ogura T, Takahashi H. Clinical analysis of eight cases with pyothorax-associated lymphoma. *Nihon Kokyuki Gakkai Zasshi* 2010;48:186–191.
179. Ansari MQ, Dawson DB, Nador R, et al. Primary body cavity-based AIDS-related lymphomas. *Am J Clin Pathol* 1996;105:221–229.
180. Banks PM, Warnke RA. Primary effusion lymphoma. In: *WHO Classification of Tumors of Hematopoietic and Lymphoid Tissues.* Swerdlow SH, Campo E, Harris NL, Jaffe ES, Pileri SA, Stein H, Thiele J, Vardiman JW, eds. Lyon: IARC Press; 2001: 179–180.
181. Banks PM, Harris NL, Warnke RA. Primary effusion lymphoma. In: *WHO Classification of Tumors of the Lung, Pleura and Mediastinum*, Travis WD, Brambilla E, eds. Lyon: IARC Press; 2004.
182. Aozasa K, Ohsaw AM, Kanno H. Pyothorax-associated lymphoma: A distinctive type of lymphoma strongly associated with Epstein–Barr virus. *Adv Anat Pathol* 1997;4:58–63.
183. Gaulard P, Harris NL. Pyothorax-associated lymphoma. In: *WHO Classification of Tumors of the Lung, Pleura and Mediastinum*, Travis WD, Brambilla E, eds. Lyon: IARC Press; 2004.
184. Ibuka T, Fukayama M, Hayashi Y, et al. Pyothorax-associated pleural lymphoma. *Cancer* 1994;73:738–744.
185. Vega F, Padula A, Valbuena JR, et al. Lymphomas involving the pleura: A clinicopathologic study of 34 cases diagnosed by pleural biopsy. *Arch Pathol Lab Med* 2006;130:1497–1502.
186. Uluba G, Eynboglu FO, Simek A, Ozyilkan O. Multiple myeloma with pleural involvement: A case report. *Am J Clin Oncol* 2005;28:429–430.
187. Giuliani N, Caramatti C, Roti G, et al. Hematologic malignancies with extramedullary spread of disease. Case 1. Multiple myeloma with extramedullary involvement of the pleura and testes. *J Clin Oncol* 2003;21:1887–1888.
188. Quinquenel ML, Moualla M, Le Coz A, et al. Pleural involvement of myeloma. Apropos of two cases. *Rev Mal Respir* 1995;12:173–174.

189. Netto GJ, Epstein JI. Immunohistology of the prostate, bladder, kidney, and testis. In: *Diagnostic Immunohistochemistry: Theranostic and Genomic Applications*, 3rd ed., Dabbs DJ, ed. Philadelphia, PA: Saunders; 2010: 593–661.

190. Colwell AS, D'Cunha J, Vargas SO, et al. Synovial sarcoma of the pleura: A clinical and pathologic study of three cases. *J Thorac Cardiovasc Surg* 2002;124:828–832.

191. Yano M, Toyooka S, Tsukuda K, et al. SYT-SSX fusion genes in synovial sarcoma of the thorax. *Lung Cancer* 2004;44:391–397.

192. Rosai J, Gorich J. Pleural metastasis of malignant thymoma: a pitfall in the CT-diagnosis of pleural mesothelioma. *Am J Surg Pathol* 1990;14:819–828.

193. Attanoos RL, Galateau-Sallé F, Gibbs AR, et al. Primary thymic epithelial tumours of the pleura mimicking malignant mesothelioma. *Histopathology* 2002;41:42–49.

194. Payne CB Jr, Morningstar WA, Chester EH. Thymoma of the pleura masquerading as diffuse mesothelioma. *Am Rev Respir Dis* 1966;94:441–446.

195. Honma K, Shimada K. Metastasizing ectopic thymoma arising in the right thoracic cavity and mimicking diffuse pleural mesothelioma: An autopsy study of a case with review of the literature. *Wien Klin Wochenschr* 1986;98:14–20.

196. Moran CA, Travis WD, Rosada-de-Christenson M, et al. Thymomas presenting as pleural tumors: Report of eight cases. *Am J Surg Pathol* 1992;16:138–144.

197. Fushimi H, Tanio Y, Kotoh K. Ectopic thymoma mimicking diffuse pleural mesothelioma: A case report. *Hum Pathol* 1998;29:409–410.

198. Attanoos RL, Gibbs AR. Unusual "pseudomesotheliomatous" neoplasms: Primary pleural thymic epithelial tumours. *Histopathology* 2002;41(Suppl. 2):170–173.

199. American Joint Committee on Cancer. *Cancer Staging Manual*, 7th ed. Chicago, IL: American Joint Committee on Cancer; 2010.

200. Tsao AS, Mehran R, Roth JA. Neoadjuvant and intrapleural therapies for malignant pleural mesothelioma. *Clin Lung Cancer* 2009;10:36–41.

201. Yan TD, Welch L, Black D, Sugarbaker PH. A systemic review on the efficacy of cytoreductive surgery combined with perioperative intraperitoneal chemotherapy for diffuse malignancy peritoneal mesothelioma. *Ann Oncol* 2007;18:827–834.

202. Christensen BC, Godleski JJ, Roelofs CR, et al. Asbestos burden predicts survival in pleural mesothelioma. *Environ Health Perspect* 2008;116:723–726.

203. Weinberg RA. Multistep tumorigenesis. In: *The Biology of Cancer*, Weinkberg RA, ed. New York: Garland Science, Taylor & Francis Group LLC; 2007: 399–462, Chapter 11.

204. Dodson RF, O'Sullivan M, Corn CJ, McLarty JW, Hammar SP. Analysis of asbestos fiber burden in lung tissue from mesothelioma patients. *Ultrastruct Pathol* 1997;21:321–336.

205. Jaurand M-C. Asbestos, chromosomal deletions and tumor suppressor gene alterations in human malignant mesothelioma. *Lung Cancer* 2006;54(Supp 1):S15.

206. Neri M, Ugolini D, Dianzani I, et al. Genetic susceptibility to malignant pleural mesothelioma and other asbestos-associated diseases. *Mutat Res* 2008;659:126–136.

207. Helsinki Consensus Report. Asbestos, asbestosis and cancer: The Helsinki Criteria for diagnosis and attribution. *Scand J Work Environ Health* 1997;23:311–316.

208. Friedman GK. Clinical diagnosis of asbestos-related disease. In: *Dail and Hammar's Pulmonary Pathology*, 3rd ed., Tomashefski New York: Springer, 2008: 309–380.

209. Oury TD, Hammar SP, Roggli VL. Asbestos content of lung tissue in patients with malignant JF, Jr, ed. peritoneal mesothelioma: A study of 40 cases. *Lung Cancer* 1997;18(Suppl. 1):235–236. Abstract 923.

210. Welch LS, Acherman YI, Haile E, Sokas RK, Sugarbaker PH. Asbestos and peritoneal mesothelioma among college-educated men. *Int J Occup Environ Health* 2005;11:254–258.

211. Dodson RF, O'Sullivan MF, Huang J, Holiday DB, Hammar SP. Asbestos in extrapulmonary sites: omentum and mesentery. *Chest* 2000;117:486–493.

212. Goldberg M, Luce D. The health impact of non-occupational exposure to asbestos. What do we know? *Eur J Cancer Prev* 2009;00:1–15.

213. National Institute for Occupational Safety and Health. Report to Congress on Workers' Home Contamination Study conducted under the Workers' Family Protection Act (29 U.S.C. 671a). U.S. Department of Human and Health Services, September 1995. DHHS (NIOSH) Publication No. 95–123.

214. Hammar SP, Roggli VL, Oury TD. Moffatt EJ. Malignant mesothelioma in women. *Lung Cancer* 1997;18(Suppl. 1):236. Abstract 924.

215. Madkour MT, El Bokhary MS, Awad Allah HI, et al. Environmental exposure to asbestos and the exposure–response relationship with mesothelioma. *East Mediterr Health J* 2009;15:25–38.

216. Pan XL, Day HW, Wang W, et al. Residential proximity to naturally occurring asbestos and mesothelioma risk in California. *Am J Respir Crit Care Med* 2005;172:1019–1025.

217. Goldberg S, Rey G, Luce D, et al. Possible effect of environmental exposure to asbestos on geographical variation in mesothelioma rates. *Occup Environ Med* 2010;67:417–421.

218. Peto J, Rake C, Gilham C, Hatch J. Occupational, domestic and environmental mesothelioma risks in Britain: A case–control study. RR696 Research Report. HSE Books; Norwich: March 2009. www.hse. gov.uk.

219. Rake C, Gilham C, Hatch J, et al. Occupational, domestic and environmental mesothelioma risks in the British population: A case–control study. *Br J Cancer* 2009;100:1175–1183.

220. Maule MM, Magnani C, Dalmasso P, et al. Modeling mesothelioma risk associated with environmental asbestos exposure. *Environ Health Perspect* 2007;115:1066–1071.

221. Kurumatani N, Kumagai S. Mapping the risk of mesothelioma due to neighborhood asbestos exposure. *Am J Respir Crit Care Med* 2008;178:624–629.

222. Roggli VL, Oury TD, Sporn TA, eds. *Pathology of Asbestos-Associated Diseases*, 2nd ed. Springer: New York; 2004.

223. Hillerdal G. Mesothelioma: Cases associated with non-occupational and low dose exposures. *Occup Environ Med* 199;56:505–513.

224. Iwatsubo Y, Pairon JC, Boutin C, et al. Pleural mesothelioma: Dose–response relation at low levels of asbestos exposure in a French population-based case–control study. *Am J Epidemiol* 1998;148:133–142.

225. Rödelsperger K, Jöckel KH, Pohlabein H, et al. Asbestos and man-made vitreous fibers as risk factors for diffuse malignant mesothelioma: Results from a German hospital-based case–control study. *Am J Ind Med* 2001;39:262–275.

226. Rolland P, Ducamp S, Gramond C, et al. Risk of pleural mesothelioma: A French population-based case–control study (1998–2002). *Lung Cancer* 2006;54:S9(35).

227. World Health Organization. Environmental Health Criteria 203. *Evaluation of Health Risks of Exposure to Chrysotile Asbestos*. Geneva: World Health Organization; 1998: 137–144.

228. Hodgson JT, Darnton A. The quantitative risk of mesothelioma and lung cancer in relation to asbestos exposure. *Ann Occup Hyg* 2000;44:565–601.

229. Hodgson JT, Darnton A. Mesothelioma risk from chrysotile. *Occup Environ Med* 2010;67:432.

230. U.S. Department of Labor. Occupational exposure to asbestos, tremolite, anthophyllite and actinolite. Final rules. 29 CFR Parts 1910 and 1926. Washington, DC: Department of Labor, Occupational Safety and Health Administration; 1996: 22612–22790.

CHAPTER 8

Asbestos and Other Cancers

Samuel P. Hammar, Richard A. Lemen, Douglas W. Henderson, and James Leigh

CONTENTS

8.1 INTRODUCTION

In the early to mid-1960s, investigation of heat and frost insulators provided evidence that this heavily asbestos-exposed group had not only a greater incidence of lung cancer and mesothelioma than expected but also a potentially higher incidence of a variety of other cancers.

With the passage of time, several cancers have emerged as potentially related to asbestos causation. These include laryngeal carcinoma, oropharyngeal carcinoma, colorectal carcinoma, bile duct carcinoma, renal cell carcinoma, ovarian carcinoma, and lymphoma.

In addition, a rare form of lung cancer exists, which is referred to as *pseudomesotheliomatous carcinoma, pleural form of primary lung cancer, pseudomesotheliomatous adenocarcinoma, mesothelioma-like tumor of the pleura*, or *pseudomesotheliomatous lung cancer*.

The purpose of this chapter is to provide information on these neoplasms.

8.2 PSEUDOMESOTHELIOMATOUS LUNG CARCINOMA

Samuel P. Hammar

My (S.P.H.) experience with pseudomesotheliomatous lung cancer was somewhat serendipitous in that in the mid-1980s most cases of suspected mesotheliomas were autopsied. Cases that occurred had been diagnosed clinically as mesotheliomas, but when the tissue was further evaluated by electron microscopy, histochemistry, and/or immunohistochemistry, the pathologic findings indicated that these tumors were not mesotheliomas but were, in fact, primary lung cancers or metastatic cancers growing in a distribution that macroscopically resembled mesothelioma.

In 1976, Harwood et al.[1] reported six cases of primary lung cancer that grew in a pleural distribution and referred to them as *pseudomesotheliomatous carcinoma of the lung.* Of these six cases, five were classified at the time as bronchioloalveolar cell carcinomas and the other was diagnosed as a poorly differentiated adenocarcinoma. In two of six cases, there were intraparenchymal lung nodules, although the dominant growth pattern was that of a diffuse pleural tumor indistinguishable from the growth pattern of mesothelioma.

In reviewing the literature, there was a case reported in 1930 of a lung cancer growing in a diffuse pleural distribution in an individual who had asbestosis.[2]

In 1956, Babolini and Blasi[3] of Naples, Italy, reported on 82 cases of primary lung cancer, 5 of which were stated to have grown in a diffuse pleural distribution mimicking mesothelioma. The authors referred to these neoplasms as the *pleural form of primary cancer of the lung.* Of the five cases reported, two were described as being composed of small, undetermined cells (cases 1 and 5) and three had a morphology that fulfilled the criteria for adenocarcinoma. The macroscopic description and the clinical features described by Babolini and Blasi[3] closely resembled the clinical and macroscopic features of diffuse pleural mesothelioma. The authors cited other references explicitly describing lung neoplasms growing in a diffuse distribution.[4–8]

In 1992, Koss et al.[9] from the Armed Forces Institute of Pathology reviewed 15 cases of pseudomesotheliomatous adenocarcinomas reported in the medical literature and 15 cases they had collected at the AFIP. Koss et al.[9] published the criteria they used for diagnosing a pseudomesotheliomatous adenocarcinoma of the lung. The criteria were as follows:

> Presentation of the tumor solely or predominantly as a diffuse pleural neoplasm grossly at thoracotomy, radiographically, or at autopsy;
> Lack of a defined primary site of a neoplasm outside of the lung;
> Microscopic evidence of intracellular, glandular, neutral or slightly acidic mucin within tumor cells with or without glandular differentiation of the tumor; and
> Availability of a generous open pleural biopsy, pleural decortication specimen, or autopsy specimen.

In their combined series of 30 cases, 90% of patients were men and had mean and median ages of 63 and 61 years, respectively. Approximately 63% of patients were stated to have been cigarette smokers, most of whom had a greater than 20-pack-year history of smoking. Of interest, 17% of these patients had a history of possible or definite exposure to asbestos.

The presenting signs and symptoms of these patients were essentially identical to those seen in mesothelioma, namely, dyspnea on exertion, chest pain, weight loss, and pleural effusion. Histologic fibrosis was stated to have been observed in lung parenchyma in 6 of 30 cases, and asbestosis was identified with numerous associated ferruginous bodies consistent with asbestos bodies in one case from the AFIP series. The mean survival of the 10 AFIP patients who expired was only 7 months.

In 1993, Dr. James Robb and I (S.P.H.) reported 27 cases of pseudomesotheliomatous lung cancer.[10] Of these 27 cases, 23 were pulmonary adenocarcinomas, 2 were squamous cell lung carcinomas, 1 was a large cell undifferentiated carcinoma, and 1 was an adenosquamous carcinoma. In 17 patients where information concerning an occupational history was known, 16 were stated to have worked in an occupational setting where they were exposed to asbestos. In 10 of 27 cases, the occupational history was unknown. Asbestos digestion analysis on seven of nine cases showed elevated numbers of asbestos bodies ranging up to 13,000 per gram of wet lung tissue. The average number of asbestos bodies per gram of wet lung tissue was 807 in the right upper lobe, 1886 in the right middle lobe, 2957 in the right lower lobe, 2401 in the left upper lobe, and 1497 in the left lower lobe.

In 1994, Hartmann and Schütz[11] identified 219 diffuse pleural tumors in an autopsy series of 33,500 cases collected between 1957 and 1987. Of the 219 diffuse pleural tumors, there were 106 primary pleural mesotheliomas and 72 neoplasms they referred to as *mesothelioma-like tumors of the pleura.* Seven of 72 mesothelioma-like tumors of the pleura were metastatic to pleura and were of extrapulmonary origin. The remaining 65 cases were considered to be primary lung cancers, of which 63 were adenocarcinomas and 2 were primary squamous cell carcinomas (SCCs). The age range in the 63 adenocarcinomas was 68 ± 9 years. The primary signs and symptoms in these patients were dyspnea, chest pain, weight loss, and pleural effusion. The average survival in 63 patients with adenocarcinoma was 6.4 ± 5 months, which was shorter than that found in 106 patients with pleural mesothelioma who survived 11.2 ± 5 months. Two patients with pseudomesotheliomatous lung cancer had squamous carcinomas and the lung tissue showed pathologic features of asbestosis.

In 1998, Koss et al.[12] reported on another 29 cases of adenocarcinoma for which the clinical, gross, and microscopic appearance resembled diffuse malignant epithelial mesothelioma. Fifteen cases were stated to have had a history of cigarette smoking, and six had a history of possible or definite exposure to asbestos. Three of 14 lung specimens contained asbestos bodies and two cases showed pathologic asbestosis. Twenty-five of 29 patients presented with unilateral pleural effusions, and 20 were stated to have undergone pleural stripping. Most patients received radiation and chemotherapy without much beneficial effect. The median survival rate was 8 months, and 13% had a survival of >18 months. The diagnosis was confirmed by histochemistry and immunohistochemistry. Koss et al.[12] concluded that these adenocarcinomas simulating mesothelioma were an aggressive variant of a peripheral adenocarcinoma with a poor prognosis and showed evidence of asbestos exposure in a subset of cases.

The largest, most recent series of pseudomesotheliomatous carcinomas was reported by Attanoos and Gibbs[13] in 2003 during a 10-year evaluation of cases submitted to the Environmental Lung Disease Research Group in Cardiff. Forty-seven of 53 cases were primary lung carcinomas, and 7 were metastatic carcinomas. Forty of 53 cases were stated to have had a history of exposure to asbestos. Attanoos and Gibbs[13] concluded the high incidence of exposure to asbestos was due to selection bias.

Me (S.P.H.), Dr. Henderson, Dr. Leigh, Dr. Dodson, and several others are in the process of investigating a large series of pseudomesotheliomatous lung cancers.[14] To date, we have approximately 160 cases of which 141 were men, 17 were women, and 2 cases in which the sex was unknown. The age range was between 38 and 96 years, with a mean age of 62.8 years and a median age of 66.5 years. Of the 141 male cases, 78 were cigarette smokers and 17 were nonsmokers. Of the 17 female cases, 9 were smokers and 1 was a nonsmoker. The smoking history in the remaining cases was unknown. Fifty-three patients had a greater than 20-pack-year history of cigarette smoking.

One hundred five of 160 cases had a history of occupational exposure to asbestos. Five cases had domestic/bystander exposure to asbestos (all women). Seven had no known history of exposure to asbestos. In 43 patients, the potential asbestos exposure history was unknown.

The occupational history and the number of cases with respect to job classification are shown in Table 8.1. Signs and symptoms of 93 cases where information was known are shown in Table 8.2. The radiographic changes in 103 cases where information was available are shown in Table 8.3. The histologic types of pseudomesotheliomatous lung cancer are shown in Table 8.4. Rare types of pseudomesotheliomatous lung carcinomas are shown in Table 8.5.

Evaluation was done at the Harrison Medical Center in Bremerton, Washington, between 1989 and 2005, where Dr. Hammar is a practicing pathologist. During this 6-year period, 2130 cases of lung cancer occurred of which 18 were pseudomesotheliomatous lung cancers, all 18 of which were reportedly associated with exposure to asbestos. The histologic types of lung cancer identified in this group are shown in Table 8.6. The cigarette smoking history of 1242 of 2130 cases is shown in Table 8.7. Asbestosis was seen in 45 cases of pseudomesotheliomatous lung cancer, and asbestos bodies were identified in lung tissue from 65 cases. Quantitative asbestos digestion analysis of lung tissue was done in 52 cases as shown in Table 8.8. The average number of asbestos bodies per gram of wet lung tissue in each case is shown in Table 8.9. The range of asbestos bodies per gram of wet

Table 8.1   Occupational History with Respect to Job
            Classification for Persons Diagnosed with
            Pseudomesotheliomatous Adenocarcinoma of Lung

Job Classification	No. of Cases
Asbestos brake plant worker	1
Asbestos worker, not otherwise specified	1
Boilermaker/boiler tender	6
Barber	1
Brake mechanic (automotive)	7
Bricklayer	3
Carpenter	8
Coal miner	1
Construction worker	3
Coppersmith	1
Domestic/bystander exposure	5 (all women)
Electrician	13
Engineer, not otherwise specified	2
Floor coverer	1
Foundry worker	3
Heavy equipment operator	2
HVAC technician	1
Insulator	6
Iron worker	1
Laborer	11
Longshoreman	1
Machinist	5
Maintenance man	4
Mechanic, not otherwise specified	7
Millwright	1
Painter	3
Paper mill worker	1
Pipefitter/Steamfitter	10
Pipe layer	1
Plasterer	3
Plumber	5
Railroad brakeman	1
Refinery worker	2
Sand blaster	1
Sheet metal mechanic	4
Shipfitter/rigger	5
Shipyard worker, not otherwise specified	7
Truck driver	1
Welder	9

lung tissue in 52 cases was between 0 and 25,000. The mean asbestos body per gram of wet lung tissue in 52 cases was 1401. The median asbestos body per gram of wet lung tissue in 52 cases is shown in Table 8.10. Asbestos fiber analysis was performed in 20 cases.

The differential pathologic diagnoses included epithelial mesothelioma, mucin-positive epithelial mesothelioma, small cell mesothelioma, poorly differentiated mesothelioma not otherwise specified, lymphoma, and metastatic neoplasms to the pleura.

Table 8.2 Signs and Symptoms of 93 Cases of
Pseudomesotheliomatous Lung Carcinoma

Symptoms	No. of Cases
Shortness of breath	64
Chest pain, pressure, discomfort	35
Cough	28
Weight loss	8
Fever	8
Fatigue/malaise	7
Abdominal pain/distention	6
Back pain	6
Fever	3
Weakness	3
Anorexia	2
Chest congestion	2
Shoulder pain	2
Wheezing	1
Flu-like illness	1
Neck pain	1
Shoulder pain	1

Note: Many patients had more than one sign/symptom.

Table 8.3 Radiographic Changes in 103 Cases of
Pseudomesotheliomatous Lung Carcinoma

Most Common (No. of Cases)	One Case Each
Pleural effusion (71)	Abdominal mass
Pleural thickening/nodularity (33)	Ascites
Pleural plaques (26)	Bone metastasis
Lung mass (16)	Compression of lung
Atelectasis (15)	Consolidation of lung
Pleural-based lung nodules (11)	Hydropneumothorax
Asbestosis (9)	Mediastinal mass
Small irregular opacities (8)	Nodule, left lung
Interstitial fibrosis (6)	Opacification, left lower lobe
Infiltrates (8)	Paravertebral mass
Bibasilar infiltrates (4)	Pulmonary nodules
Nodular densities in lung (3)	Rib destruction
Diffuse circumferential tumor (3)	Soft tissue densities
Chest wall mass (2)	Subpleural mass
Paratracheal mass (2)	Thickening of minor fissure
Mediastinal adenopathy/mass (2)	Volume loss, right upper lobe
Hilar/perihilar mass (2)	
Solid tumor mass (2)	
Pleural calcification (2)	
COPD/Centrilobular emphysema (6)	
Costophrenic angle thickening/blunting (2)	
Apical scarring (2)	

Table 8.4   Histologic Types of Pseudomesotheliomatous Lung Carcinoma

Primary pulmonary adenocarcinoma (81)

   Mucin producing (21)
   Poorly differentiated (18)
   Tubulodesmoplastic (15)
   Acinar (5)
   Tubulopapillary (4)
   Bronchioloavelolar cell (4)
   Moderately differentiated (3)
   Signet ring (3)
   Type II pneumocyte (2)
   Deciduoid morphology (2)
   Papillary (2)
   Adenoid cystic (1)
   Epithelioid/rhabdoid (1)

Primary pulmonary adenosquamous carcinoma (10)
Primary pulmonary SCC (5)
Non–small cell lung cancer (5)
Lung carcinoma, not otherwise specified (41)

Table 8.5   Rare Types of Pseudomesotheliomatous Lung Tumor

Carcinosarcoma (sarcomatoid carcinoma) (7)
Epithelioid hemangioendothelioma (3)
Small cell lung cancer (2)
Calcifying fibrous pseudotumor of the pleura (1)
Combined meso–pseudomeso (1)
Metastatic melanoma (1)
Metastatic endometrial carcinoma (1)
Metastatic ovarian carcinoma (1)
Metastatic sarcomatoid renal cell carcinoma (1)

Table 8.6   Histologic Types of Lung Cancer

   Adenocarinoma (653)
   Small cell carcinoma (312)
   Squamous carcinoma (265)
   Non–small cell carcinoma (152)
   Large cell carcinoma (136)
   Unknown (no pathology) (62)

Table 8.7   Cigarette and Asbestos Exposure History in 1242 Cases of Lung Cancer

Cigarette Smoking History	Asbestos Exposure History
Cigarette smokers, 89.4%	Likely, 29.4%
Non–cigarette smokers, 5.5%	Possible, 21.7%
Unknown, 5.1%	Unlikely, 38.9%
	Unknown, 10%

Table 8.8 Quantitative Asbestos Digestion Analysis

52 Cases	No. of Lung Tissue Samples Evaluated
41	5 samples each
4	4 samples each
2	3 samples each
2	2 samples each
3	1 sample each

Table 8.9 Average Number of Asbestos Bodies (AB) per Gram of Wet Lung Tissue

0–9 AB	10–99 AB	100–999 AB	1000–9999 AB	>10,000 AB
0	13	100	1075	11,780
0.6	13	129	1095	11,784
1.2	17	134	1095	12,600
2	27	145	1150	
2	38	172	1425	
8	38	178	1425	
	38	182	1459	
	43	197	2160	
	46	234	2640	
	55	317	2860	
	70	324	3330	
	97	346	3330	
		346	6110	
		356		
		360		
		665		
		732		
		808		
6	**12**	**18**	**13**	**3**

Table 8.10 Median Asbestos Bodies per Gram of Wet Lung Tissue in 52 Cases

Median Range	No. of Cases
0–8	6
13–97	12
100–808	18
1075–6100	13
11,780–12,600	3

A number of additional case reports[15–24] of pseudomesotheliomatous lung cancer have been reported in the literature and are summarized in Table 8.11.

The data suggest a significant number of cases of pseudomesotheliomatous lung cancer occur in persons exposed to asbestos, some of whom have asbestosis and others of whom have asbestos bodies in their lung tissue.

8.3 LARYNGEAL CARCINOMA

Douglas W. Henderson, James Leigh, and Richard A. Lemen

The association between asbestos exposure and risk of laryngeal cancer is less extensively documented in the scientific literature than for lung cancer. As for lung cancer, it is almost universally accepted that there is a strong causal relationship between tobacco smoke and squamous cell carcinoma (SCC) of the larynx, with alcohol consumption as another risk factor. Epidemiologic evidence has varied on the issue of whether asbestos represents an additional causal factor.

Observations that support a causal-contributory role for asbestos exposure in the genesis of laryngeal cancer in some patients with substantial asbestos exposure include the following:[25]

- The larynx lies directly in the path of the inhaled air stream before it reaches the lungs, with the potential for impaction and deposition of asbestos fibers onto the laryngeal mucosa, in addition to any fibers coughed up from the lungs with sputum before expectoration or swallowing.

Table 8.11   Case Reports of Pseudomesotheliomatous Lung Cancer

Reference	Age/Sex	Histologic Type	Occupation/Asbestos Exposure History	Smoking History
Hammar et al.[14]	55/M	Lung adenocarcinoma	Not given	Regular smoker
Braganza et al.[15]	65/M	Lung adenocarcinoma (tubulodesmoplastic)	Not given	Not given
Broghamer et al.[16]	80/M	Lung adenocarcinoma	Not given	Not given
Broghamer et al.[16]	59/M	Lung adenocarcinoma	Not given	40 pack-years
Lin et al.[17]	56/M	Lung adenocarcinoma	Not given	Regular smoker
Nishimoto et al.[18]	69/M	Lung adenocarcinoma (BAC)	Asbestos exposure	Pipe and cigarette smoker
Simonsen[19]	85/M	Papillary lung adenocarcinoma	No history of asbestos exposure	30 pack-years
Simonsen[19]	75/M	Lung adenocarcinoma (tubulodesmoplastic)	Asbestos exposure	40 pack-years
Simonsen[19]	70/F	Lung adenocarcinoma	Not given	Not given
Dessy and Pietra[20]	32/M	Large cell undifferentiated lung carcinoma	Not given	Not given
Brunner-La Rocca et al.[21]	51/M	Small cell	Foundry worker	Longtime smoker
Brunner-La Rocca et al.[21]	58/M	Small cell	Not given	Longtime smoker
Brunner-La Rocca et al.[21]	59/M	Small cell	Not given	Longtime smoker
Brunner-La Rocca et al.[21]	64/M	Small cell	Not given	Longtime smoker
Falconieri et al.[22]	63/M	Poorly differentiated carcinoma	Asbestos exposure	Smoker
Falconieri et al.[22]	65/M	Poorly differentiated carcinoma	Not given	Smoker
Falconieri et al.[22]	67/M	Poorly differentiated carcinoma	Not given	Nonsmoker
Shah et al.[23]	59/M	Epithelioid hemangioendothelioma	Shipyard laborer with asbestos exposure	Not given
Shah et al.[23]	73/M	Epithelioid hemangioendothelioma	Shipyard joiner with asbestos exposure	Not given
Shah et al.[23]	33/M	Epithelioid hemangioendothelioma	Shipyard welder	Not given

- Asbestos bodies and fibers have been demonstrated in laryngeal samples from asbestos-exposed individuals. Roggli et al.[26] reported asbestos bodies in digestion studies on laryngeal samples from two of five asbestos workers with proven asbestos-associated pulmonary disease, whereas they were not found in laryngeal samples taken at autopsy from 10 control subjects. Hirsch et al.[27] found significant concentrations of chrysotile and amphibole fibers (but no detectable asbestos bodies) in normal laryngeal samples from two patients with asbestosis and associated laryngeal tumors (mean fiber length for each of the two cases was 2.4 and 3.4 μm)—one of the patients had a laryngeal polyp whereas the other had laryngeal carcinoma. In particular, the detection of asbestos bodies in/on laryngeal tissue in patients with asbestos-related lung disease raises the distinct likelihood that the bodies were related to deposition of asbestos bodies derived from lung parenchyma onto the surface of the larynx from sputum. However, Hirsch et al.[27] commented that for their two cases, the surface of the laryngeal samples had been carefully washed so that the fibers were thought to be "... intratissular and not deposited on the surface of the tissue." The simple presence of asbestos fibers in the larynx does not, by itself, prove causation; rather, these findings are adduced simply to demonstrate that in subjects with substantial asbestos exposure, asbestos fibers can penetrate laryngeal tissue at the sites where laryngeal carcinoma occurs.
- Asbestos fibers represent a known carcinogen for pleural and bronchopulmonary tissues, with no known threshold level of exposure below which there is no risk of mesothelioma or lung cancer based on cohort or case–control studies.
- Among multiple epidemiologic investigations of this issue, some case-referent[28] and cohort studies showed evidence of dose–response association between asbestos and laryngeal carcinoma after allowance for tobacco smoking and alcohol consumption (see later discussion and reference 29).
- The notion that laryngeal carcinoma is an outcome of the combined effect of tobacco smoke and asbestos fiber deposition has biological plausibility by analogy with lung cancer.

There have been multiple epidemiologic investigations concerning asbestos exposure and the development of carcinoma of the larynx[29 35] (for additional references, see the U.S. Institute of Medicine Committee on Asbestos [USIMCA][29] report published in 2006 entitled *Asbestos: Selected Cancers*). The most recent studies have varied in their findings, some supporting a causal relationship (i.e., an increased risk)[29,30,34,35] whereas others did not,[31,33] and some did not adjust for smoking, alcohol, or both (in this context, it is necessary to adjust not only for smoking but also for the diminution in risk related to cessation of smoking, as set forth in detail in the 2007 book from the International Agency for Research on Cancer [IARC][36] on *Reversal of Risk After Quitting Smoking*).

However, some epidemiological studies are deeply flawed, and in particular, the following two problems are notable, apart from the issue of adjustment for smoking and alcohol:

- First, perhaps the greatest problem for some of the epidemiologic studies is that they address *deaths* from cancer of the larynx (e.g., as shown by death certificates), as is evident in the review by Browne and Gee.[37] The problem with mortality statistics in relation to cancer of the larynx is that most patients who develop laryngeal carcinoma do *not* die from that disease, so that the use of mortality data must seriously underestimate the true incidence of the disease and hence the rate ratios (RRs). The point is that carcinoma of the larynx is treatable either by surgical resection, radiotherapy, or both (and chemotherapy in advanced-stage cases). One of the most useful resources for survival data of laryngeal carcinomas can be found in the American Joint Committee on Cancer[38] *Cancer Staging Manual*, seventh edition, 2010. Accordingly, the 5-year survival rate for stage I laryngeal carcinoma (T1, N0, M0*) is in the order of approximately 84%, falling to 35.5% for stage IV disease (T4a, M0; or any N1 or N2 disease) at 5 years. For cancer of the glottis, the 5-year survival rate ranges from 90% for stage I disease falling to 44.5% for stage IV disease.

---

* The AJCC staging system is based on the TNM system originally promulgated by the UICC: T refers to the size of the primary tumor and the extent of its local invasion, N refers to the presence or absence of lymph node metastases and (if present) the number and distribution of the lymph nodes so affected (N0 = no evidence of nodal metastases), and M refers to the presence or absence of distant metastases. This system is now standard for the staging of cancers.

Accordingly, in a recent chapter on nonthoracic cancers possibly resulting from asbestos exposure, Craighead[31] commented:

> Cancer of the larynx is a relatively uncommon disease comprising about 1% of human malignancies. It predominantly occurs in males in the later decades of life. Cancer of the larynx is usually of the squamous cell type and is readily diagnosed with a high degree of specificity by both the clinician and the pathologist. Early disease is readily amenable to treatment; thus, retrospective mortality studies using death certificate data are an unsuitable means of evaluating disease occurrence.

Having stated this, Craighead[31] opined that there was insufficient evidence to assign a causal relationship between asbestos and laryngeal cancer, although his analysis of this issue seems not to have included a detailed evaluation of all the epidemiological evidence.

Despite the limitations on mortality-based studies, Battista et al.[39] found an elevated standardized mortality ratio (SMR) of 240 (95% confidence interval [CI] = 95–505) for carcinoma of the larynx related to asbestos exposure among railway carriage construction and repair workers in Italy. Although this study was based on a "best evidence" approach whereby all clinical and pathological material for every deceased person was assessed, the study did not state specifically that it had allowed for tobacco smoking and alcohol consumption. The authors[39] stated a causal relationship between asbestos and cancer of the larynx "… cannot be conclusively proven," although this comment clearly does not rule out that relationship.

- Second, some cohort and case–control studies deal with relatively few cases of laryngeal cancer, thus limiting the power of the studies to detect small to even more substantial increased risks for laryngeal cancer as a consequence of asbestos exposure (even if such a relationship does exist). For example, in the mortality study reported by Battista et al.,[39] there were only five observed cases of laryngeal cancer. In an earlier case–control study on occupational risk factors for laryngeal cancers reported by Wortley et al.[40]—which did not find any significant increase in risk—the authors[40] commented that the power of their study "… to detect a 2-fold increase in risk for those exposed 10 years or more was 50%," so that this study had no better than a 50:50 chance of detecting a risk of 2.0 if it did exist, and even less power to detect a smaller increase in relative risk (RR).

Doll and Peto[41] suggested exposure to asbestos as a risk factor for cancer of the larynx. The IARC of the World Health Organization (WHO) reported in 1977[42] and again in 1987[43] about an excess of cancers of the larynx observed in workers exposed to asbestos.

In a review of 12 cohort studies by Chan and Gee[44] in 1988, half did not show any significant excess of laryngeal cancer and the other studies had SMRs that ranged from 1.91 to 5.41; however, the authors[44] contended that none had adjusted for confounders such as alcohol and smoking.

In an analysis of six cohorts with lung cancer RRs of 2 or more, Smith et al.[45] found two cohorts with the highest RR estimates for lung cancer of 4.06 and 3.28, which supported a causal relationship between asbestos exposure and laryngeal cancer, having RRs of 1.91 (90% CI = 1.00–3.34) and 3.75 (90% CI = 1.01–9.68). Confounders of smoking and alcohol consumption did not explain the excess.

Edelman,[46] in reviewing 13 cohort studies, found 2 of 13 studies with SMRs that showed a statistically significant increase in risk for laryngeal cancer from asbestos exposure. Parnes[47] found no causal association among 322 workers examined at a friction products manufacturing plant, although 20% with asbestos exposure had laryngitis when compared with 11% in the lower risk group. Edelman[46] concluded asbestos might act as an irritant to the larynx.

Maier and Tisch[48] found the majority of laryngeal cancers were identified in blue-collar workers exposed to a variety of hazards, including asbestos, but did not make any conclusions concerning a causal association. A case–control analysis of 112 patients in Uruguay[49] found an odds ratio (OR) of 2.4 (95% CI = 1.2–4.8) for those with more than 21 years of asbestos exposure.

In a case–control study[28] of 545 cases of squamous cell cancer of the upper gastrointestinal tract compared with 641 referents among Swedish men age 40–79 years living in two regions between 1988 and 1990, the RR for laryngeal cancer in the highest exposure group was 1.8 (95% CI = 1.1–3.0).

In a case–control study of occupational exposure to asbestos and controlled for smoking and alcohol, the authors[50] found an excess of hypopharyngeal cancer (OR = 1.8, 95% CI = 1.1–2.7), which was consistent with an IARC case–control study that found an OR of 2.1 (95% CI = 1.2–3.8) associated with cancers of the hypopharynx and epilarynx, both of which are anatomically contiguous and have similar histologic characteristics, thus making a shared etiology plausible. The highest risk was for the epilarynx at the highest asbestos exposure (OR = 2.22, 95% CI = 1.05–4.70). The authors[50] found a nonstatistical excess for laryngeal cancer, which they concluded pointed in the same direction as those significant for the subsites. The authors[50] did not find any significant interaction between smoking and asbestos for laryngeal cancer.

In a Japanese study[51] of 525 autopsy cases of asbestosis between 1958 and 1996 compared with 1,055,734 nonasbestosis cases, laryngeal cancers were significantly more frequent (6 observed vs. 3 expected, or 1.1% compared with 0.3%, χ^2 = 12.0, $p < .001$).

In a review by Browne and Gee[37] of mortality and prospective morbidity studies, the authors[37] found only one of the mortality studies had clear evidence of an excess for laryngeal cancer (8 observed vs. 3 expected; SMR = 2.7, 95% CI = 1.15–5.25), and of two morbidity studies, one study had a significant excess for those hired between 1928 and 1940 (5 observed vs. 0.9 expected; SMR = 5.5, 95% CI = 1.8–12.9), whereas those hired after 1940 did not (9 observed vs. 7.5 expected; SMR = 1.2, 95% CI = 0.55–2.28). The latter finding might reflect an inadequate latency factor for those hired after 1940. It appears the authors[37] grouped their analysis together for the 22 mortality studies, then summed the observed and expected values for all studies, and then calculated an SMR for the total to reach the conclusion that there was no causal association between asbestos and laryngeal cancer, a technique not epidemiologically valid for such analysis without weighting the studies for comparison to account for their heterogeneity. In reviewing case–control studies, the authors[37] excluded three studies because of reported methodological errors and included 17 other studies on which the authors[37] made no comment as to their methodological validity. As a result, the authors[37] concluded that the 17 studies showed no causal relationship on the basis of the nonsignificance of 15 of the studies when comparing them with two studies having statistical significance. Such analysis equating studies on the basis of only additive numerical analysis and not considering the various weights of the individual studies is misleading and represents a misapplication of the methods used for meta-analysis.

A National Institute for Occupational Safety and Health (NIOSH) study[52] of the proportionate mortality among unionized roofer and waterproofers found a statistically significant increase in cancer of the larynx with a proportionate mortality rate (PMR) of 145 (95% CI = 106–193).

Recent studies have reported elevations of laryngeal cancers among asbestos workers. A study by Musk et al.[53] in 2008 of asbestos workers at the Wittenoom crocidolite mine in Western Australia between 1943 and 1966 assessed the mortality of some 7000 male miners and millers. The authors[53] did two analyses in calculating the SMRs. The first was to calculate an SMR assuming that those lost to follow-up were alive unless they had reached 85 years of age. In this analysis, laryngeal cancers were not statistically significant with 13 observed and 8 expected (95% CI = 0.83–2.62). However, when the authors[53] censored all subjects at the date last known to be alive, the SMR rose to 2.57 (8 observed vs. 5 expected, 95% CI = 1.37–4.39). The authors[53] concluded that the true SMR was somewhere between those two estimates.

Purdue et al.[30] reported a study of some 227 cases of laryngeal carcinoma in a cohort of Swedish construction workers as well as 171 SCCs of the oral cavity and 112 pharyngeal SCCs, which found an RR of 1.9 for laryngeal SCC with 95% CI of 1.2–3.1. An excess risk of pharyngeal cancer was also found (RR = 1.9, 95% CI = 1.2–3.1); however, no occupational exposures were associated with an increased risk for oral cancer. There was no significant change to the findings after adjustment for cigarette pack-years.

One of the more persuasive case–control studies is that reported by Gustavsson et al.[28] in 1998. This study[28] represented a case–control analysis dealing with the incidence of laryngeal cancer and was based on all men aged 40–79 years who were born in Sweden and lived near Stockholm or the southern health care region, which amounted to approximately 750,000 men. The population was followed from January 1988 to January 31, 1991. The study[28] involved some 545 cases of laryngeal carcinoma for which exposure histories were obtained and 641 referents. This study adjusted for tobacco smoking, alcohol consumption, geographical region, and age. Exposure to asbestos was associated with an increased risk of laryngeal cancer with a dose–response relationship. The RR was 1.82 (95% CI = 1.1–3.0) in the highest exposure group. This study[28] also took into account cumulative asbestos exposure—not expressed as fiber-years but instead as quartiles ranging from unexposed, to Quartiles I–IV "… of increasing cumulative doses, on the basis of the quartiles of the distribution of cumulative dose among the exposed referents." Unconditional logistic regression accounted for age, region, alcohol consumption (four classes), and tobacco smoking (never/ex/current smokers). Model III (RRs adjusted for age, region, alcohol and tobacco) showed an RR of 1.16 for Quartile I, increasing to 1.35 for Quartile II, 1.56 for Quartile III, and 1.8 for Quartile IV (95% CI = 1.1–3.0). Trend testing for Model III gave a statistically significant trend in relation to a dose–response relationship (p = .02).

In this context, the USIMCA surveyed numerous epidemiologic studies representing both cohort and case-referent studies, including effects modifiers in the form of smoking and asbestos exposure, in a report published in 2006 entitled *Asbestos: Selected Cancers*.[29] In this context, the USIMCA reviewed the results for 35 cohort populations and 18 case–control studies as well as experimental evidence. In dealing with the issue of consistency, the Review document[29] stated:

> Asbestos exposure was associated with increased risk of laryngeal cancer in all nine large cohort studies (those with at least 10 cases or of deaths from laryngeal cancer and in both the cohort and case-control combined analyses). Some evidence of a dose–response relationship in risk was seen in both the cohort and the case control studies. … Several case–control studies that stratified on tobacco smoking observed higher risk among men who were exposed than in those not exposed to asbestos, although these analyses did not simultaneously stratify on asbestos, tobacco and alcohol.

In addressing the strength of association, the Institute of Medicine document[29] commented:

> The RR of laryngeal cancer among persons with any occupational exposure to asbestos compared with those who reported no exposure was 1.40 (95% CI = 1.19–1.64) in the meta-analysis of the cohort populations and 1.43 (95% CI = 1.15–1.78) in the case–control studies. … The aggregate estimates of RR in the most highly exposed subjects in either type of study ranged from 1.38 to 2.57.

In addressing coherence of the evidence, the USIMCA addressed the issue of biological plausibility and considered several limitations in that evidence, including "… the absence of clinical data documenting that asbestos fibers accumulate and persist in the larynx and the lack of experimental support from animal studies."

In the Conclusion section, the Report[29] commented:

> Considering all lines of evidence, the committee placed greater weight on the consistency of the epidemiologic studies and the biologic plausibility of the hypothesis than on the lack of confirmatory evidence from animal studies or documentation of fiber deposition in the larynx. The committee concluded that the evidence is *sufficient* to infer a causal relationship between asbestos exposure and laryngeal cancer.

Position Paper 22[32] from the Industrial Injuries Advisory Council (IIAC) in the United Kingdom on *Laryngeal Cancer and Asbestos Exposure* also surveyed some of the literature, including the U.S. Institute of Medicine Review, which is described therein as a "… high quality review carried out by the U.S. National Academy of Sciences … ." In its Conclusion section, the IIAC position paper[32] stated that although a number of epidemiological studies have "… indicated an increased risk in asbestos-exposed workers, in general risks have not been more than doubled, and have typically been less than 1.5." Because the IIAC requires an RR of 2.0 or more for attribution in cases of compensation, the document concluded that the data were "… not sufficiently robust to support prescription." However, in the final paragraph, the IIAC stated that it would keep the matter under review and would monitor further research findings. The IIAC also noted that the WHO IARC proposed to conduct a review of cancers related to asbestos exposure in 2009, "... the findings from which the Council will scrutinize."

As a follow-up to the IIAC document,[32] a preliminary/special report from the IARC[35] was published in *Lancet Oncology* in May 2009. It is notable that the IARC document[35] states:

> Sufficient evidence is now available to show that asbestos also causes cancer of the larynx and of the ovary. A meta-analysis of cohort studies reported an RR of cancer of the larynx of 1.4 (95% CI 1.2–1.6) for "any" exposure to asbestos. With different exposure metrics, the RR for "high" exposure *versus* "none" was at least 2.0 (1.6–2.5).

In addition, cancer of the larynx is now recognized in Germany for the purposes of compensation by Public Health Authorities, this regulation having been introduced in 1997[54] (see also Baur and Czuppon[55]). The basis for the German regulation was laid out in the BK-Report 1/97 *Faserjahre* (Appendix 10),[56] which reviewed the evidence and reported on an independent meta-analysis of case–control and cohort studies up to 1996.[57] The meta-analysis of cohort studies gave an overall RR of 1.5 (95% CI = 1.3–1.86). Case–control studies gave a range of ORs from 0.92 to 14.5, with most between 1 and 2. Meta-analysis gave an overall OR of 1.58 (95% CI = 1.32–1.90). When studies that did not adjust for smoking and alcohol were excluded, this became 1.4 (95% CI = 1.15–1.71).

The requirement in Germany for the probabilistic causal attribution of laryngeal cancer to asbestos exposure is cumulative exposure amounting or equivalent to 25 fibers/mL-years[54] (i.e., a cumulative exposure to asbestos equivalent to the criteria set forth for lung cancer in the Helsinki Criteria[58]). This being so, the number of asbestos-associated laryngeal cancers attributed to asbestos in Germany is small.[54] For example, Baur and Czuppon[55] indicated that about 15 cases of laryngeal carcinoma were "recognized" in 1995 in comparison with 648 cases of lung cancer.

Among the present authors, Hammar, Henderson, and Leigh consider that carcinoma of the larynx (SCC) can be attributed to substantial exposure to asbestos on the same criteria as for attribution of lung cancer according to the cumulative exposure model. Another of the authors, Dr. Lemen, has expressed concerns that such attribution on the basis of the Helsinki Consensus related to lung cancer may have an inherent methodological bias toward the impact of amphibole asbestos and thus may not be sufficiently inclusive to reflect the attribution of chrysotile asbestos to cancer. Thus, he (R.A.L.) cautions using such criteria without considerations that account for the role that short/long thin chrysotile may play in contribution to pathological responses including cancer. The case for attribution is strongest when other causal factors are absent (e.g., for one of our cases, the asbestos-exposed worker was a former light smoker with cessation of smoking 36 years before the clinical onset of his laryngeal SCC and he did not consume alcohol).

8.4 OTHER MALIGNANT DISEASES

Richard A. Lemen

8.4.1 Gastrointestinal Cancers

Gastrointestinal tract cancers, which are the most common of the other malignant diseases associated with asbestos, have RRs ranging from 0.5[59] to 3.1.[60,61] By the 1960s, epidemiological studies suggested that exposure to asbestos was the cause for the increase in gastrointestinal tract malignancies.[62–64]

Selikoff et al.[62] found stomach, colon, and rectal cancers increased three times more than expected (29 vs. 9.4; RR = 3.09, 95% CI = 2.07–4.43). Among 370 New York–New Jersey asbestos insulation workers, 12 stomach, colon, and rectal cancers were observed when 3.09 were expected (RR = 3.90, 95% CI = 2.01–6.81).[61]

At the meeting of the New York Academy of Sciences, Mancuso[65] reported during a discussion of these papers that he had located 16 additional deaths since his original publication: 5 were due to cancer—1 lung, 1 stomach, 1 colon, and 2 rectal carcinomas—which increased their earlier observation to 11 gastrointestinal cancers, whereas 4.55 had been expected. Mancuso and El-Attar[60] reported SMRs in the 25- to 44-year age group of 264 and 1235 after cumulative employment years of 2.1–7.0 and 7.1–12.0, respectively.

Selikoff[66] found increased rates for cancer of the stomach and esophagus (20 observed vs. 6.46 expected; SMR = 3.09, 95% CI = 1.89–4.78) and for cancer of the colon (23 observed vs. 7.64 expected; SMR = 3.01, 95% CI = 1.91–4.52) among 632 asbestos workers from New Jersey and New York. In a larger study of 17,800 asbestos insulation workers from the United States and Canada, Selikoff et al.[67] reported similar observations for cancer of the esophagus (18 observed vs. 7.1 expected; SMR = 2.54, 95% CI = 1.50–4.00), stomach (18 observed vs. 14.2 expected; SMR = 1.27, 95% CI = 0.75–2.00), and colon and rectum (58 observed vs. 38.1 expected; SMR = 1.52, 95% CI = 1.16–1.97).

Others have observed similar results for gastrointestinal cancers among workers exposed to asbestos in various countries.[68–70] Schneiderman,[71] then senior statistician for the National Cancer Institute, concluded that "increased exposure to inhaled asbestos particles leads to increased digestive system cancer." Newhouse and Berry[72] reported an RR of 2.11 among male asbestos factory workers with <2 years of exposure (20 observed vs. 9.5 expected; calculated 95% CI = 1.29–3.25) and of 2.32 with >2 years of exposure (19 observed vs. 8.2 expected; calculated 95% CI = 1.40–3.62). For women, the corresponding SMRs were 2.46 (14 observed vs. 5.7 expected; calculated 95% CI = 1.34–4.12) and 3.46 (9 observed vs. 2.6 expected; calculated 95% CI = 1.58–6.57), respectively.

McDonald et al.[73] reported abdominal cancer in men with 20 years latency and with cumulative dust exposures of 231.6 at 10 to <20 mppcf-years, 247.0 at 20 to <40 mppcf-years, and 383.6 at 40 to <80 mppcf-years. Nine of the 12 deaths were from colon and rectal cancers.

Enterline et al.[74] reported on the mortality of cancer in a cohort of 1074 white men followed until death and found the expected number of deaths from cancers of the stomach, large intestine, and rectum to be 30.99 when 43 were observed (SMR = 1.43, 95% CI = 1.03–1.92), with the SMR for stomach cancer being 180.4 ($p < .05$).

In a fiber-year analysis study,[75] a dose–response relationship was reported for gastrointestinal cancers with years since first exposure, increasing the SMR rate from less than unity during the first 20 years to 231 after 20–45 years, 273 after 25–29 years, and 500 after 30–34 years from first exposure.

Another review on the epidemiology of gastric cancer and its risk factors[76] pointed out that many methodological problems have cast doubt on the causal association between asbestos exposure and gastrointestinal cancers. Although such methodological errors were never discussed in the review, the authors[76] pointed to only one study[77] to dispute an association—the study by de Klerk et al.,[77] which involved heavy exposure to crocidolite with no observed excess of gastrointestinal cancers, although this study also suffered from a major demographic problem: that being more than 25% of the total cohort of 6506 were lost to follow-up. However, de Klerk et al.[77] considered their methods of follow-up would have been unlikely to have missed any excess stomach cancers and the effect of this would be slight.

Albin et al.[78] reported an RR of 3.4 (95% CI = 1.2–9.5) among asbestos cement workers with ≥40 fibers/mL-years for colon and rectal cancers. A case–control study among pipefitters and boilermakers[79] reported an OR for colon cancer of 10.7 (95% CI = 1.07–10.3).

That it was biologically plausible for fibers to pass through the human gastrointestinal mucosa under conditions in the alimentary canal was shown by Cook and Olson[80] when they demonstrated that sediment in human urine contained amphibole fibers. Asbestos fibers and asbestos body formation have been identified in tumor tissue taken from the colons of asbestos-exposed workers.[81]

Reports of gastrointestinal tract cancers associated with asbestos exposure have been reviewed by the WHO,[82] with the conclusion that "overall, [it] seems that there is a correlation between lung cancer and gastrointestinal cancer rates in occupational cohorts [exposed to asbestos] which is not due to chance." Both the Surgeon General of the United States and the Department of Health, Education, and Welfare concluded that past asbestos exposure can result in an excess of gastrointestinal cancers.[83,84]

Frumkin and Berlin[85] carried out a meta-analysis to estimate the risk of gastrointestinal cancer mortality. They divided their exposure categories for asbestos exposure into two groups: the first representing heavy asbestos exposure as defined by any cohort having an SMR of 200 or greater for lung cancer and the second representing low asbestos exposure as defined by any cohort with an SMR less than 200. In the cohort with high exposure to asbestos, all gastrointestinal cancers except esophageal cancer were significantly elevated with 95% CI that exceeded 100. For the low-exposure cohorts, all SMRs were close to 100 for all gastrointestinal cancers.

In another meta-analysis, Homa et al.[86] reported that the summarized SMR for colorectal cancer in cohorts exposed only to amphibole asbestos was 1.47 (95% CI = 1.09–2.00) as compared with those cohorts exposed to chrysotile, which was 1.04 (95% CI = 0.81–1.33).

In a study by Kang et al.,[87] death certificate data were analyzed from 4,943,566 decedents from 28 states in the United States between 1979 and 1990. The authors[87] identified 15,524 cases of gastrointestinal cancer among 12 occupational groups having elevated PMRs for mesothelioma, a sentinel tumor for exposure to asbestos, and found slightly elevated PMRs for esophageal cancer (108, 95% CI = 107–110), gastric cancer (110, 95% CI = 106–113), and colorectal cancer (109, 95% CI = 107–110). The authors[87] from the NIOSH concluded that their large death certificate study supported an association between asbestos exposure and some gastrointestinal cancers.

Results of a mortality study[88] of textile and cement pipe manufacturers between 1933 and 1980 found the mortality rate for colon cancers to be statistically significant (27 observed vs. 14.78 expected; SMR = 1.83, 95% CI = 1.20–2.66).

Stomach cancer was elevated among rubber workers who worked in the early production stages of mixing and weighing, which the authors[89] concluded might point to the role of either asbestos-contaminated talc or carbon black. However, their[89] results did not support the causal role of nitrosamines. The role of carbon black in the etiology of stomach cancer was also not supported.[90]

The risk of stomach cancer was evaluated for 12 workplace hazards, including asbestos, but no significant relationship was found.[91] The study[91] was a death certificate analysis from 24 states in the United States using exposure data from a variety of sources, including two textbooks, computerized databases from OSHA and NIOSH, unpublished industrial hygiene reports, and personal experiences. The exposure surveys on the basis of the computerized databases, while containing some quantifiable data, were mainly based on subjective interpretation by the surveyors. Any use of the two textbooks for exposure classification was questionable because of the very limited exposure data reported and the inaccuracy of converting mppcf to fibers per milliliter. As one author[92] warned, using such conversions is done "… with considerable risk to the validity of the results." Readers of the paper cannot judge the author's conclusions adequately when based on unpublished industrial hygiene data or personal experiences. Given these factors, the validity of the author's conclusions must be questioned.

Limited evidence has shown an association between gastric cancer and asbestos exposure. In a plant manufacturing fireproof textiles and friction materials, a digestive cancer registry since 1978 was analyzed. The authors[93] did not find any significant excess of digestive cancers, except for the peritoneum. However, more than expected deaths occurred for other digestive cancers, which led the authors[93] to conclude that their study provided initial evidence suggesting a relationship between occupational exposure to asbestos and risk of digestive cancer and that evidence of a dose–effect relationship was seen among the whole population at risk. An important finding of this study was that the authors[93] considered that intensity of exposure was more important than duration of exposure.

In a multicenter case–control study of gastric cancer[94] in Italy involving interviews with 640 histologically confirmed male cases and 959 controls randomly selected from the resident populations of the study areas, the authors[94] found workers with 21+ years of potential exposure had no significant increase in risk related to asbestos exposure.

In a study[95] of 1756 male workers at a nitrate fertilizer plant employed for 1 year or more between 1947 and 1980 and who used asbestos and nitrogen derivatives for surrogates of individual exposure, the authors[95] found a slight increase of stomach cancer (28 observed vs. 19.9 expected; RR = 1.41, 95% CI = 0.93–2.03).

In a study of Norwegian lighthouse keepers exposed to asbestos in their drinking water, which was collected in cisterns off roofs made of asbestos cement tile, the water was found to contain fiber concentrations ranging from 1,760 to 71,350 million fibers per liter, which was higher than that measured in the general Norwegian water supply.[96] Measurements were taken 20 years after the roof tiles were installed, and those lighthouse keepers with 20 years latency or more had a stomach cancer incidence of 11 observed when only 4.57 were expected (RR = 2.41, 95% CI = 1.20–4.31). These increases in stomach cancer occurred during a period of time when the overall rate of stomach cancer was decreasing for men and women in all age groups in Norway.[97]

Case reports have identified associations between exposure to asbestos and gastrointestinal cancer. Case reports taken alone and without connection to the numerous epidemiological studies, as discussed previously, would be mostly of clinical interest or suggestive of hypothesis; however, when connected with well-controlled and conducted epidemiological studies, they are of greater importance. In a series of five cases of double cancers involving the lung and stomach[98] and after ascertaining whether the subjects had exposure to asbestos, three were confirmed to have such occupational histories and many crocidolite fibers were found in their autopsied lungs. The authors[98] suggested that there could be an association between these three cancers and their exposures to asbestos. One case report of an 84-year-old man with pleural plaques with calcification and a history of working in shipyards with known asbestos exposure presented with cancer of the stomach and colon.[99] Asbestos bodies were found in his autopsied lung tissue. Given the epidemiological literature, the authors[99] suggested that there might be an association with exposure to asbestos. In a series of 35 primary multiple cancers confirmed at autopsy,[100] lung and stomach cancers were the main components. Twenty-five cases (71%) were proven to have exposure to asbestos and 13 cases had asbestos bodies in 5 g of autopsied wet lung tissue, which calculated to more than 1000 asbestos bodies overall. The authors,[100] given the epidemiological literature, suggested that asbestos exposure might possibly have induced a high incidence of multiple cancers. Kishimoto and Shimamoto[101] reported 10 cases of double cancers of the lung and stomach—five cases developed their cancers simultaneously whereas the other five developed their lung cancer after surgery for the stomach cancer. Eight cases had histories of asbestos exposure, and almost all had significantly high numbers of asbestos bodies in autopsied lung tissue; the fiber type found in the lungs was chrysotile only. The final case report by Kishimoto and Yamaguchi[102] described a 76-year-old man with simultaneous cancers of the lung and stomach. Histologically, the two tumors were different (stomach: well-differentiated tubular adenocarcinoma; and lung: moderately differentiated papillary adenocarcinoma). Although the stomach cancer was in an early stage, the lung cancer was stage IIIa. The man was reported to have had definite exposure to asbestos in a Japanese naval shipyard. On radiography, pleural plaques with calcification were identified, as were numerous asbestos bodies (chrysotile and tremolite) in resected lung tissue. Although the man was a heavy smoker, the authors[102] suggested that asbestos exposure and smoking were etiological factors independently and together acted synergistically for cancer development in the lung.

8.4.2 Ovarian Cancers

The first suggestion that asbestos could be associated with ovarian carcinoma was by Keal,[103] who in 1960 reported that by 1953 an impression was formed that women with pulmonary asbestosis more frequently suffered from ovarian cancers than other women in the same London hospital. Of 23 women with a diagnosis of asbestosis, 15 had died and 9 had intra-abdominal neoplasms. Of those nine, one had ovarian cancer and four had peritoneal growths possibly of ovarian origin. Keal[103] considered this to be more than just coincidence and that metastasis from an undiagnosed lung cancer seemed unlikely.

By 1967, Graham and Graham[104] made observations during clinical studies of a diagnostic procedure for detecting ovarian cancer and gave results of an experimental study between asbestos and ovarian cancers that an association between asbestos and ovarian cancer might exist. In the experimental study, Swiss mice, Syrian hamsters, guinea pigs, and Dutch rabbits received a single intraperitoneal injection of tremolite asbestos. Epithelial changes in the ovaries of the guinea pigs and rabbits occurred and were similar to those seen in patients with ovarian cancers. These findings, along with findings of birefringent crystalline material in the ovaries with early malignant changes, suggested that asbestos was an etiologic factor in ovarian cancers.

It has been difficult to draw conclusions on the basis of epidemiologic studies of ovarian cancers because, histologically, their distinction between peritoneal mesothelioma and carcinomatosis peritonei (including primary peritoneal serous papillary adenocarcinoma) is difficult. Ovarian tumors tend to grow by local extension and uncommonly metastasize through the blood stream, which is similar to tumors of mesothelial origin according to Longo and Young.[105]

Newhouse and Berry[72] evaluated the mortality of more than 900 women in an asbestos factory, but because of name changes due to marriage, these were hard to trace; thus, the vital status for only 77% was known by the end of 1971. Because the last date of entry into the cohort was 1942, all women had 30 or more years of exposure. By the end of 1975, 225 of the women had died. The company used crocidolite heavily in the textile department. The analysis, however, included all women, not just production workers but also low-exposure or no-exposure workers, including office, canteen, and other low-exposure jobs. An excess of ovarian cancers was found among women in the heavily exposed jobs with three observed and 0.74 expected ($p < .05$; calculated 95% CI = 0.84–11.85). The low percentage of follow-up might have missed significant causes of mortality for the women and thus may have underestimated their overall risk for certain diseases, including ovarian cancers. The authors[72] called their finding significant at the $p < .05$ level, but by my (R.A.L.) calculations, this was insignificant.

A study[106] of 500 female gas mask assemblers exposed to asbestos (mainly crocidolite) during World War II found an excess of ovarian cancers with 5 observed and 0.63 expected (RR = 7.9, calculated 95% CI = 2.58–18.52). The authors[106] stated that the excess of ovarian cancers was unexpected but appeared to be related to asbestos exposure.

In another study by Newhouse et al.[107] concerning the mortality of an East End of London asbestos textile and other asbestos products factory using all three major types of asbestos (crocidolite, amosite, and chrysotile), an excess of ovarian cancer was found. Only 77% of the women's vital status was known out of the 932 women in the cohort. The maximum period of follow-up was 44 years, with a minimum of 38 years. There were nine deaths from ovarian cancer. In five cases categorized to have severe exposure for more than 2 years, the excess was statistically significant at the $p < .01$ level (0.9 expected; calculated RR = 5.56, 95% CI = 1.80–12.96). As in this case, the low percentage of follow-up as well as a total mortality rate of only 39% might have missed significant causes of death and thus may have underestimated their overall risk for certain diseases, including ovarian cancers. In what appears to be a follow-up to the Newhouse et al.[107] report, Berry et al.[88] continued the follow-up of those not lost to follow-up in the original cohort. Berry et al.[88] reported nine deaths from ovarian cancer (3.56 expected)—the same as in 1985—and gave an SMR of 2.52

(95% CI = 1.16–4.80). In the first paper by Newhouse et al.,[107] it was stated that five ovarian cancers occurred in the greatest exposure group but now the number of deaths (n = 5) occurred in the same highest exposure group of >2 years duration resulting in an SMR of 5.56 (0.90 expected, 95% CI = 1.80–12.96).

In a cohort of rock salt workers in Italy, the authors[108] observed two deaths from ovarian cancer when 0.42 were expected (SMR = 4.76, 95% CI = 0.58–17.20) and one case of a benign ovarian tumor. The two deaths had latency periods of 12 and 13 years, whereas the benign case had a latency of 19 years. A periodic environmental hygiene survey found chrysotile asbestos in the boiler and in the vapor-carrying piping system. Two cases of pleural mesothelioma were identified. One hundred deaths were identified out of 487 subjects (367 men and 120 women). The authors[108] stated that the main limitations of the study were the small number of subjects and exposure defined in terms of duration of employment only.

A mortality study[109] in Germany of 616 women occupationally exposed to asbestos found two cases of ovarian cancer when 1.8 were expected, giving a standardized PMR of 1.09 (95% CI = 0.13–3.95), which was not statistically significant.

A cohort mortality study[110] of 631 women compensated for asbestosis in Italy observed an excess of ovarian cancers. Of those who worked in the textile industry, four developed ovarian cancer resulting in an SMR of 526 (95% CI = 143–1347). Of those in the asbestos cement industry, five developed ovarian cancer, resulting in an SMR of 540 (95% CI = 175–1261). Overall, the nine observed ovarian cancers resulted in an SMR of 477 (95% CI = 218–906). During this same year, Vasama-Neuvonen et al.[111] published an article on ovarian cancers in Finland and found that medium to high exposures to asbestos produced a standard incidence ratio (SIR) of 1.30 (95% CI = 0.9–1.80), which constituted a weak indication for an elevated risk.

A cohort of pulp and paper mill workers was studied[112] in Norway to evaluate the relationship between asbestos exposure and ovarian cancer. Forty-six ovarian cancers were matched with four controls each. The result was an OR of 2.02 (95% CI = 0.72–5.66), again constituting a weak indication for an elevated risk.

Crocidolite asbestos was a major type of asbestos mined and used in Australia, and the impact on women has been studied for both incidence and mortality among women and girls exposed environmentally and occupationally at Wittenoom, Western Australia. The mortality study by Reid et al.[113] in 2008 found increased mortality for ovarian cancers, but not statistically significant among women and girls living in the Wittenoom area between 1943 and 1992. The mortality of the residential women and girls accounted for nine ovarian cancer deaths for an SMR of 126 (95% CI = 0.58–2.40) for the subcohort of women lost to follow-up and censored as of December 31, 2004, whereas those in the second subcohort of women lost to follow-up and censored as of the date last known to be alive had an SMR of 1.52 (95% CI = 0.69–2.88).

In a second study by Reid et al.[114] in 2009, the incidence was assessed among residents (n = 2552) and workers (n = 416) at the Australian Blue Asbestos Industry in Wittenoom. The overall SIR for all women followed to the earliest date of diagnosis, date of death, date at age 85 years, or date last known to be alive was 1.27 (n = 11 ovarian cancers, 95% CI = 0.52–2.02). For workers with the same parameters, the SIR was 0.65 (n = 1 ovarian cancer, 95% CI = 0.02–3.64), and for residents, the SIR was 1.40 (n = 10 ovarian cancers, 95% CI = 0.53–2.28). Twenty-two percent of the women were lost to follow-up, which the authors[114] stated might have underestimated the number of gynecologic (including ovarian) and breast cancers that may have occurred among the Wittenoom women.

In observing mortality among a cohort of Italian asbestos cement workers,[33] nine ovarian cancers were observed when four expected for an SMR of 2.35 (95% CI = 1.03–4.27). Crocidolite and chrysotile asbestos were used in the factory. In looking at mortality data for wives of the same cement plant factory workers studied by Magnani et al.,[33] 11 deaths were observed when 7.7 were expected for an SMR of 1.42 (95% CI = 0.71–2.54).

Certainly, the observation by Heller et al.[115] of asbestos fibers in the ovary shows the biological plausibility of asbestos fibers to reach the ovaries. The IARC[35] concluded there was sufficient evidence in humans that asbestos can cause ovarian cancer.

8.4.3 Kidney Cancers

Auerbach et al.[116] stated that asbestos bodies have been found in the kidney, which they believed could have formed in the lung and then migrated to the kidney or that the asbestos fibers themselves may have migrated and then formed the asbestos bodies in the kidney, which is the theory the authors favored. Higher than background risks of kidney cancer have been reported among men in asbestos mining areas of Quebec.[117] Selikoff et al.[67] reported an RR of 2.3 for renal cancer among 17,800 asbestos insulators in their study.

In a discussion paper published in *Dust and Disease*, Cook[118] reported finding amphibole asbestos fibers in human urine derived from drinking water, which lead to the conclusion that asbestos fibers can translocate to the kidney.

Harber et al.,[119] in a study of 1500 asbestos-exposed workers, found malignancies of the kidney that the authors[119] considered to be related to asbestos exposure.

MacLure,[120] in a case–control study of 518 renal adenocarcinomas identified between 1981 and 1984 from 37 Massachusetts area hospitals, found the incidence of asbestos-induced renal adenocarcinoma to be 1.6, with a one-sided 95% CI of 1.0, leading MacLure[120] to conclude that asbestos was a cause of renal adenocarcinoma in his study.

Smith et al.[121] analyzed three cohorts having an RR in excess of 2 for lung cancer and found all three cohorts[68,74,122] had an excess of kidney cancers. Kidney cancer in the three cohorts had SMRs of 2.22 (95% CI = 1.44–3.30),[68] 2.76 (95% CI = 1.29–5.18),[74] and 1.63 (95% CI = 1.31–2.00).[122] Smith et al.[121] concluded that because of the results in their analysis, good evidence existed that asbestos can reach the target site for kidney cancers, and because animal evidence also supported a causal association with kidney cancer, it was probable that asbestos exposure can cause kidney cancer in humans.

Pesch et al.[123] opined that the Smith et al.[121] analysis disputed the role of asbestos in the etiology of kidney cancer, which is quite the opposite of the conclusions reached by Smith et al.[121] In a letter to the editor commenting on the Smith et al.[121] analysis, Enterline and Henderson[124] concluded that the available data pointed to asbestos as a cause of kidney cancer in humans.

In a continuing evaluation of North American insulators through 1986, Seidman and Selikoff[125] reaffirmed that the major causes of mortality continued with about the same distributions, including those for kidney cancers. In New South Wales, asbestos was found to significantly increase the risk of kidney cancer (RR = 1.62, 95% CI = 1.04–2.53).[126]

McDonald et al.[127] found elevated numbers of kidney cancers in workers having accumulated exposures of 300 mppcf-years, but with no dose–response tendency. In looking at risk factors for renal cancer in Denmark,[128] a high number of cases were reported to be related to asbestos exposure according to the authors.

An international renal cell cancer study[129] found that when looking at occupation, asbestos-exposed occupations resulted in an RR of 1.4 (95% CI = 1.1–1.8). The authors[129] stated that except for asbestos exposure, no other occupational exposure or occupation had consistently been linked with kidney cancer.

Although a review of case–control studies of asbestos exposure and renal cancers was negative, McLaughlin et al.[130] concluded the power of the studies were too limited because of the low number of workers exposed but did report two case–control studies from Denmark and Australia that showed elevated risks.

Kidney cancers were increased among deck officers of merchant seamen potentially exposed to asbestos after three years of employment (OR = 2.15, 95% CI = 1.14–4.08).[131]

In a study of male Wistar rats,[132] the control group received intratracheal injections of saline and the amosite group received intratracheal injections of amosite solution. The rats were sacrificed after 6 months, and the amosite-exposed group developed glomerulosclerosis and tubulointerstitial fibrosis. Another group exposed for 2 h per day to passive smoking developed glomerulosclerosis and tubulointerstitial fibrosis. When both exposures were combined, there appeared to be an additive effect.

In a review of the epidemiology of kidney cancers, Pascual and Borque[133] concluded that asbestos was a factor in increasing the risk of renal cell carcinoma.

Sawazaki et al.[134] reported two cases of combined renal cell carcinoma and malignant mesothelioma, one in a 66-year-old man exposed to asbestos for 43 years.

On the basis of these articles, there appears to be a causal association between kidney (renal) cell carcinoma and asbestos exposure.

8.4.4 Lymphomas

Multiple studies have reported lymphomas in persons exposed to asbestos. Lymphomas encompass more than 40 related diseases that develop from lymphocytes.[135] The American Cancer Society estimates that lymphomas account for approximately 5% of all cancers in the United States, the majority being non-Hodgkin lymphomas. One study published in 2001 reviewing the epidemiological literature from six cohort studies and 16 case–control studies published through 1999 concluded that their combined analysis indicated a low increase in risk from exposure to asbestos and that future epidemiologic studies should concentrate on defining such risks.[136]

Schwartz et al.[137] observed an association between chronic lymphocytic leukemia and asbestos exposure and concluded that because of the pattern of immunologic abnormalities occurring in asbestos-exposed persons, their observation deserved further study.

The most recent study analyzing the relationship between asbestos exposure and malignant lymphoma was a multicenter case–control study[138] in Germany and Italy. The authors[138] observed no statistically significant association between cumulative asbestos exposure and the risk of any lymphoma subtype. However, an elevated risk was found for the association between exposure to more than 2.6 fiber-years (of asbestos) and multiple myeloma (OR = 6.0, 95% CI = 1.4–25.1), although the numbers were small ($n = 3$ cases; $n = 12$ control subjects). The authors[138] concluded their study did not support an association between asbestos exposure and risk of malignant lymphoma.

8.4.5 Systemic Carcinogen

Because of multiple sites of cancer in various epidemiologic studies of asbestos-exposed persons, albeit lacking statistical significance in some instances, some have suggested the possibility that asbestos could act as a systemic carcinogen in the etiology of these cancers. In other words, asbestos itself may have other biological mechanisms not directly affecting the site of the asbestos fibers final disposition, possibly involving the immune system and overriding existing defense mechanisms. This has been suggested because of the observance of leukopenia in the peripheral blood of asbestos miners[139] as well as the effects on the immune system of asbestos workers as observed by Turner-Warwick and Parkes,[140] Lange and Skibinski,[141] Lange et al.,[142,145] and Lange.[143,144]

Goldsmith[146] presented evidence to support such a theory when he analyzed 11 cohorts of asbestos-exposed persons. Reviews of the effects on the immune system also supported such a theory.[147–149] Systemic immunity appears to occur immediately after asbestos exposure and then tends to lag behind those of the local immunity during the later depressive effects of the asbestos fibers and also tends to exhibit a dose-dependent initial enhancement.[150] Such findings may have further importance as they may help determine the identity of biomarkers. One such finding to support this concept is the systemic changes in the levels of CC16, a pneumoprotein found in smoking and nonsmoking asbestos-exposed persons.[151]

In a study by Pelclová et al.[152] of 61 asbestos-exposed patients with mean exposures of 24.6 years when compared with 39 nonexposed controls, positive antineutrophil cytoplasmic antibodies (ANCAs) were detected significantly more frequently in the asbestos-exposed group compared with the controls ($p = .034$; 21.3% in the asbestos patients vs. 5.1% in the controls). However, diseases associated with ANCAs were not more frequent in the asbestos-exposed group than in the controls. The authors[152] concluded that events other than asbestos exposure were necessary to initiate vasculitic injury such as the necrotic inflammation of blood vessels and ischemic injury of involved organs. The authors[152] found asbestos-induced ANCAs more readily than they did with silica exposure. In conclusion, the authors[152] stated that exposure to asbestos led to formation of ANCA, but with mostly unknown specificity.

Another study from the Slovak Republic by Ilavská et al.[153] concluded that immune cells appeared to be influenced by exposure to asbestos. In evaluating 61 asbestos workers with at least 5 years of asbestos exposure, the authors[153] found the workers had significantly increased levels of immunoglobulin E and concentrations of interleukin-6 and interleukin-8 compared with controls from in-plant and townsfolk as well as increased levels of soluble adhesion molecule ICAM-1. The alterations of immune parameters showed that the injury mechanism for asbestosis shared features with the hypersensitivity process.

Because of the knowledge that positive antinuclear antibody tests have been associated with asbestos workers, researchers at the University of Montana decided to look at a cohort from Libby, Montana, where exposures to vermiculite-containing tremolite asbestos were common in the W.R. Grace mining area and the surrounding community. The study[154] explored the possibility of exacerbated autoimmune responses. Age- and sex-matched sets of 50 serum samples were taken from the Libby and Missoula, Montana, populations. The Libby samples contained a significantly higher frequency of positive antinuclear antibody and extractable nuclear antigen tests. The Libby samples also had higher levels of serum IgA. The authors[154] concluded their study supported the role of asbestos and its association with autoimmune response as well as supporting the possibility that autoimmunity could play a role in the progression of asbestos-related diseases.

In 2006, Noonan et al.[155] conducted a nested case–control study between asbestos exposure and autoimmune disease in Libby, Montana. The case–control study involved 7307 current and former residents of Libby. Cases included persons reporting one of the systemic autoimmune diseases (SAIDs), including systemic lupus erythematosus, scleroderma, or rheumatoid arthritis (RA). The authors[155] found a significant relationship for RA (OR = 3.23, 95% CI = 1.31–7.96) in those ≥65 years of age and who worked for the vermiculite mining company and found elevated ORs for those having been exposed to asbestos in the military of 1.70 for SAIDs and 2.11 for RA. The ≥65 year age group also showed substantially elevated risk for SAIDs and RA, and for this group working at the company, there was a threefold greater risk for RA. Elevated ORs were reported for those who had frequent contact with vermiculite through various exposure pathways—for example, frequent play on vermiculite piles, vermiculite used in gardening, and so forth. The authors[155] stated that this study could suffer from exposure misclassification, self-reporting, or recall bias or from persons with chronic health conditions like SAIDs for overreporting past vermiculite exposures. However, the authors[155] contended their preliminary findings supported the hypothesis that asbestos exposure was associated with autoimmune disease.

Looking at the immunological effects of chrysotile asbestos, a Japanese team[156] reported that in comparison with most other solid tumors, mutation of the p53 gene is rare, but loss of the p16[INK4a] expression has been detected in most mesotheliomas and their cell lines. Under experimental conditions, these same cells undergo apoptosis after high-level, short-term expo-sures to asbestos because of the production of reactive oxygen species and reactive nitrogen species by activation of the mitochondrion apoptotic pathway. The authors[156] gave a detailed schematic summary of the immunological effects of asbestos in their report. To summarize, the authors[156] concluded that immunocompetent cells and other effects may be associated with the development of auto-immunity and the development of malignant neoplasms in asbestos-exposed persons.

8.5 SUMMARY

The USIMCA conducted an extensive review of the association between asbestos and colorec-tal, laryngeal, esophageal, pharyngeal, and stomach cancers.[29] The USIMCA included experts in biostatistics, epidemiology, mineralogy, oncology, toxicology, and cancer biology. The committee[29] reviewed the evidence from epidemiologic studies and toxicologic studies, both in vitro and in ani-mal models, specifically for each cancer. The evidence related to mineralogy of asbestos and its carcinogenicity were considered to be generally relevant for all sites, particularly with regard to the causal criterion of coherence or biologic plausibility. The committee[29] found a causal association or lack thereof between asbestos as listed below:

Cancer	Conclusion
Colorectal	Suggestive of, but insufficient
Esophageal	Inadequate
Laryngeal	Sufficient
Pharyngeal	Suggestive of, but insufficient
Stomach (gastrointestinal)	Suggestive of, but insufficient

We agree with the above findings by the U.S. Institute of Medicine Committee. We also find evidence of a causal relationship or lack thereof between the following cancers:

Cancer	Conclusion
Pseudomesotheliomatous lung carcinoma	Sufficient, depending on individual case data
Kidney/renal	Possible
Ovarian	Sufficient, depending on individual case data
Lymphoma	Insufficient
Autoimmune disease	Likely in many cases

REFERENCES

1. Harwood TR, Gracey DR, Yokoo H. Pseudomesotheliomatous carcinoma of the lung. A variant of periph-eral lung cancer. *Am J Clin Path* 1976;65:159–167.
2. Mills RG. Pulmonary asbestosis: report of a case. *Minn Med* 1930;130:495–499.
3. Babolini G, Blasi A. The pleural form of primary cancer of the lung. *Dis Chest* 1956;29:314–323.
4. Verga P, Botteri G. *Il carcinoma primitive del polmone.* Bologna: Cappelli; 1931.
5. Roussy G, Huguenin R. Essai de classification anatomo-clinique des cancers primitives du poumon. *Ann Anat Pathol* 1928;5:7.
6. Olmer D, Olmer G, Roume H. (Quoted by Liberti e Stella). *Mars Med* 1938;7:328.
7. Liberti R, Stella G. *Il cancro primitive del polmone.* Napoli: E.A.T.; 1949.

8. Eizaguirre E. *El Cancer Broncopulmonar*. Madrid: Paz Montalvo; 1952.

9. Koss M, Travis W, Moran C, Hochholzer. Pseudomesotheliomatous adenocarcinoma: A re-appraisal. *Semin Diagn Pathol* 1992;9:117–132.

10. Robb JA, Hammar SP, Yooko H. Pseudomesotheliomatous lung carcinoma. *Lab Invest* 1993;68:134A.

11. Hartmann C-A, Schutz H. Mesothelioma-like tumors of the pleura: A review of 72 autopsy cases. *J Cancer Res Clin Oncol* 1994;120:331–347.

12. Koss MN, Fleming M, Przygodzki RM, Sherrod A, Travis W, Hochholzer L. Adenocarcinoma simulating mesothelioma: A clinicopathologic and immunohistochemical study of 29 cases. *Ann Diagn Pathol* 1998;2:93–102.

13. Attanoos RL, Gibbs AR. Pseudomesotheliomatous carcinomas of the pleura: A 10-year analysis of cases from the Environmental Lung Disease Research Group, Cardiff. *Histopathology* 2003;43:444–452.

14. Hammar SP, Robb JA, Dodson RF, Henderson DW, Klebe S, Leigh J, et al. Pseudomesotheliomatous lung cancer (in preparation).

15. Braganza JM, Butler EB, Fox H, Hunter PM, Qureshi MS, Samarji W, Vallon AG. Ectopic production of salivary type amylase by a pseudomesotheliomatous carcinoma of the lung. *Cancer* 1978;41:1522–1525.

16. Broghamer WL Jr, Collins WM, Mojsejenko IK. The cyto-histopathology of a pseudomesotheliomatous carcinoma of the lung. *Acta Cytol* 1978;22:239–242.

17. Lin JI, Tseng CH, Tsung SH. Pseudomesotheliomatous carcinoma of the lung. *South Med J* 1980;73:655–657.

18. Nishimoto Y, Ohno T, Saito K. Pseudomesotheliomatous carcinoma of the lung with histochemical and immunohistochemical study. *Acta Pathol Jpn* 1983;33:415–423.

19. Simonsen J. Pseudomesotheliomatous carcinoma of the lung with asbestos exposure. *Am J Forensic Med Pathol* 1986;7:49–51.

20. Dessy E, Pietra GG. Pseudomesotheliomatous carcinoma of the lung: An immunohistochemical and ultrastructural study of three cases. *Cancer* 1991;68:1747–1753.

21. Brunner-La Rocca HP, Schlossberg D, Vogt P. Pseudomesotheliomatous carcinoma in HIV infection. *Dtsch Med Wochenschr* 1995;120:1312–1317.

22. Falconieri G, Zanconati F, Bussani R, Di Bonito L. Small cell carcinoma of lung simulating pleural mesothelioma: report of 4 cases with autopsy confirmation. *Pathol Res Pract* 1995;191:1147–1152.

23. Shah IA, Salvatore JR, Kummet T, Gani OS, Wheeler LA. Pseudomesotheliomatous carcinoma involving pleura and peritoneum: A clinicopathologic and immunohistochemical study of three cases. *Ann Diagn Pathol* 1999;3:148–159.

24. Attanoos RL, Suvarna SK, Rhead E, Stephens M, Locke TJ, Sheppard MN, Pooley FD, Gibbs AR. Malignant vascular tumours of the pleura in "asbestos" workers and endothelial differentiation in malignant mesothelioma. *Thorax* 2000;55:860–863.

25. Rolston R, Oury TD. Other neoplasia. In: *Pathology of Asbestos-Associated Diseases*, 2nd ed., Roggli VL, Oury TD, Sporn TA, eds. New York: Springer; 2004: 217–230.

26. Roggli VL, Greenberg SD, McLarty JL, Hurst GA, Spivey CG, Heiger LR. Asbestos body content of the larynx in asbestos workers: A study of five cases. *Arch Otolaryngol* 1980;106:533–535.

27. Hirsch A, Bignon J, Sebastien P, Gaudichet A. Asbestos fibers in laryngeal tissues: Findings in two patients with asbestosis associated with laryngeal tumors. *Chest* 1979;76:697–699.

28. Gustavsson P, Jakobsson R, Johansson H, Lewin F, Norell S, Rutkvist LE. Occupational exposures and squamous cell carcinoma of the oral cavity, pharynx, larynx, and oesophagus: A case–control study in Sweden. *Occup Environ Med* 1998;55:393–400.

29. Institute of Medicine Committee on Asbestos. *Asbestos: Selected Cancers*. Washington DC: National Academies Press; 2006.

30. Purdue MP, Järvholm B, Bergdahl IA, Hayes RB, Baris D. Occupational exposures and head and neck cancers among Swedish construction workers. *Scand J Work Environ Health* 2006;32:270–275.

31. Craighead JE. Nonthoracic cancers possibly resulting from asbestos exposure. In: *Asbestos and Its Diseases*, Craighead JE, Gibbs AR, eds. Oxford: Oxford University Press; 2008: 230–252.

32. Industrial Injuries Advisory Council (UK). Position Paper 22: Laryngeal cancer and asbestos exposure. IIAC 2008. http://www.iiac.org.uk.

33. Magnani C, Ferrante D, Barone-Adesi F, et al. Cancer risk after cessation of asbestos exposure: A cohort study of Italian asbestos cement workers. *Occup Environ Med* 2008;65:164–170.

34. Pira E, Pelucchi C, Piolatto PG, Negri E, Bilei T, La Vecchia C. Mortality from cancer and other causes in the Balangero cohort of chrysotile asbestos miners. *Occup Environ Med* 2009;66:805–809.
35. Straif K, Benbrahim-Tallaa L, Baan R, Grosse Y, Secretan B, El Ghissassi F, Bouvard V, Guha N, Freeman C, Galichet L, Cogliano V; WHO International Agency for Research on Cancer Monograph Working Group. Special report: a review of human carcinogens—Part C: metals, arsenic, dusts, and fibres. International Agency for Research on Cancer, WHO. *Lancet Oncol* 2009;10:453–454.
36. IARC. Reversal of risk after quitting smoking. *IARC Handbooks of Cancer Prevention: Tobacco Control*, Vol. 11. Lyon: IARC; 2007.
37. Browne K, Gee JB. Asbestos exposure and laryngeal cancer. *Ann Occup Hyg* 2000;44:239–250.
38. American Joint Committee on Cancer (AJCC). *AJCC Cancer Staging Manual*, 7th ed. New York: Springer; 2010.
39. Battista G, Belli S, Comba P, Fiumalbi C, Grignoli M, Loi F, et al. Mortality due to asbestos-related causes among railway carriage construction and repair workers. *Occup Med (Lond)* 1999;49:536–539.
40. Wortley P, Vaughan TL, Davis S, Morgan MS, Thomas DB. A case–control study of occupational risk factors for laryngeal cancer. *Br J Ind Med* 1992;49:837–844.
41. Doll R, Peto J. Other asbestos-related neoplasms. In: *Asbestos-Related Malignancy*, Antman K, Aisner J, eds. London: Grune & Stratton Inc; 1987.
42. WHO-IARC. *IARC Monographs on the Evaluation of Carcinogenic Risks to Humans. Asbestos: Summary of Data Reported and Evaluation*, Vol. 14. Lyon, France: WHO-IARC; 1977. http://www.monographs. iarc.fr
43. WHO-IARC. *IARC Monographs on the Evaluation of the Carcinogenic Risks to Humans*. Overall evaluations of carcinogenicity: An updating of IARC Monographs Volumes 1 to 42. Lyon, France: WHO-IARC; 1987. Suppl 7. http://www.monographs.iarc.fr
44. Chan CK, Gee JB. Asbestos exposure and laryngeal cancer: An analysis of the epidemiologic evidence. *J Occup Med* 1988;30:23.
45. Smith AH, Handley MA, Wood R. Epidemiological evidence indicates asbestos causes laryngeal cancer. *J Occup Med* 1990;32:499–507.
46. Edelman DA. Laryngeal cancer and occupational exposure to asbestos. *Int Arch Occup Environ Health* 1989;61:223–227.
47. Parnes SM. Asbestos and cancer of the larynx: Is there a relationship? *Laryngoscope* 1990;100:254–261.
48. Maier H, Tisch M. Epidemiology of laryngeal cancer: Results of the Heidelberg case–control study. *Acta Otolaryngol* 1997;527:160–164.
49. De Stefani E, Boffetta P, Oreggia F, Ronco A, Kogevinas M, Mendilaharsu M. Occupation and the risk of laryngeal cancer in Uruguay. *Am J Ind Med* 1988;33:537–542.
50. Marchand JL, Luce D, Leclerc A, Goldberg P, Orlowski E, Bugel I, Brugère J. Laryngeal and hypopharyngeal cancer and occupational exposure to asbestos and man-made vitreous fibers: Results of a case–control study. *Am J Ind Med* 2000;37:581.
51. Murai Y, Kitagawa M. Autopsy cases of asbestosis in Japan: A statistical analysis on registered cases. *Arch Environ Health* 2000;55:447–452.
52. Stern FB, Ruder AM, Chen G. Proportionate mortality among unionized roofers and waterproofers. *Am J Ind Med* 2000;37:478–492.
53. Musk AW, de Klerk NH, Reid A, Ambrosini GL, Fritschi L, Olsen NJ, et al. Mortality of former crocidolite (blue asbestos) miners and millers at Wittenoom. *Occup Environ Med* 2008;65:541–543.
54. Henderson DW, Rödelsperger K, Woitowitz H-J, Leigh J. After Helsinki: A multidisciplinary review of the relationship between asbestos exposure and lung cancer, with emphasis on studies published during 1997–2004. *Pathology* 2004;36:517–550.
55. Baur X, Czuppon AB. Regulation and compensation of asbestos diseases in Germany. In: *Sourcebook on Asbestos Diseases*, Vol 15, Peters GA, Peters BJ, eds. Charlottesville: Lexis; 1997: 405–419.
56. BK Report Faserjahre 1/97 Anlage 10. Hauptverband der gewerblichen Berufsgenossenschaften. Sankt Augustin; 1996.
57. Berger J, Chang-Claude J, Moehlner M, Wichmann HE. Larynxkarzinom und Asbestexposition: eine Bewertung aus epidemiologicher Sicht. *Zentralbl Arbeitsmed* 1996;46:166–186.
58. Consensus report: asbestos, asbestosis, and cancer: the Helsinki criteria for diagnosis and attribution. *Scand J Work Environ Health* 1997;23:311–316.

59. Meurman L, Kiviluoto R, Hakama M. Mortality and morbidity among the working population of anthophyllite asbestos miners in Finland. *Br J Ind Med* 1974;31:105–112.
60. Mancuso TF, El-Attar AA. Mortality patterns in a cohort of asbestos workers: A study based on employment experiences. *J Occup Med* 1967;9:147–162.
61. Selikoff IJ. Epidemiology of gastrointestinal cancer. *Environ Health Perspect* 1974;9:299–305.
62. Selikoff IJ, Churg JC, Hammond EC. Relation between exposure to asbestos and mesothelioma. *N Engl J Med* 1965;272:560–565.
63. Enterline PE. Mortality among asbestos products workers in the United States. *Ann N Y Acad Sci* 1965;132:156–165.
64. Hammond EC, Selikoff IJ, Churg J. Neoplasia among insulation workers in the United States with special reference to intra-abdominal neoplasia. *Ann N Y Acad Sci* 1965;132:519–525.
65. Mancuso TF. Discussion. *Ann N Y Acad Sci* 1965;132:590.
66. Selikoff IJ. Clinical survey of chrysotile asbestos miners and millers in Baire Verte, Newfoundland 1976: report to the National Institute of Environmental Health Sciences, December 22, USPHS, Department of Health and Human Services, Research Triangle, NC; 1977.
67. Selikoff IJ, Hammond EC, Seidman H. Mortality experience of insulation workers in the United States and Canada, 1943–1976. *Ann N Y Acad Sci* 1979;330:91–116.
68. Elmes PC, Simpson MJC. Insulation workers in Belfast: A further study of mortality due to asbestos exposure (1940–1975). *Br J Ind Med* 1977;34:174–180.
69. Kogan FM, Guselnikova NA, Gulevskaya MR. The cancer mortality rate among workers in the asbestos industry of the Urals. *Gig Sanit* 1972;37:29–32.
70. Newhouse ML, Berry G. Asbestos and laryngeal carcinoma. *Lancet* 1973;2:615.
71. Schneiderman MA. Digestive system cancer among persons subjected to occupational inhalation of asbestos particles: A literature review with emphasis on dose response. *Environ Health Perspect* 1974;9:307–311.
72. Newhouse ML, Berry G. Patterns of mortality in asbestos factory workers in London. *Ann N Y Acad Sci* 1979;330:53–60.
73. McDonald AD, Fry JS, Woolley AJ, McDonald JC. Dust exposure and mortality in an American chrysotile textile plant. *Br J Ind Med* 1983;40:361–367.
74. Enterline PE, Harley J, Henderson V. Asbestos and cancer: A cohort followed up to death. *Br J Ind Med* 1987;44:396–401.
75. Finkelstein MM. Mortality among employees of an Ontario asbestos-cement factory. *Am Rev Respir Dis* 1984;129:754–761.
76. Kelley JR, Duggan JM. Gastric cancer epidemiology and risk factors. *J Clin Epidemiol* 2003;56:1–9.
77. de Klerk NH, Armstrong BK, Musk AW, Hobbs MS. Cancer mortality in relation to measures of occupational exposure to crocidolite at Wittenoom Gorge in Western Australia. *Br J Ind Med* 1989;46:529–536.
78. Albin M, Jakobsson K, Attewell R, Johansson L, Welinder H. Mortality and cancer morbidity in cohorts of asbestos cement workers and referents. *Br J Ind Med* 1990;47:602–610.
79. Vineis P, Ciccone G, Magnino A. Asbestos exposure, physical activity and colon cancer: A case-control study. *Tumori* 1993;79:301–303.
80. Cook PM, Olson GF. Ingested mineral fibers: Elimination in human urine. *Science* 1979;204:195–198.
81. Ehrlich A, Gordon RE, Dikman SH. Carcinoma of the colon in asbestos-exposed workers: Analysis of asbestos content in colon tissue. *Am J Ind Med* 1991;19:629–636.
82. World Health Organization. *Occupational Exposure Limit for Asbestos*, WHO/OCH/89.1. Geneva: Office of Occupational Health, World Health Organization; 1989.
83. Richmond JB. Surgeon General of the United States Physicians Advisory—Health effects of asbestos. Washington, DC: United States Public Health Service, Department of Health, Education and Welfare; 1978.
84. Califano JM. Statement on asbestos, Secretary Joseph M. Califano, Jr. HEW News. Washington, DC: Department of Health, Education and Welfare; 1978.
85. Frumkin H, Berlin J. Asbestos exposure and gastrointestinal malignancy review and meta-analysis. *Am J Ind Med* 1988;14:79–84.
86. Homa DM, Garabrant DH, Gillespie GW. A meta-analysis of colorectal cancer and asbestos exposure. *Am J Epidemiol* 1994;139:1210–1222.
87. Kang SK, Burnett CA, Freund E, et al. Gastrointestinal cancer mortality of workers in occupations with high asbestos exposures. *Am J Ind Med* 1997;31:713–718.

88. Berry G, Newhouse ML, Wagner JC. Mortality from all cancers of asbestos factory workers in east London 1933–1980. *Occup Environ Med* 2000;57:782–785.
89. Straif K, Chambless L, Weiland SK, Wienke A, Bungers M, Taeger D, Keil U. Occupational risk factors for mortality from stomach and lung cancer among rubber workers: An analysis using internal controls and refined exposure assessment. *Int J Epidemiol* 1999;28:1037–1043.
90. International Agency for Research on Cancer. *Printing Processes and Printing Inks, Carbon Black and Some Nitro Compounds*. IARC Monographs on the Evaluation of Carcinogenic Risks to Humans, Vol. 65. Lyon, France: International Agency for Research on Cancer; 1996.
91. Cocco P, Ward MH, Dosemcci M. Risk of stomach cancer associated with 12 workplace hazards: Analysis of death certificates from 24 states of the United States with the aid of job exposure matrices. *Occup Environ Med* 1999;56:781–787.
92. Levy SA. Occupational pulmonary diseases. In: *Occupational Medicine—Principles and Practical Applications*, Zenz C, ed. Chicago: Year Book Medical Publishers Inc.; 1975.
93. De la Provote S, Desoubeaux N, Paris C, Letourneux M, Raffaelli C, Galateau-Salle F, Gidnouz M, Launoy D. Incidence of digestive cancers and occupational exposure to asbestos. *Eur J Cancer Prev* 2002;11:523–528.
94. Cocco P, Palli D, Buiatti E, Cipriani F, DeCarli A, Manca P, et al. Occupational exposures as risk factors for gastric cancer in Italy. *Cancer Causes Contr* 1994;5:241–248.
95. Zandjani F, Hogsaet B, Andersen A, Långard S. Incidence of cancer among nitrate fertilizer workers. *Int Arch Occup Environ Health* 1994;66:189–193.
96. Andersen A, Glattre E, Johansen BV. Incidence of cancer among lighthouse keepers exposed to asbestos in drinking water. *Am J Epidemiol* 1993;138:682–687.
97. Maartmann-Moe H, Hartveit F. On the reputed decline in gastric carcinoma: Necropsy study from western Norway. *Br Med J (Clin Res Ed)* 1985;290:103–105.
98. Kishimoto T, Okada K. The relationship between lung cancer and asbestos exposure. *Chest* 1988;94:486–490.
99. Kishimoto T, Okada K, Nagake Y, Doi K, Takusagawa Y, Ono T, Shimamoto F. A case of asbestosis complicated with double cancer of the stomach and colon. *Gan No Rinsho* 1989;35:417–420.
100. Kishimoto T, Ono T, Okada K. Evaluation of primary multiple cancer manifesting exposure to asbestos. *Gan No Rinsho* 1989;35:825–827.
101. Kishimoto T, Shimamoto F. Evaluation of double cancers in relation to previous asbestos exposure. *Gan No Rinsho* 1990;36:787–790.
102. Kishimoto T, Yamaguchi K. A case of simultaneous double cancer (lung and stomach cancer) related to asbestos exposure. *Nippon Kyobu Geka Gakkai Zasshi* 1990;28:1028–1032.
103. Keal EE. Asbestosis and abdominal neoplasms. *Lancet* 1960;3:1211–1216.
104. Graham J, Graham R. Ovarian cancer and asbestos. *Environ Res* 1967;1:115–128.
105. Longo DL, Young RC. Cosmetic talc and ovarian cancer. *Lancet* 1979;2:349–351.
106. Wegnall HK, Fox J. Mortality of female gas mask assemblers. *Br J Ind Med* 1983;39:34–38.
107. Newhouse ML, Berry G, Wagner JC. Mortality of factory workers in east London 1933–80. *Br J Ind Med* 1985;42:4–12.
108. Tarchi M, Orsi D, Comba P, De Santis M, Pirastu R, Battista G, Valiani M. Cohort mortality study of rock salt workers in Italy. *Am J Ind Med* 1994;25:251–256.
109. Rösler JA, Woitowitz HJ, Lange HJ, Woitowitz RH, Ulm K, Rödelsperger K. Mortality rates in a female cohort following asbestos exposure in Germany. *J Occup Med* 1994;36:889–893.
110. Germani D, Belli S, Bruno C, Grignoli M, Nesti M, Pirastu R, Comba P. Cohort mortality study of women compensated for asbestosis in Italy. *Am J Ind Med* 1999;36:129–134.
111. Vasama-Neuvonen K, Pukkala E, Paakkulainen H, Mutanen P, Weiderpass E, Boffetta P, et al. Ovarian cancer and occupational exposures in Finland. *Am J Ind Med* 1999;36:83–89.
112. Langseth H, Kjerheim K. Ovarian cancer and occupational exposure among pulp and paper employees in Norway. *Scand J Work Environ Health* 2004;30:356–361.
113. Reid A, Heyworth J, de Klerk N, Musk AW. The mortality of women exposed environmentally and domestically to blue asbestos at Wittenoom, Western Australia. *Occup Environ Med* 2008;65:743–749.
114. Reid A, Segal A, Heyworth JS, de Klerk NH, Musk AW. Gynecologic and breast cancers in women after exposure to blue asbestos at Wittenoom. *Cancer Epidemiol Biomarkers Prev* 2009;18:140–147.

115. Heller D, Gordon RE, Westhoff C, Gerber S. Asbestos exposure and ovarian fiber burden. *Am J Ind Med* 1996;29:435–439.

116. Auerbach O, Conston AS, Garfinkel L, Parks VR, Kaslow HD, Hammond EC. Presence of asbestos bodies in organs other than the lung. *Chest* 1980;77:133–137.

117. Graham S, Blanchet M, Rohrer T. Cancer in asbestos-mining and other areas of Quebec. *J Natl Cancer Inst* 1977;59:1139–1145.

118. Cook PM. Discussion. In: *Dust and Disease*, Lemen RA, Dement JM, eds. Park Forest, IL: Pathotox Publishers; 1979:111.

119. Harber P, Mohsenifar Z, Oren A, Lew M. Pleural plaques and asbestos-associated malignancy. *J Occup Med* 1987;29:641.

120. MacLure M. Asbestos and renal adenocarcinoma: A case-control study. *Environ Res* 1987;42:353.

121. Smith AH, Shearn VI, Wood R. Asbestos and kidney cancer: The evidence supports a causal association. *Am J Ind Med* 1989;16:159.

122. Puntoni R, Vercelli M, Merlo F, Valerio F, Santi L. Mortality among shipyard workers in Genoa, Italy. *Ann N Y Acad Sci* 1979;330:353–377.

123. Pesch B, Haerting J, Ranft U, Klimpel A, Oelschlägel B, Schill W. Occupational risk factors for renal cell carcinoma: Agent-specific results from a case-control study in Germany. *Int J Epidemiol* 2000;29:1014–1024.

124. Enterline PE, Henderson V. Asbestos and kidney cancer. *Am J Ind Med* 1990;17:645–650.

125. Seidman H, Selikoff IJ. Decline in death rates among asbestos insulation workers 1967–1986 associated with diminution of work exposure to asbestos. *Ann N Y Acad Sci* 1990;609:300–317.

126. McCredie M, Stewart JH. Risk factors for kidney cancer in New South Wales. IV. Occupation. *Br J Ind Med* 1993;50:349–354.

127. McDonald JC, Liddell FDK, Dufresne A, McDonald AD. The 1891–1920 birth cohort of Quebec chrysotile miners and millers: Mortality 1976–1988. *Br J Ind Med* 1993;50:1073–1081.

128. Mellemgaard A, Engholm G, McLaughlin JK, Olsen JH. Occupational risk factors for renal-cell carcinoma in Denmark. *Scand J Work Environ Health* 1994;20:160–165.

129. Mandel JS, McLaughlin JK, Schlehofer B, Mellemgaard A, Helmert U, Lindblad P, et al. International renal-cell cancer study. IV. Occupation. *Int J Cancer* 1995;61:601–605.

130. McLaughlin JK, Blot W, Devesa SS, Fraumeni JF. Renal cancer. In: *Cancer Epidemiology and Prevention*, Schottenfeld D, Fraumeni JF, eds. New York: Oxford University Press; 1996: 1142.

131. Saarni H, Pentti J, Pukkala E. Cancer at sea: A case-control study among male Finnish seafarers. *Occup Environ Med* 2002;59:613–619.

132. Boor P, Casper S, Celec P, Hurbánková M, Beno M, Heidland A, et al. Renal, vascular and cardiac fibrosis in rats exposed to passive smoking and industrial dust fibre amosite. *J Cell Mol Med* 2009;13:4484–4491.

133. Pascual D, Borque A. Epidemiology of kidney cancer. *Adv Urol* 2008:782381. Epub Nov 4, 2008.

134. Sawazaki H, Yoshikawa T, Takahashi T, Taki Y, Takeuchi H, Sakai Y. Renal cell carcinoma with malignant pleural mesothelioma after asbestos exposure: A case report. *Hinyokika Kiyo* 2007;53:805–808.

135. Seattle Cancer Care Alliance. *What Is Lymphoma?* Seattle, WA: Seattle Cancer Care Alliance; 2004.

136. Becker N, Berger J, Bolm-Audorff U. Asbestos exposure and malignant lymphomas—A review of the epidemiological literature. *Int Arch Occup Environ Health* 2001;74:459–469.

137. Schwartz DA, Vaughan TL, Heyer NJ, Koepsell TD, Lyon JL, Swanson GM, Weiss NS. B cell neoplasms and occupational asbestos exposure. *Am J Ind Med* 1988;14:661–671.

138. Seidler A, Becker N, Nieters A, Arhelger R, Mester B, Rossnagel K, et al. Asbestos exposure and malignant lymphoma: a multicenter case-control study in Germany and Italy. *Int Arch Occup Environ Health* 2010;83:563–570.

139. Munan L, Thouez JP, Kelly A, Gagné M, Labonté D. Relative leucopenia in the peripheral blood of asbestos miners: an epidemiologic analysis. *Scand J Haematol* 1981;26:115–122.

140. Turner-Warwick M, Parkes WR. Circulating rheumatoid and antinuclear factors in asbestos workers. *Br Med J* 1970;3:492–495.

141. Lange A, Skibinski G. T and B cells and delayed-type skin reactions in asbestos workers. *Proceedings of the Third European Immunology Meet*; 1976.

142. Lange A, Skibinski G, Garncarek D. The follow-up study of skin reactivity to recall antigens and E- and EAC-RFC profiles in blood in asbestos workers. *Immunobiology* 1980;157:1–11.

143. Lange A. An epidemiological survey of immunological abnormalities in asbestos workers: I. Nonorgan and organ-specific autoantibodies. *Environ Res* 1980;22:162–175.

144. Lange A. An epidemiological survey of immunological abnormalities in asbestos workers: II. Serum immunoglobulin levels. *Environ Res* 1980;22:176–183.

145. Lange A, Nineham LJ, Garncarek D, Smolik R. Circulating immune complexes and antiglobulins (IgG and IgM) in asbestos-induced lung fibrosis. *Environ Res* 1983;31:287–295.

146. Goldsmith JR. Asbestos as a systemic carcinogen: The evidence from eleven cohorts. *Am J Ind Med* 1982;3:341–348.

147. Hyodoh F, Kinugawa K, Ueki A. Effects of asbestos on the cell cycle of PHA-stimulated human peripheral blood lymphocytes. *Nippon Eiseigaku Zasshi* 1991;45:1074–1081.

148. Rosenthal GJ, Corsini E, Simeonova P. Selected new developments in asbestos immunotoxicity. *Environ Health Perspect* 1998;106:159–169.

149. Rosenthal GJ, Simeonova P, Corsini E. Asbestos toxicity: An immunologie perspective. *Rev Environ Health* 1999;14:11–20.

150. Rola-Pleszczynski M, Lemaire I, Sirois P, Massé S, Bégin R. Asbestos-related changes in pulmonary and systemic immune responses—Early enhancement followed by inhibition. *Clin Exp Immunol* 1982;49:426–432.

151. Petrek M, Hermans C, Kolek V, Fialová J, Bernard A. Clara cell protein (CC 16) in serum and bronchoalveolar lavage fluid of subjects exposed to asbestos. *Biomarkers* 2002;7:58–67.

152. Pelclová D, Bartůnková J, Fenclová Z, Lebedová J, Hladíková M, Benáková H. Asbestos exposure and antineutrophil cytoplasmic antibody (ANCA) positivity. *Arch Environ Health* 2003;58:662–668.

153. Ilavská S, Jahnová E, Tulinská J, Horváthová M, Dusinská M, Wsolová L, et al. Immunological monitoring in workers occupationally exposed to asbestos. *Toxicology* 2005;206:299–308.

154. Pfau JC, Sentissi JJ, Weller G, Putnam EA. Assessment of autoimmune responses associated with asbestos exposure in Libby, Montana, USA. *Environ Health Perspect* 2005;113:25–30.

155. Noonan CW, Pfau JC, Larson TC, Spence MR. Nested case-control study of autoimmune disease in an asbestos-exposed population. *Environ Health Perspect* 2006;114:1243–1247.

156. Otsuki T, Maeda M, Murakami S, Hayashi H, Miura Y, Kusaka M, et al. Immunological effects of silica and asbestos. *Cell Mol Immunol* 2007;4:261–268.

CHAPTER 9

Asbestosis

Samuel P. Hammar

CONTENTS

9.1 HISTORICAL PERSPECTIVE

Cases of severe pulmonary fibrosis in association with asbestos were first described in the early 1900s.[1] In 1914, T. Fahr, a German pathologist, described the pathological features of interstitial pulmonary fibrosis in a 35-year-old asbestos worker and attributed them to asbestos.[2] In 1924, Cooke[3] coined the term *asbestosis* and published a detailed pathological description of the disease. In 1938, Dreessen et al.[4] reported ground-glass changes in chest radiographs of 440 South Carolina textile workers and described the relationship of abnormalities to the duration and intensity of exposure to asbestos. Although their study was criticized, they concluded that if the concentration of asbestos in the air did not exceed 5 million particles per cubic foot, then no radiographic abnormalities would occur. Thus, this concentration of asbestos was adopted as the environmental standard at that time. A similar study was done by Merewether and Price,[5] who in 1930 reported on the effects of asbestos dust on the lungs and the issue of dust suppression in the asbestos industry.

Details of the history of asbestosis are provided in Chapters 1 and 5.

9.2 PATHOGENESIS OF ASBESTOSIS

The cellular–molecular basis of asbestosis has undergone an evolution on the basis of studies that have been reported since the early 1900s. As described by Rom et al.[6] and as diagramed by these authors (Figure 9.1), the asbestos fibers that bypass the upper airway defenses are initially deposited in the region of the respiratory bronchioles and alveolar ducts. This is followed by rapid accumulation in this area of pulmonary macrophages, which phagocytose the shorter asbestos fibers and attempt to phagocytose longer asbestos fibers. This causes activation of macrophages that release lysosomal enzymes and cytokines resulting in an intense inflammatory response that eventually leads to fibrosis.[7–11] The alveolar macrophages produce a variety of substances, including fibroblast growth factor, that appear to stimulate fibroblasts to produce collagen resulting in fibrosis (see Chapter 4).

With respect to the pathogenicity of asbestos in causing asbestosis, studies[12,13] have suggested that the most important factor is the total surface area of the asbestos fiber rather than their concentration in lung tissue. The importance of surface area has been discussed for other fibers as well.[14,15]

In experimental animals such as sheep whose pulmonary anatomy most closely resembles that of humans, the initial lesion caused by experimentally delivered asbestos involves the respiratory bronchioles and the alveolar ducts.[16]

Bellis et al.[17] studied the minimal pathological changes in the lungs of humans exposed to asbestos and concluded that minimal bronchioloalveolar fibrotic change with concomitant asbestos bodies could be considered a mild pneumoconiotic lesion referred to as *grade 1 asbestosis* and that similar lesions referred to as *small airway lesions* in which no asbestos bodies were found could also be regarded as an additional indicator of asbestos exposure because the concentration of asbestos in lung tissue from these two groups was essentially identical.

Harless et al.[18] reported relatively acute onset obstructive airway disease in 17 of 23 construction workers after an intense 5-month exposure to chrysotile asbestos and referred to an article published by Jodoin et al.[19] that reported asbestos could cause obstructive disease of small airways early after asbestos exposure. Harless et al.[18] stated that no possible cause for the airway obstruction other than from asbestos could be identified in six of the men. That asbestos can cause larger airways disease, including bronchiectasis and fibrotic narrowing, was reported by Jacob and Bohling.[20]

With respect to asbestos airway disease and parenchymal lung disease, one study[21] suggested that deposition of asbestos in the lung might be related to the length of the airway away from the hilum to the periphery of the lung and to the degree of branching airways. This hypothesis was

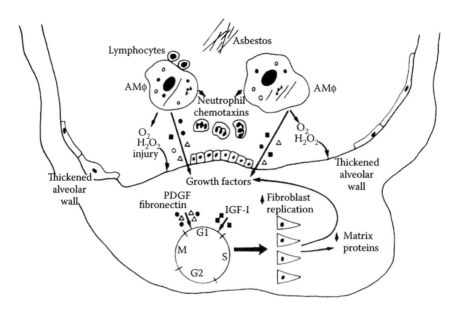

Figure 9.1 Schematic diagram of pathogenesis of asbestosis.

challenged by Delfino et al.[22] who studied 178 construction insulators and found no association between pleural abnormalities and airway geometry or length of airways.

Mossman and Churg[23] reviewed literature and concluded a multiplicity of interactions between effector cells and target cell types of injury, including bronchiolar and alveolar epithelial cells and fibroblasts that govern the pathogenesis and progression of disease. They stated that early injury to alveolar type 1 epithelial cells was regarded as an early event in fibrogenesis followed by hyperplasia and hypertrophy of type 2 alveolar lining cells. They suggested that an increase in epithelial cell proliferation was crucial to repair and regeneration and, if unchecked, could lead to fibrogenesis and carcinogenesis. They listed the mediators of inflammatory and fibrogenic responses to silica and asbestos (Table 9.1) and a hypothetical scheme of events occurring in the lung after exposure to pathogenic mineral dust.

Although not directly related to the pathogenesis of asbestosis, Attanoos et al.[24] studied a group of 188 naval dockyard workers who were stated to have been exposed to asbestos for pathological asbestosis according to the Roggli–Pratt criteria and compared them with 175 nonasbestos-exposed U.K. subjects from urban and rural areas who were stated to have died from diseases unrelated to asbestos. Attanoos et al.[24] found that mild interstitial fibrosis (grades 1 and 2 asbestosis) was more prevalent in the nonasbestos-exposed population. They stated that the excess rates of fibrosis in the asbestos-exposed cohort were observed only in grades 3 and 4 asbestosis. They suggested that fibroblastic foci suggested a diagnosis other than asbestosis. Because this was an abstract publication, detailed information such as how much asbestos the dockyard workers were exposed to (asbestos fiber/body concentration in lung tissue), the smoking history of both groups, and the occupational history of the nonexposed population was unavailable.

The observations of Attanoos et al.[24] concerning the asbestos-exposed group was markedly different than what Dodson et al.[25] found during pathological evaluation of lung tissue from 55 mostly heavily exposed individuals with mesothelioma where only three individuals had clinical asbestosis and 29 of 55 had pathological asbestosis, most of which was the College of American Pathologists–National Institutes for Occupational Safety and Health (CAP-NIOSH) grades 1 and 2. In addition, Dodson et al.[25] believed that nonspecific patchy interstitial fibrosis is not uncommon in persons occupationally exposed to asbestos.

Table 9.1 Putative Mediators of Inflammatory and Fibrogenic Responses to Silica and Asbestos

Factors	Silicosis	Asbestosis
Arachidonic acid and lipid metabolites	+	+
Cytokine-induced neutrophil chemoattractant	+	+
Epidermal growth factor	+	+
Insulin-like growth factor	+	+
Interleukin-1	+	+
Interleukin-8	+	+
Macrophage inflammatory proteins 1α and 2	+	+
Monocyte chemoattractant protein-1	+	+
Platelet-derived growth factors	+	+
Reactive nitrogen species	+	+
Reactive oxygen species	+	+
TGF-β	+	+
TGF-α	+	+
TNF-α	+	+

Note: Plus sign indicates positive association in experimental models and/or clinical studies.

The editorial by Arnold Brody[26] titled "Asbestos and Lung Disease" stated an additional piece of relative information concerning fiber deposition and translocation was that all varieties of inhaled asbestos deposited initially along all aspects of the respiratory tract. In the larger airways, Dr. Brody[26] stated that the fibers tended to accumulate at bifurcation by internal impaction, and this was where many lung cancers appeared. Dr. Brody[26] went on to state that at the alveolar level, the bronchiolar–alveolar duct junctions were the anatomic sites at which the majority of the initial fiber deposition occurred by interception. These fibers were stated to be actively translocated by type I pneumocytes to the underlying connective tissue space (interstitium). Dr. Brody[26] stated these fibers underlying the connective tissue space injured the epithelium and activated the fibrogenic growth factors that caused asbestosis. Physical elimination of chrysotile from the air surface of the lower respiratory tract was shown at one year post chronic exposure; however, many of the chrysotile fibers within the interstitium remained.[27]

Dr. Brody[26] stated that oxidants clearly play a major role in fibrotic and neoplastic asbestos-induced diseases. Transforming growth factor β (TGF-β) can be activated from its latent form by asbestos-derived reactive oxygen species. TGF-β was stated to be well known as a fibrogenic cytokine in asbestosis and could induce epithelial mesenchymal transitions as well as differentiation in interstitial lung fibroblasts. Reactive oxygen species were also stated to be generated by chrysotile and amphiboles and caused amino acid disruption in the latent associated peptides that renders TGF-β biologically inactive, thus activating TGF-β to its receptor binding active state. Dr. Brody[26] stated tumor necrosis factor α (TNF-α) up-regulated the expression of gene coating for TGF-β.

Dr. Brody's[26] final point was that alveolar macrophages, an early hallmark of inhalation of asbestos, have been shown to be activated by the fifth component of compliment (C5a) by inhaled asbestos on alveolar surfaces within minutes after the fibers were deposited. Activated compliment 5A (C5a) was stated to be a potent chemoattractant for alveolar macrophages, and these cells quickly accumulated at the site of asbestos fiber deposition. Dr. Brody[26] stated others found that these cells release TNF-α, which could explain why the developing lesions of asbestosis were initiated at the bronchoalveolar duct junctions.

In 1970, Turner-Warwick and Parkes[28] studied the presence of circulating rheumatoid factor and antinuclear antibodies in persons exposed to asbestos. It had previously been pointed out that there was an increased prevalence of rheumatoid factor in asbestos workers, especially with those having an abnormal chest radiograph. Turner-Warwick and Parkes[28] evaluated 80 patients with asbestos exposure referred to the London Pneumoconiosis Medical Panel and found antinuclear antibodies and rheumatoid factors in 28% and 27%, respectively, which was at least a fourfold increase over their incidence in the random population. The identification of these antibodies was stated to not be related to the duration of exposure but was related to the extent of the radiographic abnormality (the extent of severity of asbestosis). Turner-Warwick and Parkes[28] stated the stimulus to the formation of antinuclear antibodies and rheumatoid factors and their role in pathogenesis remained unknown, but they pointed out there appeared to be a correlation between the severity of disease and the presence of antibodies. They suggested that circulating antibodies and cellular hypersensitivity together initiated lung damage analogous to experimental allergic orchitis.

In 1973, Dr. Turner-Warwick[29] presented data at the Proceedings of the Royal Society suggesting that a greater incidence of antinuclear antibodies and rheumatoid factors were found in the Pneumoconiosis Medical Panel series where the majority of subjects had abnormal chest radiographs, which was in contrast to a near-normal incidence in the East Ham and Medical Research Unit series where the majority had no clinical or radiographic evidence of asbestos-induced lung disease. The increased prevalence of antinuclear antibody (ANA) was stated to appear to be related to the development of asbestosis and not to the concentration of exposure to asbestos dust alone. Dr. Turner-Warwick[29] stated that whether antinuclear antibodies could be used to identify an individual's susceptibility to the development of asbestosis or whether it influenced the evolution of the pathology was yet to be determined.

In 1976, in the *British Medical Journal*, investigators from Finland commented on the fact that antinuclear antibodies and rheumatoid factors in cases of asbestosis resulted from pulmonary lesions and were not evidence of an autoimmune mechanism in the pathogenesis of the disease.[30] Another probable explanation of the negative finding in their cases was that anthophyllite, owing to its different physiochemical structures, caused less destruction of lung tissue than other types of asbestos.

In 1978, Lange et al.[31] found a highly significant correlation between asbestosis and impaired responsiveness in skin reaction to intermediate and second-strength tuberculin and SK-SD. Antinuclear antibodies were found with higher frequency in asbestos workers who lacked a cutaneous response to recall antigens. In asbestosis cases, peripheral blood lymphocyte profiles demonstrated low proportions of E-RFC. An MIF test showed the impairment of the cytokine generation when lymphocytes were stimulated with SK-SD, PPD, and PHA in asbestosis cases. The lymphocyte transformation study documented an impaired response to a lower dose of PHA and ConA in asbestosis cases and in asbestos workers with antinuclear antibodies.

In 1983, a report by Lange et al.[32] suggested that asbestos workers with IgG antinuclear antibodies had the highest incidence of elevated serum immune complex levels. The exact significance of this finding is uncertain.

A report by Zone and Rom[33] in 1985 concerning circulating immune complexes, rheumatoid factor, and antinuclear antibodies stated that 25 asbestos insulation workers and 32 brick mason controls were evaluated. Ten asbestos workers had radiographic pleural or parenchymal changes consistent with asbestos exposure. There were no differences in antinuclear antibodies or rheumatoid factor between the asbestos workers and the controls. However, the asbestos workers had significantly increased levels of IgG and IgA circulating immune complexes. The significance of this finding is uncertain.

A review article by Morris et al.[34] concluded that although immune responses in asbestos-exposed individuals had not yet been adequately defined, several trends were evident. Most significant was an increase in IgG, IgM, and IgA, probably related to pulmonary asbestos burden, which served as a chronic antigenic stimulant resulting in an accompanying suppression of regulator T cells. Morris et al.[34] stated that additional studies were warranted.

In 1988, a study performed by Lahat et al.[35] concerning immunologic profiles of chest radiograph-negative, asymptomatic asbestos workers showed that increased T-cell activities in asbestos-exposed persons was unclear, and further clinical and immunological follow-up was recommended.

Jarad et al.[36] studied histocompatibility antigen in asbestos-related diseases and found no difference in prevalence of human leukocyte antigen (HLA) between asbestos workers and patients with asbestos-related disease. However, a previously reported study suggested a possible protective effect of HLA-DR5 against asbestosis.

Tamura et al.[37] studied antinuclear antibodies and rheumatoid factor in 220 employees of an asbestos plant. They studied the relationship of the appearance of two factors to sex, smoking habit, duration of asbestos exposure, and asbestos exposure levels. In 207 employees who had chest radiographs, the relationship of these two factors to pulmonary and pleural lesions was examined. Of the 220 employees, 33 (15%) had a positive ANA and 7 (3.2%) had a positive rheumatoid factor. The ANA-positive rate in the asbestos plant employees was significantly higher than that in the controls. Factors significantly correlating to their appearance could not be demonstrated.

Marczynski et al.[38] studied the incidence of DNA double-strand breaks and anti-dsDNA antibodies in blood of workers occupationally exposed to asbestos. They concluded that workers occupationally exposed to asbestos had distinctly more double-strand breaks and that anti-dsDNA antibodies could mean that an increased incidence of DNA-fragments might be important as an indicator in the chronic effect of asbestos-associated carcinogenesis.

Nigam et al.[39] studied humoral immunological profiles of workers exposed to asbestos in asbestos mines and suggested that immunological changes were associated with asbestos exposure and could play an important role in the pathogenesis of asbestos-induced diseases.

Pfau et al.[40] studied autoimmune responses associated with asbestos exposure in Libby, Montana. They performed a case–control epidemiologic study and concluded that asbestos exposure was associated with autoimmune responses and suggested a relationship existed between these responses and asbestos-related disease processes.

Finally, Pfau et al.[41] reported on asbestos-induced autoimmunity in C57BL/6 mice. The purpose of the study was to test the hypothesis that asbestos could lead to a specific pattern of autoantibodies and pathological findings indicative of systemic autoimmune disease. Female C57BL/6 mice were instilled intratracheally with 2 doses × 60 μg/mouse of amphibole asbestos (tremolite), wollastonite (a nonfibrogenic control fiber), or saline alone. Serum samples were collected, and urine was checked for protein biweekly for 7 months. By 26 weeks, the asbestos-instilled animals had a significantly higher frequency of positive ANA tests compared with wollastonite and saline groups. The majority of positive ANAs showed homogeneous or combined homogeneous/speckled patterns and tested positive for antibodies to dsDNA and SSA/Ro 52. Serum isotyping showed no significant changes in IgM, IgA, or IgG subclasses. However, there was an overall decrease in the mean IgG serum concentration in asbestos-instilled mice. IgG immune complex deposition was demonstrated in the kidneys of asbestos-instilled mice, with evidence of glomerular and tubule abnormalities suggestive of glomerulonephritis. Flow cytometry demonstrated moderate changes in the percentages of CD25+ T-suppressor cells and B1a B-cells in the superficial cervical lymph nodes of the asbestos-instilled mice. The data indicated that asbestos leads to immunologic changes consistent with the development of autoimmune disease.

There appears to be a significant amount of data to suggest that asbestos causes abnormalities in the immune system. The most recent studies suggest that asbestos causes an increase in antinuclear antibodies (ANA), which may be involved in the pathogenesis of asbestosis.

9.3 MORPHOLOGY OF ASBESTOSIS

The 1982 document by Craighead et al.[42] provided the most comprehensive pathological description of asbestosis. Roggli and Shelburne,[43] Roggli,[44,45] and Becklake[46] also provided reviews of the morphologic features of asbestosis.

The simplest definition of asbestosis is *pulmonary fibrosis caused by accumulation of airborne asbestos in the lungs*. The term *pleural asbestosis* has sometimes been used to refer to scarring of the pleura caused by asbestos, but in my (S.P.H.) opinion, the term *pleural asbestosis* should be avoided because it adds confusion to an already confusing area—asbestos terminology. Not infrequently, medical scientists use the terms *asbestos* and *asbestosis* improperly. *Asbestosis* is a scarring disease of lung tissue that has a dose–response relationship and is probably related to host factors. As discussed by Warnock and Isenberg[47] in 1986 concerning lung cancer and asbestosis, the degree of fibrosis in a person's lungs with the same concentrations of asbestos varies significantly. As discussed later in this chapter, cigarette smoke may influence the development of asbestosis, although the exact relationship between asbestosis and cigarette smoking in causing pulmonary fibrosis is unclear.

The macroscopic morphology of asbestosis depends on the severity of the disease. Persons with histologic grades 1 and 2 asbestosis typically show no gross abnormalities. As fibrosis becomes more severe, the pleura often becomes somewhat nodular because of scarring of the septa separating the secondary lobules. There are streaks and foci of grayish-white fibrous tissue within the parenchyma, usually in a subpleural location. With progression, there are additional deposits of scar tissue in the peripheral parts of the lung and honeycombing may occur (Figure 9.2). Asbestosis is often accompanied by visceral pleural fibrosis.

Asbestosis is typically stated to begin in and be most severe in the lower lobes, although I (S.P.H.) am is not convinced of that finding. In a study published by me (S.P.H.) and Winterbauer et al.[48]

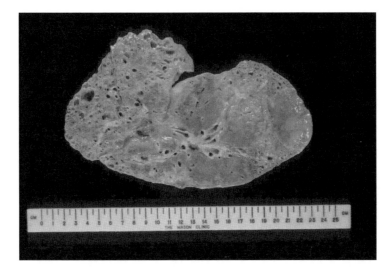

Figure 9.2 (See color insert.) "End-stage" pulmonary fibrosis with honeycombing caused by asbestos. Macroscopic features are identical to those seen in idiopathic pulmonary fibrosis.

Table 9.2   Asbestosis Grading Schema

Grade 0	No fibrosis is associated with bronchioles
Grade 1	Fibrosis involves wall of at least one respiratory bronchiole with or without extension into the septa of the immediately adjacent layer of alveoli; no fibrosis is present in more distant alveoli
Grade 2	Fibrosis appears as in grade 1, plus involvement of alveolar ducts or two or more layers of adjacent alveoli; there still must be a zone of nonfibrotic alveolar septa between adjacent bronchioles
Grade 3	Fibrosis appears as in grade 2, but with coalescence of fibrotic change such that all alveoli between at least two adjacent bronchioles have thickened, fibrotic septa; some alveoli may be obliterated completely
Grade 4	Fibrosis appears as in grade 3, but with formation of new spaces of a size larger than alveoli, ranging up to as much as 1 cm; this lesion has been termed *honeycombing*; spaces may or may not be lined by epithelium

in 1978, pulmonary fibrosis was just as severe in the upper lobes as it was in the lower lobes pathologically, although radiographically the changes appeared most severe in the lower lobes. As reported by Churg et al.[49] and Dodson et al.,[50] the concentration of asbestos in the lungs of those occupationally exposed to asbestos was just as great in the upper lobes as it was in the lower lobes.

In 1982, the panel commissioned by the CAP and the NIOSH headed by Craighead et al.[51] graded asbestosis into four categories, depending on the location of the fibrosis and its severity (see Table 9.2). As to the extent of the disease, three grades have been identified:

- Grade A (extent 1): only occasional bronchioles are involved and most show no lesion;
- Grade B (extent 2): more than an occasional bronchiole is involved, but less than half of all bronchioles in the section of lung tissue are involved; and
- Grade C (extent 3): more than half of all bronchioles are involved.

The total score of any given lung tissue section was stated to have been determined by multiplying the grade of asbestosis by the extent, in which the letter is converted to a number. This might be inappropriate because a relatively high score could be obtained by a focal area of severe fibrosis in a localized area, although this was not usually observed.

The histological grades of asbestosis are described in Table 9.3 and are shown in Figures 9.3 through 9.6.

A variety of other changes are seen in some cases of asbestosis. Occasionally, asbestos bodies are difficult to find in cases of diffuse fibrosis consistent with grade 4 asbestosis (Figure 9.7), whereas in

Table 9.3   Histological Grades of Asbestosis

Grade 1	Peribronchiolar fibrosis with possible extension into the septa of the adjacent layer of the alveoli, but with no fibrosis in the more distant alveoli (Figure 9.3). Simplified: peribronchiolar fibrosis.
Grade 2	Peribronchiolar fibrosis with involvement of alveolar ducts and two or more layers of adjacent alveoli with a zone of nonfibrotic alveolar tissue between adjacent bronchioles (Figure 9.4). Simplified: peribronchiolar fibrosis with involvement of alveolar ducts and alveoli.
Grade 3	Coalescence of fibrotic change with alveoli between at least two adjacent bronchioles showing interstitial fibrosis in addition to peribronchiolar fibrosis (Figure 9.5). Simplified: coalescence of fibrotic change between at least two bronchiolar units with obliteration of alveoli.
Grade 4	Diffuse interstitial fibrosis with honeycombing in association with asbestos bodies. The morphology is essentially identical to that of end-stage idiopathic pulmonary fibrosis with the exception that asbestos bodies are observed (Figure 9.6). Simplified: diffuse irregular interstitial fibrosis with honeycombing.

(a)

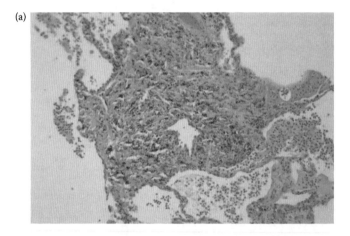

(b)

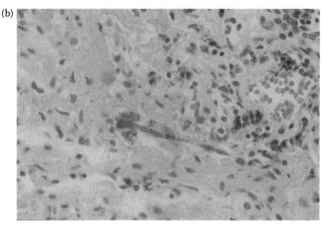

Figure 9.3   (See color insert.) (a) Grade 1 asbestosis characterized by peribronchiolar fibrosis in association with asbestos bodies and other dusts. (b) Ferruginous body morphologically consistent with an asbestos body.

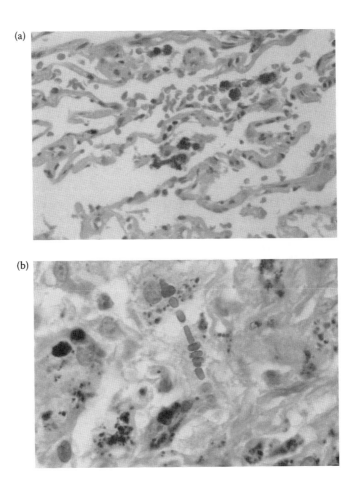

Figure 9.4 **(See color insert.)** (a) Grade 2 asbestosis characterized by mild septal fibrosis of two layers of alveoli. (b) Asbestos body is associated with other dusts.

other cases, large numbers of asbestos bodies are present (Figure 9.8) in persons with similar histories of occupational exposure to asbestos. This may be related to clearance of asbestos from the lung or to the "ability" to form asbestos bodies. Asbestos bodies are occasionally seen in the cytoplasm of multinucleated histiocytic giant cells (Figure 9.9), often being fragmented. Foci of ossification are not uncommonly seen in grade 4 asbestosis (Figure 9.10), as are blue bodies (Figure 9.11). Blue bodies are more likely related to cigarette smoking than they are to asbestos exposure. In rare cases, asteroid bodies are noted in multinucleated histiocytic giant cells but are nondiagnostic (Figure 9.12).

Alcoholic hyalin was first described in alveolar pneumocytes in a case of asbestosis[52] (Figure 9.13).

Roggli and Shelburne[43] categorized the histological changes in 100 cases of asbestosis (Table 9.4).

Several controversies exist concerning the pathological features and pathological diagnosis of asbestosis.[53] For example, Churg[54] defined asbestosis as "bilateral diffuse interstitial fibrosis of the lungs caused by exposure to asbestos" and stated that "diffuse interstitial fibrosis is the only process to which the term asbestosis should be applied." This definition, in part, may relate to his concept of whether the lesion referred to as grade 1 asbestosis (peribronchiolar fibrosis in association with asbestos bodies) should be referred to as asbestosis. As discussed by Churg and Wright[55] and Wright et al.,[56] a variety of mineral dusts, including coal, talc, mica, silica, aluminum oxide, and iron oxide as well as chrysotile and amphibole asbestos can induce small airways disease consisting

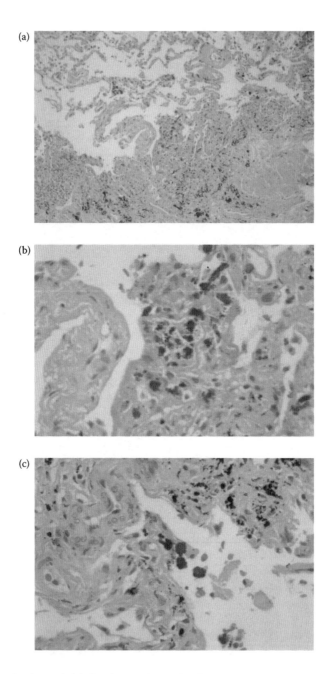

Figure 9.5 (See color insert.) (a) Grade 3 asbestosis characterized by coalescence of fibrosis with involvement of two adjacent acinar units. (b and c) Several ferruginous bodies consistent with asbestos bodies in fibrotic lung tissue.

of fibrotic thickening of the walls of the membranous bronchioles and respiratory bronchioles. They suggested the generic term *mineral dust-induced airways disease* be used to describe such lesions. As reviewed by Wright et al.,[56] part of the problem in determining whether mineral dust induces such a change is the fact that many of the persons exposed to mineral dust are cigarette smokers, and cigarette smoking can cause a similar lesion. They provided evidence that mineral dust appeared to cause membranous bronchiolar fibrosis above and beyond that caused by cigarette smoking alone.

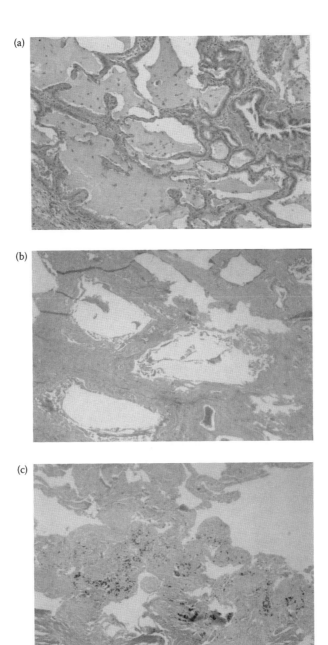

Figure 9.6 **(See color insert.)** (a and b) Grade 4 asbestosis characterized by diffuse interstitial fibrosis with honeycombing. (c and d) Fibrosis in subpleural location, the region of most severe fibrosis in grade 4 asbestosis. (e) Asbestos body in dense connective tissue. (f) Asbestos bodies seen in filter preparation made from case of grade 4 asbestosis.

As stated by Wright et al.,[56] only 4% of control (nondust-exposed) smokers showed fibrosis in the region of respiratory bronchioles, whereas this was found in 48% of respiratory bronchioles from smoking workers with asbestos exposure and 35% of the alveolar ducts from such workers. Similar changes were seen in 31% of the respiratory bronchioles and 14% of the alveolar ducts from subjects with other types of dust exposure. These latter findings would suggest that asbestos is more potent than other dusts in inducing fibrosis.

(d)

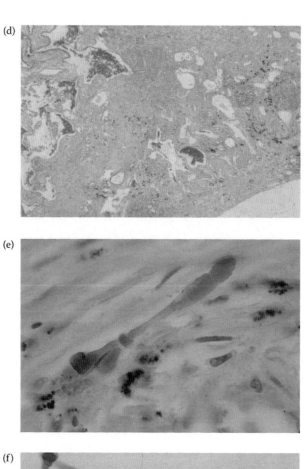

(e)

(f)

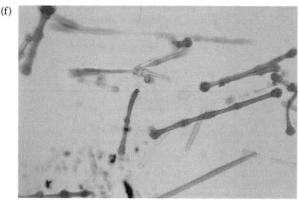

Figure 9.6 Continued.

The Helsinki Consensus Report[57] defines asbestosis as "diffuse interstitial fibrosis of the lung as a consequence of exposure to asbestos dust." The 2004 ATS document[58] defines "asbestosis as interstitial pneumonitis and fibrosis caused by inhalation of asbestos fibers."

I (S.P.H.) use the CAP-NIOSH system for grading asbestosis. However, I feel that lung scarring caused by asbestos is often patchy and of variable severity. Asbestos bodies are not infrequently seen in the walls of blood vessels (Figure 9.14). Asbestos bodies in iron-stained sections are more intensely blue than hemosiderin found in the lung (Figure 9.15).

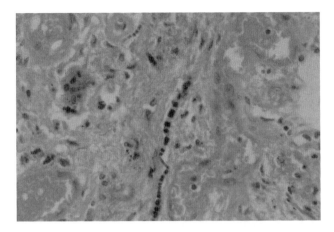

Figure 9.7 (See color insert.) In this case of grade 4 asbestosis, it was difficult to identify asbestos bodies; however, high concentrations of asbestos fibers were found in lung tissue.

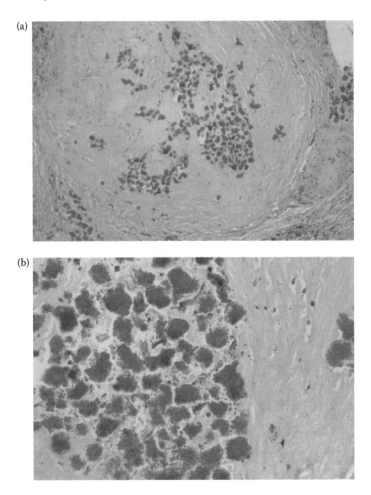

Figure 9.8 (See color insert.) In this case, the patient's lung tissue contained numerous aggregates of asbestos bodies formed on anthophyllite cores (a) Low power magnification and (b) high power magnification.

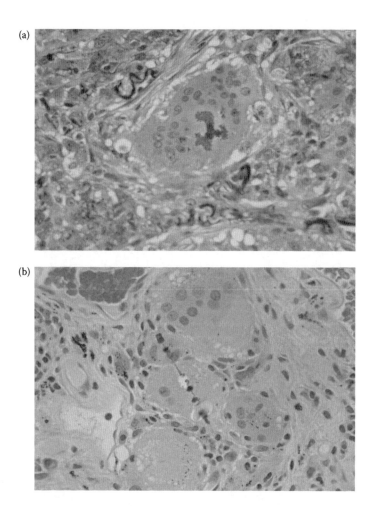

Figure 9.9 **(See color insert.)** (a and b) Asbestos bodies are occasionally found in cytoplasm of multinucle-ated histiocytic giant cells; they are often fragmented.

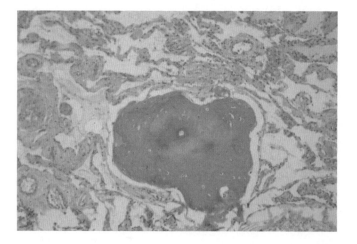

Figure 9.10 **(See color insert.)** This area of grade 4 asbestosis shows a region of ossification, a relatively frequent finding in grade 4 asbestosis.

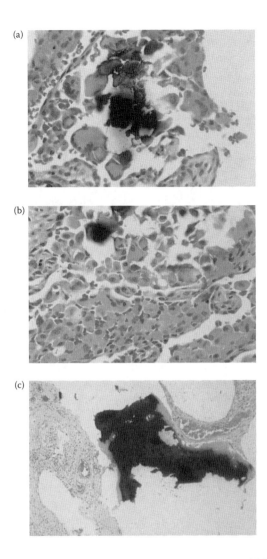

Figure 9.11 **(See color insert.)** (a) Calcified bodies are clustered in alveoli. (b) Multiple laminated irregular blue bodies are seen. (c) Multiple blue bodies present with alveolar macrophages.

9.4 MINERALOGY OF ASBESTOSIS

Asbestosis is a disease that shows a dose–response relationship, and in most instances relatively high concentrations of asbestos are needed to cause grades 3 and 4 asbestosis, although the definition of what is considered "high" has not been defined (see below). Although Wagner et al.[59] suggested that asbestosis does not occur in individuals exposed only to chrysotile asbestos, experimental studies have shown that all commercial types of asbestos cause asbestosis. A number of experimental and clinical studies have suggested that short-fiber chrysotile asbestos (<5 μm long) is nonfibrogenic.[60–67] However, there is no doubt that long-fiber chrysotile asbestos causes asbestosis in asbestos miners and millers and in asbestos textile workers.[68,69] As mentioned throughout this book, short fibers cannot be disregarded as potential contributors to disease in lung tissue where they are the predominant form or certainly in extrapulmonary sites where asbestos-induced changes occur.[70] Short fibers of all types of asbestos are cleared from the lung more readily than longer fibers

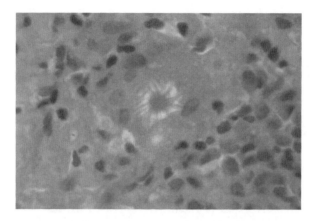

Figure 9.12 **(See color insert.)** Asteroid body. Stellate inclusion, measuring 10 to 15 micrometers, in the upper right corner of a multinucleated giant cell.

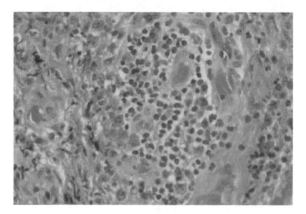

Figure 9.13 **(See color insert.)** Cytoplasmic hyaline in alveolar cells. Dense ropelike glassy inclusion is surrounded by clear space in enlarged alveolar cells in center and upper right.

Table 9.4   Histological Features Found in 100 Cases of Asbestosis

Histological Feature	Percentage
Always present	
Asbestos bodies	100
Peribronchiolar fibrosis	100
Often present	
Alveolar septal fibrosis	82
Occasionally present	
Honeycomb changes	15
Foreign-body giant cells	15
Pulmonary adenomatosis	10
Cytoplasmic hyaline	7
Desquamative interstitial pneumonitis-like areas	6
Rarely present	
Osseous metaplasia (dendriform pulmonary ossification)	2
Pulmonary blue bodies	1

Source: Roggli, V.L., Shelburne, J.D. *Semin. Respir. Med.* 4,128–138, 1982.

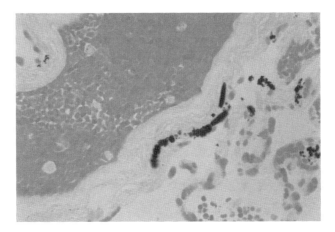

Figure 9.14   (See color insert.) In many persons exposed to asbestos, asbestos bodies are frequently seen in the wall of blood vessels (iron stain).

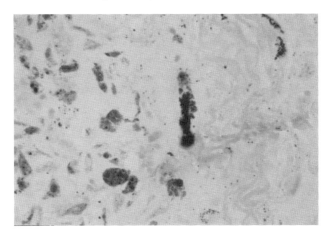

Figure 9.15   (See color insert.) Not infrequently, abundant hemosiderin is present in lung tissue. In iron-stained sections, asbestos bodies are typically more intensely blue than the surrounding hemosiderin (iron stain).

of the same type, but it is also known that these same short fibers are the ones most readily found in extrapulmonary sites and even in mesothelial tissue.[71,72]

The statement is often made that asbestos can be found in the lungs of most adult men between age 50 and 55 years in industrialized nations, and therefore by itself is not a specific marker for asbestosis. However, in 1999 Dodson et al.[73] reported the majority of persons younger than 20 years had no asbestos bodies or asbestos fibers in their lungs when evaluated by digestion analysis.

In general, the concentration of asbestos in dry lung is approximately 10 times that in wet lung because the wet weight:dry weight ratio is usually about 1:10. However, there often is significant variation in asbestos body/fiber concentration in lung tissue as determined by different laboratories.[74]

Roggli and Shelburne[43] reviewed the asbestos content of lung tissue in four reported series of patients with asbestosis (Table 9.5) and reported on the asbestos body count in the lungs of 76 patients with histologically confirmed asbestosis (Figure 9.16). In Roggli and Shelburne's report, the median asbestos body count for patients with asbestosis was 37,800 per gram of wet lung tissue, whereas the median values for patients with idiopathic pulmonary fibrosis was 16 asbestos bodies per gram of wet lung tissue, and for the control group it was 0.4 asbestos bodies per gram of wet

Table 9.5   Asbestos Content of Lung Tissue in Reported Series of Patients with Asbestosis[a]

Source	No. of Cases	Method	Asbestos Bodies per Gram of Dry Lung	Uncoated Fibers per Gram of Dry Lung
Ashcroft and Heppleston	22	PCLM	12.2 (0.49–192)	32 (1.3–493)
Roggli	76	SEM[b]	0.378 (0.006–16)[c]	3.3 (0.18–125)[c]
Wagner et al.	100	PCLM	–	1.5 (0.001–31.6)
	170	TEM	–	372 (<1.0–10,000)
Warnock et al.	22	TEM[b]	0.123 (0.001–7.38)	5.68 (1.6–121)
Whitwell et al.	23	PCLM	–	8 (1.0–7.0)

Notes: PCLM, phase contrast light microscopy; TEM, transmission electron microscopy; SEM, scanning electron microscopy.

[a] Values reported are the median counts for millions (10^6) of asbestos bodies or uncoated fibers per gram of dried lung tissue, with ranges indicated in parentheses, except for the study of Wagner et al., where only the mean value could be obtained from the data presented.

[b] In these two studies, asbestos bodies were counted by conventional light microscopy.

[c] Values multiplied by a factor of 10 (approximate ratio of wet to dry lung weight) for purposes of comparison.

Source: Roggli, V.L., Shelburne, J.D. *Semin. Respir. Med.* 4,128–138, 1982.

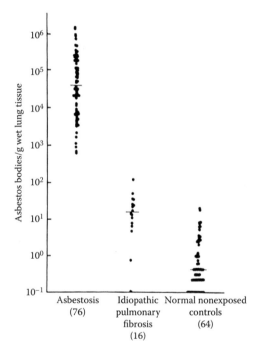

Figure 9.16   Number of asbestos bodies in lung tissue in patients with asbestosis compared with patients with idiopathic pulmonary fibrosis and normal nonasbestos-exposed controls.

lung tissue. Roggli and Shelburne[43] found that in 95% of asbestosis cases, the asbestos body count was ≥1700 asbestos bodies per gram of wet lung tissue. They stated that when this concentration of asbestos is present in lung tissue, one can usually, but not always, see several asbestos bodies in a 2×2-cm iron-stained section. As illustrated by Roggli and Shelburne[43] in Figure 9.17, asbestosis best correlates with the content of uncoated asbestos fibers in lung tissue. They found very few patients with alveolar septal fibrosis (total score of 4 or higher) to have uncoated fiber counts of less than 100,000 per gram of dry lung tissue.

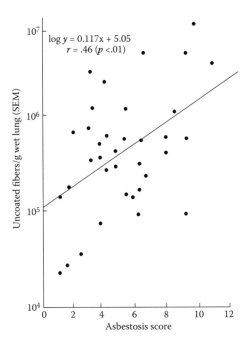

$$\log y = 0.117x + 5.05$$
$$r = .46 \ (p < .01)$$

Uncoated fibers/g wet lung (SEM)

Asbestosis score

Figure 9.17 Correlation of asbestos score (asbestos grade times extent of disease) with concentration of uncoated fibers in lung tissue.

Table 9.6 Correlation of Histological Grade of Asbestosis with Tissue Asbestos Content and Other Parameters

	Correlation Coefficient (*r*)	*p*
Uncoated fibers/gram (>5 µm), SEM	.46	<.0l
Total fibers per gram (coated and uncoated), SEM	.44	<.01
Asbestos bodies per gram by light microscopy	.26	Insignificant
Smoking history (pack-years)	.22	Insignificant
Age (years)	.12	Insignificant
Duration of exposure (years)	.06	Insignificant

Note: SEM, scanning electron microscopy; pack-years = number of packs smoked daily × number of years smoked.
Source: Roggli, V.L., Shelburne, J.D. *Semin. Respir. Med.* 4,128–138, 1982.

As reported by Churg[75] and by Bellis et al.,[17] it takes considerably less asbestos to cause grade 1 asbestosis. Bellis et al.[17] found evidence of grade 1 asbestosis in some patients with fiber counts as low as 1000 to 10,000 fibers per gram of dry lung tissue; and of the 15 patients they reported with grade 1 asbestosis, 13 had fiber counts less than 100,000 per gram of dry lung tissue.

Roggli and Shelburne[43] correlated the histologic grade of asbestosis with tissue asbestos content and other parameters (Table 9.6) and found that only the uncoated fibers (>5 µm long as determined by scanning electron microscopy) and the total fibers per gram of lung tissue (coated and uncoated) had the highest correlation coefficients and were statistically significant. Asbestos bodies per gram of lung tissue, smoking history, age, and duration of exposure to asbestos had correlation coefficients between .26 and .06 and were not statistically significant. Our findings are different than Roggli and Shelburne's and correspond to those reported by Warnock and Isenberg.[47]

9.5 ASBESTOS, ASBESTOSIS, AND CIGARETTE SMOKING

A major problem in determining the exact relationship between cigarette smoke and asbestos in causing interstitial fibrosis is that many persons who have been occupationally exposed to asbestos and who have developed asbestosis have also been chronic cigarette smokers. Churg et al.[76] studied the effect of cigarette smoke on the retention of amosite fibers in the lungs of guinea pigs and found that smoking caused a marked increase in the number of fibers found in macrophages in the lung but did not appear to change the size of the fibers in the macrophage or the phagocytic capacity of the macrophages. Their[76] data suggested that cigarette smoke decreased macrophage removal via the mucociliary escalator and that macrophage mobility was impaired. McFadden et al.[77] found that cigarette smoke increased the penetration of UICC amosite asbestos fibers into airway walls in guinea pigs, resulting in an increased concentration of fibers in the interstitium.

Clinical studies evaluating the effect of cigarette smoke on the development of small opacities in chest radiographs of asbestos-exposed workers have recorded variable findings. These have been reviewed in published reports by Barnhart et al.[78] and by Blanc and Gamsu.[79] Barnhart et al.[78] concluded the cumulative evidence supported that in the setting of exposure to asbestos and tobacco smoke, asbestos exposure and not cigarette smoke was the necessary risk factor for the development of roentgenographic small opacities. They also concluded that cigarette smoking appeared to add to the risk, particularly for lesser degrees of roentgenographic small opacities, and it was uncertain whether roentgenographic small opacities represented interstitial fibrosis. Blanc and Gamsu[79] found no correlation between high-resolution computed tomography (HRCT) scan abnormalities and asbestosis and cigarette smoking. They concluded that HRCT scan analysis of lung might be the best method for separating the radiographic abnormalities caused by asbestos and those caused by cigarette smoke. A somewhat different conclusion was reached by Weiss[80] concerning cigarette smoking and small irregular opacities in the lungs. Weiss[80] concluded that the data from his study suggested that abnormalities observed in 181 workers not exposed to asbestos were directly related to age and smoking habits among workers who were not exposed to hazardous dusts. Weiss[81] previously suggested cigarette smoke might be responsible for the development of radiographically detected small irregular opacities in the lung and suggested that cigarette smoke caused pulmonary fibrosis.

The 2004 ATS document[58] on environmental and occupational health issues stated that asbestosis was more prevalent and more advanced for a given duration of exposure in cigarette smokers, presumably because of reduced clearance of asbestos fibers from the lung. Although some studies suggested that smokers without dust exposure showed occasional irregular radiographic opacities on chest films, smoking alone was stated to not cause changes of asbestosis. However, smokers and ex-smokers were stated to have a higher frequency of asbestos-related opacities on their chest radiographs than did nonsmoking asbestos workers in all profusion categories. The 2004 ATS document[58] further stated that cigarette smoking did not affect asbestos-induced pleural fibrosis.

9.6 CLINICAL FEATURES OF ASBESTOSIS

The clinical features of asbestosis depend on the severity of the disease. Those persons with pathological grades 1 and 2 asbestosis may have no symptoms or radiographic abnormalities. Patients with grade 4 asbestosis (diffuse interstitial fibrosis with honeycombing) are usually symptomatic, with the most common symptom being dyspnea on exertion.[82] There is an increased incidence of clubbing of the fingers, although the diagnostic usefulness of this finding is minimal. Most patients with pathological grade 4 asbestosis have basilar rales, frequently described as "velcro" rales. Pulmonary function tests usually show restrictive lung disease changes with a decrease in total lung capacity and forced vital capacity. Hypoxemia may be present at rest or may develop with exercise. The diffusing capacity is usually decreased. In 1986, the American Thoracic Society[82] proposed the following criteria for the clinical diagnosis of asbestosis:

(1) A reliable history of exposure to asbestos;
(2) An appropriate latent interval between exposure and detection of disease;
(3) Chest roentgenographic evidence of type "s," "t," or "u" small, irregular opacifications with a profusion of 1:1 or greater;
(4) A restrictive pattern of lung impairment with forced vital capacity below the lower limit of normal;
(5) A diffusing capacity below the lower limit of normal; and
(6) Bilateral late or pan-inspiratory crackles at the posterior lung bases, not cleared by coughing.

The 2004 ATS document[58] lists the criteria for diagnosis of nonmalignant lung disease related to asbestos and commented on the 1986 criteria (Table 9.7).

In the report by Huuskonen[83] of 202 patients diagnosed as having asbestosis by the Institute of Occupational Health between 1934 and 1976, 88.7% had breathlessness, 71.4% had persistent sputum production, 58% had crepitations, and 32.3% had clubbing of their fingers. Of the 174 men registered as having asbestosis, 56 died, whereas the expected number of deaths among men of the same age in the Finnish general population was 23.4. Of the 62 patients who died before 1977, the cause of death was (1) asbestosis, 26 patients (41.9%); (2) lung cancer, 20 patients (32.2%); (3) other malignant diseases, 4 patients (6.5%); and (4) other causes, 12 patients (19.4%).

9.7 APPROACH TO THE DIAGNOSIS, PATHOLOGICAL DIFFERENTIAL DIAGNOSIS, AND CONTROVERSIES

The pathological criteria for diagnosing asbestosis have been previously reviewed.[84] In general, the pathological diagnosis is simply defined as fibrosis in association with asbestos bodies or fibers. The 1982 CAP-NIOSH Committee[51] required two asbestos bodies in association with fibrosis to diagnose asbestosis. Tissue sections are insensitive for detecting asbestos bodies, and chrysotile asbestos does not readily form asbestos bodies because most of the chrysotile that is inhaled is of insufficient fiber length. As observed in the article by Dodson et al.[25] in 1997 where only 1 of approximately 900 ferruginous bodies had a chrysotile core, one could never make a diagnosis of asbestosis on the basis of the 1982 CAP-NIOSH Committee criteria for diagnosing asbestosis even in people with high levels of chrysotile in their lung tissue because chrysotile fibers are not typically formed on cores.

In my (S.P.H.) experience, there are cases of asbestosis in which asbestos bodies are not easily identified. In a situation in which there is a strong history of occupational exposure to asbestos in association with pulmonary fibrosis but no observable asbestos bodies in hematoxylin and eosin (H&E) or iron-stained sections, one should attempt to perform asbestos fiber analysis on the tissue. Examples of asbestosis have been reported in which asbestos bodies have not been recognized in lung tissue but in which asbestos fibers have been found in great enough concentrations to cause asbestosis.[85–87]

In the proper clinical context, analysis of bronchoalveolar lavage fluid can strongly suggest the diagnosis of asbestosis by containing an increased number of neutrophils and eosinophils in the fluid[88] (Figure 9.17) and in some instances can be relatively specific by containing asbestos bodies or fibers (Figures 9.18 through 9.20). Likewise, the identification of asbestos bodies in sputum (Figure 9.21) or in transbronchial biopsy specimens (Figure 9.22) can strongly suggest the diagnosis of asbestosis given the proper clinical setting (see Chapter 3).

Table 9.7   Criteria for Diagnosis of Nonmalignant Lung Disease Related to Asbestos

1986 Guidelines	2004 Guidelines	Comparison and Notes
	Evidence of structural change, as demonstrated by one or more of the following:	Demonstrates the existence of a structural lesion consistent with the effects of asbestos. The criteria outlined in the 1986 guidelines were most explicit for asbestosis.
Chest film (irregular opacities)	• Imaging methods	Chest film, HRCT, and possibly future methods based on imaging. The 1986 guidelines specified ILO classification 1/1.
Pathology (CAP)	• Histology (CAP)	Criteria for identifying asbestosis on microscopic examination of tissue are unchanged.
Consistent time interval	Evidence of plausible causation, as demonstrated by one or more of the following:	
Occupational and environmental history	• Occupational and environmental history of exposure (with plausible latency) • Markers of exposure (e.g., pleural plaques)	
Asbestos bodies or fibers in lung tissue	• Recovery of asbestos bodies	The 2004 guidelines are not limited to lung tissue, consider the role of BAL to be established, and de-emphasize fibers because they are difficult to detect and a systematic analysis for asbestos fibers is not generally available.
Rule out other causes of interstitial fibrosis or obstructive disease	Exclusion of alternative diagnoses	The 1986 guidelines primarily addressed asbestosis but mentioned smoking as a cause of obstructive disease. Implicit in the article, however, is that nonmalignant diseases presenting similarly to asbestos-related disease should also be ruled out.
"Evidence of abnormal test"	Evidence of functional impairment, as demonstrated by one or more of the following:	Functional assessment is not required for diagnosis but is part of a complete evaluation. It contributes to diagnosis in defining the activity of disease and the resulting impairment.
Crackles, bilateral, not cleared by cough	• Signs and symptoms (including crackles)	Signs and symptoms are not specific for diagnosis but are valuable in assessing impairment.
Restrictive disease	• Change in ventilatory function (restrictive, obstructive patterns in context or disease history)	The 1986 criteria admitted the possibility of obstructive disease; the 2004 criteria address this specifically.
Reduced diffusing capacity	• Impaired gas exchange (e.g., reduced diffusing capacity)	
	• Inflammation (e.g., by bronchoalveolar lavage)	The 1986 guidelines noted possible utility of bronchoalveolar lavage and gallium scanning but considered them to be experimental techniques. The 2004 guidelines exclude gallium scanning, suggest that additional indicators of active inflammation may become useful in future.
	• Exercise testing	

Note: BAL, bronchoalveolar lavage; HRCT, high-resolution computed tomography; ILO, International Labour Organization.
Source: Guidotti, T.L., Miller, A., Christiani, D., Wagner, G., Balmes, J., Harber, P., et al. *Am. J. Respir. Crit. Care Med.* 170, 691–715, 2004.

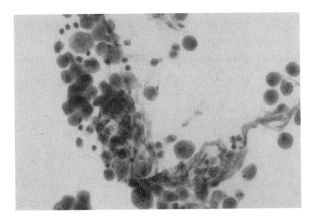

Figure 9.18 **(See color insert.)** Representative region of cytocentrifuge preparation of bronchoalveolar lavage fluid from a patient with clinical features of asbestosis. Note the increased number of neutrophils.

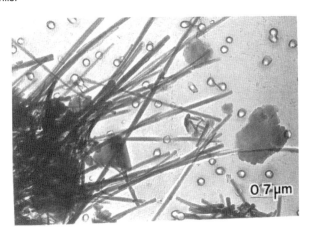

Figure 9.19 Bundle of long chrysotile fibers found in lavage sample that contained chrysotile-cored ferruginous bodies (transmission electron microscopy).

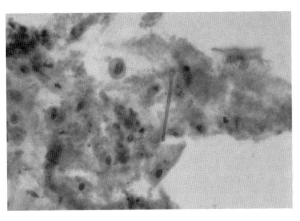

Figure 9.20 **(See color insert.)** Amosite-cored ferruginous body obtained from digested lavage sample from individual occupationally exposed to this form of asbestos (transmission electron microscopy).

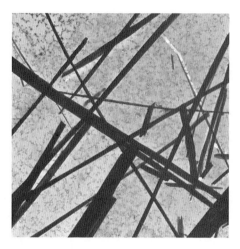

Figure 9.21 Lavage material from occupationally exposed individuals such as seen in Figure 9.20 also contained uncoated amosite fibers such as this (transmission electron microscopy).

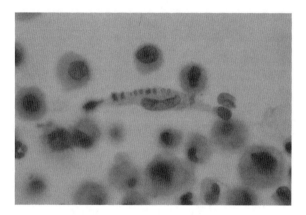

Figure 9.22 **(See color insert.)** Thin section of embedded sputum shows ferruginous body with associated macrophages and mucous material (transmission electron microscopy).

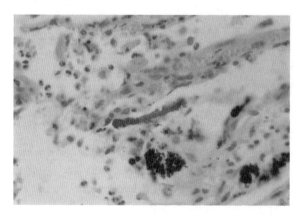

Figure 9.23 **(See color insert.)** Transbronchial biopsy specimen from patient with clinical features of asbestosis shows a ferruginous body consistent with an asbestos body.

The primary pathological differential diagnosis of asbestosis is usual interstitial pneumonia (UIP; idiopathic pulmonary fibrosis). This differential diagnosis occurs in cases in which there is a history of exposure to asbestos but in which the lung tissue sections show no asbestos bodies. As stated, one must always be aware of cases in which asbestos bodies are in low numbers or are not observed in H&E or iron-stained histological sections but in which there is a significantly elevated fiber concentration. As previously discussed, asbestosis correlates best with the total content of uncoated asbestos fibers. Gaensler et al.[89] reported on 176 asbestos-exposed persons in which lung tissue was available for analysis and identified 9 cases in which the clinical features were consistent with asbestosis but in which the histological sections did not show asbestos bodies and there was no evidence of increased numbers of asbestos fibers. They concluded the following:

(1) The American Thoracic Society criterion of "a reliable history of exposure" is sometimes difficult to define;
(2) Asbestos bodies are seen in tissue sections only when exposure has been reasonably high, and given the proper clinical setting, the presence of diffuse fibrosis and asbestos bodies in tissue sections is sensitive and specific criteria for the diagnosis of asbestosis; and
(3) The prevalence of 5.1% nonasbestos-induced interstitial lung disease among asbestos-exposed persons is artifactually high because of atypical case selection.

They further concluded that because asbestosis was a disappearing disease, cases of "idiopathic" pulmonary fibrosis in persons with a history of asbestos exposure will increase.

Roggli[90] came to a somewhat similar conclusion in his study of 24 cases of diffuse pulmonary fibrosis of unknown cause. Roggli found that patients with advanced pulmonary fibrosis whose tissue samples did not meet the histologic criteria for asbestosis usually did not have asbestos-induced fibrosis. However, as discussed by Roggli,[90] there was concern whether cases 23 and 24 in his series represented idiopathic pulmonary fibrosis or asbestosis. In case 23, the asbestos mineral fiber content was below the 95% confidence limit for diffuse asbestosis (grade 9 total score), although it was well within the range of milder asbestosis, which may have been obscured by superimposed radiation-associated fibrosis. Case 24 concerned an 85-year-old man who developed fatal pulmonary fibrosis 20 years after retiring as a brakeline grinder. In that case, the uncoated fiber content was low, although asbestos body content by light microscopy and scanning electron microscopy was within the range expected in cases of asbestosis.

Monso et al.[91] evaluated 25 patients diagnosed as having idiopathic pulmonary fibrosis by standard examination and found two cases with a high number of asbestos fibers (>100 fibers per scanning electron microscopy field). Monso et al.[91] concluded that standard pathological techniques overdiagnosed idiopathic pulmonary fibrosis in a few cases in which asbestos bodies were not found with the optical microscope.

I (S.P.H.) have seen several cases of CAP-NIOSH grade 4 asbestosis in persons with relatively low concentrations of asbestos bodies (<100–200 AB per gram) and less than 100,000 fibers per gram of dry lung tissue.

Persons who are occupationally exposed to asbestos are sometimes exposed to other dusts that can cause pulmonary fibrosis. These dusts include silica, talc, nonasbestos silicates, and welding fumes, all of which may cause fibrosis. In some instances, the pattern of fibrosis, for example, silicosis, allows for the easy differentiation from asbestosis. Also, one can identify "pseudoasbestos" bodies in some lung tissue sections, which suggest a nonasbestos cause for the fibrosis.

A recent update has been published by the Asbestosis Committee of the College of American Pathologists and Pulmonary Pathology Society.[92] This document provides a significant amount of useful information but also illicits controversies about certain aspects of *asbestosis*. Roggli et al.[92] define *asbestosis* as diffuse pulmonary fibrosis caused by the inhalation of excessive amounts of asbestos fibers. They point out that all types of asbestos have been implicated to a greater or lesser degree in causing asbestosis, and there appears to be a dose–response relationship between the concentration of fibers in the lung and the severity of asbestosis. They stated asbestosis typically occurs in individuals with prolonged and heavy exposures to asbestos and the disease may progress even after exposure has ceased. There is no definition of what "heavy" is. The diagnosis of asbestosis is usually based on the exposure history, clinical findings, and radiographic findings. Roggli et al.[92] do not point out what their definition of "excessive" is with respect to the amount of asbestos fibers and they do not point out the fact that although there is a dose–response relationship as pointed out by me and Dr. Ronald F. Dodson (S.P.H.), one can be exposed to very high concentrations of asbestos and not develop asbestosis and vice versa—be exposed to much lower concentrations of asbestos but still develop asbestosis. This was pointed out in our (S.P.H., R.F.D) 1997 article[25] in which we evaluated cases of patients with mesothelioma and found that 29 of 55 individuals had asbestosis, but only three had clinical asbestosis and most of the other cases had grades 1 and 2 asbestosis. Of more interest was that there were a significant number of patients with mesothelioma who had incredibly high concentrations of asbestos in their lung tissue who did not develop asbestosis. Likewise, there were cases that occurred where the concentrations of asbestos were relatively low who developed asbestosis. This is similar to what was published by Warnock and Isenberg[47] in 1986.

According to this manuscript, Roggli et al.[92] stated that with respect to the clinical aspects, when asbestosis is symptomatic and progressive, the clinical features are similar to those encountered in diffuse interstitial lung disease such as UIP. Most cases of asbestosis are stated to be diagnosable on the basis of clinical and radiographic findings without having to obtain a biopsy. The criteria for diagnosing asbestosis as listed in the manuscript were as follows:

(1) A history of moderate to heavy asbestos exposure typically, but not always, occupational and often protracted for many years. Asbestosis is stated to not invariably be an outcome of substantial or even heavy asbestos exposure. In general, when the cumulative exposure has been substantial to heavy, the likelihood of clinical asbestosis and its severity are correspondingly greater. (My (S.P.H.) note: Once again, there is no definition of what "substantial" and "heavy" is and there is no definition of what "likelihood" means.)
(2) Clinical signs of interstitial fibrosis in the form of end-inspiratory crackles on auscultation of the lung fields, especially in the lower zones.
(3) Detection of reticular-linear diffuse opacities in the lower zones of the lung fields by radiologic examination.
(4) Classic, restrictive impairment of lung function.
(5) Usually, but not always, associated with parietal pleural fibrous plaques and/or diffuse pleural fibrosis.

Roggli et al.[92] pointed out that according to published literature, lung volume measurements have low specificity and sensitivity, the lack of sensitivity being explicable in part by the wide range of reference values.

The article by Roggli et al.[92] stated that histological diagnosis of asbestosis was most useful as follows:

(1) When the clinical or radiologic features are atypical or nondiagnostic, for example, when the history of asbestos exposure is equivocal and a biopsy of lung is carried out (optimally, a wedge biopsy);
(2) When histologic examination shows lung parenchyma remote from the lung cancer or mesothelioma in surgical resection specimens; or
(3) At autopsy.

Chest radiograph and imaging findings in asbestosis are discussed by Dr. Friedman in Chapters 12 and 13.

The American College of Chest Physicians Consensus Statements on the Respiratory Health Effects of Asbestos: Results of a Delphi Study[93] stated there was consensus agreement as to the following:

(1) A history of asbestos exposure of sufficient duration, dose, and latency is likely the cause of interstitial fibrosis in the absence of other explanations (consensus statement no. 10).
(2) Identification of asbestos fibers in lung specimens is integral to the histological diagnosis of asbestosis (consensus statement no. 12). (My (S.P.H.) note: In most cases of asbestosis, one does not see asbestos fibers. These are too thin and almost transparent. What the consensus statement probably should have stated was "the identification of asbestos *bodies* in lung specimens is integral to the histological diagnosis of asbestosis.")
(3) The chest radiograph, an HRCT scan, is a more sensitive method for detecting asbestos-related pleural and parenchymal disease (consensus statement no. 16).

The study[93] stated there was consensus disagreement as to the following:

(1) Chest radiographs are a sensitive method to diagnose interstitial disease attributable to asbestos exposure (consensus statement no. 1); and
(2) Asbestos exposure, in the absence of interstitial fibrosis, leads to COPD (consensus statement no. 5).

The differential diagnosis of asbestosis includes UIP/idiopathic pulmonary fibrosis and nonspecific interstitial pneumonia (NSIP). The features of UIP, asbestosis, and NSIP are listed in Table 9.8.

Perhaps the most significant issue in the pathological diagnosis of asbestosis in the manuscript by the Asbestosis Committee[92] is how many asbestos bodies must be present in a certain area of lung tissue to be diagnostic of asbestosis. According to the article by Roggli et al.,[92] two or more asbestos bodies per square cm of a 5-μm-thick lung section in combination with interstitial fibrosis of the appropriate pattern are necessary for diagnosing asbestosis. They pointed out that fewer asbestos bodies did not necessarily exclude a diagnosis of asbestosis; however, evidence of excess asbestos would then require quantitative studies be performed on lung digest specimens. Of interest, they did not reference the article by Warnock and Isenberg[47] published in Chest in January 1986, which dealt with the concentration of asbestos in lung tissue necessary to cause lung cancer and asbestosis.

Table 9.8 Differential Diagnosis of Asbestosis versus Idiopathic Interstitial Pneumonia

Histological Feature	UIP	NSIP	Asbestosis
Asbestos bodies	Absent	Absent	Frequent, although in a small percentage of cases, asbestos bodies are not easily demonstrable. Fiber analysis is indicated in such cases when the exposure history is compelling.
Distribution	Subpleural accentuation, lower lung zones	Diffuse	Peribronchiolar with subpleural accentuation
Fibroblastic foci	Conspicuous	Inconspicuous	Rare
Honeycomb changes	Common	Uncommon	Uncommon except in advanced cases
Inflammation	Minimal, typically localized to honeycomb foci	Variable	Minimal
Parietal pleural plaques and/or diffuse visceral pleural fibrosis	Uncommon	Uncommon	Common

In the report by Warnock and Isenberg,[47] the number of asbestos bodies found to cause asbestosis ranged from 0 to 1.97 per cm^2 in seven subjects with grossly visible fibrosis. Thus, the number of asbestos bodies used to pathologically diagnose asbestosis used by the Asbestosis Committee of the College of American Pathologists and the Pulmonary Pathology Society would be less than two asbestos bodies per square centimeter of lung tissue. Warnock and Isenberg[47] pointed out that "asbestos bodies were sometimes very infrequent in histologic sections [as seen in Table 9.9] and stated their correlation coefficient for extracted and histologic asbestos bodies (0.9, Spearman rank test) was considerably lower than that of Roggli and Pratt,[94] who employed many correction factors to obtain their good correlation; but no matter how good the correlation is, the variation in the ratios of uncoated to coated fibers (4:1 to 136,000) precludes the use of asbestos bodies as the standard for diagnosing asbestosis."

It is my (S.P.H.) opinion that the statement by Warnock and Isenberg[47] is correct on the basis of my own experience, which is that two asbestos bodies per square centimeter of lung tissue is too high and that a more reliable number—0.5 asbestos bodies per square centimeter—as used by Warnock and Isenberg[47] and as stated verbally by Dr. William R. Salyer,[95] is sufficient. Case in point, I (S.P.H.) recently evaluated the case of a 67-year-old woman with a history of paraoccupational exposure to asbestos from her father between approximately 1945 and 1955. The woman unfortunately developed a predominantly epithelial biphasic pleural mesothelioma and subsequently died from that condition. Autopsy tissue was obtained and bilateral hyaline pleural plaque characteristic of plaque caused by asbestos was identified. Iron-stained sections showed a total of 19 asbestos bodies (1 in block A6, 1 in block A7, 6 in block A8, 5 in block A9, and 6 in block A10). Repeat iron stains showed a total of 6 asbestos bodies (1 in block A5, 1 in block A6, 1 in block A7, 1 in block A8, and 2 in block A10). The H&E-stained sections showed mild diffuse interstitial fibrosis without asbestos bodies. This analysis is of significance in that the first specimens analyzed for asbestos bodies in iron-stained sections showed 5.6 asbestos bodies per square centimeter of lung tissue, whereas on the second go-around using exactly the same blocks but on deeper cut, 1.77 asbestos bodies per square centimeter were identified. This points out that asbestos is not evenly distributed and, if one used the "magic number" of two asbestos bodies per square centimeter, one would make a diagnosis of asbestosis in the first go-around but not in the second. This also points out something that had been stated several years previous by Bellis et al.[17] when evaluating patients with grade 1 asbestosis compared with small airways disease with the criteria for asbestosis—specifically, that there are approximately equal numbers of asbestos bodies and asbestos fibers in tissue that showed grade 1 asbestosis versus tissue that did not show grade 1 asbestosis but did show some scarring in the peribronchiolar region without association with

Table 9.9 Asbestos Bodies in Tissue Sections from Seven Subjects in Group 2 with Grossly Visible Fibrosis[a]

Case	Asbestos Bodies/Gram	AC Fibers/ Gram	Asbestos Bodies Counted	Total Area per cm^2	Asbestos Bodies per cm^2
1	444	284,000	1	6.96	0.14
2	825	128,000	0	9.12	0
3	1400	202,000	1	6.96	0.14
4	4000	461,000	1	5.08	0.2
5	5640	210,000	12	6.47	1.85
6	8000	949,000	4	8.36	0.48
7	13,000	412,000	14	7.1	1.97

Note: [a]TAAG fibers ranged from 97,000 to 699,000/g except for two cases that had 2.05 million and 3.43 million/g. All cases had 1+ fibrosis, except cases 4 and 5, which had 3+ fibrosis.

asbestos bodies. Once again, this points out the fallacy that it takes a precise amount of asbestos to cause asbestosis on the basis of histological sections using iron stains.

A report by Wick et al.[96] in 2009 tried to determine if certain morphologic features were more likely to be present in asbestosis than in nonasbestos-induced fibrosis. They stated the interstitial connective tissue response in asbestosis might be fibroelastic rather than fibrotic, and for that reason they performed a comparative characterization of the connective tissue response in cases of asbestosis and other forms of interstitial lung disease. They used archival open lung biopsies or autopsy specimens featuring interstitial connective tissue abnormalities (15 of asbestosis, 21 of organizing pneumonia, 15 of usual interstitial pneumonitis/idiopathic pulmonary fibrosis, 9 with organizing diffuse alveolar damage, 9 with "nonspecific interstitial pneumonitis, 4 with sarcoidosis, 3 each of desquamative interstitial pneumonia and chronic amiodarone toxicity, 2 with cryptogenic organizing pneumonias, and 1 each of chronic hypersensitivity pneumonitis and chronic eosinophilic pneumonitis [85 total]). They stained the tissue with H&E, Perl method for asbestos bodies, Gomori's trichrome procedure, and the Verhoeff–van Gieson technique. Representative subsets of the cases ($n = 20$) were also studied immunohistochemically using an antibody to elastin. Fibroelastosis in each of the samples was assessed for the degree of response and its location using a three-tiered scale. The degree of fibroelastosis in the 15 cases of asbestosis was variable with the pattern being peribronchial and perivascular in all instances, and at least two asbestos bodies were identified in fibroelastotic foci in each of the 15 cases as highlighted with Perl's stain. Forty-seven cases (71%) of nonasbestotic lung disease showed interstitial fibrosis with a variable (usually modest) amount of mixed elastic tissue, and when present, the elastic fibers were distributed in a diffuse interstitial pattern with or without perivascular accentuation. All cases of idiopathic pulmonary fibrosis also showed areas of fibroelastosis, but those foci were confined to regions of honeycomb change. No asbestos bodies were identified in any of the diseases except asbestosis. A predominantly peribronchial pattern of fibroelastosis was not identified in any nonasbestotic interstitial lung disease in this study. Wick et al.[96] concluded that this type and pattern of pulmonary connective tissue response in interstitial lung disease might provide additional diagnostic clues to the pathological diagnosis of asbestosis.

REFERENCES

1. Selikoff IJ, Lee DHK. *Asbestos and Disease*. New York: Academic Press; 1978.
2. Craighead JE. Eyes for the epidemiologist: The pathologist's role in shaping our understanding of asbestos-associated diseases. *Am J Clin Pathol* 1988;89:281–287.
3. Cooke WE. Pulmonary asbestosis. *Br Med J* 1927;2:1024–1025.
4. Dreessen WC, Dallavalle JM, Edward TI, Miller JM, Sayers RR. A study of asbestos in the asbestos textile industry. *Public Health Bulletin No. 24*. Washington, DC: U.S. Treasury Department; 1938: 1–126.
5. Merewether ERA, Price CW. *Report on the Effects of Asbestos Dust on the Lungs and Dust Suppression in the Asbestos Industry*. London: HM Stationery Office; 1930: 1–34.
6. Rom WN, Travis WD, Brody AR. Cellular and molecular basis of asbestos-related diseases. *Am Rev Respir Dis* 1991;143:408–422.
7. Hartman DP. Immunological consequences of asbestos exposure. *Immunol Rev* 1985;4:65–68.
8. Kagan E. The alveolar macrophage: Immune derangement and asbestos-related malignancy. *Semin Oncol* 1980;8:258–267.
9. Spurzem JR, Saltini C, Rom W, Winchester RJ, Crystal RG. Mechanism of macrophage accumulation in the lungs of asbestos subjects. *Am Rev Respir Dis* 1987;136:276–280.
10. Dubois CM, Bissonnette E, Rola-Pleszycynski M. Asbestos fibers and silica particles stimulate rat alveolar macrophages to release tumor necrosis factor. *Am Rev Respir Dis* 1989;139:1257–1264.
11. Lemaire I, Beaudoin H, Massé S, Grondin C. Alveolar macrophage stimulation of lung fibroblast growth in asbestos-induced pulmonary fibrosis. *Am J Pathol* 1986;122:205–211.
12. Hansen K, Mossman BT. Generation of superoxide from alveolar macrophages exposed to asbestiform and nonfibrous particles. *Cancer Res* 1987;47:1681–1686.

13. Timbrell V, Ashcroft T, Goldstein B, Heyworth F, Meurman LO, Rendall REG, et al. Relationships between retained amphibole fibers and fibrosis in human lung tissue specimens. In: *Inhaled Particles VI*. Dodgson J, McCallum RI, Bailey MR, Fisher DR, eds. Oxford: Pergamon Press; 1988: 323–340.

14. Oberdörster G, Maynard A, Donaldson K, Castranova V, Fitzpatrick J, Ausman K, et al. Principles for characterizing the potential health effects from exposure to nanomaterials: Elements of a screening strategy. *Particle Fibre Toxicol* 2005;2:8.

15. Oberdorster G, Oberdorster E, Oberdorster J. Nanotoxicology: An emerging discipline evolving from studies of ultrafine particles. *Environ Health Perspect* 2005;113:823–839.

16. Begin R, Masse S, Bureau MA. Morphologic features and function of the airways in early asbestosis in the sheep model. *Am Rev Respir Dis* 1982;126:870–876.

17. Bellis D, Andrion A, Delsedime L, Mollo F. Minimal pathologic changes of the lung and asbestos exposure. *Hum Pathol* 1989;20:102–106.

18. Harless KW, Watanabe S, Renzetti AD. The acute effects of chrysotile asbestos exposure on lung function. *Environ Res* 1978;16:360–372.

19. Jodoin G, Gibbs GW, Macklem PT, McDonald JC, Becklake MR. Early effects of asbestos exposure on lung function. *Am Rev Respir Dis* 1971;104:525–535.

20. Jacob G, Bohling H. Das verhalten des bronchialbaumes bei der asbestaublunge. *Arch Gewerbepathol Gewerbehyg* 1960;18:247–257.

21. Pinkerton KE, Plopper CG, Mercer RR, Roggli VL, Patra AL, Brody AR, Crapo JD. Airway branching patterns influence asbestos fiber location and the extent of tissue injury in the pulmonary parenchyma. *Lab Invest* 1986;55:688–695.

22. Delfino R, Ernst P, Bourbeau J. Relationship of lung geometry to the development of pleural abnormalities in insulation workers exposed to asbestos. *Am J Ind Med* 1989;15:417–425.

23. Mossman BT, Churg A. Mechanisms in the pathogenesis of asbestosis and silicosis. *Am J Respir Crit Care Med* 1998;157:1666–1680.

24. Attanoos RL, Gibbs AR, Corrin B. The dilemma of "asbestosis" or lung fibrosis: A case referent necropsy study of 188 asbestos exposed naval dockyard workers and 175 UK non-exposed "control" subjects. *Mod Pathol* 2006;1:302A.

25. Dodson RF, O'Sullivan M, Corn CJ, McLarty JW, Hammar SP. Analysis of asbestos fiber burden in lung tissue from mesothelioma patients. *Ultrastruct Pathol* 1997;21:321–336.

26. Brody A. Asbestos and lung disease. *Am J Respir Cell Mol Biol* 2010;42:131–132.

27. Pinkerton KE, Pratt PC, Brody AR, Crapo JD. Fiber localization and its relationship to lung reaction in rats after chronic inhalation of chrysotile asbestos. *Am J Pathol* 1984;117:484–498.

28. Turner-Warwick M, Parkes WR. Circulating rheumatoid and antinuclear factors in asbestos workers. *Br Med J* 1970;3:492–495.

29. Turner-Warwick M. Immunological mechanisms in occupational disorders. *Proc R Soc Med* 1973;66: 927–930.

30. Toivanen A, Salmivalli M, Molnar G. Pulmonary asbestosis and autoimmunity. *Br Med J* 1976;20:691–692.

31. Lange A, Smolik R, Chmielarczyk W, Garncarek D, Gielgier Z. Cellular immunity in asbestosis. *Arch Immunol Ther Exp (Warsz)* 1978;26:899–903.

32. Lange A, Nineham LJ, Garncarek D, Smolik R. Circulating immune complexes and antiglobulins (IgG and IgM) in asbestos-induced lung fibrosis. *Environ Res* 1983;31:287–295.

33. Zone JJ, Rom WN. Circulating immune complexes in asbestos workers. *Environ Res* 1985;37:383–389.

34. Morris DL, Greenberg SD, Lawrence EC. Immune responses in asbestos-exposed individuals. *Chest* 1985;87:278–279.

35. Lahat N, Sobel E, Djerassi L, Kaufman G, Horenstein L, Gruener N. Immunological profile of chest x-ray-negative, asymptomatic asbestos workers. *Am J Ind Med* 1988;13:473–482.

36. Al Jarad N, Uthayakumar S, Buckland EJ, Green TS, Ord J, Newland AC, Rudd RM. The histocompatibility antigen in asbestos related disease. *Br J Ind Med* 1992;49:826–831.

37. Tamura M, Liang D, Tokuyama T, Yoneda T, Kasuga H, Narita N, et al. Study on the relationship between appearance of autoantibodies and chest x-ray findings of asbestos plant employees. *Sangyo Igaku* 1993;35:406–412.

38. Marczynski B, Czuppon AB, Marek W, Reichel G, Baur X. Increased incidence of DNA double-strand breaks and anti-ds DNA antibodies in blood of workers occupationally exposed to asbestos. *Hum Exp Toxicol* 1994;13:3–9.

39. Nigam SK, Suthar AM, Patel MM, Karnik AB, Dave SK, Kashyap SK, Venkaiah K. Humoral immuno-logical profile of workers exposed to asbestos in asbestos mines. *Indian J Med Res* 1993;98:274–277.

40. Pfau JC, Sentissi JJ, Weller G, Putnam EA. Assessment of autoimmune responses associated with asbestos exposure in Libby, Montana, USA. *Environ Health Perspect* 2005;113:25–30.

41. Pfau JC, Sentissi JJ, Li S, Calderon-Garciduenas L, Brown JM, Blake DJ. Asbestos-induced autoimmunity in C57BL/6 mice. *J Immunotoxicol* 2008;5:129–137.

42. Craighead JE, Abraham JL, Churg A, Green FH, Kleinerman J, Pratt PC, et al. The pathology of asbestos-associated diseases of the lungs and pleural cavities: Diagnostic criteria and proposed grading schema. Report of the Pneumoconiosis Committee of the College of American Pathologists and the National Institute for Occupational Safety and Health. *Arch Pathol Lab Med* 1982;106:544–596.

43. Roggli VL, Shelburne JD. New concepts in the diagnosis of mineral pneumoconiosis. *Semin Respir Med* 1982;4:128–138.

44. Roggli VL. Pathology of human asbestosis: A critical review. *Adv Pathol* 1989;2:31–60.

45. Roggli VL. Asbestosis. In: *Pathology of Asbestos-Associated Diseases*, Roggli VL, Greenberg SD, Pratt PC, eds. Boston: Little Brown; 1992: 77–108.

46. Becklake MR. Asbestos-related diseases of the lung and other organs: Their epidemiology and implications for clinical practice. *Am Rev Respir Dis* 1976;114:187–227.

47. Warnock ML, Isenberg W. Asbestos burden and the pathology of lung cancer. *Chest* 1986;89:20–26.

48. Winterbauer RH, Hammar SP, Hallman KO. Diffuse interstitial pneumonitis: Clinicopathologic correlations in 20 patients treated with prednisone/azathioprine. *Am J Med* 1978;65:661–672.

49. Churg A, Sakoda N, Warnock ML. A simple method of preparing ferruginous bodies for electron microscopic examination. *Am J Clin Pathol* 1976;68:513–517.

50. Dodson RF, Williams MG, Corn CJ, Brollo A, Bianchi C. Asbestos content of lung tissue, lymph nodes and pleural plaques from former shipyard workers. *Am Rev Respir Dis* 1990;142:843–847.

51. Craighead JE, Abraham JL, Pratt PC, et al. The pathology of asbestos-associated diseases of the lungs and pleural cavities: diagnostic criteria and proposed grading schema. Report of the Pneumoconiosis Committee of the College of American Pathologists and the National Institute for Occupational Safety and Health. *Arch Pathol Lab Med* 1982;106:544–596.

52. Kuhn C, III, Kuo TT. Cytoplasmic hyalin in asbestosis: A reaction of injured alveolar epithelium. *Arch Pathol* 1973;95:190–194.

53. Hammar SP. Controversies and uncertainties concerning the pathologic features and pathologic diagnosis of asbestosis. *Semin Diagn Pathol* 1992;9:102–109.

54. Churg A. Non-neoplastic diseases caused by asbestos. In: *Pathology of Occupational Lung Diseases*, Churg A, Green FHY, eds. New York: Igaku-Shoin; 1988: 253–277.

55. Churg A, Wright JL. Small airway lesions in patients exposed to nonasbestos mineral dusts. *Hum Pathol* 1983;14:688–693.

56. Wright JL, Cagle P, Churg A, Colby TV, Myers J. Diseases of the small airways. *Am Rev Respir Dis* 1992;146:240–262.

57. Helsinki Consensus Report. Asbestos, asbestosis, and cancer: The Helsinki Criteria for diagnosis and attribution. *Scand J Work Environ Health* 1997;23:311–316.

58. American Thoracic Society. Diagnosis and initial management of nonmalignant diseases related to asbestos. *Am J Respir Crit Care Med* 2004;170:691–715.

59. Wagner JC, Newhouse ML, Corrin B, Rossiter CE, Griffiths DM. Correlation between fibre content of the lung and disease in East London asbestos factory workers. *Br J Ind Med* 1988;45:305–308.

60. Davis JMG, Jones AD. Comparisons of the pathogenicity of long and short fibres of chrysotile asbestos in rats. *Br J Exp Pathol* 1988;69:717–737.

61. Vorward AJ, Durkan TM, Pratt PC. Experimental studies of asbestosis. *Arch Ind Hyg Occup Med* 1951;3:1–43.

62. Wright GW, Kuschner M. The influence of varying length of glass and asbestos fibers on tissue response in guinea pigs. In: *Inhaled Particles IV*, Walton WH, ed. Oxford: Pergamon Press; 1977: 455–474.

63. Davis JMG, Beckett ST, Bolton RE, Collings P, Middleton AP. Mass and the number of fibers in the pathogenesis of asbestos-related lung disease in rats. *Br J Cancer* 1978;37:673–688.

64. Crapo JD, Barry BE, Brody AR, O'Neil JJ. Morphological, morphometric and x-ray microanalytical studies on lung tissue of rats exposed to chrysotile asbestos in inhalation chambers. In: *Biological Effects of Mineral Fibers*, Wagner JC, ed. Lyon, France: IARC Scientific Publications; 1980: 273–283.

65. Davis JMG, Addison J, Bolton RE, Donaldson K, Jones AD, Smith T. The pathogenicity of long versus short fibre samples of amosite asbestos administered to rats through inhalation and intraperitoneal injection. *Br J Exp Pathol* 1986;67:415–430.

66. Adamson IYR, Bowden DH. Response of mouse lungs to crocidolite asbestos. I. Mineral fibrotic reaction to short fibers. *J Pathol* 1987;152:99–107.

67. Adamson IYR, Bowden DH. Response of mouse lungs to crocidolite asbestos. II. Pulmonary fibrosis after long fibres. *J Pathol* 1987;152:109–117.

68. Holden J, Churg A. Asbestos bodies and the diagnosis of asbestosis in chrysotile workers. *Environ Res* 1986; 39:232–236.

69. McDonald AD, Fry JS, Woolley AJ, McDonald JC. Dust exposure and mortality in an American chrysotile textile plant. *Br J Ind Med* 1983;40:361–367.

70. Dodson RF, Atkinson MAL, Levin JL. Asbestos fiber length as related to potential pathogenicity: A critical review. *Am J Ind Med* 2003;44:291–297.

71. Suzuki Y, Yuen SR. Asbestos tissue burden study on human malignant mesothelioma. *Ind Health* 2001;39:150–160.

72. Suzuki Y, Yuen SR. Asbestos fibers contributing to the induction of human malignant mesothelioma. *Ann N Y Acad Sci* 2002;982:160–176.

73. Dodson RF, Williams MG, Huang J, Bruce JR. Tissue burden of asbestos in nonoccupationally exposed individuals from East Texas. *Am J Ind Med* 1999;35:281–286.

74. Gylseth B, Churg A, Davis JM, Johnson N, Morgan A, Mowe G, et al. Analysis of asbestos fibers and asbestos bodies in tissue samples from human lung: An international interlaboratory trial. *Scand J Work Environ Health* 1985;11:107–110.

75. Churg A. Asbestos fiber content of the lungs in patients with and without asbestos airways disease. *Am Rev Respir Dis* 1983;127:470–473.

76. Churg A, Tron V, Wright JL. Effects of cigarette smoke exposure on retention of asbestos fibers in various morphologic compartments of the guinea pig lung. *Am J Pathol* 1987;129:385–393.

77. McFadden D, Wright J, Wiggs B, Churg A. Cigarette smoke increases the penetration of asbestos fibers into airway walls. *Am J Pathol* 1986;123:95–99.

78. Barnhart S, Thornquist M, Omen GS, et al. The degree of roentgenographic parenchymal opacities attributable to smoking among asbestos-exposed subjects. *Am Rev Respir Dis* 1990;141:1102–1106.

79. Blanc PD, Gamsu G. The effect of cigarette smoking on the detection of small radiographic opacities in inorganic dust diseases. *J Thorac Imaging* 1988;3:51–56.

80. Weiss W. Cigarette smoking and small irregular opacities. *Br J Ind Med* 1991;48:841–844.

81. Weiss W. Smoking and pulmonary fibrosis. *J Occup Med* 1988;30:33–39.

82. American Thoracic Society. The diagnosis of nonmalignant diseases related to asbestos. *Am Rev Respir Dis* 1986;134:363–368.

83. Huuskonen MS. The clinical features, mortality and survival of patients with asbestosis. *Scand J Work Environ Health* 1978;4:265–274.

84. Becklake MR. Asbestosis criteria. *Arch Pathol Lab Med* 1984;108:93.

85. Churg A, Warnock ML. Analysis of the cores of ferruginous (asbestos) bodies from the general population. III. Patients with environmental exposure. *Lab Invest* 1979;40:622–626.

86. Warnock ML, Wolery G. Asbestos bodies or fibers and the diagnosis of asbestosis. *Environ Res* 1987;44:29–44.

87. Dodson RF, Williams MG, O'Sullivan MF, Corn CJ, Greenberg SD, Hurst GA. A comparison of the ferruginous body and uncoated fiber content in the lungs of former asbestos workers. *Am Rev Respir Dis* 1985;132:143–147.

88. Robinson BWS, Rose AH, James A, Whitaker D, Musk AW. Alveolitis of pulmonary asbestosis: Bronchoalveolar lavage studies in crocidolite- and chrysotile-exposed individuals. *Chest* 1986;90:396–402.

89. Gaensler EA, Jederline PJ, Churg A. Idiopathic pulmonary fibrosis in asbestos-exposed workers. *Am Rev Respir Dis* 1991;144:689–696.

90. Roggli VL. Scanning electron microscopic analysis of mineral fiber content of lung tissues in the evaluation of diffuse pulmonary fibrosis. *Scanning Microsc* 1991;5:71–83.

91. Monso E, Tura JM, Morell F, Ruiz J, Morera J. Lung dust content in idiopathic pulmonary fibrosis: A study with scanning electron microscopy and energy-dispersive x-ray analysis. *Br J Ind Med* 1991;48:327–331.

92. Roggli VL, Gibbs AR, Attanoos R, Churg A, Popper H, Cagle P, et al. Pathology of asbestosis: An update of the diagnostic criteria. Report of the Asbestosis Committee of the College of American Pathologists and Pulmonary Pathology Society. *Arch Pathol Lab Med* 2010;134:462–480.

93. Banks DE, Shi R, McLarty J, Cowl CT, Smith D, Tarlo SM, et al. American College of Chest Physicians Consensus Statement on the respiratory health effects of asbestos: Results of a Delphi Study. *Chest* 2009;135:1619–1627.

94. Roggli VL, Pratt PC. Numbers of asbestos bodies on iron-stained tissue sections in relation to asbestos body counts in lung tissue digests. *Hum Pathol* 1983;14:355–361.

95. Salyer WR. Berkeley, CA: PSI/Pathology Services, Inc. [verbal communication with Samuel P. Hammar].

96. Wick MR, Kendall TJ, Ritter JH. Asbestosis: demonstration of distinctive interstitial fibroelastosis: A pilot study. *Ann Diagn Pathol* 2009;13:297–302.

CHAPTER 10

Asbestos-Induced Pleural Disease

Samuel P. Hammar

CONTENTS

10.1 INTRODUCTION

Asbestos causes a variety of pleural changes. These include benign asbestos-induced pleural effusion (BAPE), fibrosing pleuritis (fibrous pleurisy), diffuse visceral or localized visceral pleural scarring, round atelectasis, hyaline pleural plaques, and a condition referred to as fibrothorax.

10.2 BENIGN ASBESTOS-INDUCED PLEURAL EFFUSION

There are many causes of benign pleural effusions (see Chapter 30 in *Dail and Hammar's Pulmonary Pathology*, Third Edition).[1] With respect to BAPE, most occur in older men who were usually last exposed to asbestos 15–20 years before the development of their pleural effusion. BAPEs are frequently hemorrhagic and have features of an exudate. They may be painful and superimposed on parietal pleural plaques and asbestosis. They are usually unilateral but may be bilateral. They can last several months, occasionally are recurrent, and usually cause chest pain.[2–6] The pleural fluid typically contains leukocytes and especially eosinophils (Figure 10.1).[2] Pleural effusions are characteristically seen as a presenting finding in pleural mesothelioma and are more frequent than BAPEs. In 1982, Epler et al.[7] reported 34 benign effusions among 1135 asbestos-exposed workers and compared them with otherwise unexplained effusions among 717 unexposed control subjects. The prevalence of BAPE was dose related with 7%, 3.7%, and 0.2% associated with severe, indirect, and peripheral asbestos exposure, respectively. The latency period (time from first exposure to asbestos to the time of disease development) was shorter for asbestos-induced pleural effusions than it was for other asbestos-related conditions and was the most common asbestos-related abnormality identified in the first 20 years after exposure to asbestos. The final conclusion of Epler et al.[7] was that inquiries should be made as to possible exposures to asbestos in persons with "idiopathic" pleural effusions.

In 1971, Gaensler and Kaplan[8] reviewed their files of 4077 patients evaluated in their laboratory between 1951 and 1969 and identified 91 patients with pleural effusions. Of the 4077 patients, 57 had asbestosis or asbestos exposure and 24 had pleural effusion. Twelve patients (21.1%) with asbestosis or asbestos exposure were diagnosed with BAPE.

10.2.1 Clinical Manifestations of Asbestos-Induced Pleural Effusions

As reported by Collins[9] and Mattson and Ringqvist,[10] most patients with BAPE had exudative effusions without signs or symptoms of other disease. Mattson[11] later reported 25 persons with monosymptomatic exudative pleurisy of unknown etiology and found that 11 patients had been

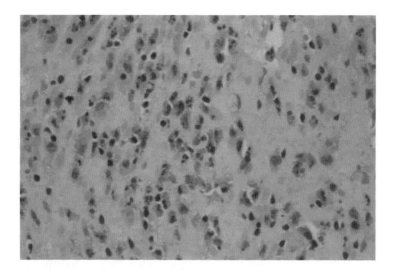

Figure 10.1 This asbestos-induced pleural effusion specimen contained a mixture of inflammatory cells, including frequent eosinophils.

exposed to asbestos. No other cause of the pleural effusion was noted in these 11 men during an observation period of 4–8 years. Diffuse pleural fibrosis may develop in patients with BAPE and progress to fibrothorax.

Eisenstadt[12] reported on a 54-year-old male insulator suffering from acute left hemithorax chest pain and who had an asbestos pleural effusion. The patient subsequently developed similar symptoms and evidence of a right pleural effusion, which over a period of time progressed to pleural thickening requiring decortication. Eisenstadt[12] commented that benign asbestos pleurisy resembled tuberculosis in that its appearance was apparently a self-limited disease that could progress to fibrosis.

In Gaensler and Kaplan's[8] report, all patients were symptomatic. Several had dyspnea possibly related to asbestosis, one had joint pain and lumps on their elbows, and another had fatigue. This is in contrast to the report of Epler et al.[7] in which 66% of patients were asymptomatic and to Hillerdal and Ozesmi's report[13] in which 47% were asymptomatic, 34% had chest pain, 6% had dyspnea, and the remainder had a variety of other symptoms.

10.2.2 Characteristics of Pleural Fluid

The pleural fluid in BAPE is characteristically serous/serosanguinous and generally has an elevated white blood count of greater than 12,000 per microliter. The differential white blood count typically shows a predominance of polys, lymphocytes, and eosinophils.

10.2.3 Pathological Features and Pathogenesis of Asbestos Pleural Effusion

In most cases of BAPE, the pleura is usually abnormal and shows either an acute pleuritis with increased vascularity, an infiltrate of acute inflammatory cells, and a layer of fibrin on the outer surface of the pleura (Figure 10.2) or will show a predominantly chronic inflammatory cell infiltrate (Figure 10.3). As time progresses, the exudate has a tendency to become more fibrotic (Figure 10.4).

The pathogenesis of BAPE is not well understood but may relate to asbestos fibers in the pleural space or pleural tissue that causes inflammation and irritation. As previously discussed, asbestos has a variety of biologic properties and results in release of various cytokines from inflammatory cells, which may be important in the generation of the fluid. Why there is a relatively long latent period in many cases is unknown.

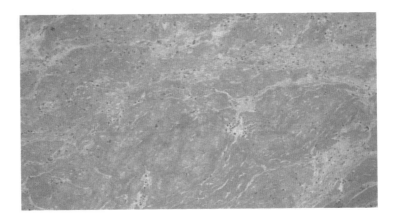

Figure 10.2   Pleural biopsy from patient with benign acute asbestos-induced pleural effusion shows pleural thickening from fibrin deposition with mild acute inflammation.

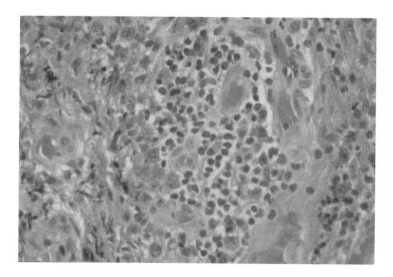

Figure 10.3 Open lung biopsy from 78-year-old retired refinery worker who presented with bilateral pleural effusion; markedly thickened pleura with predominantly chronic inflammatory cell infiltrate.

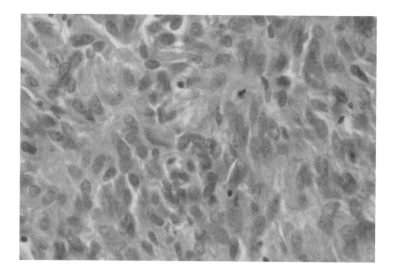

Figure 10.4 This pleural biopsy shows reactive fibrosis caused by multipotential subserosal proliferation with varying degrees of inflammation and vascular proliferation.

10.3 HYALINE PLEURAL PLAQUES

Hyaline pleural plaques are discrete, white to yellow-white, irregularly shaped, frequently calcified, raised structures involving the parietal pleura (Figure 10.5). In persons occupationally exposed to asbestos, hyaline pleural plaques occur most frequently on the parietal pleura covering the diaphragm and commonly between the fifth and eighth ribs in the posterior and lateral portions of the chest, characteristically sparing the apices and costophrenic angles. Plaques are occasionally seen on the visceral pleural surface (Figure 10.6) and may be seen on the visceral or parietal pericardium, adventitia of the aorta, peritoneal serosal surface, and on the capsule of the spleen and liver.[14–17]

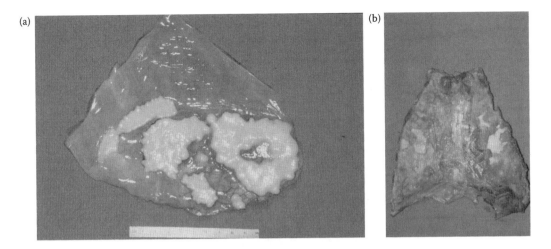

Figure 10.5 (a and b) Representative appearance of hyaline pleural plaques. (a) Plaque on diaphragmatic surfaces. (b) Plaques on parietal pleural surface of anterior chest wall from patient with malignant mesothelioma.

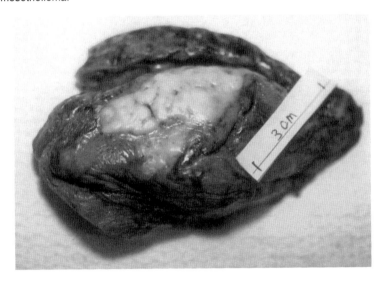

Figure 10.6 Hyaline pleural plaque involved visceral pleural surface of lung, a relatively uncommon location for asbestos-induced plaques.

Microscopically, hyaline pleural plaques have a characteristic histological appearance, being composed of dense, relatively hypocellular connective tissue that often exhibits a basket weave pattern (Figure 10.7). Hyaline pleural plaques may be associated with focal chronic inflammation and sometimes in association with mesotheliomas or pseudomesotheliomas.

10.3.1 Incidence of Hyaline Pleural Plaques

The exact incidence of pleural plaques is uncertain. Wain et al.[16] reported 25 cases of pleural plaques in 434 autopsies performed over a 2 ½-year period. Schwartz[17] reviewed 16 separate autopsy studies and identified pleural plaques in 857 of 7085 routine autopsies (12.2%; range = 0.5%–30.3%). Rogan et al.,[18] in the late 1980s, and Miller and Zurlo,[19] in the mid-1990s, found the incidence of pleural plaques consistent with those caused by asbestos in 2.3% of U.S. men.

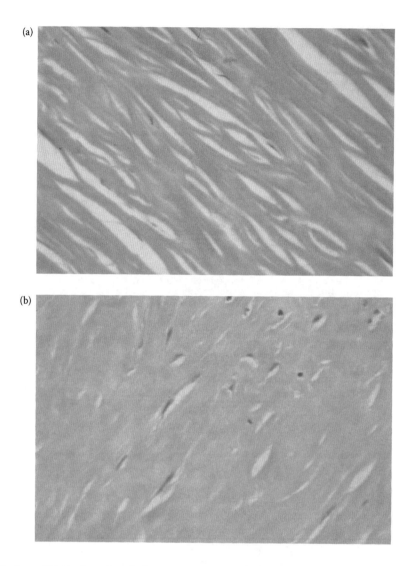

Figure 10.7   (a and b) Hyaline pleural plaques are composed of dense, relatively hypocellular connective tissue that exhibits a basket weave histological pattern.

In 2008, Paris et al.[20] identified that 474 (46.9%) of 1011 patients had pleural plaques and 61 (6.0%) had interstitial changes compatible with asbestosis on CT scan. Time since first exposure ($p < .0001$) and either cumulative or mean exposure ($p < .0001$) showed independent associations with pleural plaques and asbestosis prevalence and pleural plaques incidence. Modeling incidence of pleural plaques showed a 0.8% to 2.4% yearly increase for a mean exposure of 1 fiber/mL. Paris et al.[20] stated that their findings confirmed the role played by time since first exposure and dose, but not duration, in asbestos-related diseases.

In 2009, Paris et al.[21] analyzed a population of 5545 subjects and found that the time since first exposure to asbestos ($p < .0001$) and the cumulative exposure to asbestos ($p = .02$, or level, depending on the models used) were independently associated with the frequency of pleural plaques. Only cumulative exposure ($p < .001$) or level of exposure ($p = .02$) was significantly associated with asbestosis. Both time–response and dose–response relationships were demonstrated for pleural plaques, whereas only dose–response relationships were demonstrated for asbestosis.

Sichletidis et al.[22] reported three dentists who presented with roentgenographic pleural plaques secondary to occupational exposure to asbestos while manipulating wet asbestos tape during casting operations. Chrysotile was stated to have been used in dentistry since 1930 when it was introduced as a lining material for casting rings. All three patients had radiographic pleural plaques identified on chest radiograph and CT scans. The dentists had worked as dentists for 35–45 years. Sichletidis et al.[22] used the membrane filter method and phase-contrast optical microscopy to evaluate asbestos fiber concentration in material used to make fire-resistant molds and melt gold inside them. Dry asbestos sheets were scanned and showed 0.008 fibers/mL during the sampling period. Sichletidis et al.[22] concluded everyday occupational exposure for many years, even at low levels, under poor ventilation conditions in a closed space could result in the development of pleural plaques.

More than 80% of persons occupationally exposed to asbestos develop hyaline pleural plaques as identified at autopsy, most frequently occurring on the diaphragmatic surfaces. In our experience, all patients with plaques have had elevated numbers of asbestos bodies or fibers in their lung tissue.

10.3.2 Association of Plaques with Asbestos

As stated previously, hyaline pleural plaques are seen predominantly in persons exposed to asbestos. As reported by Wain et al.,[16] asbestos bodies were identified in lung digests from 25 patients with pleural plaques and exceeded the normal range for their laboratory (20 asbestos bodies per gram of wet lung tissue) in 14 cases. In the 25 patients with plaques, 3 had definite exposure to asbestos, 7 had probable exposure to asbestos, 9 had possible exposure to asbestos, and 6 were considered unlikely to have been exposed to asbestos.

Hourihane et al.[23] reported hyaline pleural plaques in 4.2% of 381 autopsies (16 cases). They stated that they had not personally attended all the autopsies and wondered if the incidence was lower than expected.

An evaluation of all autopsies performed at the Department of Forensic Medicine between January and March 1965 found that 15 (11.2%) of 134 necropsies showed hyaline pleural plaques with many individuals having metastatic lung neoplasms or primary diffuse malignant mesothelioma.[23] In 115 routine autopsies, asbestos bodies were found in 28 cases (24.3%). In contrast, asbestos bodies were found in all 56 cases of patients with hyaline pleural plaques. Hourihane et al.[23] stated that the association between plaques and asbestos bodies in the lungs was statistically significant ($p <$ .01) when compared with the control series, whether asbestosis was or was not present. Using phase-contrast microscopy, four incinerated plaques were found to contain asbestos bodies.

Warnock et al.[24] reviewed epidemiologic studies and found that all types of asbestos were incriminated in the development of plaques. Likewise, some plaques developed in persons exposed to talc,[25] which may have been due to asbestos fibers such as tremolite in talc. Warnock et al.[24] found plaques most frequently in persons age 60–80 years with a latency in the range of 20 years, although there were cases of reported plaques with a latency as short as 5–6 years after initial exposure.[26] Warnock et al.[24] found a significantly higher concentration of amosite and crocidolite fibers in the lung tissue of persons with plaques as compared with the control group. They also found focal minimal areas of asbestosis in three patients with plaques with the highest concentration of amosite in their lung tissue. In the control patients, they found the fibers to consist mostly of chrysotile, tremolite, actinolite, and anthophyllite, with relatively few amosite and crocidolite fibers. In subjects with plaques, most amosite and crocidolite fibers had high aspect ratios, which led Warnock et al.[24] to conclude that the fibers were of commercial origin.

Sebastien et al.[27] analyzed lung tissue from two groups of patients with pleural plaques and found 10^7 fibers/cm^3 in those with asbestosis and 10^6 fibers/cm^3 in those without asbestosis. Whitwell et al.[28] found a correlation between pleural plaques and asbestos fibers in lung tissue with 55% of subjects with more than 20,000 fibers/g dry lung tissue having plaques and only 5.5% of those with fewer than 20,000 fibers/g dry lung tissue having pleural plaques. Sebastien et al.[27] and Whitwell et al.[28] did not provide information concerning asbestos fiber types in lung tissue.

Churg,[29] in a study of 29 patients with pleural plaques at autopsy, found that the average number of asbestos bodies in the plaque group was 1732 asbestos bodies per gram of wet lung tissue and 42 asbestos bodies per gram of wet lung tissue in the control group. Fiber analysis showed the plaque group to have a concentration of asbestos fibers similar to that of the control group (114,000 vs. 99,000/g wet lung tissue) and similar numbers of chrysotile fibers (51,000 vs. 68,000/g wet lung tissue) and noncommercial amphiboles (13,000 vs. 29,000/g wet lung tissue). The number of commercial amphiboles identified in the plaque group was significantly higher (50,000/g wet lung tissue) than in the control group (1000/g wet lung tissue). Churg[29] found certain asbestos exposure in 16 of 29 plaque patients and concluded that half of patients in the general autopsy population who developed plaques had a history of asbestos exposure while the etiology of the plaques in the other half was unclear. Churg[29] concluded that pleural plaques correlated with an approximately 50-fold increase in the number of high-aspect-ratio commercial amphiboles in lung tissue but did not correlate with the number of chrysotile fibers, noncommercial amphiboles, or the total number of asbestos fibers.

Churg and dePaoli[30] compared asbestos concentrations in four men 70 years or older who had pleural plaques and lived near Thetford Mines in Quebec but who did not work in the asbestos mining/milling industry. Lung asbestos content of these four men was compared with nine persons living in the same vicinity who did not have pleural plaques. Churg and dePaoli[30] found an equal concentration of chrysotile in the four men with plaques versus the nine persons without plaques but found a fourfold elevation in the median tremolite content of the four men with plaques versus the nine persons without plaques. Churg and dePaoli[30] concluded that environmental pleural plaques in this region of Quebec were caused by tremolite or titanium oxide of environmental origin.

Kishimoto et al.[31] studied the concentration of asbestos bodies in 400 autopsy lungs and found 71 cases in which asbestos bodies were significantly elevated. In all 71 cases, hyaline pleural plaques were identified.

Others have found chrysotile to be the dominant fiber type in pleural plaques.[32–36]

10.3.3 Pathogenesis of Hyaline Pleural Plaques

The pathogenesis of pleural plaques remains uncertain. Asbestos fibers that are not removed from the larger conducting airways and which reach the alveolar parenchyma are cleared primarily by the lung lymphatic channels.[37,38] Fibers in the vicinity of the parenchymal lymphatic plexus drain to mediastinal lymph nodes, whereas fibers in the network of the pleural lymphatic plexus drain to the periphery of the lung and collect in a subvisceral pleural location. Most investigators have been unable to identify asbestos bodies in pleural plaques.[39] Rosen et al.[40] and Roberts[41] identified asbestos bodies in some pleural plaques, and Sebastien et al.[27] identified asbestos bodies in most plaques they examined. LeBouffant et al.[42] and Dodson et al.[43] identified chrysotile fibers in plaques by electron microscopy and concluded that short chrysotile was the most common form of asbestos found within the plaques in their studies. Warnock et al.[24] identified chrysotile in several plaques but stated that no chrysotile was found in most plaques.

Kiviluoto[44] and Meurman[38] suggested that pleural plaques develop from local inflammation of the parietal pleura caused by asbestos fibers that protrude from the visceral pleura and directly "irritate" the parietal pleura. No pathological evidence has been found to support this theory. Asbestos fibers have been identified in pleural effusions of persons occupationally exposed to asbestos.[45] Wang[46] described preformed lymphatic stoma on the surface mesothelium of the parietal pleura connecting the pleural cavity and the lymphatics of the parietal pleura. Wang[46] suggested that asbestos fibers gain access to the parietal pleura via this route. A study concerning the pathogenesis of mesothelioma[47] showed that fibers directly injected into the pleural cavity accumulated around the lymphatic stoma where they caused an inflammatory reaction. Taskinen et al.[48] suggested asbestos fibers reached the parietal pleura via retrograde lymphatic flow from mediastinal lymph nodes through the retrosternal and intercostal lymphatic channels.

Of potential importance with respect to which asbestos fiber type causes hyaline pleural plaques, Wagner et al.[49] exposed rats via inhalation for 1 day up to 24 months to comparable daily doses of chrysotile and amphibole asbestos to determine the concentration of asbestos as measured by silica content in the dust isolated from the rat lungs. Wagner et al.[49] found a direct correlation between the concentration of amphiboles, but not chrysotile, in the rats' lungs with the dose given. In the rats exposed to asbestos for 24 months, the weight of the amphiboles was 35 times that of the chrysotile. Despite this, asbestosis and neoplasms such as mesothelioma developed just as frequently in the animals exposed to chrysotile asbestos as in those exposed to amphiboles. As stated by Warnock et al.,[24] one must be extremely careful in interpreting low concentrations of chrysotile in the lungs of persons occupationally exposed to asbestos because it may not rule out the possibility that chrysotile was responsible for the disease.

10.4 DIFFUSE PLEURAL FIBROSIS

Diffuse pleural fibrosis is relatively common in patients occupationally exposed to asbestos. The exact incidence of diffuse pleural fibrosis is not well documented although in our experience is significantly less frequent than localized hyaline pleural plaques. Diffuse pleural fibrosis has a latency period of about 15–40 years with a dose–response relationship.

10.4.1 Morphology and Location of Diffuse Pleural Fibrosis

The morphology of pleural fibrosis is variable and depends on the severity of change. Visceral pleural fibrosis frequently involves the costophrenic angles but may be relatively diffuse (Figure 10.8). The condition may involve the apical region of the upper lobes.[50] In some instances, this condition is severe, with fusion of the visceral and parietal layers of the pleura producing a condition

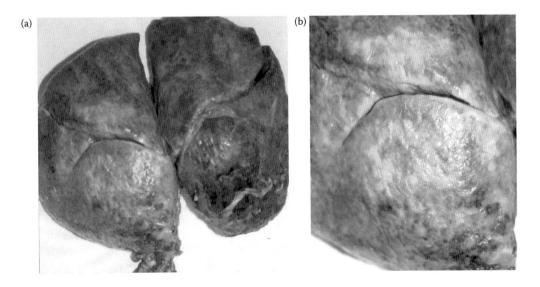

Figure 10.8   (a and b) Lungs from asbestos insulation worker show diffuse visceral pleural scarring. Normally transparent visceral pleura becomes opacified by scarring.

known as *fibrothorax* in which the pleural cavity is obliterated by dense fibrous tissue (Figure 10.9). Histologically, the fibrous tissue often shows increased vascularity and inflammation (Figure 10.10).

10.4.2 Pathogenesis of Diffuse Pleural Fibrosis

The pathogenesis of diffuse pleural fibrosis is poorly understood. Factors involved in the formation of hyaline pleural plaques may be involved in the production of visceral pleural fibrosis. As reviewed by Schwartz,[17] visceral pleural fibrosis may be a direct extension of parenchymal fibrosis and may begin as an inflammatory process initiated by asbestos with the progressive development of scarring. Asbestos has been reported to be somewhat preferentially restricted to the periphery of the lung below the pleural surface.[24] We observed several cases of diffuse visceral–parietal

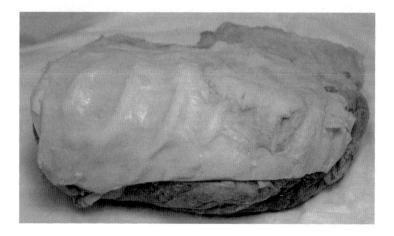

Figure 10.9 Lungs and pleura from a man occupationally exposed to asbestos for many years show diffuse thickening and fusion of visceral–parietal pleura, resulting in fibrous obliteration of pleural cavity referred to as fibrothorax.

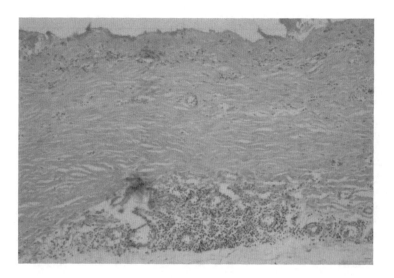

Figure 10.10 Fibrothorax represents fused visceral and parietal pleura composed mostly of dense fibrous tissue sometimes having the appearance of hyaline pleural plaque.

pleural fibrosis that had been diagnosed radiographically as asbestosis. Many, if not most, of these cases show some degree of subpleural parenchymal fibrosis (Figure 10.11) and could be diagnosed as asbestosis. However, this is an area of controversy in asbestos-induced pleuropulmonary disease.[50]

Stephens et al.[51] reviewed the pathological and mineralogical features of seven cases of diffuse pleural fibrosis in persons with known asbestos exposure, all of whom had a significant asbestos exposure history ranging from 2 to 25 years. In all seven cases, the histologic features were those of a basket weave pattern of thickened pleural tissue and dense subpleural parenchymal interstitial fibrosis with fine honeycombing extending to a depth of 1 cm into the underlying lung tissue. Crocidolite and amosite concentrations in lung tissue were elevated in six of seven patients, and chrysotile concentration was elevated in four cases. Stephens et al.[51] concluded that diffuse pleural fibrosis was a specific asbestos entity of uncertain pathogenesis, with lung tissue containing asbestos mineral fiber concentrations between those found in plaques and those found in minimal asbestosis (2.4–28 × 10^6 fibers of amosite or crocidolite per gram of dry lung tissue).

Gibbs et al.[52] studied lung tissue from 13 cases of diffuse pleural fibrosis in persons with a history of asbestos exposure. Samples were taken from the visceral pleura and central and subpleural lung zones for histopathologic and mineralogical studies. Gibbs et al.[52] found an increased concentration of amphibole fiber counts in a concentration similar to that seen in cases of pleural plaques, mild asbestosis, and mesothelioma. Gibbs et al.[52] found a wide case-to-case variation with no significant difference between the central and the subpleural lung zones, whereas the pleura had low asbestos counts and the asbestos in the pleura consisted mostly of short chrysotile fibers. Within the lung tissue, more than 45% of the asbestos fibers were long (>4 μm) and thin (<0.25 μm) amphibole fibers, which they interpreted to suggest that the longer, thinner fibers were important in the pathogenesis of diffuse pleural fibrosis. The conclusion by Gibbs et al.[52] that amphiboles rather than chrysotile fibers are retained in the lungs may be correct, although whether or not it implies that amphiboles are necessarily responsible for the observed changes remains uncertain.

As reviewed by Schwartz[17] and as reported by Kilburn and Warshaw,[53] diffuse pleural fibrosis is associated with signs and symptoms of respiratory disease and with abnormal pulmonary function tests.

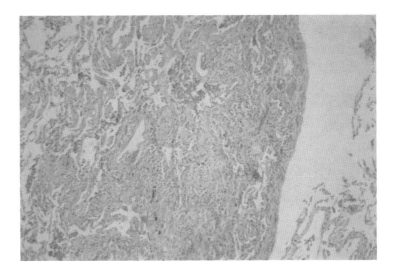

Figure 10.11 In this case of diffuse visceral pleural fibrosis there was significant subpleural parenchymal interstitial fibrosis.

10.5 ROUND (ROUNDED) ATELECTASIS

Round (rounded) atelectasis is a condition most frequently observed by radiologists in persons occupationally exposed to asbestos. Round atelectasis is usually asymptomatic and radiographically shows a unilateral round peripheral density in the lower lobe of the lung, usually the right lower or middle lobe, with one or more curvilinear shadows that radiate from this density toward the hilum of the lung (Figure 10.12) and which may be misinterpreted as a neoplasm.

Loeschke[54] in 1928 observed localized atelectasis in association with a pleural effusion. Hanke[55] reported a similar condition in 1971 that he called "round atelectasis." Blesovsky[56] in 1966 described the condition in the English literature as "folded lung," and Dernevik et al.[57] reported on 28 patients with similar radiographic and histologic features they termed "shrinking pleuritis with atelectasis." Round atelectasis has also been reported as Blesovsky's syndrome,[58] pleuroma,[59] and pulmonary pseudotumor.[60]

10.5.1 Pathological Features of Round Atelectasis

Macroscopically, the visceral pleura shows localized irregular fibrosis and may be fused with a thickened parietal pleura. Below the area of pleural fibrosis is an infolding of the pleura causing one or more areas of invagination. Histologically, the pleural fibrosis is superficial to the outer layer of visceral pleural elastic tissue, and the portion of the visceral pleura consisting of the internal and external layers of elastic tissue are thrown into variably-sized, complex wrinkles that extend downward into the underlying lung tissue for a variable distance (Figure 10.13). The lung tissue under the area of invagination of the visceral pleura may be normal or may show compressive atelectasis and/or interstitial fibrosis.

10.5.2 Etiology of Round Atelectasis

Chung-Park et al.[61] reviewed 107 cases of round atelectasis reported in the literature and found that 61 (57%) had a history of asbestos exposure. The remaining 46 had no history of exposure to asbestos or evidence of asbestosis, but developed localized atelectasis apparently from other factors

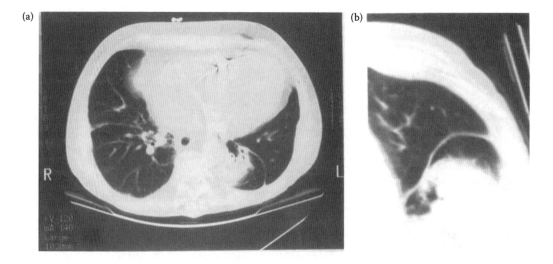

Figure 10.12 CT scan of chest shows curvilinear density raising from pleura and radiating toward hilum of left lung. Note the mass effect caused by this process.

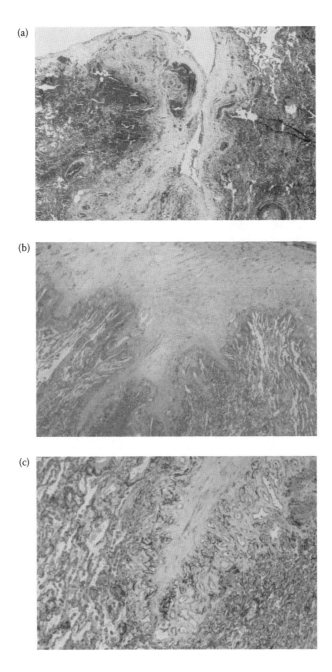

Figure 10.13 (a–c) Representative regions of round atelectasis from right lower lobe of asbestos-exposed individual. Note thickening and infolding of visceral pleura, with invagination into underlying lung tissue.

such as tuberculosis, exudative pleural infection, congestive heart failure, myocardial infarction, or trauma. In three cases reported by Chung-Park et al.,[61] two had recurrent or longstanding pleural effusion from congestive heart failure and chronic renal failure, and the third had remote fibrocaseous tuberculosis. Two were former coal miners who had mixed-dust exposure with elevated numbers of asbestos bodies in their lung tissue indicating the potential role of asbestos as a contributing factor in pleural fibrosis.

10.5.3 Pathogenesis of Round Atelectasis

As discussed by Menzies and Fraser[62] concerning the pathogenesis of round atelectasis, Loeschke,[54] Hanke,[55] and Kretzschmar[60] proposed that round atelectasis began with the development of a pleural effusion large enough to result in a separation of the visceral pleural-covered lung from the parietal pleura. According to their theory, focal collapse of the lung parenchyma occurred because the effusion formed a groove or cleft in the lung tissue with folding of this lung tissue upon itself, causing an area of invagination (Figure 10.14). Organization of the fibrinous exudate on the pleural surface resulted in mature fibrous tissue being formed, which then fixed the area of fold and maintained the underlying atelectasis. An alternative theory proposed by Blesovsky[56] and Dernevik et al.[57] is shown in Figure 10.15, as illustrated by Menzies and Fraser.[62] According to their theory, the pleural fibrous tissue matures and contracts, pulling the underlying pleura with it. Because the pleura can only be minimally compressed, there is no alternative other than for it to buckle into the lung tissue in accordion fashion, which leads to collapse of the lung parenchyma with the associated thickened pleura. I have seen many cases similar to that described by Chung-Park et al.,[61] which they refer to as shrinking pleuritis, in which patients exposed to asbestos developed pleural fibrosis and/or pleural effusion, with the understanding the pleural fibrosis may be a consequence of organization of the pleural fluid.

10.6 PLEURAL BLACK SPOTS

In 1966, Boutin et al.[63] described preferential accumulation of long amphibole asbestos fibers in regions of carbonaceous dust deposits in the parietal pleura that they referred to as "black spots."

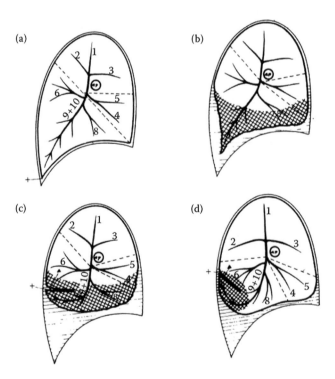

Figure 10.14 (a–d) "Folding" theory of pathogenesis of round atelectasis. (a) Normal lung and pleura. Pleural effusion causes the lung to float, (b) collapse, and (c) eventually fold about itself . Because of adhesions within cleft, one region remains collapsed as the remainder of the lung (d) reexpands.

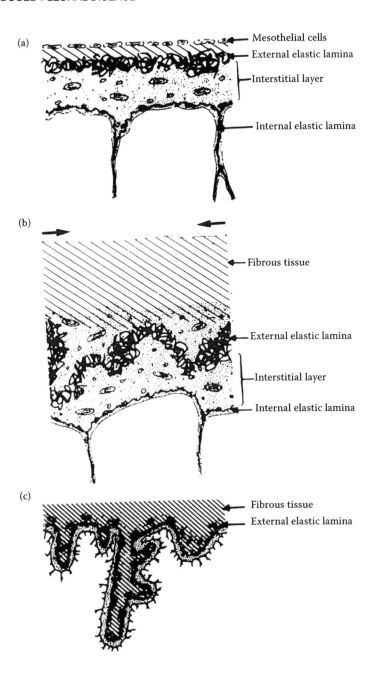

Figure 10.15 (a–c) "Fibrosing" theory of round atelectasis. (a) Normal pleura. Fibrous tissue in superficial pleura contracts, causing (b) wrinkling and eventually (c) folding of pleura, associated with collapse of the underlying parenchyma.

These "black spots" were hypothesized to be the starting point for asbestos-related neoplastic and inflammatory conditions. Boutin et al.[63] specifically suggested that mesotheliomas may originate from these black spots as a response to asbestos fibers (in this case amphiboles) at these anatomical sites. It is of interest that 77% of the amphiboles found in the black spots were <5 μm.

Mitchev et al.[64] evaluated the entire parietal pleura of 150 consecutive necropsies of urban dwellers for the prevalence, anatomic distribution, and macroscopic distribution of black spots and hyaline pleural plaques. Black spots consisted of deposits of opaque particulate material located under an intact mesothelial layer often in association with chronic inflammatory cells. Black spots were found predominantly in the lower paravertebral zones on the spine or close to it, on the central tendinous parts of both diaphragms, and around the anterior axillary lines. Black spots were observed in 92.7% of cases and more frequently in males and those persons of advanced age. In contrast, hyaline pleural plaques were observed in nineteen men and two women (14%). Plaques were bilateral in twelve cases and unilateral in nine cases.

Asbestos body concentration was greater than 1000 per gram of dry lung in 15 of 97 cases evaluated. Twelve cases (80%) with asbestos body concentration greater than 1000 g/dry lung had pleural plaques. Asbestos body lung concentration was greater than 5000 asbestos bodies per gram of dry lung tissue in four cases, all of whom had bilateral pleural plaques. The sites of predominance were different for black spots and pleural plaques, although black spots and pleural plaques were observed close to each other in 12 cases. The difference in the mean scores reflecting the total black material burden in the pleura in those with and without plaques was stated to not be statistically significant ($p = .062$).[64]

Mitchev et al.[64] concluded that there was no correlation between the locations of anthracotic spots and pleural plaques. Pleural plaques were observed predominantly in areas of the parietal pleura with a lower prevalence of black spots. Black spots were stated to be related to the structures responsible for lymphatic drainage of the pleural cavity and specifically reflected the "clogged sewage system" marking the places of maximal pleural resorption. Mitchev et al.[64] stated that their observations did not exclude the possibility that black spots could be the starting point for malignant mesothelioma because black spots concentrated asbestos fibers (in this study including some longer amphibole fibers) together with carbonaceous material.

The article by Muller et al.[65] concerning black spots stated that black spots on the parietal pleura developed in close correlation to lymphatic channels and blood vessels. The black spots were composed of fibrous tissue and inflammatory cells with foreign particles such as aluminum and silicone. Muller et al.[65] concluded that although there were hints for an increased proliferation of mesothelial cells in some areas with black spots, their findings did not support the classification of black spots as an obligate precursor in the development of malignant mesothelioma. The study by Muller et al.[65] did not report finding asbestos fibers within the black spots that were evaluated by transmission electron microscopy.

I (S.P.H.) have evaluated approximately 7000 cases of mesothelioma, including approximately 3000 autopsy tissue cases, and have yet to identify parietal pleural black spots.

10.7 ASBESTOS PLEURAL DISEASE—CLINICOPATHOLOGIC CORRELATION—APPROACH TO THE DIAGNOSIS

Recent articles by Cugell and Kamp,[66] Kamp,[67] and Heintz et al.[68] provide molecular biology studies concerning essentially all asbestos-related diseases.

10.7.1 Pleural Effusion—Acute Pleuritis

Pleural effusions are typically unilateral and are not uncommonly associated with a significant number of eosinophils in pleural fluid. BAPEs frequently disappear slowly and spontaneously over a period of several months. It can be very difficult to differentiate mesothelioma from BAPE, clinically. With respect to the article by Cugell and Kamp,[66] asbestos-induced pleural effusions have no specific prognostic implications with respect to subsequent development of pleural plaques and mesothelioma.

10.7.2 Hyaline Pleural Plaques

Pleural plaques may cause functional impairment.[69] A conventional chest film is a sensitive and an appropriate imaging method for plaques, although it may identify abnormalities that resemble plaques but are not.

According to the American Thoracic Society,[69] high-resolution CT scanning is not a practical screening method for demonstrating plaques because of the separation between the sections, the high-radiation exposure, and the lack of access to the test in some locations.

A substantial portion of plaques found at postmortem examination or by CT scan are missed by plain radiographs. High-resolution CT scans are thought to be superior to any other radiographic method in identifying plaques. Some large cohorts have shown a significant reduction in lung function attributable to plaques, averaging about 5% of forced vital capacity, even when asbestosis is absent radiographically.[70–73]

Paris et al.[20] conducted a CT scan screening program to select the most relevant exposure variables for the prediction of pleural plaques and asbestosis to guide clinicians in their use of CT scans. They recommended that the use of precise assessments of asbestos exposure be obtained by occupational hygiene measurements and a job-exposure matrix, including time since first exposure, duration, intensity, and cumulative exposure to asbestos in high-risk populations suitable for screening of these diseases. They concluded short periodicity of survey of pleural plaques by CT scan seemed unwarranted.

Circumscribed plaques have been associated with restrictive impairment and diminished diffusion capacity on pulmonary function testing and in the absence of radiographic asbestosis.[74,75]

Lilis et al.[76] stated that the functional relevance of pleural fibrosis, especially circumscribed pleural fibrosis, was controversial. They stated that stepwise regression analysis showed a significant inverse relationship between the forced vital capacity and the integrative index of pleural fibrosis. In those persons with parenchymal and pleural fibrosis, the pleural index made a significant contribution to a decrease in forced vital capacity.

Pleural plaques may be associated with severe pain as described by Bicer et al.[77] Kilburn and Warshaw[53] concluded that asbestos-induced pleural disease was associated with significant pulmonary dysfunction in men who never smoked as well as current and ex-smokers who had additional dysfunction even after adjusting for duration of smoking.

Most people with pleural plaques and no other lung abnormalities have normal lung function.

There is no association between the development of lung cancer and mesothelioma in persons who have pleural plaques.[67]

REFERENCES

1. Hammar SP. Non-neoplastic pleural disease. In: *Dail and Hammar's Pulmonary Pathology*, 3rd ed., Tomashefski, Jr, JF, ed. New York: Springer; 2008: Chapter 30.
2. Hillerdal G, Ozesmi M. Benign pleural effusion: 73 exudates in 60 patients. *Eur J Respir Dis* 1987;71:113–121.
3. Robinson BWS, Musk AW. Benign asbestos pleural effusion: Diagnosis and course. *Thorax* 1981;36:896–900.
4. Lilis R, Lerman Y, Selikoff IJ. Symptomatic benign pleural effusions among asbestos insulation workers: Residual radiographic abnormalities. *Br J Ind Med* 1988;45:443–449.
5. Miller A, Miller JA. Diffuse pleural thickening superimposed on circumscribed pleural thickening and related to asbestos exposure. *Am J Ind Med* 1993;23:859–871.
6. Miller A. Chronic pleuritic pain in four patients with asbestos induced pleural fibrosis. *Br J Ind Med* 1990;47:147–153.

7. Epler GR, McCloud TC, Gaensler EA. Prevalence and incidence of benign asbestos pleural effusion in a working population. *JAMA* 1982;247:617–622.
8. Gaensler EA, Kaplan AI. Asbestos pleural effusion. *Ann Intern Med* 1971;74:178–191.
9. Collins TFB. Pleural reaction associated with asbestos exposure. *Br J Radiol* 1968;41:655–661.
10. Mattson S, Ringqvist T. Pleural plaques and exposure to asbestos. *Scand J Respir Dis* 1970;75(Suppl):1–41.
11. Mattson S. Monosymptomatic exudative pleurisy in persons exposed to asbestos dust. *Scand J Respir Dis* 1975;56:263–272.
12. Eisenstadt HB. Asbestos pleurisy. *Dis Chest* 1964;46:78–81.
13. Hillerdal G, Ozesmi M. Benign asbestos pleural effusion: 73 exudates in 60 patients. *Eur J Respir Dis* 1987;71:113–121.
14. Fondimare A, Duwoos H, Desbordes J, Perrotey J, Tayot J. Plaques fibroyalines calcifiees du foie dans l'asbestose. *Nouv Presse Med* 1974;3:893.
15. Andrion A, Pira E, Mollo F. Peritoneal plaques and asbestos exposure. *Arch Pathol Lab Med* 1983;107:609–610.
16. Wain SL, Roggli VL, Foster WL Jr. Parietal pleural plaques, asbestos bodies, and neoplasia: A clinical, pathologic and roentgenographic correlation of 25 consecutive cases. *Chest* 1985;86:707–713.
17. Schwartz DA. New developments in asbestos-induced pleural disease. *Chest* 1991;99:191–198.
18. Rogan WJ, Gladen BC, Regan NB, Anderson HA. US prevalence of occupational pleural thickening: A look at x-rays from the First National Health and Nutrition Examination Survey. *Am J Epidemiol* 1987;126:893–900.
19. Miller JA, Zurlo JV. Asbestos plaques in a typical veterans hospital population. *Am J Ind Med* 1996;30:726–729.
20. Paris C, Martin A, Letourneux M, Wild P. Modelling prevalence and incidence of fibrosis and pleural plaques in asbestos-exposed populations for screening and follow-up: A cross-sectional study. *Environ Health* 2008;7:30.
21. Paris C, Thierry S, Brochard P, Letourneux M, Schorle E, Stoufflet A, et al. Pleural plaques and asbestosis: dose– and time–response relationships based on HRCT data. *Eur Respir J* 2009;34:72–79.
22. Sichletidis L, Spyratos D, Chloros D, Michailidis K, Fourkioutou I. Pleural plaques in dentists from occupational asbestos exposure: A report of three cases. *Am J Ind Med* 2009;52:926–930.
23. Hourihane DO, Lessof L, Richardson PC. Hyaline and calcified pleural plaques as an index of exposure to asbestos: A study of radiological and pathological features of 100 cases with a consideration of epidemiology. *Br Med J* 1966;1:1069–1074.
24. Warnock ML, Prescott BT, Kuwahara TJ. Numbers and types of asbestos fibers in subjects with pleural plaques. *Am J Pathol* 1982;109:37–46.
25. Rohl AN. Asbestos in talc. *Environ Health Perspect* 1974;9:129–132.
26. Hillerdal G. Pleural plaques in a health survey material: Frequency, development and exposure to asbestos. *Scand J Respir Dis* 1978;59:257–263.
27. Sebastien P, Fondimare A, Bignon J, Monchaux G, Desbordes J, Bonnaud G. Topographic distribution of asbestos fibres in human lung in relation to occupational and non-occupational exposure. In: *Inhaled Particles*, Vol. 4, Walter WH, McGovern B, eds. New York: Pergamon Press; 1977: 435–444.
28. Whitwell F, Scott J, Grimshaw M. Relationship between occupations and asbestos fibre content of the lungs in patients with pleural mesothelioma, lung cancer, and other diseases. *Thorax* 1977;32:377–386.
29. Churg A. Asbestos fibers and pleural plaques in a general autopsy population. *Am J Pathol* 1982;109:88–96.
30. Churg A, dePaoli L. Environmental pleural plaques in residents of a Quebec chrysotile mining town. *Chest* 1988;94:58–60.
31. Kishimoto T, Ono T, Okada K, Ito H. Relationship between numbers of asbestos bodies in autopsy lung and pleural plaques on chest x-ray film. *Chest* 1989;95:549–552.
32. Dodson RF, Williams MG Jr., Corn CJ, Brollo A, Bianchi C. A comparison of asbestos burden in lung parenchyma, lymph nodes, and plaques. *Ann N Y Acad Sci* 1991;643:53–60.
33. Sebastien P. Jason X., Gaudichet A, Hirsch A, Bingnon J. Asbestos retention in human respiratory tissues: comparative measurements in lung parenchyma and in parietal pleura. In: *Biological Effects of Mineral Fibers*, Wagner JC, ed. Lyon: IARC; 1980: 237–246.

34. Suzuki Y, Kohyama N. Translocation of inhaled asbestos fibers from the lung to other tissues. *Am J Ind Med* 1991;19:701–704.

35. Suzuki Y, Yuen SR. Asbestos tissue burden study on human malignant mesothelioma. *Ind Health* 2001;39:150–160.

36. Suzuki Y, Yuen SR. Asbestos fibers contributing to the induction of human malignant mesothelioma. *Ann N Y Acad Sci* 2002;982:160–176.

37. Lauweryns JM, Baert JH. Alveolar clearance and the role of the pulmonary lymphatics. *Am Rev Respir Dis* 1977;115:625–683.

38. Lee KP. Lung response to particles with emphasis on asbestos and other fibrous dusts. *CRC Crit Rev Toxicol* 1985;14:33–86.

39. Meurman L. Asbestos bodies and pleural plaques in a Finnish series of autopsy cases. *Acta Pathol Microbiol Scand* 1966;181(Suppl):7–107.

40. Rosen P, Gordon P, Savino A, Melamed M. Ferruginous bodies in benign fibrous plural plaques. *Am J Clin Pathol* 1973;60:608–617.

41. Roberts GH. The pathology of parietal pleural plaques. *J Clin Pathol* 1961;24:348–353.

42. LeBouffant L, Martin JC, Durif S, Daniel H. Structure and composition of pleural plaques. In: *Biological Effects of Asbestos*, Bogovski P, Gilson JC, Timbrell V, Wagner JC, eds. Lyon, France: International Agency for Research on Cancer; 1973: 249–257.

43. Dodson RF, Williams MG Jr., Corn CJ, Brollo A, Bianchi C. Asbestos content of lung tissue, lymph nodes, and pleural plaques from former shipyard workers. *Am Rev Respir Dis* 1990;142:843–847.

44. Kiviluoto R. Pleural calcification as a roentgenologic sign of nonoccupational endemic anthophyllite asbestosis. *Acta Radiol* 1960;194(Suppl):1–67.

45. Hillerdal G. The pathogenesis of pleural plaques and pulmonary asbestosis: Possibilities and impossibilities. *Eur J Respir Dis* 1980;61:129–138.

46. Wang NS. The preformed stomas connecting the pleural cavity and the lymphatics in the parietal pleura. *Am Rev Respir Dis* 1975;111:12–20.

47. Moalli PA, MacDonald JL, Goodglick LA, Kane AB. Acute injury and regeneration of the mesothelium in response to asbestos fibers. *Am J Pathol* 1987;128:426–445.

48. Taskinen E, Ahlmon K, Wiikeri M. A current hypothesis of the lymphatic transport of inspired dust to the parietal pleura. *Chest* 1973;64:193–196.

49. Wagner JC, Berry G, Skidmore JW, Timbrell V. The effects of the inhalation of asbestos in rats. *Br J Cancer* 1974;29:252–269.

50. Hammar SP. Controversies and uncertainties concerning the pathologic features and pathologic diagnosis of asbestosis. *Semin Diagn Pathol* 1992;9:102–109.

51. Stephens M, Gibbs AR, Pooley FD, Wagner JC. Asbestos-induced diffuse pleural fibrosis: Pathology and mineralogy. *Thorax* 1987;42:583–588.

52. Gibbs AR, Stephens M, Griffiths DM, Blight BJN, Pooley FD. Fiber distribution in the lungs and pleura of subjects with asbestos-related diffuse pleural fibrosis. *Br J Ind Med* 1991;48:762–770.

53. Kilburn KH, Warshaw R. Pulmonary functional impairment associated with pleural asbestos disease: Circumscribed and diffuse thickening. *Chest* 1990;98:965–972.

54. Loeschke H. Storungen des Lufgehalts der Lunge. In: *Hanke-Lubarsch Hanbuch der Spezielleu Pathologischen Anatomie and Histologie*. 3. Bd, I. Teil. Berlin: Springer; 1928: 599.

55. Hanke R. Rundatelektasen (Kugel and Walzenatelektasen): Ein bietrag zur differential diagnosis intrapulmonaler rundherde. *Roefo* 1971;114:164–183.

56. Blesovsky A. The folded lung. *Br J Dis Chest* 1966;60:19–22.

57. Dernevik L, Gatzinsky P, Hultman E, Selin K, William-Olsson G, Zettergren L. Shrinking pleuritis with atelectasis. *Thorax* 1982;37:252–258.

58. Payne CR, Jaques P, Kerr IH. Lung folding simulating peripheral pulmonary neoplasm (Blesovsky's syndrome). *Thorax* 1980;35:936–940.

59. Sinner WN. Pleuroma. A cancer-mimicking atelectactic pseudotumor of the lung. *Roefo* 1980;133:578–585.

60. Kretzschmar R. Uber atelaktatische pseudotumoren der Lunge. *Roefo* 1975;122:19–29.

61. Chung-Park M, Tomashefski JF, Jr., Cohen AM, El-Gazzar M, Cotes EE. Shrinking pleuritis with lobar atelectasis: A morphologic variant of "round atelectasis." *Hum Pathol* 1989;20:382–387.

62. Menzies R, Fraser R. Round atelectasis: pathologic and pathogenetic features. *Am J Surg Pathol* 1987;11:674–681.
63. Boutin C, Dumorlier P, Rey F, Viallat JR, De Vuyst P. Black spots concentrate oncogenic asbestos fibers in the parietal pleura: Thoracoscopic and mineralogic study. *Am J Respir Crit Care Med* 1996;153:444–449.
64. Mitchev K, Dumortier P, DeVuyst P. "Black spots" and hyaline pleural plaques on the parietal pleura of 150 urban necropsy cases. *Am J Surg Pathol* 2002;26:1198–1206.
65. Müller KM, Schmitz I, Konstantinidis K. Black spots of the parietal pleura: Morphology and formal pathogenesis. *Respiration* 2002;69:261–267.
66. Cugell DW, Kamp DW. Asbestos and the pleura: A review. *Chest* 2004;125:1103–1117.
67. Kamp DW. Asbestos-induced lung diseases: An update. *Transl Res* 2009;153:143–152.
68. Heintz NH, Janssen-Heininger YM, Mossman BT. Asbestos, lung cancers, and mesotheliomas: From molecular approaches to targeting tumor survival pathways. *Am J Respir Cell Mol Biol* 2010;142:133–139.
69. Kilburn KH, Warshaw RH. Abnormal pulmonary function associated with diaphragmatic pleural plaques due to exposure to asbestos. *Br J Ind Med* 1990;47:611–614.
70. American Thoracic Society. Diagnosis and initial management of nonmalignant diseases related to asbestos. *Am J Respir Crit Care Med* 2004;170:691–715.
71. Rockoff SD, Chu J, Rubin LJ. Special reports: Asbestos-induced pleural plaques; a disease process associated with ventilatory impairment and respiratory symptoms. *Clin Pulmon Med* 2002;9:113–124.
72. Schwartz DA, Fuortes LJ, Galvin JR, Burmeister LF, Schmidt LE, Leistikow BN, et al. Asbestos-induced pleural fibrosis and impaired lung function. *Am Rev Respir Dis* 1990;141:321–326.
73. Jarvolm B, Sanden A. Pleural plaques and respiratory function. *Am J Ind Med* 1986;10:419–426.
74. Hjorstberg U, Orbaek P, Aborelios M Jr, Ranstam J, Welinder H. Railroad workers with pleural plaques. I. Spirometric and nitrogen washout investigation on smoking and nonsmoking asbestos-exposed workers. *Am J Ind Med* 1988;14:635–641.
75. Oliver LC, Eisen EA, Green R, Sprince NL. Asbestos-related pleural plaques and lung function. *Am J Ind Med* 1988;14:649–656.
76. Lilis R, Miller A, Godbold J, Chan E, Selikoff IJ. Pulmonary function and pleural fibrosis: Quantitative relationships with an integrative index of pleural abnormalities. *Am J Ind Med* 1991;20:145–161.
77. Bicer U, Kurtas O, Ercin C, Gundogmus UN, Colak B, Paksoy N. Pain-driven suicide due to pleural plaques associated with asbestos exposure. *Saudi Med J* 2006;27:894–896.

CHAPTER 11

Uncommon Nonmalignant Asbestos-Induced Conditions

Samuel P. Hammar

CONTENTS

11.1 INTRODUCTION

The mechanism by which asbestos causes injury is complex and not completely understood, although early studies have suggested inflammatory mechanisms may play a contributing role.[1,2] With the passage of time, additional information has been published concerning mechanisms of disease. Articles have recently been published showing asbestos is extensively involved in the immune system.[3–19] A wide range of nonneoplastic lymphoid lesions occur in the lung.

11.1.1 Bronchial-Associated Lymphoid Tissue

An overview of lymphoid tissue and lymphoid inflammatory conditions is provided as a prerequisite to understanding some specific nonneoplastic conditions caused by asbestos. Lymphoid tissue is inconspicuous or absent in most normal adult human lung tissue. There has been significant debate as to whether bronchial-associated lymphoid tissue (BALT) is seen in normal adult human lungs.[20] Exogenous or endogenous antigenic stimulation of a variety of types causes lymphoid tissue to appear in human lung tissue, and in most instances it occurs in a fairly distinct anatomic location, namely, in association with bronchi and bronchioles. It is referred to as *BALT*. In nonsmoking adults, lymphoid tissue is seldom seen in the lung and when present occurs as small aggregates usually found at bronchial divisions and adjacent to respiratory bronchioles. In smokers, there is a significant increase in BALT with occasional large lymphoid follicles, some of which have germinal centers.[21]

As reviewed by Swigris et al.,[22] BALT is part of a larger system referred to as *mucosal-associated lymphoid tissue* and is uncommonly seen in the normal adult lung but commonly seen in other mammals such as rats, rabbits, and sheep. The lymphoid tissue is usually poorly organized and consists of aggregates of lymphocytes around small bronchi and at bronchial divisions. Some lymphocytes reside in the bronchial epithelium between epithelial cells. Lymphoid cells populate these areas by contact of cell surface homing receptors such as integrins or specific intrapulmonary vascular adhesion molecules in postcapillary vascular endothelial cells. Approximately 60% of BALT is composed of B lymphocytes and the remaining of T lymphocytes. BALT is thought to play an essential role in the prevention of infection of inhaled microorganisms and is a site for lymphoid differentiation where lymphocytes come in contact with inhaled antigens to become antigen-specific memory or immune effector cells. When primed by antigen, these lymphoid cells are thought to circulate throughout the BALT and remaining lung parenchyma and are ready to react to exposure to antigens such as asbestos. There are other cells involved in the immunologic response such as dendritic macrophages (Langerhans cells). The respiratory epithelium overlying the BALT usually contains relatively few goblet cells and ciliated cells. The BALT-associated epithelial cells are surfaced by microvilli. The epithelium is infiltrated by predominantly CD8-positive lymphocytes and occasionally CD4-positive lymphocytes. According to Swigris et al.,[22] BALT does not express the secretory component of IgA and differs from other mucosal-associated lymphoid tissue such as that seen in the GI tract. Bienenstock et al.[23] were the first to provide information on the morphologic and functional characteristics of BALT.[23,24]

The majority of nonneoplastic and neoplastic lymphoid infiltrates in the lung are related to BALT. In neoplasia, BALT proliferations can explain most neoplastic pulmonary lymphoid diseases. As stated previously, it is often difficult to distinguish between neoplastic and nonneoplastic lymphoid lesions. In many instances, molecular biology techniques such as gene rearrangement and T-cell evaluations are necessary to prove malignancy.[25,26]

11.1.2 Benign Pulmonary Conditions with Frequent "Haphazard" Lymphoid Infiltrates

A variety of recognizable benign conditions of the lung are associated with lymphoid infiltrates that seem haphazardly oriented. These include usual interstitial pneumonia (UIP); desquamative interstitial pneumonia (DIP); some cases of collagen vascular-associated lung disease; nonspecific interstitial pneumonia, cellular phase; hypersensitivity pneumonitis; the early phase of sarcoidosis; Wegener's granulomatosis; Churg–Strauss granulomatosis; microscopic polyarteritis nodosa; and infiltrates associated with certain drugs such as sulfasalazine.

Detailed information concerning most lymphoproliferative diseases of the lung is provided by Colby,[27] Fraser and Paré,[28] Jaffe et al.,[29] Nicholson,[30] and Yousem.[31]

11.1.3 Hyperplasias of BALT

Most pulmonary lymphoid lesions represent hyperplasias of BALT and neoplastic lymphoproliferative disorders arising from BALT. Kradin and Mark[32] discarded the terms *pseudolymphoma* and *lymphocytic interstitial pneumonia* (LIP) and replaced them with nodular and diffuse *hyperplasias of BALT*. As discussed in detail by Koss,[33] localized hyperplasias of BALT (also termed *follicular bronchitis/bronchiolitis*) represents a proliferation of BALT in the region of small bronchi and bronchioles. This proliferation can be seen in a number of different clinical conditions, including chronic infections, congenital immune deficiency syndromes, obstructive pneumonias, and collagen vascular diseases. Pathologically, BALT hyperplasias are characterized by collections of lymphoid nodules with or without germinal centers in a peribronchial/peribronchiolar distribution.

Nodular lymphoid hyperplasia of BALT has replaced the term *pseudolymphoma* and is characterized by a reactive lymphoid proliferation that characteristically shows numerous lymphoid follicles with large germinal centers usually occurring in middle-aged people, most of whom are asymptomatic. Approximately 10%–15% of patients with nodular lymphoid hyperplasia have a collagen vascular disease such as systemic lupus erythematosus or an immune disease of uncertain etiology and frequently exhibit polyclonal gammopathy. Pathologically, the condition is characterized by aggregates of well-defined lymphoid nodules with germinal centers. Polytypic plasma cells are common. Marker studies show a mixed population of CD4- and CD8-positive T cells. Most cases occur as solitary nodules and reoccur in up to 15% of surgically excised cases.

LIP is currently thought to be a diffuse hyperplasia of BALT.[34] It is thought to be a response to a variety of stimuli, including a wide spectrum of autoimmune diseases; systemic immunodeficiency states; alogenetic bone marrow transplantation; pulmonary alveolar microlithiasis; uncommon infections such as *Legionella* pneumonia, tuberculosis, mycoplasma, and *Chlamydia*; dilantin use; and pulmonary alveolar proteinosis. Most patients who develop LIP are women between the ages of 40 and 70 years. They may present with a variety of symptoms such as fever, hemoptysis, arthralgias, weight loss, fever, and pleuritic chest pain. Some have Sjogren's syndrome or myasthenia gravis. Chest radiographs usually show a diffuse reticular or reticulonodular infiltrate with occasional nodular lesions. Some patients have hypergammaglobulinemia, and approximately 10% of adult patients have hypogammaglobulinemia. If LIP patients have a monoclonal gammopathy, it is usually due to a coexistent lymphoma. A significant number of patients with LIP respond to steroids, although approximately 30%–50% succumb to the disease within 5 years, frequently from infectious complications and some as a result of treatment. Some patients develop lymphoma and immunoblastic sarcomas.

11.1.4 Nodular Lymphoid Infiltrates of Uncertain Etiology

Nodular lymphoid lesions of uncertain etiology can occur in the lung. These include plasma cell granulomas, pulmonary hyalinizing granulomas, and an entity referred to as *benign lymphocytic angiitis and granulomatosis* (BLAG).

Plasma cell granulomas, also referred to as *myofibroblastic tumors or inflammatory pseudotumors*, occur predominantly in the lung of younger individuals and have been observed in a wide variety of organs and tissues, including trachea, thyroid, heart, stomach, liver, pancreas, spleen, lymph nodes, kidney, retroperitoneum, mesentery, bladder, pelvic soft tissue, breast, spinal cord meninges, and orbit.[34] The term *granuloma* may be somewhat misleading, unless one understands that this term has been used loosely to describe a mass of inflammatory tissue similar to that observed in Wegener's and lymphomatoid granulomatosis. Histologically, these nodules are composed of lung tissue with an associated intense inflammatory infiltrate composed predominantly of plasma cells and a proliferation of myofibroblasts.

Pulmonary hyalinizing granulomas occur most frequently in younger individuals as single or, occasionally, multiple nodules. Some individuals are asymptomatic and others have cough, shortness of breath, chest pain, and/or weight loss. Histologically, the dominant finding is one of dense lamellar collagen bundles oriented parallel to one another and, not infrequently, an associated lymphoid infiltrate frequently in a bronchial distribution.

BLAG was described in 1977 by Saldana et al.[35] and by Israel et al.[36] BLAG was described as being less common than Wegener's granulomatosis and lymphomatoid granulomatosis. Most patients are middle aged and in most instances have multiple lesions. Histologically, the nodules are composed of a dense lymphoid infiltrate with occasional giant cells, including multinucleated histiocytic giant cells but without well-defined granuloma formation. Lymphoid infiltrates around arteries and veins are frequent, and lymphocytes invade vessel walls and occasionally produce occlusion of vascular lumina. Differential diagnosis includes lymphocytic lymphoma and LIP when the lesions are multiple.

11.2 LYMPHOCYTIC INTERSTITIAL PNEUMONIA ASSOCIATED WITH ASBESTOS EXPOSURE

Rom and Travis[37] reported lymphocytic interstitial pneumonia (LIP) in two patients who were stated to have been occupationally exposed to asbestos. In my opinion, the changes described by Rom and Travis[37] were similar to those seen in hypersensitivity pneumonitis and the cellular phase of chronic nonspecific interstitial pneumonia,[38] which is currently thought to be one of the mechanisms by which asbestos causes injury. In my study with Hallman,[39] we described a patient who developed a lymphoid interstitial inflammatory infiltrate (Figures 11.1 and 11.2), which in our opinion was essentially identical to that reported by Rom and Travis.[37] The patient in our case[39] was stated radiographically to have grade 4 asbestosis, which was not seen pathologically. As stated earlier, there are numerous studies suggesting that asbestos has an effect on the immune system, including the development of hypersensitivity reactions.[3–19]

11.3 LOCALIZED MASSES—ASBESTOMAS, BRONCHIOLITIS OBLITERANS WITH ORGANIZING PNEUMONIA (BOOP) CHANGES

Although asbestos is usually not thought to produce nonmalignant localized parenchymal masses, Hillerdal and Hemmingson[40] reported 10 patients who developed localized visceral pleural fibrosis and fibrosis of the underlying lung parenchyma that caused the development of a pseudotumor. Lynch et al.[41] identified 16 localized masses (9 intraparenchymal and 7 subpleural) in 260 asbestos-exposed individuals that were evaluated radiographically. A case reported in the clinicopathologic correlation section of the *New England Journal of Medicine* in 1961[42] suggested that asbestos could cause a localized bronchiolitis obliterans with organizing pneumonia-like pulmonary lesion (BOOP). In that case, a 61-year-old man developed a localized consolidation in his left

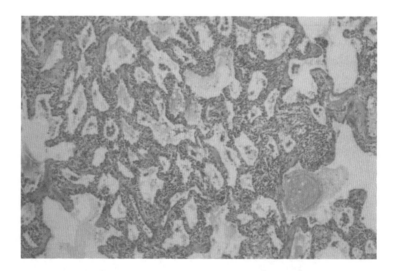

Figure 11.1   Lung tissue shows diffuse mild thickening of alveolar septa with interstitial infiltrate of lymphocytes and plasma cells resembling LIP (low power magnification).

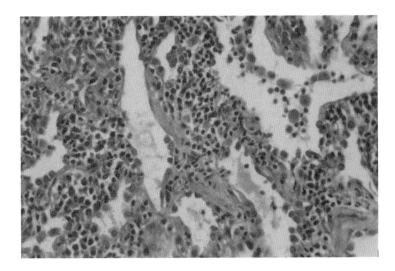

Figure 11.2 Lung tissue shows diffuse mild thickening of alveolar septa with interstitial infiltrate of lymphocytes and plasma cells resembling LIP (high power magnification).

upper lobe that histologically showed changes of organizing pneumonia in which numerous asbestos bodies were identified. In that case,[42] a secondary infection was suggested, although was never proven. In 1981, Saldana[43] described four men whose chest radiographs showed localized infiltrates in the absence of diffuse changes that had the histologic features of bronchiolitis obliterans with asbestos bodies and organizing masses of granulation tissue occluding the bronchi. There were a large number of histiocytes and confluent granulomata, lymphocytic angiitis, a dense lymphoplasmacytic cellular infiltrate, and varying degrees of organizing pneumonia and fibrosis. Saldana[43] referred to these changes as *localized asbestos pneumonia*. Roggli[44] reported observing organizing pneumonia in several asbestos-exposed patients who underwent thoracotomy for suspected malignancy. Likewise, Spencer[45] also described organizing pneumonia as a primary pathologic feature of asbestosis. In 1993 we[39] reported four cases of organizing pneumonia with focal bronchiolitis obliterans in patients occupationally exposed to asbestos who had significantly elevated concentrations of asbestos in their lung tissue and in which no other obvious cause of BOOP was identified.

Keith et al.,[46] while studying asbestos in rats using intratracheally injected UICC Canadian chrysotile-B asbestos, observed alveolar and interstitial edema at 1, 3, and 6 months after treatment and found bronchiolitis obliterans in 33%–45% of the bronchioles examined.

In the cases reported by us[39] of organizing pneumonitis, patients were usually asymptomatic and presented with nodular masses identified radiographically (Figure 11.3). Histologically, the masses showed the pathologic features of bronchiolitis obliterans with organizing pneumonia (BOOP). Nodular masses of moderately cellular, somewhat loose myxomatous granulation tissue filled the alveolar spaces and bronchioles (Figure 11.4) and were associated with frequent ferruginous bodies consistent with asbestos bodies (Figure 11.5). In one case, a fairly distinct nodule was composed predominantly of edema fluid and proteinaceous material within alveolar spaces in association with many inflammatory cells and showed foci of organization (Figure 11.6). We[39] wondered if the changes in this case may have represented an early phase of bronchiolitis obliterans with organizing pneumonia (BOOP).

We[39] also observed other nodular masses composed of randomly dispersed, dense fibrous tissue with varying numbers of inflammatory cells and frequent asbestos bodies (Figures 11.7 through 11.10). These changes were recently referred to as *asbestomas*.[47]

More recently, Cavazza et al.[48] described a case of BOOP in a 65-year-old man who was previously treated for gastric lymphoma and who had a history of asbestos exposure. The patient presented with fever and two nodular opacities in the left lower lobe. Histologically, examination

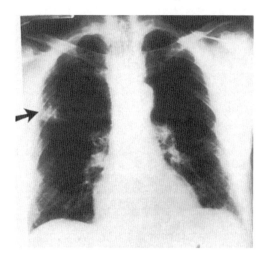

Figure 11.3 Chest radiograph shows nodular mass in right upper lobe that was interpreted radiographically as likely representing a primary lung neoplasm.

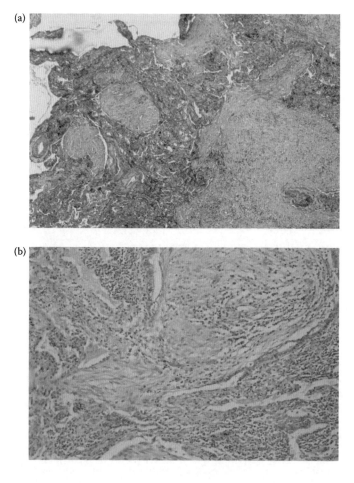

Figure 11.4 (a and b) Nodular mass shows bronchiolitis obliterans with organizing pneumonitis (BOOP) characterized by inflammation and fibrosis in distal airways.

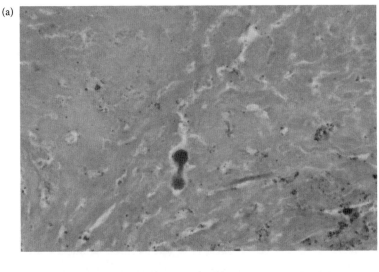

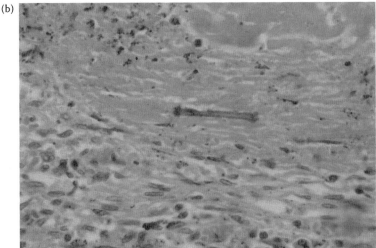

Figure 11.5 (a) Heavily coated and (b) lightly coated ferruginous bodies morphologically consistent with asbestos bodies in organizing connective tissue.

revealed BOOP. Cavazza et al.[48] suggested that patients exposed to asbestos may rarely present with localized inflammatory pulmonary lesions and that the possible etiopathogenic role of asbestos needed further studies.

We have seen one case of acute fibrinous and organizing pneumonia (AFOP) as described by Beasley et al.[49] in which there was fibrin in alveolar spaces (Figure 11.11) that was organizing and in which we found asbestos bodies (Figure 11.12). In that case, the organizing tissue also evolved into areas of ossification (Figure 11.13). This finding would suggest asbestos can cause this type of injury and might explain why it is fairly common to see areas of ossification in patients with asbestosis (Figure 11.14).

11.4 DESQUAMATIVE INTERSTITIAL PNEUMONITIS-LIKE CHANGES

In 1965, Liebow et al.[50] reported on 40 cases of a lung condition they referred to as *DIP*. As described by Liebow et al.,[50] DIP was characterized by filling of alveolar spaces with cells that, at

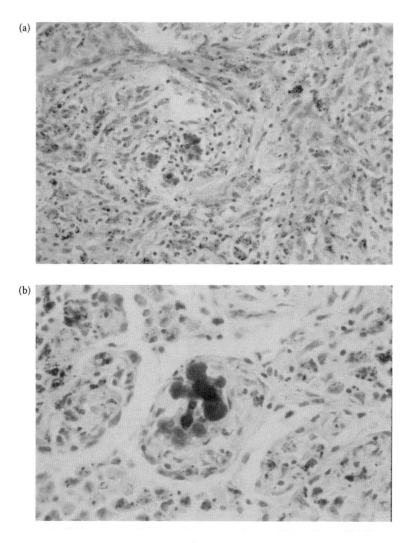

Figure 11.6 (a and b) Nodular mass composed of dense, disorganized connective tissue with scattered inflammatory cells. Ferruginous bodies morphologically consistent with asbestos bodies are easily identified.

that time, were thought to represent alveolar type II pneumocytes although later were shown to be macrophages. DIP was associated with varying degrees of interstitial fibrosis. Not uncommonly, the individuals with DIP had fever and other symptoms. DIP was subsequently found to be associated with respiratory bronchiolitis, a condition characterized by fibrosis around respiratory bronchioles and alveolar ducts in which there were smoker's macrophages in alveolar ducts and respiratory bronchioles. See Chapter 9 (Asbestosis) for a discussion concerning usual interstitial pneumonia versus grade IV asbestosis.

In 1972, Corrin and Price[51] reported a case of DIP in a 53-year-old man who smoked 10 cigarettes per day until 1 year before his illness. Asbestos bodies were identified within intraalveolar macrophages.

In 1991, Freed et al.[52] reported a case of DIP in a man with a 32-year history of working in the drywall construction trade and who had a three-pack per day cigarette smoking history. In that case,[52] a single asbestos body was identified in the frozen section of the lung tissue specimen. Asbestos digestion analysis showed 4666 asbestos bodies per gram of wet lung tissue (our

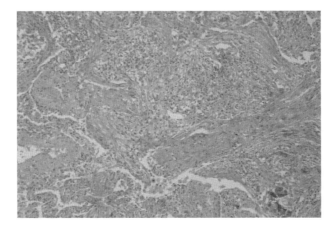

Figure 11.7 Nodular masses composed of randomly dispersed, dense fibrous tissue with varying number of inflammatory cells (low power magnification).

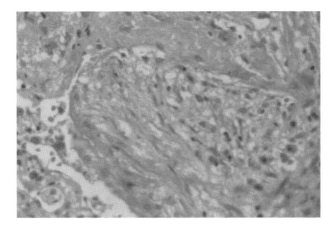

Figure 11.8 Nodular masses composed of randomly dispersed, dense fibrous tissue with varying number of inflammatory cells (high power magnification).

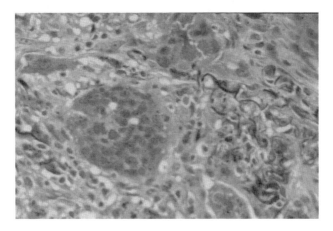

Figure 11.9 Frequent asbestos bodies. These were recently referred to as *asbestomas*.

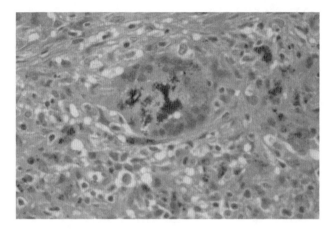

Figure 11.10 Asbestoma composed of fibroinflammatory tissue with intracytoplasmic asbestos bodies in multinucleated macrophage giant cells.

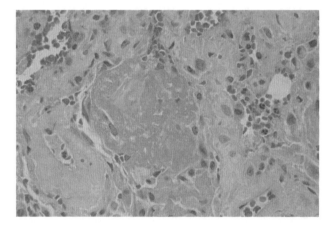

Figure 11.11 AFOP with fibrin in alveolar spaces.

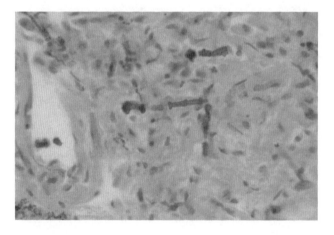

Figure 11.12 AFOP with asbestos bodies.

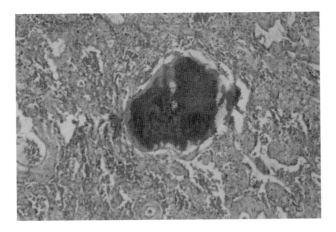

Figure 11.13 AFOP with areas of ossification.

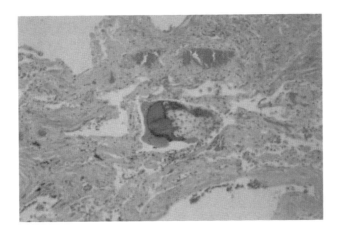

Figure 11.14 AFOP with areas of ossification and asbestos bodies.

background of "normal" is 20 asbestos bodies per gram of wet lung tissue), 819 million chrysotile fibers per gram of dry lung tissue, and 20 million tremolite asbestos fibers per gram of dry lung tissue.

In our study[39] published in 1993, we observed one patient who had DIP changes in which asbestos bodies were easily identified in the tissue, specifically in macrophages that filled alveolar spaces (Figures 11.15 and 11.16).

Over the last 17 years, Hallman and I have observed approximately 10 cases of what we currently refer to as *asbestos–cigarette-smoke-induced interstitial lung disease*. These cases show large numbers of smoker's macrophages within alveolar spaces and perhaps more severe interstitial fibrosis than would be observed in typical cases of DIP (Figures 11.17 and 11.18). We believe that there is a spectrum of DIP that ranges from relatively mild interstitial fibrosis to fairly severe interstitial fibrosis. In some cases, we observed asbestos bodies in alveolar macrophages (Figure 11.19) and fibrotic lung tissue (Figure 11.20).

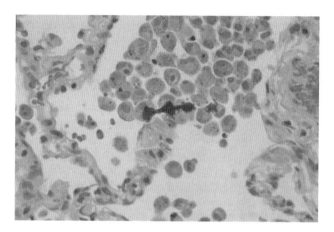

Figure 11.15 Representative regions of lung biopsy specimen show desquamative-type infiltrate of macrophages.

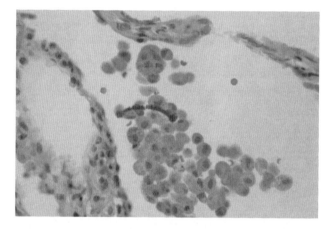

Figure 11.16 Ferruginous bodies morphologically consistent with asbestos bodies are noted in the cytoplasm of macrophages.

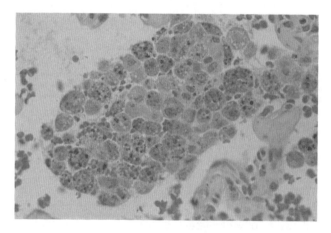

Figure 11.17 More severe fibrosis is seen in this case of asbestos–cigarette-smoke-induced interstitial lung disease than seen in typical cases of DIP (high power magnification).

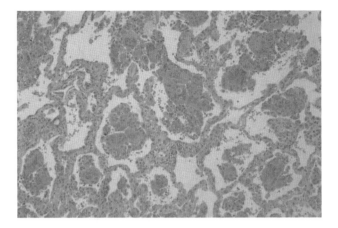

Figure 11.18 More severe fibrosis is seen in this case of asbestos–cigarette-smoke-induced interstitial lung disease than seen in typical cases of DIP (low power magnification).

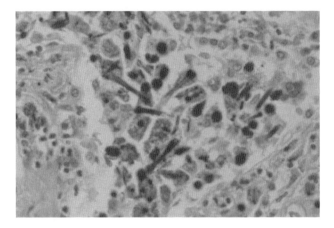

Figure 11.19 Relatively frequent asbestos bodies are observed in alveolar macrophages and fibrotic lung tissue in this case of DIP.

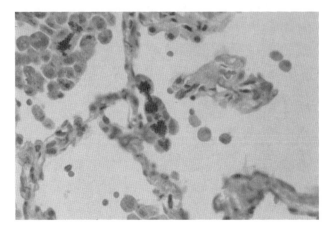

Figure 11.20 Two asbestos bodies are observed in alveolar macrophages and fibrotic lung tissue in this case of DIP.

11.5 *ASPERGILLUS*-INDUCED LUNG CHANGES

Aspergillus involvement in the lung is typically seen in a couple of different settings, namely, in individuals who are immunocompromised hosts and in individuals who have bronchiectasis, usually because of cigarette-smoke-induced lung disease.

Hillerdal and Heckscher[53] reported *Aspergillus* infection in the lungs of four asbestos-exposed persons, two of whom reportedly had localized lung masses. A case of aspergilloma in association with asbestosis was reported by Hinson et al.[54] They suggested that asbestos could cause cylindric bronchiectasis and fibrotic narrowing of the bronchi. Hillerdal and Heckscher[53] suggested that asbestos could potentially lead to immune dysfunction and perhaps result in an opportunistic infection caused by *Aspergillus* organisms. Roggli et al.[55] mentioned five cases in which *Aspergillus* was identified in the lungs of persons occupationally exposed to asbestos.

In our study (Hammar and Hallman[39]) of eight patients with localized masses, we found one in which there was focal *Aspergillus* infection in association with a relatively localized nodular area of fibrosis (Figure 11.21) in which asbestos bodies were commonly seen in the tissue (Figure 11.22). This patient had a history of occupational exposure to asbestos while working at the Puget Sound Naval Shipyard in Bremerton, Washington. In our[39] case, there was no evidence of allergic bronchopulmonary aspergillosis, and the patient was not asthmatic. We[39] have subsequently observed seven additional cases of focal aspergillosis in association with asbestos-induced pulmonary fibrosis, the most recent being in an asbestos-exposed person who had mild asbestosis in which there were several foci of *Aspergillus* infection (Figure 11.23).

11.6 GRANULOMATOUS INFLAMMATORY CHANGES

Granulomatous inflammation is seen in a variety of different conditions in the lung, including infections such as tuberculosis and fungal infections, and also in various other conditions such as hypersensitivity pneumonia, pulmonary angiitis, and granulomatosis (e.g., Wegener's granulomatosis).

Histiocytic giant cells containing asbestos bodies/fibers are occasionally seen in the lungs of persons occupationally exposed to asbestos. Occasionally, small nodular aggregates of histiocytes

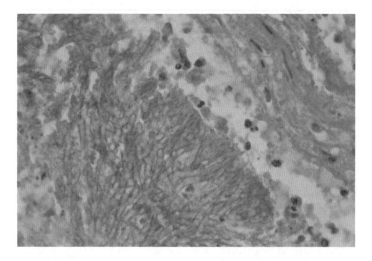

Figure 11.21   Nodule composed mostly of dense fibrous tissue with focal necrosis with *Aspergillus* organisms (high power magnification).

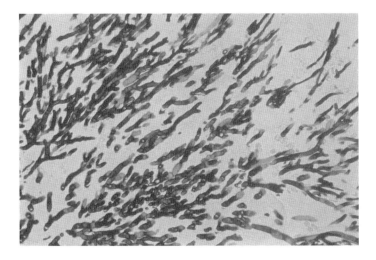

Figure 11.22 Nodule composed mostly of dense fibrous tissue with focal necrosis with *Aspergillus* organisms Methenamine silver stained section.

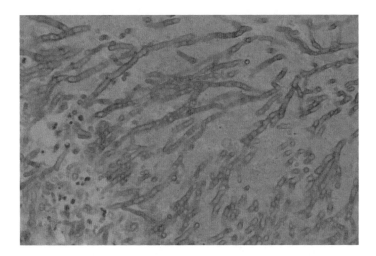

Figure 11.23 Asbestos-exposed individual with mild asbestosis in which there were several foci of *Aspergillus* infection.

consistent with nonnecrotizing granulomata are seen in the lungs of persons exposed to asbestos. In one case that we reported (Hammar and Hallman[39]), a fairly striking granulomatous inflammation was localized in the lung in which we identified asbestos bodies in giant cells forming granulomata (Figures 11.24 and 11.25). The patient in whom we observed these changes had a history of rheumatoid arthritis, although had a negative rheumatoid factor and had no clinical or laboratory evidence of sarcoidosis.

With respect to granulomatous inflammation induced by asbestos, Monseur et al.[56] reported an asbestos factory worker who developed a granulomatous inflammatory reaction in his urinary bladder and whose prostate tissue contained asbestos fibers.

De Vuyst et al.[57] reported granulomatous inflammation in the lung of a 32-year-old chemist who worked for 8 years in a dusty environment containing aluminum powders. De Vuyst et al.[57] stated the pathologic changes observed in the lung biopsy of that patient were similar to those seen in berylliosis and sarcoidosis. The patient, however, did not have either of those diseases.

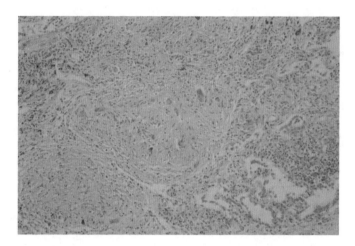

Figure 11.24 Representative region of lung tissue from shipyard worker with asbestos exposure. Tissue shows fairly extensive regions of granulomatous inflammation resembling sarcoidosis.

(a)

(b)

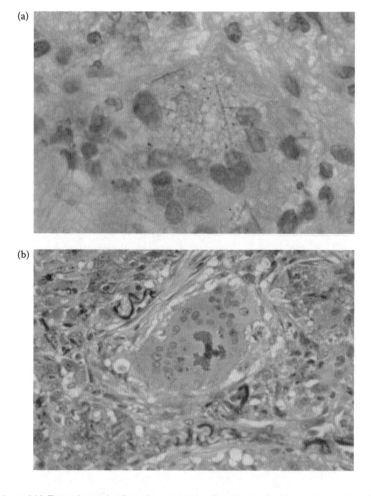

Figure 11.25 (a and b) Ferruginous bodies characteristic of asbestos bodies and asbestos fibers are often seen in or are closely associated with multinucleated histiocytic giant cells.

We reviewed pathology materials from two patients occupationally exposed to aluminum dust who developed granulomatous inflammation in open lung biopsies. These observations suggested that asbestos, aluminum dust, and beryllium can cause a granulomatous inflammatory reaction in the lung that can be confused with sarcoidosis or an infectious process.

11.7 CONCLUSION

One should be aware that asbestos can cause a variety of nonneoplastic inflammatory tissue reactions in the lung. Although these findings are uncommon, they do occur.

REFERENCES

1. Garcia Joe GN, Gray LD, Dodson RF, Callahan KS. Asbestos-induced endothelial cell activation and injury: Demonstration of fiber phagocytosis and oxidant-dependent toxicity. *Am Rev Respir Dis* 1988;138:958–964.
2. Kennedy TP, Dodson RF, Rao NV, Ky H, Hopkins C, Baser M, et al. Dusts causing pneumoconiosis generate OH and produce hemolysis by acting as Fenton catalysts. *Arch Biochem Biophys* 1989;269:359–364.
3. Lemaire I, Beaudoin H, Masse S, Grondin C. Alveolar macrophage stimulation of lung fibroblast growth in asbestos-induced pulmonary fibrosis. *Am J Pathol* 1986;122:205–211.
4. Kamp DW. Asbestos-induced lung diseases: An update. *Transl Res* 2009;153:143–152.
5. Heintz NH, Janssen-Heininger YMW, Mossman BT. Asbestos, lung cancers, and mesotheliomas: From molecular approaches to targeting tumor survival pathways. *Am J Respir Cell Mol Biol* 2010;42:133–139.
6. Brody AR. Asbestos and lung disease. *Am J Respir Cell Mol Biol* 2010;42:131–132.
7. Currie GP, Watt SJ, Maskell NA. An overview of how asbestos exposure affects the lung. *Br Med J* 2009;339:b3209.
8. Turner-Warwick M, Parkes WR. Circulating rheumatoid and antinuclear factors in asbestos workers. *Br Med J* 1970;3:492–495.
9. Turner-Warwick M. Immunological mechanisms in occupational disorders. *Proc R Soc Med* 1973;66:927–930.
10. Toivanen A, Salmivalli M, Molnar G. Pulmonary asbestosis and autoimmunity. 1976;691–692.
11. Morris DL, Greenberg SD, Lawrence EC. Immune responses in asbestos-exposed individuals. *Chest* 1985;87:278–280.
12. Jarad NA, Uthayakumar S, Buckland EJ, Green TS, Ord J, Newland AC, Rudd RM. The histocompatibility antigen in asbestos-related disease. *Br J Ind Med* 1992;49:826–831.
13. Tamura M, Liang D, Tokuyama T, Yoneda T, Kasuga H, Narita N, et al. Study on the relationship between appearance of autoantibodies and chest x-ray findings of asbestos plant employees. *Sangyo Igaku* 1993;35:406–412.
14. Nigam SK, Suthar AM, Patel MM, Karnik AB, Dave SK, Kashyap SK, Venkaiah K. Humoral immunological profile of workers exposed to asbestos in asbestos mines. *Indian J Med Res* 1993;98:274–277.
15. Marczynski B, Czuppon AB, Marek W, Reichel G, Baur X. Increased incidence of DNA double-strand breaks and anti-ds DNA antibodies in blood of workers occupationally exposed to asbestos. *Hum Exp Toxicol* 1994;13:3–9.
16. Pfau JC, Sentissi JJ, Weller G, Putnam EA. Assessment of autoimmune responses associated with asbestos exposure in Libby, Montana, USA. *Environ Health Perspect* 2005;113:25–30.
17. Miura Y, Nishimura Y, Katsuyama H, Maeda M, Hayashi H, Dong M, et al. Involvement of IL-10 and Bcl-2 in resistance against an asbestos-induced apoptosis of T-cells. *Apoptosis* 2006;11:1825–1835.
18. Otsuki T, Maeda M, Murakami S, Hayashi H, Miura Y, Kusaka M, et al. Immunological effects of silica and asbestos. *Cell Mol Immunol* 2007;4:261–268.
19. Pfau JC, Sentissi JJ, Li S, Calderon-Garciduenas L, Brown JM, Blake DJ. Asbestos-induced autoimmunity in C57BL/6 mice. *J Immunotoxicol* 2008;5:129–137.

20. Tschernig T, Pabst R. Bronchus-associated lymphoid tissue (BALT) is not present in the normal adult lung but in different disease. *Pathobiology* 2000;68:1–8.

21. Richmond I, Pritchard GE, Ashcroft T, Avery A, Corris PA, Walters EH. Bronchus associated lymphoid tissue (BALT) in human lungs: its distribution in smokers and nonsmokers. *Thorax* 1993;48:1130–1134.

22. Swigris JJ, Berry GJ, Raffin TA, Kuschner WG. Lymphoid interstitial pneumonia: A narrative review. *Chest* 2002;122:2150–2164.

23. Bienenstock J, Johnston N, Perey DYE. Bronchial lymphoid tissue: I. Morphologic characteristics. *Lab Invest* 1973;28:686–692.

24. Bienenstock J, Johnston N, Perey DYE. Bronchial lymphoid tissue: II. Functional characteristics. *Lab Invest* 1973;28:693–698.

25. Pisani RJ, Witzit TE, Li CY, Morris MA, Thibodeau SN. Confirmation of lymphomatous pulmonary involvement by immunophenotypic and gene rearrangement analysis of broncho-alveolar lavage fluid. *Mayo Clin Proc* 1990;65:651–656.

26. Kuroso K, Yumo T, Rom WN, Takiguchi Y, Jaishree J, Nakata K, et al. Oligoclonal T cell expansions in pulmonary lymphoproliferative disorders: Demonstration of the frequent occurrence of oligoclonal T cells in human immunodeficiency virus-related lymphoid interstitial pneumonia. *Am J Respir Crit Care Med* 2002;165:254–259.

27. Colby TV. Lymphoproliferative diseases. In: *Pulmonary Pathology Tumors*, Dail DH, Hammar SP, Colby TV, eds. New York: Springer Verlag; 1995: 343–368.

28. Fraser RS, Paré PD. Lymphoproliferative disorders and leukemia. In: *Diagnosis of Diseases of the Chest*, 4th ed., Fraser RS, Müller NL, Colmann N, Paré PD, eds. Philadelphia: WB Saunders Company; 1999: 1269–1330.

29. Jaffe ES, Harris NL, Stein H, Vardiman JW. *Genetics of Tumours of Hematopoietic and Lymphoid Tissues.* Lyon: IARC Press; 2001.

30. Nicholson AG. Lymphoproliferative lung disease. In: *Pathology of Lung Tumors*, Corrin B, ed. New York: Churchill Livingstone; 1997: 213–223.

31. Yousem SA. Lung tumors in the immunocompromised host. In: *Pathology of Lung Tumors*, Corrin B, ed. New York: Churchill Livingstone; 1997: 189–212.

32. Kradin RL, Mark EG. Benign lymphoid disorders of the lung with a theory regarding their development. *Hum Pathol* 1983;14:857–867.

33. Koss MN. Pulmonary lymphoid disorders. *Semin Diagn Pathol* 1995;12:158–171.

34. Dail DH. Uncommon tumors. In: *Pulmonary Pathology*, 2nd ed., Dail DH, Hammar SP, eds. New York: Springer-Verlag; 1994: 1329–1336.

35. Saldana MJ, Patchfsky AS, Israel HL, Atkinson GN. Pulmonary angiitis and granulomatosis: The relationship between histologic features, organ involvement and response to treatment. *Hum Pathol* 1977;8:391–409.

36. Israel HL, Patchfsky AS, Saldana MJ. Wegener's granulomatosis, lymphomatoid granulomatosis and benign lymphocytic angiitis and granulomatosis of lung: recognition and treatment. *Ann Intern Med* 1977;87:691–699.

37. Rom WN, Travis WD. Lymphocyte-macrophage alveolitis in non-smoking individuals occupationally exposed to asbestos. *Chest* 1992;101:779–786.

38. Katzenstein A-L A, Myers JL, Mazur MT. Acute interstitial pneumonia: A clinicopathologic, ultrastructural, and cell kinetic study. *Am J Surg Pathol* 1986;10:256–267.

39. Hammar SP, Hallman KO. Localized inflammatory pulmonary disease in persons occupationally exposed to asbestos. *Chest* 1993;103:1792–1799.

40. Hillerdal G, Hemmingson A. Pulmonary pseudotumors and asbestos. *Acta Radiol Diagn* 1980;21(Facs. 5):615–620.

41. Lynch DA, Gamsu G, Ray CS, Aberle DR. Asbestos-related focal lung masses: Manifestations on conventional and high-resolution CT scans. *Radiology* 1988; 169:603–607.

42. Case Records of the Massachusetts General Hospital. Case 73–1961. *N Engl J Med* 1961;265:745–751.

43. Saldana MJ. Localized asbestos pneumonia. *Lab Invest* 1981;44:57–58A [abstract].

44. Roggli VL. Pathology of human asbestosis: A critical review. *Adv Pathol* 1989;2:31–60.

45. Spencer H. The pneumoconioses and other occupational lung diseases. In: *Pathology of the Lung*, 3rd ed. Spencer H, ed. Oxford: Pergamon Press; 1977: 427–429.

46. Keith I, Day R, Lemaire S, Lemaire I. Asbestos-induced fibrosis in rats: Increase in lung mast cells and autocoid contents. *Exp Lung Res* 1987;13:311–327.

47. American Thoracic Society. Diagnosis and initial management of nonmalignant diseases related to asbestos. *Am J Respir Crit Care Med* 2004;170:691–715.

48. Cavazza A, Nigrisoli E, De Marco L, Paci M, Annessi V, Agostini L, Gardini G. Bronchiolitis obliterans-organizing pneumonia (BOOP) containing asbestos bodies: Clinico-pathological study of a case. *Pathologica* 2001;93:681–684.

49. Beasley MB, Franks TJ, Galvin JR, Gochuico B, Travis WD. Acute fibrinous and organizing pneumonia: A histologic pattern of lung injury and possible variant of diffuse alveolar damage. *Arch Pathol Lab Med* 2002;126:1064–1070.

50. Liebow AA, Steer A, Billingsley JG. Desquamative interstitial pneumonia. *Am J Med* 1965;39:369–404.

51. Corrin B, Price AB. Electron microscopic studies in desquamative interstitial pneumonia associated with asbestos. *Thorax* 1972;27:324–331.

52. Freed JA, Miller A, Gordon RE, Fischbein A, Kleinerman J, Langer AM. Desquamative interstitial pneumonia associated with chrysotile asbestos fibers. *Br J Ind Med* 1991;48:332–337.

53. Hillerdal G, Heckscher T. Asbestos exposure and *Aspergillus* infection. *Eur J Respir Dis* 1982;63:420–424.

54. Hinson KFW, Moon AJ, Plummer NS. Bronchopulmonary aspergillosis. *Thorax* 1952;7:317–333.

55. Roggli VL, Johnson WW, Kaminsky DB. Asbestos bodies in fine needle aspirates of the lung. *Acta Cytol* 1984;28:493–498.

56. Monseur J, Leguene B, Lebouffant L, Tichoux G. Asbestose du col vesical et de la prostate. *J Urol* 1986;92:17–21.

57. De Vuyst P, Dumortier P, Schandene L, Esenne M, Verhest A, Yernault J. Sarcoid-like lung granulomatosis induced by aluminum dusts. *Am Rev Respir Dis* 1987;135:493–497.

CHAPTER 12

Clinical Diagnosis and Management of Nonmalignant Asbestos-Related Diseases

Gary K. Friedman

CONTENTS

12.1 INTRODUCTION

Asbestos-related diseases have the potential for necessitating costly medical care, causing impairment, reducing life expectancy, and having major societal impact. The importance of appropriate diagnosis and management is emphasized by the numerous position statements issued by various professional societies and the volumes of peer-reviewed medical literature devoted to asbestos-related medical issues.

In the past decade, approximately 750,000 reported cases of asbestos-related disease have been filed as claims for compensation. More than 70 major U.S. corporations have been driven into bankruptcy. However, recent events in the legal system have raised serious questions concerning the reliability of many of these diagnoses.[1] Increased utilization of high-resolution computed tomography (HRCT) and increased awareness by physicians has resulted in the diagnosis of previously undetected cases. A 2004 report by the Centers for Disease Control and Prevention (CDC) indicated that asbestosis was the only pneumoconiosis to document increases in deaths decade over decade.[2] In 2009, the CDC reported 2705 mesothelioma deaths for 2005, with a death rate of 14 per million, which was identical to that in 1999.[3] Although the diagnostic criteria and clinical aspects of most illnesses are relegated to the purview of physicians and scientists, asbestos-related diseases have become a topic of heated debate for the courts, employers, insurers, and legislative bodies at the state and federal levels. Texas, Ohio, and Florida have passed state legislation with medical criteria requiring proof of impairment before a nonmalignant case may be eligible to seek compensation in the Tort System.

During the past 10 years, the following official statements and guidelines have been published, which have had significant impact on the diagnosis and management of asbestos-related nonmalignant disease:

1. American Thoracic Society (ATS), Diagnosis and Initial Management of Nonmalignant Diseases Related to Asbestos.[4]
2. The *Guidelines for the Use of the ILO International Classification of Radiographs of Pneumoconiosis*, Revised Edition, 2000.[5]
3. ATS/European Respiratory Society (ERS) Task Force:
   a. Standardization of Lung Function Testing[6]
   b. Standardization of Spirometry[7]
   c. Standardization of Single-Breath Determination of Carbon Monoxide Uptake in the Lung[8]
   d. Standardization of the Measurement of Lung Volumes[9]
   e. Standardization of Interpretive Strategies of Lung Function Tests[10]
4. American Medical Association (AMA), *Guides to the Evaluation of Permanent Impairment*, Fifth[11] and Sixth Editions[12]
5. American College of Chest Physicians (ACCP) Consensus Statement on the Respiratory Health Effects of Asbestos[13]

Many patients diagnosed with nonmalignant asbestos-induced disease may be seeking second opinions, require monitoring for progression of their disease, or have concerns about the possible development of malignant complications. This and the following chapter are written for the clinician who may be called upon to address these issues.

12.2 A BRIEF OVERVIEW OF THE HISTORY OF CLINICAL ASBESTOS-RELATED DISEASE

It is traditional to provide a history of the use of asbestos and the chronology of scientific advances in asbestos-related disease. The finer details of the past 100 years of the history of asbestos are left to others.[14] A relationship between asbestos exposure and pulmonary fibrosis has been recognized since the late 1800s. Sufficient knowledge of the relationship between asbestos and pulmonary injury existed by 1918, which caused certain insurance companies to deny life insurance to asbestos workers.[15] The term *asbestosis* was first used by Cooke[16] in 1927, who published a postmortem examination of a 33-year-old woman who began working at the age of 13 years in the carding room of an asbestos factory. In 1930, a report from the Mayo Clinic[17] detailed clinical aspects of asbestosis, including the radiographic findings, the clinical symptoms, the latency, the description of asbestos bodies (previously described by McDonald),[18] the potential for progression, the lack of satisfactory treatment, the relationship between pulmonary asbestosis and pulmonary hypertension, cor pulmonale, and the potentially fatal outcome of the disease.

A report associating lung cancer and asbestos exposure (asbestosis) was authored in 1935 by Lynch and Smith.[19] By 1948, Lynch and Cannon[20] stated, "carcinoma of the lung was also of such prominence as to require continued consideration as possibly inducible in a susceptible subject by severe asbestosis until disproved by further investigation." In 1955, Sir Richard Doll[21] reported a cohort documenting the carcinogenicity of asbestos and the development of lung cancer.

A few case reports of mesothelioma associated with asbestos exposure appeared in the late 1940s and early 1950s. Eisenstadt[22] provided a case report originating in Texas refinery settings in the late 1950s. Wagner et al.[23] reported 33 cases of diffuse pleural mesothelioma in patients exposed to crocidolite asbestos in the Asbestos Hills northwest of Cape Province South Africa and clearly established the relationship between asbestos and this uncommon tumor.

Reports within the medical and industrial hygiene literature led to recommendations for standards limiting asbestos exposure. On May 29, 1969, asbestos exposure limits previously recommended by the American Conference of Government Industrial Hygienists were incorporated into federal regulation under the Walsh Healey Act, which applied to work practices of federal contractors. The Occupational Safety and Health Administration (OSHA) was established the following year with one of its first priorities being the promulgation of an emergency standard regulating the industrial use of asbestos in 1971. The passage of the permissible exposure limit by OSHA had the goal of reducing the risk of asbestosis to less than one per thousand workers during a 45-year working lifetime of exposure. Over the next 15 years, progressively stringent regulatory standards were issued, further reducing the allowable exposures to asbestos.[24]

Medical evidence, new regulatory standards, and employer concerns over compensable work-related injury resulted in a marked decline in the utilization of asbestos in the United States by the early 1970s. All asbestos-related diseases exhibit a dose–response relationship as one of the factors in their causation. A reduction in asbestos exposure has occurred during the past 35 years, and both the incidence and the severity of nonmalignant respiratory diseases have declined. An understanding of the differences in the levels of asbestos exposure that have occurred during different periods of time and in different occupations and working conditions is critical for the clinician in his assessment of a given case.

12.3 ASBESTOS EXPOSURE

Between 1940 and 1979, it was estimated that 27,500,000 U.S. workers were occupationally exposed to asbestos.[25] No other occupational lung disease has been the subject of as many peer-reviewed articles or epidemiological studies. The literature has identified the occupations, industries, and other circumstances where significant exposure to asbestos may occur.[25–28] The spectrum of diseases that may result from asbestos exposure and the occurrence of impairment, disability, or death resulting from each of these diseases have been described by many authors.

As asbestos utilization in the United States has fallen, subsequent exposures were typically much lower than historic levels, which caused severe impairment and deaths reported in the asbestos literature of prior years. Engineering controls, use of respiratory protection, and other factors affecting asbestos exposure have resulted in a decline in the incidence and severity of asbestos-induced diseases. Because different asbestos-related diseases are associated with different levels of exposure and latency, each case deserves careful individual evaluation and an understanding of the evolving and dynamic nature of asbestos-induced diseases.

With reduced exposure, a substantial decrease in incidence of most asbestos-related diseases (with the exception of mesothelioma) was anticipated to have occurred by the mid-1990s. Thus, the recent "epidemic" of hundreds of thousands of cases of asbestosis diagnosed within the past decade poses new challenges to the clinician. There are some within the medical and legal communities who have raised questions concerning the soundness of the methodology[29] used and the reliability of the diagnosis in some cases. Others point out that there may be additional cases that have gone undiagnosed. Hopefully, the following will provide assistance to many physicians who will face the challenges of providing appropriate future medical care and in properly addressing the questions and concerns of their patients with asbestos-induced diseases.

12.4 HOW ASBESTOS MEASUREMENTS ARE USED IN CLINICAL PRACTICE

The measurement of levels of airborne asbestos is within the purview of industrial hygiene and is discussed elsewhere in this book. Such measurements are rarely available to the clinician. Nicholson et al.[30] used the levels of asbestos exposure within certain industries and occupations in an attempt to project future risks for mesothelioma and lung cancer. The National Institute for Occupational Safety and Health (NIOSH) has used job descriptions to stratify risks of asbestos exposure.[31] The ATS[32] states that exposure levels are rarely available to the clinician and, when available, the significance is often not well understood. The ATS stresses the importance of a detailed occupational history over measured levels of exposure and, when necessary, consultation with an occupational physician or other resource.[32]

Asbestos exposure is frequently referred to in terms of total or cumulative dose. The dose is a product of the duration of exposure (in years) and the intensity of exposure as defined by average workplace air concentration in fibers per cubic centimeter. Only fibers greater than 5 µm in length are counted. The OSHA permissible exposure limit[24] is 0.1 fibers/cm^3. This is designed to limit future deaths from asbestosis but does not protect against the malignant complications of asbestos exposure.

The Helsinki consensus criteria statement on asbestos, asbestosis, and lung cancer states that asbestosis "may occur" at 25 fiber-years.[33] There is a doubling of the risk of lung cancer at this dose. Increased risk of disease may occur at lesser exposure levels. There is no compelling evidence that asbestosis occurs at less than 10 fiber-years of exposure.

12.4.1 Occupation and Exposure

The analysis of exposure in some occupations such as brake repair is more complex. Consideration must be given not only to fiber counts but also to fiber type, fiber size, and conversion to forsterite as a result of friction-induced heat. Nicholson et al.[30] documented a substantially lower risk of asbestos-related disease for brake mechanics than insulators for equal duration of exposure. Additional examples of specific occupational exposures are covered in Chapter 5.

12.5 LATENCY

Latency is the period of time between the first exposure to asbestos and the appearance of an asbestos-induced disease. The median latency period for asbestosis is in the range of 25–30 years. The incidence of benign asbestos pleural disease is dependent upon the duration of time since exposure and, to a lesser degree, on dose. Shorter latencies described historically were attributed to very high levels of exposure that occurred in the remote past.[34] An exception to the above is benign asbestos effusion, which may occur in the first decade after exposure. The unique issues relating to latency are discussed under each disease.

12.6 DIAGNOSTIC STUDIES

12.6.1 Chest X-Ray: Standard X-Ray Interpretations versus "B" Reading

The chest radiograph is the most widely used among the objective studies performed for the diagnosis of asbestos-related diseases. Although clinicians are familiar with the typical radiographic narrative interpretations rendered by clinical radiologists, asbestosis and other pneumoconioses are frequently reported in the literature by using a standardized system developed by the International Labor Office (ILO; Revised 2000)[5] (Figure 12.1). The system was originally developed for epidemiology and research in Black Lung disease, and the radiographic reports are referred to as "B" readings. The American College of Radiology in conjunction with NIOSH offers instruction on the use of this system. NIOSH administers an examination to certify physicians as "B" readers as proof of proficiency in reading pneumoconiosis chest radiographs using the ILO system.

For the purpose of ILO interpretation, only the posterior–anterior (PA) view is used. A series of numerical values, letters, and symbols are used to characterize various aspects of the PA radiograph. The ILO publishes a set of 22 standard radiographic films for purposes of comparison. The degrees of fibrosis are measured by profusion (concentration) of small irregular opacities. Standard

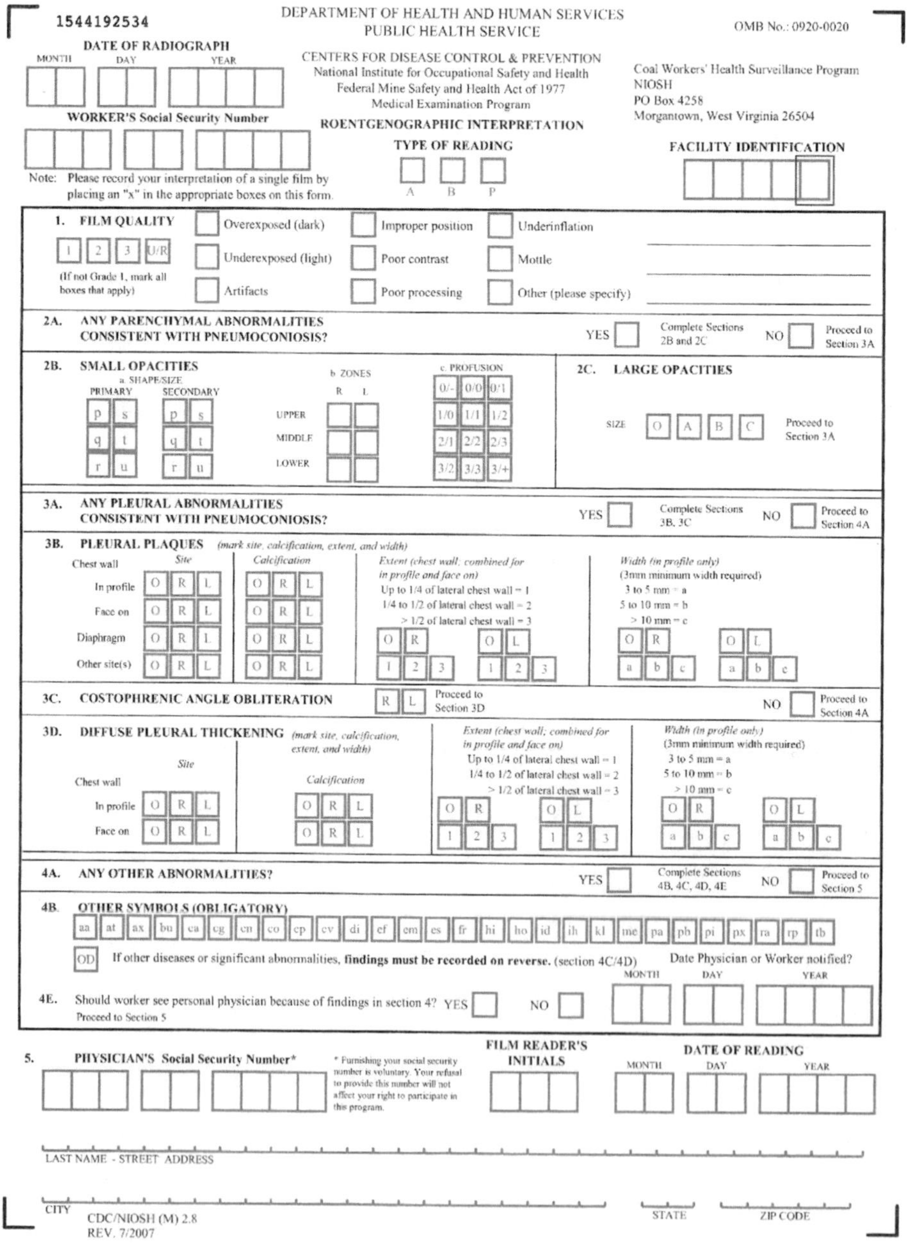

1544192534

DEPARTMENT OF HEALTH AND HUMAN SERVICES
PUBLIC HEALTH SERVICE
CENTERS FOR DISEASE CONTROL & PREVENTION
National Institute for Occupational Safety and Health
Federal Mine Safety and Health Act of 1977
Medical Examination Program
ROENTGENOGRAPHIC INTERPRETATION

OMB No.: 0920-0020

Coal Workers' Health Surveillance Program
NIOSH
PO Box 4258
Morgantown, West Virginia 26504

DATE OF RADIOGRAPH — MONTH DAY YEAR

WORKER'S Social Security Number

TYPE OF READING — A B P

FACILITY IDENTIFICATION

Note: Please record your interpretation of a single film by placing an "x" in the appropriate boxes on this form.

1. FILM QUALITY — 1 2 3 U/R (If not Grade 1, mark all boxes that apply)
Overexposed (dark) | Improper position | Underinflation
Underexposed (light) | Poor contrast | Mottle
Artifacts | Poor processing | Other (please specify)

2A. ANY PARENCHYMAL ABNORMALITIES CONSISTENT WITH PNEUMOCONIOSIS? YES — Complete Sections 2B and 2C; NO — Proceed to Section 3A

2B. SMALL OPACITIES
a. SHAPE/SIZE — PRIMARY: p s q t r u; SECONDARY: p s q t r u
b. ZONES — R L — UPPER, MIDDLE, LOWER
c. PROFUSION — 0/- 0/0 0/1; 1/0 1/1 1/2; 2/1 2/2 2/3; 3/2 3/3 3/+

2C. LARGE OPACITIES — SIZE: O A B C — Proceed to Section 3A

3A. ANY PLEURAL ABNORMALITIES CONSISTENT WITH PNEUMOCONIOSIS? YES — Complete Sections 3B, 3C; NO — Proceed to Section 4A

3B. PLEURAL PLAQUES (mark site, calcification, extent, and width)
Chest wall — Site / Calcification: In profile O R L / O R L; Face on O R L / O R L; Diaphragm O R L / O R L; Other site(s) O R L / O R L
Extent (chest wall; combined for in profile and face on): Up to 1/4 of lateral chest wall = 1; 1/4 to 1/2 of lateral chest wall = 2; > 1/2 of lateral chest wall = 3 — O R 1 2 3; O L 1 2 3
Width (in profile only) (3mm minimum width required): 3 to 5 mm = a; 5 to 10 mm = b; > 10 mm = c — O R a b c; O L a b c

3C. COSTOPHRENIC ANGLE OBLITERATION — R L — Proceed to Section 3D; NO — Proceed to Section 4A

3D. DIFFUSE PLEURAL THICKENING (mark site, calcification, extent, and width)
Chest wall — Site / Calcification: In profile O R L / O R L; Face on O R L / O R L
Extent (chest wall; combined for in profile and face on): Up to 1/4 of lateral chest wall = 1; 1/4 to 1/2 of lateral chest wall = 2; > 1/2 of lateral chest wall = 3 — O R 1 2 3; O L 1 2 3
Width (in profile only) (3mm minimum width required): 3 to 5 mm = a; 5 to 10 mm = b; > 10 mm = c — O R a b c; O L a b c

4A. ANY OTHER ABNORMALITIES? YES — Complete Sections 4B, 4C, 4D, 4E; NO — Proceed to Section 5

4B. OTHER SYMBOLS (OBLIGATORY)
aa at ax bu ca cg cn co cp cv di ef em es fr hi ho id ih kl me pa pb pi px ra rp tb
OD If other diseases or significant abnormalities, **findings must be recorded on reverse.** (section 4C/4D)
Date Physician or Worker notified? MONTH DAY YEAR

4E. Should worker see personal physician because of findings in section 4? YES NO
Proceed to Section 5

5. PHYSICIAN'S Social Security Number* — * Furnishing your social security number is voluntary. Your refusal to provide this number will not affect your right to participate in this program.

FILM READER'S INITIALS

DATE OF READING — MONTH DAY YEAR

LAST NAME - STREET ADDRESS

CITY — STATE — ZIP CODE

CDC/NIOSH (M) 2.8
REV. 7/2007

Figure 12.1 NIOSH Roentgenographic Interpretation ("B" reader) form 2000.

4961192530

4C. MARK ALL BOXES THAT APPLY: (Use of this list is intended to reduce handwritten comments and is optional)

Abnormalities of the Diaphragm
☐ Eventration
☐ Hiatal hernia

Airway Disorders
☐ Bronchovascular markings, heavy or increased
☐ Hyperinflation

Bony Abnormalities
☐ Bony chest cage abnormality
☐ Fracture, healed (non-rib)
☐ Fracture, not healed (non-rib)
☐ Scoliosis
☐ Vertebral column abnormality

Lung Parenchymal Abnormalities
☐ Azygos lobe
☐ Density, lung
☐ Infiltrate
☐ Nodule, nodular lesion

Miscellaneous Abnormalities
☐ Foreign body
☐ Post-surgical changes/sternal wire
☐ Cyst

Vascular Disorders
☐ Aorta, anomaly of
☐ Vascular abnormality

4D. OTHER COMMENTS

Public reporting burden of this collection of information is estimated to average 3 minutes per response, including time for reviewing instructions, searching existing data sources, gathering and maintaining the data needed, and completing and reviewing the collection of information. An agency may not conduct or sponsor, and a person is not required to respond to a collection of information unless it displays a currently valid OMB control number. Send comments regarding this burden estimate or any other aspect of this collection information, including suggestings for reducing this burden to CDC, Project Clearance Officer, 1600 Clifton Road, MS E-11, Atlanta, GA 30333, ATTN: PRA (09020-0020). Do not send the completed form to this address.

Figure 12.1 Continued.

radiographs also demonstrate examples of pleural abnormalities. The "B" reader is instructed to compare the patient's chest radiograph against the ILO standard radiographs that most closely resemble the subject's radiograph. The results are then recorded in a systematic fashion on a special form (Figure 12.1). The ILO publishes the guidelines for interpretation of the radiographs as a handbook,[5] which accompanies the set of standard x-rays.

Films are graded for technical quality. Films of very poor quality are deemed unreadable and should not be used for the purpose of ILO interpretation. The fibrosis of asbestosis is represented radiographically as irregular opacities and is characterized by the following symbols denoting the dominant size of the opacity: S (fine—like a piece of thread), T (medium thickness—like a piece of string), and U (coarse—like a piece of heavy twine).

The profusion (concentration) of small irregular opacities is quantified along a continuous 12-point scale. A zero indicates the absence of small irregular opacities or a profusion less than that demonstrated on a Category 1 ILO standard chest radiograph. The chest radiographs within Category 1 (e.g., standard film 1/1) indicate a mild profusion of small irregular opacities, Category 2 (e.g., standard film 2/2) indicate a moderate profusion, and Category 3 indicate a severe profusion (e.g., standard film 3/3).

Because the subject's chest radiograph often does not perfectly match the standard film, two numbers are assigned to the radiograph. The first number represents the category to which the reader believes to be present and the second number represents the category to which the reader gave serious consideration as an alternative. For example, if a physician was convinced a chest radiograph was mildly abnormal and matched a standard 1/1 radiograph, that symbol would be marked on the ILO form. However, if the subject's chest radiograph was felt to approximate a Category 1 profusion but showed substantially less concentration of small irregular opacities than on the 1/1 standard film and consideration was given to the film being normal (Category 0), the 1/0 would be used. The ILO indicates this would be a chest radiograph that was "classified as Category 1 after having seriously considered Category 0 as an alternative."[35]

The 1986 ATS statement on asbestos cautioned that "the prevalence of lesser degrees of interstitial fibrosis is not well known. Considerable caution has to be exercised in attributing all such phenomena to asbestos exposure either known or occult."[32] The 2004 ATS[4] statement on asbestos uses 1/0 as the boundary between normal and abnormal films for asbestosis. However, the 2004 ATS statement qualifies the description of 1/0 as being "presumptively diagnostic but not unequivocal." Furthermore, the positive predictive value of a 1/0 film for diagnosing asbestosis "may fall below 30% when exposure to asbestos has been infrequent and exceed 50% when it has been prevalent."[4]

12.6.2 HRCT and Chest X-Ray Interpretation

Recent technical advances in HRCT have increased its utility in the diagnosis of nonmalignant asbestos-related diseases. This is especially true at lower levels of profusion. The ATS noted that "when radiographic abnormalities were indeterminate, HRCT is often useful in revealing characteristic parenchymal abnormalities." The recent ACCP Consensus Statement[13] agreed "in the setting of a 1/0 radiograph, the HRCT scan would increase the specificity of these radiographic findings." The ACCP was in consensus that chest radiographic changes of 1/0 small irregular opacities are a good screening tool but lack specificity for an accurate diagnosis of asbestosis. HRCT should be performed to increase the specificity of these chest radiographic findings. There was ACCP consensus that a 1/1 profusion of S, T, and U irregular opacities were of recognized value in the diagnosis of asbestosis.

Pleural abnormalities are defined as either discrete (plaques) or diffuse areas of pleural thickening. They are characterized as to location (site), including the chest wall, mediastinum, diaphragm, and costophrenic angle. The left and right sides of the chest are recorded separately. Calcification of plaques is also to be noted on the ILO form.

Diffuse pleural thickening refers to thickening of the visceral pleura. Under the most recent ILO (2000) classification,[5] pleural thickening with a minimum width of 3 mm extending up the lateral chest wall is recorded as diffuse thickening only in the presence of continuity with a blunted or obliterated costophrenic angle. The 1980 ILO Classifications[35] identify the importance of costophrenic angle blunting in asbestos-related disease. It also comments on its potential as a nonspecific finding, especially when unilateral.

Under the ILO system, a substantial number of obligatory symbols must be completed. These include the radiographic presence of changes suggesting cancer, emphysema, pneumothorax, tuberculosis, mesothelioma, pleural effusion, rib fracture, abnormality of the cardiac silhouette, and a number of other findings.[5]

12.6.3 Purpose and Limitations of the ILO Classification

The ILO classification was originally designed for epidemiologic purposes. The ILO specifically stated the object was to codify the radiographic abnormalities of the pneumoconiosis in a simple reproducible manner. The Guidelines for the Use of ILO International Classification of Radiographs of Pneumoconiosis[35,5] states: "The classification neither defines pathological entities nor takes into account working capacity." "It does not imply legal definitions of pneumoconiosis for compensation purposes and does not set or imply a level at which compensation is payable." The importance of the differential diagnosis of any chest radiographic abnormality is addressed as: "No radiographic features are pathognomonic of dust exposure. Some radiographic features that are unrelated to inhaled dust may mimic those caused by dust."[5]

12.6.4 Conventional Film Chest Radiographs versus Digital Radiographs

As of June 2009, NIOSH and the CDC stated only conventional screen film chest radiographs should be used for the purpose of ILO interpretation, stating: "Until the ILO endorses the use of digital standards, however, readers must continue to use the current ILO reference films and conventional chest radiographs for classifying using the ILO system."[36]

Digital diagnostic imaging is rapidly being used worldwide. There is an increasing demand for adaptation of the ILO classification system to a digital format. A thorough review of this topic is contained in a NIOSH Workshop dated July 2008 (NIOSH Publication No. 2008-139: Application of the ILO International Classification of Radiographs of Pneumoconiosis To Digital Chest Radiographic Images),[37] which states that radiographic imaging is an imperfect tool and is not a diagnostic gold standard and functional impairment does not always correlate with imaging. Furthermore, one cannot provide certainty about the etiology of observed findings due to the limited number of ways in which the lung may respond.

According to Dr. Igor Fedatov[37] (ILO) (Fedatov I. Personal Communication. Geneva: World Health Organization; 2008), the advantage of digital imaging includes a better quality of image, and digital images can be manipulated to help with interpretation. Digital imaging makes it easier to access image is cheaper to store, and the images are less subject to loss and are more readily adaptable for use with telemedicine. However, at this time, the hardware and the software are not standardized. Additional trials are needed to determine the comparability of conventional chest films with digital radiographs and to develop digital standard images for ILO comparison purposes, which are currently unavailable.

Continued investigation is underway by the ILO and NIOSH in hopes of rapidly resolving these issues. The NIOSH Web site ("B" reader information for medical professionals) section entitled "Digital Radiography" states: "Thus, until provisions for use of digital images have been specified, readers using the ILO classifications *for all purposes* should continue to use traditional film screen radiographs and standards." As of June 2010, the ILO and the NIOSH continue to investigate the difficulties in standardizing both digital x-rays and HRCT. Currently, there is no system similar to the ILO for systematic reporting of CT or HRCT.

12.7 PULMONARY FUNCTION TESTS

Pulmonary function tests (PFTs) represent a battery of studies with each component assessing a different aspect of lung function. A detailed guide for pulmonary function laboratory management and procedures was published by the ATS in 1998[38] and has been updated. The ATS/ERS Task Force has published a series of statements that set forth criteria for the performance of pulmonary function testing.[6–10] PFTs are used in several different capacities in evaluating asbestos-related disease (Table 12.1).

Table 12.1   Utilization of Pulmonary Function Testing

- Diagnosis—the reduction below lower limits of normal for FVC and DLCO is of value in supporting the diagnosis of asbestosis[32]
- Impairment rating—to document impairment of lung function[36,43–45]
- Monitoring to determine the progression or improvement of lung function over a period of time (improvement suggests an etiology other than asbestos)
- Preoperative evaluation
- Disability determination[36,43–46]
- Certification for respirator use
- Assessment of symptoms

Table 12.2   Spirometry—Acceptability Criteria

- Free from artifact (cough, variable effort, leak, etc.)
- Good start of test (back extrapolation) (ATS/ERS—expiratory volume <5% FVC or 0.15 L, whichever is greater)
- Satisfactory end of study—minimum 6 sec exhalation time and/or plateau in the volume time curve or patient cannot or should not continue
- Minimum of three acceptable studies
- Submission of at least three time volume curves/flow volume loops for inspection

Source: ATS/ERS Task Force, *Eur. Resp. J.*, 26, 319–338, 2005.

The most recent published standards for pulmonary function testing come from a series of statements published by the ATS/ERS Task Force on Standardization of Lung Function Testing.[6] These supersede the prior ATS Statement on Pulmonary Function Testing. Topics include the ATS/ERS Task Force Statement on Standardization of Spirometry;[7] the ATS/ERS Standardization of the Single Breath Determination of Carbon Monoxide Uptake in the Lung;[8] the ATS/ERS Standardization of Lung Function Testing: Standardization of the Measurement of Lung Volumes;[9] and the ATS/ERS Standardization of Lung Function Testing: Interpretive Strategies for Lung Function Tests.[10] For pulmonary functions performed before 2005, the ATS Standardization of Spirometry 1994 would be appropriate[39] as would the ATS Single-Breath Carbon Monoxide Diffusing Capacity (Transfer) Statement[40] and the ATS Lung Function Testing: Selection of Reference Values and Interpretive Strategies.[41]

12.7.1 Spirometry, Acceptability, and Reproducibility

Spirometry is the most commonly performed study and measures inhaled and exhaled volumes of air as measured over time (flow). The actual volume, which the patient can exhale with maximal effort from a maximum inhalation, is the forced vital capacity (FVC). The maximum amount that can be expelled during the first second of exhalation is the forced expiratory volume in one second (FEV_1). Peak expiratory flows, slow vital capacities, and exhaled volumes at various increments of time can also be measured. The study provides important information concerning airflow obstruction and possible restriction. The studies must be performed in compliance with the appropriate ATS or ATS/ERS criteria cited above.

The results of these tests are dependent, in part, upon the patient's effort, the accuracy of the measuring device, and the skill of the technician. Therefore, it is important for the clinician to determine whether or not a valid study was obtained before assigning clinical significance to the results. The physician should review time volume curves and flow volume loops to check for artifact, back-extrapolation, or other factors that can affect the results of the study. Brief summaries of the ATS/ERS guidelines that may prove useful in the clinician's determination of reliability of the test results are shown in Tables 12.2 and 12.3.

Table 12.3   Reproducibility Criteria

After three acceptable spirograms have been obtained:

- Two largest FVC must be within 150 cc of each other
- The two largest FEV$_1$s must be within 150 cc of each other
- The patient should repeat these studies until either acceptability and reproducibility have been achieved or a total of eight tests have been performed or if the subject cannot continue.
- The best three studies should be saved with appropriate notations made by the technician as to the reason the study was discontinued.

Source: ATS/ERS Task Force, *Eur. Resp. J.,* 26, 319–338, 2005.

Table 12.4   ATS/ERS Criteria for DLCO

- Use of proper quality controlled equipment
- Inspired volume of greater than 85% of vital capacity in less than 4 sec
- A stable breath hold of 10 ± 2 sec with no evidence of leak, valsalva, or Muller maneuvers
- Expiration in less than 4 sec with appropriate clearance of dead space and proper sampling analysis of alveolar gas
- Alveolar volumes should be measured
- At least two acceptable tests must be performed
- Reproducibility of the two best acceptable tests within 10% or 3 mL of CO

Source: ATS/ERS Task Force, *Eur. Resp. J.,* 26, 720–735, 2005.

12.7.2 Contraindications to Spirometry

Relative contraindications to spirometry include hemoptysis; pneumothorax; unstable cardiovascular status; thoracic, cerebral, or abdominal aneurysms; recent eye surgery; vomiting; and recent abdominal or thoracic surgery.[38]

12.7.3 Diffusion Capacity

The diffusing capacity of the lung for carbon monoxide (DLCO) measures the transfer of gas across the alveolar capillary interface. The test uses a low concentration of inspired carbon monoxide inhaled by the patient. The breath is held for 9–11 sec, and an exhaled volume is collected. Pulmonary diseases that affect the alveolar–capillary interface either by destruction of the alveolar wall, as in emphysema, or thickening of the barrier, as in interstitial lung disease, may reduce the DLCO. There are numerous factors that can affect the diffusion capacity other than injury to the alveolar wall. Nonpulmonary factors including reduced hemoglobin concentration, reduced cardiac output, exogenous sources of carbon monoxide (such as smoking), chronic renal failure, and others may cause a decrease in diffusion capacity. Increases in diffusion capacity have been reported with polycythemia, pulmonary hemorrhage, left to right heart shunts, and exercise.[40]

A summary of the ATS/ERS[8] criteria for performance of the diffusion capacity is shown in Table 12.4.

The volume of collection should be 0.5–1 L and collected in less than 4 sec. The use of supplemental oxygen should be discontinued at least 5 min before beginning the test. Cigarette smoking affects test results in at least two different ways:

1. Emphysema with destruction of alveolar units reduces the diffusion capacity.
2. Recent cigarette smoking elevates carboxyhemoglobin levels. This will adversely affect gas transfer and artificially reduce the DLCO. Smoking cessation is recommended for 24 h before the performance of this study.[40,8]

There should be at least 4 min between DLCO test efforts to allow for complete elimination of the test gas before repeating the study.[40] Two acceptable studies must be obtained and reproducibility criteria achieved.

12.8 AIRWAY OBSTRUCTION AND BRONCHODILATORS

When airway obstruction is present, the ATS recommends the use of bronchodilators to determine reversibility. Bronchodilators are recommended when the FEV_1 is less than 70% of predicted.[38] Relative contraindications for bronchodilator testing include a known adverse reaction to a specific bronchodilator or unstable cardiovascular status such as arrhythmias, elevated blood pressure, or other diseases that could be aggravated by beta agonist stimulation.[42,43] Contraindication to the use of bronchodilator should be noted in the technician's comments. Additional recommendations for the performance and interpretation of bronchodilator studies are available.[44,45] Use of bronchodilators as proscribed under the AMA *Guides to the Evaluation of Permanent Impairment*[12] and Social Security Disability[42] should be performed as required.

12.8.1 Total Lung Capacity

Methods for determining lung volume are defined in detail in the ATS/ERS Task Force: Standardization for Measurement of Lung Volumes,[9] and because of the various techniques and complexity of the methodologies, the reader is referred to the ATS/ERS Statement for more information. The total lung capacity (TLC) represents the sum of the residual volume (RV) and the FVC or can be measured as the sum of the inspiratory capacity plus functional residual capacity (FRC). TLC is used in determining restrictive defect[41] (especially in the presence of obstruction) and, in the alternative, to demonstrate hyperinflation. FRC can be measured by gas dilution using helium and may be measured by collecting nitrogen, which has been washed out of the lung by 100% oxygen (nitrogen washout method).

Plethysmography measures the gas volume within the thorax and is another means of measuring TLC. The patient sits in a tightly sealed, specially constructed chamber (body box). The patient breathes or pants against a shutter attached to a mouthpiece. A variation of Boyle's law measures changes in the patient's mouth pressure and the pressure in the sealed box. A "loop" is created on a graph plotting mouth pressure against change in volume (change in box pressure). The tangent of the loop is measured and corresponds to lung volume with the mouth shutter closed (FRC).[46] Plethysmography is considered to be the preferred method to measure RV, FRC, and TLC. Nitrogen and helium methods may underestimate volumes, especially when significant airway obstruction is present or if noncommunicating air spaces such as cysts, large bullae, and so forth, prevent thorough gas distribution.

12.8.2 PFT Interpretation

After determining a study meets the performance criteria, the physician must then interpret the study. Guidelines have been established for selecting reference values and interpretive strategies.[41,10] The results of the patient's PFTs are compared against those of "normal individuals" of same height, sex, age, and race, all of which have been found to be important determinants of lung function. Several reference equations are available in the peer-reviewed literature for predicted normal values. The reference equations most suitable for the laboratory's patient population should be used. Predicted values developed by the NIOSH and the CDC during the National Health and Nutrition Examination Survey III and reported by Hankinson et al.[47] were derived for three separate ethnic groups (Caucasian, African American, and Mexican American, aged 8–80 years). These predicted values are available for clinical use and are incorporated in the AMA *Guides to the Evaluation of Permanent Impairment*, Sixth Edition, and are recommended by the ATS/ERS.[12]

12.8.3 Normal versus Abnormal (Lower Limits of Normal)

The 1986 ATS Statement on Impairment and Disability Secondary to Respiratory Disorders has defined impairment as less than 80% of predicted for FVC or FEV$_1$, or DLCO.[48] The AMA *Guides to the Evaluation of Permanent Impairment* adopted the same criteria in 1990.[49] These guides are used for the purpose of impairment for worker compensation in at least 40 states or districts within the United States.

In aged individuals or those at the extremes of height, the use of 80% of predicted does not always equate to the lower limit of normal (LLN) when the latter is defined as the lower fifth percentile. In 1991, the ATS stated that the use of 80% of predicted for a lower limit in adult PFTs was not recommended[41] and normal ranges should be based on the fifth percentile (LLN). In 2001, the AMA *Guides to the Evaluation of Permanent Impairment*, Fifth Edition,[11] adopted the use of the LLN to define impairment. The current ATS/ERS guidelines employ the LLN.[10]

12.9 THE SPECTRUM OF ASBESTOS-RELATED NONMALIGNANT DISEASES

Asbestos causes inflammatory reaction, fibrosis, and malignancy in the lung and pleura. Cellular injury occurs long before disease becomes apparent. Details of such injury are beyond the scope of this chapter and are discussed elsewhere in this book. Asbestos-induced diseases occur along a "spectrum" reflecting levels of asbestos exposure, latency, and other factors. Nonmalignant asbestos-related diseases are summarized in Table 12.5.

12.10 PLEURAL DISEASES

The pleura is the most common site of clinical findings in asbestos-exposed individuals. Pleural abnormalities may occur at lower levels of exposure than those that cause asbestosis. The pathogenesis and method of transport to the pleura is poorly understood and has been summarized by others.[50] Theories on causation include mechanical irritation and hypersensitivity reaction. Asbestos may cause changes in the visceral or parietal pleura, involving the lateral chest walls, the diaphragm, the pericardium, and the mediastinum. Pleural diseases may occur individually or in combination with other benign or malignant asbestos-related diseases.

12.10.1 Pleural Plaques on Chest Radiograph

Pleural plaques (Figure 12.2) represent the single most common radiographic finding in individuals exposed to asbestos. In surveillance studies of large groups of individuals exposed to asbestos, the occurrence of pleural plaques in the absence of interstitial fibrosis is a far more common finding

---

Table 12.5 Nonmalignant Pulmonary and Pleural Manifestations of Asbestos Exposure

- Benign asbestos effusion
- Hyaline plaques
- Calcified plaques
- Diffuse pleural thickening (requires pleural thickening of the lateral chest wall of at least 3 mm thickness contiguous with blunting of a costophrenic angle)
- Rounded atelectasis
- Asbestos pleuritis
- Pulmonary asbestosis
- Asbestos-related small airway disease

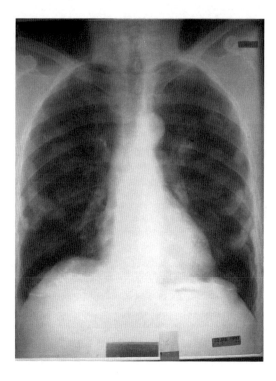

Figure 12.2   Bilateral calcified pleural plaques—both chest walls and diaphragms.

than the finding of pulmonary asbestosis in the absence of plaques. In individuals with pulmonary asbestosis, 60% or more of reported cases have accompanying pleural findings.[51–53]

Pleural plaques are discrete areas of circumscribed pleural thickening most frequently involving the parietal pleura. They most often occur on the diaphragm and posterolateral chest walls in the lower-half of the chest. They frequently parallel the course of the ribs (Figure 12.3) and typically have markedly irregular margins, which are sometimes likened to a holly leaf in appearance. They may be flat or have a more nodular morphology, which can be mistaken for a pleural-based density on chest radiograph. Plaques have a unique tendency to involve the parietal pleura covering the diaphragm (Figure 12.4), especially in the region of the central tendon. They may involve the mediastinal pleura and the pericardium. They tend to spare the apices and the costophrenic angles. Calcification may be a good indicator of the age of the plaque as radiographically apparent calcification usually does not appear until 20 years or more after initial exposure. Although calcification may be dramatic in its extent, it only occurs in less than 10% of plaques and, by itself, neither significantly increases impairment nor does it increase the risk of malignancy.

In the ILO classification, plaques seen on the lateral chest wall are described as being "in profile" (Figure 12.2). Formation of plaques on the anterior or posterior chest wall is a less common occurrence.[45] In this position, they are perpendicular to the x-ray beam on PA projection and, because of their typically thin profile, may only present as a somewhat hazy or milky shadow and are described as being seen face on or "en face." To confirm the presence of such plaques, oblique views and CT scan may detect plaques not easily seen on PA projection.

12.10.2 Exposure and Latency

Pleural plaques may occur at substantially lower levels of asbestos exposure than does parenchymal disease (pulmonary asbestosis). Their growth and progression is dependent upon elapsed

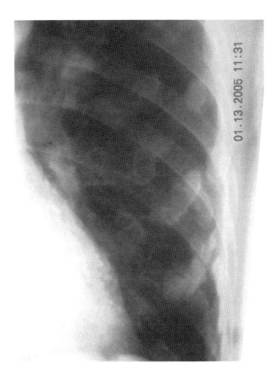

Figure 12.3 Calcified plaques paralleling the ribs (close-up).

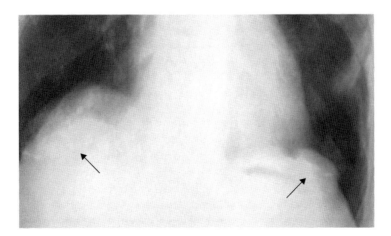

Figure 12.4 Diaphragmatic plaques—multiple punctuate calcifications in plaque on right and calcified plateau-shaped plaque on the left.

time from exposure and, to a lesser extent, level of exposure.[54] Radiographically, they are rarely evident less than 15 years from first exposure and typically are not radiographically apparent in most cases until at least 20 years or more after initial exposure. Thereafter, the probability of growth and developing calcification increases with time.[55]

Although most pleural plaques are the result of occupational exposure to asbestos, they have been reported in household contacts of asbestos workers. This has been most commonly reported in spouses who washed a worker's asbestos-contaminated clothing over a prolonged period of time.[56] Environmental exposures to asbestos have been reported to cause pleural disease in Turkey, Finland, and Greece where forms of asbestos occur naturally in the soil. In Turkey, erionite, a form of fibrous zeolite (an asbestiform fiber), has been used in whitewash on walls of homes leading to a high incidence of pleural plaque and mesothelioma in that population.

Epler et al.[57] reported an increased incidence of plaques over time after occupational exposure. Plaques were found in 10% of exposed workers with less than 20 years of latency and almost 60% by 49 years of latency. These data probably represent substantially heavier exposure than experienced in the past three decades, as Epler's cohort had exposure dating back to 1933.

The 2009 ACCP statement group could not reach consensus as to whether extent of exposure correlates with presence and extent of pleural abnormalities.[13]

12.10.3 Differential Diagnosis

Plaque with calcification, the plateau-shaped plaque on the diaphragm, or bilateral areas of discrete pleural thickening with sparing of the costophrenic angles usually do not pose a diagnostic dilemma in the presence of an occupational history of asbestos exposure with adequate latency. However, in some cases of circumscribed pleural thickening, the differential diagnosis can be more difficult.

The most common source of mistaken diagnosis is subpleural fat.[58] Subpleural fat tends to involve the apical and axillary region and may extend all the way down into the lower one-third of the chest but does not involve the costophrenic angle. Mid-chest wall bilateral symmetric areas of smooth pleural thickening with tapering or indistinct borders may also represent subpleural fat. Serratus anterior muscle shadows have a sawtooth appearance, which can mimic pleural thickening or plaque formation in some individuals. Skin folds, breast tissue, pectoral muscle shadows, and other soft tissue shadows must be excluded as a potential source of confusion for en face or in-profile plaque formation.

The common sources of circumscribed pleural thickening on the lateral chest wall are chest tube insertion sites, other postoperative change, or penetrating chest wound. Postoperative changes from cardiac surgery, hiatal hernia, or subdiaphragmatic surgery may cause diaphragmatic irregularities that can be confused with plaque. Careful inspection of the thorax on physical examination with correlation of the position of surgical scars with the appearance of pleural irregularities on chest radiograph is important. Rib fracture and callous formation with adjacent pleural thickening must be distinguished from pleural plaque. Tuberculosis may result in pleural calcification, which may mimic asbestos-related changes. However, this usually is accompanied by other radiographic stigmata of tuberculosis. Eventration of the diaphragm may mimic diaphragmatic plaques.

Silica may cause areas of pleural thickening, which are described as having a candle wax appearance. The typical rounded opacities involving the upper lung zones, hilar adenopathy, and other manifestations of silica exposure help establish the etiology. Talc may cause pleural plaques and some of the earliest descriptions of calcified plaques occurred among talc workers.[59] Talc pleurodesis is a common mimic of pleural change because of asbestos. Talc is often contaminated with asbestos (usually tremolite). Careful inquiry into these and other causes of pleural disease combined with the physical examination should result in the proper clinical diagnosis.

12.10.4 Incidence: Pleural versus Pulmonary

In asbestos-exposed populations, regardless of industry or occupation, there is a substantially higher incidence of pleural disease compared with pulmonary asbestosis. Kishimoto et al.[60] studied chest radiographs of 2951 construction workers in Japan and confirmed his findings by CT scan. Eighty-five patients had pleural plaques alone, 9 had asbestosis alone, and 74 had pleural plaques and asbestosis. In 11 subjects, pleural plaques were suggested on chest radiograph but were not confirmed on CT scan.

In 1986, Sider et al.[56] screened 117 wives of insulation workers by chest radiograph. No abnormalities were noted among women under age 40. Eighteen (19.4%) of 93 women older than 40 years demonstrated pleural changes, 6 of whom had diaphragmatic plaque. There was no evidence of parenchymal disease. The only significant variable predicting the finding of these radiographic changes was the elapsed time from first exposure to asbestos. The mean latency was 32.8 years. The intensity and the duration of exposure appeared to be less significant than latency.

Bresnitz et al.[61] reported a series of 91 elevator construction workers exposed to asbestos during refurbishment of older buildings. All had more than 20 years of employment in the industry. Twenty workers (22%) had pleural disease, but none had an interstitial process consistent with asbestosis. Fifteen had bilateral circumscribed plaques and five had unilateral plaque. Cases of diffuse pleural thickening or pleural effusion were not described.

In 1994, Miller et al.[62] reported radiographic findings of 2611 long-term insulators with heavy exposure to asbestos. Those with only pleural abnormalities (633, 24%) exceeded those with only parenchymal disease (301, 11.5%). In 1996, Miller et al.[63] studied 1245 sheet metal workers with at least 20 years in the trade and compared them with insulators. They noted a substantially lower incidence of asbestosis (1/0) among sheet metal workers compared with insulators (17.5% vs. 59.5%). Also noted with lower exposure was a lower incidence of pleural disease (36% vs. 75%). Pleural abnormalities outnumbered parenchymal changes by a 2:1 ratio.

In 1994, Welch et al.[64] investigated a larger group of sheet metal workers (9605) with 20 years or more in the trade. The median age was 57 years, and there was an average of 32 years in the industry. Radiographically, 18.8% demonstrated pleural disease, whereas 6.6% had parenchymal changes (1/0 or greater). Of 2552 workers with 40 or more years since entering the sheet metal trade, 24.2% had pleural abnormalities, 7.7% had parenchymal changes, and 9.6% had both.

In 1991, Oliver et al.[65] studied 120 public school custodians and found that 40 (33%) had pleural plaque and 3 (2.5%) had parenchymal disease of 1/0.

NIOSH[31] investigated sequelae of asbestos exposure at a petrochemical refinery at the request of a union. Investigators performed a detailed analysis stratified by occupation and length of exposure. The stratification identified those with high levels of asbestos exposure such as insulators, pipefitters, and boilermakers; moderate levels of exposure such as construction carpenters, riggers, welders, and so forth; and those with lesser levels of exposure such as those working security. Regardless of occupation, pleural disease predominated over parenchymal abnormalities by a 2:1 ratio or greater. Prominence of pleural over parenchymal changes on chest radiographs was demonstrable regardless of length of employment and held true for both retirees and current employees.

Rosenstock et al.[66] studied 681 plumbers and pipefitters and found 17% had pleural disease, 7% had parenchymal changes, and 12% had both.

Sepulveda and Merchant[67] studied 266 railroad workers (75% were older than 60 years) and found 49 (23%) had pleural changes, 3 (1.5%) had parenchymal changes, and 3 (1.5%) had both.

Epler et al.[68] reported the incidence of benign asbestos pleural effusion (BAPE) and stated that there was a greater incidence of pleural disease than pulmonary fibrosis in subjects with substantial asbestos exposure in all latency periods ranging from 3 to 49 years.

Jones et al.[69] studied 5000 American marine engineers and found 12% with either plaque or diffuse pleural thickening, whereas only 1.2% had interstitial small opacities. They described pleural plaque and calcification as the most common manifestation of asbestos exposure, which may be seen after relatively brief or low-dose exposures.

Dement et al.[70] studied 2602 Department of Energy workers and found 5.4% had 1/0 or greater profusion of small irregular opacities whereas 23.1% had pleural changes. Of these, 2% had only parenchymal changes (1/0 or greater), 20% had only pleural changes, and 3% had pleural and parenchymal changes.

Peipins et al.[71] studied 7000(+) residents of the Libby, Montana, area after alleged environmental exposure to tremolite-contaminated vermiculite. Their methodology for radiographic interpretation included oblique and PA views. Positive results included unilateral pleural disease. Their cohort had a significantly elevated body mass index. They reported radiographic changes but rendered no opinion as to diagnosis or causation. They reported pleural abnormalities in 17% and parenchymal changes in <1% of the residents examined.

Substantially more pleural plaques are found at autopsy than are visible on chest radiograph. Hillerdal and Lindgren[72] reported the correlation between occupational history and radiographic observation of plaques. At autopsy, using a strict criteria for plaques, only 12.5% were seen on chest radiograph. Hillerdal's criteria for definite pleural plaques included bilateral pleural changes in the chest wall or diaphragm with at least 5-mm thickness and progression in a 5-year period if serial chest radiographs were available for examination. When Hillerdal used a more liberal radiographic criteria, the number of false-positive cases exceeded the previously undetected negatives.

12.10.5 Anatomic Site—Predominance

Historically, there have been reports of left-sided predominance for benign pleural disease, which is unexplained. A study by Gallego[73] in 1998 reported on CT scans performed on 40 subjects with asbestos exposure and pleural plaque. Gallego calculated the surface area of each plaque and the sum of these areas. Gallego found a lack of statistically significant predominance for either side.

12.10.6 CT Scan and Plaques

Almost since its advent, CT scan has been reported to identify pleural plaques, which were not readily identifiable on chest roentgenogram.[74] In 1984, Sluis-Cremer et al.[75] studied 19 men, 8 of whom had exposure to amphiboles, and concluded that "CT did not consistently demonstrate either parenchymal or pleural change earlier than conventional films." Further, pleural plaques were missed on CT when visible on conventional films. They concluded that CT and conventional chest radiographs were complimentary. With the introduction of HRCT and refinement of other advanced imaging techniques, the ability to detect pleural and parenchymal diseases has improved. CT scan is useful in distinguishing the density of subpleural fat from fibrotic pleural thickening or plaque. The 2009 ACCP Delphi Panel could not reach consensus as to whether CT scanning of the chest should be used to screen populations at risk for asbestos-related diseases. However, they concluded that HRCT was useful for further evaluation of radiographs with lesser degrees of profusion of opacities (such as 1/0).[13] The 2004 ATS Statement on Diagnosis and Management of Nonmalignant Asbestos-Related Disease uses HRCT in its criteria[4] as supportive evidence for exposure.

12.10.7 Malignancy and Pleural Plaques

Sanden and Jarvholm[76] evaluated 3893 shipyard workers in an attempt to identify predictors for mesothelioma risk. The authors did not find any distinction between exposure parameters versus presence of pleural plaque and increased risk of mesothelioma. Studies cite pleural plaque as a common occurrence in pleural mesothelioma. Dodson et al.[77] performed fiber burden analysis on lung tissue from 55 individuals with pathologic mesothelioma. Fifty patients were reported to have pleural plaque. Forty-six had ferruginous body concentrations of more than 1000 per gram of dry weight of lung tissue. The majority of ferruginous bodies had cores of amosite. The ATS 2004[4] Statement on the Diagnosis and Management of Nonmalignant Asbestos-Related Disease identifies pleural plaques as a marker of increased risk of malignancy, especially lung cancer, compared with others with similar exposure and without plaques. The 2009 ACCP Consensus Statement disagrees with that conclusion.[13] The ACCP cites Weiss' opinion that "lung cancer risk is not elevated among individuals with asbestos-related pleural plaques in the absence of asbestosis." The ACCP did reach consensus that patients with plaques were at an increased risk for mesothelioma.

12.10.8 Symptoms of Plaques

Pleural plaques are usually considered to be painless and, as a rule, are asymptomatic. Jarvholm and Larsson[78] studied 130 subjects with pleural plaques and compared them with a large control population without plaques. No difference in thoracic pain was found between the two groups. When severe pain is present, the clinician should be alerted to the possibility of mesothelioma, cancer metastatic to the pleura, inflammatory or infectious pleuritis, or some etiology other than pleural plaque. Unless extensive surface area is involved, plaques usually do not result in impairment sufficient enough to cause dyspnea. When significant dyspnea is present, underlying interstitial disease or other etiology should be ruled out.

12.10.9 Smoking and Pleural Plaques

There is no causal relationship between pleural plaques and smoking.[79]

12.10.10 PFT and Pleural Plaques

Because pleural plaques predominantly affect the parietal pleura, they have no effect on lung function or one which is usually less than that seen with diffuse pleural thickening involving the visceral pleura. Jarvholm and Sanden[80] investigated 202 nonsmoking shipyard workers with varying degrees of asbestos exposure. The majority had normal pulmonary function, and there was no evidence that plaques alone caused impairment. They reported that 87 workers with plaques and no other radiographic abnormalities had, on average, 6.9% lower FVC than those without plaques. This difference was largest for those with heaviest exposure to asbestos. Jarvholm and Sanden[80] hypothesized this decrease was possibly due to subroentgenographic pulmonary fibrosis or decrease in chest wall mobility in cases where plaques covered large surface areas.

Ohlson et al.[81] questioned whether change in lung function of asbestos cement workers was due to plaque per se or was the result of heavier asbestos exposure. Jarvholm and Sanden[80] opined that a possible distinction between their findings and those of Ohlson et al.[81] was reflective of levels of exposure in the shipyard workers of Jarvholm and Sanden[80] versus the cement workers of Ohlson et al.[82]

Rosenstock et al.[82] studied spirometric values of 684 plumbers and pipefitters and evaluated radiographic evidence of parenchymal fibrosis, pleural thickening, and cigarette smoking. In chest radiographs, 17% had only pleural abnormalities, 7% had only parenchymal abnormalities, and 12% had both pleural and parenchymal abnormalities. Pleural abnormalities were associated with a slight lowering of FVC independent of pulmonary fibrosis at low profusion (1/0 or less). Mean values of FVC and FEV_1 were 95% and 91% of predicted values, respectively. Functional changes were only slightly greater for those with diffuse pleural disease than those with plaque only. The population with pleural findings was small. Of 684 exposed workers, 48 patients had bilateral discrete pleural thickening whereas 63 demonstrated diffuse pleural thickening. Four-hundred eighty reportedly had no pleural abnormalities.

Baker et al.[83] found a reduction in FVC in sheet metal workers with greater than 30 years employment who had evidence of pleural disease, including pleural plaque after "controlling for potential confounding effects of age, smoking, and employment duration."

Most patients with plaques have well-preserved lung function. The ATS 2004 Statement reports that some large cohorts have shown reduction in lung function attributable to plaques, averaging approximately 5% of FVC even when interstitial fibrosis (asbestosis) was absent roentgenographically. However, the loss of function was not a consistent finding, and longitudinal studies have not shown a more rapid decline in lung function.[4] The ACCP Consensus Statement disagreed with the opinion that "pleural plaques alter lung function to a clinically significant degree."[13]

12.10.11 Physical Examination

There are no specific physical findings that identify pleural plaques, and they are not associated with a pleural rub. A palpable mass in the chest wall should alert the physician to the possibility of mesothelioma or other malignant process as a cause for a pleural-based abnormality.

12.11 ASBESTOS PLEURAL EFFUSION AND PLEURITIS

Benign asbestos pleural effusion (BAPE) is one of the few pathologic responses to asbestos that occurs within 10 years of first exposure. Epler et al.[68] reported such effusions to be bilateral or recurrent in 50% of their cases and sanguineous in one-third. Epler et al. defined benign asbestos pleural effusion with the following criteria:

(1) Exposure to asbestos
(2) Confirmation of effusion by radiograph or thoracentesis
(3) Exclusion of other more probable disease
(4) The appearance of no malignant tumor within 3 years.

The latter is required to exclude those cases where the pleural effusion is attributable to mesothelioma, lung cancer, or metastatic disease, which was not detected at the time of the initial clinical evaluation. Interestingly, two-thirds of Epler's patients reported no symptoms at the time the effusion was discovered.

One of the first descriptions of asbestos-related pleural effusion came from Eisenstadt,[84] an astute internist in Port Arthur, Texas, where numerous large chemical plants, refineries, and shipyards resulted in substantial asbestos exposure. In 1962, during the course of his private practice, Eisenstadt observed "asbestos pleuritis" and asbestos pleurisy. He reported benign asbestos pleurisy was a "frequent disease" among welders, pipefitters, insulators, boilermakers, and others employed in shipyards and oil refineries. He described the disease as having an acute, subacute, recurrent, or chronic course, which could be followed by mesothelioma many years later. Eisenstadt described effusions as clear, cloudy, or bloody.[22]

Gaensler and Kaplan[85] reported pleural effusion occurred in 21% of all patients with asbestosis seen in their practice. Their paper described the pathologic findings from six decortication cases and one autopsy case.

Scully, in a CPC[86] from Massachusetts General Hospital in 1987, described a 48-year-old gentleman with a pleural effusion. Scully opined that pleural effusion was the most common asbestos-related disease during the first two decades after exposure. It may recur on either side, may be hemorrhagic or clear, and may be accompanied by rather mild symptoms. Blunting of the costophrenic angle is a common sequelae. BAPE may be part of the pathogenesis for the later development of diffuse pleural thickening, which by definition requires associated blunting of the costophrenic angle.

12.12 DIFFUSE PLEURAL THICKENING

12.12.1 Description

Unlike pleural plaques, diffuse pleural thickening originates in the visceral pleura. Typically, it is a bilateral process. Because it is usually more extensive in surface area, involves the visceral pleura, and is adherent to the pulmonary parenchyma, it is more likely to cause impairment of lung function than discrete plaques. Some opine diffuse pleural thickening represents residua from prior benign effusions.[87,88] Others suggest that diffuse pleural thickening is the fibrotic result of inflammatory pleuritis, which may be dry and unassociated with effusion. Coalescence of pleural plaques has been suggested as another theory in the etiology of diffuse fibrosis.[87] However, this would not explain the blunting of the costophrenic angles or involvement of the visceral pleura. Historically, diffuse pleural thickening was felt to represent a continuation to the pleura of an underlying process of interstitial fibrosis or is frequently associated with such fibrosis histologically.[89] On HRCT scan, interstitial fibrosis (pulmonary asbestosis) is frequently associated with diffuse pleural thickening.[87] Hillerdal[90] suggested the possibility of an immunologic pathogenesis, noting elevation of sedimentation rate in diffuse pleuritic reactions but not plaques. Stephens et al.[91] concluded that diffuse pleural fibrosis was a specific asbestos-associated entity "of uncertain pathogenesis" whose asbestos fiber counts fell between those with plaques and those with minimal asbestosis.

12.12.2 Latency—Diffuse Pleural Thickening

Typically, diffuse pleural fibrosis occurs 20 or more years from the time of exposure and the incidence increases over time.

12.12.3 Chest Radiograph—Diffuse Pleural Thickening

The ILO definition[5] of diffuse pleural thickening requires blunting of at least one costophrenic angle with contiguous pleural thickening of at least 3-mm width (Figure 12.5) seen on the lateral chest wall. In the ILO classification, the extent of the pleural thickening is defined as Category 1 if it involves up to one-fourth of the projection of the lateral chest wall, Category 2 from one-fourth to one-half of the projection of the lateral chest wall, and Category 3 with thickening of the pleura greater than one-half of the projection of the lateral chest wall. The letters A, B, and C represent the width of the pleural thickening. Calcification may occur usually greater than 25 years after exposure.

12.12.4 Smoking and Diffuse Pleural Thickening

There is no proven association between smoking and diffuse pleural fibrosis.[92]

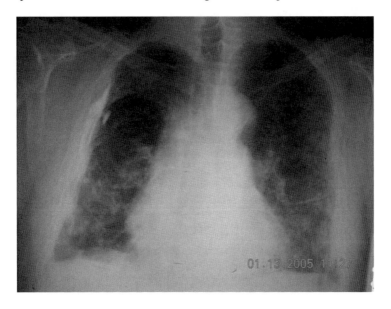

Figure 12.5 Diffuse pleural thickening with calcification bilaterally.

12.12.5 PFT and Diffuse Pleural Thickening

Thickening of the visceral pleura may affect chest wall compliance and impede expansion of the underlying parenchyma, which becomes entrapped by the thickened pleura. Impairment of lung function, in part, is related to the extent of diffuse pleural thickening. However, costophrenic angle blunting often results in similar degrees of functional impairment regardless of the presence or extent of radiographic contiguous pleural thickening.[4] Blunting of the costophrenic angle in diffuse pleural thickening is now deemed important both radiographically and functionally. In some cases of diffuse pleural thickening, a restrictive defect may occur in the absence of radiographically apparent pulmonary fibrosis. Reduction in diffusion capacity has been reported and attributed to possible underlying interstitial disease.[93] However, in many cases, the DLCO is normal when corrected for alveolar volume.

12.12.6 Symptoms and Complications

Given that diffuse pleural thickening may result in impairment of lung function and in reduction of compliance, shortness of breath (especially with exertion) is the most common complaint. With active pleuritis, pain and chest wall discomfort may occur.

With diffuse pleural thickening (especially when bilateral or extensive), the degree of functional impairment may result in disability in the absence of underlying asbestosis.[94] Wright et al.[93] stated that if diffuse pleural thickening caused reduction in lung function with resulting symptoms, disability could occur without asbestosis and compensation might be appropriate for this complication of asbestos exposure. Wright studied six patients with circumferential pleural thickening and no evidence of asbestosis and found that four of six demonstrated reduction in diffusion capacity and lung volumes. Miller et al.[95] described seven patients with severe chest wall restriction caused by asbestos-induced pleural fibrosis. Four died from respiratory failure and one was near death at the time of publication. At autopsy, these patients either had minimal or no accompanying interstitial fibrosis, and the severe impairment was attributed to extensive pleural disease.

12.12.7 Physical Examination

Physical examination may reveal diminished breath sounds and dullness to percussion in severe cases. Diminished respiratory excursion may be apparent when there is circumferential thickening or trapped lung. When acute pleuritis is present, a rub may be heard, but in my experience is uncommon. Typically, the disease is diagnosed long after its inception; thus, acute findings are lacking. If a chest wall mass is palpable, malignancy must be excluded as a cause for the diffuse pleural disease. Evidence of prior blunt trauma, thoracic surgery, or penetrating wounds may be found on physical examination suggesting another more probable cause for the pleural abnormality. Skin or joint manifestations of autoimmune disease, thrombophlebitis suggesting pulmonary emboli, pneumonia, empyema, or extrapulmonic manifestations of systemic disease should also be sought on physical examination.

12.12.8 Diagnosis

The diagnosis of diffuse pleural thickening is one of exclusion. Given a history of significant asbestos exposure and adequate latency along with exclusion of other causes for the radiographic findings, the diagnosis can usually be made clinically without biopsy. Unilateral pleural thickening may occur, but diagnosis is more problematic as such findings are less specific and the differential diagnosis is far broader than for bilateral disease. If pleural effusion is present and the etiology is uncertain, thoracentesis and pleural biopsy are recommended. Given the increased risk for lung cancer and mesothelioma in asbestos-exposed individuals, an aggressive approach to pleural effusions is recommended. If a definitive diagnosis cannot be made, their clinical course should be monitored carefully because of the increased risk of malignancy.

Because of the risk of mesothelioma, if the pleura appears unusually thickened or has a "lumpy-bumpy" or irregular appearance, or if a mass is suspected on imaging, then video-assisted thoracoscopy or open biopsy should be strongly considered in the event a diagnosis is not obtained by other means.

12.12.9 Treatment

Extensive pleural thickening should be treated as in other causes of fibrothorax. Decortication has proven beneficial in select cases. However, surgical success may be limited by the technical difficulties of dissecting the adherent visceral pleura from the lung. Underlying pulmonary fibrosis may prevent reexpansion of the lung and limit the benefits of decortication. Those with diffuse pleural disease of recent onset are more likely to benefit from surgery than those with longstanding or chronic fibrothorax. A thorough preoperative evaluation is mandatory.

12.13 ROUNDED ATELECTASIS

Rounded atelectasis is a benign process associated with asbestos exposure, which may be difficult to distinguish radiographically from a solitary nodule of malignant origin. It occurs as a peripheral lesion within the lung because of fibrosis of the visceral pleura, which folds inward to bend or roll upon itself. The invaginated thickened visceral pleura causes atelectasis of the lung parenchyma, producing a structure resembling a comet tail, which is referred to as a "comet tail sign" on imaging studies. Rounded atelectasis most commonly occurs in the inferior lobes posteriorly. This condition is often seen to better advantage on HRCT than on chest radiograph if sufficient slices are obtained to visualize the attachment to the pleura.

Hillerdal[96] reported on 74 patients with rounded atelectasis, 64 of whom had previous asbestos exposure. Thirteen cases resulted from slowly increasing pleural fibrosis; however, in 39 patients, rounded atelectasis was a sudden finding.

Bayeux et al.[97] reported on 286 patients suffering from benign asbestos pleural disease and found a diagnosis of rounded atelectasis in 26 patients on computerized tomography. Their criteria included a rounded opacity of less than 7 cm in diameter situated at the periphery of the lung in contact with thickened pleura, reduction of lung volume on the side of the atelectasis, and presence of a comet tail sign.

Doyle and Lawler[98] described eight major and five minor signs of rounded atelectasis in three patients studied with CT scan (see Table 12.6).

The primary importance of rounded atelectasis is that it must be distinguished from lung cancer, mesothelioma, or other pleural-based mass. Serial chest radiographs may be of benefit in demonstrating

Table 12.6   Major Signs of Rounded Atelectasis

- A rounded mass of 4–7 cm in diameter in the lung periphery
- The mass is never completely surrounded by lung
- Mass is most dense in its periphery
- Mass forms an acute angle with the pleura
- Pleural scarring is usually present
- Vessels and bronchi curve toward the mass
- At least two sharp margins are present
- "Comet tail" sign
- Air bronchogram is usually seen in the central part of the mass

Source: Modified from Doyle, T.C., Lawler, G.A. *Am. J. Roentgenol.* 143(2), 225–228, 1984.

the evolution process. Recognition of asbestos as a common cause of rounded atelectasis requires its inclusion in the differential diagnosis of solitary pulmonary nodules in the asbestos-exposed worker.

12.14 PLEURAL DISEASE AND CANCER

There is no evidence that either pleural plaque or diffuse pleural thickening evolves into mesothelioma or lung cancer. The risk of developing mesothelioma and lung cancer is reported by some to be higher among asbestos-exposed workers with pleural disease than among equally exposed controls with no evidence of pleural abnormality.[83] Selikoff et al.[99] opined pleural fibrosis (even in the absence of parenchymal disease) was a "bad omen," with higher death rates from lung cancer and mesothelioma than in an asbestos-exposed group without pleural fibrosis.

Hillerdal[100] reported individuals with pleural plaque possess an increased risk for developing lung cancer and recommended surveillance for early detection. He found the risk of primary lung cancer was four times more than that of matched controls.

In 1987, Harber et al.[101] studied pleural plaques and their relation to asbestos-related malignancy in a nested case–control study of 1500 asbestos workers. They concluded there was no association between the pleural plaques and the risk of asbestos-associated malignancies that were independent of other factors such as duration of exposure, age, and cigarette smoking. However, Harber et al.[101] stated that the presence or absence of plaques should not be used to allocate cancer screening resources, stating that "if workers are known to have significant exposure it appears unwise to deny them appropriate examinations which they might otherwise receive simply because pleural plaque is not detected." The most recent ATS statement on asbestos[4] adopts the position that the presence of pleural plaque is associated with a greater risk of mesothelioma and lung cancer compared with subjects with comparable histories of asbestos exposure lacking plaques. The ATS identifies plaques as a "marker for elevated risk of malignancy" and such risk may be higher than exposure history might suggest.

I (G.K.F.) am of the opinion that pleural plaques are a reliable objective indicator of nontrivial asbestos exposure and that asbestos-exposed individuals with pleural plaques or diffuse asbestos-related pleural thickening are at an increased risk for asbestos-related malignancies.

12.15 PULMONARY ASBESTOSIS

Asbestosis is pulmonary interstitial fibrosis caused by the inhalation of airborne fibers of asbestos that are of respirable size. The pathologic findings and grading of asbestosis are discussed in Chapter 9. Before 1986, there was considerable confusion in the application of the terminology "asbestosis." Many authors used the term pleural asbestosis to indicate pleural plaque, pleural thickening, asbestos pleuritis, and other stigmata of asbestos exposure.[102–111] In 1986, the ATS recommended the term *asbestosis* be reserved for diffuse interstitial fibrosis of the pulmonary parenchyma caused by asbestos. The ATS cited significant differences between pleural abnormalities and interstitial fibrosis in regard to epidemiology, pathology, and prognosis.[32] The most recent ATS Statement on the Diagnosis and Management of Nonmalignant Asbestos-Related Disease (2004)[4] likewise reserves the term "asbestosis" for interstitial fibrosis and specifically excludes pleural changes. The ACCP also defines asbestosis as an interstitial process.[13]

12.15.1 Exposure

Asbestosis is not caused by trivial exposures to asbestos and does not occur as a result of levels encountered in the ambient air in an urban setting. There is a dose–response relationship between cumulative exposure and development of disease.

Although cellular injury occurs at low exposures, there probably is a threshold below which clinical asbestosis does not occur. There is no reliable evidence that clinically detectable asbestosis occurs with less than 10 fiber-years of exposure. The Helsinki criteria[33] states that the risk of asbestosis detectable on a PA chest radiograph may occur at a 25-fiber-year level. The fiber burden necessary to cause microscopic change is beyond the scope of this chapter and is discussed elsewhere in this book. The clinical expression of dose–response relationship is mirrored in pathologic studies, which show a substantially higher burden of uncoated asbestos fibers in patients with pulmonary asbestosis than in exposed workers without asbestosis or in those with only pleural plaques. Exposure to high levels of airborne asbestos for periods of 1 year or less may be sufficient to cause asbestosis.[33]

12.15.2 Latency

Exposure levels experienced during the past three decades typically have a minimum latency of 20 years or longer, in my experience. The latency period for asbestosis is inversely related to the dose of exposure, such that lower levels of exposure have substantially longer latencies.[112]

12.15.3 Symptoms

Asbestosis may be present without respiratory symptoms or with only minimal dyspnea on exertion. As the disease progresses, dyspnea becomes the most common symptom. Pain is typically not a symptom of asbestosis and may suggest some other etiology. Because of the increased risk for lung cancer and mesothelioma, persistent or severe chest pain in a patient with asbestosis merits further investigation to rule out a malignant process. Also, because of hypoxemia and pulmonary hypertension, cardiac origin of chest pain should be another consideration. Some patients may present with a dry cough, but in my experience this is not often a prominent presenting symptom. Hemoptysis is not a common feature of asbestosis and should lead the clinician to investigate for lung cancer, laryngeal cancer, or another etiology. Hoarseness is not a manifestation of asbestosis but warrants further evaluation for possible laryngeal cancer or involvement of the laryngeal nerve by a malignancy.

12.15.4 Physical Examination

Historically, bibasilar inspiratory rales are reported to occur in approximately 40% of patients with asbestosis. Rales may precede roentgenographic findings. Rales are typically end inspiratory, often heard in the area of the posterior axillary line immediately above the diaphragm, and do not clear with coughing. They are often referred to as dry crackles. They must be distinguished from rales of pulmonary edema, rhonchi, and other adventitious sounds.

Although clubbing is historically a reported feature of asbestosis, it is now a much less common finding than may have been observed in the remote past. A lower incidence of clubbing is probably attributable to the reduced incidence of severe asbestosis resulting from lower exposures. When clubbing is present, care should be taken to exclude hypertrophic pulmonary osteoarthropathy, which may reflect a malignancy in the asbestos-exposed patient. As in any patient with severe pulmonary disease, physical examination should include a careful inspection of the jugular venous pulse, prominent second heart sound, hepatomegaly, pedal edema, or other stigmata of current or impending cor pulmonale. Likewise, cyanosis could be a possible indicator of the need for supplemental oxygen. Stigmata of chronic renal or liver disease, autoimmune disease, sarcoidosis, amyloidosis, and systemic illnesses known to cause increased interstitial markings should be excluded at the time of physical examination.

12.15.5 Chest Radiograph

In asbestosis, the PA view of the chest demonstrates (Figure 12.6) bilateral increase in fine reticular (also described as linear or irregular) markings in the lower one-third of the lungs (Figure 12.7) during the early stages of the disease. If the lower lobes are spared or if there is diffuse involvement of the lungs at low profusion (especially in the absence of pleural disease), a thorough search to exclude other more probable causes should be undertaken. Pleural plaque or diffuse pleural thickening is found in approximately 60% or more of cases. The ATS 2004 Statement[4] emphasizes pleural plaques as supportive evidence of causation. As the disease progresses and profusion increases, middle and upper lobe involvement may occur. Rare cases of massive upper lobe fibrosis attributable to asbestosis have been reported.[113,114] The appearance of honeycombing is indicative of far-advanced disease and is usually accompanied by respiratory symptoms.

The chest radiograph may be submitted to a "B" reader for interpretation. The NIOSH sponsored B-reading program has come under criticism in recent years[115] and NIOSH has published a "B" Reader Code of Ethics.[116] A subcommittee of the American College of Occupational and Environmental Medicine has suggested that "B" readings should not be used for the clinical diagnosis of a specific case of asbestosis and the use of that system is more appropriate for epidemiologic and research purposes.[117] Current inability to perform "B" readings on digital x-rays is discussed in Section 12.6.4.

Gitlin[29] reported on 492 chest radiographs interpreted by "B" readers involved in asbestos litigation purporting to show asbestosis. A blinded panel of six "B" readers reviewed these films. The panel concurred that a 1/0 profusion or greater was present in 4.5% of 2952 readings. Questions concerning the initial "B" readings were raised as these discrepancies could not be explained by interreader variability.

In 1988, an analysis of the practices of 23 "B" readers interpreting 105,000 radiographs were reviewed.[118] A marked difference was observed between "B" readers for the frequency of perceived "definite parenchymal abnormalities." Ducatman et al.[118] felt that "B"-reader certification should not be the only quality assurance for radiographic surveillance programs, medical decision making,

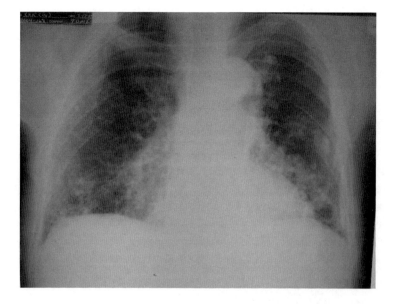

Figure 12.6 Pulmonary asbestosis: basilar fibrosis with bilateral plaques (some calcified).

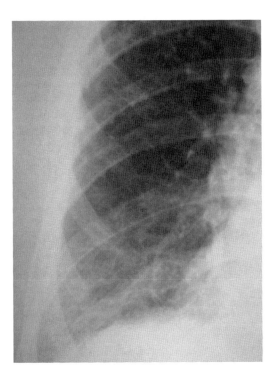

Figure 12.7   Asbestosis—lower lobe interstitial fibrosis (a close-up view).

or related legal activities. A follow-up study by Ducatman[119] suggested the formation of quality assurance panels for "B" readers to provide feedback and recommended the dropping of outliers.

Many diagnoses of asbestosis were made under the 1980 ILO system.[35] In January 2004, a newer version (2000 Revision) was instituted.[5]

12.15.6 Radiographic Technique and Profusion

Overestimation of the profusion of small opacities is encountered in obese individuals and those with elevated diaphragms because of compression of lower lobe markings. Poor inspiratory effort and underpenetration of the chest radiograph may account for increased markings. Compression from large bullae, scoliosis, and other conditions can enhance markings and compress interstitium. On the other hand, overpenetration of the chest radiograph may cause a false-negative interpretation. Severe pleural disease may mask the underlying interstitial fibrosis, making diagnosis difficult. Histopathologic evidence of asbestosis may appear before radiographic evidence of the disease. Selikoff[24] stated he had seen individuals who had difficulty walking across the room when little abnormality was detected on chest radiograph. However, the ATS[32] warns that caution should be taken in diagnosing asbestosis in the face of a normal chest radiograph.

12.15.7 1/0 versus 1/1 in the Diagnosis of Asbestosis

The 1986 ATS criteria[32] opined that chest radiographic findings of small irregular opacities having a profusion of 1/1 or greater to be of proven value. However, these criteria came under substantial criticism.[120] The ATS committee subsequently clarified their statement,[121] and Weill[122] later stated that 1/1 was simply to be considered a level that was "illustrative of a film compatible with asbestosis, so might also a Category 1/0 film; it depends on the reader." The Helsinki criteria recommended using the ILO criteria and required the use of the ILO standard films. They regard a 1/0 as an "early stage of asbestosis" for screening and epidemiologic purposes.[33] The 2004 ATS[4] statement on asbestos indicates a Category 1/0 profusion on chest radiograph is "presumptive but not unequivocal" for the diagnosis of asbestosis.

The 2009 ACCP Consensus Statement[13] was in agreement that "1/0 small irregular opacities are a good screening tool, but lack specificity for an accurate diagnosis of asbestosis. HRCT scanning should be performed to increase the specificity of these chest radiographic findings." The distinction between 1/0 and 1/1 is emphasized by the ACCP Consensus Statement showing agreement that "chest radiographic changes of profusion 1/1 small irregular opacities or greater or HRCT scanning images in the prone position at lung bases indicating interstitial fibrosis are of value in detecting asbestosis."[13]

12.15.8 CT Scan in Asbestosis

With the advent of CT scans in the 1970s, application of its use for the diagnosis of interstitial and other pulmonary disease has been investigated. Initially, there were technical limitations because of resolution. With the advent of HRCT using thin 1 mm sections and other technical advances, significant improvement in clarity and diagnostic accuracy has increased the utility of the study in the diagnosis of pulmonary disease. There is no widely accepted standard for HRCT interpretation similar to the ILO system for the chest radiograph. There are those who have argued that such a program is not appropriate at this time because it may encounter the same problems that occurred in the B-reader program for plain films.[117] Standardization of equipment has proved challenging.

Huuskonen et al.[123] proposed a semiquantitative HRCT fibrosis score. Six hundred two asbestos-exposed workers and 49 controls had HRCT findings compared with ILO interpretations for the same patients. Using three radiologists, there was good inter- and intraobserver agreement in the interpretation of the scans, and positive findings correlated with occupation and age. They reported specificity and sensitivity substantially greater than that reported by the ILO method and felt that application of an international classification for HRCT could possibly be adopted.

Biscaldi et al.[124] compared HRCT findings with those of chest radiographs interpreted according to the ILO classification and came to the conclusion that "high resolution chest tomography does not appear to be an indispensable test for the diagnosis" but may contribute to the evaluation of pleural thickening. Murray et al.[125] studied 49 patients exposed to asbestos and used HRCT in the prone position at specific preselected levels and found a relatively high level of accuracy could be obtained with a single prone scan. The results of the studies were improved when additional images were used. Murray et al.[125] opined that using a limited number of preselected prone HRCT images could be applicable for screening a large patient group for asbestosis. Kraus et al.[126] proposed a classification system for CT/HRCT and opined it was practical in more than 2000 patients they had studied. Harkin et al.[127] studied the use of HRCT to better differentiate normal versus abnormal chest radiographs among those with low profusion scores on the ILO system, attempting to distinguish between 0/1 and 1/0 radiographs. They studied 37 asbestos-exposed individuals using the ILO classification and combined it with HRCT, respiratory symptom questionnaires, PFTs, and bronchoalveolar lavage (BAL). A normal HRCT was an excellent predictor of normality, as demonstrated by completely normal pulmonary function studies with no evidence of inflammatory cells on BAL. When HRCT and ILO abnormalities were jointly found, there was a diminution in the FEV_1/FVC ratio and diffusion capacity, and an alveolitis by BAL was noted, which was consistent with asbestosis.

Staples et al.[128] studied 169 asbestos-exposed workers with normal chest radiographs (ILO less than 1/0) and found that HRCT was normal or near normal in 76 subjects, indeterminate in 36, and abnormal with suggestive asbestosis in 57. They found significant reductions in vital capacity and diffusion capacity in those with an abnormal HRCT but a normal chest radiograph.

The ATS[4] has included HRCT as an imaging study that can be used to document structural change in the diagnosis of asbestosis. They recommend its use over routine CT as being more sensitive for detecting parenchymal fibrosis. However, it is acknowledged that because of the high degree of sensitivity of HRCT, an abnormal finding may have "uncertain prognostic significance."

12.16 PULMONARY FUNCTION IN ASBESTOSIS

Pulmonary function testing (PFT) plays several important roles in the diagnosis and management of asbestosis (Table 12.1). First, it can provide information useful in supporting the diagnosis when used in conjunction with other criteria. Impairment ratings are dependent upon pulmonary function testing rather than radiographic findings or patient symptomatology. PFTs are useful in monitoring physiologic progression of asbestosis when serial studies are performed. PFTs can provide objective support for subjective complaints such as dyspnea.

The ATS (1986)[32] states that a restrictive pattern of lung impairment with an FVC and reduced vital capacity below the LLN are of recognized value in making the diagnosis of asbestosis. Although in advanced asbestosis the physiologic pattern is typically one of restrictive lung disease, early in the disease, small airway obstruction may be noted. There is no indication that asbestos causes reversible airway obstruction. When there is reduction of the FEV_1/FVC ratio and in the absence of medical contraindication, bronchodilators should be administered to assess for reversibility.

A dose–response relationship between asbestos exposure and impairment of function has been suggested by Weill et al.[129] They reported that small airway obstruction with impaired flow at low lung volumes may occur in preradiographic stages of asbestosis. Other causes of small airway obstruction, especially that associated with cigarette smoking, must also be given careful consideration as etiologic factors in a given case. The ATS 2004[4] discusses airway obstruction at length and opines that although such changes attributable to asbestos are minor, when superimposed on underlying chronic obstructive pulmonary disease or other advanced pulmonary disease, the obstructive contribution from asbestos could be clinically significant. The ACCP 2009 Consensus Statement could not reach a consensus that "a decline in small airway flow rate in a nonsmoker can be attributed to asbestos exposure." On the other hand, they did reach a consensus disagreeing with the statement that "A decline in small airway flow rate in a smoker can be attributed to asbestos exposure."[13]

Reduction in TLC is of benefit in confirming a restrictive defect, especially when airway obstruction is present. If TLC is unavailable, reduction in FVC below the LLN with normal or elevated FEV_1/FVC ratio is strongly suggestive of restriction.[42] Extrapulmonic causes of reduced lung volumes including exogenous obesity, neuromuscular weakness, chest deformity, and other causes of loss of volume should be excluded before attributing such abnormalities to asbestosis. Asbestosis may occur with normal lung function.

12.17 THE PREDICTIONS FOR THE FUTURE INCIDENCE OF ASBESTOSIS

With markedly lower levels of exposure to asbestos in the 35 years following 1973 than in the three decades preceding 1973, a significant decline in the incidence of asbestos-related diseases was predicted. In 1978, Selikoff and Lee[130] noted that the majority of the previously reported cases "had their origin in past years when dust levels generally were much higher than they are today. We would expect that with improvement in working conditions, the number of new cases would be less and that a longer time would elapse before the disease reaches the stage of being radiologically detectable."[130] They further opined this would be especially true for asbestosis but less apparent for pleural calcification.

In 1982, Nicholson et al.[30] opined that only the heaviest and longest exposed individuals would suffer serious nonmalignant disease in the future. They projected mesothelioma deaths would exceed deaths from asbestosis and the incidence of asbestosis would peak in 1997 and decline thereafter.

In 1983, Walker et al.[131] from the Harvard School of Public Health performed a detailed analysis attempting to project asbestos-related disease between the years 1980 and 2009. Using the incidence of mesotheliomas, they projected there would be 11,400 patients with asbestosis who would be alive between the years 2000 and 2004. However, they opined there could conceivably be many additional cases which "would include many people with few or no symptoms whose asbestosis would be detected by physical or radiologie examination only." It was opined the number of future patients with asbestosis would depend upon the diagnostic criteria which were used and might reflect nonmedical influences.

In 1990, Seidman and Selikoff[132] reported the decline in death cases among insulation workers associated with reduction in asbestos exposure. They reported diminution of exposure between 1967 and 1986. There was a significant decline in the death rate from lung cancer, peritoneal mesothelioma, and asbestosis in men with less than 40 years from onset of exposure. For those with greater than 40 years from first exposure (1946 or earlier), these declines were not observed.

Despite these predictions, the CDC[133] reported a significant increase in asbestosis deaths between 1980 and 2000 when compared with the preceding two decades. The possible causes for this increase included: (1) change in coding, (2) increased awareness of the disease, (3) litigation, and (4) improved diagnostic techniques.

12.17.1 Diagnosis of Asbestosis

In 1986, the ATS published an Official Statement on the Diagnosis of Nonmalignant Asbestos-related Disease.[32] In 2004, the ATS published an updated statement entitled "Diagnosis and Initial Management of Nonmalignant Diseases Related to Asbestos."[4] In 2009, the ACCP published a Consensus Statement on the Respiratory Health Effects of Asbestos.[13] My (G.K.F.) criteria for diagnosing asbestosis is summarized in Table 12.7 and is more fully described in items 1–6 below.

1. Asbestos exposure history: A chronological history should be obtained from the patient identifying all sources of asbestos exposure and, where possible, identifying the duration, intensity, and circumstances under which the exposure occurred. Specific job duties should be described in addition to occupational titles. In addition to the work practices of the patient, bystander exposure should be identified, as should household or potential environmental exposure. In addition, the history should include any other fibrogenic dusts, gases, fumes, or other occupational or nonoccupational sources of exposure that could cause or contribute to interstitial fibrosis on a chest x-ray.
2. Latency: On the basis of levels of exposure commonly experienced in the past three decades, a typical latency period is 20 years or longer from the time of initial exposure.

Table 12.7   Criteria for Diagnosis of Asbestosis

Required
1. Adequate asbestos exposure history
2. Latency
3. Evidence of structural pathology (interstitial fibrosis)
   a) imaging studies or
   b) pathologic changes
4. Evidence of causation by asbestos
5. Exclusion of alternative causes for interstitial fibrosis or obstructive disease

Supportive evidence
Rales

Clubbing

Pulmonary function abnormalities

3. Evidence of structural pathology (interstitial fibrosis) consistent with asbestos-related disease as documented by imaging or histology.

   a. Imaging studies: chest radiograph and/or HRCT—The 1986 ATS criteria identified a 1/1 profusion as being of "proven value." The 2004 ATS indicates that "A profusion of irregular opacities at the level of 1/0 is used as the boundary between normal and abnormal in the evaluation of the film" (p. 700). However, the definition of "boundary" is vague and subject to interpretation. "A critical distinction is made between films that are suggestive but not presumptively diagnostic as 0/1 and those that are presumptively diagnostic but not unequivocal (1/0). This dividing point is generally taken to separate films that are considered to be 'positive' for asbestosis from those that are considered to be 'negative,' however, profusion itself is continuous"[4] (p. 696).

   The ACCP 2009 Consensus Statement aligns itself more closely with the ATS 1986 position, stating that a 1/0 profusion should be further evaluated using HRCT and that "profusion 1/1 small irregular opacities or greater or HRCT scanning images in the prone position of lung bases indicating interstitial fibrosis are of value in detecting asbestosis." The ACCP further states that "Radiographic changes of a profusion level 1/0 small irregular opacities are a good screening tool but lack specificity for an accurate diagnosis of asbestosis."[13] The ACCP Consensus Statement concurs that HRCT is a more sensitive method for detecting both pleural and parenchymal disease attributable to asbestos.

   b. Pathologic changes (see Chapter 9).

4. Evidence of causation by asbestos.[4]

   a. Occupational and environmental history

   b. Markers of exposure (usually pleural plaque)

   c. Demonstration of asbestos bodies or elevated asbestos fibers in lung tissue

5. Exclusion of alternative causes for interstitial fibrosis or obstructive disease—The ATS 2004 criteria document states that "Nonmalignant diseases presenting similarly to asbestos-related disease should also be ruled out." They require "exclusion of alternative plausible causes for the findings."

6. Supportive evidence: The 1986 ATS[32] identified PFT abnormalities and physical findings as of "proven value." The ATS 2004[4] indicates that these supportive findings are not required but contribute to the diagnosis of asbestosis in defining activity of disease and resulting impairment. ATS 2004 (p. 700) states that "Specificity of the diagnosis of asbestosis increases with the number of consistent findings on chest film, the number of clinical features present, and the significance and strength of the history of exposure."

   a. Pulmonary function testing: "Asbestos exposure independently contributes to accelerated decline in airflow over time whether or not asbestos exposure ceases"[4] (p. 708). The ACCP 2009 Consensus Statement disagrees with the position that asbestos exposure in the absence of interstitial fibrosis leads to chronic obstructive pulmonary disease and likewise disagrees that a decline in small airway flow rates in a smoker can be attributed to asbestos exposure (p. 1623).[13] Pulmonary function testing is not required in the diagnosis of asbestosis. Following diagnosis, pulmonary function testing is required to determine impairment.[4]

   b. Rales.

   c. Clubbing.

12.18 DIFFERENTIAL DIAGNOSIS OF ASBESTOSIS

Evaluation of asbestosis requires familiarity with the differential diagnosis of interstitial lung diseases. A detailed history from the patient should include careful inquiry into all prior pulmonary illnesses and injuries; presence or absence of autoimmune disease, such as scleroderma,[134] lupus,[135] and rheumatoid arthritis,[136] which may cause interstitial lung disease; and medications, including chemotherapeutic agents,[137] amiodarone,[138] methotrexate,[139] gold,[140] furadantin,[141] and other drugs that have been implicated in causing interstitial fibrosis. Inquiry concerning use of illicit drugs, including inhaled and intravenous substances, may prove rewarding.[142] Heroin and other injectables may be cut with talc or other impurities that can cause fibrosis and granulomatous reactions. Crack cocaine[142] has been associated with pulmonary sequelae. Paraquat sprayed on marijuana has caused interstitial damage.

Specific disease entities including sarcoidosis, amyloidosis,[143] and other infiltrative diseases should be considered. Hepatitis C[144] and inflammatory bowel disease[145] may be accompanied by interstitial fibrosis. The group of diseases including usual interstitial pneumonia (UIP), fibrotic phase of nonspecific interstitial pneumonia (NSIP), and fibrotic phase of hypersensitivity pneumonia (HP) identified as idiopathic pulmonary fibrosis may cause severe interstitial fibrosis and honeycombing, as seen with asbestosis.[146,147] A diagnosis of idiopathic pulmonary fibrosis is usually not rendered in patients with an adequate history of occupational asbestos exposure and appropriate latency unless there is compelling evidence to the contrary. Pleural plaques or diffuse pleural thickening are considered supportive evidence for asbestosis. Pathologic evidence is considered decisive if available and adequate specimens have been obtained.

The clinician must inquire as to all other occupational exposures that may have occurred within the same setting or during a different employment. Pneumoconiosis including silicosis, talcosis, aluminum oxide, berylliosis, coal miner's pneumoconiosis, hard metal pneumoconiosis, arc welder's pneumoconiosis, and other inorganic mineral exposures should be explored. Fumes and chemicals such as vinyl chloride have been shown to cause pulmonary fibrosis. Many workers may have worked in agriculture or other industries where they may have contracted hypersensitivity pneumonitis, which also may be of occupational origin.[148] Occupational and therapeutic exposures to high levels of radiation also merit consideration.[149]

Prior surgery, sepsis, or shock resulting in ARDS, pneumonias, mycobacterial, fungal, and other pulmonary infections should be routine components of inquiry. Lymphomas and lymphangitic spread of tumor usually are distinguishable by history or other diagnostic studies.

The preceding paragraphs give only a partial list of examples in the differential diagnosis. There are numerous review articles and texts that provide a more detailed discussion of interstitial lung disease.[150]

12.18.1 Smoking

There are conflicting reports concerning the contributory role smoking plays in asbestosis. Some studies report a higher prevalence of interstitial disease among asbestos-exposed workers who smoke.[151] Selikoff et al.[152] failed to find statistically significant increases in such changes among smokers. Barnhart et al.[153] attempted to determine the relationship between ILO roentgenographic classification of pneumoconiosis, spirometric values, and effects of cigarette smoking. A positive association between smoking and level of ILO parenchymal abnormality was demonstrated, especially in those with the heaviest cumulative smoking history. There is biologic plausibility that smoking would increase the risk of asbestosis given that cigarette smoke adversely affects clearance mechanisms. On the other hand, mucus production from smoking along with chronic coughing due to bronchitis may actually enhance clearance. Pulmonary injury and associated diseases caused by smoking such as desquamative interstitial pneumonia, respiratory bronchiolitis and pulmonary Langerhans cell histiocytosis, as well as the more common complications of emphysema and chronic bronchitis, are present in asbestos-exposed workers as they are in other populations.[154-156]

Cigarette smoking may cause increased bronchovascular markings and the appearance of "dirty lungs."[157] The ATS 2004 Statement[4] (p. 700) states that smoking alone rarely causes irregular opacities of 1/0 and "Therefore, does not result in a chest film with the characteristics of asbestosis." However, according to a review from the Mayo Clinic,[158] smoking has been linked to desquamative interstitial pneumonia, pulmonary Langerhans cell histiocytosis, and respiratory bronchiolitis associated interstitial lung disease where most cases are considered caused by smoking. Smoking may be a risk factor for the incidence and severity of interstitial lung disease in asbestos-exposed individuals.

12.18.2 Airway Obstruction

Smoking and asbestos may cause small airway disease. There is no convincing proof that asbestos causes emphysema or bronchoreactive disease. Attempting to assess the contributions of tobacco use requires obtaining a detailed smoking history, including age of onset, duration, pack-years, and objective findings on chest radiograph examination and pulmonary function testing.

The ATS[4] states that assessment of functional impairment of clinical significance should generally be based on the restrictive findings associated with asbestosis because these are more likely to be disabling. However, the opposing effects of hyperinflation attributable to obstruction and the restrictive effect from fibrosis, which may end in a net zero change in TLC, may compromise utilization of TLC to measure restriction.[4,159]

Churg[160] previously described asbestos-related small airway disease as an entity separate from asbestosis, which is a fibrotic process initially affecting the respiratory bronchioles and the alveolar ducts. He opined that the abnormality was of "questionable functional significance" and was not a radiographically visible lesion. Nevertheless, he opined small airway disease could represent a marker of "parenchymal damage even in the absence of diffuse fibrosis." The Helsinki Consensus Report includes small airway disease as one of the clinical findings which may occur in asbestosis.[33]

12.18.3 Recommendations for the Clinician Concerning Care of the Patient Diagnosed with Asbestosis

1. Notify the patient there is no treatment or therapy which either cures the disease or prevents progression.
2. Secondary prevention—patient should be informed of the synergistic effects between asbestos and cigarette smoking in increasing the risk of lung cancer and should be advised to stop smoking completely and immediately.
3. Prognosis has been correlated with the level of profusion on chest radiograph at the time of diagnosis.
4. The prognosis for individuals with asbestosis, in part, reflects the increased risk for developing an asbestos-related malignancy. Patients should be notified of the increased risk of lung cancer, mesothelioma, and other asbestos-related malignancies.
5. Patients should be advised to undergo yearly checkups by their treating physicians with emphasis on the respiratory and GI tract in keeping with OSHA recommendations.
6. Chest radiographs—OSHA recommends yearly chest radiographs for employees over age 40 and with asbestos exposure at least 10 years prior.[24,28] The ATS[4] recommends chest radiographs every 3–5 years. Chest radiographs should be performed more often if there is a change in clinical symptoms.
7. Periodic screening for colon cancer should be performed according to the criteria established by the UICC International Workshop on Facilitating Screening for Colorectal Cancer[161–163] as well as the guidelines of the American Cancer Society.[164] Change in bowel habit or detection of blood in the stool would call for additional testing. Guidotti[165] and other members of the ATS 2004 Committee opine a relationship between asbestos exposure and colon cancer.
8. Screening for lung cancer and mesothelioma—there is no proof at this time that either chest radiograph or sputum cytology alters survival and no major health organization recommends routine screening for lung cancer or mesothelioma. Low-dose CT scan has shown some promise and improvement over routine x-ray, but there is insufficient data at this time to recommend for or against its use in screening.[164] The risk of morbidity and mortality associated with false-positives appears to offset any benefit.
9. Patient should receive appropriate inoculations for:
   a. Influenza vaccine
   b. Pneumococcal pneumonia vaccine
10. Individuals with asbestosis should be advised to avoid any future exposure to high concentrations of asbestos or other fibrogenic dusts including coal, silica, and so forth.
11. Individuals with asbestosis should be advised to exercise caution in the use of pharmacologic agents known to cause interstitial fibrosis such as bleomycin, furadantin, amiodarone, methotrexate, and so forth.

12. If there is evidence of household or environmental asbestos exposure, patient should be properly informed so as to avoid future exposure.

13. The patient should be notified if he or she has a condition that may be compensable.

14. The patient should be notified of pulmonary function results. If appropriate criteria are fulfilled, the patient should be notified of disability.

15. The physician should report to the appropriate state agencies as required by law.

16. For the patient who is found not to have asbestosis, strong reassurance should be given as to the absence of the disease. Clear distinctions between pleural plaque and asbestosis should be explained. Appropriate information should be provided as to the need for proper follow-up and that smoking cessation is mandatory.

12.19 SUMMARY

Because no radiographic finding is pathognomonic of asbestosis, the physician must evaluate all other available data, including exposure history, latency, physical findings, pulmonary function, and a detailed medical and occupational/paraoccupational history (including chronology of the disease). Review of prior radiographs and medical records, when available, is necessary to render a proper diagnosis in some cases.

In evaluating asbestos-related diseases, the physician must consider multiple variables in each case. Studies have shown that cumulative exposures experienced by insulators may be very different than that experienced by other trades. Latency has a significant impact on the timing of the appearance of various asbestos-related diseases. Many other fibrogenic agents within the workplace and nonoccupational causes for interstitial fibrosis and pleural disease can consume an entire text. Smoking and occupational carcinogens may either enhance the effects of asbestos or act independently.

The impact of OSHA regulations on mandatory respiratory protection and safeguards during abatement and removal has affected workplace exposure. New attempts to treat or slow progression of disease are in their infancy. The criteria for diagnosing nonmalignant asbestos diseases have evolved. Within the past 5 years, the ATS published new guidelines for the diagnosis and management of nonmalignant asbestos diseases, the ILO has revised the guidelines for the interpretation of pneumoconiosis chest radiographs, the ATS/ERS issued new guidelines for the performance of pulmonary function testing, the AMA redefined the criteria for pulmonary impairment, and the ACCP has issued a Delphi Study Consensus Statement.[13]

The physician should keep in mind that asbestosis is a potentially serious disorder that has no satisfactory treatment and can progress even after exposure ceases. Likewise, the diagnosis may adversely affect the patient's employability and insurability. Accordingly, the same diligent care should be taken in diagnosing asbestosis as would be undertaken with any other medical illness that is nontreatable and may result in disability or death.

The level of the skills of the clinician required to properly evaluate asbestos-related diseases must be matched by the level of dedication to provide scientifically sound information and the best care for their patients.

REFERENCES

1. Jack J. In the United States District Court for the Southern District of Texas, Corpus Christi Division. In *Re: Silica Product Liability Litigation*, MDL Docket No. 1553; 2005.

2. Centers for Disease Control and Prevention. Changing patterns of pneumoconiosis mortality, United States, 1968–2002. *MMWR Morb Mortal Wkly Rep* July 23, 2004;53(28):627–632.

3. Centers for Disease Control and Prevention. Malignant mesothelioma mortality—United States 1999–2005. *MMWR Morb Mortal Wkly Rep* April 22, 2009;58(15):393–396.

4. American Thoracic Society. Diagnosis and initial management of nonmalignant diseases related to asbestos. *Am J Respir Crit Care Med* 2004;170(6):691–715.

5. International Labor Office. *The Guidelines for the Use of ILO International Classification of Radiographs of Pneumoconiosis.* Revised ed. Geneva: International Labor Office; 2000.

6. ATS/ERS Task Force. Standardization of lung function testing. *Eur Respir J* 2005;26:153–161.

7. ATS/ERS Task Force. Standardization of spirometry. *Eur Respir J* 2005;26:319–338.

8. ATS/ERS Task Force. Standardization of the single breath determination of carbon monoxide uptake in the lung. *Eur Respir J* 2005;26:720–735.

9. ATS/ERS. Standardization of lung function testing: Standardization of the measurement of lung volumes. *Eur Respir J* 2005;26:511–522.

10. ATS/ERS. Standardization of lung function testing: Interpretive strategies for lung function tests. *Eur Respir J* 2005;26:948–968.

11. American Medical Association. *Guides to the Evaluation of Permanent Impairment,* 5th ed. Chicago, IL: AMA Press; 2001.

12. American Medical Association. *Guides to the Evaluation of Permanent Impairment,* 6th ed. Chicago, IL: AMA Press; 2007.

13. Banks DE, Shi R, McLarty J, Cowl CT, Smith D, Tarlo SM, et al. ACCP consensus statement on the respiratory health effects of asbestos: Results of a Delphi study. *Chest* 2009;135:1619–1627.

14. Brooks SM. *Environmental Medicine.* St. Louis, MO: Mosby-Yearbook Inc.; 1995: 440.

15. Hoffman FL. Mortality from respiratory diseases in the dusty trades [inorganic dusts]. *Bulletin of the United States Bureau of Labor Statistics,* Bureau of Labor Statistics Report 231. Washington, DC: Bureau of Labor Statistics; 1918: 172–180.

16. Cooke WE. Pulmonary asbestosis. *Br Med J* 1927;2:1024–1025.

17. Mills RG. Pulmonary asbestosis: Report of a case. *Minn Med* July 1930:495–499.

18. McDonald S. Histology of pulmonary asbestosis. *Br Med J* December 3, 1927:1025–1026.

19. Lynch KM, Smith WA. Pulmonary asbestosis: III. Carcinoma of lung in asbestos-silicosis. *Am J Cancer* 1935;24:56–64.

20. Lynch KM, Cannon WM. Asbestosis: VI analysis of 40 necropsied cases. *Chest* November–December 1948:874–884.

21. Doll R. Mortality from lung cancer in asbestos workers. *Br J Ind Med* 1955;12(2):81–86.

22. Eisenstadt HB. Malignant mesothelioma of the pleura. *Dis Chest* 1956;30(5):549–556.

23. Wagner JC, Sleggs CA, Marchand P. Diffuse pleural mesothelioma and asbestos exposure in the North Western Cape Province. *Br J Ind Med* 1960;17:260–271.

24. Federal Register 29 CFR Parts 1910 and 1926: Part II. Occupational exposure to asbestos, tremolite, anthophyllite and actinolite. Final rules, vol. 51 (No. 119). Washington, DC: Occupational Safety and Health Administration, Department of Labor; June 20, 1986.

25. Delclos GL, Buffler PA, Greenberg SD, Key MM, Perrotta DM, Alexander C, Wilson RK. Asbestos-associated disease: A review. *Tex Med* 1989;85(5):50–59.

26. Becklake MR. Asbestos-related diseases of the lung and other organs: The epidemiology and implications for clinical practice. *Am Rev Respir Dis* 1976;114(3):192–227.

27. Hammar SP, Dail DH. *Pulmonary Pathology,* 2nd ed. New York: Springer-Verlag; 1994:904–906.

28. McLemore TL, Greenberg SD, Wilson RK, Buffler PA, Roggli VL, Mace M. Update on asbestos-associated pulmonary disease. *Tex Med* 1981;77(6):38–46.

29. Gitlin JN, Cook LL, Linton OW, Garrett-Mayer E. Comparison of "B" readers' interpretations of chest radiographs for asbestos-related changes. *Acad Radiol* 2004;11(8):843–856.

30. Nicholson WJ, Perkel G, Selikoff IJ. Occupational exposure to asbestos: Population at risk and projected mortality—1980–2030. *Am J Ind Med* 1982;3(3):259–311.

31. Liveright T, Gann P, McAna J. HHE Report No. HETA-81-372-1727, Exxon Corporation, Bayway Refinery and Chemical Plant, Linden, New Jersey. NIOSH 1986.

32. American Thoracic Society. The diagnosis of nonmalignant diseases related to asbestos. *Am Rev Respir Dis* 1986;134:363–368.

33. Helsinki Consensus Report. Asbestos, asbestosis, and cancer: The Helsinki criteria for diagnosis and attribution. *Scand J Work Environ Health* 1997;23(4):311–316.

34. Morgan WKC, Seaton A. *Occupational Lung Diseases,* 3rd ed. Philadelphia: W.B. Saunders & Company; 1995:313.

35. International Labor Office. *The Guidelines for the Use of ILO International Classification of Radiographs of Pneumoconiosis.* Revised ed. Geneva: International Labor Office;1980.
36. CDC NIOSH. Chest radiography. Issues in classification of chest radiographs and "B" reader information for medical professionals. Available at: CDC.gov/NIOSH/topics/chestradiography/breader-info.html
37. Fedatov I. Application of the ILO International Classification of Radiographs of Pneumoconiosis to Digital Chest Radiographic Images: a NIOSH Scientific Workshop (ILO Perspective). NIOSH Publication No. 2008-139;2008. Available at: www.cdc.gov/niosh/docs/2008-139/Fedatov-ILOPerspect.html
38. Wanger J, Crapo RO, Irvin CG. *Pulmonary Function Laboratory Management and Procedure Manual.* New York: American Thoracic Society; 1998.
39. American Thoracic Society. Standardization of spirometry: 1994 update. *Am J Respir Crit Care Med* 1995;152(3):1109–1136.
40. American Thoracic Society. Single-breath carbon monoxide diffusing capacity (transfer factor). *Am J Respir Crit Care Med* 1995;152(6 Pt. 1):2185–2198.
41. American Thoracic Society. Lung function testing: Selection of reference values and interpretative strategies. *Am Rev Respir Dis* 1991;144(5):1202–1218.
42. U.S. Department of Health and Human Services. A guide to pulmonary function studies under the social security disability program—Social security administration. Publication No. 64-055. Washington, DC: U.S. Department of Health and Human Services; 1994.
43. American Association for Respiratory Care. Clinical practice guidelines spirometry: 1996 update. *Respir Care* 1996;41:629–636.
44. American Thoracic Society. Guidelines for the evaluation of impairment disability in patients with asthma, Medical Section of the American Lung Association. *Am Rev Respir Dis* 1993;147(4):1056–1061.
45. National Asthma Education Program. Expert panel report—Guidelines for diagnoses and management of asthma. NIH Publication No. 91-3042A; 1991.
46. Wanger J, Crapo RO, Irvin CG, in collaboration with the American Thoracic Society. *Pulmonary Function, Laboratory Management and Procedure Manual.* New York: American Thoracic Society; 1998: 13, Chapter 8.
47. Hankinson JL, Odencrantz JR, Fedan KB. Spirometric reference values from a sample of the general U.S. population. *Am J Respir Crit Care Med* January 1999;159(1):179–187.
48. American Thoracic Society Ad Hoc Committee on Impairment/Disability Criteria. Evaluation of impairment/disability secondary to respiratory disorders. *Am Rev Respir Dis* 1986;134:1205–1209.
49. American Medical Association. *Guides to the Evaluation of Permanent Impairment,* 3rd revised ed. American Medical Association; 1990: 125.
50. Roggli VL, Greenberg D, Pratt PC. *Pathology of Asbestos-Associated Diseases.* Boston: Little, Brown & Company; 1992: 166.
51. Dement JM, Welch L, Bingham E, Cameron B, Rice C, Quinn, Ringen K. Surveillance of respiratory diseases among construction and trade workers at Department of Energy nuclear sites. *Am J Ind Med* 2003;43(6):559–573.
52. Barnhart S, Keogh J, Cullen MR, Brodkin C, Liu D, Goodman G, et al. The CARET asbestos-exposed cohort: Baseline characteristics and comparison to other asbestos-exposed cohorts. *Am J Ind Med* 1997;32(6):573–581.
53. Garcia-Closas M, Christiani DC. Asbestos-related diseases in construction carpenters. *Am J Ind Med* 1995;27(1):115–125.
54. Jones RN, Diem JE, Hughes JM, Hammad YY, Glindmeyer HW, Weill H. Progression of asbestos effects: A prospective longitudinal study of chest radiographs and lung function. *Br J Ind Med* 1989;46(2):97–105.
55. Selikoff IJ. The occurrence of pleural calcification among asbestos insulation workers. *Ann N Y Acad Sci* 1965;132(1):351–367.
56. Sider L, Holland EA, Davis TM Jr, Cugell DW. Changes on radiographs of wives of workers exposed to asbestos. *Radiology* 1987;164(3):723–726.
57. Epler GR, McLoud TC, Gaensler EA. Prevalence and incidence of benign asbestos pleural effusion in a working population. *JAMA* 1982;247(5):617–622.
58. Sargent EN, Boswell WD Jr, Rails PW, Markovitz A. Subpleural fat pads in patients exposed to asbestos: Distinction from non-calcified pleural plaques. *Radiology* 1984;152(2):273–277.
59. Porro FW, Patton JR, Hobbs AA. Pneumoconiosis in the talc industry. *Am J Roentgenol* 1942;47:507.

60. Kishimoto T, Morinaga K, Kira S. The prevalence of pleural plaque and/or pulmonary changes among construction workers in Okayama, Japan. *Am J Ind Med* 2000;37(3):291–295.

61. Bresnitz EA, Gilman MJ, Gracely EJ, Airoldi J, Vogel E, Gefter W. Asbestos-related radiographic abnormalities in elevator construction workers. *Am Rev Respir Dis* 1993;147(6 Pt. 1):1341–1344.

62. Miller A, Lilis R, Godbold J, Chan E, Wu X, Selikoff IJ. Spirometric impairment in long-term insulators. Relationships to duration of exposure, smoking, and radiographic abnormalities. *Chest* 1994;105(1):175–182.

63. Miller A, Lilis R, Godbold J, Wu X. Relation of spirometric function to radiographic interstitial fibrosis in two large work forces exposed to asbestos and evaluation of the ILO profusion score. *Occup Environ Med* 1996;53(12):808–812.

64. Welch LS, Michaels D, Zoloff R. National Sheet Metal Worker Asbestos Disease Screening Program: radiologic findings. *Am J Ind Med* 1994;25(5):635–648.

65. Oliver LC, Sprince NL, Greene R. Asbestos-related disease in public school custodians. *Am J Ind Med* 1991;19(3):303–316.

66. Rosenstock L, Barnhart S, Heyer NJ, Pierson DJ, Hudson LD. Relation among pulmonary function chest x-ray abnormalities and smoking status in an asbestos-exposed cohort. *Am Rev Respir Dis* 1988;138(2):272–277.

67. Sepulveda MJ, Merchant JA. Roentgenographic evidence of asbestos exposure in a select population of railroad workers. *Am J Ind Med* 1983;4(5):631–639.

68. Epler GR, McLoud TC, Gaensler EA. Prevalence and incidence of benign asbestos pleural effusion in a working population. *JAMA* 1982;247(5):617–622.

69. Jones RN, Diem JE, Ziskand MM, Rodriguez M, Weill H. Radiographic evidence of asbestos effects on American marine engineers. *J Occup Med* 1984;26(4):281–284.

70. Dement JM, Welch L, Bingham E, Cameron B, Rice C, Quinn P, Ringen K. Surveillance of respiratory diseases among construction and trade workers at Department of Energy nuclear sites. *Am J Ind Med* 2003;43(6):559–573.

71. Peipins LA, Lewin M, Campolucci S, Lybarger JA, Miller A, Middleton D, et al. Radiographic abnormalities and exposure to asbestos-contaminated vermiculite in the community of Libby, Montana, USA. *Environ Health Perspect* 2003;111(14):1753–1760 .

72. Hillerdal G, Lindgren A. Pleural plaques: Correlation of autopsy findings to radiographic findings in occupational history. *Eur J Respir Dis* 1980;61(6):315–319.

73. Gallego JC. Absence of left-sided predominance in asbestos-related pleural plaques: A CT study. *Chest* 1998;113(4):1034–1036.

74. Kreel L. Computer tomography in the evaluation of pulmonary asbestosis. Preliminary experiences with the EMI general purpose scanner. *Acta Radiol Diagn (Stockh)* 1976;17(4):405–412.

75. Sluis-Cremer GK, Thomas RG, Schmamen IB. The value of computerized axial tomography in the assessment of workers exposed to asbestos. *Am J Ind Med* 1984;6(1):27–35.

76. Sanden A, Jarvholm B. A study of possible predictors of mesothelioma in shipyard workers exposed to asbestos. *J Occup Med* 1991;33(7):770–773.

77. Dodson RF, O'Sullivan M, Corn CJ, McLarty JW, Hammar SP. Analysis of asbestos fiber burden in lung tissue from mesothelioma patients. *Ultrastruct Pathol* 1997;21(4):321–336.

78. Jarvholm B, Larsson S. Do pleural plaques produce symptoms? A brief report. *J Occup Med* 1988;30(4):345–347.

79. Kennedy SM. Air flow obstruction among asbestos-exposed insulators associated with pleural thickening. *Am Rev Respir Dis* 1989;139(4):A209.

80. Jarvholm B, Sanden A. Pleural plaques and respiratory function. *Am J Ind Med* 1986;10(4):419–426.

81. Ohlson CG, Bodin L, Rydman T, Hogstedt C. Ventilatory decrements in former asbestos cement workers: A four-year follow up. *Br J Ind Med* 1985;42(9):612–616.

82. Rosenstock L, Barnhart S, Heyer NJ, Pierson DJ, Hudson LD. The relation among pulmonary function, chest roentgenographic abnormalities and smoking status in an asbestos-exposed cohort. *Am Rev Respir Dis* 1988;138(2):272–277.

83. Baker EL, Dagg T, Greene RE. Respiratory illness in the construction trades: I. The significance of asbestos-associated pleural disease among sheet metal workers. *J Occup Med* 1985;27(7):483–489.

84. Eisenstadt HB. Pleural asbestosis. *Am Pract* 1962;13:573.

85. Gaensler EA, Kaplan AI. Asbestos pleural effusion. *Ann Intern Med* 1971;74(2):178–191.

86. Scully RE. Weekly clinocopathological exercises: Case 4—1987. A 50-year-old man with recurrent pleuro-pulmonary abnormalities. Case records of the Massachusetts General Hospital. *N Engl J Med* 1987;316(4):198–208.

87. McLoud TC, Woods BO, Carrington CB, Epler GR, Gaensler EA. Diffuse pleural thickening in an asbestos-exposed population: Prevalence and causes. *Am J Roentgenol* 1985;144(1):9–18.

88. Gibbs AR, Seal RME, Wagner JC. Pathological reaction of the lung to dust. In: *Occupational Lung Diseases*, 2nd ed., Morgan WKC, Seaton A, eds. Philadelphia: Saunders; 1984: 129–162.

89. Rockoff SD, Kagan E, Schwartz A, Kriebel D, Hix W, Rohatgi P. Visceral pleural thickening in asbestos exposure: the occurrence and implications of thickened interlobar fissures. *J Thorac Imag* 1987;2(4):58–66.

90. Hillerdal G. Pleural changes and exposure to fibrous minerals. *Scand J Work Environ Health* 1984;10(6):473–479.

91. Stephens M, Gibbs AR, Pooley FD, Wagner JC. Asbestos-induced pleural fibrosis: Pathology and mineralogy. *Thorax* 1987;42(8):583–588.

92. Lilis R, Selikoff IJ, Lerman Y, Seidman H, Gelb SK. Asbestosis: Interstitial pulmonary fibrosis and pleural fibrosis in a cohort of asbestos insulation workers: Influence of cigarette smoking. *Am J Ind Med* 1986;10(5–6):459–470.

93. Wright PH, Hanson A, Kreel L, Capel LH. Respiratory function changes after asbestos pleurisy. *Thorax* 1980;35(1):31–36.

94. McGavin CR, Sheers G. Diffuse pleural thickening in asbestos workers: Disability and lung function abnormalities. *Thorax* 1984;39(8):604–607.

95. Miller A, Teirstein AS, Selikoff IJ. Ventilatory failure due to asbestos pleurisy. *Am J Med* 1983; 75(6):911–919.

96. Hillerdal G. Rounded atelectasis. Clinical experience with 74 patients. *Chest* 1989;95(4):836–841.

97. Bayeux MC, Letourneux M, Brochard P, Raffaelli C, Pairon JC, Iwatsubo Y, Ameille J. Rolled atelectasis. Apropos of 26 patients. *Rev Mal Respir* 1998;15(3):281–286.

98. Doyle TC, Lawler GA. CT features of rounded atelectasis of the lung. *Am J Roentgenol* 1984;143(2):225–228.

99. Selikoff IJ, Willis R, Seidman H. Predictive significance of parenchymal and/or pleural fibrosis for subsequent death of asbestos-associated disease. NIH Grant No. E00298. New York: American Cancer Society. p. R53.

100. Hillerdal G. Pleural plaques and risk for cancer in the County of Uppsala. *Eur J Respir Dis Suppl* 1980;107:111–117.

101. Harber P, Mohsenifar Z, Oren A, Lew M. Pleural plaques and asbestos-associated malignancy. *J Occup Med* 1987;29:641–644.

102. Selikoff IJ, Lee DHK. *Asbestos and Disease*. New York: Academic Press Inc.; 1978.

103. al Jarad N, Poulakis N, Pearson MC, Rubens MB, Rudd RM. CT scan versus x-ray estimations to the extent of pleural asbestosis. *Am Rev Respir Dis* 1989;139(4):A211.

104. Silberschmid M, Sabro ES, Andresen J, et al. Light asbestos exposure–dose index is a measure for exposure in dose–effect studies. In: *Occupational Lung Disease*, Gee JB, ed. New York: Raven Press; 1984: 212.

105. Lewinsohn HC. Early malignant changes in pleural plaques due to asbestos exposure: A case report. *Br J Dis Chest* 1974;68(2):121–127.

106. Rom WM. *Environmental and Occupational Medicine*, 1st ed. Boston, MA: Little, Brown & Company; 1983: 165.

107. International Labor Office (ILO). *Encyclopedia of Occupational Health and Safety*, 3rd revised ed. Geneva: International Labor Office; 1988.

108. Fletcher DE, Edge JR. The early radiological changes in pulmonary and pleural asbestosis. *Clin Radiol* 1970;21(4):355–365.

109. Segarra F, Monte MB, Ibanez LP, Nicolas JP. Asbestosis in a Barcelona fiber cement factory. *Environ Res* 1980;23:292–300.

110. Solomon A, Webster I. The visceral pleura in asbestosis. *Environ Res* 1976;11:128–134.

111. Beritic T. Asbestos-related disease without asbestosis: Why not pleural asbestosis? *Am J Ind Med* 1985;8:517–520 [editorial].

112. Smither WJ. Asbestos, asbestosis and mesothelioma of the pleura. *Proc R Soc Med* 1966;59:57. In: *Asbestos and Disease*, Selikoff IJ, Lee DHK, eds. New York: Academic Press; 1978: 215.

113. Hillerdal G. Asbestos exposure and upper lobe involvement. *Am J Roentgenol* 1982;139(6):1163–1166.

114. Hillerdal G. Pleural and parenchymal fibrosis mainly affecting the upper lung lobes in persons exposed to asbestos. *Respir Med* 1990;84(2):129–134.

115. Mulloy KB, Coultas DB, Samet JM. Use of chest radiographs in epidemiological investigations of pneumoconiosis. *Br J Ind Med* 1993;50(3):273–275.

116. CDC/NIOSH. Chest radiography ethical considerations for "B" readers. Available at: www.cdc.gov/niosh/topics/chestradiography/breader-ethics.html

117. NIOSH B Reader Program, ACOEM News. January–February 2004:3. Available at www.acoem.org/gov

118. Ducatman AM, Yang WN, Forman SA. "B-readers" and asbestos medical surveillance. *J Occup Med* 1988;30(8):644–647.

119. Ducatman AM. Variability in interpretation of radiographs for asbestosis abnormalities: Problems and solutions. *Ann N Y Acad Sci* 1991;643:108–120.

120. Franzblau A, Lilus R. The diagnosis of nonmalignant diseases related to asbestos. *Am Rev Respir Dis* 1987;136(3):790–791.

121. Murphy RL Jr. The diagnosis of nonmalignant diseases related to asbestos. *Am Rev Respir Dis* 1987;136(6):1516–1517.

122. Weill H. Diagnosis of asbestos-related diseases. *Chest* 1987;91(6):802–803.

123. Huuskonen O, Kivisaari L, Zitting A, Taskinen K, Tossavainen A, Vehmas T. High-resolution computed tomography classification of lung fibrosis for patients with asbestos-related disease. *Scand J Work Environ Health* 2001;27(2):106–112.

124. Biscaldi G, Fonte R, Paita L, Vittadini G, Caprotti M. High resolution computerized tomography in the diagnosis of asbestosis. *G Ital Med Lav Ergon* 1999;21(4):271–277.

125. Murray KA, Gamsu G, Webb WR, Salmon CJ, Egger MJ. High resolution computed tomography sampling for detection of asbestos-related lung disease. *Acad Radiol* 1995;2(2):111–115.

126. Kraus T, Raithel HJ, Lehnen G. Computer-assisted classification system for chest x-ray and computed tomography findings in occupational lung disease. *Int Arch Occup Environ Health* 1997;69(6):482–486.

127. Harkin TJ, McGuinness G, Goldring R. Differentiation of the ILO boundary chest roentgenograph (0/1 to 1/0) in asbestosis by high-resolution computed tomography scan, alveolitis, and respiratory impairment. *J Occup Environ Med* 1996;38(1):46–52.

128. Staples CA, Gamsu G, Ray CS, Webb WR. High resolution computed tomography and lung function in asbestos-exposed workers with normal chest radiographs. *Am Rev Respir Dis* 1989;139(6):1502–1508.

129. Weill H, Ziskind MM, Waggenspack C, Rossiter CE. Lung function consequences of dust exposure in asbestos cement manufacturing plants. *Arch Environ Health* 1975;30(2):88–97.

130. Selikoff IJ, Lee DHK. *Asbestos and Disease*. New York: Academic Press; 1978: 215.

131. Walker AM, Loughlin JE, Friedland ER, Rothman KJ, Dreyer NA. Projections of asbestos-related disease 1980–2009. *J Occup Med* 1983;25(5):409–425.

132. Seidman H, Selikoff IJ. Decline in death rates among asbestos insulation workers 1967–1986 associated with diminution of work exposure to asbestos. *Ann N Y Acad Sci* 1990;609:300–317 [discussion 317–318].

133. Centers for Disease Control and Prevention. Changing patterns of pneumoconiosis mortality—United States, 1968–2000. *MMWR Morb Mortal Wkly Rep* 2004;54(28):627–632.

134. Owens GR, Follansbee WP. Cardiopulmonary manifestations of systemic sclerosis. *Chest* 1987;91(1):118–127.

135. Eisenberg H, Dubois EL, Sherwin RP, Balchum OJ. Diffuse interstitial lung disease in systemic lupus erythematosus. *Ann Intern Med* 1973;79(1):37–45.

136. Garcia JG, James HL, Zinkgraf S, Perlman MB, Keogh BA. Lower respiratory tract abnormalities in rheumatoid interstitial lung disease. Potential role of neutrophils in lung injury. *Am Rev Respir Dis* 1987;136(4):811–817.

137. Luna MA, Bedrossian CW, Lichtiger B, Salem PA. Interstitial pneumonitis associated with bleomycin therapy. *Am J Clin Pathol* 1972;58(5):501–510.

138. Martin WJ, II, Rosenow EC, III. Amiodarone pulmonary toxicity. Recognition and pathogenesis (Part I). *Chest* 1988;93(5):1067–1075.

139. Elsasser S, Dalquen P, Soler M, Perruchoud AP. Methotrexate-induced pneumonitis: appearance four weeks after discontinuation of treatment. *Am Rev Respir Dis* 1989;140;(4):1089–1092.

140. Agarwal R, Sharma SK, Malaviya AN. Gold-induced hypersensitivity pneumonitis in a patient with rheumatoid arthritis. *Clin Exp Rheumatol* 1989;7(1):89–90.

141. Rosenow EC, III, DeRemee RA, Dines DE. Chronic nitrofurantoin pulmonary reaction. Report of 5 cases. *N Engl J Med* 1968;279(23):1258–1262.
142. Haim DY, Lippmann ML, Goldberg SK, Walkenstein MD. The pulmonary complications of crack cocaine: A comprehensive review. *Chest* 1995;107(1):233–240.
143. Gertz MA, Greipp PR. Clinical aspects of pulmonary amyloidosis. *Chest* 1986;90(6):790–791.
144. Chin K, Tabata C, Satake N, Nagai S, Moriyasu F, Kuno K. Pneumonitis associated with natural and recombinant interferon alpha therapy for chronic hepatitis C. *Chest* 1994;105(3):939–941.
145. Tarlo SM, Broder I, Prokipchuk EJ, Peress L, Mintz S. Association between celiac disease and lung disease. *Chest* 1981;80(6):715–718.
146. American Thoracic Society. Idiopathic pulmonary fibrosis: diagnosis and treatment. International Consensus Statement, American Thoracic Society (ATS), and the European Respiratory Society (ERS). *Am J Respir Crit Care Med* 2000;161(2 Pt. 1):646–664.
147. Katzenstein AL, Myers JL. Idiopathic pulmonary fibrosis: Clinical relevance of pathologic classification. *Am J Respir Crit Care Med* 1998;157(4 Pt. 1):1301–1315.
148. Richerson HB, Bernstein IL, Fink JN, Hunninghake GW, Hovey HS, Reed CE, et al. Guidelines for the clinical evaluation of hypersensitivity pneumonitis. Report of the Subcommittee on Hypersensitivity Pneumonitis. *J Allergy Clin Immunol* 1989;84:839–844.
149. Gibson PG, Bryant DH, Morgan GW, Yeates M, Fernandez V, Penny R, Breit SN. Radiation-induced lung injury: a hypersensitivity pneumonitis? *Ann Intern Med* 1988;109(4):288–291.
150. Schwartz MI, King TE. *Interstitial Lung Disease*, 4th ed. Hamilton, London: BC Decker Inc.; 2003.
151. Pearle JL. Smoking and duration of asbestos exposure in the production of functional and roentgenographic abnormalities in shipyard workers. *J Occup Med* 1982;24(1):37–40.
152. Selikoff IJ, Nicholson WJ, Lilis R. Radiological evidence of asbestos disease among ship repair workers. *Am J Ind Med* 1980;1(1):9–22.
153. Barnhart S, Thornquist M, Omenn GS, Goodman G, Feigl P, Rosenstock L. The degree of roentgenographic parenchymal opacities attributable to smoking among asbestos-exposed subjects. *Am Rev Respir Med* 1990;141:1102–1106.
154. Flaherty KR, Martinez FJ. Cigarette smoking in interstitial lung disease: concepts for the internist. *Med Clin North Am* 2004;88(6):1643–1653, xiii.
155. Davies G, Wells AU, du Bois RM. Respiratory bronchiolitis associated with interstitial lung disease and desquamative interstitial pneumonia. *Clin Chest Med* 2004;25(4):717–726, vi.
156. Heyneman LE, Ward S, Lynch DA. Respiratory bronchiolitis, respiratory bronchiolitis-associated interstitial lung disease, and desquamative interstitial pneumonitis: Different entities or part of the spectrum of the same disease process? *Am J Roentgenol* 1999;173(6):1617–1622.
157. Guckel C, Hansell DM. Imaging the "dirty lung"—Has high resolution computed tomography cleared the smoke? *Clin Radiol* 1998;53(10):717–722.
158. Ryn JH, Hartman TE, Vasallo R. Smoking-related interstitial lung diseases: A concise review. *Eur Respir J* 2001;17:122–132.
159. Barnhart S, Hudson LD, Mason SE, Pierson DJ, Rosenstock L. Total lung capacity. An insensitive measure of impairment of patients with asbestosis and chronic obstructive pulmonary disease? *Chest* 1988;93(2):299–302.
160. Churg A. Current issues in the pathologic and minéralogie diagnosis of asbestos-induced disease. *Chest* 1983;84(3):278.
161. Boyle P, Vainio H, Smith R. Workgroup I: criteria for screening. UICC International Workshop on Facilitating Screening for Colorectal Cancer, Oslo, Norway (June 29 and 30, 2002). *Ann Oncol* 2005;16(1):25–30.
162. Patnick J, Ransohoff D, Atkin W, et al. Workgroup III: Facilitating screening for colorectal cancer: Quality assurance and evaluation. UICC International Workshop on Facilitating Screening for Colorectal Cancer, Oslo, Norway (June 29 and 30, 2002). *Ann Oncol* 2005;16(1):34–37.
163. Levin B, Smith RA. The Global Challenge of Colorectal Cancer. Reports from the UICC International Workshop on Facilitating Screening for Colorectal Cancer: an international agenda. *Ann Oncol* 2005;16(1):23.
164. Smith RA, Mettlin CJ, Davis KJ, Eyre H. American Cancer Society Guidelines for the early detection of cancer. *CA Cancer J Clin* 2000;50:34–49.
165. Guidotti TL, Miller A, Christiani DC, Wagner G, Balmes J, Harber P, et al. Nonmalignant asbestos-related disease: diagnosis and early management. *Clin Pulm Med* 2007;14:82–92.

CHAPTER 13

Malignant Diseases Attributed to Asbestos Exposure

Gary K. Friedman

CONTENTS

13.1 INTRODUCTION

Asbestos has been recognized as a human carcinogen for more than 50 years, and the International Agency for the Research of Cancer (IARC) has classified asbestos as a class 1A human carcinogen. The IARC has stated "all commercial forms of asbestos tested are carcinogenic in mice, rats, hamsters, and rabbits."[1] Dose–response relationships have been established, and numerous epidemiologic studies in humans have documented a significant increase in cancer risk following asbestos exposure from a wide variety of products, occupations, and industrial settings. The American Thoracic Society, the American Cancer Society, the American College of Chest Physicians (ACCP), the Occupational Safety and Health Administration (OSHA), the Environmental Protection Agency (EPA), the National Institute for Occupational Safety and Health (NIOSH), the Agency for Toxic Substances and Disease Registry, the Centers for Disease Control and Prevention, and other governmental agencies and professional societies also recognize asbestos as a human carcinogen. Elevated cancer risk for a variety of organ systems has been reported by numerous authors throughout the decades.

Not surprisingly, because the primary route of exposure is through inhalation, the malignancies of the respiratory system have the strongest cancer risk after exposure. Shortly after the documentation of increased risk of lung cancer in workers exposed to asbestos, there was recognition of an increased risk of mesothelioma.[2] The malignant pulmonary and pleural sequelae of asbestos exposure are listed in Table 13.1.

As epidemiologic studies were performed on insulation workers and other cohorts with significant asbestos exposure, increased risk of gastrointestinal, kidney, laryngeal, and other malignancies were detected in asbestos-exposed populations.[3] The 2009 ACCP Consensus Statement reported agreement among the participants that "asbestos exposure causes other neoplasms in addition to lung cancer and mesothelioma."[4] Extrathoracic malignancies showing increased risk after exposure to asbestos as reported in the peer reviewed literature are listed in Table 13.2. However, there is continued controversy concerning asbestos causation in regard to several of those malignancies.

Historically,[5] increased risk for esophageal carcinoma and stomach cancer have been attributed to asbestos exposure. OSHA and EPA considered risks for these malignancies when formulating policy. Recent reports have raised questions concerning the role of asbestos and the magnitude of increased risk[6] in the causation of extrathoracic malignancy other than mesothelioma and laryngeal cancer.

Table 13.1   Malignant Pulmonary and Pleural Manifestations of Asbestos Exposure

Lung cancer

Adenocarcinoma

Squamous cell carcinoma

Large cell undifferentiated carcinoma

Small cell lung carcinoma

Malignant mesothelioma

Epithelial

Sarcomatoid

Mixed

Other (rare)

Table 13.2   Extrathoracic Malignancies Reported to Have Increased Risk after Asbestos Exposure

Laryngeal carcinoma

Gastrointestinal carcinoma (e.g., esophageal, stomach, colon)

Peritoneal mesothelioma

Pericardial mesothelioma

Mesothelioma of the tunica vaginalis

Guidotti et al.[7] associated colon cancer with asbestos exposure. Certain pathologic entities including multicystic mesothelioma,[8] well-differentiated papillary mesothelioma, and deciduoid mesothelioma[9] have been reported to occur in the absence of known asbestos exposure, especially in young adults and women.

13.2 LUNG CANCER

Lung cancer represents the most common cause of cancer deaths in both men and women in the United States. The American Cancer Society[10] reported that 90,490 men and 73,020 women (a total of 163,510) died of cancer of the lung and bronchus in 2005. It was estimated that there were 172,570 new cases of lung cancer diagnosed in 2005, which accounted for 13% of all cancer diagnoses. Alberg and Samet[11] noted that the rise and the decline in the incidence of lung cancer paralleled the trends in cigarette smoking. The incidence of lung cancer has been declining since 1991 at the rate of approximately 1.9% per year. However, a similar decline in the utilization of asbestos began to occur approximately 35 years ago. Given the latency of asbestos-related lung cancer, this may likewise have contributed to the decline.

13.2.1 Pulmonary Carcinogens

In an occupational setting, exposure to established human carcinogens must be considered if causation of a lung cancer is in question. Table 13.3 lists carcinogens for lung cancer in humans.

13.2.2 Geographic Patterns

Lung cancer is more common in the United States than in developing countries. In the United States, an increased risk of lung cancer has been reported in coastal areas. This geographic distribution was hypothesized, in part, to reflect employment in the shipbuilding industry with increased cancer risk attributed to asbestos utilization.

Table 13.3   Carcinogens for Lung Cancer in Humans

- Arsenic
- Asbestos
- Beryllium
- Bischloromethyl ether (BCME)
- Cadmium
- Chromium (VI) compounds
- Nickel compounds
- Silica (crystalline)
- Talc containing asbestiform fibers
- Tobacco smoke carcinogens, *N*-nitrosamines, metals including polonium 210, and polycyclic aromatic hydrocarbons and others
- Radon
- Cool tars and coal pitches

13.2.3 A Brief Historical Perspective of Asbestos and Lung Cancer

In 1935, Lynch and Smith[12] reported a possible association between asbestos and lung cancer. In 1949, Merewether, the Chief Inspector of Factories in England and Wales, observed that 13.2% of patients found to have asbestosis at autopsy also suffered from an intrathoracic malignancy. Between 1935 and 1954, 90 cases of lung cancer were found at autopsy in asbestos workers as published in 26 separate reports. Most workers also suffered from asbestosis.[13]

In 1955, Doll[14] reported 11 deaths in a cohort of British asbestos textile workers where 0.8 were expected (standard mortality ratio [SMR] = 14.0). Subsequent to that time, numerous studies of various designs conducted on asbestos-exposed workers in a variety of industries have reconfirmed carcinogenicity of asbestos for lung cancer. In 1986, OSHA[15] stated "lung cancer constitutes the greatest health risk for American asbestos workers."

Selikoff et al.[16] studied 632 insulators who entered the trade before 1943 and followed through 1962. Forty-five died from cancer of the lung or pleura (mesothelioma), whereas only 6.6 such deaths were expected. Selikoff et al.[16] also reported increased cancer risk of the gastrointestinal system, larynx, and other organ systems. In 1980, McDonald[17] reviewed 18 epidemiologic studies and applied the criteria of Sir Austin Bradford Hill[18] to identify features by which a causal hypothesis could be judged. McDonald stated: "I believe we may fairly conclude that it has been demonstrated beyond reasonable doubt that asbestos of the types used commercially is a cause of human lung cancer. Other agents such as tobacco may enhance the effect, but the carcinogenicity of asbestos is independent of them." Furthermore, McDonald found "irrespective of the nature of the exposure, results have consistently shown some excess mortality from lung cancer" (p. 374).[17] The incidence between asbestos exposure and lung cancer reached a "threefold risk and much higher."

13.2.4 Cell Type and Tumor Location

Occupational exposure to asbestos is associated with increased risk of all major histological types of lung cancer. The cell type cannot be used as an argument for or against the involvement of asbestos in a given case. Churg[19] reviewed eight studies totaling 471 patients and determined squamous carcinomas accounted for 43% of tumors, small cell for 28%, adenocarcinoma for 19%, and large cell for 10%. The Helsinki Criteria[20] reported that all four major cell types of lung cancer were related to asbestos exposure. The location of the tumor within the lung did not distinguish an asbestos-related tumor from lung cancer attributed to other causes. Weill[21] noted that there was no specific histologic type of lung tumor linked to asbestos exposure nor could the location of the tumor within the lung be used to support or exclude causation by asbestos. Bronchoalveolar cell carcinomas (sometimes referred to as "scar cancers") are more strongly associated with areas of fibrosis and less strongly linked to smoking than other cell types. However, there is strong evidence that scarring in primary pulmonary adenocarcinoma may be caused by the neoplasm rather than developing in a scar. A review of the literature does not demonstrate any epidemiologic confirmation of increased risk for carcinoid tumors or sarcomas (other than sarcomatoid mesotheliomas) being attributable to asbestos.

13.2.5 Fiber Type

Amosite, crocidolite, tremolite, and chrysotile are all considered carcinogens for lung cancer. Although there is evidence for greater carcinogenicity of amphiboles over chrysotile with respect to mesothelioma, the establishment of a clear gradient in the carcinogenicity of fiber types is unproven at this time as it relates to lung cancer. A review by Henderson et al.[22] suggested different attribution criteria (greater cumulative exposure) are more appropriate for some chrysotile-only exposures and chrysotile mining and milling than for amphibole or mixed exposures.

13.2.6 Exposure: Dose–Response Relationship

Lung cancer risk attributed to asbestos is related to cumulative exposure. Weill[23] noted "The risks for the development of lung cancer in asbestos-exposed workers are clearly related to exposure dose." A linear relationship between the cumulative asbestos exposure and the development of lung cancer has been described. However, there is some question whether a threshold exists below which excess risk for lung cancer does not occur.[23] At ordinary ambient levels of asbestos exposure, there is no objective data that demonstrate increased risk for lung cancer. At very low levels of exposure, theoretical risk assessments have been developed, which assume a linear, no threshold model extrapolating from health effects at higher levels of exposure reported in occupational settings. Hughes and Weill[24] assessed theoretical risks at low-level asbestos exposure for students with 6-year average enrollment in schools containing asbestos products. The students' cancer risks were substantially less than risk of death from activities of daily living such as riding a bicycle or playing high school football. Governmental agencies and regulatory bodies erring on the side of caution assumed a zero threshold when developing public policy. The Department of Labor Asbestos Work Group stated that there was no level of exposure to asbestos below which clinical effect did not occur and recommended a permissible exposure limit (PEL)[15] on the basis of the limits of current technology for measuring airborne concentrations of asbestos without distinction of fiber type.

Efforts have been made to quantify the relationship between fiber-years of cumulative exposure and relative risk of lung cancer. The Helsinki Criteria[20] states that the increase in risk is estimated to be between 0.5% and 4% for each fiber-year of cumulative exposure. Using the upper boundary of this range, cumulative exposure of 25 fiber-years would double the risk of lung cancer. At this level, clinical asbestosis may or may not occur. This equates to a tissue fiber burden of approximately 5000–15,000 asbestos bodies per gram of dry tissue. Because chrysotile fibers undergo clearance with time, some experts feel that occupational history is a better indicator of lung cancer risk than is measurement of chrysotile fiber burden.[20] According to the Helsinki Criteria, attribution to asbestos as a substantial contributing factor in a specific case of lung cancer could be stated with probability at the 25-fiber-year exposure level. Lower levels of exposure may be associated with an increased risk of lung cancer, but to a lesser extent.

OSHA, in the Final Rules on Asbestos[15] (p. 22644, Table 6), demonstrates a dose–response relationship on the basis of years of exposure and asbestos fiber concentration. Excess relative risk of lung cancer is expressed as mortality per 100,000 exposed individuals. At 0.1 fiber-years

(0.1 fibers/mL for 1 year exposure), the risk of lung cancer is 7.2 per 100,000 exposed. The highest calculated risk is for those with a 10-fiber/mL exposure for 45 years (450 fiber-year exposure) where the risk rises to 18,515 per 100,000. There is a nonlinear increase in the risk at 45 years of exposure because of other competing causes of death in an aging population.

From a pragmatic standpoint, as noted in the ATS 1986 statement on the diagnosis of nonmalignant diseases related to asbestos,[25] the physician rarely has industrial hygiene measurements of fiber levels, and reliance must be placed on a detailed chronologic occupational history.

The risk of asbestos-related lung cancer may vary between occupations or exposure settings as the asbestos content of products, work practices, intensity, and duration of asbestos exposure may differ by occupation and specific job descriptions. For example, the risk of lung cancer is dramatically different for an insulator than it is for a brake mechanic.[26] Thus, a detailed exposure history is essential in estimating risk or attribution.

13.2.7 Low Levels of Asbestos Exposure and Increased Risk of Lung Cancer

McLemore et al.[27] cited increased cancer risk after asbestos exposure for periods as short as 1 month of employment at an amosite factory. The risk of lung cancer increased both with exposure and latency because "retained asbestos in lung tissues constitutes a continuing exposure." These in situ or residential exposures are of concern for cancer as well as asbestosis. "In this type of exposure model, the direct dose as well as the time in situ are determinants of the disease response."

Seidman et al.[28] studied an amosite factory in Patterson, New Jersey, reporting that "work exposure to amosite asbestos for as short a period as one month was associated with an increased cancer risk. The risk of cancer increased with longer direct exposure (e.g., two months, three months, or six months) and the length of time after onset of work. With very brief, direct exposure, cancer risk was increased only after 25 to 35 years emphasizing that with lighter (or brief) direct exposure, prolonged follow-up is necessary to evaluate asbestos-associated health effects."

13.2.7.1 OSHA Final Rules, 1986—Health Effects

OSHA's[15] assessment of the carcinogenic threat of asbestos in the workplace is confirmed by the statement: "OSHA is aware of no instance in which exposure to a toxic substance has more clearly demonstrated detrimental health effect on humans than has asbestos exposure. The diseases caused by asbestos exposure are life-threatening or disabling. Of all of the diseases caused by asbestos, lung cancer constitutes the greatest health risk for American asbestos workers. Lung cancer has been responsible for more than half of the excess mortality from asbestos exposure in some occupational cohorts." In 1980, a joint NIOSH/OSHA asbestos work group concluded that there was "no level of exposure to asbestos below which clinical effects did not occur" and recommended a PEL of 0.1 fibers/cm^3 on the basis of the limitation of current technology for measuring airborne concentrations of asbestos (p. 22616).[15]

OSHA[15] (p. 22620) described the evidence as "exceptionally strong" for a "dose–response relationship between asbestos and an excess risk of either lung cancer or mesothelioma" citing numerous studies and concluded "Cumulative exposure levels of asbestos below that permitted by lifetime exposure to the 2 fibers/cc PEL results in excess mortality from lung cancer and mesothelioma." They further noted the Seidman, Finkelstein, and Selikoff studies "clearly indicate that workers exposed for a relatively short period of time experience significant excess mortality from lung cancer and from all asbestos diseases." On the basis of these and additional studies from Zoloth and Michel, "OSHA concludes that well conducted studies demonstrate a substantially increased rate of lung cancer and mesothelioma mortality among workers having low cumulative exposures to asbestos."

13.2.8 Latency

Authors of the Helsinki Criteria cite a minimum of 10 years from first exposure before attributing lung cancer to asbestos.[20] A 15- to 20-year or longer minimum latency period is more commonly reported. The latency can be affected by level of asbestos exposure, synergy, and cocarcinogens. The risk of lung cancer increases with time and appears to peak approximately 30 to 35 years after exposure.[29]

13.2.9 Clinical Approach to Asbestos-Related Lung Cancer

Approximately 85%–90% of patients diagnosed with lung cancer die from that disease. Malignant transformation of cells occurs years before the disease becomes clinically apparent. In the early stages of lung cancer, the disease is typically asymptomatic and there is a tendency for early metastatic spread. In most cases, the tumor has either spread beyond the lung or involves critical structures within the chest, preventing surgical resection at the time of diagnosis.

When symptoms are present, these may include a persistent cough, chest pain (especially when there is bone involvement), hemoptysis, and shortness of breath. When the tumor has spread beyond the chest, presenting symptoms may reflect metastatic spread. Seizure disorder, paralysis, or other neurological complaints indicate tumor spread to the brain. Back pain, pelvic pain, and so forth, may indicate metastatic spread to bone. Paraneoplastic syndromes are occasionally present.

There is nothing unique about the cell type, tumor location, growth pattern, metastatic tendencies, or response to therapy that distinguishes an asbestos-related lung cancer (Figure 13.1). Therefore, the clinical approach to the diagnosis and management of these tumors is similar to that of nonasbestos-exposed individuals except for factors cited in Table 13.4.

13.3 ATTRIBUTION AND APPORTIONMENT OF LUNG CANCER TO ASBESTOS

The clinician is sometimes called upon to render an opinion concerning the causation of lung cancer in a given patient. In the individual case, the probability that asbestos was a contributing factor relies in part upon the dose–response relationship between cumulative exposure and causation of lung cancer. Because the cumulative levels of exposure that cause asbestosis in some patients is similar to that which causes lung cancer, some authors[30,31] require asbestosis before attributing causation to asbestos in a given case. Other authors[32–34] have argued that asbestos is a carcinogen and that fibrogenicity (asbestosis) as an intermediate process is not required.

There may be more than one mechanism for the causation of lung cancer in asbestos-exposed individuals. Dr. Margaret Becklake[35] suggests that some asbestos-related cancers may arise from scars, whereas other cancers such as squamous cell carcinomas often occur in association with only minimal fibrosis, are centrally located, and are usually seen in workers who smoke. Dr. Becklake notes that pulmonary fibrosis may predate the appearance in "some but not all subjects who later died of cancer." Dr. Becklake stated: "These findings are also not inconsistent with the possibility of more than one etiologic mechanism operating in the production of asbestos-related lung cancer."

13.3.1 Incidence of Lung Cancer Due to Asbestos

LaDou[36] opined that 5%–7% of all lung cancers are due to asbestos exposure (8500–12,000 per annum). Andrew Churg[37] cites Doll and Peto,[145] who estimated that "asbestos contributes to the development of some 5000 to 10,000 cases of lung cancer per year in the United States."

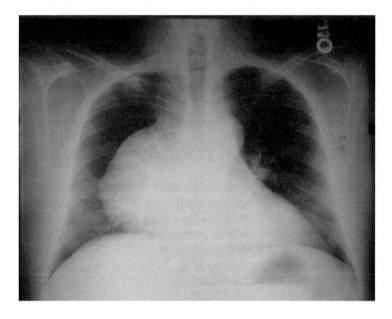

Figure 13.1   Nonsmall-cell lung cancer in person with lengthy history of heavy asbestos exposure.

Table 13.4   Asbestos-Related Lung Cancer—Special Issues

1. The need to distinguish between lung cancer and mesothelioma.
2. The presence of underlying asbestosis may affect lung function to an extent that impacts decisions concerning resectability, selection of chemotherapeutic agents, or radiation therapy that may be fibrogenic.
3. Rounded atelectasis must be distinguished from pulmonary nodules or pleural-based masses.
4. Lymphangitic spread of tumor may cause radiographic appearance that is similar to interstitial disease.
5. Issues may arise as to whether interstitial fibrosis was present preceding treatment of the tumor or whether such fibrosis was caused by treatment of the tumor itself.

In 2001, Haus et al.[38] reviewed excess risk of lung cancer attributable to occupational and environmental causes. They stated that approximately 4% (7000) of all lung cancers diagnosed annually in the United States are attributable to asbestos.

In 1996, Steenland et al.[39] at NIOSH reviewed 20 asbestos-exposed cohort studies and found that the combined relative risk for lung cancer was 2.0 compared with an unexposed population. Six studies identified that the combined relative risk for developing lung cancer of individuals with asbestosis (rather than just exposure) was 5.91.

13.3.2 Asbestos Bodies, Asbestos Fibers, Asbestosis, and Lung Cancer

Roggli et al.[40] found the asbestos body content in patients with lung cancer to be variable. Roggli et al.[41] demonstrated substantially higher fiber counts in 48 patients with lung cancer and asbestosis as compared with 25 patients with pleural plaque and lung cancer or 70 patients who only had histories of asbestos exposure. They reported a separate group of six nonsmoking asbestos workers with lung cancer but without plaques or asbestosis. Four of these demonstrated tissue asbestos fiber content above the range of normal for their laboratory with a fiber analysis demonstrating approximately 30,000 uncoated fibers per gram of wet lung. They opined that asbestos was a substantial contributing factor in the development of lung cancer even in the absence of asbestosis.

Warnock and Isenberg[42] studied 75 men with lung cancer and reported the results of fiber burden and pulmonary fibrosis. All but eight patients had some history of asbestos exposure. After measuring fibers per gram of dry lung, they reported that a substantial number of subjects with the highest fiber burden did not have asbestosis. Warnock and Isenberg[42] opined that because large burdens of asbestos did not always cause pulmonary fibrosis, asbestosis may in fact be a poor marker of fiber-related lung cancer. They opined a concentration of 1000 or more asbestos bodies per gram of dried tissue, or a combined fiber count of amosite and crocidolite totaling 100,000 or more fibers per gram of dried tissue could be used as an indicator of a relationship between lung cancer and asbestos exposure.

Wagner et al.[43] reported that the pathologic grade of asbestosis in rats was related to lung neoplasms. There was an excess of tumors in rats with slight asbestosis even when exposure was as minimal as 1 day, but there was no excess of tumors when asbestosis was absent. It is to be noted that after reviewing these studies and others, Sluis-Cremer[44] concluded that it was "unreasonable" to demand proof of the presence of asbestosis before attributing a bronchial cancer to inhalation of asbestos dust.

13.3.3 Radiographic Evidence of Asbestosis and Lung Cancer

Wilkinson et al.[45] reviewed chest radiographs for fibrosis and obtained occupational and smoking histories from 271 lung cancer patients compared with 678 controls. After correction for age, sex, and smoking, the odds ratio (OR) was 2.03 for those with an International Labour Organization (ILO) score of 1/0 or greater and 1.56 for those with an ILO score of 0/1 or less. Wilkinson et al.[45] opined that workers from occupations with high probability of asbestos exposure were at increased risk of lung cancer even in the absence of radiographically apparent asbestosis.

IARC[46] concluded an excess incidence of bronchial carcinoma existed in those exposed to asbestos without concomitant radiologic signs of asbestosis. In 1972, Kannerstein and Churg[47] stated that they were unable to accept fibrogenesis as an intermediate essential causal phase in the development of lung cancer in asbestos-exposed individuals. Although Kipen et al.[48] found some element of pulmonary fibrosis histologically in all members of a cohort of lung cancer patients, they reported that 10%–15% did not have radiographic asbestosis. Kipen et al.[48] stated that the probability that interstitial fibrosis will not be radiologically detectable in a sizeable proportion of cases of cancer is of considerable significance. Whether or not asbestosis histologically always preceded lung cancer was unresolved.

The Helsinki Criteria[20] indicates that 1 year of heavy exposure, such as demolition of old buildings, manufacturing or insulation work, or 5 to 10 years of moderate exposure such as construction and shipbuilding, may cause a greater than a doubling of the risk of lung cancer. This consensus statement opines that a cumulative exposure of 25 fiber-years may likewise double the risk. At these levels of cumulative exposure, asbestosis may or may not be present. The author concluded: "Heavy exposure in the absence of radiologically diagnosed asbestosis is sufficient to increase the risk of lung cancer."

The ACCP Consensus Statement on Respiratory Health Effects of Asbestos[4] reached agreement stating: "In an exposed worker without asbestosis and with lung cancer, the recognition of asbestosis among coworkers with similar exposures is sufficient to attribute the worker's lung cancer to asbestos exposure." Consensus was also reached concerning the statement that "workers who have significant asbestos exposure (but who do not have asbestosis) are at increased risk of bronchogenic carcinoma."

13.4 SMOKING AND LUNG CANCER

13.4.1 Smoking Risk Factors: Intensity, Duration, and Age

Peto[49] opined that there was a stronger effect attributable to the duration of smoking rather than the amount smoked per day. Alberg and Samet[11] noted "The risk of lung cancer among cigarette smokers increases with the duration of smoking and the number of cigarettes smoked per day." A tripling of the number of cigarettes smoked per day was estimated to triple the risk, whereas a tripling of the duration of smoking was estimated to increase the lung cancer risk one hundred fold.[11] Alberg stated: "Thus, those who initiate smoking earlier in life are most likely to develop lung cancer and are most likely to do so at younger ages." Historical statistics concerning smoking and lung cancer may be obtained from reports by the American Cancer Society[50] and from the U.S. Surgeon General report on the health consequences of smoking.[51]

13.4.2 Smoking Abstinence

Abstinence from smoking diminishes the risk of lung cancer but does not return to the baseline of a lifetime nonsmoker. This decline first appears after approximately 10 years of smoking cessation and continues to decline with continued cessation. After 15 to 20 years, the risk approaches that of a nonsmoker.[51]

13.4.3 Low Tar and Nicotine Filters

The Institute of Medicine (IOM) report concluded that "smoking lower yield products had not been shown to benefit the health of smokers."[11] The National Cancer Institute monograph on risks associated with smoking cigarettes with low machine-measured yields of tar and nicotine found that "compensatory changes in smoking patterns reduce any theoretical benefit of lower yield products."[11] They further concluded changes in cigarette design and manufacturing over the last 50 years "had not benefited public health."

13.4.4 Smoking, Asbestos, and Lung Cancer

13.4.4.1 Smokers versus Nonsmokers

Hammond et al.[52] reported approximately a fivefold increase in lung cancer risk among smoking and nonsmoking insulators. Although carcinogens in asbestos and cigarettes may each independently cause lung cancer, exposure to both results in an increase in risk that is greater than the additive sum of the lung cancer risks. This is referred to as *multiplicative synergism*. For example, if asbestos increased the risk of lung cancer fivefold in a nonsmoking asbestos worker (example: insulators) and smoking increased the lung cancer risk 11-fold in a smoking nonasbestos-exposed individual, the synergistic effects in a smoking insulator could result in a 55-fold (5 × 11) increase in risk.

The relative risk for lung cancer attributable to asbestos exposure is similar in smokers and nonsmokers.[52–54] Weill,[23] citing Enterline, stated: "If the relative risk is similar for nonsmokers and smokers (although the excess cases are far greater among smokers), one can clearly disregard smoking in attempting to determine the role of asbestos exposure in an individual case. We are still left with the burden of assessing asbestos dose."

Liddell[55] reviewed the additive and multiplicative models for lung cancer risk due to the interaction of asbestos and smoking and concluded that the relative risk of asbestos-induced lung cancer was approximately twice as high in nonsmokers compared with smokers.

Berry et al.[56] reviewed six epidemiologic studies and found a relative risk of nonsmokers to smokers of 1.8 (1.1–2.8), 95% confidence interval (CI).

Reid et al.[57] studied crocidolite miners to determine if the risk of lung cancer declined with increasing time since ceasing exposure to asbestos and quitting smoking and to determine the relative asbestos effect between nonsmokers and current smokers. They concluded that persons exposed to asbestos and tobacco but who subsequently quit smoking remained at increased risk for lung cancer up to 20 years after smoking cessation compared with never smokers. They stated: "although the relative risk of lung cancer appears higher in never and ex-smokers than in current smokers, those who both smoke and have been exposed to asbestos have the highest risk."

Lee[58] performed an analysis of 23 studies assessing the relationship between asbestos exposure, smoking, and lung cancer and found that asbestos multiplied the risk of lung cancer in nonsmokers and smokers by a similar factor. Lee opined that the combined relationship of asbestos exposure and smoking was multiplicative rather than additive.

In 2004, Berry and Liddell[59] published a study on the interaction between asbestos and smoking in causation of lung cancer. They used the term *modified relative asbestos effect* as the ratio of the excess relative risk in nonsmokers to that of smokers. They concluded that the modified relative asbestos effect was 3.19 with 95% CI (1.67–6.13).

13.4.4.2 Synergistic Effect of Asbestos and Cigarette Smoking in Causation of Lung Cancer

Asbestos and cigarette smoking are carcinogens each capable of causing lung cancer. With exposures to asbestos and cigarette smoking, the carcinogenic effect is reported to be multiplicative as opposed to additive. The mechanism by which the synergism occurs has been the subject of some debate. One theory is that smoking enhances retention of asbestos fibers.[60] Another theory is that the carcinogens in cigarette smoke (such as alpha-1 benzpyrene, nitrosamines, arsenic, etc.) adhere to the surface of the asbestos fibers, which increases their retention in the lung.[27,60]

The synergy between asbestos and smoking was computed by Hammond et al.[52] They noted that asbestos exposure increased the risk of lung cancer in smokers fivefold and likewise increased the risk of lung cancer in nonsmokers approximately fivefold. Asbestos workers who were nonsmokers had a mortality ratio of 5.17 for lung cancer, whereas those who smoked had a mortality ratio of 53.24. The Surgeon General of the United States, C. Everett Koop, MD, stated: "Of particular concern for lung cancer risk is the synergistic relationship that exists between smoking and certain occupational agents such as asbestos and possibly radioactive aerosols. Asbestos workers who smoke cigarettes have five times the risk of lung cancer as smokers without asbestos exposure, and more than fifty times the risk of individuals who neither smoke nor work with asbestos."[61]

Rom[62] states: "McDonald concluded that the relative risk for nonsmokers exposed to asbestos is at least as great as that for smokers and that in absolute terms most asbestos-related cancers occur in those who have smoked." Rom reported that Selikoff and Hammond found lung cancer mortality was approximately one-third for asbestos insulators who stopped smoking compared with that of their workmates who continued to smoke after 10 years of follow-up.

Selikoff et al.[63] reported that "of 283 workmen with a history of regular cigarette smoking, 24 died of bronchogenic carcinoma although only three were expected to die of this disease. Calculations suggest that asbestos workers who smoke have approximately 92 times the risk of dying of bronchogenic carcinoma as men who neither work with asbestos nor smoke cigarettes." McLemore et al.[27] appeared to support this statistic stating: "Cigarette smokers who experience long term exposure to asbestos have a marked increase in lung cancer incidence (10- to 92-fold) compared with the unexposed nonsmoking population." Neither author reports a requirement for underlying asbestosis.

OSHA[15] (p. 22616) cites Selikoff, Hammond, and others: "Here asbestos exposure greatly multiplied the already high risk that would have been present with cigarette smoking alone ..." There is no indication that OSHA required underlying asbestosis. Rather, OSHA states: "Asbestos exposure acts synergistically with cigarette smoking to multiply the risk of developing lung cancer."

A joint committee between NIOSH and the pneumoconiosis panel of the American College of Pathologists issued a statement on the pathology of asbestos-related disease in 1982 in which they recognized the synergistic effect between asbestos exposure and cigarette smoking, stating that the risk of lung cancer was increased "greater than fifty-fold in asbestos workers who smoked compared with nonsmokers who lacked exposure to asbestos."[64]

Because of all independent variables relating asbestos and cigarette smoking, a precise formula for risk and apportionment is difficult. The ACCP could not reach a consensus as to whether or not "a reasonable scheme can be developed to apportion the individual attributability of smoking and exposure in a cigarette smoking asbestos exposed worker with lung cancer."[4]

In 2004, the ATS[65] warned of the risk of the interaction between smoking and asbestos exposure in the causation of lung cancer but did not quantify the risk. Smoking cessation was encouraged.

13.4.4.3 Guidelines for Attribution of Causation of Lung Cancer

The following represents my (G.K.F.) opinions and may prove helpful in assessing the role of asbestos as a carcinogen in the causation of the major cell types of lung cancer (squamous cell, adenocarcinoma, small cell, large cell undifferentiated carcinoma, and mixed tumors of the above cell types). The following also assumes a 15-year or greater latency unless there is compelling evidence of unusually heavy exposure.

- If clinical or pathologic asbestosis is present, lung cancer is attributed to asbestos.
- If diffuse pleural thickening (as defined by ILO 2000 Revised) caused by asbestos is present, lung cancer is attributed to asbestos (Helsinki Criteria).
- If there is radiographic or HRCT evidence of bilateral pleural plaques, lung cancer is attributed to asbestos when a significant supportive asbestos exposure history is documented.
- In the absence of objective clinical evidence of asbestos exposure and if adequate pathology is not available for review, if a history of cumulative asbestos exposure of 25 fiber-years or greater can be documented, then lung cancer is attributed to asbestos.
- If there is no evidence of asbestosis, but the patient has a significant occupational history of asbestos exposure, and asbestosis is recognized among coworkers with similar exposures, lung cancer can be attributed to asbestos.[4]
- If there is no evidence of asbestosis, but there is pathologic evidence of findings of asbestos bodies or a fiber burden sufficient to cause asbestosis, lung cancer can be attributed to asbestos.
- If adequate pathologic material is available which fails to show evidence of asbestos-related pathology, a significant asbestos body, or fiber burden, attribution of the cancer to asbestos cannot be given regardless of exposure history. In rare cases, asbestos bodies may not be seen, but asbestos fibers may be found in very high concentration. Dodson et al.[66] reported tissue samples from 12 asbestos workers. Digested samples from two workers demonstrated no ferruginous bodies on light microscopy but contained 780,000 and 1.2 million uncoated amphibole fibers per gram.
- If the patient is a lifetime nonsmoker and no other carcinogenic exposures are identified, and if a significant history of asbestos exposure can be documented, attribution may be possible based on the level of exposure, latency, and other specifics in the medical history.
- In asbestos-related malignancies, consideration must be given to co-carcinogens based on exposure histories.

13.5 FUTURE RISK OF LUNG CANCER

When confronted with a patient who had significant exposure to asbestos or who had recently been diagnosed with asbestosis, the physician should be prepared to answer questions concerning future risk of cancer. To properly counsel the patient who has asbestos exposure or an asbestos-related nonmalignant disease, the assessment of cancer risk is multidimensional. The physician must take into consideration the level of asbestos exposure, the presence or absence of benign asbestos-related diseases that might help quantify prior exposure, the presence of risk factors from other carcinogens (including smoking), the potential for the synergistic interaction between asbestos and such carcinogens, the patient's age, and other competing risk factors.

13.5.1 Background Risk of Lung Cancer

An "increased risk" of cancer suggests the physician has some knowledge or understanding of the background risk of lung cancer in the absence of asbestos exposure. The lifetime odds of dying of lung cancer are approximately 7.5% for men and 6.25% for women (American Cancer Society). The estimate for new cases of lung cancer during 2009 is 219,440, with 116,090 occurring in men and 103,350 in women. Estimates suggest that tobacco smoking causes or contributes to at least 87% of lung cancer deaths.[67]

13.5.2 Occupations, Asbestos Exposure, and Risk of Lung Cancer and Nonmalignant Disease

Historically, many references cite the study of Selikoff et al.[63] on cancer risk in 17,800 U.S. and Canadian asbestos insulation workers. A group of 9590 cigarette smoking men had 25 lung cancer deaths predicted and 134 observed (relative risk = 5.34). Among a select group of 370 New York–New Jersey insulation workers, there was one lung cancer death among 87 nonsmokers and 41 lung cancer deaths among 283 smokers (relative risk = 12.39). Kleinfeld et al.[68] reported on 152 asbestos workers with more than 15 years exposure before 1965 and found that 10 of 46 deaths were due to lung cancer as compared with the expected 1.43. Selikoff and Lee[69] noted a ratio of observed versus expected deaths with a relative risk of 6.29 for workers in an amosite factory and 3.21 for those working in a chrysotile factory.

In 1982, Nicholson et al.[26] projected mortalities from asbestos-related diseases covering the years 1980–2030. They estimated future cancer projections attributable to prior asbestos exposure for a number of different occupations and industries. They identified fiber contents of various products and potential exposure levels in different occupational settings. They reviewed lengths of employment within the occupations, primary source of asbestos exposures, and estimated indices of relative asbestos exposure between selected occupations and industries. By example, in primary manufacturing, they estimated the average fiber concentration to be 20–40 fiber/mL of air, insulation work 15 fiber/mL, ship building and repair (exclusive of insulators) 2 fiber/mL, and auto maintenance 0.1–0.3 fibers/mL. From these numbers, they determined a relative risk of lung cancer in primary manufacturing to be up to 6.1, among insulators to be 4.8, and among chemical plant and refinery maintenance workers to be 1.5. They did not attribute any increased risk of lung cancer or mesothelioma to automotive maintenance workers.

Minimum employment was 20 years for all industries except automotive maintenance, which was calculated at 10 years because of employee turnover. Comparing the relative risk of lung cancer of other occupations to insulation work after 25 years of employment, it was revealed that shipbuilders and repair workers (except insulators) had half the risk, and the construction trade (except insulators) had between 0.15 and 0.25 the risk of lung cancer experienced by insulators. Auto maintenance workers had a 0.04 relative risk of malignancy compared with insulators. These opinions were based on the prevalence of nonmalignant chest radiographic abnormalities among these populations when studied. Specific occupations within the industries may exhibit levels of risk differing from the industry as a whole.

Miller et al.[70] compared insulators and sheet metal workers (a trade recognized as having substantial risk of asbestos exposure), observing that the incidence of radiographic findings of sheet metal workers with asbestosis was only 29% that of insulators. Their risk of pleural disease was less than half that of insulators. They concluded that despite having similar age, duration of exposure, and smoking histories, the sheet metal workers had less severe radiographic findings, which were "consistent with a less intense exposure to asbestos as may be expected from the nature of their work compared with insulators."

Koskinen et al.[71] conducted a study of asbestos-induced occupational diseases in Finland between 1990 and 2000 for the Finnish Institute of Occupational Health. They analyzed specific occupations with descriptions of actual job duties and created an expert evaluated cumulative asbestos exposure index. Radiographic abnormalities of asbestosis as indicators of asbestos-related cancer risk among construction workers were evaluated. Different weights were assigned to asbestos exposure occurring before 1976 and after 1977. Likewise, different scores were assigned for levels of asbestos exposure to different trades. Of 16,696 male Finnish construction workers, 249 cases of lung cancer were observed. Of the lung cancers, 150 had pleural plaques and 32 had an ILO profusion of 1/0 or greater. A dose–response relationship was documented on the basis of the cumulative exposure index. Using a univariate analysis, insulators had a relative risk of 5, plumbers 2.4, and electricians 1.8. A strong relationship between an asbestos exposure index and malignancy was observed. Koskinen et al.[71] opined that pleural plaques alone did not identify a group with an elevated risk of lung cancer, whereas lung fibrosis, category 1/0 or higher, identified a twofold risk and the expert evaluated cumulative exposure index imparted a threefold relative risk of lung cancer.

In 1990, Seidman and Selikoff[72] reported a reduction in mortality associated with diminished occupational exposure and observed a decline in death rates among insulators in recent years. There is a decline in the risk of development of lung cancer approximately 40 years after first asbestos exposure.[73]

13.5.3 Presence of Nonmalignant Respiratory Disease

The relationship between pleural plaque and risk of lung cancer is discussed in Chapter 12. It is widely accepted that when asbestosis is present, the risk of lung cancer is significantly increased. In 1965, Buchanan[74] performed a study for the medical branch of Her Majesty's Inspectorate of Factories of the Ministry of Labor. The study involved workers previously diagnosed with asbestosis and who had expired before 1964. More than 50% of men with asbestosis who died between 1961 and 1963 also had an intrathoracic neoplasm as found in 42 of 77 patients with asbestosis, 4 of which were recorded as mesothelioma. However, lesser death rates were recorded during other time periods.

Berry[75] reviewed workers registered with a British pneumoconiosis panel between 1952 and 1976 as having been certified as suffering from asbestosis. Of 665 men, 283 died (39% from lung cancer and 9% from mesothelioma). The SMR for lung cancer was 9.1. The incidence of lung cancer was related to the severity of the underlying asbestosis at the time of initial reporting as measured by percentage disability. It should be noted that these studies are of historic interest, demonstrating the carcinogenicity of asbestos with exposure levels prevalent during the time of the above cohorts' employment.

The studies that have been performed in more recent years reflect the effects of reductions of exposure to asbestos that occurred in the 1970s and may be more appropriate for many patients with recently diagnosed asbestosis. Hillerdal[76] studied 1596 men with pleural plaques from 1963 through 1985. The relative risk for lung cancer among individuals with pleural plaques and asbestosis (when adjusted for smoking) was 2.3, whereas those who only had plaques had a relative risk of 1.4.

A recent report from Poland[77] assessed the risk of asbestos-related malignancies in 907 men and 490 women previously diagnosed with asbestosis between 1970 and 1997 and followed through December 1999. Of the 300 male deaths, 39 were attributed to lung cancer (13%). Szeszenia-Dabrowska et al.[77] opined that increased risk of lung cancer and mesothelioma occurred in persons exposed to a dose more than 25 fiber-year/mL. Men had an SMR of 168 for lung cancer, whereas women had an SMR of 621. In addition to lung cancer, mesothelioma was found in three men and three women.

Oksa et al.[78] reported radiographic progression of asbestosis as a predictor for the development of lung cancer. They studied 85 patients with asbestosis who were followed radiographically between 1978 and 1987. Those who progressed in one major or two minor ILO categories were identified as having progressive disease. Of 24 men with radiographically progressive small opacities, 11 (46%) developed lung cancer. Five (9%) of 54 men without progression developed lung cancer. The SIR for lung cancer was 37 (95% CI = 18–66) for the progressors and 4.3 (95% CI = 1.4–9.9) for the nonprogressors. Oksa et al.[78] concluded that progression of pulmonary fibrosis might be an independent risk factor for lung cancer risk in addition to smoking history and intensity of asbestos exposure.

Hughes and Weill[30] performed a prospective mortality study on 839 men employed in manufacturing asbestos cement products in 1969 and followed through 1983. Workers were studied for lung cancer risk in relation to radiographic evidence of pulmonary fibrosis, controlling for age, smoking, and asbestos exposure. Twenty or more years after hire, no excess cancer was found among those without radiographically detectable pulmonary fibrosis. Workers with a 1/0 or greater profusion had an SMR of 3.6.

The age of the patient is important in considering future cancer risk. An individual at age 50 years has a far greater period at risk for developing a future malignancy than does an individual at age 80 years. Also, the length of time since initial exposure is important as there is some reduced risk of lung cancer 40 years after exposure. Competing risks for mortality are important. For example, an individual with asbestosis who also has hypertension, diabetes, a prior history of coronary artery disease, and/or cerebrovascular disease is less likely to die from a future lung cancer than is a patient with asbestosis of similar age who lacks any such competing factors. Prostate cancer and other non-asbestos-related malignancies likewise pose significant competing risk in an elderly population.

13.6 MALIGNANT MESOTHELIOMA

Malignant mesothelioma is a rare malignancy arising from the serosal surface. The most common origin is from the pleura followed by peritoneal mesothelioma and rarely from the pericardial surface or the tunica vaginalis. The association between asbestos exposure and occurrence of mesothelioma is so well established that the finding of a pleural mesothelioma may act as a "sentinel tumor" or as a "signal malignancy" serving as an epidemiologic marker for asbestos exposure.

Dail and Hammar[79] reviewed the association between asbestos exposure and incidence of mesothelioma. They cited 14 studies where the incidence of asbestos exposure ranged from 13% of cases to 100%. In 11 of 14 studies, more than 50% of the mesothelioma cases had asbestos exposure. The Helsinki consensus report[20] states that asbestos exposure can be identified in approximately 80% of mesotheliomas. The incidence of mesothelioma in women is approximately one to two per million, which some suggest may reflect the background risk of the tumor. However, it is probable that some cases represent household exposure or other nonoccupational exposure to asbestos. In men, the incidence has varied from 0.65 per million[80] to 17 per million. The difference in incidence of occurrence between men and women is largely attributable to the male dominance in occupations where asbestos exposure is most likely to occur.

The number of mesotheliomas reported annually has been increasing. Possible explanations include the following:

(1) True increase in incidence due to length of latency from heavy exposures in the remote past;
(2) Improvement in immunohistochemical and other pathologic techniques resulting in increased recognition of the disease; and
(3) Increased awareness of the public and physicians due to litigation and articles published in the peer-reviewed literature and the media.

13.6.1 Latency

Although mesotheliomas have been reported in an isolated number of pediatric cases, its occurrence in individuals younger than 50 years is rare. The latency for mesothelioma, although rarely as short as 15 years, usually exceeds 30–40 years. The occurrence of mesothelioma with latencies of less than 15 years and some cases reported in young females raises the possibility of deciduoid mesothelioma, multicystic mesothelioma, and well-differentiated papillary epithelial mesothelioma of the peritoneum, which have been reported in the absence of asbestos exposure.

13.6.2 Risk Factors for Mesothelioma

The risk factors for mesothelioma are listed in Table 13.5. There is a dose–response relationship that is linear with no threshold. For crocidolite, it has been stated that the threshold must be less than 0.015 fiber-years.[81] The risk increases exponentially with time. Thus, time may be a more crucial factor than dose. It is recognized that amphiboles are more carcinogenic than chrysotile in the causation of mesothelioma. Among the amphiboles, crocidolite is more carcinogenic than amosite. There is evidence that the carcinogenicity of some chrysotile may, in part, be due to a component of tremolite, which has been found in commercial chrysotile.

13.6.3 Pleural Mesothelioma—Clinical Manifestations

Mesothelioma typically presents with symptoms of chest pain, shortness of breath, and/or a pleural effusion.[82] The effusion may be sanguineous and have a high protein content. The diagnosis may be difficult to establish and reliance upon cytology, fine needle aspiration biopsy, and Tru-Cut needle biopsy specimens may be fraught with difficulty.[83] The tumor grows in a contiguous fashion along the pleural surface, encapsulating the lung and resulting in reduced lung volume. Involvement of the mediastinum and pericardium is common and may result in pericardial effusion, extrinsic compression of the esophagus, and compromise of other mediastinal structures.

Patients with mesothelioma often experience marked weight loss, fever, sweating, cachexia, and hypoxia. The pain associated with mesothelioma may be severe and unrelenting, requiring significant amounts of analgesics, including narcotics. Although the growth of mesothelioma is usually contiguous, it may exhibit metastatic spread and may grow through the diaphragm to involve the liver or peritoneum. Conversely, peritoneal mesotheliomas may penetrate upward through the diaphragm causing pleural effusion.

13.6.4 Prognosis

The prognosis for mesothelioma (both pleural and peritoneal) is grim, and life expectancy for pleural mesothelioma is typically 9–18 months from the time of presentation with symptoms. Ribak

---

Table 13.5   Asbestos Exposure and Mesothelioma

- Eighty percent of pleural mesotheliomas have identifiable asbestos exposure.
- Latency: risk increases exponentially with elapsed time since first exposure.
- Dose–response relationship: linear.
- Fiber type: amphiboles are substantially more carcinogenic than chrysotile for mesothelioma.
- Location: peritoneal mesotheliomas are usually the result of lengthy high-dose exposures to amphiboles. However, the highest incidence of peritoneal mesotheliomas occurs in insulators who had high exposures to both amphiboles and chrysotile.
- Histologic characteristics: deciduoid, multicystic, and well-differentiated papillary epithelial mesotheliomas have been reported in the absence of asbestos exposure in a significant number of cases in young females.

and Selikoff[84] reported a mean of 11.4 months from presentation until death for pleural mesothelioma and 7.4 months for peritoneal mesothelioma in 457 consecutive fatal cases of mesothelioma in asbestos insulation workers.

13.6.5 Chest X-Ray in Mesothelioma

Chest radiographic findings in cases of mesothelioma may begin with a unilateral pleural effusion, minimal nonspecific pleural thickening, or blunting of the costophrenic angle. The initial finding is often described as a pleural-based density or pleural-based mass (Figure 13.2). As the disease progresses, the chest radiograph typically shows marked pleural thickening, which may begin anywhere along the pleural surface (including mediastinum) and in some cases may extend circumferentially resulting in compression and areas of atelectasis. The pleura typically has an irregular or nodular surface and is sometimes described as having a "lumpy-bumpy" appearance (Figure 13.3). As the disease progresses, there is volume loss. Opacification of a hemithorax may occur as a result of either pleural effusion or tumor growth complicated by atelectasis or underlying pneumonia. Radiographic pleural plaques or asbestosis may be seen on x-ray or CT scan but are not mandatory for diagnosis.

13.6.6 Laboratory: Hematologic Abnormalities

Increased incidence of thrombocytosis has been reported in association with mesothelioma. Although the pathogenesis is unclear, in approximately 25% of cases tumor cells produced large amounts of interleukin-6.[85] Tumors may secrete small amounts of granulocyte macrophage colony stimulating factor.[86] Leukocytosis may develop. Yoshimoto et al.[86] reported a case in which the white count increased from 8600 to 53,600 (93% neutrophils) within 17 months. C-reactive protein was also elevated. Granulocyte macrophage colony stimulating factor had increased to 36.0 pg/dL (normal less than 5.0 pg/dL). Interleukin-6 had risen to 197 pg/dL with normal less than 4.0 pg/dL. The patient suffered from a malignant pleural mesothelioma, and tumor cells were positive for the

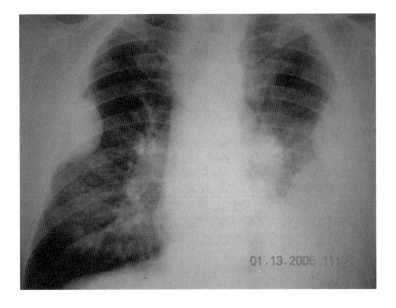

Figure 13.2 Malignant mesothelioma with bilateral pleural-based masses.

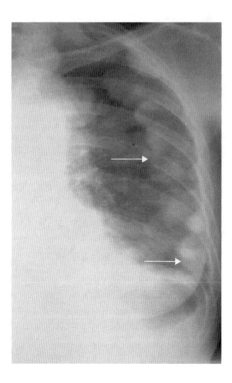

Figure 13.3   "Lumpy-bumpy" appearance of mesothelioma.

above factors as well as other cytokines. Thrombocytosis appears to be a common occurrence in peritoneal mesothelioma.[87]

Anemia is commonly observed in cases of malignant mesothelioma. Selleslag et al.[88] reported a Coombs positive autoimmune hemolytic anemia associated with malignant peritoneal mesothelioma in two case reports. Red blood cells were found coated with IgG and C3D. Selleslag et al.[88] opined that a guanidine-type mechanism of hemolysis could be responsible for the Coombs positive hemolytic anemia. Anemia of chronic disease in the absence of iron deficiency or evidence of marrow metastatic disease may occur. Finally, anemia is a frequent complication of chemotherapeutic agents that typically have little success in the treatment of this disease.

13.6.7 Diagnosis of Pleural Mesothelioma

The diagnosis of pleural mesothelioma requires pathologic confirmation. The pathologic distinction between mesothelioma and lung cancer (especially adenocarcinoma) metastatic to the pleura may be difficult and requires the use of immunohistochemical staining and, rarely, electron microscopic evaluation. The U.S.–Canadian Mesothelioma Panel[83] stresses the importance of being familiar with the gross features of the tumor either as seen radiographically or as described by the surgeon. Because small pleural biopsies and cytology may be misleading, specimens obtained by video-assisted thoracoscopic surgery or thoracotomy provide a more reliable diagnosis. At the time of surgery, the surgeon often describes extensive pleural thickening or studding of the visceral and parietal pleura by tumor. Tumor invasion of parietal and visceral pleura may make dissection of the lung from the chest wall virtually impossible. In some cases, diagnosis may not be made until autopsy.

Care must be taken in distinguishing benign pleural reactions from mesothelioma.[89] Many immunohistochemical stains are of little value in distinguishing benign from malignant processes.

This is especially true in differentiating reactive mesothelial hyperplasia from invasive epithelial mesothelioma and desmoplastic mesothelioma from fibrosing pleuritis. Here, a pathologist's familiarity with mesothelioma may be essential in making the distinction. Documentation of tumor invasion is the most important pathologic feature separating benign from malignant processes. Further complicating this issue is the fact that mesothelioma may present with a variety of pathologic patterns. Dail and Hammar[79,90] discuss the spectrum of benign and malignant pleural diseases and identify the various pathologic presentations of mesothelioma and the difficulties in differentiating pseudomesotheliomatous carcinoma from mesothelioma.

13.7 PERITONEAL MESOTHELIOMA

Peritoneal mesothelioma arises from the serosal surface of the abdomen. It is an extremely rare tumor, representing approximately 10%–20% of all mesotheliomas, and the diagnosis requires pathologic confirmation. Sugarbaker et al.[91] reported 51 patients with peritoneal mesothelioma whom they had treated. Typical presenting symptoms include abdominal pain or distention either with ascites or tumor mass. Fever may be present in some cases.[87] Because the tumor involves the serosal surface of the abdominal cavity, gastroesophagoscopy, colonoscopy, and contrast studies are normal/nondiagnostic. CT scan may be of benefit in visualizing the extraluminal tumor. Often, the diagnosis is not made until the patient develops ascites, bowel obstruction, palpable abdominal mass, or other sequelae of the tumor. At that time, laparoscopy or laparotomy is performed, and the diagnosis is rendered. In women, clinically distinguishing mesothelioma from ovarian carcinoma and certain other tumors of gynecologic origin may be difficult.

13.7.1 Asbestos Fibers and Peritoneal Mesothelioma

The fact that asbestos fibers can be recovered from the omentum and mesentery has been reported by Dodson et al.[92] Twenty individuals with mesothelioma had tissue from lung, omentum, and mesentery analyzed for asbestos bodies/fibers. Uncoated fibers were found in the lungs of 19, of which 17 had fibers in at least one extrapulmonary site. Dodson et al.[92] found amosite to be the most common fiber type and stated that fibers in the peritoneum could be predicted on the basis of the type and concentration of fibers in the lung.

Peritoneal mesotheliomas are typically associated with lengthy exposures to amphiboles. Because peritoneal mesotheliomas are associated with high cumulative levels of amphibole exposure, they are more frequently accompanied by pleural plaques and pulmonary asbestosis than are pleural mesotheliomas. Although there is little proof that chrysotile causes peritoneal mesothelioma, there are several case reports suggesting chrysotile can cause peritoneal mesothelioma. Mancuso et al.[93] reported four peritoneal mesotheliomas occurring in workers in the manufacture of brake linings. Godwin and Jagatic[94] reported a similar case of peritoneal mesothelioma in a man who worked as a young adult for 3 years with brake linings made from chrysotile. Dement et al.[95] reported one peritoneal mesothelioma in a chrysotile textile production worker. Morinaga et al.[96] reported a peritoneal mesothelioma in a 54-year-old design engineer whose lung tissue contained only chrysotile asbestos. Oury et al.[97] reported asbestos content of lung tissue in patients with malignant peritoneal mesothelioma in a study of 40 cases. Of 36 men and 4 women, 18 had histologically confirmed asbestosis and 21 of 33 had pleural plaques (unknown in seven cases). The vast majority of fibers were commercial amphiboles. Chrysotile was present at levels above background in only one case.

Welch et al.[98] examined 40 cases of primary peritoneal mesothelioma in which 30 patients had attended college. There was an OR of 6.6 for asbestos exposure among this group of primary peritoneal mesothelioma cases with relatively slight asbestos exposure. Light microscopy and histochemical staining were performed on all cases to confirm the diagnosis of mesothelioma. The cases were matched to controls by sex and age within 2 years. Patients or next of kin were interviewed. The report focused on 24 male peritoneal mesothelioma cases. The group had a relative mean age of 53 years. Welch et al.[98] cautioned that their case series was not a cohort; however, an excess risk for asbestos exposure among those peritoneal mesothelioma cases was consistent with the hypothesis that peritoneal cancers occur in less highly exposed groups than had previously been reported. A review of the asbestos exposures suggests that 21 (88%) of the 24 cases had been involved in at least one of nine activities where there was potentially heavy asbestos exposure. A numerical scoring of asbestos exposure used by the authors may have some limitations and result in imprecision of exposure estimates.

Peritoneal mesothelioma in individuals younger than 40 years requires careful pathologic review to determine whether the tumor represents multicystic mesothelioma, well-differentiated papillary mesothelioma, or deciduoid mesothelioma, which have been reported to occur in the absence of asbestos exposure. Pancreatic cancer, ovarian cancer, and other intraperitoneal extraluminal cancers should be excluded through appropriate pathologic evaluation.

13.7.2 Household, Familial, and Environmental Exposure

Mesothelioma may occur with low levels of asbestos exposure (Figure 13.4). Nonoccupational sources of asbestos exposure have been reported among household contacts, from environmental pollution, and from community contamination. In 1965, Newhouse and Thompson[99] reported 76 cases of mesothelioma in the London area. Nine of these occurred as household contacts of family members, and there were 11 cases whose only known source of exposure was living within half a mile of an asbestos factory. In 1978, Chen and Mottet[100] reported malignant mesothelioma in a 50-year-old executive with minimal asbestos exposure. They used energy dispersive x-ray analysis to confirm the presence of asbestos bodies and fibers. A case of pleural mesothelioma in a 56-year-old computer executive whose only known asbestos exposure was cutting crocidolite gaskets during a summer job in high school was recently evaluated.[101] All other potential sources of occupational,

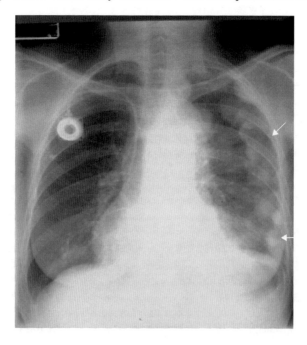

Figure 13.4   Malignant mesothelioma in the wife of an insulator (household contact).

environmental, and household exposures were eliminated. Despite the limited exposure history, high levels of crocidolite fibers and asbestos bodies were confirmed on fiber analysis of a pneumonectomy specimen.

In 1976, Anderson et al.[102] reviewed the literature from nine countries and reported a series of 37 cases of mesothelioma attributed to household exposure. In 1979, Anderson et al.[103] studied radiologic findings in 326 household contacts of asbestos workers and found that 16% had only pleural changes, 11% had parenchymal fibrosis of low profusion, and 8% had combined pleural and parenchymal change. Anderson suggested that nonmalignant asbestos-related findings observed on x-ray might provide supportive information for appearance of malignant disease among household contacts. In 1980, Epler et al.[104] reported four individuals with asbestos-related disease attributed to household exposure. Three had benign pleural disease and one developed malignant pleural mesothelioma. In 1978, Vianna and Polan[105] studied a series of 52 female New York State residents who developed mesothelioma between the years 1966 and 1977. When compared with controls, they found a 10-fold increased risk of mesothelioma in those with household exposure to asbestos. Occupational histories revealed that six patients might have had occupational exposure to asbestos. The majority of household contacts worked as insulators and all female patients had routinely hand-laundered their fathers' and husbands' clothing.

Dodson et al.[106] studied the asbestos burden in women with mesothelioma using autopsy material in 15 women with a pathologic diagnosis of mesothelioma. Exposures ranged from direct exposure to asbestos-containing products to household exposure (paraoccupational exposure) from contaminated work clothing. Two of 15 women had confirmed asbestosis. Seven had more than 1000 ferruginous bodies per gram of dry weight, whereas no ferruginous bodies were found in two. Analysis of the ferruginous bodies confirmed that 55 contained an amosite core whereas 4 had crocidolite and 3 had tremolite. The ratio of asbestos fibers to ferruginous bodies demonstrated great variability ranging from 19:1 to 2686:1. Dodson compared these 15 females to a group of 55 males with mesothelioma whom he had studied. Fourteen female cases had asbestos burdens that fell in the lower one-third of the male concentrations for asbestos bodies and uncoated asbestos fibers.

Roggli et al.[107] reported on malignant mesothelioma in women noting that 86% had pleural mesothelioma. Pleural plaques were found in half of the women for whom that information was available. Asbestosis was found in 16%. Over half had household contact with asbestos workers, whereas 19% had occupational exposure. In those women for whom fiber analysis was available, 70% demonstrated increased asbestos burden with the primary fiber type being amosite followed by tremolite and chrysotile.

Although mesothelioma may occur at low levels of exposure, dose–response relationships have been documented, and those with the highest levels of exposure have the greatest increased risk of disease.[108]

Questions concerning genetic predisposition to development of mesothelioma have been raised. Hammar et al.[109] reported two families with familial mesothelioma and cited five reports from the literature of familial mesothelioma occurring in two or more family members. Hammar reported on three brothers who worked with asbestos insulation and developed mesothelioma. He also reported on a father who was occupationally exposed to asbestos and died of peritoneal mesothelioma and whose son later died from the identical histologic type of peritoneal mesothelioma (tubulopapillary). In 1978, Li et al.[110] reported on familial mesothelioma in which a father who installed asbestos insulation in shipyards developed asbestosis and lung cancer. His wife, who hand-washed his clothing, developed mesothelioma at the age of 50 years and his daughter developed mesothelioma at the age of 34 years.

There are multiple references within the literature to mesothelioma arising from environmental exposure among inhabitants living near asbestos mines, asbestos manufacturing plants, shipyards, and similar industries. Magnani et al.[111] opined that household exposure to asbestos or exposure from significant levels of environmental exposure carries a measurable risk of malignant pleural mesothelioma.

The Helsinki Criteria Consensus Group identifies environmental and household exposure as recognized causes of mesothelioma.

13.7.3 Asbestos in Schools and Mesothelioma in Young Adults

The risk of asbestos exposure in schools was widely debated in the 1980s. In 1987, the Committee on Environmental Hazards for the American Academy of Pediatrics[112] reported that mesothelioma risk is proportional to a power of time since first exposure. Such risk significantly increases when time since first exposure exceeds 40 years. Therefore, the committee expressed concerns about early childhood exposures and cited an EPA risk estimate that between 100 and 7000 excess deaths were anticipated to occur as a result of exposure to asbestos in schools over a 30-year period (1980–2010). They stated: "the most reasonable estimate is approximately 1000 premature deaths." It was opined that 90% of those deaths were expected to occur among persons exposed to asbestos as school children. The Asbestos Health Emergency Response Act became federal law requiring schools to conduct inspections in May 1988 and implement management plans for removal or abatement of asbestos by July 1989.[113] At least three other risk assessment studies provided evidence that a major health threat was not present in building exposure.[113]

The occurrence of mesothelioma in pediatric patients and young adults raises special questions concerning latency and causation. McDonald et al.[114] described 115 men and 13 women who were 50 years or younger and who were diagnosed with malignant mesothelioma. Occupational histories were obtained and related to lung tissue concentration of asbestos fiber by type. McDonald et al.[114] found that the predominant occupations were carpenters, plumbers, electricians, and insulators in the construction industry and that the mesotheliomas were predominantly attributable to amphibole exposure.

Mesotheliomas in children are so rare they are usually presented as case reports. Brenner et al.[115] from the Memorial Sloan-Kettering Cancer Center reported seven cases of pediatric mesothelioma and conducted a review of the literature identifying 49 cases of malignant mesothelioma that had been reported by 1981. Of 148 patients with mesothelioma seen between 1950 and 1980, only 7 (5%) were younger than 20 years.

13.8 TREATMENT

Multiple modalities of therapy have been attempted for both pleural and peritoneal mesotheliomas. Although some recent chemotherapeutic advances appeared promising, they have only extended life expectancy by a few months and have had no significant effect on mortality. Radiation may provide palliative relief when there is intercostal nerve and bone involvement but is not a curative measure. It may extend survival when selectively applied in combination with surgery.

Extrapleural pneumonectomy (EPP) is an aggressive surgical procedure that typically involves removal of the involved lung, parietal pleura, portions of the chest wall, pericardium, and diaphragm requiring reconstruction. Although there have been reports of success with this procedure,[116] the surgery is extensive and the probability of cure is low. Sugarbaker et al.[117] described the prevention and management of complications they observed in 496 patients treated with EPP. In a subset of 328 patients, 198 (60.4%) experienced major or minor postoperative complications. A postoperative mortality rate of 3.4% was noted. This group of patients had a median age of 58 years. Treasure and Sedrakyan[118] raised questions concerning the effectiveness of this approach and cautioned to avoid "futile and distressing treatment."

Trimodality therapy with radiation, chemotherapy, and surgery has been advocated. With the exception of the occasional case report, there is little convincing evidence of long-term success. Weder et al.[119] reported 19 patients who preoperatively were considered to be "completely resectable" and underwent complete EPP including pericardium and diaphragm. Neoadjuvant chemotherapy with gemcitabine and cisplatin was given. EPP was performed on 16 patients, with major surgical complications occurring in 6 patients. Thirteen received postoperative radiotherapy. The median survival was 23 months.

Janne and Baldini[120] reported a 45% 5-year survival rate for patients with "early stage" disease with epithelial histology and absence of mediastinal nodal involvement who were treated with EPP. They noted that, unfortunately, most patients presented with more advanced disease and optimum treatment had yet to be defined. They stated that adjuvant therapy with radiation, intrapleural and intravenous chemotherapy, and brachytherapy failed to show consistent benefit. New approaches with radiation and chemotherapy including heated intrapleural cisplatin were discussed.

Chang and Sugarbaker[121] investigated intraoperative, intracavitary chemotherapy with high-dose cisplatin. Pistolesi and Rusthoven[122] published a review on current knowledge and recent discoveries in malignant pleural mesothelioma. They cited various new markers such as folic acid receptor alpha, cyclooxygenase 2, and others suggesting a potential avenue for new therapeutic approaches. To date, the value of these markers remains unproven.

In 2007, Rice et al.[123] at the M.D. Anderson Cancer Center reported their experiences for outcomes after EPP and intensity-modulated radiation therapy (IMRT). They studied 100 consecutive patients undergoing EPP. Sixty-three patients received IMRT. Chemotherapy was not routinely administered. One-third of patients were nonepithelioid. Perioperative mortality was 8%, and median overall survival was 10.2 months. For those receiving IMRT, the median overall and 3-year survival was 14.2 months and 20%. Of those patients who had negative lymph nodes at the time of surgery and had epithelioid histology ($N = 18$), they had a median and a 3-year survival of 28 months and 41%. Although IMRT provided good local control for malignant pleural mesothelioma, distant metastases remained a significant problem and limited survival. Rice et al.[123] concluded that the study provided a strong rationale for combining aggressive local regimens with systemic therapy.

The complications of these treatment modalities are well known. It is my opinion that quality of life is more important than extending life a few months while the patient experiences not only the consequences of their disease but also the iatrogenic complications of our well-intended attempts to render treatment. In most cases, only palliative treatment and supportive care are recommended. In the case where early and localized disease can be documented after thorough staging workup, I recommend referral to a cancer center with experience in treating these cases.

13.9 OTHER ASBESTOS-RELATED CANCERS

Although the strongest associations between asbestos exposure and cancer risk have been established for lung cancer and malignant mesothelioma, asbestos fibers have been documented in other organs, and epidemiologic studies have reported increased risk for extrathoracic cancers after asbestos exposure. In 2006, a committee of the IOM reviewed evidence relevant to causation of cancers of the pharynx, larynx, esophagus, colon, and rectum for the purpose of determining whether there was sufficient evidence to infer a causal association with asbestos exposure. The five specified sites were drawn directly from proposed Senate Bill No. 852, The Fairness in Asbestos Injury Resolution (FAIR Act), the purpose of which was to establish a $140 billion asbestos trust fund.[6]

The IOM had four levels for classifying the strength of evidence for causal inference: sufficient, suggestive, inadequate, or suggestive of no causal association. To attribute causation, the committee required evidence to reach the level of sufficient.[6] The IOM found sufficient evidence to infer a causal relationship for laryngeal cancer and to be "suggestive" for pharyngeal, stomach, and colorectal cancers. Some authors have reported stronger associations between asbestos exposure and malignancy for some of these organs, whereas others have found the results inconclusive.

In addition to the above organ systems, asbestos exposure has been reported by some authors to cause increased risk for developing renal carcinoma.

13.9.1 Gastrointestinal Cancers

Kolonel et al.[124] reported a doubling of the risk of gastrointestinal cancer (SMR = 2.2, 95% CI = 1.1–4.0) in Pearl Harbor Naval shipyard workers with greater than 30 years latency and less than 15 years exposure. This may have been an aberration as those with greater than 15 years exposure and 30+ years latency did not show a similar increase. Sanden et al.[125] reported an OR of 2.3 for lung cancer and 1.4 for gastrointestinal cancer in 365 deceased shipyard workers who reportedly had "heavy asbestos exposure."

Increased risk of gastrointestinal malignancy was noted by Selikoff et al.[126] during the course of their study of heat, frost, and insulation workers. Selikoff et al.[126] reported 29 deaths from cancer of the gastrointestinal tract with 9.7 expected. They noted there were 17 deaths from cancer of the colon and rectum compared with 5.2 expected.

Becklake, in her 1976 state-of-the-art article on asbestos-related diseases,[5] noted that lung cancer showed the greatest relative risk followed by cancers of the gastrointestinal tract: "The excess of gastrointestinal cancers is evident in all series whatever the reference population used to calculate expected numbers of death with one exception, namely workers exposed to Anthophyllite mining" (p. 214). Dr. Becklake further stated that by 1976 the pathologic effect of asbestos exposure in man, including neoplasms of the gastrointestinal tract, was "established" (p. 189).[5]

In 1986, OSHA[15] determined that there was an increased risk of esophageal, stomach, colorectal, kidney, and other cancers and instructed physicians to include the gastrointestinal system in their asbestos surveillance physical examinations. Currently, OSHA regulation 1926.1101(M)(2) for medical examinations and consultations as part of mandated surveillance requires a medical and work history with special emphasis including the gastrointestinal system. OSHA concluded in the 1986 Final Rules and Regulations for Asbestos[15] (p. 22620) that after reviewing 12 epidemiologic studies of a variety of occupational cohorts exposed to asbestos, an excess mortality from gastrointestinal cancers was found. Seven of ten studies found statistically significant excesses and OSHA concluded the findings "constitutes substantial evidence of an association between asbestos exposure and a risk of incurring gastrointestinal cancer." Accordingly, OSHA included gastrointestinal malignancies in formulating its risk assessments.

Hillerdal[127] investigated whether a population of patients with gastrointestinal carcinoma had an increased incidence of pleural plaque on chest radiograph compared with a control group. Such plaques were seen in 3.4% of tumor patients and only 1.7% of controls. This doubling of risk was felt to be significant. In his study, plaques were most commonly found in patients with carcinoma of the stomach. Hillerdal noted his findings were in accord with "many other reports" in which exposure to asbestos had been linked to approximately double the risk of gastrointestinal malignancy.

Morgan and Seaton[128] reported that gastrointestinal malignancies were a frequent cause of death in asbestos-exposed populations. Finkelstein[129] reported an SMR of 240 for gastrointestinal cancers. Harber et al.[130] identified malignancies of the larynx, pharynx, lung, kidney, and gastrointestinal tract to be asbestos related.

The EPA, in a supporting document for the final rule on asbestos in school buildings,[131] stated that the hazards of asbestos exposure identified by epidemiologic research included the esophagus, stomach, rectum, larynx, kidney, and so forth.

Vineis et al.[132] studied the association between colon cancer and occupation in the automobile industry and found no association between colon cancer and any job in the automotive industry. However, they did find an excess risk of colon cancer among men in job titles involving putative exposure to asbestos. Pipefitters and boilermakers had an OR of 10.7 with a CI of 1.07–103. However, this was based on only three cases and one control.

Ehrlich et al.[133] reported that epidemiological studies indicated an increased incidence of carcinoma of the colon in asbestos workers. They evaluated colon tissue for asbestos burden by light and electron microscopic analysis in patients with a history of occupational asbestos exposure and colon cancer. Asbestos fibers and/or asbestos bodies were identified in 14 of 44 workers studied. A mean fiber count of 2,517,823 fibers per gram of wet weight was described. No asbestos fibers were found in the colons of 20 controls who had colon cancer but no history of asbestos exposure. In a study of asbestos factory workers in London, Berry et al.[134] reported an excess of colon cancer with 27 observed and 15 expected.

The ACCP Consensus Statement[4] reached an agreement that there is increased risk for cancers other than lung cancer and mesothelioma but does not define the cancers.

The ATS 2004 statement on asbestos[65] initially reported that studies suggested that after asbestos exposure, there may be an elevation in the risk of colon cancer, although this association remains controversial. This opinion was shortly thereafter amended by Guidotti (chairman) and the members of the ATS Committee.[7] Guidotti et al.[7] reported that epidemiologic studies of workers exposed to asbestos were "generally consistent in demonstrating an elevated risk" of colon cancer. To support this opinion, the committee cites Homa et al.,[135] Gerhardsson et al.,[136] and four additional studies that demonstrate a "relatively large and significant relative risk." In addition, the committee cites two authors who disagreed with this position, including Gamble[137] and Morgan et al.[138] In a study by Garabrant et al.,[139] there was stated to be no elevated risk of colon cancer after asbestos exposure. Guidotti et al.[7] felt "the weight of evidence suggests a likely association between asbestos exposure and risk of colon cancer" and recommended screening for same.

One argument against an increased risk of gastrointestinal malignancy after asbestos exposure is the possibility of misdiagnosis of peritoneal mesothelioma for gastrointestinal malignancy. Such an error might overestimate the incidence of primary gastrointestinal malignancy.

In reviewing studies concerning the risk of colon cancer (and gastrointestinal malignancies), it is noted that most studies only identify patients with "asbestos exposure." Studies were not identified where the incidence of colon cancer was limited to those patients with sufficient exposure to cause asbestosis. If the cohort were limited to those patients who suffered from asbestosis, it is reasonable to anticipate that the SMRs might be significantly higher.

Opinion: It is reasonable to attribute colon cancer to asbestos in those patients who also have asbestosis rather than granting attribution to all patients who simply had asbestos exposure regardless of degree. Furthermore, other more probable cause for colon cancer requires exclusion.

13.9.2 Laryngeal Cancer

Laryngeal cancer is a relatively uncommon cancer in the United States. According to the American Cancer Society,[140] approximately 9500 new cases of laryngeal cancer are diagnosed per annum, resulting in 3740 deaths in 2006. Laryngeal cancer includes cancer of the glottis, superglottis and subglottis. It occurs four times more frequently in men than in women, and the risk increases with age. The most common risk factors are the use of tobacco products and alcohol consumption. Exposure to both products frequently occurs in combination. Risk increases with the number of cigarettes smoked and the duration of smoking.[6]

The IOM reports that the combination of tobacco smoking and heavy drinking causes a much larger increase in laryngeal cancer than would be expected from the sum of the relative risk estimates that would occur with separate exposures.

As the gateway to the respiratory tract, the laryngeal structures are among the first impacted by inhalation of asbestos fibers and other inhaled toxins. The relationship between asbestos exposure and cancer of the larynx has been reported in numerous cohort and case–control studies,[6] and several of these studies have documented an SMR of 2.0 or greater.

IARC states that laryngeal cancer has been considered in two case–control studies resulting in risk ratios of 2.4 and 2.3 in shipyard work and unspecified exposure. A risk ratio of 3.2 was reported among chrysotile miners. Two correlation studies also indicated a relationship between asbestos exposure and laryngeal cancer.[141]

In patients with asbestosis, Karjalainen et al.[142] reported that the standardized incidence ratio of mesothelioma had a relative risk of 32 and a lung cancer relative risk of 6.7. The relative risk of laryngeal cancer was 4.2 (with a 95% CI = 1.4–9.8) in men but not women.

The IOM[6] investigated cases with the heaviest exposure by definition and found 11 cohorts in which information was available. In each individual cohort, the relative risk exceeded 1.0, and the aggregate relative risk for laryngeal cancer estimate in the most highly asbestos-exposed subjects was 2.57 (95% CI = 1.47–4.49) for the strongest association reported and 2.02 (95% CI = 1.64–2.47) for the weakest association reported. For those cohorts simply identifying any exposure to asbestos, the relative risk was 1.40 (95% CI = 1.19–1.64). The IOM concluded larger cohort studies "consistently show increased risk of laryngeal cancer in asbestos-exposed workers in a wide array of industries and in a large cohort of workers with asbestosis." The IOM opined that there was some evidence of a dose–response relationship.

After reviewing 35 cohort populations and 18 case–control studies in a wide array of industries and occupations, some of which were controlled for confounding by tobacco smoking and alcohol consumption, the IOM concluded that the evidence was sufficient to infer a causal relationship between asbestos exposure and laryngeal cancer.

The EPA[131] states that hazards of asbestos exposure included cancer of the larynx.

Doll and Peto[143] stated: "On the present evidence, we conclude that asbestos should be regarded as one of the causes of laryngeal cancer." The relative risk, however, is less than that for lung cancer and the absolute risk is much less.

Stell and McGill[144] studied 119 patients with histologically proven squamous carcinoma of the larynx and compared them with a control group without carcinoma of the larynx. A history of asbestos exposure and smoking was obtained from both groups. Of the patients with laryngeal carcinoma, 27.7% had significant exposure to asbestos compared with 2.5% of the control group. The maximum age of onset of the carcinoma in patients with asbestos exposure was a decade less than those who had no history of exposure. There was a greater smoking history among the cancer cases than among the controls.

Newhouse and Berry[145] reported two deaths from laryngeal cancer from a population of 4000 employees in an asbestos textile and cement factory. Only 0.37 deaths were expected. Likewise, there was an increased risk of lung cancer where 56 deaths occurred and only 13 were expected.

Shettigara and Morgan[146] studied 43 pairs of patients with matched controls and reported a substantial association between asbestos exposure and laryngeal cancer.

13.9.2.1 Asbestos Bodies and Laryngeal Cancer

Roggli et al.[147] reported that asbestos exposure had been associated with laryngeal cancer, but no studies had been performed to quantify asbestos fiber content in laryngeal tissue. They studied larynges from five men with proven asbestos-associated disease using tissue digestion. Three had exposure through asbestos pipe insulation and two were from patients with asbestosis, lung cancer, and pleural mesothelioma. All five patients were cigarette smokers, and two had consumed alcohol in moderate amounts. Asbestos bodies were recovered from two of the five larynges and none from 10 autopsy control subjects.

Hirsch et al.[148] found significant concentrations of asbestos fibers in the laryngeal tissue from two patients with a past history of exposure to asbestos and associated asbestosis. One patient had laryngeal carcinoma and the other had a polyp on a vocal cord. Hirsch et al.[148] opined that the findings could provide indication of a local carcinogenic effect of asbestos fibers in laryngeal tissue.

On the basis of all available evidence, I (G.K.F.) concur with the position of the IOM that there is sufficient evidence to render an opinion that asbestos is a cause of laryngeal cancer. However, because high levels of exposure are required, attribution should only be given in those cases where the patient has asbestosis or asbestos-related pleural disease and a history of asbestos exposure similar to that rendered for asbestosis.

Heller et al.[149] recovered asbestos fibers from ovarian tissue and fallopian tubes and stated that the evidence suggested an increased risk of ovarian cancer with asbestos exposure. When studied by analytic electron microscopy, there was 71.4% agreement between the fallopian tube and the ovary for the presence of asbestos. In 2007, Langseth et al.[150] reported an elevated risk of ovarian cancer in Norwegian pulp and paper workers possibly exposed to asbestos in the course of their occupation. Of 46 women diagnosed with ovarian cancer, 2 were found to have asbestos fibers in ovarian tissue after digestion analysis by transmission electron microscopy. Langseth et al.[150] confirmed that asbestos fibers may reach the ovaries but could not draw any firm conclusions about an association between occupational exposure to asbestos and ovarian cancer in this cohort. I (G.K.F.) concur with Langseth's position concerning ovarian cancer.

REFERENCES

1. *IARC Monograph on the Evaluation of Carcinogenic Risks to Humans*, Vol. 14. Asbestos. Lyon, France: IARC; 1977. [Updated 03/26/98].
2. Wagner JC, Sleggs CA, Marchand P. Diffuse pleural mesothelioma and asbestos exposure in the North Western Cape Province. *Br J Ind Med* 1960;17:260–271.
3. Selikoff IJ, Lee DHK. *Asbestos and Disease*. New York: Academic Press Inc.; 1978.
4. Banks, Shi R, McLarty J, Cowl CT, Smith D, Tarlo SM, et al. American College of Chest Physicians consensus statement on the respiratory health effects of asbestos. *Chest* 2009;135:1619–1627.
5. Becklake MR. Asbestos-related diseases of the lung and other organs: The epidemiology and implications for clinical practice. *Am Rev Respir Dis* 1976;114(3):192–227.
6. Institute of Medicine. *Committee on Asbestos: Selected Health Effects*. Washington, DC: National Academy Press; 2006.
7. Guidotti TL, Miller A, Christiani DC, Wagner G, Balmes J, Harber P, et al. Nonmalignant asbestos-related disease: Diagnosis and early management. *Clin Pulm Med* 2007;14(2):82–92.
8. Weiss WS, Tavassori FA. Multicystic mesothelioma. An analysis of pathologic findings and biologic behavior in 37 cases. *Am J Surg Pathol* 1988;12(10):737–746.
9. Attanoos RL, Gibbs AR. Pathology of malignant mesothelioma. *Histopathology* 1997;30(5):403–418.
10. American Cancer Society. Cancer Facts and Figures 2005. Atlanta: American Cancer Society; 2005.
11. Alberg AJ, Samet JM. Epidemiology of lung cancer. *Chest* 2003;123(1):21–49S.
12. Lynch KM, Smith WA. Pulmonary asbestosis III carcinoma of lung in asbestos-silicosis. *Am J Cancer* 1935;24:56–64.
13. Antman K, Eisner J. *Asbestos-Related Malignancy*. Orlando: Gruen and Stratton, Inc.; 1987: 57–59.
14. Doll R. Mortality from lung cancer in asbestos workers. *Br J Ind Med* 1955;12(2):81–86.
15. Federal Register 29 CFR Parts 1910 and 1926: Part II. Occupational exposure to asbestos, tremolite, anthophyllite and actinolite. Final rules. Washington, DC: Occupational Safety and Health Administration, Department of Labor; 1986.
16. Selikoff IJ, Churg J, Hammond EC. Asbestos exposure and neoplasia. *JAMA* 1964;252(1):91–95.
17. McDonald JC. Asbestos and lung cancer: Has the case been proven? *Chest* August 1980;78 (2 Suppl.):374–376.
18. Hill AB. *A Short Textbook of Medical Statistics*. London: Hodder and Stoughton; 1977: 285–296.
19. Churg A. Lung cancer cell type in asbestos exposure. *JAMA* 1985;253(20):2984–2985.
20. Helsinki Consensus Statement. Asbestos, asbestosis, and cancer: The Helsinki Criteria for diagnosis and attribution. *Scand J Work Environ Health* 1997;23(4):311–316.
21. Weill H. Asbestos-associated diseases: Science, public policy, and litigation. *Chest* 1983;84(5): 601–608.

22. Henderson DW, Rodelsperger K, Woitowitz HJ, Leigh J. After Helsinki: A multidisciplinary review of the relationship between asbestos exposure and lung cancer, with emphasis on studies published during 1997–2004. *Pathology* 2004;36:517–550.
23. Weill H. Basis for clinical decision making. *Chest* 1980;78(2):382–383.
24. Hughes JM, Weill H. Asbestos exposure. Quantitative assessment of risk. *Am Rev Respir Dis* 1986;133(1):5–13.
25. American Thoracic Society. The diagnosis of nonmalignant diseases related to asbestos. *Am Rev Respir Dis* 1986;134:363–368.
26. Nicholson WJ, Perkel G, Selikoff IJ. Occupational exposure to asbestos: Population at risk and projected mortality—1980–2030. *Am J Ind Med* 1982;3(3):259–311.
27. McLemore TL, Greenberg SD, Wilson RK, Buffler PA, Roggli VL, Mace M. Update on asbestos-associated pulmonary disease. *Tex Med* 1981;77(6):38–46.
28. Seidman H, Selikoff IJ, Hammond EC. Short term asbestos work and long term observations. *Ann N Y Acad Sci* 1979;330:61–69.
29. Hillerdal G, Henderson DW. Asbestos, asbestosis, pleural plaques and lung cancer. *Scand J Work Environ Health* 1997;23(2):93–103.
30. Hughes JM, Weill H. Asbestosis as a precursor of asbestos-related lung cancer: Results of a prospective mortality study. *Br J Ind Med* 1991;48(4):229–233.
31. Browne K. Is asbestos or asbestosis the cause of the increased risk of lung cancer in asbestos workers? *Br J Ind Med* 1986;43(3):145–149.
32. Henderson DW, DeKlerk NH, Hammar SP, et al. Asbestos-related lung cancer: Is it attributable to asbestosis or to asbestos fiber exposure? In: *Tumors of the Lung: Contemporary Issues*, Corrin B, ed. Edinburgh: Churchill Livingstone; 1997: 83–118.
33. Abraham JL. Asbestos inhalation, not asbestosis, causes lung cancer. *Am J Ind Med* 1994;26(6):839–842.
34. Roggli VL, Hammar SP, Pratt PC, et al. Does asbestos or asbestosis cause carcinoma of the lung? *Am J Ind Med* 1994;26(6):835–838.
35. Becklake M. Asbestos-related disease of the lung and pleura. *Am Rev Respir Dis* 1982;126:187–189 [editorial].
36. LaDou J. The asbestos cancer epidemic. *Environ Health Perspect* 2004;112(3):285–290.
37. Churg A. Current issues in the pathologic and minéralogie diagnosis of asbestos-induced disease. *Chest* 1983;84(3):278.
38. Haus BM, Razavi H, Kuschner WG. Occupational and environmental causes of bronchogenic carcinoma. *Curr Opin Pulm Med* 2001;7(4):220–225.
39. Steenland K, Loomis D, Shy C, Simonsen N. Review of occupational lung carcinogens. *Am J Ind Med* 1996;29(5):474–490.
40. Roggli VL, Pratt PC, Brody AR. Asbestos content of lung tissue in asbestos-associated diseases: A study of 110 cases. *Br J Ind Med* 1986;43(1):18–28.
41. Roggli VL, Greenberg DS, Pratt PC. *Pathology of Asbestos-Associated Diseases*. Boston: Little, Brown & Company; 1992: 324–329.
42. Warnock ML, Isenberg W. Asbestos burden and the pathology of lung cancer. *Chest* 1986;89(1):20–26.
43. Wagner JC, Berry G, Skidmore JW, Timbrell V. The effects of the inhalation of asbestos in rats. *Br J Cancer* 1974;29:252.
44. Sluis-Cremer GK. The relationship between asbestosis and bronchial cancer. *Chest* August 1980;78(2, Suppl.):380–381.
45. Wilkinson P, Hansell DM, Janssens J, et al. Is lung cancer associated with asbestos exposure when there are small opacities on the chest radiograph? *Lancet* 1995;345(8957):1074–1078.
46. IARC, Monographs on the Evaluation of Carcinogenic Risk of Chemicals to Man—Asbestos Volume 14. International Agency for Research on Cancer. Lyon France; 1977.
47. Kannerstein M, Churg J. Pathology of carcinoma of the lung associated with asbestos exposure. *Cancer* 1972;30(1):14–21.
48. Kipen HM, Lilis R, Suzuk Y, Valciukas JA, Selikoff IJ. Pulmonary fibrosis in asbestos insulation workers with lung cancer: A radiologie and histopathological evaluation. *Br J Ind Med* 1987;44(2):960–100.
49. Peto R. *Influence of Dose and Duration of Smoking on Lung Cancer Rates*. IARC Science Publication No. 7420. Lyon, France: WHO IARC; 1986: 22–33.

50. Jemal A, Tiwari RC, Murray T, et al. American Cancer Society, Cancer statistics, 2004. *CA Cancer J Clin* 2004;54(1):8–29.
51. Koop CE, Luoto J. The health consequences of smoking: Cancer. Overview of a report of the Surgeon General. Public Health Report 1982;97:318–324.
52. Hammond EC, Selikoff IJ, Seidman H. Asbestos exposure, cigarette smoking and death rates. *Ann N Y Acad Sci* 1979;330:473–490.
53. Enterline PE. Attributability in the face of uncertainty. *Chest* August 1980;72(2 Suppl.):377.
54. Brooks SM, Locke JE, Harber P. Occupational lung diseases. *Clin Chest Med* May 1981;2(2):194.
55. Liddell FD. The interaction of asbestos and smoking in lung cancer. *Ann Occup Hyg* 2001;45(4):341–356.
56. Berry G, Newhouse ML, Antonis P. Combined effect of asbestos and smoking on mortality from lung cancer and mesothelioma in factory workers. *Br J Ind Med* 1985;42:12–18.
57. Reid A, deKlerk NH, Ambrosini GL, Berry G, Musk AW. The risk of lung cancer with increasing time since ceasing exposure to asbestos and quitting smoking. *Occup Environ Med* 2006;63(8):509–512.
58. Lee PN. Relation between exposure to asbestos and smoking jointly, and the risk of lung cancer. *Occup Environ Med* 2001;58:145–153.
59. Berry G, Liddell FD. The interaction of asbestos and smoking in lung cancer: A modified measure of effect. *Ann Occup Hyg* 2004;48(5):459–462.
60. Churg A, Stevens B. Enhanced retention of asbestos fibers in the airways of human smokers. *Am J Respir Crit Care Med* 1995;151:1409–1413.
61. Koop CE Luoto J. The health consequences of smoking: Cancer. Overview of a report of the Surgeon General. *Public Health Rep* July–August 1982;197(4):318–325.
62. Rom WM. *Environmental and Occupational Medicine*, 1st ed. Boston, MA: Little, Brown & Company; 1983: 165.
63. Selikoff IJ, Hammond EC, Churg J. Asbestos exposure, smoking, and neoplasia. *JAMA* 1968;204(2):106–112.
64. Craighead JE, Abraham JL, Churg A, Green FH, Kleinerman J, Pratt PC, et al. The pathology of asbestos-associated diseases of the lungs and pleural cavities: Diagnostic criteria and proposed grading schema. *Arch Pathol Lab Med* 1982;106(11):544–596.
65. American Thoracic Society. Diagnosis and initial management of nonmalignant diseases related to asbestos. *Am J Respir Crit Care Med* 2004;170(6):691–715.
66. Dodson RF, Williams MG Jr, O'Sullivan MF, Corn CJ, Greenberg SD, Hurst GA. A comparison of the ferruginous body and uncoated fiber content in the lungs of former asbestos workers. *Am Rev Respir Dis* July 1985;132(1):143–147.
67. American Cancer Society. Cancer Facts and Figures 2009. Atlanta: American Cancer Society 2009. Available at: www.oralcancerfoundation.org/facts/pdf/Us_Cancer_Facts.pdf.
68. Kleinfeld M, Messite J, Kooyman O. Mortality experience in a group of asbestos workers. *Arch Environ Health* 1967;15(2):177–180.
69. Selikoff IJ, Lee DHK. *Asbestos and Disease*. New York: Academic Press; 1978: 327.
70. Miller A, Lilis R, Godbold J, Wu X. Relation of spirometric function to radiographic interstitial fibrosis in two large workforces exposed to asbestos: An evaluation of the ILO profusion score. *Occup Environ Med* 1996;53(12):808–812.
71. Koskinen K, Pukkala E, Martikainen R, Reijula K, Karjalainen A. Different measures of asbestos exposure in estimating risk of lung cancer and mesothelioma among construction workers. *J Occup Environ Med* 2002;44(12):1190–1196.
72. Seidman H, Selikoff IJ. Decline in death rates among asbestos insulation workers 1967–1986 associated with diminution of work exposure to asbestos. *Ann N Y Acad Sci* 1990;609:300–317 [discussion 317–318].
73. Selikoff IJ, Hammond EC, Seidman H. Latency of asbestos disease among insulation workers in the United States and Canada. *Cancer* 1980;46(12):2736–2740.
74. Buchanan WD. Asbestosis and primary intrathoracic neoplasms. *Ann N Y Acad Sci* 1965;132(1):507–518.
75. Berry G. Mortality of workers certified by pneumoconiosis medical panels as having asbestosis. *Br J Ind Med* 1981;38(2):130–137.
76. Hillerdal G. Pleural plaque and risk for bronchial carcinoma and mesothelioma: A prospective study. *Chest* 1994;105(1):144–150.

77. Szeszenia-Dabrowska N, Urszula W, Szymczak W, Strzelecka A. Mortality study of workers compensated for asbestosis in Poland 1970–1997. *Int J Occup Med Environ Health* 2002;15(3):267–278.
78. Oksa P, Klockars M, Karjalainen A, et al. Progression of asbestosis predicts lung cancer. *Chest* 1998;113(6):1517–1521.
79. Dail DH, Hammar SP. *Pulmonary Pathology*, 2nd ed. New York: Springer-Verlag; 1994: 1489.
80. McDonald AD, Harper A, Elattan DA, McDonald JC. Epidemiology of primary malignant mesothelial tumors in Canada. *Cancer (Philadelphia)* 1970;26:914–919.
81. Roggli VL. Environmental asbestos contamination: What are the risks? *Chest* 2007;131(2):336–338.
82. Ribak J, Lilis R, Suzuki Y, Penner L, Selikoff IJ. Malignant mesothelioma in a cohort of asbestos insulation workers: clinical presentation, diagnosis, and causes of death. *Br J Ind Med* 1988;45(3):182–187.
83. McCaughey WT, Colby TV, Battifora H, et al. Diagnosis of diffuse malignant mesothelioma: Experience of a U.S./Canadian Mesothelioma Panel. *Mod Pathol* 1991;4(3):342–353.
84. Ribak J, Selikoff IJ. Survival of asbestos insulation workers with mesothelioma. *Br J Ind Med* 1992;49(10):732–735.
85. Higashihara M, Sunaga S, Tange T, Oohashi H, Kurokawa K. Increased secretion of interleukin-6 in malignant mesothelioma cells from a patient with marked thrombocytosis. *Cancer* 1992;70(8):2105–2108.
86. Yoshimoto A, Kasahara K, Saito K, Fujimura M, Nakao S, et al. Granulocyte colony-stimulating factor-producing malignant pleural mesothelioma with expression of other cytokines. *Int J Clin Oncol* 2005;10(1):58–62.
87. dePangher MV. Malignant peritoneal mesothelioma. *Tumori* 2005;91(1):1–5.
88. Selleslag DL, Geragty RJ, Ganesan TS, Slevin ML, Wrigley PF, Brown R. Autoimmune hemolytic anemia associated with malignant peritoneal mesothelioma. *Acta Clin Belg* 1989;44(3):199–201.
89. Churg A, Colby TV, Cagle P, et al. The separation of benign and malignant mesothelial proliferations. *Am J Surg Pathol* 2000;24(9):1183–1200.
90. Hammar SP. The pathology of benign and malignant pleural disease. *Chest Surg Clin N Am* 1994;4(3):405–430.
91. Sugarbaker PH, Acherman YI, Gonzalez-Morano S, et al. Diagnosis and treatment of peritoneal mesothelioma: The Washington Cancer Institute experience. *Semin Oncol* 2002;29(1):51–61.
92. Dodson RF, O'Sullivan MF, Huang J, Holiday DB, Hammar SP. Asbestos in extrapulmonary sites: omentum and mesentery. *Chest* 2000;117(2):486–493.
93. Mancuso TF, Coulter EJ. Methodology of industrial health studies: The cohort approach with special reference to an asbestos company. *Arch Environ Health* 1963;6:210–226.
94. Godwin MC, Jagatic G. Asbestos and mesothelioma. *JAMA*, 1968;204(11):1009.
95. Dement JM, Harris RL Jr, Symons MJ, Shy CM. Exposure and mortality among chrysotile asbestos workers: Part II. Mortality. *Am J Ind Med* 1983;4:421–33.
96. Morinaga K, Kohyama N, Yokoyama K, Yasui Y, Hara I, Sasaki M, et al. Asbestos fiber content of lungs with mesothelioma in Osaka, Japan: A preliminary report. *IARC Sci Publ* 1989;90:438–443.
97. Oury TD, Hammar SP, Roggli VL. Asbestos content of lung tissue in patients with malignant peritoneal mesothelioma: a study of 40 cases. *Lung Cancer* 1997;18(Suppl):235–236 [Abstract 923].
98. Welch LS, Acherman YI, Haile E, Sokas RK, Sugarbaker PH. Asbestos and peritoneal mesothelioma among college-educated men. *Int J Occup Environ Health* 2005;11:254–258.
99. Newhouse ML, Thompson H. Mesothelioma of pleura and peritoneum following exposure to asbestos in the London area. *Br J Ind Med* 1965;22:161.
100. Chen WJ, Mottet NK. Malignant mesothelioma with minimal asbestos exposure. *Hum Pathol* 1978;9(3):253–258.
101. Dodson RF, Hammar SP, Poye LW, Friedman GK. Mesothelioma in an individual following exposure to crocidolite-containing gaskets as a teenager [submitted for publication].
102. Anderson HA, Lilis R, Daum SM, Fischbein AS, Selikoff IJ. Household-contact asbestos neoplastic risk. *Ann N Y Acad Sci* 1976;271:311–323.
103. Anderson HA, Lilis R, Daum SM, Selikoff IJ. Asbestosis among household contacts of asbestos factory workers. *Ann N Y Acad Sci* 1979; 330:387–399.
104. Epler GR, Fitz Gerald MX, Gaensler EA, Carrington CB. Asbestos-related disease from household exposure. *Respiration* 1980;39(4):229–240.
105. Vianna NJ, Polan AK. Non-occupational exposure to asbestos and malignant mesothelioma in females. *Lancet* 1978;1(8073):1061–1063.

106. Dodson RF, O'Sullivan M, Brooks DR, Hammar SP. Quantitative analysis of asbestos burden in women with mesothelioma. *Am J Ind Med* 2003;43(2):188–195.

107. Roggli VL, Oury TD, Moffatt EJ. Malignant mesothelioma in women. *Anat Pathol* 1997;2:147–163.

108. Iwatsubo Y, Pairon JC, Boutin C, et al. Pleural mesothelioma: Dose–response relation at low levels of asbestos exposure in a French population-based case–control study. *Am J Epidemiol* 1998;148(2):133–142.

109. Hammar SP, Bockus D, Remington F, Freidman S, LaZerte G. Familial mesothelioma: A report of two families. *Hum Pathol* 1989;20(2):107–112.

110. Li FP, Lokich J, Lapey J, Neptune WB, Wilkins EW Jr. Familial mesothelioma after intense asbestos exposure at home. *JAMA* 1978;240(5):467.

111. Magnani C, Agudo A, Gonzalez CA, et al. Multicentric study on malignant pleural mesothelioma and non-occupational exposure to asbestos. *Br J Cancer* 2000;83(1):104–111.

112. American Academy of Pediatrics Committee on Environmental Hazards. Asbestos exposure in schools. *Pediatrics* 1987;79(2):301–305.

113. Garrahan K. Friable asbestos in schools must be found by May 1988, removal plan must start by 1989. *JAMA* 1987;257(12):1570–1571.

114. McDonald JC, Edwards CW, Gibbs AR, et al. Case-referent survey of young adults with mesothelioma: II. Occupational analyses. *Ann Occup Hyg* 2001;45(7):519–523.

115. Brenner J, Sordillo PP, Magill GB. Malignant mesothelioma in children: Report of seven cases and review of the literature. *Med Pediatr Oncol* 1981;9:367–373.

116. Chang MY, Sugarbaker DJ. Extrapleural pneumonectomy for diffuse malignant pleural mesothelioma: Techniques and complications. *Thorac Surg Clin* 2004;14(4):523–530.

117. Sugarbaker DJ, Jaklitsch MT, Bueno R. Prevention, early detection, and management of complications after 328 consecutive extrapleural pneumonectomies. *J Thorac Cardiovasc Surg* 2004;128(1):138–146.

118. Treasure T, Sedrakyan A. Pleural mesothelioma: Little evidence, still time to do trials. *Lancet* 2004;364(9440):1183–1185.

119. Weder W, Kestenholz P, Taverna C, et al. Neoadjuvant chemotherapy followed by extrapleural pneumonectomy in malignant pleural mesothelioma. *J Clin Oncol* 2004;22(17):3451–3457.

120. Janne PA, Baldini EH. Patterns of failure following surgical resection for malignant pleural mesothelioma. *Thorac Surg Clin* 2004;14(4):567–573.

121. Chang MY, Sugarbaker DJ. Innovative therapies: Intraoperative intra-cavitary chemotherapy. *Thorac Surg Clin* 2004;14(4):549–556.

122. Pistolesi M, Rusthoven J. Malignant pleural mesothelioma: Update, current management, and newer therapeutic strategies. *Chest* 2004;126(4):1318–1329.

123. Rice DC, Stevens CW, Correa AM, Vaporciyan AA, Tsao A, Forster KM, et al. Outcomes after extrapleural pneumonectomy and intensity modulated radiation therapy for malignant pleural mesothelioma. *Ann Thorac Surg* November 2007;84(5):1685–1692.

124. Kolonel LN, Yoshizawa CN, Hirohata T, Myers BC. Cancer occurrence in shipyard workers exposed to asbestos in Hawaii. *Cancer Res* 1985;45:3924–3928.

125. Sanden A, Naslund PE, Jarvholm B. Mortality in lung and gastrointestinal cancer among shipyard workers. *Int Arch Occup Environ Health* 1985;55:277–283.

126. Selikoff IJ, Churg J, Hammond EC. Asbestos exposure and neoplasia. *JAMA* 1964;188:22–26.

127. Hillerdal G. Gastrointestinal carcinoma and occurrence of pleural plaques on pulmonary x-ray. *J Occup Med* 1980;22:806–809.

128. Morgan WKC, Seaton A. *Occupational Lung Diseases*, 2nd ed. Philadelphia: W.B. Saunders and Company; 1984: 333.

129. Finkelstein MM. Mortality among employees of an Ontario asbestos-cement factory. *Am Rev Respir Dis* 1984;129:754–761.

130. Harber P, Mohsenifar Z, Oren A, Lew M. Pleural plaque and asbestos-associated malignancy. *J Occup Environ Med* 1987;29(8):641–644.

131. EPA Support Document for Final Rule on Friable Asbestos-Containing Materials in School Buildings. Washington, DC: Office of Toxic Substances, U.S. Environmental Protection Agency; January 1982.

132. Vineis P, Ciccone G, Magnino A. Asbestos exposure, physical activity and colon cancer: A case control study. *Tumori* 1993;79(5):301–303.

133. Ehrlich A, Gordon RE, Dikman SH. Carcinoma of the colon in asbestos exposed workers: Analysis of asbestos content in colon tissue. *Am J Ind Med* 1991;19(5):629–636.

134. Berry G, Newhouse ML, Wagner JC. Mortality from all cancers of asbestos factory workers in east London, 1933–1980. *Occup Environ Med* 2000;57(11):782–785.

135. Homa DM, Garabrandt DH, Gillespie. A meta analysis of colorectal cancer and asbestos exposure. *Am J Epidemiol* 1994;139:1210–1222.

136. Gerhardsson de Verdier M, Plato N, Steinbeck G, Peters JM. Occupational exposures and cancers of the colon and rectum. *Am J Ind Med* 1992;22:291–303.

137. Gamble JF. Asbestos and colon cancer: A weight-of-the-evidence review. *Environ Health Perspect* 1994;102:1038–1050.

138. Morgan RW, Foliart DE, Wong O. Asbestos and gastrointestinal cancer: A review of the literature. *West J Med* 1985;143:60–65.

139. Garabrant DH, Peters RK, Homa DM. Asbestos and colon cancer: Lack of association in a large-case control study. *Am J Epidemiol* 1992;135:843–853.

140. Jemal A, Siegel R, Ward E, Murray T, Xu J, Smigal C, Thun MJ. Cancer statistics 2006. *CA Cancer J Clin* 2006;56:106–130.

141. IARC. Summaries and evaluations—Asbestos. Supplement 7; 1987. Available at: www.inchem.org/documents/iarc/suppl7/asbestos.html.

142. Karjalainen A, Pukkala E, Kauppinen T, Partanen T. Incidence of cancer among finish patients with asbestos-related pulmonary or pleural fibrosis. *Cancer Causes Control* 1999;10(1):51–57.

143. Doll R, Peto J. Other asbestos-related neoplasms. In: *Asbestos-related Malignancy*, Antman K, Aisner J, eds. Orlando: Grune and Stratton, Inc.; 1987: 90–91.

144. Stell PM, McGill T. Exposure to asbestos and laryngeal carcinoma. *J Laryngol Otol* 1973;59(25): 513–517.

145. Newhouse ML, Berry G. Asbestos and laryngeal carcinoma. *Lancet* 1973;2:615.

146. Shettigara T, Morgan RW. Asbestos, smoking and laryngeal carcinoma. *Environ Health* 1975;30(10):517–519.

147. Roggli VL, Greenberg SD, McLarty JL, Hurst GA, Spivey CG, Heiger LR. Asbestos body content of the larynx in asbestos workers. *Arch Otolaryngol* 1980;106:533–535.

148. Hirsch A, Bingnon J, Sebastien, Gaudichet A. Asbestos fibers in laryngeal tissues: Findings in two patients with asbestosis associated with laryngeal tumors. *Chest* 1979;76(6):697–699.

149. Heller DS, Gordon RE, Katz N. Correlation of asbestos fiber burdens in fallopian tubes and ovarian tissue. *Am J Obstet Gynecol* 1999;181(2):346–347.

150. Langseth H, Johansen BV, Nesland JM, Kjaeheim K. Asbestos fibers in ovarian tissue from Norwegian pulp and paper workers. *Int J Gynecol Cancer* 2007;17(1):44–49.

CHAPTER 14

Core Curriculum for Practicing Physicians Related to Asbestos

Jeffrey L. Levin and Paul P. Rountree

CONTENTS

14.1 INTRODUCTION

There have been thousands of publications in scientific journals and other venues regarding asbestos. In spite of its recognized health hazard, like so many other occupational causes of illness and injury in the United States and around the world, asbestos is frequently overlooked in the clinical setting. There are many complex factors and explanations that account for this rather routine oversight. Chief among them is the relative lack of emphasis that occupational causes of disease command in medical training programs at the graduate and postgraduate levels.

The American Board of Preventive Medicine is a Member Board of the American Board of Medical Specialties.[1] The board was created in 1948 and was authorized to certify specialists in occupational medicine in 1955. In spite of a long history of certifying physicians, in 1990 it was estimated that occupational medicine specialists numbered fewer than 1500, with a deficit of physicians having special competence in the field of almost 5500.[2] In 2000, the Council on Graduate Medical Education noted that in-depth data on physicians in the public health workforce were in short supply.[3] In addition to proposing the collection of more comprehensive data, a second recommendation focused on increased funding for training physicians in preventive medicine. The Institute of Medicine likewise concluded that "the continuing burden of largely preventable occupational diseases and injuries and the lack of adequate occupational safety and health (OSH) services in most small and many larger workplaces indicate a clear need for more OSH professionals at all levels."[4] In 2009, a search of the directory of the American Board of Preventive Medicine yielded fewer than 3600 specialists certified in Occupational Medicine,[5] with 2638 physicians certified between 1985 and 2007.[6]

The deficiency of educating health care professionals, particularly physicians, may be more fundamental. In 1991, the Institute of Medicine reported that only 66% of U.S. medical schools specifically teach occupational medicine as a part of the required curriculum.[7] Approximately half of these dedicate an average of 4 h over a 4-year period. Among departments of internal medicine, roughly 20% offered clinical occupational medicine experience to residents, mostly on an elective basis. Family medicine is one of the few areas of residency that requires the incorporation of occupational medicine into the training. The Accreditation Council for Graduate Medical Education Residency Review Committee for Family Medicine requires that programs provide residents with a structured curriculum, which includes "population epidemiology and the interpretation of public health statistical information, environmental illness and injury, community-based disease screening/prevention/health promotion, and occupational medicine including disability determination, employee health, and job-related illness/injury."[8] A recent review revealed that 68.2% of residency training programs in family medicine offer specific training in occupational medicine.[9] However, only one-half of these had faculty with occupational medicine experience.

It is not surprising that health care providers, particularly physicians, have little comfort with occupational and environmental issues such as asbestos-induced disease. This is also true of postgraduate trainees embarking upon residency programs in preventive medicine and occupational medicine. It is incumbent upon such programs, and textbooks such as this one, to impart essential and practical knowledge to these individuals as reference tools for achieving a level of competence that will permit quality practice in this arena.

In addition to general competencies required by the Accreditation Council for Graduate Medical Education, the Residency Review Committee for Preventive Medicine specifies a number of academic core content areas, which must also address health services administration, biostatistics, epidemiology, clinical preventive medicine, behavioral aspects of health, and environmental health.[10] The study of pragmatic issues related to asbestos is in keeping with occupational medicine knowledge content areas and patient care competencies that should be achieved for effective practice in occupational medicine. These are listed in Table 14.1.

As it relates to asbestos, what then constitutes pragmatic and essential knowledge and skills for the residency trainee and practitioner? An understanding of the scope of asbestos-induced diseases and the impact of asbestos on future human health is critical. Some might suggest the topic is passé and hardly worth the effort. There are numerous ongoing attempts to pass legislation at the federal level to curtail the legal implications of injury associated with a history of occupational and environmental contamination and human exposure to asbestos. Yet, the number of asbestos claims persist and its widespread implications continue to grow. Stallard, for example, estimated that 400,000 to 500,000 personal injury claims would be filed during 2000–2049.[11]

Paramount is some understanding of the basic pathophysiology of the diseases caused by asbestos along with the fundamentals of diagnosis and treatment strategies, particularly of a preventive nature. Finally, residents and practitioners who deal with asbestos-exposed patients should develop a facility with regulatory requirements associated with medical surveillance of exposed workers and with the essential medical–legal considerations that face the individual serving as an expert.

Table 14.1   Occupational Medicine Knowledge Content Areas and Patient Care Competencies

Occupational medicine knowledge content areas

Disability management and work fitness

Workplace health and surveillance

Hazard recognition, evaluation, and control

Clinical occupational medicine

Regulations and government agencies

Environmental health and risk assessment

  Health promotion and clinical prevention

  Management and administration

  Toxicology

Occupational medicine patient care competencies

Manage the health status of individuals who work in diverse work settings

  Adequate supervised time in direct clinical care of workers, from numerous employers and employed in more than one work setting, must be provided to ensure competency in mitigating and managing medical problems of workers

  Residents must be able to assess safe/unsafe work practices and to safeguard employees and others on the basis of clinic and worksite experience

Monitor/survey workforces and interpret monitoring/surveillance data for prevention of disease in workplaces and to enhance the health and productivity of workers

Active participation in several surveillance or monitoring programs, for different types of workforces, is required to learn principles of administration and maintenance of practical workforce and environmental public health programs. Residents must plan at least one such program

Manage worker insurance documentation and paperwork for work-related injuries that may arise in numerous work settings

Initially learn worker insurance competencies under direct supervision of faculty and demonstrate competency to "open," "direct," and "close" injury/illness cases

Recognize outbreak events of public health significance as they appear in clinical or consultation settings

  Residents should understand the concept of sentinel events and know how to assemble/work with a team of fellow professionals who can evaluate and identify worksite public health causes of injury and illness

  Residents must be able to recognize and evaluate potentially hazardous workplace and environmental conditions, and recommend controls or programs to reduce exposures, and to enhance the health and productivity of workers

  Reliance on toxicological and risk assessment principles in the evaluation of hazards must be demonstrated

Report outcome findings of clinical and surveillance evaluations to affected workers as ethically required; advise management concerning summary (rather than individual) results or trends of public health significance

Source: Accreditation Council for Graduate Medical Education. Program requirements for preventive medicine, effective July 2007. Available at: http://www.acgme.org/acWebsite/downloads/RRC_progReq/380pr07012007.pdf. Accessed 2009.

14.2 BACKGROUND

Asbestos is a generic term applied to a group of six naturally occurring fibrous silicate minerals that have been used extensively in commercial products.[12] These minerals are more commonly found in their nonfibrous form. The crystalline fibrous minerals are grouped into two categories: serpentine and amphibole. Chrysotile is serpentine asbestos made up of flexible fibers, which can be woven. Amphiboles are made up of brittle fibers and include amosite, crocidolite, and fibrous forms of tremolite, anthophyllite, and actinolite. Both categories may give rise to separable, long, and thin fibers, which may persist in lung tissue. The vast majority of the asbestos commercially used in the United States has been chrysotile. The physical and chemical properties of these minerals have resulted in their widespread applications and distribution in construction and industry, including their important use as a thermal insulating material. Although use of asbestos has steadily declined over the last two decades in the United States largely because of health reasons, the circumstances of prior exposure and its rather ubiquitous persistence create ongoing health concerns. Disturbance of asbestos-containing materials may result in the release of fibers, which can be suspended for long periods and which may travel long distances.

The earliest uses of asbestos date back to ancient times.[13] However, the first death due to pulmonary asbestosis was not described in the scientific medical literature until 1924, when Cooke reported on the death of Nellie Kershaw from fibrosis of the lungs due to inhalation of asbestos dust from work in asbestos factories in Britain.[14] In 1930, Merewether and Price conducted an investigation of the condition of workers in asbestos textile factories in Britain.[13] They demonstrated a direct relationship between exposure intensity and the speed of onset and severity of fibrosis. By 1955, Doll[15] showed convincing evidence of the relationship between asbestos exposure and lung cancer. In 1960, Wagner et al.[16] published on pleural mesotheliomas in individuals associated with crocidolite asbestos in South Africa. Selikoff and others demonstrated the relationship between asbestos exposure and neoplasia among building trades insulation workers in a landmark article in 1964.[17] The association between asbestos and nonmalignant and neoplastic diseases among insulation workers in the United States and Canada has been confirmed in subsequent analyses.[18] In spite of the "early" and clear recognition of occupationally induced disease, unprotected exposure was ongoing as illustrated in Figures 14.1 and 14.2.

Asbestos production continues in many countries throughout the world, particularly in developing countries, where extensive commercial utilization of asbestos is ongoing.[19] The majority of asbestos is currently consumed in Eastern Europe, Latin America, and Asia. Despite a decline in use in the United States, the U.S. Department of Labor estimates that there are 3.2 million workers who encounter asbestos as a function of building renovation, maintenance, custodial work, and similar activities and who are subject to the requirements of the current construction standards of that agency. These circumstances of exposure give rise to the notion of a "third wave" of asbestos disease.[20] The first phase of asbestos disease was associated with work in the mining and milling of ore and the manufacture of asbestos products. The second phase of disease was recognized among users of these products such as insulators. The third wave of disease relates to exposure to asbestos in place. The potential for bystander exposure exists for each of these circumstances (e.g., in the households of these workers). Although many applications have been phased out of production, a partial list of uses is included in Table 14.2.[21]

It should be noted that asbestos could be a contaminant of other products such as vermiculite (used in gardening or landscaping products and home insulation) and talc (used in cosmetics).

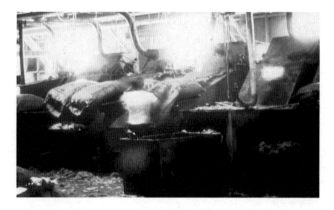

Figure 14.1 Worker in pipe insulation manufacturing facility operating from 1954 to 1972. Note the lack of respiratory protection and the qualitatively visible haze as he opens and empties burlap bags containing amosite asbestos.

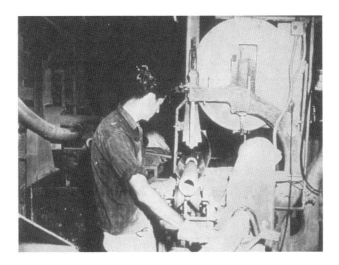

Figure 14.2   Worker in same facility as in Figure 14.1. Again note the absence of respiratory protection as he prepares to cut the cured pipe insulation in half along its length.

On a worldwide basis, asbestos is being used increasingly in countries where previously there has been little use or manufacture.[22] This is not an unusual pattern of events where developing countries "import disease" as a function of their industrialization. This is a matter of particular concern as it relates to cancer where the disease is considered to be epidemic in nature, with mortality projections in the millions.[23] Some have suggested that banning use often does not occur until after the costs exceed profitability. In developing countries, the lack of control measures to prevent disease is such that the equation remains profitable, at least for now.

14.3 BASIC PATHOPHYSIOLOGY

Any discussion of human exposure to a toxic substance merits a brief review of route of entry and factors that may determine dose. Inhalation is, no doubt, the primary route of entry for asbestos fibers, although there is transfer of inhaled fibers from the lung to the gastrointestinal (GI) tract as well as ingestion of fibers from drinking water. Concern for asbestos exposures in the GI system is mostly related to the suspicion of increased risk for GI cancers.[12] This remains a controversial matter. Dermal exposure in and of itself appears to be of lesser import in that the only adverse health effect associated with this route of exposure is the formation of small "warts" or corns, presumably associated with skin penetration by macroscopic spicules.

Fibrous particles (e.g., asbestos) are those whose length substantially exceeds their diameter.[24] The so-called aspect ratio of length to diameter is variably defined for fibers, but 3:1 has been widely adopted by pathologists and researchers. Certainly, aerosols are rarely monodisperse but are made up of a range of compact and fibrous particles. The deposition of particles is largely determined by mean aerodynamic diameter and distribution of particle diameter. Deposition in the respiratory tract occurs when a particle comes in contact with an airway or alveolus. Other factors such as size, density, and shape of particles as well as respiratory volume are important determinants of deposition. Larger particles tend to inertially impact within the large airways. In the smaller airways and alveoli, flow velocity is low and gravitational sedimentation plays a greater role for those particles and fibers that are small enough to reach this level. Fibrous particles such as asbestos are particularly affected by interception, where aerodynamic diameter is especially important. Fibers that are long with a high aspect ratio, but of sufficiently narrow diameter (<3.5 μm), are axially entrained in the air stream and

Table 14.2   Applications and Uses of Asbestos

Current commercial uses

Brake pads
Automobile clutches
Roofing materials
Vinyl tile
Imported cement pipe/corrugated sheeting
Contaminated commercial products (such as vermiculite in potting soil/home insulation)

Former commercial uses

Boilers and heating vessels
Cement pipe
Clutch, brake, and transmission components
Conduits for electrical wire
Corrosive chemical containers
Electric motor components
Heat-protective pads
Laboratory furniture
Paper products
Pipe covering
Roofing products
Sealants and coatings
Insulation products
Textiles (including curtains)

Homes and buildings

Duct and home insulation
Fire protection panels
Fireplace artificial logs or ashes
Fuse box liners
Gypsum wallboard
Hair dryers
Toasters
Heater register tape and insulation
Joint compounds
Patching and spackling compounds
Pipe or boiler insulation
Pot holders and ironing board pads
Sheet vinyl or floor tiles
Shingles
Textured acoustical ceiling
Textured paints
Underlayment for flooring and carpets

Source: Tucker, P. Case studies in environmental medicine (CSEM): asbestos toxicity. Atlanta, GA: Agency for Toxic Substances and Disease Registry (ATSDR); 2007. Available at: http:// www.atsdr.cdc.gov/csem/asbestos/cover2.html. Accessed 2009.

avoid impaction and sedimentation until reaching the walls of terminal and respiratory bronchioles, particularly at bifurcations. Not all fibers that are deposited, however, are retained. Many are efficiently eliminated by cough, mucociliary clearance, and acinar clearance (Figure 14.3). These clearance mechanisms may be altered by a number of factors, particularly cigarette smoking.[25]

Particles larger than 10 μm in diameter are mostly removed in the nasal chamber.[26] The penetration of particles and deposition in the respiratory tract from sedimentation occurs mostly in the diametric range of 0.5–5 μm, with those penetrating to and deposited in the pulmonary airspaces having a maximum value between 1 and 2 μm. Some of these fibers may be quite long (Figure 14.4).

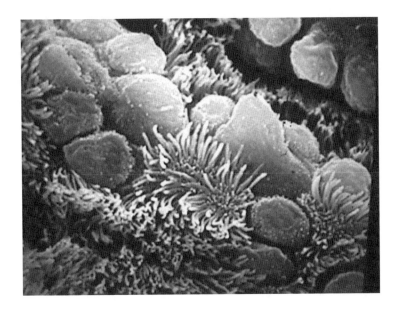

Figure 14.3   View of bronchiolar ciliated columnar epithelial surface by scanning electron microscopy. (Courtesy of Ronald F. Dodson, PhD.)

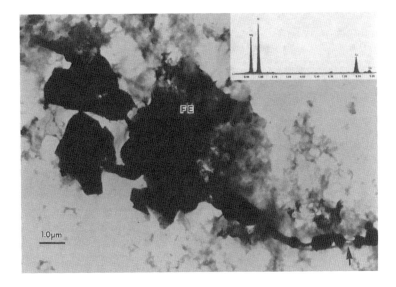

Figure 14.4   Long coated chrysotile asbestos fiber from digested lung tissue of an exposed individual. This is a transmission electron micrograph of a ferruginous body on a chrysotile asbestos core. The inset demonstrates a characteristic x-ray energy dispersive analytic spectrum of chrysotile asbestos fibers. FE, ferruginous material; arrow, fiber core. (Courtesy of Ronald F. Dodson, PhD.)

The clearance, fate, pathologic effect, and implications of various coated and uncoated fiber types and sizes within the lung and sputum are described in detail elsewhere in this textbook. Relocation of fibers occurs to lymph nodes, pleura, and omentum and mesentery, presumably by way of the pulmonary interstitium or lymphatics.[27,28]

A brief discussion of the asbestos body (AB) is worthwhile. The AB represents an asbestos fiber that has been phagocytized by pulmonary macrophages and partially or completely coated by an iron-rich protein.[29] Their shape is variable and classically appears like a dumbbell or drumstick by light and electron microscopies (Figures 14.5 and 14.6). An important feature of the AB is its controversial implication for tissue diagnosis of asbestosis using light microscopy. There are people who argue "the minimal features that permit the diagnosis are the demonstration of discrete foci of fibrosis in the walls of respiratory bronchioles associated with accumulations of ABs."[30] Although ABs confirm past asbestos exposure, they typically form on asbestos fibers that are ≥8 μm in length, with other fiber characteristics also determining which of the longer fibers will be coated.[31] In most studies, the majority of cores analyzed are amphiboles.[32–36] Theoretically, because of physical characteristics of the fibers, chrysotile has a larger aerodynamic diameter than amphibole fibers. As a result, the opportunity for entrapment of chrysotile in the upper airways combined with the view that it may fragment or "dissolve" over time[37] would support the idea that presence of ABs indicates exposure to amphiboles[38] or correlation with amphibole exposure.[39]

Clearly, the physical and chemical properties of asbestos fibers are important in environmental and occupational exposures in relation to the pathophysiology of penetration, retention, and tissue response. This may be particularly true in the case of pleural malignancy as demonstrated by Stanton and Wrench in the early 1970s.[13] Their experiments involving the placement of refined and sized asbestos and manmade mineral fibers into the pleural space of laboratory animals led to Stanton's hypothesis, suggesting that the diameters and lengths of the fibers or fibrils were largely responsible for the development of cancer. These physicochemical properties have remained of considerable interest as demonstrated by recent efforts by the National Institute for Occupational Safety and Health (NIOSH) to develop a *Roadmap* of research strategies which will help to reduce existing scientific uncertainties and inform future policy initiatives pertaining to determinants of toxicity, health risks of exposure, and sampling and analytic methods for asbestos fibers and other elongated

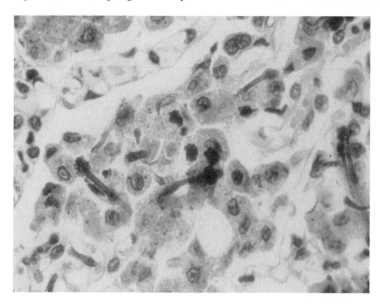

Figure 14.5 Alveolar architecture disrupted by the presence of inflammatory cells and fibrosis. Note the presence of numerous coated asbestos fibers of variable size and shape, some resembling a dumbbell or drumstick. (Courtesy of Ronald F. Dodson, PhD.)

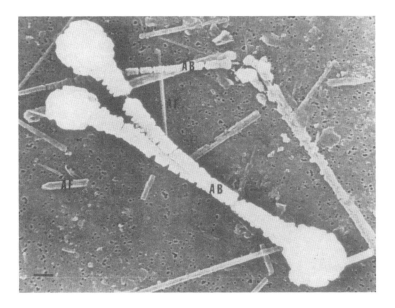

Figure 14.6 Scanning electron micrograph of coated asbestos fibers or ABs from digested lung tissue of an exposed individual. Note that exposure of limited portions of the long thin fibers would permit their identification as asbestos through use of sophisticated identification techniques. (Courtesy of Ronald F. Dodson, PhD.)

mincral particles. At present, this *Roadmap*, initiated by an internal workgroup at NIOSH, has been subject to public and expert peer scrutiny and was published in 2009 as a Revised Draft NIOSH Current Intelligence Bulletin, which is undergoing continued review.[40,41]

14.4 FUNDAMENTALS OF CLINICAL DIAGNOSIS

As with most clinical diagnoses, much emphasis should be placed on obtaining medical history. This includes occupational and environmental history taking, a measure that is frequently overlooked in clinical practice.[42] "Most environmental and occupational diseases either manifest as common medical problems or have nonspecific symptoms. Yet environmental factors rarely enter into the clinician's differential diagnosis. As a result, clinicians miss the opportunity to make correct diagnoses that might influence the course of disease" by stopping or avoiding exposure.[43] This component of history taking can be pivotal in appropriately uncovering an etiology. An exposure history, taking only a few minutes, should be obtained on every patient. There are many important areas to cover including an exposure survey and a work history (Table 14.3). Exposures and their effects may be acute or chronic. The latency period from exposure to manifestation of symptoms or disease can range from immediate to delayed (hours to days) to prolonged (years). Therefore, exploring past as well as current exposures is important. Elucidating a chronology of work and examining temporal and activity patterns related to occupational and environmental disease is the key. It should also be emphasized that listing of job titles alone is inadequate, but a description of work activities offers potential exposure information. Hobbies should not be overlooked for their potential exposure concerns. Additional information concerning obtaining an exposure history is available from the Agency for Toxic Substances and Disease Registry. A case study program is available on the Internet at http://www.atsdr.cdc.gov/csem/exphistory/ehcover_page.html.

In relation to asbestos, it is important to consider the range of commercial products previously noted to contain this material (Table 14.2) and the many trades and construction or maintenance occupations where exposure may occur (e.g., insulating, sheet metal work, pipefitting, firefighting, custodial

Table 14.3   Occupational Profile
Fill in the table below listing all jobs you have worked, including short term, seasonal, part-time
employment, and military service. Begin with your most recent job. Use additional paper if necessary.

Dates of Employment	Job Title and Description of Work	Exposures*	Protective Equipment

*List the chemicals, dusts, fibers, fumes, radiation, biologic agents (i.e., molds or viruses), and physical agents (i.e., extreme heat, cold, vibration, or noise) that you were exposed to at this job.
Source: Yu, D. Case studies in environmental medicine: taking an exposure history. Atlanta, GA: Agency for Toxic Substances and Disease Registry (ATSDR); 2008. Available at: http://www.atsdr.cdc.gov/csem/exphistory/ehcover_page.html. Accessed 2009.

work, etc.).[19] Routine medical history regarding dyspnea, cough, sputum, chest pain, and respiratory infections may be nonspecific. A smoking history is particularly important in the case of asbestos, where exposure interactions relative to disease are known to exist. Asbestos-related conditions often manifest themselves for the first time 20 years and more after first exposure. Military service may be especially important given the historical and vast application of asbestos in this arena. Reviewing the work history of family members living in the home (parents, spouse, etc.) may be pertinent to uncover bystander exposure.[20] A physical examination focused on the respiratory, cardiovascular, and GI systems targets the organs most likely affected by asbestos and is included in the medical surveillance requirements of various regulatory standards (e.g., 29 CFR 1910.1001 for asbestos exposure in general industry and 29 CFR 1926.1101 for asbestos exposure in the construction trades). The asbestos diseases of the lung are generally separated into nonmalignant and malignant categories. Each category can affect the pleural surfaces or the lung parenchyma and bronchial tree.

14.4.1 Nonmalignant Diseases

In 1986, the American Thoracic Society (ATS) outlined the criteria for the diagnosis of various nonmalignant diseases related to asbestos. This organization suggested that it was necessary to include a reliable history of exposure, an appropriate latency period, and clinical criteria including chest x-ray evidence, pulmonary function changes, and physical findings.[44] The guidelines for diagnosis and management of these disorders were more recently updated.[45] The nonmalignant processes affecting the lung are largely fibrotic in nature. Asbestosis is a pneumoconiosis characterized by diffuse interstitial fibrosis of the lungs caused by the inhalation of asbestos fibers.[12] All fiber types are considered to be fibrogenic, although there may be some differences in potency. Like other asbestos-related diseases, there is an extended period of latency from the time of first exposure to the onset of disease. Although the period of latency may vary inversely with the intensity of exposure, the severity of the disease varies proportionately. It is notable that asbestosis is the only major pneumoconiosis to demonstrate increased mortality over the period 1982–2000.[46] This is largely explained by the fact that peak asbestosis mortality occurs 40–45 years after initial occupational exposure. Asbestos consumption in the United States increased substantially during and after the Second World War, reaching its height in 1973.[47] Consequently, it is anticipated that asbestosis-related mortality will continue to climb in years to come.

Cugell and Kamp provided a review of asbestos-related pleural diseases.[48] The most common nonmalignant pleural changes are lesions referred to as pleural plaques. These are discrete areas of collagen deposited on the pleural surface. Diffuse thickening and fibrosis of the pleura may also occur, as can benign pleural effusions and rounded areas of atelectasis.[19]

14.4.2 Malignant Diseases

It is now well accepted that asbestos can lead to increased risk of lung cancer and pleural mesothelioma.[12] Both are associated with chronic exposure. There is evidence to suggest that shorter

Table 14.4   **Synergistic or Multiplicative Interaction between Asbestos and Smoking in Lung Cancer Mortality**

Group	Standard Mortality Ratio from Lung Cancer
Controls	1.00
Asbestos workers only	5.17
Smoking only	10.85
Smoking asbestos workers	53.24

Source: Hammond, E.C., Selikoff, I.J., Seidman, H. *Ann. N.Y. Acad. Sci.*, 330, 472–490, 1979.

exposures may also induce these neoplasms. Asbestos exposure may also pose a risk for cancers of the GI tract and laryngeal cancers. The latter remain controversial.[12,18]

Although case reports of lung cancer among asbestos-exposed workers surfaced in the 1930s, an association was firmly established by Doll, who reported the first epidemiologic study in 1955. Later, investigators noted that 17.6% of workers with more than 20 years of asbestos exposure died of lung or pleural cancer.[17] LaDou estimated that 5%–7% of all lung cancer is due to asbestos exposure.[23] Currently, approximately one (14.3%) of every seven individuals with asbestosis are expected to develop lung cancer.[49] The latent period between exposure and disease onset is approximately 20 years.[19] All major lung cancer cell types have been noted, very similar to the general population with no history of exposure to asbestos. Although lung cancers occur with increased frequency throughout the lung after asbestos exposure, they have been reported to occur with greatest frequency peripherally in the lower lung zones. Recent studies of lung cancer distributions found no difference in anatomical site between those associated with asbestos exposure and those related to cigarette smoking. A synergistic or multiplicative relationship between cigarette smoking and asbestos exposure has been identified, which greatly increases the risk for development of lung cancer as demonstrated in Table 14.4.[50]

Mesothelioma is a tumor that typically involves the pleura and less frequently occurs in the peritoneal cavity or in other locations such as the pericardial cavity and tunica vaginalis. Mesothelioma is most often associated with exposure to amphibole forms of asbestos but may occur after chrysotile exposure. An estimated 2000–3000 new cases are diagnosed each year in the United States,[51] and it is believed that approximately 250,000 will die of this disease in Western Europe during the next three decades.[23] Patients typically complain of chest pain and dyspnea but may have other systemic symptoms such as weight loss, night sweats, and fever. The cancer is locally aggressive and may metastasize. In most reported case series, survival averages vary from 4 to 18 months.[52] Multimodality treatments may include surgery, chemotherapy, and radiation therapy, but the overall results are poor and the prognosis is grim. Several authors have reviewed various therapeutic strategies.[51,52] Despite trials using a combination of treatment approaches, no regimen appears to have demonstrated an improvement in survival.[53]

14.4.3 Diagnostic Tools

As previously discussed, a thorough history with a focus on occupational, paraoccupational, and environmental exposures as well as a careful physical examination are the cornerstones in the diagnosis of asbestos-related health problems. The physician may use a variety of tools to recognize diverse forms of disease due to asbestos. It must be remembered that measurable abnormalities will not necessarily be present in early or mild cases. Ohar et al.[54] noted that in recent times patients are more likely to have fewer radiographic changes, long latent periods, and a normal or obstructive pattern on pulmonary function tests (PFTs). Explanations for obstructive physiologic abnormalities have been offered elsewhere.[45] Some patients may have an entirely normal examination; whereas, those with more advanced disease may show signs and symptoms of severe pulmonary effects such as cough, dyspnea, rales, or clubbing of the fingers.

Radiography is an essential component in the evaluation of an asbestos-exposed patient. Asbestos is capable of causing numerous changes in the lungs and pleura, which can be detected by either chest x-ray or computerized tomography (CT). These findings most commonly include pleural thickening, plaques, or effusions, but atelectasis and parenchymal fibrotic changes may also occur. In asbestosis, patients may have interstitial disease characterized by small, irregular opacifications of variable profusion. In addition, as noted, a variety of neoplasms are associated with exposure.

In an effort to standardize discussions about the radiographic abnormalities that are associated with various dust diseases of the lungs, the International Labour Organization (ILO) established a system for reporting abnormalities. For a physician to demonstrate competence in the use of this ILO classification system, the NIOSH administers a test called the NIOSH B-Reader Certification Examination to interested physicians.[55] The certified B-reader examines films and specifically grades the size and type of parenchymal opacities (e.g., fine, medium, and coarse opacities may be termed as s, t, and u, respectively), their location, and their profusion or extent (graded 0 for normal, 1 for mild, 2 for moderate, and 3 for severe). Comparison is made with a standard set of chest radiographic films. A similar approach is taken with regard to pleural changes and the presence of calcification. The B-reader then issues a standardized report concerning all abnormalities. In this report, the B-reader includes an opinion about the types of small parenchymal opacities that predominate (primary) and those that are present in lesser degree (secondary). Along with this assessment, two profusion scores are provided: the first indicates the extent of disease compared with the standard set of films and the second represents a possible score for the film. For example, a patient may have t and t opacities with profusion of 2/1 (Figure 14.7).

The revised edition (2000) of the *Guidelines for the Use of the ILO International Classification of Radiographs of Pneumoconioses* has been in use for several years and NIOSH has updated the B-Reader Program to reflect changes in guidelines and technology.[55] A new Roentogenographic Interpretation Form is available from NIOSH, which reflects the changes in the Guidelines. Regarding the comparison standard set of images, a new "Quad Set" consisting of 14 radiographs of enhanced quality became available with the 2000 revisions.

Advances in digital radiography have stimulated questions regarding their application to classification of pneumoconioses.[55] Hospitals and clinics have embraced digital technology because of convenience and cost. In fact, it is becoming difficult to obtain traditional chest radiographs in some areas. Current regulation related to the Coal Workers' X-Ray Surveillance Program requires that B-readers use standard film-screen radiographs for this purpose. Digital chest radiographs can be read as "soft copy" images on a monitor or "hard copy" images printed on film. NIOSH is presently comparing classifications performed on digital and standard film-screen images, and in 2008 NIOSH hosted a workshop to address issues such as image acquisition and presentation as well as file interchange, in consideration of the transition of radiologic surveillance from standard to digital images.[55,56]

There can be considerable variability among B-readers' interpretations. Gitlin et al.[57] performed a study comparing the reports of "B" readers retained by plaintiffs' attorneys with results from independent consultants who reviewed the same films. The findings suggested that the magnitude of differences was too great to be attributed to interobserver variability. In spite of this variability, the ILO reading is widely accepted, and its use is required in mandatory medical surveillance programs.

Patients with little or no change on chest radiograph are not necessarily proven to be free of disease.[58] Other investigators have estimated that 10%–20% of cases of asbestosis are reported to have normal chest radiographs.[59] The use of a film "triad" including a postero-anterior (PA) view with right and left lateral oblique films increases validity and reliability.[60]

There is a good deal of evidence to suggest that smoking enhances the presence and profusion of small irregular opacities on chest radiograph.[19] However, the ability of smoking to independently produce such a radiographic appearance has been debated.

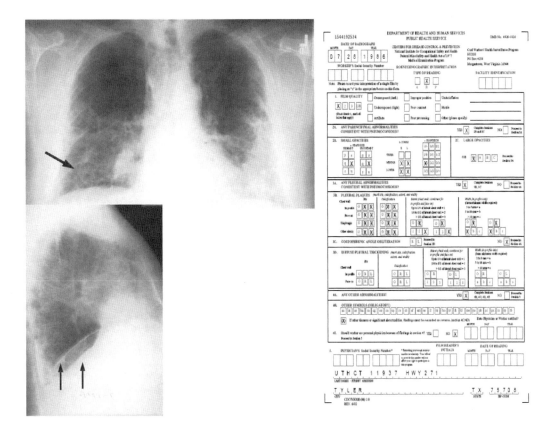

Figure 14.7 PA and lateral chest x-ray views of a patient with asbestosis and bilateral calcified pleural plaque disease. The arrow in the PA view demonstrates irregular opacities in the lower lung zones, whereas the arrows in the lateral view demonstrate bilateral calcified diaphragmatic plaques. An accompanying B-reading has been conducted on an ILO form showing small parenchymal opacities of "t" size and shape and profusion score of 2/1. (ILO reading courtesy of Dr. David Finlay, Professor and Chair of Radiology, The University of Texas Health Science Center at Tyler.)

CT and high-resolution CT scans are considered to be the most sensitive radiographic methods of detection[61,62] and are associated with less variability of interpretation.[58,63] However, they are too expensive and time consuming for routine surveillance purposes. CT scans can be useful in the diagnosis of benign and malignant disease (Figures 14.8 and 14.9).

PFTs are extremely important in the evaluation of the patient with asbestos exposure. PFT results are effort dependent and, to be credible, these tests should be performed with appropriate equipment operated by a technician who has successfully received NIOSH-certified training, with strict adherence to guidelines published by the ATS.[64] The ATS has suggested that asbestosis is a restrictive lung disease characterized by a decline in the forced vital capacity (FVC), with a preserved ratio of the forced expiratory volume at 1 second (FEV$_1$) to the FVC (also referred to as the FEV$_1$/FVC ratio or FEV 1%).[44] More recent published studies,[54] however, suggest that nowadays, patients are likely to be older and have reduced levels of exposure. More patients are found to have normal pulmonary function, and when abnormalities exist, they are more likely to reveal obstruction rather than restriction. Pulmonary function studies typically include measurement of the forced expiratory flow rate at mid-expiration (25–75) and may include a diffusion study (DLCO) to detect gas exchange abnormalities.

Bronchoalveolar lavage has been used to identify asbestos bodies (ABs). ABs are considered a marker of exposure to asbestos and may be a diagnostic aid. However, the absence of an AB in

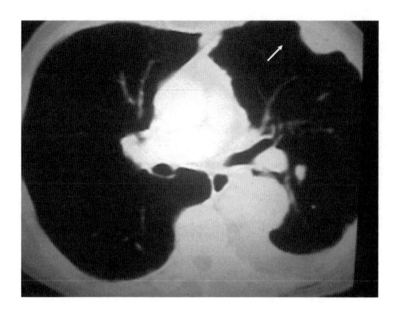

Figure 14.8   CT scan of asbestos-exposed patient with pleural plaque disease. Arrow, circumscribed pleural plaque, left anterior parietal pleura.

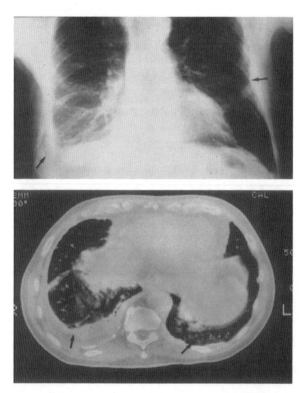

Figure 14.9   Patient with military and occupational exposure to asbestos, diagnosed with pleural mesothelioma. Upper image is a PA chest radiograph with diffuse pleural changes and blunting of the right costophrenic angle (arrow) and left-sided pleural plaque disease (arrow). The lower image is a CT slice showing interstitial fibrotic changes (asbestosis) at the left base (arrow) and thickened pleural rind on the right (arrow) consistent with the diagnosis of pleural mesothelioma.

bronchoalveolar lavage fluid does not exclude the diagnosis. There is considerable variability in the ratio of ABs and parenchymal fiber burden. Such studies may be of limited usefulness in the clinical evaluation of exposed patients.[65] Spontaneous or induced sputum examination may be useful in detecting ABs and is less invasive.[66] Their identification in sputum is specific for significant tissue burden but is not sensitive.[67]

14.5 TREATMENT

Unfortunately, there is limited effective treatment for the patient with asbestosis. Prevention of exposure to asbestos and early identification of affected individuals is essential. Corticosteroids and immunosuppressants have had little effect on symptoms or survival.[68] Prevention of infectious complications through appropriate vaccination should be considered. It is extremely important for the physician to warn the asbestos-exposed patient of the dangerous synergism that exists with concomitant exposure to tobacco smoke. The approach to the management of cancer is uniform regardless of the contribution of asbestos. Unfortunately, an occupational history is frequently overlooked when new cases of cancer are diagnosed (Stuart D. Personal communication, 2004.)

14.6 CONSENSUS ITEMS AND CONTROVERSIES

Although a number of issues remain unresolved, there is general agreement between scientists and health agencies regarding several health effects from asbestos.[12] These consensus items are outlined in Table 14.5 along with key unresolved issues. The American College of Chest Physicians released a consensus statement on the respiratory health effects of asbestos.[69] This was accomplished through an interactive technique known as the Delphi method, in which a systematic and iterative approach is applied to achieve consensus among an expert panel regarding asbestos and respiratory health on questions for which disagreement remains. The physician who becomes engaged as an expert in these matters should become very familiar with these consensus items and controversies and the conclusions, discussions, and scientific literature surrounding them.

14.7 MEDICAL SURVEILLANCE AND ESSENTIAL REGULATORY ISSUES

Until now, this chapter has focused on the diagnosis of disease, mostly when it has become clinically manifested in individual patients. In contrast, medical surveillance is "the systematic collection, analysis, and dissemination of data on groups of workers and workplaces for the prevention of illness and injury."[70] This prevention (secondary prevention) frequently takes place at a subclinical level resulting in early disease intervention and potential application to the larger group of workers. A component of this surveillance activity is the Sentinel Health Event Occupational or SHE(O). The SHE(O) is "a disease, disability, or untimely death that is occupationally related and whose occurrence may provide the impetus for evaluations and interventions to prevent future cases."[70] Mesothelioma serves as a SHE(O) or heralding event given its unique association with asbestos exposure and its accompanying morbidity and mortality.

As with many other regulatory standards under the Occupational Safety and Health Administration (OSHA) and similar federal agencies, medical surveillance is an important component of monitoring the individual worker while monitoring the workforce. Surveillance is driven by risk, and in the case of asbestos regulations, workers who are subject to medical surveillance activities are those who are exposed at the action level which, presently, is equal to the permissible exposure limit (0.1 fibers/cm^3, 8-h time-weighted average). Although there are subtle differences

Table 14.5   Consensus and Unresolved Issues Regarding Health Effects from Asbestos

Consensus issues

Exposure to any asbestos type (i.e., serpentine or amphibole) can increase the likelihood of lung cancer, mesothelioma, and nonmalignant lung and pleural disorders.

Important determinants of toxicity include exposure concentration, exposure duration and frequency, and fiber dimensions and durability.

Fibers of amphibole asbestos such as tremolite, actinolite, and crocidolite are retained longer in the lower respiratory tract than chrysotile fibers of similar dimension.

Pulmonary interstitial fibrosis associated with deposition of collagen, progressive lung stiffening and impaired gas exchange, disability, and death occurred in many asbestos workers.

Most cases of asbestosis or lung cancer in asbestos workers occurred 15 years or more after their initial exposure to asbestos.

Asbestos-exposed tobacco smokers have greater than additive risks for lung cancer than do asbestos-exposed nonsmokers.

The time between diagnosis of mesothelioma and the time of initial occupational exposure to asbestos commonly has been 30 years or more.

Cases of mesotheliomas have been reported after household exposure of family members of asbestos workers and in individuals without occupational exposure who live close to asbestos mines.

Unresolved issues

Does exposure to asbestos increase the risk for GI cancer?

Are chrysotile fibers (or amphibole asbestos fibers) primarily responsible for mesotheliomas in certain groups of workers predominantly exposed to chrysotile?

Are amphibole asbestos types more potent than chrysotile in inducing asbestosis and lung cancer?

Should the U.S. regulatory definition of an asbestos fiber (length ≥ 5 μm with aspect ratio $\geq 3:1$), established for purposes of quantifying exposure levels, be changed?

What are the molecular events involved in the development of asbestos-induced respiratory and pleural effects and how are they influenced by fiber dimensions and mineral type?

What are the actual risks for malignant or nonmalignant respiratory disease that may exist at exposure levels below air concentrations (0.1–0.2 fiber/mL) established as recent occupational exposure limits?

Can lung cancer be attributed to asbestos exposure (regardless of fiber type) in the absence of pulmonary fibrosis?

Source: Syracuse Research Corporation, Toxicological Profile for Asbestos (Update), Contract 205-1999-00024, prepared for the U.S. Department of Health and Human Services, Public Health Service, Agency for Toxic Substances and Disease Registry, September, 2001, Appendix F.

in the requirements surrounding and content of preplacement, periodic, and termination examinations, they are similar for the general industry, the construction trades, the shipyard industry, and those categories of government or municipal employees and other workers covered under rules set forth by the U.S. Environmental Protection Agency. Conformance with OSHA's respirator standard (29 CFR 1910.134) is essential. Table 14.6 outlines the applicable federal regulatory standards and the general content of examinations required for asbestos medical surveillance. Individual states may have additional state-specific rules.

From a medical standpoint, systematic review of relevant evidence has resulted in recommendations that, "although screening the general population for asbestosis is not warranted," consideration should be given to "screening for asbestosis in patients with occupations at high risk for asbestos exposure."[71] Similarly, consideration of "lifelong health surveillance in persons with significant current or prior airborne asbestos exposure," including annual respiratory symptom review, physical examination, and pulmonary function studies in such high-risk patients, accompanied by periodic chest radiography with frequency on the basis of duration since first asbestos exposure, have been suggested. The rationale for such screening is one of early detection and further exposure prevention. The role of serum markers in screening for mesothelioma in patients at high risk may be considered (e.g., serum mesothelin-related protein, osteopontin), but at present their measurement is not routinely recommended.[53,72–74]

Table 14.6   Medical Surveillance for Asbestos: Relevant Federal Regulatory Standards and General Content of Examinations

Relevant federal regulatory standards with medical surveillance components for asbestos
29 CFR 1910.1001—OSHA, general industry
29 CFR 1926.1101—OSHA, construction industry
29 CFR 1915.1001—OSHA, shipyard industry
40 CFR 763—Environmental Protection Agency, state and local government employees (like schools)
General medical surveillance examination content for asbestos
Medical and work history
Standardized questionnaire (initial or periodic)
Physical examination with emphasis on respiratory, cardiovascular, and digestive systems
Spirometry
FVC
FEV_1
Calculation of FEV_1/FVC ratio (FEV_1 percent)
Comparison with predicted values
Chest radiograph
PA film (PA view)
At physician discretion; General Industry—at preplacement and periodically based on age and years since onset exposure
Reviewed in accordance with ILO
Other tests at physician's discretion

14.8 THE CLINICIAN IN THE COURTROOM: ESSENTIAL MEDICAL–LEGAL CONSIDERATIONS

Since the 1993 landmark Daubert decision by the U.S. Supreme Court, trial courts have evaluated scientific evidence with greater rigor. U.S. courts are now required to evaluate for themselves whether testimony or evidence is relevant and reliable rather than depending solely upon the credibility of purported experts. In other words, they must determine whether the scientific methodology is reliable and the science valid.

On the matter of reliability, the U.S. Supreme Court offered a list of factors to guide lower courts when judging a "novel" scientific theory or methodology (Table 14.7).[75] However, it has become standard procedure for defendants to seek this analysis in toxic and occupational exposure cases even when classic rather than novel approaches have been used. The trial courts have become "gatekeepers" and judges "junior scientists" to block "junk science" from entering the courtroom. As to relevance, the determination to be made is that the methodology used by the expert must "fit" the type of scientific inquiry at hand. If one accepts the premise that an expert's opinion has a reliable basis in the knowledge and experience of his or her discipline, then the focus relies on the "fit" of the methodological approach and the reliability as judged by the guidance given by the Supreme Court. This is a complex matter beyond the scope of this book, but it is worth mentioning two specific methodological considerations as they relate to asbestos and drawing conclusions about causality.

First is the matter of concluding a causal link between exposure and chronic disease using traditional epidemiologic and public health principles (Table 14.8). The reader should consider these factors carefully in determining whether he or she can conclude a causal link between asbestos, the circumstances surrounding exposure, and the disease end point in question. Second, the use of differential diagnosis is considered an acceptable methodology assuming that techniques such as history and physical examination, reliable laboratory data, and consideration of alternative causes were used. The clinician should ascribe to ethical principles outlined by established bodies of peers

Table 14.7   U.S. Supreme Court in Daubert, Nonexclusive List of Factors to Determine Reliability of "Novel" Scientific Theory or Methodology

Nonexclusive List of Factors
Testability
Peer review
Known error rate
Operational standards and controls
General acceptance of method or theory in the profession

Source: Guidotti, T.L., Rose, S.G., Eds., *Science on the Witness Stand: Evaluating Scientific Evidence in Law, Adjudication and Policy*, OEM Press, Beverly Farms, MA, 2001, p. 81.

Table 14.8   Epidemiologic Criteria for Judging Causality in Public Health

Criteria
Strength of the association or high relative risk
Dose–response relationship
Consistency of findings
Biological plausibility, including experimental evidence
Temporal cogency
Control of confounding and bias
Specificity
Overall coherence

Source: Guidotti, T.L., Rose, S.G., Eds., *Science on the Witness Stand: Evaluating Scientific Evidence in Law, Adjudication and Policy*, OEM Press, Beverly Farms, MA, 2001, pp. 60–62.

and be prepared to answer the question at hand by explaining why and offering the evidentiary basis for reaching that conclusion in the citable scientific literature.

14.9 THE INTERPLAY BETWEEN SCIENCE AND HISTORY: A BRIEF INSTRUCTIVE CASE EXAMPLE

Given amosite asbestos' role as the predominant commercial amphibole in the United States, its contribution to disease burden among exposed individuals has remained of particular interest.[76] As exposures to commercial asbestos have rarely involved a single fiber type, historical situations where this has occurred in the occupational setting, partly as a matter of chance, have created circumstances to evaluate the implications epidemiologically.

During the Second World War, a plant in Patterson, New Jersey, produced amosite asbestos insulation for use in shipbuilding and repair in the U.S. Navy. That factory closed in 1954. In the same year, a successor amosite asbestos insulation plant opened in Tyler, Texas (Figure 14.10). The facility was in operation until 1972, when it closed after citations from the OSHA because of worker exposures in excess of the regulatory standard at the time. Of note is the availability of actual air monitoring data collected in the facility on multiple occasions.

The most recent mortality analysis conducted on this cohort of workers was published in 1998, and current follow-up analysis 10 years later is presently underway. "The uniqueness of this asbestos cohort lies with the fact that people working in the Tyler plant were from a rural environment, sheltered from adjacent industrial complexes, and exposed to a single asbestiform mineral during plant operations."[76] The data confirmed a strong link between amosite asbestos and respiratory malignancy as well as mesothelioma. Follow-up analysis continues to reveal additional deaths from asbestos-related diseases.

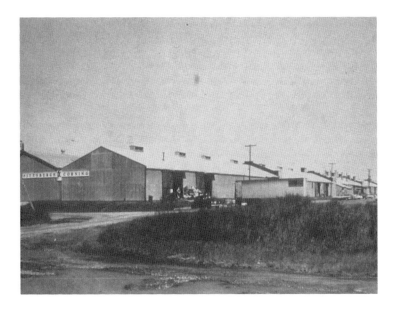

Figure 14.10 Amosite asbestos insulation manufacturing facility in Tyler, Texas.

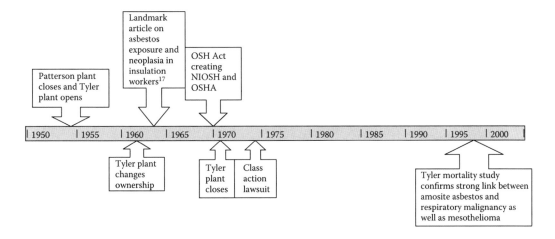

Figure 14.11 Timeline of plant operations at the Tyler, Texas, amosite asbestos insulation manufacturing facility.

Although the former Tyler asbestos plant remains of continued scientific importance for these reasons, it is also instructive for practicing clinicians and trainees in occupational medicine to briefly mention a few key historical and social factors that came together at the time the plant closed its doors. Many of these are recounted in an investigative novel entitled *Expendable Americans*[77] and illustrated in the timeline in Figure 14.11. In particular, 1970 represents a landmark year with passage of the federal Occupational Safety and Health Act, which provided for creation of the OSHA and the NIOSH. Massing scientific evidence of the health implications of occupational exposure to asbestos, prodding by organized labor, champions from numerous settings willing to persist and confront strong forces at multiple levels, and a recognition of important industrial hygiene principles related to exposure came together in this new regulatory framework to effect change in protecting the safety and health of workers. Occupational exposure to asbestos had made its way

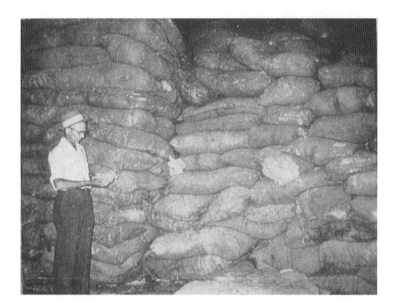

Figure 14.12 Burlap bags containing imported amosite asbestos. Burlap bags were later sold in large quantity to local rose nursery operations where additional occupational exposure occurred.

beyond the confines of the plant. The asbestos had been imported in burlap bags (see Figure 14.12), which were later sold in large quantity to rose nursery operations in Tyler. It is interesting that the Tyler asbestos plant ceased operation after rather modest fines, but on the heels of this event, in January 1974 "a $100 million class action lawsuit, the largest in recent history, was filed in Tyler's U.S. District Court on behalf of former employees" (p. 249).[77] A new era was ushered in.

REFERENCES

1. American Board of Preventive Medicine (ABPM). History. Available at: http://www.abprevmed.org/infobook.cfm. Accessed 2009.
2. Castorina JS, Rosenstock L. Physician shortage in occupational and environmental medicine. *Ann Intern Med* 1990;113(12):983–986.
3. Council on Graduate Medical Education. Update on the physician workforce. U.S. Department of Health and Human Services, Health Resources and Services Administration; August 2000.
4. Institute of Medicine. *Safe Work in the 21st Century: Education and Training Needs for the Next Decade's Occupational Safety and Health Personnel*. Washington, DC: National Academy Press; 2000: 1–15.
5. American Board of Preventive Medicine (ABPM). Search the diplomate directory; 2009. Available at: https://www.theabpm.org/directory_search.cfm. Accessed 2009.
6. American Board of Preventive Medicine (ABPM). Examination pass rates; 2009. Available at: https://www.theabpm.org/pass_rates.cfm. Accessed 2009.
7. Institute of Medicine. Addressing the physician shortage in occupational and environmental medicine. Publication No. 91-03. Washington, DC: National Academy of Sciences; 1991: 14–15.
8. Accreditation Council for Graduate Medical Education. Program requirements for graduate medical education in family medicine, effective July 1, 2007. Available at: http://www.acgme.org/acWebsite/downloads/RRC_progReq/120pr07012007.pdf. Accessed 2009.
9. Michas MG, Iacono CU. Overview of occupational medicine training among US family medicine residency programs. *Fam Med* 2008;40(2):102–106.
10. Accreditation Council for Graduate Medical Education. Program requirements for preventive medicine, effective July 2007. Available at: http://www.acgme.org/acWebsite/downloads/RRC_progReq/380pr07012007.pdf. Accessed 2009.

11. Stallard E. Product liability forecasting for asbestos-related personal injury claims: A multidisciplinary approach. *Ann N Y Acad Sci* 2001;954:223–244.
12. Syracuse Research Corporation. Toxicological profile for asbestos (update). Contract No. 205-1999-00024. Prepared for the U.S. Department of Health and Human Services, Public Health Service, Agency for Toxic Substances and Disease Registry, September 2001.
13. Kilburn KH. Asbestos and other fibers. In: *Maxcy-Rosenau-Last Public Health and Preventive Medicine*, 14th ed., Wallace RB, Last JM, eds. New York: McGraw-Hill; 1998: 459–474.
14. Selikoff IJ, Greenberg M. A landmark case in asbestosis. *JAMA* 1991;265(7):898–901.
15. Doll R. Mortality from lung cancer in asbestos workers. *Br J Ind Med* 1955;12:81–86.
16. Wagner JC, Sleggs CA, Marchand P. Diffuse pleural mesothelioma and asbestos exposure in the north-western cape province. *Br J Ind Med* 1960;17:260–271.
17. Selikoff IJ, Churg J, Hammond EC. Asbestos exposure and neoplasia. *JAMA* 1964;188:22–26.
18. Selikoff IJ, Seidman H. Asbestos-associated deaths among insulation workers in the United States and Canada, 1967–1987. *Ann N Y Acad Sci* 1991;643:1–14.
19. Levin SM, Kann PE, Lax MB. Medical examination for asbestos-related disease. *Am J Ind Med* 2000;37:6–22.
20. Landrigan PJ. The third wave of asbestos disease: exposure to asbestos in place, public health control, preface. *Ann N Y Acad Sci* 1991;643:xv–xvi.
21. Tucker P. Case studies in environmental medicine (CSEM): Asbestos toxicity. Atlanta, GA: Agency for Toxic Substances and Disease Registry (ATSDR); 2007. Available at: http://www.atsdr.cdc.gov/csem/asbestos/cover2.html. Accessed 2009.
22. Frank AL. Global problems from exposure to asbestos. *Environ Health Perspect* 1993;101(Suppl. 3):165–167.
23. LaDou J. The asbestos cancer epidemic. *Environ Health Perspect* 2004;112(3):285–290.
24. Parkes WR. Aerosols: Their deposition and clearance. In: *Occupational Lung Disorders*, 3rd ed., Parkes WR, ed. Oxford: Butterworth Heinemann; 1994: 35–49.
25. Stanley PJ, Wilson R, Greenstone MA, MacWilliam L, Cole PJ. Effect of cigarette smoking on nasal mucociliary clearance and ciliary beat frequency. *Thorax* 1986;41:519–523.
26. Glenn RE, Craft BF. Air sampling for particulates. In: *Occupational Respiratory Diseases*, Merchant JA, ed. Publication DHHS (NIOSH) 86-102. Washington, DC: U.S. Government Printing Office; 1986: 69–82.
27. Dodson RF, Williams MG, Corn CJ, Brollo A, Bianchi C. A comparison of asbestos burden in lung parenchyma, lymph nodes, and plaques. *Ann N Y Acad Sci* 1991;643:53–60.
28. Dodson RF, O'Sullivan MF, Huang J, Holiday DB, Hammar SP. Asbestos in extrapulmonary sites: Omentum and mesentery. *Chest* 2000;117(2):486–493.
29. Hammar SP, Dodson RF. Asbestos. In: *Pulmonary Pathology*, 2nd ed., Dail DH, Hammar SP, eds. New York: Springer Verlag Inc.; 1994: 901–983.
30. Craighead JE, Abraham JL, Churg A, Green FH, Kleinerman J, Pratt PC, et al. The pathology of asbestos-associated diseases of the lungs and pleural cavities: Diagnostic criteria and proposed grading schema. *Arch Pathol Lab Med* 1982;106:544–596.
31. Dodson RF, Williams MG, Hurst GA. Method for removing the ferruginous coating from asbestos bodies. *J Toxicol Environ Health* 1983;11:959–966.
32. Churg A, Warnock ML. Analysis of the cores of ferruginous (asbestos) bodies from the general population: I. Patients with and without lung cancer. *Lab Invest* 1977;37:280–286.
33. Churg A, Warnock ML. Analysis of the cores of asbestos bodies from members of the general population: patients with probable low-degree exposure to asbestos. *Am Rev Respir Dis* 1979;120:781–786.
34. Churg A, Warnock ML. Asbestos and other ferruginous bodies. *Am J Pathol* 1981;102:447–456.
35. Churg A, Warnock ML, Green N. Analysis of the cores of ferruginous (asbestos) bodies from the general population. *Lab Invest* 1979;40:31–38.
36. Dodson RF, O'Sullivan MF, Williams MG, Hurst GA. Analysis of cores of ferruginous bodies from former asbestos workers. *Environ Res* 1982;28:171–178.
37. Mossman BT, Bignon J, Corn M, Seaton A, Gee JBL. Asbestos: Scientific developments and implications for public policy. *Science* 1990;247:294–301.
38. Churg A, Warnock ML. Asbestos fibers in the general population. *Am Rev Respir Dis* 1980;122:669–678.

39. Albin M, Johansson L, Pooley FD, Jakobsson K, Attewell R, Mitha R. Mineral fibres, fibrosis, and asbestos bodies in lung tissue from deceased asbestos cement workers. *Br J Ind Med* 1990;47:767–774.

40. National Institute for Occupational Safety and Health (NIOSH). Asbestos fibers and other elongated mineral particles: state of the science and roadmap for research. Revised Draft NIOSH Current Intelligence Bulletin, Department of Health and Human Services, Centers for Disease Control and Prevention, January 20, 2009.

41. National Institute for Occupational Safety and Health (NIOSH). Safety and health topic: asbestos. Available at: http://www.cdc.gov/niosh/topics/asbestos. Accessed 2009.

42. Politi BJ, Arena VC, Schwerha J, Sussman N. Occupational medical history taking: how are today's physicians doing? A cross-sectional investigation of the frequency of occupational history taking by physicians in a major U.S. teaching center. *J Occup Environ Med* 2004;46(6):550–555.

43. Yu D. Case studies in environmental medicine: Taking an exposure history. Atlanta, GA: Agency for Toxic Substances and Disease Registry (ATSDR), 2008. Available at: http://www.atsdr.cdc.gov/csem/exphistory/ehcover_page.html. Accessed 2009.

44. American Thoracic Society. The diagnosis of nonmalignant diseases related to asbestos. *Am Rev Respir Dis* 1986;134:363–368.

45. American Thoracic Society. Diagnosis and initial management of nonmalignant diseases related to asbestos. *Am J Respir Crit Care Med* 2004;170:691–715.

46. Centers for Disease Control and Prevention. Changing patterns of pneumoconiosis mortality in the United States, 1968–2000. *MMWR* 2004;53(28):627–632.

47. Virta RL. Asbestos: geology, mineralogy, mining, and uses. Open-File Report 02-149. U.S. Geological Survey. Available at: http://pubs.usgs.gov/of/2002/of02–149/. Accessed 2009.

48. Cugell DW, Kamp DW. Asbestos and the pleura: A review. *Chest* 2004;125(3):1103–1117.

49. American Cancer Society. Asbestos. Available at: http://www.cancer.org/docroot/PED/content/PED_1_3X_Asbestos.asp?sitearea=PED. Accessed 2009.

50. Hammond EC, Selikoff IJ, Seidman H. Asbestos exposure, cigarette smoking and death rates. *Ann N Y Acad Sci* 1979;330:472–490.

51. Tomek S, Manegold C. Chemotherapy for malignant pleural mesothelioma: Past results and recent developments. *Lung Cancer* 2004;45(Suppl. 1):S103–S119.

52. Stewart DJ, Edwards JG, Smythe WR, Waller DA, O'Byrne KJ. Malignant pleural mesothelioma: An update. *Int J Occup Environ Health* 2004;10(1):26–39.

53. O'Reilly KMA, McLaughlin AM, Beckett WS, Sime PJ. Asbestos-related lung disease. *Am Fam Physician* 2007;75:683–688, 690.

54. Ohar J, Sterling DA, Bleeker E, Donohue J. Changing patterns in asbestos-induced lung disease. *Chest* 2004;125(2):744–753.

55. National Institute for Occupational Safety and Health (NIOSH). Safety and health topic: Chest radiography. Available at: http://www.cdc.gov/niosh/topics/chestradiography/breader-info.html#d. Accessed 2009.

56. National Institute for Occupational Safety and Health (NIOSH). Application of the ILO International Classification of Radiographs of Pneumoconioses to Digital Chest Radiographic Images. NIOSH Publication No. 2008–139. Available at: http://www.cdc.gov/niosh/docs/2008–139/. Accessed 2008.

57. Gitlin JN, Cook LL, Linton OW, Garrett-Mayer E. Comparison of "B" readers' interpretations of chest radiographs for asbestos related changes. *Acad Radiol* 2004;11:843–856.

58. Lebedova J, Dlouha B, Rychla L, Neuwirth J, Brabec M, Pelclova D, Fenclova Z. Lung function impairment in relation to asbestos-induced pleural lesions with reference to the extent of lesions and the initial parenchymal fibrosis. *Scand J Work Environ Health* 2003;29(5):388–395.

59. Rockoff SD, Schwartz A. Roentgenographic underestimation of early asbestosis by International Labor Organization classification: Analysis of data and probabilities. *Chest* 1988;93(5):1088–1091.

60. Lawson CC, LeMasters MK, Lemasters GK, Reutman SS, Rice CH, Lockey JE. Reliability and validity of chest radiograph surveillance programs. *Chest* 2001;120(1):64–68.

61. Aberle DR, Gamsu G, Ray CS. High-resolution CT of benign asbestos-related diseases: Clinical and radiographic correlation. *Am J Roentgenol* 1988;151(5):883–891.

62. Harkin TJ, McGuinness G, Goldring R, Cohen H, Parker JE, Crane M, et al. Differentiation of the ILO boundary chest roentgenograph (0/1 to 1/0) in asbestosis by high-resolution computed tomography scan, alveolitis, and respiratory impairment. *J Occup Environ Med* 1996;38(1):46–52.

63. Begin R, Ostiguy G, Filion R, Colman N, Bertrand P. Computed tomography in the early detection of asbestosis. *Br J Ind Med* 1993;50(8):689–698.

64. American Thoracic Society. Standardization of spirometry: 1994 update. *Am J Respir Crit Care Med* 1995;152:1107–1136.

65. Schwartz DA, Galvin JR, Burmeister LF, Merchant RK, Dayton CS, Merchant JA, Hunninghake GW. The clinical utility and reliability of asbestos bodies in bronchoalveolar fluid. *Am Rev Respir Dis* 1991;144(3 Pt. 1):684–688.

66. Paris C, Galateau-Salle F, Creveuil C, Morello R, Raffaelli C, Gillon JC, et al. Asbestos bodies in the sputum of asbestos workers: correlation with occupational exposure. *Eur Respir J* 2002;20(5):1167–1173.

67. Roggli VL, Greenberg SD, Pratt PC, eds. *Pathology of Asbestos-Associated Diseases*. Boston: Little, Brown and Company; 1992: 238–244.

68. Mossman BT, Churg A. Mechanisms in the pathogenesis of asbestosis and silicosis. *Am J Respir Crit Care Med* 1998;157(5 Pt. 1):1666–1680.

69. Banks DE, Shi R, McLarty J, Cowl CT, Smith D, Tarlo SM, et al. American College of Chest Physicians consensus statement on the respiratory health effects of asbestos: Results of a Delphi study. *Chest* 2009;135:1619–1627.

70. McCunney RJ, ed. *A Practical Approach to Occupational and Environmental Medicine*, 3rd ed. Philadelphia: Lippincott Williams and Wilkins; 2003: 283–288, 582.

71. Millar JS, Morrissey BM, Chan AL. Asbestosis. American College of Physicians—Physicians' Information and Education Resource (pier). Available at: http://pier.acponline.org/physicians/diseases/d848/d848.html. Accessed 2008.

72. Hassan R, Pass HI. Mesothelioma. American College of Physicians—Physicians' Information and Education Resource (pier). Available by protected access at: http://pier.acponline.org/physicians/diseases/d1010/d1010.html. Accessed 2009.

73. Robinson BWS, Creaney J, Lake R, Nowak A, Musk AW, de Klerk N, et al. Mesothelin-family proteins and diagnosis of mesothelioma. *Lancet* 2003;362(9396):1612–1616.

74. Pass HI, Lott D, Lonardo F, Harbut M, Lui Z, Tang N, et al. Asbestos exposure, pleural mesothelioma, and serum osteopontin levels. *N Engl J Med* 2005;353:1564–1573.

75. Guidotti TL, Rose SG, eds. *Science on the Witness Stand: Evaluating Scientific Evidence in Law, Adjudication and Policy*. Beverly Farms, MA: OEM Press; 2001.

76. Levin JL, McLarty JW, Hurst GA, Smith AN, Frank AL. Tyler asbestos workers: Mortality experience in a cohort exposed to amosite. *Occup Environ Med* 1998;55:155–160.

77. Brodeur P. *Expendable Americans*. New York: The Viking Press; 1974.

CHAPTER 15

Asbestos Regulations and Their Applications

Daniel T. Crane and Adele Cardenas Malott

CONTENTS

15.1 INTRODUCTION

The three federal agencies who regulate asbestos and asbestos-containing materials (ACMs) in the United States are the Occupational Safety and Health Administration (OSHA), the Mine Safety and Health Administration (MSHA), and the Environmental Protection Agency (EPA). OSHA is required to protect employees from harmful working conditions when handling asbestos and ACMs in most workplaces. MSHA is required to protect employees from harmful working conditions when handling asbestos or ACMs in mines and mills. The EPA is required to protect human health and the environment through rules and regulations, which provide standards for handling asbestos and ACMs that enter the environment, resulting in some form of exposure.

Each agency is responsible for different population sectors, and their respective regulations have definitions that are not the same, partly as a result of differences in individual rulemaking. It is important to assess what each agency intends and not assume that even fundamental definitions are universal.

15.2 OSHA—OCCUPATIONAL EXPOSURE TO ASBESTOS IN GENERAL INDUSTRY, CONSTRUCTION INDUSTRY, AND SHIPYARDS (29 CFR 1910.1001, 29 CFR 1926.1101, AND 29 CFR 1915.1001)*

The OSHA has a long history of regulation of asbestos in the workplace. Indeed, among the strongest arguments made in favor for passage of the Williams–Steiger Act of 1970 were those describing the exposure of workers to asbestos and the resultant ravages of asbestos-related disease. Both NIOSH and OSHA were established by that Act and have worked collaboratively on this and many other occupational health and safety issues.

A permissible exposure limit (PEL) of 12 fibers per cubic centimeter of air (f/cc) or 2 million particles per cubic foot of air (mppcf) for asbestos was among the first exposure levels adopted by OSHA in 1971. It was based on the levels from the Walsh-Healey and Public Contracts Acts of 1969. In December 1971, OSHA promulgated an Emergency Temporary Standard of 5 f/cc, and asbestos was the very first expanded health standard promulgated by OSHA in 1972. An expanded standard contains specific information and compliance instruction about a particular substance in addition to the PEL. The PEL was set at 5 f/cc as an 8-h time-weighted average. This rulemaking provided for a delayed decrease of the PEL to 2 f/cc in 1976 to allow time for industry to comply. In late 1983, OSHA issued an Emergency Temporary Standard that lowered the PEL to 0.5 f/cc. This was overturned by the U.S. Circuit Court of Appeals in early 1984. In 1986, using a quantitative risk assessment, the PEL was reduced to 0.2 f/cc with the promulgation of two separate standards, one for construction industry and one for general industry. Responding to issues raised in challenges to that rulemaking, OSHA lowered the PEL to 0.1 f/cc in 1994. OSHA issued this PEL in three separate rules: one for shipyard (29 CFR 1915.1001), one for construction (29 CFR1926.1101), and another for general industry (29 CFR 1910.1001). Although all three specify the same PEL, each industry segment has some unique work practices and statutory requirements. Shipyard industries are defined in 29 CFR 1915.4, construction industries are defined in 29 CFR 1910.12(b), and general industry includes all the rest.

Each of the three standards contains work practices and statutory language specific to the applicable industries, yet the general requirements are essentially the same. In particular, the construction and shipyard requirements and work practices are very similar, with the shipyard standard including elements of both construction and general industry.

15.2.1 Discussion of Common Elements of the Three OSHA Standards

Asbestos, as defined by OSHA, includes chrysotile, Amosite, crocidolite, tremolite asbestos, anthophyllite asbestos, actinolite asbestos, and any of these minerals that have been chemically treated and/or altered. ACM means any material containing more than 1% asbestos. If a building

---

* Available at: www.osha.gov (accessed April 20, 2010).

was constructed before 1980, it is assumed to contain some asbestos. Such thermal systems insulation is called presumed ACM (PACM). It is the employer's responsibility to either treat this material as if it were asbestos or provide analytical evidence to rebut the presence of ACM.

Each standard establishes a PEL of 0.1 f/cc as an 8-h time-weighted average and an excursion level (EL) of 1 f/cc over a 30-min time period. The concentration must never exceed the EL. The standards require personal air sampling in the breathing zone of employees to demonstrate compliance. Results of monitoring must be made available to employees. The nexus between the PEL and the quantitative risk assessment imposed a requirement to limit the uncertainty in the analysis. OSHA provided the OSHA Reference Method (ORM) in Appendix A for all three standards. It is a list of requirements necessary to limit uncertainty in the analysis. It includes measures known to limit variability and requires quality control and formal training of analysts. Air samples are required to be analyzed by phase-contrast microscopy (PCM) by a method equivalent to the requirements given in the ORM. Currently, only OSHA's ID-160 and NIOSH 7400 (when it is used within the limits of Appendix A) are recognized as equivalent to the ORM. OSHA Method ID-160 was included in all standards as Appendix B.

The standards include OSHA method ID-191 as an appendix, which is a method for the analysis of bulk asbestos materials. Where sampling of bulk insulation is required, it should be analyzed by a laboratory accredited for asbestos analysis. Accrediting bodies of this sort are represented, for example, by the National Voluntary Laboratory Accreditation Program (NVLAP) or the American Industrial Hygiene Association (AIHA).

The standards require initial and ongoing or periodic monitoring of asbestos operations to establish the baseline exposure and to evaluate whenever an operational change might result in a change in the exposure.

The standards require that an employer establish a regulated area wherever there is a potential for the PEL to be exceeded. The standards indicate how the regulated areas are to be demarcated, access limited, and to control behavior in the area such as smoking, eating, respirator use, and so forth.

Each standard provides for general and specific methods of compliance that, if followed, should limit employee's exposure to asbestos fibers. These methods include wet cleanup, dust extraction on power hand tools, prohibition of the use of compressed air for blowdown, written compliance program, and prohibition of employee rotation to achieve exposure below the PEL. In addition, all standards have specific requirements for housekeeping to limit the generation of asbestos-containing dust.

A respiratory protection requirement is included in each standard that defines what kinds of respirator can be used, when and how they can be used, and requires employers to have a respirator program in place that is compliant with 29 CFR 1910.134.

Each standard contains instructions on protective clothing and equipment. Take-home exposure to family was recognized as a significant and measurable risk. This part of the standards is established to mitigate that risk. It provides that the employer must provide clothing and laundry facilities along with change rooms, showers, and the means to assure decontamination of employees and equipment. It also requires employees have areas to rest and eat where the concentration of asbestos is below the PEL.

The standards have extensive requirements for hazard communication to provide disclosure to employees, other employers, and cotenants as to the extent and nature of any asbestos hazard. Specific labeling is required on products or materials that clearly indicate the danger and hazard of generating asbestos dust. They include industry and task-specific training for employees who work with and around asbestos and ACM.

Medical surveillance is required by all of the standards to include initial, subsequent, and terminal medical examinations, including prescribed elements such as questionnaires, pulmonary function tests, and chest roentgenograms interpreted by a B-reader. These examinations are to be provided by the employer at no cost to the employee.

Records of air monitoring, building testing, and medical examinations are required to be kept for at least 30 years past employment. Building information must be transferred to subsequent owners.

15.2.2 Discussion of Industry-Specific Requirements

15.2.2.1 General Industry 29 CFR1910.1001

General industry includes manufacturing of asbestos and asbestos-containing articles and materials, brake-shoe service, custodial work around installations of ACM, and all employers not covered by either the construction or the shipyard standards. Such businesses tend to be, but are not always, in a fixed location. In the general industry standard, more emphasis is placed on controlling exposure by use of engineering controls so as to limit the need to use respirators. Respirators may only be used when it can be demonstrated that engineering control is infeasible.

Air monitoring is required initially and whenever a process is changed that might lead to a change in asbestos exposure.

Building owners are required to survey their facilities to determine the presence and extent of any asbestos or ACM and communicate this to their employees and any employers that occupy the facility. They are required to keep and post records of these surveys and make them available.

Specific work practices are given for brake-shoe service that includes wet methods to limit the generation of dust during brake-shoe service.

15.2.2.2 Construction Industry 29 CFR 1926.1101 and Shipyard Industry 29 CFR 1915.1001

The construction and shipyard industry standards are essentially the same. The shipyard standard contains instructions on brake-shoe service that may take place in shipyards. In addition, both standards require a person, called a "competent person" in the construction standard and a "qualified person" in the shipyard standard, to have the training, the knowledge, and the authority to establish and enforce the regulated areas.

Work covered by the construction standard is usually of a transitory nature and is designated as Unclassified, Class I, Class II, Class III, or Class IV, depending upon the nature of the material. Any work containing less than 1% asbestos is considered unclassified. Class I work is with thermal system insulation such as pipe wrap and sprayed-on or troweled ACM or presumed ACM insulation. Class II work includes ACM such as flooring or roofing with less potential for fiber release. Class III work includes small repair or maintenance jobs that can generally be contained in a single glove bag. Class IV work is custodial in nature in a construction setting where ACM is being cleaned up.

An employer is required to perform an initial negative exposure assessment (NEA) to determine whether or not the project can be completed without exceeding the PEL. Unless it can be shown the work will not exceed the PEL, the specific requirements of the particular class work are triggered. An employer can rely on objective data that the material cannot release fibers above the PEL or historic data that a substantially equivalent operation has never released fibers above the PEL. Daily monitoring is required for Class I and Class II. In addition to notifying employees, the employer must inform the building owner and other affected employers of the final monitoring results within 10 days of project completion.

Class I work is often performed in a negative pressure enclosure to contain the asbestos fibers. Regardless of the class of work, the employer must assure the concentration outside the regulated area is below the PEL.

All affected parties must be informed of the work being performed. This includes other employers and tenants in the building or facility.

Energetic work practices such as high-speed abrasive saws, non-HEPA vacuums, and sanders are prohibited.

15.3 OSHA—RESPONSIBILITY WITHIN THE NATIONAL RESPONSE FRAMEWORK

The *National Response Framework* presents the guiding principles that enable all response partners to prepare for and provide a unified national response to disasters and emergencies— from the smallest incident to the largest catastrophe. The framework is administered by the Federal Emergency Management Agency (FEMA) and establishes a comprehensive, national, all-hazards approach to domestic incident response.[*]

OSHA has the responsibility as the U.S. Department of Labor Representative to provide worker safety advice, assistance, and policy support for debris removal, building demolition, and other emergency support function activities defined by the Public Works and Engineering Annex 3.[†] An extensive discussion of OSHA's responsibilities in this role can be found on OSHA's Web site.[‡,§] Also available are many easily accessible resources to help employers and the general public to respond safely during disaster or emergency.

OSHA provides technical assistance and support for response and recovery worker safety and health in the changing requirements of domestic incident management to include preparedness, prevention, response, and recovery actions. Activities within the scope of this function include development of health and safety plans; identifying, assessing, and controlling health and safety hazards; conducting response and recovery exposure monitoring; collecting and managing data; providing technical assistance and support for personal protective equipment programs, incident-specific response and recovery worker training, and medical surveillance; providing exposure and risk management information; and providing technical assistance to include industrial hygiene expertise, occupational safety and health expertise, engineering expertise, and occupational medicine expertise.

The U.S. infrastructure was built using millions of tons of ACM as structural, insulating, and decorative elements such as roofing shingles, siding, thermal barriers, and in concrete. In the event of a natural disaster or other emergency and the ensuing cleanup and remediation, the potential for exposure to asbestos as well as lead, crystalline silica, high levels of dust, and event-specific materials can be significant. OSHA provides measurements and assessments of these substances along with guidance on safe and healthful practices during these activities as described in the Annex administered by FEMA.[¶]

15.4 MSHA—OCCUPATIONAL EXPOSURE TO ASBESTOS IN SURFACE METAL AND NONMETAL MINES, UNDERGROUND METAL AND NONMETAL MINES, AND SURFACE WORK AREAS OF UNDERGROUND COAL MINES (30 CFR PARTS 56, 57, AND 71)

The history of U.S. Federal regulation of safety in the mining industry began in 1891 where, among other issues, ventilation regulations and child labor restrictions were given by statute for mines. In 1910, the Bureau of Mines was established within the Department of the Interior to address the more than 2000 annual deaths in coal mining.[**] The authority to enter mines was granted in 1941, and in 1947 the first Federal regulations for mine safety were codified.

---

[*] Available at: http://www.fema.gov/emergency/nrf/aboutNRF.htm (accessed April 20, 2010).
[†] Available at: http://www.fema.gov/emergency/nrf/aboutNRF.htm nrf-esf-03 (accessed April 20, 2010).
[‡] Available at: http://www.osha.gov/SLTC/emergencypreparedness/osha_support.html (accessed April 20, 2010).
[§] Available at: http://www.fema.gov/pdf/emergency/nrf/nrf-support-wsh.pdf (accessed April 20, 2010).
[¶] Available at: http://www.fema.gov/pdf/emergency/nrf/nrf-support-wsh.pdf (accessed April 20, 2010).
[**] Available at: http://www.msha.gov/mshainfo/mshainf2.htm (accessed October 19, 2009).

In 1973, the Secretary of the Interior, through administrative action, created the Mining Enforcement and Safety Administration as a departmental agency separate from the Bureau of Mines.[*]

The Congress passed the Federal Mine Safety and Health Act in 1977, which established the MSHA, transferring the activities of the former Mining Enforcement and Safety Administration to the Department of Labor. The Mine Act strengthened and expanded the rights of miners and enhanced the protection of miners from retaliation for exercising such rights.[†]

MSHA and its predecessor's asbestos regulations date back to 1967 and are based on the Bureau of Mines standard of 5 mppcf. In 1969, the Bureau proposed and promulgated a standard of 2 mppcf and 12 f/cc. In 1970, the Bureau proposed to lower the standard to 5 f/cc, which standard was promulgated in 1974. MSHA issued a standard of 2 f/cc in 1976 for coal mining (41 FR 10223) and in 1978 for metal and nonmetal mining (43 FR 54064).[‡]

In 2008, MSHA lowered the 8-h time-weighted PEL to 0.1 f/cc consistent with the PEL promulgated by the OSHA.[§] In addition to the PEL, the regulations established a 30-min EL of 1 f/cc. The asbestos air concentration must never exceed this level. The regulations apply to three mining segments: metal and nonmetal mines, surface coal mines, and surface areas of underground coal mines. The specific regulations that apply to airborne contaminants are as follows:

30 CFR Part 56: Safety and Health Standards—Surface Metal and Nonmetal Mines Sections 56.5001, 5002, and 5005;

30 CFR Part 57: Safety and Health Standards—Underground Metal and Nonmetal Mines Sections 57.5001, 5002, and 5005; and

30 CFR Part 71: Mandatory Health Standards—Surface Coal Mines and Surface Work Areas of Underground Coal Mines Sections 71.700, 701, and 702.

All three regulations require mine operators to control dust such that employees are not exposed above levels adopted by the American Conference of Industrial Hygienist. The levels were adopted by reference from the 1972 American Conference of Industrial Hygienists threshold limit values for Part 71[¶] and 1973 for Parts 56 and 57.[**]

All three regulations have a harmonized definition for asbestos. For example, at 30 CFR Part 56.5001 (b)(1), the definitions are given as:

Asbestos is a generic term for a number of hydrated silicates that, when crushed or processed, separate into flexible fibers made up of fibrils. As used in this part—*Asbestos* means chrysotile, cummingtonite–grunerite asbestos (Amosite), crocidolite, anthophyllite asbestos, tremolite asbestos, and actinolite asbestos. *Fiber* means a particle longer than 5 micrometers (μm) with a length-to-diameter ratio of at least 3-to-1.

Air concentration measurements for these standards are made using PCM followed by a confirmation by transmission electron microscopy when the PCM shows the possibility of an overexposure.

15.5 EPA—ASBESTOS WORKER PROTECTION STANDARD (40 CFR 763 SUBPART G)

The Asbestos Worker Protection Standard under section 6(a) of the Toxic Substances Control Act (TSCA) provides protection to certain state and local government employees who are not protected by the Asbestos Standards of the Occupational Safety and Health (OSHA) Act of 1970.

---

[*] Ibid.
[†] Ibid.
[‡] Available at: http://www.msha.gov/regs/unified/December2003/1219-AB24.HTM (accessed 19 October 2009).
[§] Federal Register, Friday, February 29, 2008;73(41):284–11304.
[¶] Threshold limit values for chemical substances in workroom air adopted by ACGIH for 1972.
[**] Threshold limit values for chemical substances in workroom air adopted by ACGIH for 1973.

The rule, which was issued in 1985 and amended in 1987, applied to asbestos abatement projects only. This subpart applies the OSHA Asbestos Standards in 29 CFR 1910.1001 and 29 CFR 29 1101 to these state and local employees.

The EPA Worker Protection Standard was amended in November 2000 to apply not only to the OSHA Asbestos Construction Industry Standard but also to the Asbestos General Industry Standard for state and local government employees who were not protected by the Asbestos Standards of OSHA. EPA provides exemptions to those states seeking to implement their own asbestos worker protection plan.

15.6 EPA—ASBESTOS HAZARD EMERGENCY RESPONSE ACT OF 1986: ACMS IN SCHOOL, RULES 1987

EPA's asbestos program for schools, mandated by the Asbestos Hazard Emergency Response Act (AHERA), and its regulations for schools and other buildings are founded on the principle of "in-place" management of ACM. This approach is designed to prevent asbestos exposure by teaching people to recognize ACMs and actively monitor them.

The Asbestos Hazard Emergency Act (AHERA), a provision of the TSCA, became law in 1986. AHERA requires local education agencies to inspect their schools for asbestos-containing building materials and to prepare management plans to prevent or reduce asbestos hazards.

Public school districts and nonprofit private schools (collectively called local education agencies) are subject to AHERA's requirements. EPA provides local education agencies, parents, and teachers with information about AHERA asbestos-in-schools requirements through mailings and other outreach mechanisms.

The requirements of AHERA are published in the Code of Federal Regulations, Chapter 40, Part 763, Subpart E. The rules require local education agencies to take the following actions: perform an original inspection and reinspection of ACM every three years; develop, maintain, and update an asbestos management plan; keep a copy of the plan at the school; provide yearly notification to parents, teachers, and employee organizations regarding the availability of the schools' asbestos management plan and any asbestos abatement actions taken or planned in the school; designate a contact person to ensure the responsibilities of the local education agency are properly implemented; perform periodic surveillance of known or suspected asbestos-containing building materials; ensure that properly accredited professionals perform inspections and response actions and prepare management plans; and provide custodial staff with asbestos awareness training.

In addition to the requirements pursuant to AHERA, local education agencies need to comply with the Asbestos National Emission Standards for Hazardous Air Pollutants (NESHAP), found at 40 CFR Part 61, Subpart M. It requires that owners or operators of facilities notify the appropriate authority (usually the state designated agency for asbestos) before demolishing or renovating facilities. If minimum amounts of regulated asbestos (1% or more asbestos) will be removed or disturbed, the owner/operator must adequately wet and carefully remove the asbestos components by keeping them wet until collected for disposal and then disposing of the asbestos waste in accordance with the regulations.

Several resources can be found on the EPA Web site, including the ABC's of asbestos in schools. If assistance is needed in obtaining information on asbestos in schools, please contact EPA's National Program Chemicals Division at 202-566-0500. Anyone can request more information on the AHERA requirements from the Toxic Substances Control Act (TSCA) assistance information service at 202-554-1404, or from the Asbestos Ombudsman at 1-800-368-5888.

The EPA maintains 10 regional offices to implement federal environmental programs around the country. These regional offices cooperate with federal, state, interstate, tribal, and local agencies as well as with industry, academic institutions, and other private groups to ensure that regional needs are addressed and that federal environmental laws are upheld. Within each region, regional asbestos coordinators and NESHAP asbestos coordinators oversee asbestos efforts.

15.7 EPA—MANUFACTURE, IMPORTATION, PROCESSING, AND DISTRIBUTION IN COMMERCE PROHIBITIONS: "THE ASBESTOS BAN AND PHASE OUT RULE"

On May 18, 1999, the EPA provided clarification regarding the asbestos materials ban, stating the following:

1. This clarification presents correct information with regard to the status of asbestos products that are banned by the U.S. EPA at this time as well as categories of asbestos-containing products that are NOT subject to a ban;
2. The clarification is needed because EPA finds that there are misunderstandings about its bans on ACMs and products or uses. Numerous newspaper and magazine articles, Internet information, even some currently available (but outdated) documents from the EPA and other federal agencies may contain statements about an EPA asbestos ban that are incorrect;
3. EPA asbestos regulations fall primarily under the authority of two different federal laws and their resulting implementations:
   - The Clean Air Act (e.g., Asbestos NESHAP) rules; and
   - The TSCA (e.g., Asbestos Ban and Phaseout) Asbestos rules.

Note that the U.S. Consumer Product Safety Commission also developed bans on use of asbestos in certain consumer products such as textured paint, wall patching compounds, and so forth. For more detailed information, contact the Consumer Product Safety Commission Hotline at 1-800-638-2772.

The Clean Air Act Authority states the EPA Asbestos NESHAP bans usage of certain ACMs in facilities regulated by the NESHAP Rule (Nov. 1990 Revision; 40 CFR 60, Subpart M) as follows:

Most Spray-Applied Surfacing ACM
   - 1973 NESHAP, banned for fireproofing/insulating
   - 1978 NESHAP, banned for "decorative" purposes

Note that the Nov. 1990 revised asbestos NESHAP prohibits spray-on application of materials containing more than 1% asbestos to buildings, structures, pipes, and conduits unless the material is encapsulated with a bituminous or resinous binder during spraying and the materials are not friable after drying. The revised NESHAP still allows, on equipment and machinery, spray-on application of materials that contain more than 1% asbestos where the asbestos fibers in the materials are encapsulated with a bituminous or resinous binder during spraying and the materials are not friable after drying, or for friable materials, where either no visible emissions are discharged to the outside air from spray-on application, or specified methods are used to clean emissions containing particulate asbestos material before they escape to, or are vented to, the outside air.

Thermal system insulation
   - 1975 NESHAP, banned installation of wet-applied and preformed (molded) asbestos pipe insulation.
   - 1975 NESHAP, banned installation of preformed (molded) asbestos block insulation on boilers and hot water tanks.

Is there a NESHAP ban on troweled-on surfacing ACM?

No, that particular application was not banned by the most recent NESHAP revision (November 1990).

The TSCA authority states the following:

1. July 1989 EPA rule commonly known as the "Asbestos Ban and Phaseout Rule" (40 CFR 763 Subpart I, Sec. 762.160–763.179) (Note: Much of the original rule was vacated and remanded by the U.S. Fifth Circuit Court of Appeals in 1991. Thus, the original 1989 EPA ban on the U.S. manufacture,

importation, processing, or distribution in commerce of many asbestos-containing product categories was set aside and did not remain in effect.)

2. Federal Register (FR), Nov. 5, 1993 (58 FR 58964), factual determinations:

"Continuing restrictions on certain asbestos-containing products." In this FR notice, EPA stated its position regarding the status of its ban on various asbestos-containing product categories, which is briefly summarized as follows:

Products still banned: Six asbestos-containing product categories that are still subject to the asbestos ban include corrugated paper, roll board, commercial paper, specialty paper, flooring felt, and new uses of asbestos.

Products not banned: Asbestos-containing product categories no longer subject to the 1989 TSCA ban include asbestos-cement corrugated sheet, asbestos-cement flat sheet, asbestos clothing, pipeline wraps, roofing felt, vinyl-asbestos floor tile, asbestos-cement shingle, millboard, asbestos-cement pipe, automatic transmission components, clutch facings, friction materials, disc brake pads, drum brake linings, brake blocks, gaskets, and roofing and nonroofing coatings.

3. Federal Register, June 28, 1994 (59 FR 33208):

"Technical Amendment in Response to Court Decision on Asbestos; ..." revised the language of the asbestos ban rule to conform to the 1991 Court decision. Contains definitions, manufacturing and importation prohibitions, processing, and distribution in commerce prohibitions. Also clarifies labeling requirements for specified asbestos-containing products. (Note: These FR notices can be found on the EPA OPPT asbestos page under "Laws and Regulations.")

In summary, the following is clarified:

1. Bans on some ACM products and uses remain in place at this time (April 1999). What are they?

Under the Clean Air Act:

- Most spray-applied surfacing ACM.
- Sprayed-on application of materials containing more than 1% asbestos to buildings, structures, pipes, and conduits unless the material is encapsulated with a bituminous or resinous binder during spraying and the materials are not friable after drying.
- Wet-applied and preformed asbestos pipe insulation and preformed asbestos block insulation on boilers and hot water tanks.

Under the TSCA:

Corrugated paper, roll board, commercial paper, specialty paper, flooring felt, and new uses of asbestos.

2. The EPA has no existing bans on most other asbestos-containing products or uses. EPA does *not* track the manufacture, processing, or distribution in commerce of asbestos-containing products. It would be prudent for a consumer or other buyer to inquire as to the presence of asbestos in particular products.

Possible sources of that information include query of the dealer/supplier or manufacturer, referring to the product's "material safety data sheet," or considering having the material tested for the presence of asbestos by a qualified laboratory.

For further information, contact the TSCA Assistance Information Service at 202-554-1404, or your EPA Regional Asbestos Coordinator for the state in which you live which can be found on the EPA Web site.

15.8 EPA—THE NESHAP, ASBESTOS NESHAP 40 CFR 61 SUBPART M

A summary of the EPA's asbestos regulations under NESHAP is as follows. Relevant sections of the regulations are bracketed for reference.

The regulations are in the Code of Federal Regulations at 40 C.F.R. Part 61, Subpart M.

The asbestos NESHAP regulations apply to the following:

- All public, commercial, industrial, or institutional structures
- Ships
- Active or inactive waste disposal sites
- Residential buildings with more than four units
- Single family homes to be burned for training purposes
- Two or more single family homes on a single site to be demolished or renovated for commercial purposes

The NESHAP regulations apply jointly to owners and operators at a facility. Worker health and safety regulations also apply to asbestos projects. Other federal, state, and local agencies may have asbestos management requirements. Schools are subject to additional EPA requirements under the AHERA. The asbestos worker and inspector certification requirements referenced below can be found in the Asbestos Model Accreditation Plan (MAP), at 40 C.F.R. Part 763, Subpart E, Appendix C.

Definition of Regulated ACM (RACM): Friable asbestos material; nonfriable material that has become friable; nonfriable asbestos material that has been or will be subject to sanding, grinding, cutting, or abrading; or nonfriable asbestos material that has a high probability of becoming crumbled, pulverized, or reduced to powder by the forces expected to act on the material in the course of demolition or renovation.

Before/during demolition or renovation of a "facility":

1. Thoroughly inspect all areas that will be affected by the renovation or demolition operation. Inspection and sampling must be performed by an AHERA Certified Inspector. [61.145(a)]
2. Submit notification form to EPA 10 working days (Monday through Friday) before starting work [61.145(b)]. Notify for any demolition project (removal of load bearing member or structure), even if no asbestos is present. Notify for renovations involving removal or disturbance of more than 260 linear feet or 160 square feet of RACM.
3. Remove all RACM from the affected areas [61.145(c)]. RACM must be removed by AHERA certified workers, and a certified asbestos supervisor must be on site. RACM must be removed using wet methods, and no visible emissions are allowed during removal.

If a building is to be demolished by intentional burning and more than 260 linear feet or 160 square feet of ACM (friable or nonfriable) is present in the building, all ACM, including nonfriable asbestos, must be removed in accordance with the NESHAP before burning.

Waste Disposal [61.150]:

1. No visible emissions to the outside air are allowed during collection, packaging, transportation, or disposal of asbestos-containing waste material.
2. RACM must remain adequately wet until placed in a sealed, leak-tight container that is marked with the OSHA required warning label and must be labeled with the waste generator's name and the location at which the waste was generated.
3. Vehicles used to transport asbestos-containing waste material must be marked during loading and unloading. Signs must conform to [61.149(d)].
4. Maintain waste shipment records for all asbestos-containing waste material.
5. Dispose of all asbestos-containing waste material at a certified asbestos landfill operated in compliance with [61.154]. A copy of the waste shipment record must be provided to the disposal site operator at the time the waste is delivered.

This information can be found on an agency fact sheet that is intended to provide general information only. It should not in any way be interpreted to alter or replace the actual regulations.

15.9 EPA—ASBESTOS AT SUPERFUND SITES: FRAMEWORK FOR INVESTIGATING ASBESTOS-CONTAMINATED SUPERFUND SITES, OSWER DIRECTIVE 9200-68, SEPTEMBER 2008

Asbestos is the name given to a number of naturally occurring fibrous silicate minerals that have been mined for their useful properties such as thermal insulation, chemical and thermal stability, and high tensile strength. Asbestos is used in many commercial products, including insulation, brake linings, and roofing shingles. Past practices have led to environmental contamination and subsequent action under the Superfund (CERCLA) program.

A framework was developed and provides guidance for assessing sites contaminated with asbestos that are being addressed under the authority of Superfund. The framework implements the August 2004 directive by recommending a risk-based, site-specific approach for site evaluation on the basis of current asbestos science. This guidance provides recommended flexible framework for investigating and evaluating asbestos contamination at Superfund removal and remedial sites. The document also provides remedial/removal managers, remedial project managers, on-scene coordinators, site assessors, and other decision makers with information that should assist in the evaluation of asbestos risks at Superfund sites along with information to facilitate site decisions under conditions of incomplete characterization and to accommodate the varied nature of environmental asbestos contamination. A full copy of the Framework can be found on the EPA Web site under Addressing Asbestos at Superfund Sites.

15.10 EPA—GUIDANCE FOR CATASTROPHIC EMERGENCY SITUATIONS INVOLVING ASBESTOS, OECA DECEMBER 23, 2009, REPLACEMENT OF THE GUIDELINES FOR CATASTROPHIC EMERGENCY SITUATIONS INVOLVING ASBESTOS ISSUED IN 1992

The EPA, when involved in catastrophic events, calls upon its trained agency staff to perform a variety of activities as specified by the FEMA. It is the mission of the agency being activated to provide services to support those government agencies in the field. Catastrophes do not discriminate and communities both large and small may be impacted, especially when building destruction occurs. The age of most buildings across the country varies from pre-World War I to present day construction. Buildings are evaluated by field evaluators in order to determine, either visually or through a collection of samples, what materials were used for building, which may include ACMs. During these catastrophes, communities want to be able to redevelop in a timely fashion and community members want to return to these areas with their families. Over the years, the EPA has taken lessons learned to expedite the process of providing communities reentry to these devastated communities and surrounding areas that have been impacted the most. The importance of determining the environmental impact, which include ACMs in residential and commercial properties, is essential when determining the ramifications, both environmental and in public safety, of demolishing these properties. It is through joint oversight of state and federal partners engaged in the community's vision by preparing community leaders regarding the potential hazards of these asbestos-containing buildings, which still exist across the country. This new guidance document provides support to those first responders on the ground immediately following a catastrophe. The areas the EPA is most concerned about during these situations are as follows:

- Exposure concerns for the emergency responders and others in the immediate area;
- Cleanup and disposal of debris that may be contaminated with asbestos;
- Demolition and renovation of buildings during recovery efforts; and
- Transport and disposal of material that may contain asbestos.

This document is intended as a reference for EPA first responders and others who may also be involved in first response.

Index

Note: Page numbers followed by "*f*" and "*t*" denote figures and tables, respectively.

A

AB, *see* Asbestos bodies
ACCP, *see* American College of Chest Physicians
Accreditation Council for Graduate Medical
    Education, 594
Actinolite, 81, 85, 189, 231, 595
    chemical composition of, 2*t*
    in chrysotile-containing products, 44
    EDS x-ray spectra for, 31*f*
    exposure associated with mesothelioma, 83
    uses of, 59
Acute fibrinous and organizing pneumonia (AFOP), 507
    with areas of ossification, 511*f*
    with asbestos bodies, 510*f*, 511*f*
    with fibrin in alveolar spaces, 510*f*
Adenocarcinoma, 155, 421; *see also* Cancer; Carcinoma
    chrysotile exposure associated with, 198
    GI tract, 359
    lung
        and epithelioid pleural mesothelioma, markers for
            differentiating between, 389
    metastatic
        cytologic discriminants of, 388*t*
    pulmonary, 359, 362*f*, 363*f*
        mucin-producing, 363*f*
    renal, 437
        k-ras mutations associated with, 122
    smoking and, 270
Adenoid cystic/cystic mesothelioma, 330, 331*f*, 332*f*; *see
        also* Mesothelioma
Adenomatoid tumors, 366
    pleural, 366
    ultrastructural morphology of tumor cells in, 367*f*
    uterine, 366*f*
Adipose tissue, 313*f*
AFOP, *see* Acute fibrinous and organizing pneumonia
Agency for Toxic Substances and Disease Registry,
    562, 601
AHERA, *see* Asbestos Hazard Emergency Response Act
    of 1986
Air, measuring asbestos in, 33*t*, 35–37, 36*t*
Air Hygiene Foundation, *see* Industrial Hygiene
    Foundation
Airway obstruction, 448, 549, 553
    bronchodilators for, 532–533
    normal *vs.* abnormal, 533
    pulmonary function testing for, 533
Alcoholism and laryngeal cancer, 426–430, 585, 586
Alveolar architecture disruption, 600, 600*f*
Alveolar level, architecture of, 52, 54*f*
Alveolar macrophages, 448, 461*f*, 510*f*, 511*f*; *see also*
    Macrophages
    -mediated lung clearance, impaired, 56
Alveoli, call up macrophages, 52–53, 54*f*

American Board of Preventive Medicine, 593
American Cancer Society, 438, 553, 562, 563, 570,
    573, 585
American College of Chest Physicians (ACCP), 544, 562,
    572, 607
    Consensus Statement on the Respiratory Health
        Effects of Asbestos, 473, 523, 528, 536, 538,
        539, 548–551, 554, 562, 569, 585
American Joint Commission, 58
American Medical Association Council on Occupational
    Health, 162
American Society for Testing and Materials (ASTM), 24,
    27, 27*f*,
    Method D5755–02, 37, 38*t*
    Method D5756–02, 37, 38*t*
    Method D6281–98, 35–36
    Method D6480–99, 37, 38*t*
    Method D7200–06, 29, 31
American Thoracic Society (ATS), 471, 497, 528, 562, 602
    Diagnosis and Initial Management of Nonmalignant
        Diseases Related to Asbestos, 523, 525
    diagnostic criteria
        of asbestosis, 467
        of nonmalignant lung disease related to
            asbestos, 468*t*
American Water Works Association (AWWA), 24, 37, 37*t*
Amosite, 6*t*, 595
    chemical composition of, 2*t*
    cigarette smoke extracts and, 275
    compound exposures to, 56
    -cored ferruginous bodies, 469*f*
    EDS x-ray spectra for, 31*f*, 60, 61*f*
    exposure associated with mesothelioma, 12, 154
    fibers
        exposure associated with hyaline pleural
            plaques, 487
        uncoated, 470*f*
    -induced alveolar epithelial cell injury
    from lower respiratory system, transfer of, 58
    in sputum, 73
    toxicity of, 193–195
    uses of, 59
Analytical transmission electron microscopy (ATEM);
        see also Electron microscopy; Transmission
        electron microscopy
    for analysis of tissue digestion, 80
    asbestos fibers, 64, 87–89, 97, 233
    for determining asbestos burden in tissue, 72, 79–82
    ferruginous bodies, 70, 77
ANCAs, *see* Antineutrophil cytoplasmic antibodies
Anemia, 386, 578
Angiosarcoma of the pleura, 393–394
Anthophyllite
    chemical composition of, 2*t*
    EDS x-ray spectra for, 31*f*